Oxford Textbook of
Philosophy and Psychiatry

Oxford Textbook of
Philosophy and Psychiatry

K.W.M. (Bill) Fulford
Department of Philosophy and the Medical School,
University of Warwick, Coventry; and Department of Psychiatry,
University of Oxford, UK

Tim Thornton
Professor of Philosophy and Mental Health, Centre for Ethnicity
and Health, University of Central Lancashire, UK;
formerly, Senior Lecturer in Philosophy, Department of Philosophy
and the Medical School, University of Warwick, Coventry, UK

George Graham
Department of Philosophy, Wake Forest University,
Winston-Salem, USA

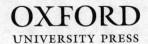

OXFORD
UNIVERSITY PRESS

OXFORD

UNIVERSITY PRESS

Great Clarendon Street, Oxford OX2 6DP

Oxford University Press is a department of the University of Oxford.
It furthers the University's objective of excellence in research, scholarship,
and education by publishing worldwide in

Oxford New York

Auckland Cape Town Dar es Salaam Hong Kong Karachi
Kuala Lumpur Madrid Melbourne Mexico City Nairobi
New Delhi Shanghai Taipei Toronto

With offices in

Argentina Austria Brazil Chile Czech Republic France Greece
Guatemala Hungary Italy Japan Poland Portugal Singapore
South Korea Switzerland Thailand Turkey Ukraine Vietnam

Oxford is a registered trade mark of Oxford University Press
in the UK and in certain other countries

Published in the United States
by Oxford University Press Inc., New York

British Library Cataloguing in Publication Data

Data available

Library of Congress Cataloging in Publication Data

Data available

Typeset by Newgen Imaging Systems (P) Ltd, Chennai, India
Printed in Great Britain on acid-free paper by
CPI Antony Rowe, Chippenham, Wiltshire

ISBN 978 0 19 852694 0 (hbk)
ISBN 978 0 19 852695 7 (pbk)

10 9 8 7 6 5 4 3

Contents

Detailed Contents

Acknowledgements

All best efforts to find copyright holders have been made, but this has not always been possible. Please accept our apologies if we have infringed copyright in any way, and please contact the Medicine Editorial department of Oxford University Press.

2.1: Extract from page 9 of 'A Distinction is not a Dichotomy' by H. Puttnam in *The Collapse of the Fact/Value Dichotomy and Other Essays* Cambridge Mass: Harvard University Press, Copyright © 2002 by the President and Fellows of Harvard College

2.2: Extract from pages 113–14 of 'The Myth of Mental Illness' by T. S. Szasz in *American Psychologist* (15, 113–118). Reprinted with permission from the American Psychological Association.

2.3: Extracts from pages 305–6, 306, 309, 310, 314, and 315 of 'The concept of disease and its implications for psychiatry' by R. E. Kendell in the *British Journal of Psychiatry* (127) (1975). Reprinted with permission from the Royal College of Psychiatrists.

4.1: Extracts from page 3 of 'A Plea for Excuses' by J. L. Austin in *Proceedings of the Aristotelian Society* Vol. LVII (1956–7). Reprinted by courtesy of the Editor of the Aristotelian Society: © 1956–7.

4.2: Extract from pages 4–6 of the Introduction from *J. L. Austin* by G. J. Warnock (1989). Reprinted with permission from Routledge.

4.3: Extract from pages 49–68 of 'On the distinction between disease and illness' by C. Boorse in *Philosophy and Public Affairs* (5) (1975). Reprinted with permission form Blackwell Publishing.

4.4: Extracts from pages 174–7 and 184–5 of 'The Body as Expression of Speech' in *Phenomenology of Perception* by Maurice Merleau-Ponty (trans. Colin Smith) (1962). Reprinted with permission from Routledge.

4.5: Extract from pages xlv–xlvi of 'Introduction: The Pursuit of Being' in *Being and Nothingness* by Jean-Paul Sartre (trans. Hazel E. Barnes) (1956). Copyright © 1956 Philosophical Library. A Citadel Press book. All rights reserved. Reprinted by arrangement with Kensington Publishing Corp.

4.6: Extract from pages 37 and 41–2 of 'Hermeneutic Method and Reflective Philosophy' in *Freud and Philosophy* by Ricoeur (trans. D. Savage 1970). Reprinted with permission from Yale University Press.

4.7: Extract from pages 43–44 and 48 of *Real People: Personal Identity Without Thought Experiments* by K. V. Wilkes (1988). Reprinted with permission from Oxford University Press.

5.3: Extract from pages 38–9 of 'The Runabout Inference-Ticket' by A. N. Prior in *Analysis* (21) (1960). Reprinted with permission form Blackwell Publishing.

6.1: Extract from pages 237–9 of 'The Value of Philosophy' in *The Problems of Philosophy* by Bertrand Russell (1912). Reprinted with permission from Oxford University Press and the Bertrand Russell Peace Foundation.

6.2: Extract from pages xx of section 6.51–7 in *Tractatus Logico-Philosophicus* by Ludwig Wittgenstein (trans. D. F. Pears and B. F. McGuinness) (1981). Reprinted with permission from Routledge.

6.3: Extract from page 9 of the Introduction to 'An Inquiry into Meaning and Truth', the William James lectures delivered at Harvard University by B. Russell (1940). Penguin Books 1962. Reprinted with permission of Taylor & Francis and the Bertrand Russell Peace Foundation.

6.4: Extract from page 23 of 'The Archimedean Point' in *Ethics and the Limits of Philosophy* by B Williams Cambridge Mass: Harvard University Press, Copyright © 1985 by Bernard Williams.

6.5 & 6.6: Extract from pages 111–17 and 121–6 of *Language of Morals* by R. M. Hare (1972). Reprinted with permission from Oxford University Press.

6.7: Extract from pages 83–4 and 97–100 from 'Moral Beliefs' by P. Foot in *PAS* 59 (1958/9). Reprinted by courtesy of the Editor of the Aristotelian Society: © 1958/9.

6.9: Extracts from pages 95–96, 96–97, 100, and 101 of 'The Construction of Definitions of Illness' in *Symptoms and Illness: The Cognitive Organisation of Disorder* by D. Locker (1981). Reprinted with permission from Routledge.

6.10: Extract from pages 115–119 of 'Illness in Action' from *Moral Theory and Practice* by K. W. M. Fulford (1989). © Cambridge University Press. Reproduced with permission of the author and publisher.

6.11: Extracts from pages 62–3, 63, 66–67, 70–71 of 'The Body' in *The Meaning of Illness: A Phenomenological Account of the Different Perspectives of Physician and Patient* by S. Kay Toombs (1993). Reprinted with kind permission from Springer Science and Business Media.

6.12: Extract from pages 126–7 of 'Illness in Action' from *Moral Theory and Practice* by K. W. M. Fulford (1989). © Cambridge University Press. Reproduced with permission of the author and publisher.

6.13: Extract from pages 135–6 of 'Illness in Action' from *Moral Theory and Practice* by K. W. M. Fulford (1989). © Cambridge University Press. Reproduced with permission of the author and publisher.

6.14: Extract from page 3 of 'A plea for excuses' by J. L. Austin in *PAS* 57 (1956–7). Reprinted by courtesy of the Editor of the Aristotelian Society © 1956–7.

7.1: Extract from page 7 of 'Matters Historical' in *The History of Mental Symptoms* by G. E. Berrios (1996). Reprinted with permission from G. E. Berrios and Cambridge University Press.

7.2: Extract from opening page of 'Mental Health in Plato's Republic' by A. J. P. Kennedy © The British Academy 1970. Reproduced by permission from *Proceedings of the British Academy* 55; 1969.

7.3: Extract from pages 287–8 of 'The Stoic Conception of Mental Disorder: The Case of Cicero' by L. Nordenfelt in *Philosophy, Psychiatry & Psychology* (1997; 4:4). © The John Hopkins University Press. Reproduced with permission of The John Hopkins University Press.

7.4: Extract from *Wild Beasts and Idle Humors* by Daniel Robinson, p.325, Cambridge, Mass,: Harvard University Press, Reprinted by permission of the publisher. Copyright © 1996 by the President and Fellows of Harvard College

7.5 & 7.6: Extracts from 'Malleus Maleficarum' Kramer, H & Sprenger, J (1996) trs by Summers, M

7.7: Extract from pages *A History of Medical Psychology* by Gregory Zilboorg and George W. Henry. Copyright 1941 by W. W. Norton & Company, Inc. Copyright © renewed 1969 by Margaret Stone Zilboorg and George W. Henry. Used by permission of W. W. Norton & Company, Inc.

7.8: Extract from page 325 of *A History of Psychiatry*, Edward Shorter (1997). Copyright © 1997 John Wiley and Sons Ltd. Reproduced with permission.

8.1: Extract from Jaspers, K 'Causal and 'Meaningful' Connections between Life History and Psychosis' (an extract from Jaspers, K (1913) 'Kausale und verständliche Zusammenhänge zwischen Schicksal und Psychose bei der Dementia praecox' (Schizophrenie), Z Neurol, 14, 158–263, trs Hoenig, J in Hirsch, S R & Shepherd, M (1974) 'Themes and Variations in European Psychiatry'

8.2: Extract from pages 1313–23 of 'The Phenomenological Approach in Psychopathology' by K. Jaspers (anon. trans of 'Die Phänomenologische Forschungrichtung in der Psychopathologie') in the *British Journal of Psychiatry* (114) (1968). Reprinted with permission from the Royal College of Psychiatrists.

9.1: Extract from pages 1313–23 of 'The Phenomenological Approach in Psychopathology' by K. Jaspers (anon. trans of 'Die Phänomenologische Forschungrichtung in der Psychopathologie') in the *British Journal of Psychiatry* (114) (1968). Reprinted with permission from the Royal College of Psychiatrists.

9.2: Extract from pages 248–266 of *Logical Investigations, Volume II* by Edmund Husser (trans. J. N. Findlay) (1970). Reprinted with permission from Routledge.

10.2: Extract from Jaspers, K 'Causal and 'Meaningful' Connections between Life History and Psychosis' (an extract from Jaspers, K (1913) 'Kausale und verständliche Zusammenhänge zwischen Schicksal und Psychose bei der Dementia praecox' (Schizophrenie), Z Neurol, 14, 158–263, trs Hoenig, J in Hirsch, S R & Shepherd, M (1974) 'Themes and Variations in European Psychiatry'

10.4: Extract from Roscher and Kines: the Logical Problems of Historical Economics by Max Weber, translated by Guy Oakes. Copyright © 1975 by The Free Press. All rights reserved. Reprinted with permission of The Free Press, a division of Simon & Schuster Adult Publishing Group.

10.5: Extract from page 99 of *Weber, Sections on Translation* (1978) by W. G. Runciman (trans. Eric Matthews). Reprinted with permission from W. G. Runciman and Cambridge University Press.

11.1: Extract from pages xiv–xv and 1–6 of *Clinical Psychology*, Mayer-Gross et al (3rd edn) (1969). Copyright © 1969. Reprinted with permission from Elsevier.

11.2: Extract from the Introduction of *Diagnostic and Statistical Manual of Mental Disorders* (4th edn, text revision) Copyright 2000, published by the American Psychiatric Association. Reprinted with permission from the Diagnostic and Statistical Manual of Mental Disorders, Copyright 2000. American Psychiatric Association.

11.3: Extract from 'Signs and Symptoms of Mental Disorder' of *The Oxford Textbook of Psychiatry* edited by M. G. Gelder, G. Gath, and R. A. M. Mayou (1983). Reprinted with permission from Oxford University Press.

11.4: Extract from pages 295–297 Sigmund Freud © Copyrights, The Institute of Psychoanalysis and the Hogarth Press for permission to quote from *Project for a Scientific Psychology* from *The Standard Edition of the Complete Psychological Works of Sigmund Freud* translated and edited by James Strachey. Reprinted by permission of The Random House Group Ltd.

11.5: Extract from pages 41, 45–49 Sigmund Freud © Copyrights, The Institute of Psychoanalysis and the Hogarth Press for permission to quote from *Project for a Scientific Psychology* from *The Standard Edition of the Complete Psychological Works of Sigmund Freud* translated and edited by James Strachey. Reprinted by permission of The Random House Group Ltd.

11.6: Extract from pages 60–63 Sigmund Freud © Copyrights, The Institute of Psychoanalysis and the Hogarth Press for permission to quote from *Project for a Scientific Psychology* from *The Standard Edition of the Complete Psychological Works of Sigmund Freud* translated and edited by James Strachey. Reprinted by permission of The Random House Group Ltd.

11.7: Extract from pages 57, 69, 93, 94, 149–150 Sigmund Freud © Copyrights, The Institute of Psychoanalysis and the Hogarth Press for permission to quote from *Project for a Scientific Psychology* from *The Standard Edition of the Complete Psychological Works of Sigmund Freud* translated and edited by James Strachey. Reprinted by permission of The Random House Group Ltd.

11.8: Extract from pages 87–93 of 'Chapter 2: Energetics and Hermeneutics in The Interpretation of Dreams' in *Freud and Philosophy* by Ricoeur (trans. D. Savage 1970). Reprinted with permission from Yale University Press.

11.10: Extract from pages 131–6 of 'Wish' in *Irrationality and the Philosophy of Psychoanalysis* by S. Gardner (1993). Reprinted with permission from S. Gardner and Cambridge University Press.

12.1: Extract from pages vii and viii of the Preface in *Measurement and Classification of Psychiatric Symptoms* (1974) by M. C. Wing, J. E. Cooper, and N. Sartorius. Reprinted with permission from the authors and Cambridge University Press.

12.2: Extract from pages 145 and 147 in *The Aim and Structure of Physical Theory* by Pierre Duhem (© 1954 Princeton University Press, 1982 renewed PUP). Reprinted with permission from Princeton University Press.

12.3: Extract from pages 8–10 of *Scientific Realism and the Plasticity of Mind* by P. Churchland (1979). Reprinted with permission from P. Churchland and Cambridge University Press.

12.5: Extract from page 25 of *What Is This Thing Called Science?* by A. F. Chalmers (1999). Reprinted with permission from the University of Queensland Press.

13.15: Extract from page 207 of *On the Current Status of Scientific Realism* by R. Boyd (1983). Reprinted with permission from Springer Science and Business Media.

13.16: Extract from pages 38–9 of 'The Reality of Causes in a World of Instrumental Laws' by Nancy Cartwright (1980) in *PSA* (vol. 2). Reprinted with permission from Nancy Cartwright and the PSA.

13.17: Extract from Ian Hacking, 'Experimentation and Scientific Realism' from Philosophical Topics 13 (1982). Used with the permission of the University of Arkansas Press, www.uapress.com

13.18: Two-page extract from pages 83–107 of 'The Natural Ontological Attitude' by Arthur Fine printed in *Scientific Realism* by J. Leplin (ed) (© 1984). Reprinted with permission from the Regents of the University of California and Professor Arthur Fine.

14.1: Extract from pages 47–69 of 'Philosophy of Natural Science' 1e © 1967. Electronically reproduced by permission of Pearson Education, Inc, Upper Saddle River, New Jersey.

14.3: Extract from page 324–5 of 'The pragmatics of explanation' by B. Van Fraassen in *American Philosophical Quarterly* (14) (1977). Reprinted with permission from the University of Pittsburgh Press.

14.5: Extract from pages 46–7 of 'The Priority of Paradigms' by T. S. Kuhn in *The Structure of Scientific Revolutions* (1962). Reprinted with permission from The University of Chicago Press.

14.6: Extract from pages 152 and 154 of 'Phenomenological and criteriological diagnosis' by A. Kraus in *Philosophical Perspectives on Psychiatric Diagnostic Classification* by John Z. Sadler et al. © 1994. Reproduced with permission from The John Hopkins University Press.

15.1: Extract from pages 315–17 of 'Causal Reasoning and the Diagnostic Process' by D. A. Rizzi in *Theoretical Medicine* (15) (1994). Reprinted with permission from Springer Science and Business Media.

15.2: Extract from pages 63–4 and 74–5 of *Enquiries Concerning Human Understanding* by D. Hume (1975). Reprinted with permission from Oxford University Press.

15.3: Extract from two pages of 'Causes and Conditions' by John L. Mackie in *American Philosophical Quarterly* (2/4) (1965). Reprinted with permission from the University of Pittsburgh Press.

15.5: Extract from pages 23–5 of How *the Laws of Physics Lie* by N. Cartwright (1983). Reprinted with permission from Oxford University Press.

15.6: Extract from *Mind and the World* by John McDowell, pages 70–72, Cambridge, Mass,: Harvard University Press, Reprinted by permission of the publisher. Copyright © 1994 by the President and Fellows of Harvard College.

15.7: Extract from pages 233–8 of 'Depression and Loss' in *Social Origins of Depression* by G. W. Brown and T. O. Harris (1978). Reprinted with permission from Routledge.

16.1: Extract from pages 220–25 of 'Closing the gap between research and practice' by J. R. Geddes and P. J. Harrison in the *British Journal of Psychiatry* (171) (1997). Reprinted with permission from the Royal College of Psychiatrists.

16.2: Extract from pages 37–8 of *Enquiries Concerning Human Understanding* by D. Hume (1975). Reprinted with permission from Oxford University Press.

16.3: Extract from pages 7–9 of *Objective Knowledge* by K. Popper (1972). Reprinted with permission from Oxford University Press.

16.4: Extract from pages 91–6 of 'Falsification and the methodology of scientific research programmes' by I. Lakatos in *Criticism and the Growth of Knowledge* by I. Lakatos and A. Musgrave (eds) (1970). Reprinted with permission form J. Worrall and Cambridge University Press.

16.5: Extract from pages 4–6 of 'Logic of discovery or psychology of research' by T. S. Kuhn in *Criticism and the Growth of Knowledge* by I. Lakatos and A. Musgrave (eds) (1970). Reprinted with permission from Cambridge University Press.

16.6: Extracts from pages 1–3 of 'The Strong Programme in the Sociology of Knowledge' in *Knowledge and Social Imagery* by D. Bloor (1976). Reprinted with permission from Dr. D. Bloor.

16.7: Extracts from pages 254–5 of 'Introduction' and pages 263–8 of 'Induction' in *The Warrant of Induction*, Chapter 15, in David Mellor, *Matter of Metaphysics* (1991), originally published in *The Warrant of Induction*, Cambridge University Press (Inaugural Lecture, published by Cambridge University Press in 1988). Reprinted with permission from David Mellor and Cambridge University Press.

17.1: Extract from page 184 of Dependency: the foundational value in medical ethics by A.V Campbell in *Medicine and Moral Reasoning* by Fulford, Gillett and Soskice (eds) (1994). Reprinted with permission from Cambridge University Press.

17.2: Extract from page 694 of 'Ethics of Psychiatry Practice: Consent, Compulsion, and Confidentiality' by A. Okasha in *Current Opinion in Psychiatry* (13(6)) (2000). Reprinted with permission from Lippincott Williams & Wilkins, Medical Research, a division of Wolters Kluwer Health.

17.3: Extracts from pages 85–6 and 89–90 of 'The virtues in a professional setting' by W. F. May in *Medicine and Moral Reasoning* by Fulford, Gillett, and Soskice (eds) (1994). Reprinted with permission from W. F. May and Cambridge University Press.

17.4: Extract from pages 29–31 of 'How Should We Measure Need?' by M. Marshall in *Philosophy, Psychiatry, and* Psychology (1:3 (1994)). © The John Hopkins University Press. Reproduced with permission of The John Hopkins University Press.

17.6: Extract from pages 228–9 of the Report of the Committee on Mentally Abnormal Offenders, Cmnd., 6244 (1975). Reprinted with permission of the Office of Public Sector Information.

18.2: Extract from page 210, a definition of 'Hippocratic Oath' from *Dorland's American Illustrated Medical Dictionary* (25th edn) (1974). Reprinted with permission from Elsevier.

18.3 and 18.4: Two extracts from pages 684–6 and 688–9 from Psychiatric Ethics: a Bioethical Ugly Duckling? by K. W. M. Fulford and T. Hope in *Principles of Health Care Ethics*, Raanan Gillon (ed.) (1993). Copyright © 1993 John Wiley and Sons Ltd. Reproduced with permission.

18.5: Extract from pages 21–37, two pages from 'Case Method and Casuistry: the Problem of Bias' by L. M. Kopelman in *Theoretical Medicine* (15) (1994). Reprinted with permission from Springer Science and Business Media.

18.6: Extract from page 181 of 'Quality of life and health care' by R. Crisp in *Medicine and Moral Reasoning* (1994) by Fulford, Gillett, and Soskice (eds). Reprinted with permission from R. Crisp and Cambridge University Press.

18.7: Extract from pages 28–9 of 'The philosophical basis of psychiatric ethics' reprinted from *Psychiatric Ethics* edited by S. Bloch and P. Chodoff from 'Essays on Bioethics' edited by R. M. Hare (1993). Reprinted with permission from Oxford University Press.

18.8: Extract from pages 802–3 of 'Concepts of Disease and the Abuse of Psychiatry in the USSR' by K. W. M. Fulford, A. Y. U. Smirnov, and E. Snow in the *British Journal of Psychiatry* (162)

(1993). Reprinted with permission from the Royal College of Psychiatrists.

18.9: Extract from Evidence-Based Medicine: how to practise and teach EBM (2e) by D.L. Sackett, S.E. Strauss, W. Scott Richardson, W. Rosenberg and R.B. Haynes (2000). Reprinted with permission of the authors.

19.2: Extract from page 335, the Consent Form, in *Health Care Law: text and materials* by J. McHale, M. Fox, and J. Murphy (1999). Reprinted with permission from Sweet and Maxwell.

19.3: Extract from pages 269–71 of 'Consent' in *Health Care Law: text and materials* by J. McHale, M. Fox, and J. Murphy (1999). Reprinted with permission from Sweet and Maxwell.

19.4: Extracts from 'Tests of competency to consent to treatment' and 'The case of Re C (Adult: Refusal of Treatment)'. Reprinted with permission from Her Majesty's Stationery Office.

19.5: Extract from pages 341–51 of *Health Care Law: text and materials* by. McHale, M. Fox, and J. Murphy (1999). Reprinted with permission from Sweet and Maxwell.

19.6a: Extract from pages 11–13 of 'The Key Principles: Capacity, Best Interests, and the General Authority to Act Reasonably' in Who Decides? Making Decisions on Behalf of Mentally Incapacitated Adults, Cmnd., 3803 (1997). Reprinted with permission from the Office of Public Sector Information.

19.6b: Extracts from pages 663 and 664 of 'Mental Health Legislation is now a harmful anachronism' by G. Szmukler and F. Holloway in *Psychiatric Bulletin* (22) (1998). Reprinted with permission from the Royal College of Psychiatrists.

19.6c: Extracts from pages 666, 667, and 668 of 'Replacing the Mental Health Act 1983? How to change the game without losing the baby with the bath water or shooting ourselves in the foot' by K. W. M. Fulford in *Psychiatric Bulletin* (22) (1998). Reprinted with permission from the Royal College of Psychiatrists.

19.6d: Extract from page 669 of 'Transcending mental health law' by L. Sayce in *Psychiatric Bulletin* (22) (1998). Reprinted with permission from the Royal College of Psychiatrists.

19.7: Extract from one page of *In Two Minds: a casebook of psychiatric ethics* by D. Dickenson and K. W. M. Fulford (2000). Author's own material.

20.1: Extract from pages 109–111 of *In Two Minds: a casebook of psychiatric ethics* by D. Dickenson and K. W. M. Fulford (2000). Author's own material.

20.2 Extract from page 112 of *In Two Minds: a casebook of psychiatric ethics* by D. Dickenson and K. W. M. Fulford (2000). Author's own material.

20.3: Extract from pages xv of *Diagnostic and Statistical Manual of Mental Disorders* (4th edn, text revision) Copyright 2000, published by the American Psychiatric Association. Reprinted with permission from the Diagnostic and Statistical Manual of Mental Disorders, Copyright 2000. American Psychiatric Association.

20.4: Extract from pages xxi and xxii of *Diagnostic and Statistical Manual of Mental Disorders* (4th edn, text revision)

Copyright 2000, published by the American Psychiatric Association. Reprinted with permission from the Diagnostic and Statistical Manual of Mental Disorders, Copyright 2000. American Psychiatric Association.

20.5: Extract from page 630 of *Diagnostic and Statistical Manual of Mental Disorders* (4th edn, text revision) Copyright 2000, published by the American Psychiatric Association. Reprinted with permission from the Diagnostic and Statistical Manual of Mental Disorders, Copyright 2000. American Psychiatric Association.

20.6: Extract from page 523 of *Diagnostic and Statistical Manual of Mental Disorders* (4th edn, text revision) Copyright 2000, published by the American Psychiatric Association. Reprinted with permission from the Diagnostic and Statistical Manual of Mental Disorders, Copyright 2000. American Psychiatric Association.

20.7 Extract from pages 59–60 of *In Two Minds: a casebook of psychiatric ethics* by D. Dickenson and K. W. M. Fulford (2000). Author's own material.

20.8: Extract from pages 193–224 from Psychiatric diagnosis as an ethical problem by W. Reich (1999) in *Psychiatric Ethics* 3rd edn (ed S. Bloch, P. Chodoff and S. Green). Reprinted with permission from Oxford University Press.

21.1: Extract from pages 194 and 197 of 'Recent Criticism of Psychiatric Nosology: A Review' by J. Radden in *Philosophy, Psychiatry, and* Psychology (1:3 (1994)). © The John Hopkins University Press. Reproduced with permission of The John Hopkins University Press.

21.2: Extract from pages 195–6 from Psychiatric diagnosis as an ethical problem by W. Reich (1999) in *Psychiatric Ethics* 3rd edn (ed S. Bloch, P. Chodoff and S. Green). Reprinted with permission from Oxford University Press.

21.3: Extract from 'A proposal to classify happiness as a psychiatric disorder' R.P. Bentall (1992) Journal of Medical Ethics, 18: 94–98. Reprinted with permission from the BMJ Publishing Group.

22.8: Extract from pages 16–19 of *Descartes: Meditations on First Philosophy With Selections from the Objections and Replies* by John Cottingham (ed) (1996). Reprinted with permission from John Cottingham and Cambridge University Press.

22.9: Extract from pages 53–5 of 'Discourse 4' in *Discourse on Method and Meditations* by Rene Descartes (1968) (trans. F. E. Sutcliffe). Reprinted with permission from Penguin Group UK.

22.10: Extract from pages 122–126 of 'The Philosophical Writings of Descartes, 2' edited and translated by J Cottingham, R Stoothoff and D Murdoch (1985). Reprinted with permission from Cambridge University Press.

22.12 & 22.13: Extracts from pages 17–20 and 119–120 'The Concept of Mind' by G. Ryle, ([1949]1963), London, Penguin Books. Reproduced by permission of Taylor & Francis Books UK. With the permission of the Principal, Fellows and Scholars of Hertford College in the University of Oxford.

23.1: Extract from pages 673–4 of 'Seeing the Mind' by M. I. Posner in *Science* (1993). Reprinted with permission from AAAS and M. I. Posner.

23.3: Extract from pages 247–8 and 250 of 'Mental Events' by D. Davidson in *Experience and Theory* by Foster and Swanson (1980). Reprinted with permission from University of Massachusetts Press.

24.1: Extract from pages 143–6 of 'Recognising and Understanding Spoken Words' in *Human Cognitive Neurophysiology: a textbook with readings* by A. Ellis and A. Young (1996). Reprinted with permission from Taylor & Francis.

24.3 and 24.4: Two extracts from 'Meaning and the World Order' in *Psychosemantics* by J. A. Fodor. Reprinted with permission from MIT Press.

25.1: Extract from pages 145–149 of 'The Alzheimer's Disease Sufferer as a Semiotic Subject' in *Philosophy, Psychiatry, and* Psychology (1 (1994)), pages 75–90. © The John Hopkins University Press. Reproduced with permission of The John Hopkins University Press.

25.2: Extract from pages 340–1 of 'True Believers: The Intentional Strategy and Why It Works' in *The Intentional Stance* by D. Dennett (1987). Reprinted with permission from MIT Press.

25.3: Extracts from pages 125–6, 127–8, and 136–7 of 'Radical Interpretation' by D. Davidson in *Dialectica* (27: 1973). Reprinted with permission from Blackwell Publishing.

25.5: Extract from pages 158–61 of *Subject, Thought and Context* edited by J. McDowell et al (1986). Reprinted with permission from Oxford University Press.

25.6: Extract from pages 150–152 of 'The Alzheimer's Disease Sufferer as a Semiotic Subject' in *Philosophy, Psychiatry, and* Psychology (1 (1994)), pages 75–90. © The John Hopkins University Press. Reproduced with permission of The John Hopkins University Press.

26.1: Extract from 'Free Will in the Light of Neuropsychiatry' by S. A. Spence in *Philosophy, Psychiatry, and* Psychology (3:2 (1996)), pages 75–90. © The John Hopkins University Press. Reproduced with permission of The John Hopkins University Press.

26.2: Extract from pages 62–6 of ''The Will' in *Concept of Mind* by G. Ryle (1963). Reprinted with permission from Taylor & Francis. With the permission of the Principal, Fellows and Scholars of Hertford College in the University of Oxford.

26.4: Extract from pages 296–8 of 'Paradoxes of Irrationality' by D. Davidson in *Philosophical essay on Freud* by Wollheim and Hopkins (eds) (1982). Reprinted with permission from Cambridge University Press.

26.5: Extract from pages 108–13 of 'Why reasons may not be causes' by J. Tanney in *Mind and Language* (11) (1995). Reprinted with permission form Blackwell Publishing.

27.1: Extract from pages 12–13 of *Descartes: Meditations on First Philosophy With Selections from the Objections and Replies* by

John Cottingham (ed) (1996). Reprinted with permission from John Cottingham and Cambridge University Press.

27.4: Extract from pages 1–2 of *Psychosemantics* by J. A. Fodor (1987). Reprinted with permission of MIT Press.

27.6: Extract from pages 131–4 of 'The mental stimulation debate: a progress report' by T. Stone and M. Davies in *Theories of mind* by P. Carruthers and P Smith (eds) (1996). Reprinted with permission from T. Stone, M. Davies and Cambridge University Press.

28.1: Extract from *An Essay Concerning Human Understanding* by John Locke, edited by P. Nidditch (1979). Reprinted with permission from Oxford University Press.

Reading Guides

Preface

A proactive textbook

This is a proactive textbook. Most textbooks report on their field. This textbook aims to give you the skills to contribute to the field.

Philosophy is about argument. Hence, through a case study approach, the reader is engaged actively in a series of both traditional and emerging lines of argument around key topics on the shared agenda of philosophy and mental health, thus developing his or her own skills to contribute to the field.

Although a large book, and covering a good deal of ground, the case study approach of the book means that while there is a strong overall structure, each chapter can be read, up to a point, independently. Thus, a reader interested in, say, personal identity, could read Chapter 28 in Part V (Philosophy of mind) without reading the whole of that part, or indeed the whole of the book. Similarly, a philosopher who wants nothing more than an introduction to psychopathology and the classification of psychiatric disorders, could get this from Chapter 3; though our hope is that he or she would then get drawn into reading other chapters to fill out particular topics.

As the basis, on the other hand, of a comprehensive course in philosophy and mental health, the book's strong overall structure supports progressive development of knowledge and skills, running from key concepts (Part I), through the philosophical history of these concepts (Part II), to topics in the philosophy of science relevant to each stage of the clinical encounter, psychopathology, diagnosis, treatment, etc. (Part III), through ethics and the 'added value' for practice from philosophical value theory (Part IV), and so, finally, in Part V, to specific areas of psychopathology and the two-way connections between these and some of the deepest problems in the philosophy of mind.

If philosophy is about argument, it is also about change. Philosophy provokes change. But it also gives us the skills of open and flexible thinking needed to engage with and manage change in a positive and problem-solving way. Mental health in many countries is currently experiencing revolutionary changes, driven in part by the growing power and authority of the 'user voice', in part by the development of new models of service delivery (user-led, community-based, multidisciplinary, and multiagency), and in part by the promise of the new neurosciences (such as behavioural genetics and functional neuroimaging). The five main parts of the book are thus geared directly to different, although related, aspects of the change management process:

- Part I (*Core concepts in philosophy and mental health*) puts *people's individual experiences of mental distress and disorder* on an equal footing with the generalized knowledge and skills of professionals;

- Part II (*A philosophical history of psychopathology*) brings *empathic understanding of subjective meanings* back into clinical assessment alongside causal explanations;

- Part III (*Philosophy of science and mental health*) enriches our understanding of observational science to show the importance of *subjectivity and judgement* (including *clinical judgement*) based on tacit knowledge alongside objectivity and induction (including the inductive inferences of *evidence-based practice*) based on explicit knowledge;

- Part IV (*Values, ethics, and mental health*) focuses on the importance of *differences of values* alongside the 'framework' shared values prescribed by ethics and law. Values-Based Practice, as the approach derived from philosophical value theory in Part IV is called, involves clinical skills training and a model of service delivery that supports balanced decision-making in situations (such as those involving involuntary hospitalization and treatment) where values conflict;

- Part V (*Philosophy of mind and mental health*) broadens our understanding of rationality to include *personal and interpersonal processes* alongside the subpersonal processes on which the cognitive and behavioural sciences have traditionally focused.

The case study approach of the book, and our aim of proactively contributing to service change, mean that we have been unable to do justice equally to all those whose work in many and diverse areas of scholarship has made often crucial contributions to the new philosophy of psychiatry. We take this opportunity to acknowledge our debt to the many colleagues around the world—academic, practice-based, administrative and political—who have contributed in so many different ways to the development of the field. Large parts of this book are based on materials from a Masters programme in the Philosophy and Ethics of Mental Health (PEMH) developed in the Department of Philosophy at Warwick University. Again, our debt to the many colleagues and students who contributed to the course will be evident throughout the book. We are grateful particularly to Richard Gipps, Matthew Philpott, Chris Walker, Ian Lyne, Paul Sturdee, Mark Bratton and Paul Hoff, who contributed key materials to particular chapters (as detailed in the Table of Contents). Our particular thanks go also to Greg Hunt and to Michael Luntley, as successive Heads of the Philosophy Department, to Martin Warner as Chair of the PEMH Steering Group, and to Jonathan Nichols as University Registrar, for their unstinted support and always wise guidance during the development of the PEMH programme.

It is always invidious to mark out particular individuals for special thanks. But we believe that everyone involved with the PEMH programme will wish to join us in acknowledging the central contribution of Paul Sturdee, as the first PEMH Programme Manager, and as the founder (by way of a generous and substantial donation from his personal library) of the PEMH Resource Base. Without Paul's energy, entrepreneurial skills and wide-ranging scholarship, there would have been no PEMH Masters Programme, and, hence, no Oxford Textbook of Philosophy and Psychiatry.

Bill Fulford
Tim Thornton
George Graham

Foreword (from the voluntary sector)

Lord Victor Adebowale CBE

In 2004 I was asked to speak at the annual conference of Psychiatry 2004 in Madrid. On receiving my invite I was of course flattered but also curious about why I had been asked other than being a peer of the realm and having a career in social care and housing. What qualified me to speak to several hundred psychiatrists? I guessed that being a member of the House of Lords has a certain cache at such gatherings but it's not exactly a qualification in psychiatry, although it is a qualification (of sorts) in making speeches. So I said I would and put my mind to thinking about what I wanted to say.

I needed to rely on my experience of the mental health world from the point of view of those who have used it, over a twenty year career in social care management. I have worked in communities whose access to good mental health care is minimal, unless someone is in extremis, and then they become subject to the Mental Health Act, the legal framework for compulsion in England. I have also worked in settings where people's experience of mental health has led them to self medicate using alcohol and other drugs. My own experience of mental health has been mercifully robust but at the back of my mind as a black man I have the same fear that many minority ethnic people in the United Kingdom report, that is, I have a fear of the system. I hold my mental health dear to me because I know that should it slip from my grasp the system that I may be subject to will diagnose me on the basis of its own values, not necessarily my own or my culture's. What can be more frightening than to be subject to the confusion of your own mind while being at the mercy, however learned, of the diagnosis of others?

I made my contribution to the Madrid conference against a back drop in the UK of mistrust of psychiatry. The press had latched onto the grim details of murder committed by people released into the community. The press did not make the distinction between personality disorder, psychosis, what is treatable and what is manageable, the struggles of diagnosis and the challenge of finding the balance between the resources of care and the assessment of change in a troubled individual. In short, psychiatry was being caricatured

as being out of touch with society's reasonable desire for safety. This crude view was not helped by the growing cry from members of the black and minority ethnic communities in the UK about the feeling that psychiatry was not applying the same rules to black people as it applied to white people. Psychiatrists like Sulman Fernandez and academics like Professor Kamlesh Patel were producing the evidence to back up the suspicion. The death of David 'Rocky' Bennett had sparked a self examination of a system that the investigating judge had termed institutionally racist. I was asked to co-chair with the Minister of State for Health, Rosie Winterton, the national black and minority ethnic mental health strategy as part of the Department of Health's response to the Rocky Bennett tragic death and the feelings of injustice this had generated in the ethnic minority community.

While the structures of mental health struggled to come to terms with challenges from patients and society, psychiatry and psychiatrists were seen as being at the top of the mental health tree, the holders of the rings of power and the process of diagnosis. Psychiatrists had prozac and a model that was based on the biological and social sciences. The question that I felt society was asking was 'is this paradigm enough?' I came to the conclusion that psychiatry was in trouble and I think it was fair to say so at the conference as a manager of mental health services and as someone who knew the users of those services. It was clear to me that psychiatry was of value only if it could examine how it could relate to the perceptions of its users. It is not that psychiatry needed attack from me or anyone else, there are enough anti psychiatry websites and groups around to do that job. My view was (and still is) that debate about psychiatry is not just about the profession but about what we understand to be mental health and what are the concepts that guide our approach to its treatment of those with mental health challenges.

As I prepared my speech I came across the work of Professor Bill Fulford and his colleagues. As a non-psychiatrist it seems to me that an examination of the values on which judgments are made may give some clearer understanding of what shapes perception of both professionals and the users of the services those professionals provide. The challenge is to create a dialogue that allows the examination of the self as an instrument of clinical judgement. In other words the question needs to be asked, do the values of the psychiatrist, mental health workers, psychologist, and psychotherapist have some play in the relationship with the patient. I think this is a fundamental question that drives to the heart of the challenges that psychiatry is faced with. If this question can be faced and answered then a major contribution to the field can be made. The issue of values-based psychiatry cannot be examined in isolation; by definition, it needs an international input with which it can debate its approach. It is only through the creation of a constant process of critique, a critique applicable in clinical settings, that psychiatry can take on the challenge of difference not just in the UK but internationally.

I do not know where values-based psychiatry will lead us but in my view this may be a good thing. The tyranny of certainty can create the biggest block to change. I am impressed by the idea that perhaps the skills of psychiatry can be enhanced by the concept of applied philosophy in some ways. This may be apt given that the roots of mental health lie in the ideas of philosophy. The Lunatic Act was an attempt to end a debate which will simply not go away as long as there are people in the world who are challenged by mental ill health and yet are determined not to give up intellectual freedom in the face of prevailing ideas. The production of this work is a major step forward in creating a new paradigm for psychiatry to contribute to the understanding of mental health. It is overdue but very welcome by those of us who are not psychiatrists and yet want psychiatry to use its authority to lead the way.

The story of my speech to the international conference in Madrid ends quite simply. I said pretty much what I have written here. The response? Well, 50% of the audience liked what I had to say, the other half wanted me 'sectioned'.

Lord Victor Adebowale CBE
Chief Executive, Turning Point
House of Lords
February, 2006

Foreword (from clinical practice)

Professor Ahmed Okasha

A psychiatrist has said that he did not want to burden himself with philosophy .. but the exclusion of philosophy would.. be disastrous for psychiatry.

(Karl Jaspers, 1963)

I never imagined that I should find myself writing a Foreword on Philosophy and Psychiatry but I am delighted to welcome this unprecedented textbook. Karl Jaspers, writing at the start of the twentieth century, during what has become known as psychiatry's first biological phase, was keenly aware of the importance of philosophy as a partner to the neurosciences underpinning our discipline. Yet for much of the twentieth century, psychiatry has lost touch with philosophy. It is all the more exciting, then, that as we enter the twenty-first century, and with it psychiatry's second biological phase, this book, and the new philosophy of psychiatry that it embodies, promises, finally, to fulfil Jaspers' vision.

The World Psychiatric Association, along with many other national and subject-based groups around the world, has strongly embraced the emerging discipline of philosophy of psychiatry by establishing a new section for the field. There are many reasons why philosophy is important in psychiatry. First, there are the deep dichotomies by which we are challenged every day in our clinical work and research: the dichotomy of mind and body, of course, to which I return below; but also, and equally important though less well recognised, the dichotomies of universality versus specificity and of collectivity versus individuality.

Second, is the importance of individual and cultural differences. While researchers, intellectuals, scientists and physicians continue their attempts to find formulaic interpretations summarizing our universal human nature, such formulae usually amount more to a series of exceptions than to a "common" description of the world. It is not surprising that the more we move from the pragmatic and scientific to the humanitarian, the more exceptions come to the forefront. Among the many factors involved here, in resisting generalisations, culture is probably the most prominent. But psychiatry is also the one branch of medicine and science in which the uniqueness of individuals can never be overlooked. Each and every school of psychiatry is characterised by a vision of life, and of individual human nature, that differentiates it from other schools, even if this is not acknowledged by

the advocates of the school in question. Psychiatrists and mental health professionals in general, therefore, while never abandoning their attempts to identify a shared explanatory vision of the world, must always proceed without jeopardizing the individuality not only of different cultural regions, but also of individual persons. Understanding the individual is indispensable to understanding human nature. Descriptive generalizations alone do not suffice.

A third reason for the importance of philosophy in psychiatry today, is the growing complexity of our subject. In a typical clinical interaction psychiatrists are centrally concerned with both subjective, mental, first person constructs, and with objective, third person brain states. In such settings the psychiatrist traverses many times the "mind-brain" divide (Kendler, 2001). Therefore, as a discipline, psychiatry should be deeply interested in the mind-body problem, the answer to which, if there is one, cannot be sought without help from philosophy. Unfortunately training in biomedicine is likely to produce impatience with philosophical discourse in this area. Such impatience is driven by the strongly held desire to find *the* explanation for individual psychiatric disorders, a desire that, although fully understandable, is misplaced and may be counterproductive. Our current knowledge, although incomplete, strongly suggests that all major psychiatric disorders are complex and multifactorial. The best that we can hope for, in consequence, is many small explanations, from a variety of different explanatory perspectives, each addressing part of the complex processes underlying "normality" or disorder. Similarly, there are no simple linear models where one thing leads to another and then to another in a one-way causal direction. Etiological pathways are complex and interacting, more like networks than linear pathways.

Recent decades have witnessed the rise in psychiatry of a biological-reductionist perspective. Multilevel models, especially those including mental and social explanatory perspectives, are typically rejected or accepted only with the caveat, explicit or implicit, that all the "real" causal effects occur at the level of basic biology (Bickle, 2003). This is understandable up to a point. After all, if we agree that there are no mental processes that are independent of brain functioning, then should not all the causes of psychiatric disorders be reducible, at least in principle, to brain processes? This reductionist perspective is understandable sociologically as a reaction to earlier radically mentalistic programs within psychiatry. It is also appealing because of the ease with which it fits into a medical model. But the biological-reductionist approach is too narrow to encompass the range and complexity of causal processes that are operative in psychiatric disorders.

In place of biological reductionism, Engel (1977), McHugh and Slavney (1986) and others, have been strong advocates of explanatory pluralism, in which mutually informative perspectives—social and psychological as well as biological—are combined in approaching natural phenomena. This is a powerful approach. Yet each of these perspectives assumes the natural science paradigm that Jaspers termed "explanation". This brings us, therefore, to a fourth reason for embracing philosophy in psychiatry. For psychiatry needs a pluralistic approach that engages not only with the explanatory paradigms of natural science, but also, as Jaspers insisted, with the paradigms of human understanding.

The need for a fully pluralistic approach in psychiatry, an approach fully encompassing Jaspers' twin demands for human understanding as well as for scientific explanation, has never been more urgent, both at an individual and at a cultural level. At an individual level, a long clinical tradition and much empirical evidence point to the importance of first person mental processes in the aetiology of psychiatric disorders. Loss, for example, cannot be dealt with adequately without understanding the meaning of loss for a particular grieving person, whatever explanatory insights we may have into its underlying basic neurobiological mechanisms (Kendler et al., 2003).

At the level of culture, the importance of human understanding as well as scientific explanation is reflected in a large body of descriptive literature showing that cultural processes affect psychiatric illnesses. Culture gives *meaning* to events, where the same event may mean different things in different settings. The importance of cultural differences has been neglected even in bioethics (Okasha, 2000). Here, perhaps, it is understandable, although certainly to be resisted; and the strongly international nature of the new philosophy of psychiatry, drawing equally on the mutual strengths of different traditions around the world (Fulford et al., 2004), is very much to be welcomed in this respect. But that cultural differences should have been so marginalized in the biosciences is surely remarkable. There is, no doubt, a sense in which culture ultimately exists as belief systems in the brains of individual members of a cultural group. But it is unlikely in the extreme that the cultural forces that shape psychopathology will ever be efficiently understood at the level of brain biology. After all, even chemistry, although today reducible in principle to physics, cannot be efficiently explained in terms of interactions between electron shells!

And chemistry, correspondingly, continues to thrive as a discipline that is deeply connected with, but still independent of, physics.

Scientific explanation and human understanding are not incompatible, of course. The pluralistic approach has sometimes been wrongly interpreted as a model in which disparate factors act independently to affect risk. However, even at the level of scientific explanation, the reality is more complex. The actions of basic biological risk factors for psychiatric illnesses are modified by forces acting at higher levels of cultural abstraction, such as the rearing environment, stressful life experiences and exposure to other cultural forces. Furthermore, environmental risk factors modulate the effect of biological risk factors in causing illness. For example, genetic risk factors for major depression increase the probability of interpersonal and marital difficulties, which are themselves known risk factors for depression. The relationships between causes (explanation) and meanings (understanding) in psychiatric illness are thus not one to one. Genetic risk factors can predispose to a range of different psychiatric disorders, depending on the action of other factors, including the meaning and significance of events for an individual, creating a many-to-many aetiological linkage rather than a one-to-one pattern (Kendler, 2005).

Critical processes in the mind-brain system therefore, as Jaspers so clearly recognised, can only be captured through an understanding of the higher organizational levels of these goal directed systems. This means that working in the field of psychiatry inevitably involves us in some of the most important and perplexing questions facing the human race. But it also means that, with Karl Jaspers at the start of the twentieth century, our hope at the start of the twenty-first century should continue to be for the development of psychiatry as a genuinely humanitarian discipline that will in turn allow us to use future scientific advances to good effect in helping our patients and their families. We have to be modest while being challenged by the complexity of the human brain-mind interaction, and with great humility accept that full understanding thereof, if at all possible, will call for the integration of multiple disciplines and perspectives. This book will take us an important step towards achieving that goal.

Professor Ahmed Okasha
MD, PhD, FRCP, FRCPsych, FACP (Hon.)
Director, WHO Coordinating Center for
Research and Training in Mental Health,
President WPA
Cairo, September, 2005

References

Bickle J. (2003). Philosophy and Neuroscience: A ruthlessly reductive account. Boston, Kluwer Academic.

Engel GL. (1977). The need for a new medical model: a challenge for biomedicine. Science 196: 129–136.

Fulford, K.W.M., Stanghellini, G. and Broome, M. (2004). What can philosophy do for psychiatry? Special Article for *World Psychiatry* (WPA), Oct 2004, pps 130–135.

Japers K. (1963). General Psychopathology. Chicago, University of Chicago Press.

Kendler KS, Hettema JM, Butera F, Gardner CO, Prescott CA. (2003). Life event dimensions of loss, humiliation, entrapment and danger in the prediction of onsets of major depression and generalized anxiety. Arch Gen Psychiatry 60: 789–796.

Kendler KS. (2001). A psychiatric dialogue on the mind-body problem. Am J Psychiatry, 158: 989–1000.

Kendler KS. (2005). Toward a philosophical structure for psychiatry. Am J Psychiatry, 162: 433–440.

McHugh PR, Slavney PR. (1986). The Perspectives of psychiatry. Baltimore, Johns Hopkins University Press.

Okasha, A. (2000). Ethics of Psychiatric Practice: Consent, Compulsion and Confidentiality. *Current Opinion in Psychiatry*. Vol 13, 693–698.

Foreword (from philosophy)

Baroness Warnock

The publication of the *Oxford Textbook of Philosophy and Psychiatry* marks a step forward in the practical interaction between philosophy and medicine, especially psychiatric medicine. Through the growth of teaching in Bioethics (as well as of research and publication), the overlap between philosophical theory and medical advance has become an accepted phenomenon. However, largely because of the success of the pioneering work of Beauchamp and Childress (Beauchamp, T.L. and Childress, J.F. Principles of Biomedical Ethics NY: OUP 1989) bioethics has become somewhat hidebound, a matter almost of received dogma. Their widely adopted four principles, Beneficence, Non-maleficence, Autonomy and Justice have been repeatedly cited as giving the framework for ethical decisions in medicine, without due recognition of the vagueness and imprecision of the principles. All are in need of interpretation in order to provide guidance in particular cases. The merit of the *Textbook* is its insistence that dialogue between patient and doctor lies at the heart of good treatment, and that such dialogue must rely on insight into the way a particular patient experiences the world and the significance for him or her of these experiences. The four principles may be accepted: but what is essentially required in good practice is a realization of what it is to gain access to another mind.

There are, it seems to me, three features of the *Textbook* that are of peculiar importance. First, there is its insistence, as I have suggested, on the crucial place of discourse in psychiatry. At a common-sense level, we are all still at risk of adopting a version of Cartesian dualism, a division between mind and body. Such dualism is deeply ingrained in ordinary language, in the dichotomy we tend to accept between the mental and the physical, the inner and the outer. This leads to an artificial anxiety about how it is possible to communicate with one another. After all, in Descartes' view, all we can really know is our own sensations and perceptions. These include the visual, auditory and tactile ideas we have of other people; but it cannot include any knowledge of their minds. We are aware of our own inner life but not of theirs. We

may therefore fall into a pessimistic view of true communication; we may tend to rely on behaviouristic or perhaps physiological symptoms as a way of understanding the problems other people may suffer. The ways out of this anxiety were illuminatingly explored in the initial volume of the series on International Perspectives in Philosophy and Psychiatry (Nature and Narrative edited by Bill Fulford, Katherine Morris, John Sadler and Giovanni Stanghellini, Oxford 2003), especially in the essays by Rom Harré and Grant Gillett, and are further pursued at a more immediately practical level in the *Textbook*. The crucial insight derives originally from the phenomenology of Brentano and Husserl, and thence from Wittgenstein's view of language as essentially a shared and public connexion between 'us' (people in the same boat, experiencing the world together and part of that world), not a private attempt to describe our inner experiences. Language, then, being intrinsically for communication, needs to have particular attention paid to it in the discourse between patient and doctor.

Secondly, the *Textbook* insists on the importance of discovering the values usually embedded in the language of this discourse, carefully unravelling the areas where values may be disguised as facts (though, perhaps I should add, the areas also where values and facts are inextricably linked. The Oxford philosopher, J.L. Austin, an inspiration for this book, used as an example of such linkage the aesthetic terms 'dainty' and 'dumpy'). It also insists on the importance of thereafter uncovering where the values of the participants in the dialogue may differ. For example it may be assumed by a physician that it is always in the best interests of a patient to stay alive, and that a disposition towards suicide must always be pathological; whereas for a patient, life may not be the highest value.

Thirdly, and perhaps most importantly of all, the *Textbook* highlights those problems about personal identity that have always been at the centre of philosophy. In the seventeenth century the philosopher John Locke distinguished what made someone the same person from what made him the same man. 'Person' he argued was a forensic term, essentially an issue of what someone could be held responsible for in a court of law; 'man' on the other hand was a matter simply of physical continuity from the cradle to the grave. Since then philosophers have wrestled with the problem of what it means to be an individual person, what it is that the pronoun 'I' refers to. It has long been understood that psychiatric 'cases' of multiple personality and amnesia have light to throw on this question. In my view there is no area where the interlocking of psychiatry and philosophy is of more practical (and of course moral and legal) significance than here. Our unthinking common language may conceal but can sometimes prove adequate for the distinctions we ought to draw. Once again, the *Textbook* should be an invaluable starting point for enhanced understanding.

Baroness Warnock
House of Lords
January, 2006

CHAPTER 1

Progress in five parts

The Oxford philosopher, J.L. Austin, on whose work we will be drawing particularly in Part I of this book, once described philosophy as unique among academic disciplines in being concerned with problems not only without solutions but without even agreed methods for finding solutions. Philosophy is in this sense an 'edge discipline'. It is concerned with problems at the edge of our understanding. However, for many philosophical problems of this edge kind, there is a practical counterpart edge problem just below the surface of day-to-day practice or research in mental health: the problem of free-will, for example, is just below the surface of the addictive disorders, volition is just below the surface of obsessional disorders, knowledge of other minds is at the heart of childhood autism, disturbances of personal identity are central to the experiences of people with schizophrenia, problems of rationality are at the heart of the clinical concept of delusion, responsibility and issues of 'mad or bad?' are central concerns in forensic psychiatry, and, not least, the wider issues of the relationship between mind and brain are raised in acute new ways by functional neuroimaging research.

This book explores a series of edge problems shared between philosophy and mental health in five key topic areas, concepts of disorder, the philosophical history of psychopathology, philosophy of science, ethics and philosophical value theory, and philosophy of mind. Adopting a case study approach, the aim is depth not breadth. Each chapter takes the reader along one or more lines of argument around a given 'edge problem' shared between philosophy and mental health, testing and challenging the ideas presented through guided readings and other exercises aimed at developing the sharp thinking skills that are at the heart, equally, of both disciplines.

The extent of the shared agenda between philosophy and mental health is such that our selection of case studies is inevitably partial and incomplete. A number of important topic areas are covered in other books, some of them, as noted in Box 1.1, within this series: contemporary phenomenology, for example, although

introduced in this book, will be the particular focus of Joseph Parnas, Louis Sass, and Giovanni Stanghellini's (forthcoming) *The Vulnerable Self: the clinical phenomenology of the schizophrenic and affective spectrum disorders*. However, there are other areas, such as the praxis-based Eastern philosophies, the meditative, Islamic and other spiritual traditions, and an emerging African philosophy, all of which, as noted in chapter 4, although offering potentially important resources for philosophy and mental health, await substantive treatment within the newly emerging field.

Box 1.1 Core companion literature for the *Oxford Textbook of Philosophy and Psychiatry*

The book as a whole

- Parnas, J., Sass, L., Stanghellini, G., and Fuchs, T. (forthcoming). *The Vulnerable Self: the clinical phenomenology of the schizophrenic and affective spectrum disorders*. Oxford: Oxford University Press

- Radden, J. (ed.). (2004). *The Philosophy of Psychiatry: a companion*. New York: Oxford University Press.

- The journal, *Philosophy, Psychiatry, & Psychology* (published in Baltimore, MD, USA, by The Johns Hopkins University Press).

Part I Core concepts in philosophy and mental health

- Caplan, A.L., Engelhardt, T., and McCartney, J.J. (ed.) (1981). *Concepts of Health and Disease: interdisciplinary perspectives*. Reading, MA: Addison-Wesley Publishing Co.

- Fulford, K.W.M. (1989, reprinted 1995 and 1999). *Moral Theory and Medical Practice*. Cambridge: Cambridge University Press.

♦ Tyrer, P. and Steinberg, D. (2005). *Models for Mental Disorder: conceptual models in psychiatry*, (3rd). Chichester: John Wiley and Sons.

Part II A philosophical history of psychopathology

♦ Berrios, G.E. (1996). *The History of Mental Symptoms*. Cambridge: Cambridge University Press.

♦ Berrios, G.E. and Porter, R. (1992). *A History of Clinical Psychiatry: the origin and history of mental disorders*. London: Athlone Press.

Part III The philosophy of science and mental health

♦ Boyd, R., Gasker, P., and Trout, J.D. (1999). *The Philosophy of Science*. Cambridge, MA: MIT Press.

♦ Sadler, J.Z., Wiggins, O.P., and Schwartz, M.A. (ed.) (1994). *Philosophical Perspectives on Psychiatric Diagnostic Classification*. Baltimore, MD: Johns Hopkins University Press.

Part IV Values, ethics, and mental health

♦ Bloch, S., Chodoff, P., and Green, S. A. (1999). *Psychiatric Ethics*, (3rd edn). Oxford: Oxford University Press.

♦ Dickenson, D. and Fulford, K.W.M. (2000). *In Two Minds: a casebook of psychiatric ethics*. Oxford: Oxford University Press.

♦ Sadler, J.Z. (ed.) (2002). *Descriptions & Prescriptions: values, mental disorders, and the DSMs*. Baltimore: Johns Hopkins University Press.

♦ Sadler, J.Z. (2004). *Values and Psychiatric Diagnosis*. Oxford: Oxford University Press.

♦ Woodbridge, K. and Fulford, K.W.M. (2004). *Whose Values? A workbook for values-based practice in mental health care*. London: Sainsbury Centre for Mental Health.

Part V Philosophy of mind and mental health

♦ Graham, G. and Stephens, G.L. (1994). *Philosophical Psychopathology*. Cambridge, MA: The MIT Press.

♦ Rosenthal, D. (ed.) (1991). *The Nature of Mind*. Oxford: Oxford University Press.

Consistently with the edge nature of the problems on the shared agenda of philosophy and mental health, there are no 'grand unified theories' in this book, no claims to 'explanations' of consciousness or of free will, or to 'solutions' of the mind–body problem. The temptation to come up with 'answers' is real enough. As we describe more fully in the concluding chapter of this book, 'Histories of the future', during the twentieth century philosophy and mental health both suffered stigmatizing negative attitudes arising from their respective failures to come up with 'answers'. A natural response to such attitudes is to take short-cuts, to collapse complex problems to solutions that, although perhaps simple and easy to understand, are wrong. In philosophy such short-cuts are relatively harmless. However, in mental health they lead to ideologically-driven foreclosures on this or that particular model of service delivery, which, in constraining the rich diversity of human experience and behaviour to a one-size-fits-all diagnostic or therapeutic system, became the basis of some of the worst abuses in twentieth century mental health care.

We should not be *too* chary of progress, on the other hand. On the contrary, as each part of the book illustrates in different ways, progress of a modest kind (albeit not in the form of incontestable or final 'answers') is already being made across a number of topics within the interdisciplinary field of philosophy and mental health.

Part I, on *Core Concepts in Philosophy and Mental Health*, focuses on the concept of mental disorder as the concept at the interface between philosophy and mental health. Three chapters draw out the characteristic features, respectively, of philosophical problems, methods, and results, as these bear particularly on mental health research and practice. There is also a chapter introducing psychiatric classification and descriptive psychopathology for philosophers, and a chapter introducing philosophical logic for practitioners.

It may seem inconsistent with the shared status of philosophy and mental health as 'edge' disciplines, to be talking of characteristically philosophical problems and methods, let alone results. The storyline of Part I, however, runs from an opening up of complex conceptual problems through methodological pluralism to results that amount to a more complete view of the original conceptual difficulties. Again, no grand unified theory emerges from this process, no claim to a full or final account of the complex concept of mental disorder. However, the more complete view to which we come provides a framework that is rich enough to support the user-centred and multidisciplinary models of service delivery of modern mental health practice.

Part II, *A Philosophical History of Psychopathology*, starts with a short sharp chapter, a 20-minute history of the shifting boundary between medical and moral understandings of mental disorder since classical times. The Part follows with an account of the foundational work of the German philosopher-psychiatrist Karl Jaspers on descriptive psychopathology in the early twentieth century, and then goes deep with two chapters on the influence on Jaspers respectively of Husserl's phenomenology and of the nineteenth century debate on methods in the human sciences, the *Methodenstreit*.

Throughout Part II, although focusing on the history of ideas behind modern descriptive psychopathology, our eye will be fixed very much on the future. Understanding how we came to current systems of psychopathology may help to guide future developments particularly as these are driven by advances in the neurosciences. Although covered in more detail in other books in this series, we include in Part II sections on 'phenomenology today' and on the 'modern methodenstreit', the range of rigorous methods now available for the study of subjective meanings and significance alongside the methods available from the neurosciences for studying causal pathways in the brain.

With *Part III, Philosophy of Science and Mental Health*, we move into a series of in-depth case studies organized broadly around the stages of the clinical encounter: (1) the implications of the failure of logical empiricism for careful observation as the basis of clinical work; (2) diagnosis, classification, and realism in science; (3) clinical judgement and tacit knowledge; (4) the relationship between reasons and causes and theories of aetiology; and (5) the nature of progress in science and the role of evidence-based medicine in guiding treatment choice.

It is here above all, in the philosophy of science, that the 'edge' nature of the problems in mental health research and practice is most clearly evident. In the opening chapter of Part III, for example, a series of short excerpts from one of Freud's extended early case studies (the case of Dora) anticipates each of the key innovations in late twentieth century philosophy of science that we study in detail in later chapters. The scientific status of psychoanalysis, indeed of psychiatry itself, is a matter of continuing philosophical debate. But the message of Part III, a message that is captured most decisively by the problems of psychiatric classification explored in Chapter 13, is that psychiatric science is not a deficient, but, simply, a *difficult* science, closer perhaps in the rich mix of conceptual and empirical difficulties with which it is concerned, and the role that this gives to individual judgement in the scientific process, to theoretical physics than to the biological models underpinning traditional medicine.

Part IV, on *Values, Ethics and Mental Health*, starts with the familiar ethical issues of involuntary treatment and confidentiality but rapidly moves into the relatively unfamiliar territory of philosophical value theory. The storyline of Part IV is that the tools of traditional bioethics, effective as they have been up to a point in general medicine, are not well adapted to the conceptually more complex edge-of-understanding problems of mental health.

Part IV illustrates the way in which, even in an edge discipline, a discipline concerned with complex problems for which there is as yet no settled methodology, progress of a modest kind is still possible, not through 'solving' the big problems of philosophy, but by running with the breaks, by discovering a way in which some small part of a complex problem can be made tractable through new instrumentation or by way of a novel conceptual insight. Thus, a small but practically important part of the extra conceptual complexity of mental health ethics is the diversity of the values involved. This is because in mental health we are concerned with areas of human experience and behaviour—emotion, desire, volition, belief, identity, sexuality, and so forth—in which human values are highly variable. Philosophical value theory, introduced in Part I, makes this aspect of the added conceptual difficulty of mental health ethics tractable. Values-Based Practice, as the practical counterpart of philosophical value theory is called, is introduced in

Part IV and its philosophy-into-practice applications (primarily through clinical skills training) are described, including its central importance for diagnostic assessment, an aspect of clinical practice that is of primary importance in all areas of health care and yet has been almost entirely ignored by traditional bioethics.

With *Part V*, on *Philosophy of Mind and Mental Health*, the final part of the book, we move into the metaphysical deeps of the philosophy of mind. As the natural bed-fellow of mental health research and practice, the philosophy of mind, in both analytic and Continental (especially phenomenological) traditions, has been an area of particularly active cross-disciplinary work in philosophy and mental health. The chapters in Part V thus cover case studies in the mind–body problem and organic psychiatry (in the case of Mrs Lazy whose brain tumour altered her personality 'for good'), in free will and volitional disorders, in autism and Knowledge of Other Minds, in personal identity and the disturbances of consciousness in schizophrenia, and in the relationship generally between reasons (of the kind we give for the things we do) and causes (of the kind offered by neuroscientists by way of explanations for the things we do).

Part V illustrates a further and crucial feature of the shared status of philosophy and mental health as disciplines at the edge of understanding. Through Parts I–IV most of the trade between the two disciplines has (thus far) been from philosophy to mental health: Values-Based Practice, for example, is a direct draw-down into mental health policy and practice from philosophical value theory. In the philosophy of mind, by contrast, there is an important trade the other way. Philosophy of mind does have implications for research and practice in mental health: Matthew Philpott's work, for example, described in Part II, draws on Merleau Ponty's phenomenology to explain the surface phenomena of dyslexia in terms of underlying differences in the temporal structuring of experience. However, in this area, much of the trade is the other way, the rich variety of psychopathology providing a crucial real-world resource for philosophy. A number of philosophers have recognized this. The Oxford philosopher of mind, for example, the late Kathleen Wilkes, made the resources of psychopathology the central theme of her seminal book, *Real People: personal identity without thought experiments*.

As noted earlier, the difficulties of making progress in both philosophy and mental health, as disciplines working at the edge of understanding, were consistently misconstrued throughout much of the twentieth century as deficiencies in the disciplines themselves, and philosophy and mental health were thus alike in being the butt of negative stigmatizing attitudes. The progress already made in the new interdisciplinary field points to a very different future in the twenty-first century. We return to this theme, to the trajectory of the interdisciplinary field of philosophy and mental health, at the end of this book, in chapter 29. Our conclusion will be that, contrary to the stigmatizing attitudes of the twentieth century, the new interdisciplinary field of philosophy and mental health is leading the way in the development of a model of twenty-first century health care that is equally science-based and person-centred.

PART I

Core concepts in philosophy and mental health

Part contents

Introduction to Part I

In this first part we explore some of the difficulties surrounding the concept of mental disorder. These difficulties are at the heart of the interdisciplinary field of philosophy and mental health: as we will see, they define the overlap between, on the one hand, the problems of traditional philosophy, and, on the other, the problems faced by those involved practically in mental health, as users and as providers of services, as policy makers and as researchers.

Exploring these difficulties, therefore, in this part, in addition to introducing each side to the other—philosophers to practitioners and practitioners to philosophers—will provide a framework of ideas within which the more specific materials of later parts of the book will be set, materials drawn respectively from the history of ideas in Part II, from the philosophy of science in Part III, from ethics and philosophical value theory in Part IV, and from the philosophy of mind in Part V. (*Note*: In this book we use the term 'practitioner' to mean anyone with practical experience of mental health issues. This includes not only professionals of various kinds, policy makers, and researchers, but also, and centrally, users (or consumers) of services, i.e. patients, informal carers, their families and the wider community.)

Introductory, yes, elementary, no

Part I, then, is in this sense introductory: it outlines the key conceptual difficulties by which the interdisciplinary field between philosophy and mental health practice is defined.

If Part I is an introduction, however, it is anything but elementary. On the contrary, in starting with the difficulties surrounding the concept of mental disorder, we will be diving straight in at the deep end. For these difficulties, as we will see, combine some of the trickiest problems of traditional philosophy with the urgency of practical necessity: in mental health, as in other practical disciplines, philosophical no less than empirical research is directly driven by the real problems faced by real people in the real world.

The structure of Part I

Part I has five chapters covering, broadly, problems, methods, and outputs. Thus,

♦ *Chapters 2 and 3* set out the *problem of mental disorder* in its conceptual, i.e. philosophical, aspects. Chapter 2 shows that the difficulties surrounding the concept of mental disorder in everyday practice reflect deeper (if largely unacknowledged) difficulties in the conceptual structure of medicine and health care as a whole. Chapter 3 fills out the specific features, the range and diversity of psychopathological states, that any philosophical analysis of the conceptual structure of medicine and health care must seek to explain.

♦ *Chapters 4 and 5* are concerned with methods of philosophical enquiry. Chapter 4 shows the need for both analytic and 'Continental' methods in philosophy and mental health. Chapter 5 introduces modern logic as a 'toolkit' for clear thinking and for assessing the validity of arguments.

♦ *Chapter 6*, as the final chapter in Part I, brings us to *outputs*, to the results we should expect from philosophical work in mental health. We will see that both too much and too little has been claimed for philosophy. Chapter 6 avoids both extremes, arguing that, for the interdisciplinary field at least, a key output from philosophical research is to give us a more complete understanding of the meanings of the core concepts—mental illness, disease, etc.—by which the field itself is shaped and defined.

Difficult, yes, intractable, no

With the deep problems of general philosophy—mind and brain, freedom, truth and so forth—the game, as they say, will perhaps always be more in the playing than in (ultimate) success. The plain difficulty of these problems is perhaps why philosophy is so widely characterized as failing to make progress.

In mental health too, then, to the extent that the conceptual difficulties we face reflect these same problems, we should not expect (ultimate) success. But progress, at least, can be made. The more complete understanding of the meanings of our concepts, to which philosophical enquiry leads, is a small step, certainly, to resolving the difficulties with which these concepts are associated. But it is a step in the right direction. For as we will see in later parts of the book, notably in Part IV (on philosophical value theory), improved understanding of concepts of disorder, derived from work in the new interdisciplinary field, is already making a number of distinct contributions to practice, in the development of policy, in new skills-training programmes for frontline staff, and in the organization of services.

CHAPTER 2

Philosophical problems in mental health practice and research

Chapter contents

It is a remarkable fact that philosophers, in a sense the experts on rationality, should have taken so little interest in irrationality.

Anthony Quinton (1985)

Things have changed a lot since Anthony Quinton, a British philosopher, formerly at Oxford and then a member of the House of Lords, made this observation in a lecture to the Royal Institute of Philosophy (Quinton, 1985). Philosophers are nowadays actively interested in a wide range of topics from mental health practice and research. Conversely, mental health practitioners (including both professionals and users of services) are actively interested in a wide range of philosophical topics. Indeed, the explosive growth in cross-disciplinary contact in the last few years (see Reading Guide) has been as remarkable as the earlier long period of mutual neglect.

The years of neglect have left a legacy, though, in the form of a communication gap. Philosophers coming for the first time to a problem in mental health often lack the background knowledge, the first-hand 'craft' experience, to tap into the philosophically relevant aspects of mental health problems in a practically relevant way. Practitioners, on the other hand, coming to philosophy for the first time, often have little understanding of what philosophers do and of how they go about doing it.

Part I of this book is designed to throw a bridge across the communication gap between philosophy and mental health. In this chapter, we start the process of bridge-building with a look at the nature of philosophical problems in mental health. We examine how and where they arise, and the ways in which they differ from the empirical (or scientific) problems with which practitioners are usually more familiar.

Structure of the chapter

This chapter is divided into four sessions:

* *Session 1*: What is philosophy? What is psychiatry?

* *Session 2*: Fact, value, and the concept of mental disorder.

* *Session 3*: Antipsychiatry and the debate about mental illness.

* *Session 4*: The medical model (and beyond).

Session 1 introduces both sides, philosophers and practitioners, to the nature of philosophical problems in mental health. Then, in *Sessions 2–4*, we tackle what is perhaps the central philosophical problem in mental health, i.e. how the very *concept* of mental disorder should be understood. Session 2 sets out the terms of reference of the problem in the form of a conceptual 'map' of the key features of mental disorder. Session 3 looks at antipsychiatry and how this measures up to the need to explain the conceptual features of mental disorder. Session 4 repeats this process for pro-psychiatry.

Taking the results of Sessions 3 (antipsychiatry) and 4 (pro-psychiatry) together will give us a deeper understanding of the problem of how the concept of mental disorder is to be understood. Chapter 3 will build on this, filling out the details of the wide variety of mental disorders covered by the conceptual

map of psychiatry introduced here in Session 2. This in turn will pave the way for an introduction to philosophical methods, the topic we will be taking up in Chapters 4 and 5.

Session 1 What is philosophy? What is psychiatry?

What philosophy is, is a problem with which philosophers themselves have been much concerned—there are whole books on the subject, and many introductions to philosophy start with a section on this question.

Psychiatrists have not in general been much concerned with what psychiatry is. Most textbooks make some simple opening statement about it being a branch of medicine concerned with disorders of the mind. Other groups, however, psychologists, mental health nurses, users of services, and carers, have often been critical of psychiatry's self-image as a branch of medicine. As we will see later in this chapter, they have adopted different, although not necessarily incompatible, models of mental health.

A clinical case history

So, there is a problem about what philosophy is; and there also is a problem about what psychiatry is. Let's start with an example.

EXERCISE 1   (20 minutes)

First, think of a problem case, preferably one where involuntary treatment was an issue. If you have practical experience of mental health, there may be a case known to you personally, either in a professional capacity or as a user of services. Any case will do: but write down brief details, covering the problem, how it was assessed (including the 'diagnosis'), management, and outcome. (Obviously, if you are working in a group, you need to be careful to anonymize the story to ensure confidentiality.) If you are a philosopher, or otherwise do not have access to a suitable case, here is an example . . .

Example case: Mr AB, Age 48, bank manager

Presented in casualty with low mood, biological symptoms of depression (he had been waking early and had lost weight), and a hypochondriacal delusion (that he had brain cancer). He had a past history of a serious suicide attempt. He had come to casualty complaining of pain in his face and asking for something to 'help him sleep'. He was diagnosed as suffering major depression but refused to stay in hospital for treatment. On an application from his wife, he was admitted as an involuntary patient under the Mental Health Act, 1983 (applicable at the time in England and Wales). He made a full recovery on antidepressant medication. At follow-up a few weeks later, he admitted that he had been planning to kill himself when he believed he had brain cancer and had been feeling so depressed.

(We will be returning to Mr AB's story several times in this and later sessions. It is described more fully in Fulford, 1989.)

Now, think about the problem presented by Mr AB when he was refusing treatment (or your own equivalent case). This is an 'everyday' clinical problem. But is it a *philosophical* problem?

As we will see, there are a number of ways in which Mr AB could be said to present a philosophical problem. Before going on, think about this for yourself:

1. list as many philosophical problems presented by Mr AB as you can think of, and

2. contrast these with the way his problem would ordinarily be formulated clinically.

Everyday clinical assessment

In everyday clinical practice, the assessment of a person such as Mr AB would be 'summed up' in a *diagnosis*, e.g. 'major depression', as in the vignette. This is based on a wide range of information derived from: (1) taking a 'clinical history' (from the patient and from 'other witnesses', e.g. Mrs AB); (2) from an examination of 'the *mental state*'; and (3) from a physical examination. We will be returning to this in Chapter 3. Briefly, the Mental State Examination (or MSE) is a structured review of the patient's appearance, behaviour, and speech, especially as these reflect their mental state. It also covers the form and content of their thoughts; their mood (happy, sad, etc.), beliefs (including delusions), and perceptions (including hallucinations); their 'cognitive functioning' (which in this context means orientation in time and for place and person; attention; short- and long-term memory; and general intellectual level, or IQ); and their insight into the problem. Detailed accounts of psychiatric assessment, including examination of the mental state, can be found in any of the textbooks listed in the reading guides to this chapter and to Chapter 3 (the introduction to psychopathology).

The large amount of information gathered about the patient, from the history, MSE, and physical examination, now has to be summarized and organized into what is called a *formulation*. A formulation sets out in note form the key information about the patient under four main headings:

1. *Differential diagnosis*: this covers (a) the patient's *symptoms* (the precise form of which may be important—we look at a number of particular delusions, hallucinations, and disorders of thinking in more detail in later sessions), and (b) the *pattern* of symptoms and the extent to which these fit the 'disease entities' or particular disorders defined in psychiatric classifications. A differential diagnosis takes the form of a list of possible diagnoses with a summary of the points from the clinical history, etc., for and against each of them. In Mr AB's case, the list would include not only major depression, but, e.g. atypical facial pain, and indeed, brain cancer.

2. *Aetiology*: the causal factors that may be operating, usually divided into predisposing, precipitating, maintaining and protective, i.e. strengths or positive factors.

3. *Treatment*: the management plan, building on the person's own strengths and resources to produce the particular combination of psychological, social, and physical interventions (e.g. antidepressant drugs), appropriate to the individual's needs, but also including (a) *explanation* (i.e. the understanding of the problem to which the practitioner has come with the patient), and (b) plans for *follow up*.

4. *Prognosis*: i.e. an estimate of the likely outcome.

Points arising: empirical and conceptual

The process of gathering and organizing all this information may be highly problematic in straightforwardly empirical (or fact-gathering) ways. In more technological areas of medicine, *most* of the problems of assessment are empirical. In primary care, though, and in mental health in particular, some of the most difficult problems arise not so much from disagreements about the *facts*, as from disagreements about how the facts should be *understood* or *interpreted*.

Mr AB: a clinical conceptual problem

This is well illustrated by Mr AB. Most psychiatrists reading the facts of his case (as in the vignette) think that it is obvious what should be done, i.e. that Mr AB should be treated as an involuntary patient under the relevant mental health legislation. Other groups, however, disagree with this, rejecting involuntary treatment on grounds of human freedom and dignity. We will be returning to involuntary treatment in detail later (in Part IV). The essential *clinical* difficulty with involuntary treatment, however, is not the facts but how the facts should be interpreted or understood. If we understand Mr AB's condition (defined by his sadness, beliefs, pain, etc.) to be a mental illness (or other form of mental *disorder*), then involuntary treatment may be appropriate in view of the risk of suicide. If we do *not* take his condition to be a mental illness, then involuntary treatment is *not* appropriate (though other *non*-medical preventive interventions may still be made, on, e.g. humanitarian or religious grounds).

So the critical clinical issue in Mr AB's case (and this is an *everyday* clinical case, remember) is not the facts but how the facts are interpreted. This is where philosophy comes in. Broadly speaking, where science is concerned with facts, philosophy is concerned with concepts, with the general framework of ideas within which facts have to be interpreted or understood.

No sharp divide

We will see later, especially in Part III, that this way of putting it suggests too sharp a divide: science is not, merely, fact-gathering, whatever some scientists may think; philosophy, similarly, cannot proceed in a fact-free world, whatever its pretensions in that direction. There are no 'theory-free facts': all concepts are contingent (dependent on the way things are), even if only developmentally (i.e. in the way we come to grasp them). All the same, the distinction as formulated perhaps most clearly by the eighteenth century Prussian philosopher Immanuel Kant, between form (concepts) and content (facts), still serves well in many areas. (We return latter in detail in Part II.)

Philosophy and clinical cases

Where does this leave Mr AB? What is 'philosophical' about his problem? The term 'philosophy', understood as a concern with concepts, is used in three main ways, ranging from (1) one's overall '*Weltanschauung*', or scheme of life, through (2) various specific branches of philosophy (such as ethics), to (3) more detailed conceptual analytic concerns with clarifying meanings and implications. Mr AB can be understood as raising philosophical problems in all three senses of the term.

1. *Weltanschauung*. There is an issue of '*Weltanschauung*'. Should Mr AB be regarded as someone who is ill and, to this extent, not responsible? Or does he have a spiritual or moral problem? Many religions would not condone suicide even for someone who believes he has brain cancer. Issues of courage, of free will, come in. We all bring a general 'philosophy of life' of some kind to our understanding of human behaviour. Given Mr AB's story as described here, it is more (or less) natural to think of him as ill. However, suppose he had raped someone? Issues of responsibility are especially emotive in forensic psychiatry.

2. *Specific areas of philosophy*. Several philosophical disciplines are relevant to the clinical problem presented by Mr AB. At one level, the problem is *ethical*—the ethical problem is between Mr AB's right to autonomous choice and the responsibility of the doctor to use his skills with the patient's best interests in mind. (We will return to this in Part IV). But there is also an *epistemological* (or theory of knowledge) question at the heart of the case (is his belief *really* a delusion); a *jurisprudential* issue (of the legal grounds for taking Mr AB to be not responsible for his own choices, however foolish); there is a *phenomenological* issue (just how do we 'understand' Mr AB's experience, how should his mental states—his wishes, motives, and so forth—be properly described? This is an area to which Continental philosophy is especially relevant). There are also issues of a *political philosophical* kind. Michel Foucault, writing in the Continental tradition, argued on historical grounds that the incarceration of the mentally ill reflected the 'work ethic' of the industrial revolution and the need to preserve social order. This tension, between moral (or social) and medical interpretations of cases such as Mr AB, has a long history. So the *history* of *ideas* is important, as we explore in Part II. Finally, Mr AB's case also raises a range of deeper *metaphysical* issues: if he has a *mental* illness, how should we understand the relationship between mind and brain? (The mind–body problem is explored in detail later, in Part V.)

3. *Conceptual analysis*. At the heart of all these issues, though, as we saw a moment ago, is a conceptual problem, namely, just what is meant by saying that Mr AB is mentally ill. We will return to this in more detail in Part IV, where we will see that involuntary psychiatric treatment depends on two conditions being satisfied: the person concerned must be (1) at *risk* (to themselves or others), but also, (2) suffering from a *mental disorder*. In Mr AB's case, as noted in the vignette, the relevant legislation was the UK Mental Health Act, 1983: but there is similar legislation in most countries around the world. In all legislations, the second condition, that the person concerned is suffering from a mental disorder, is crucial (see, e.g. Fulford and Hope, 1996). Yet the key terms here, 'mental disorder', 'mental illness', and so on, are not defined legally.

Neglect of conceptual difficulties

So the law is not much help on the central conceptual issue raised by Mr AB. Surprisingly, perhaps, neither is psychiatry. Medical textbooks define particular mental disorders, but they rarely attempt to define what, in general, makes a disorder a *mental* disorder, let alone the still more general question of what makes a condition a *disorder* in the first place. A notable exception is the American Psychiatric Association's (APA) classification of mental disorders, the DSM; however, this explicitly precludes its use in medico-legal contexts (APA, 1994, pp. xxiii–xxiv). Thus, we can indeed map Mr AB's symptoms (early waking, weight loss, low mood) on to the criteria in the textbooks for 'major depression'. But this simply begs the question of why these 'symptoms' should be regarded as 'symptoms', and Mr AB's condition as a mental illness, and hence as a mental *disorder* as required by the Mental Health Act.

The scope of philosophy and mental health

Philosophy in all three senses of the term is therefore relevant to our understanding of Mr AB's case, and thus, by implication (his case being an *everyday* clinical case), to mental health generally.

In this book, it is with sense 2 (specific philosophical areas) and sense 3 (conceptual analysis) that we will be mainly concerned. This is because it is philosophy in these two senses of the term that allows joint work focused at a level of detail sufficient for effective interdisciplinary exchange: thus,

- *Conceptual analysis*. This provides the most general point of contact between psychiatry and philosophy, at least as practised in the Anglo-American tradition. The great philosopher–psychologist, William James, writing early in this century, described philosophy as '…an unusually stubborn effort to think clearly' (James, 1987, p296). It is the lack of clear meaning, the need for conceptual clarification, which is at the heart of psychiatry's need for philosophy.

◆ *Specific philosophical areas*. It is the problems in specific areas of philosophy, on the other hand, which are at the heart of philosophy's need for psychiatry. This is because, as in Mr AB's case, the practical problems of everyday research and practice in mental health provide concrete and specific instances of the metaphysical problems studied in general philosophy.

The *Weltanschauung* (sense 1 of 'philosophy', as above) is also important, however. So long as the mind-sets of philosophers and practitioners were incompatible, they could not 'see' their mutual dependence. It is the change in *Weltanschauung* in the decade since Anthony Quinton's observation (with which we started this chapter) that has allowed both sides, practitioners and philosophers, to recognize that far from ignoring each other, we are now on the brink of a partnership potentially as fruitful as the well-established partnership between clinical practice and science.

Reflection on the session and self-test questions

Run over the materials we have covered in this session, the clinical case history, of Mr AB; the 'points arising', as we called them, empirical and conceptual; and their implications for the scope of the interdisciplinary field of philosophy and psychiatry. What key points do you think should be taken from these materials?

We list a number of our own suggested key points at the end of the book. However, remember that as with all the exercises in this book, drawing on your own background experience and skills, you may spot very different key points from us. So, write your own ideas down first and then try answering the following questions:

1. With what kinds of disorders is psychiatry particularly concerned?

2. What is covered by a psychiatric diagnostic formulation?

3. How does the subject matter of philosophy differ from that of science?

4. What broad areas or kinds of philosophy are there?

5. What concepts are at the interface between philosophy and psychiatry?

Session 2 Fact, value, and the concept of mental disorder

In the first session in this chapter, we identified an important general point of contact between philosophy and mental health in the problems raised by the concept of mental disorder. In this session, we start to look at these problems in more detail.

The aim will be to set out more explicitly just what it is about mental disorder that makes it more problematic conceptually than bodily disorder. Gilbert Ryle, an Oxford philosopher writing in the 1940s and 50s, and the author of an important book on the philosophy of mind, *The Concept of Mind* (1949/1963), described this setting out process as mapping the 'logical geography'. We will come back to the importance of this in Chapter 4, when we consider philosophical methods. However, the basic idea is to get a picture of the *features shown by a given concept or set of concepts as they are actually used in a given area*, these being the features that a philosophical analysis of the meanings of the concepts in question must explain. This 'mapping out' process will prepare us for looking at two very different explanations of the meaning of mental disorder in the remaining two sessions in this chapter.

A conceptual map of mental disorder

In Exercise 2, then, we are going to start building up a map (a conceptual map, remember) of mental disorder. As we emphasized in Session 1, you will get a lot more out of this if you don't cheat; i.e. try the exercise for yourself *before* reading on.

EXERCISE 2	(20 minutes)

This is a two-stage exercise.

Stage 1 (15 minutes)
Write a list of mental disorders—Write down as many examples of the different main categories of mental disorder as you can think of. If you are working in a group, this exercise is best done in philosopher–practitioner pairs. If you are working on your own, a good way to 'brainstorm' a suitable list is to start with you own list, and then check through the relevant chapters and/or index of a textbook of psychiatry.

Stage 2 (5 minutes only)
Make a map—Reorganize your list to make a map showing the extent to which you think the different kinds of mental disorder are more or less like bodily disorders. In doing this, don't think too hard about just why a particular mental disorder is like or unlike a bodily disorder (we will be covering this in detail later in this part). Just make a quick 'guts-feel' global judgement of the extent to which you feel the mental disorder in question is 'like a disease'.

Now, look at the 'map' in Figure 2.1. There may well be differences between this map and yours. But the overall pattern people come up with is usually (though not invariably!) more or less the same.

For those not from a mental health background, the numbers on the map can be cross-referenced to the glossary of examples in Box 2.1. As noted above, we will be looking at the details of all these conditions in Chapter 3.

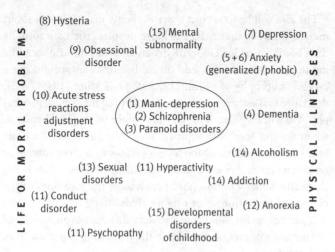

Fig. 2.1 A conceptual map of mental disorder. The different kinds of mental disorder can be set out schematically, as in this 'map'. Although not representing a well established classification of these disorders, the map illustrates a number of the features of the conceptual terrain of psychiatry which any theory of the meaning of mental illness must explain. The numbers refer to the illustrative case vignettes given in the accompanying glossary (Box 2.1). (Adapted from Fulford, K.W.M. (1993). Value, action, mental illness, and the law. In *Action and Value in Criminal Law* (ed. S. Shute, J. Gardner, and J. Horder). Oxford: Oxford University Press, pp. 279–310).

Box 2.1 A glossary of examples of mental disorder—brief definitions and examples of pyschological disorder

(*All cases based on real patients but with biographical details disguised. Further examples and details of psychopathology are given in chapter 3.*)

1. Manic-depressive illness

(a) Depressed type

Psychotic disorder with depressed mood. The psychoses are severe disorders typically with loss of insight shown characteristically by delusions, hallucinations, and certain forms of thought disorder (e.g. thought insertion—*see case 2*).

> **Mr SD, age 38—senior manager.** Presented in casualty (with his wife) with a 3-week history of 'biological' symptoms of depression 'early waking, weight loss, fixed diurnal variation of mood' and delusions of guilt 'believed he caused the war in former Yugoslavia'. History of attempted suicide during previous similar episode. Denied that he was depressed but said he needed something to help him sleep.

(b) Manic type

Psychotic disorder with elevated mood.

> **Miss HM, age 25—novice nun.** Brought by superiors for urgent out-patient appointment as they were unable to contain her bizarre and sexually disinhibited behaviour (running away from convent and soliciting 'for the Lord'). Showed pressure of speech (continuous talking), grandiose

delusions (that her minor charities are saintly acts of 'great and enduring moral worth'), and auditory hallucinations (female voices telling her she is Mary Magdalene).

2. Schizophrenia

Psychotic disorder with specific delusions, hallucinations, and disorders of thought ('first-rank' symptoms), together with a large number of other disturbances, especially of affect and volition.

> **Mr. S, age 18—student.** Emergency psychiatric admission from his college. Behaving oddly (found wandering, in bemused and agitated state). Complained that people were talking about him. Showed thought insertion (John Major 'using my brain for his thoughts') but no cognitive impairment (*see case 4*).

3. Paranoid disorders, e.g. Othello syndrome

Psychotic disorders with well-developed delusional symptoms (not necessarily of persecution) and little other pathology. In the Othello syndrome the paranoid system is built round delusions of infidelity.

> **Mr A, age 47—publican.** Seen by general practitioner initially because his wife was depressed. However, Mr A complained of anxiety and impotence. GP suspected alcohol abuse. After some discussion, Mr A suddenly announced that 'the problem' was that his wife was 'a tart'. Once started, he went on at length about her infidelity, drawing on a wide range of evidence, some of it bizarre (that she washed their towels on a different day; pattern of cars parked in street had changed).

4. Dementia

Psychotic disorder with progressive impairment of 'cognitive' functions—namely memory, attention, orientation (time, place, person), and general IQ—caused by gross brain pathology, hence sometimes called 'organic psychosis'. Acute (and usually reversible) disturbances of cognitive functions occur in confusional states (e.g. after blow to the head, or with intoxication). Visual hallucinations are common.

> **Mrs GM, age 65—shopkeeper.** Referred by general practitioner when her customers complained that she had started to forget their orders. Family confirmed she had become forgetful and at times seemed confused. She had been complaining of seeing rats in her storeroom but there was no evidence of these. Initially denied problem but on cognitive function testing unable, e.g. to recall a simple name and address after a gap of 5 minutes.

5. Anxiety disorder—generalized

Sustained periods of anxiety with associated bodily symptoms in absence of appropriate cause.

> **Mrs B, age 35—teacher.** Presented to general practitioner complaining of a constant sense of anxiety for which she

could give no reason, developing over about 3 months. Had always been a worrier but coped well with a stressful job. Had difficulty getting to sleep and bodily symptoms (palpitation and difficulty swallowing).

6. Anxiety disorder-phobic

Pathological anxiety related to a specific object or situation and leading to avoidance.

Mrs RD, age 23—housewife. Visited by district nurse at home as she had failed to attend for postnatal follow-up. She explained that she had become afraid to go out because of a fear of thunder. This had been a lifelong fear but had become worse since she gave up work to have her baby. Even approaching the front door produced feelings of panic with bodily symptoms (palpitation, hyperventilation, tingling in her fingers).

7. Depression—non-psychotic

Pathological depression of mood without psychotic features.

Mr RJ, age 32—bricklayer. Presented to general practitioner complaining of feeling miserable and difficulty getting to sleep. For some months he had lost his enjoyment of life and tended to lie awake at night worrying about the future, even though he had no particular problems at present. Physical examination was normal and he had not lost weight.

8. Hysterical disorders

Physical symptoms (e.g. paralysis, blindness, memory loss) with psychological causes.

Miss HP, age 30—secretary. Admitted to neurology ward and transferred to psychiatry under protest. Unable to move right hand. No evidence of physical lesion. History of depression and self-injury.

9. Obsessive-compulsive disorder

Recurrent mental content (obsession) or behaviour (compulsion) typically recognized by patient to be irrational and resisted but unsuccessfully (like a bad case or getting a tune 'stuck in your head').

Mr OC, age 27—bank clerk. Three-year history of progressive slowness. Referred with recent depression and anxiety following suspension from work. Showed severe and progressive compulsive checking, which he saw as 'ridiculous', but was unable to stop.

10. Acute reaction to stress

Marked psychological reaction to sudden stressful stimulus. Adjustment disorders are corresponding reactions to more chronic situations, e.g. a grief reaction which becomes excessively extended. These disorders are in many respects the psychological counterpart of physical trauma or wounds.

Mr JB, age 55—doctor. Involved in serious car accident while returning from an emergency call-out late at night. No head injury. Was unable to recall the accident. Felt anxious, distressed, and unable to cope with his work for several days. Then developed a brief, self-limiting manic reaction.

11. Psychopathic personality disorder

Personality disorders differ from illnesses in being more or less fixed features of the way a person feels, thinks, or behaves. With psychopathy the disorder is manifested mainly in repeated delinquency. The conduct disorders of childhood have similar manifestations but are self-limiting. Hyperkinetic syndrome of childhood is pathological overactivity.

Mr PP, age 23—unemployed. Seen in casualty by duty psychiatrist. Brought in by girlfriend because he was threatening to kill a rival. Had been drinking. History of repeated criminal assaults. Promiscuous.

12. Anorexia nervosa

Pathological disorder of eating in which patient refuses to eat, may exercises excessively, and/or abuses laxatives. Self-induced vomiting is common. Typically perceive themselves as fat, despite extreme emaciation, together with physiological and other changes of starvation.

Miss AN, age 21—student. Four-year history of intermittent anorexia. Currently seriously underweight, exercising, and using laxatives; amenorrhoeic. Refusing admission on the grounds that she is 'too fat'.

13. Sexual disorders

These may involve (a) pathological changes in sexual drive and/or function, or (b) disorders of sexual-object choice (e.g. sadism, paedophilia).

Mr RP, age 24—postgraduate student. Attended student counselling service complaining of difficulty maintaining an erection. Had a steady girlfriend and normal sexual interest and drive. Struggling to finish his doctoral thesis.

14. Alcoholism and drug addiction

Abuse of alcohol or drugs which is out of the patient's control. There is often denial of the problem.

Mr AR, age 38—shopkeeper. Self-referral to general practitioner from Relate (marriage guidance counselling). Over several years had increased his alcohol consumption and was now drinking a bottle of spirits and several pints of beer every day. Without a drink in the morning his hands shook. His wife was threatening to divorce him and he had lost many of his customers. However, he was ambivalent about the referral, arguing that he had the problem 'under control'.

15. Mental subnormality and developmental disorders of childhood

With mental subnormality there is pathologically low IQ together with varying degrees of emotional and behavioural abnormality persisting from birth. The developmental disorders of childhood include delays in reaching normal milestones, e.g. persistent urinary incontinence ('bed wetting'), delayed walking, talking, or reading.

Maps of the kind shown in Figure 2.1 can be used as Rylean 'logical geographies'. They incorporate a number of important features of the concept of mental disorder (as explored in the next exercise). Hence, any philosophical theory of mental disorder that purports to give us a better understanding of the *meaning* of mental disorder must explain at least these features. In this respect, these features (as set out in the 'Rylean' map) are like the data of a scientific theory—the better the theory, the more 'data' (the more features of the map) it will explain.

This is not to say that the theory must *endorse* these features. A philosophical theory of the meaning of mental disorder must explain, either why the concept of mental disorder *has* the features it has, or why it only *appears* to have these features. Either way, though, *some* theory of these features (as summarized in the map) is required.

Four features of the map of mental disorder

So, what are the features of 'mental disorder', set out in this way? We will be looking at four features in all, starting with, (1) *diversity*, and (2) variable conceptual *distance from bodily disorder*—these are the two features we concentrated on in Exercise 2. These two features lead, in turn, to two further features: (3) variable *status as illnesses*, especially in the extent to which a mental disorder is an excusing conditions in law, rendering the sufferer 'not responsible', and (4) variable *degree of value-ladenness*.

Start with your own ideas

We will be looking at each of these features in detail, in particular Feature 4, the value-ladenness of mental disorder. Before going on, however, it is important to think about them a bit further for yourself.

EXERCISE 3	(15 minutes)

Go back to your own map and the map in Figure 2.1. Think about the four features just listed:

1. What do they mean?

2. Are they really features of mental disorder?

3. Are they features specifically of mental disorder (i.e. more so than bodily disorder)?, and

4. Why do they matter?

Note: At this stage, you may feel you have no idea what we are talking about, what we mean, for example, by 'diversity' or 'conceptual distance': don't be put off! At this stage, this is all to the good. It makes it all the more important to think for yourself about these features of mental disorder before going on. Remember, this book is all about acquiring new skills through your own active engagement with the line of argument. It is not about passively acquiring other people's ideas.

We are now ready to look together at the first of the four features of the conceptual map of mental disorder, diversity.

Feature 1 of mental disorder: diversity

Diversity, straightforwardly, is the plain variety of mental disorder. At first glance it may seem odd to claim that diversity is a feature specifically of mental disorder. After all, if you flick through a *medical* textbook, you will find just as many different categories of disorder as there are mental disorders in a *psychiatry* textbook, and covering a wide range of systems (cardiovascular, gastrointestinal, etc.).

There is one important respect, though, in which mental disorders really are more diverse than bodily disorders, namely, in the form of their *symptoms*. The details of this will take us, later on in this part, into the whole question of the relationship between illness and disease. For now, though, the point is this. The symptoms of bodily disorders are largely confined to sensations (nausea, dizziness, bodily pains, etc.), movements (abnormal movements such as tics; or paralysis), and perceptions (especially failures of perception, such as blindness or deafness).

Symptoms of mental disorder, on the other hand, as the glossary in Box 2.1 indicates, although occurring in each of these categories, also include disturbances of emotion (anxiety, depression), volition ('made impulses', in schizophrenia; compulsive actions, e.g. handwashing); desire (addictions, sexual disorders); appetite (anorexia, bulimia); motivation (hysteria); belief (delusions); perception (hallucinations); and thought (obsessive thoughts; also thought insertion, withdrawal and broadcasting, in schizophrenia). Mental disorders also include wider disturbances of personal identity (e.g. multiple personality disorder), of relationships based on empathic understanding (autism), and of behaviour (e.g. in personality disorder).

The diversity of psychopathology is important practically—you will remember from Session 1, that psychiatrists do a full 'mental state examination' (or MSE), covering all of these areas; and for each area, we need to be aware of the precise features of all the possible 'symptoms' that may be present. But the diversity of psychopathology is also important philosophically. As a key feature of the 'Rylean' map, any philosophical analysis of the concept of mental disorder must explain the diversity of its constituent symptoms compared with those of bodily disorder.

Feature 2 of mental disorder: conceptual distance from bodily disorder

Most people recognize that some mental disorders are more, and others less, intuitively like bodily disorders. Psychiatrists, being the most medical of mental health practitioners, have traditionally emphasized the similarities between mental and bodily disorders, while antipsychiatrists, as you might expect, have emphasized the differences between them. Even in this 'debate about mental illness', though, both sides have to start from the fact (a fact of the 'logical geography' of mental disorder) that there are both similarities and differences between them. The trick is to show, in the terms of reference of this debate, whether it is the similarities (for psychiatrists) or the differences (for antipsychiatrists) that are the more important.

We will be returning to the debate about mental illness in detail in the next two sessions (Session 3 for the antipsychiatrists, Session 4 for the psychiatrists). If, though, we combine the fact that there are both similarities and differences between mental and bodily disorders, with Feature 1, the diversity of mental disorders, we see that the starting point for the debate has to be less polarized. Some mental disorders are more and others less like bodily disorders. Hence there is no global 'mental disorder' that either is or is not relevantly similar (psychiatrists) or dissimilar (antipsychiatrists) to 'bodily disorder'.

The need for a less polarized starting point in the psychiatry/antipsychiatry debate is brought out clearly by our map. Thus, the dementias are generally placed nearest to bodily medicine, these disorders indeed being included among what are often called the 'organic' psychoses (though, as emphasized in Chapter 3, the term 'organic' in this context is defined by reference to particular *symptoms*, not to knowledge of underlying bodily causes). Next to the dementias, most people put the functional psychoses (schizophrenia, manic-depressive disorder, and the paranoid psychoses). After this, there is more variability: the disease 'status' of some disorders is highly contentions (e.g. anorexia is 'obviously' a disease for some, 'obviously not' for others); but by and large, depression, anxiety disorders and the addictions, tend to be placed closer to 'disease', with hysteria, reactions to stress (such as post-traumatic stress disorder, or PTSD), personality disorder, and sexual disorders, all further away.

A note on terminology

The diversity of mental disorders (Feature 1), and their variable conceptual distance from bodily disorders (Feature 2), is reflected in the somewhat confused and inconsistent terminology employed in this area. 'Mental disorder' is the most popular generic term for everything on the map, the implication being that all these conditions are in some way different from just plain 'distress'. The term 'mental *illness*' is probably best used for those disorders that are intuitively most like bodily illness (or disease) and, yet, mental rather than bodily. This of course implies

everything that is built into the mind–brain problem! (We return to the mind-brain problem later in the book, in Part V.)

This usage is broadly reflected in most mental health legislation. Thus, in the UK's Mental Health Act, 1983, 'mental disorder' is defined as 'mental illness, arrested or incomplete development of mind, psychopathic disorder and or any other disorder or disability of the mind'. We will follow this convention in the rest of this book. Terminological inconsistencies in this area, it should be said, reflect real underlying conceptual difficulties, although, as we will see later, they have certainly contributed to some of the avoidable confusions in the debate about mental illness.

Feature 3 of mental disorder: illness status

This brings us to the third feature of the map of mental disorder, its variable status as illness. This feature of mental disorder, like the last, is differentially spread across the map. These two features, indeed, tend to go hand in hand—the further from bodily disorders a condition is on the map, the more disagreement there is likely to be about its status as a mental illness. Thus personality disorder and hysteria, as conditions the illness status of which is highly contentious, are both conceptually further from bodily illness than the organic psychoses, like dementia.

The two features, however, the conceptual distance of mental disorders from bodily disorders (Feature 2) and their illness status (Feature 3), are not fully co-extensive. This is clear if we look at an important feature of illness, namely that it is an *excuse*. Thus, illness excuses from responsibility. As a feature of illness in general, bodily as well as mental, this has been emphasized especially by sociologists, for example by Talcott Parsons in his early, and now classic, study of deviance (1951): if I am ill, it is not my fault that, say, I fail to turn up for work (hence the need for an 'off work' medical certificate). The status of m*ental* illness as an excuse is important especially in forensic contexts. The intuitive basis of this is that someone who is mentally ill, or at any rate severely mentally ill, is not responsible for their actions. They are 'irrational', as we say. This is also closely related to the ethical justification of involuntary psychiatric treatment. Someone who is irrational, our intuitions suggest, may not be competent to choose for themselves whether or not they should have treatment. (We return to both aspects of the 'excusing' status of mental illness in Part IV.)

It is because illness in general, bodily as well as mental, excuses, that, as noted above, the illness status of mental disorders (Feature 3), runs closely with their conceptual distance from bodily disorders (Feature 2). But as also just noted, the two features are not fully co-extensive. Thus, dementia is intuitively closest to bodily disorders; however, in some administrations, it is excluded from the legal provision for involuntary treatment. The *functional psychoses*, on the other hand, although intuitively further from bodily disorders, are the paradigm cases both of mental illness as an excuse (especially with delusions—see later in this part) and of (justified) involuntary treatment (see Part IV).

It is the centrality of the functional psychoses in this respect that led the radical antipsychiatrists (such as Thomas Szasz and

R.D. Laing—see Session 3), to focus their attacks on such conditions as schizophrenia. If schizophrenia falls (as a genuine illness), they argued, the concept of mental illness falls with it! On the other hand, personality disorder is both intuitively distant from bodily disorders and highly contentious as an excuse in law; addiction is equivocal (for example, Aristotle (1980, p. 60, lines 1113^{b}20–1114^{a}6) argued in the *Nichomachean Ethics* that a crime committed when drunk, far from being excused, deserves a double punishment); and hysteria is often written off as mere malingering.

Feature 4 of mental illness: value-ladenness

This fourth feature of mental disorder also runs broadly parallel with Features 2 and 3. That is to say, the further from bodily disorders a mental disorder is, and the more contentious is its status as a mental illness, the more overtly value-laden is it likely to be.

The value-ladenness of mental disorder is a crucially important feature of its logical geography. It is central to many of the issues in the psychiatry/antipsychiatry debate, for example, as we will see. Before going on, then, it will be worth looking at it in a little more detail, starting with the meaning of the term 'value'.

EXERCISE 4   (5 minutes)

Before going on, write down as many senses of the term 'value' (or 'evaluative') as you can think of. Which of these applies to mental disorders?

The meaning of value

Like many important terms in philosophy, 'value' is used in everyday language with a variety of meanings: to put a monetary value on, to roughly estimate, to evaluate as opposed to exactly measure, to evaluate a (mathematical) equation, and so on. In the context of the debate about mental illness, however, value is used to mean good/bad in contrast to facts (or evaluation in contrast to description). In this good/bad sense of value, we say 'this is a good pencil' (a value judgement evaluating the pencil) in contrast to 'this is a blue pencil' (a statement of fact, describing the pencil).

Like many other important terms in philosophy, there are also whole philosophies on what 'value', even in the good/bad sense of the term, actually means! Think about these for yourself before going on.

EXERCISE 5   (10 minutes)

Write down a few more examples of the good/bad use of value terms and then pair them with value-free, factual examples. Now think about two questions:

1. Are all your examples of value terms of the same general kind, or can good/bad uses of value terms be further subdivided or classified?

2. How easy is it to distinguish fact from value?

The point of this exercise is to start you thinking about value terms in anticipation of some of the work we will be doing in Session 3 and later in this part.

The varieties of values

You may have noticed from your further examples

1. That even good/bad uses of the term 'value' (as opposed to the other uses of the term noted a moment ago) come in varieties— there are moral ('he is a wicked man'), aesthetic ('this is a beautiful rose'), prudential ('he is a foolish man'), etc., varieties of value. This will be important especially when we come to consider specifically medical value (e.g. in relation to involuntary psychiatric treatment). Philosophers have tended to neglect the varieties of value, but see G.H. von Wright's *The Varieties of Goodness* (1963) for a notable exception.

2. That there is no easy distinction between value and fact. Everyday language is a rich tapestry, with fact and value (as well as many other linguistic threads) woven into it. This does not mean that it is impossible to unpick the threads, or that it is always a mistake to do so; however, it does mean we need to proceed carefully.

This last point, in particular, will be important when we start to work on the implications of the more value-laden nature of mental disorders compared with bodily disorders.

No dichotomy—but a distinction

Before moving on, though, it will be worth spending a moment or two on the fact/value (or description/evaluation) distinction itself. It is sometimes suggested, more in philosophical than non-philosophical circles, that the distinction between fact and value, along with other widely debated distinctions (analytic/synthetic, see Chapter 5; mind/brain, see Part V; and so on), is otiose, that no self-respecting philosopher would nowadays talk in these terms at all.

The American philosopher, Hilary Putnam, for example, actually called his recent collection of essays *The Collapse of the Fact/Value Dichotomy* (2002). But what did Putnam actually mean by this?

EXERCISE 6   (15 minutes)

Read the short section from page 9 of:

Putnam, H. (2002). The Empiricist background. Chapter 1 in *The Collapse of the Fact/Value Dichotomy and other Essays*. Cambridge, MA: Harvard University Press.

Link with Reading 2.1

◆ What do you take Putnam to mean by the distinction he draws between distinctions and dichotomies (or dualisms)?

Putnam's point, which he attributes to the American pragmatist John Dewey, is that a distinction is not a dichotomy (or dualism). A dichotomy applies across the board, all cases (of the relevant kind) falling on one side or the other (fact *or* value, analytic *or* synthetic, mind *or* brain). A distinction is considerably more modest. A distinction may be helpfully drawn, Putnam says, 'for certain purposes' without implying a dualism, i.e. that it can be drawn in all cases of the relevant kind.

Thus, to take a non-medical example, 'above' and 'below' is a distinction that may be helpfully drawn for some purposes, but that clearly cannot be drawn in all cases (because there will be cases of equality). Similarly, then, we will be arguing in this part that for certain purposes in health care it may helpful to distinguish fact from value (or description from evaluation). We will be suggesting, in particular, that there are concepts (such as the concept of disease) that, although widely taken to fall firmly on the fact side of the distinction, are none the less (in part) evaluative in meaning. Recognizing this evaluative element in the meaning of such concepts, we will further suggest, is helpful (in Putnam's terms) not only for theory but also for practice. It is helpful for theory in that it allows us to explain certain otherwise inexplicable features of the way these terms are actually used (the features of their 'ordinary usage', as we will call it in Chapter 4). It is helpful for practice in that it leads to an enriched model of healthcare decision-making in which description and evaluation have equal and complementary roles (values-based practice, see Part IV, especially Chapters 18 and 21). But all this is very far from claiming, and certainly does not require, that the distinction can be driven all the way back, that it can be established, to use Putnam's term again, as a dichotomy. To the contrary, as one of us has argued elsewhere (Fulford, 1989, chapter 10), psychopathology itself (specifically, the remarkable logical range of delusions, see chapter 3), gives a uniquely clear signal that the fact/value *distinction* does *not* go all the way back, that it is not, in Putnam's terms, a *dichotomy*.

Returning, then, to our map of mental disorder, it is in the good/bad sense of value, and recognizing what Putnam goes on to call the entanglement of fact and value in ordinary usage, that the parts of the map of mental disorder farthest from bodily disorders are the more value laden. We can see this in a number of ways:

1. *Medicine merges with morals*: many of the conditions at the edge of the map of mental disorder are close to moral conditions in differential diagnosis (e.g. psychopathic personality disorder is close to delinquency; alcoholism to drunkenness, hysteria to malingering).

2. *Excuses merge with no excuse*: this means that peripheral conditions are more likely to be understood in terms of moral responsibility, both in situations involving involuntary treatment and in respect of mental illness as an excuse in law (in both types of case, as we have seen, it is usually psychotic conditions, shown here at the centre of the map, that are considered paradigmatic).

3. *Mental disorders are defined (in part) by moral criteria*: even in 'scientific' classifications, the criteria by which some conditions near the edge of the map are (partly) defined, are social-evaluative rather than scientific-factual. For example, in the American classification, The Diagnostic and Statistical Manual, 'Conduct Disorder' is defined as 'a repetitive and persistent pattern of behaviour in which the basic rights of others or major age-appropriate *societal norms or rules are violated*' (APA, 1994, p. 290, emphasis added), and the paraphilias (disorders of sexual object choice) are defined in terms of behaviour that brings the individual '*into conflict* with sexual partners or society' (ibid., p. 280, emphasis added). We look at these again in Part III. (We return to classification in detail in Part III and IV.)

The four features and the philosophical problem of mental disorder

In all, then, there are four features of mental disorder for which any philosophical analysis of the concept must account: (1) diversity; (2) distance from bodily disorder; (3) variable status as illness; and (4) degree of value-ladenness.

In the next two sessions, we will examine two broad approaches to explaining these features of mental disorder: the non-medical (usually antipsychiatric approach), and the medical (usually pro-psychiatric approach), respectively. We will find that neither approach is able to explain the features of the map *as a whole*. This will bring us, by the end of this chapter, to a deeper understanding of the 'problem of mental illness' as a philosophical problem, and of the nature of philosophical problems in general.

Reflection on the session and self-test questions

Write down your own reflections on the materials in this session drawing out any points that are particularly significant for you. As with Session 1, the last exercise in this session involves reflecting on the material we have covered and drawing out your own key 'take away' points. As we said at this point in Session 1, it is important to think about and write down your own points before turning to the one's we selected (listed at the end of the book). The points that are significant from your particular perspective may be unique to you!

However, among the points to consider are:

1. Whose metaphor did we use to describe the conceptual map of mental disorders in Figure 2.1? What is its significance for philosophical theory?

2. What are the main areas (the main groups of conditions) in the conceptual map of mental disorder?

3. List the four conceptually significant features of the map that we identified (you may have thought of others)

4. In Putnam's view, is there a fact/value distinction or a fact/value dichotomy?

5. There are three ways in which mental disorders are in general more value-laden than bodily disorders. What are they?

Session 3 Antipsychiatry and the debate about mental illness

Since the 1960s there has been a wide-ranging and at times polemical debate about the validity of the concept of mental illness. In this session we look at a selection of the many different views falling broadly under the flag of 'antipsychiatry'. In Session 4 we will consider the opposing 'pro-psychiatry' view. What will emerge, though, from the two sessions taken together, is not so much the differences (important as these are) as the extent of the *similarities* between the arguments of many on both sides in this debate.

These similarities have not been well recognized (Fulford, 1989, chapter 1). Yet they are the key to a deeper understanding of the nature of the 'problem of mental illness'; and hence of this problem as illustrating the nature of philosophical problems in general.

Thomas Szasz, philosophy, and antipsychiatry

Although Thomas Szasz has always resisted the description 'antipsychiatrist', he was one of the first to attack psychiatry primarily on the *conceptual* grounds that mental disorders are

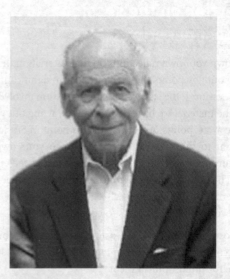

Fig. 2.2 Thomas Szasz

not, properly, medical disorders. In attacking the very *concept* of mental illness, Szasz was the most explicitly philosophical of the early antipsychiatrists (in the sense of the term 'philosophy' as used in this book; although Szasz himself never claims to 'be' a philosopher). We will thus start with a careful look at Szasz' arguments against the concept of mental illness before considering the wider antipsychiatry movement.

| **EXERCISE 7** | (60 minutes) |

Read the opening section, page 113–114, from:

Szasz, T. (1960). The myth of mental illness. *American Psychologist*, 15: 113–118

Link with Reading 2.2

Spend some time on this, thinking about Szasz's argument, as it runs from problem, to method, to conclusion.

♦ What, exactly, are his objections to people being said to be mentally ill?

♦ What dangers does he see in this?

♦ How does he seek to show that the very concept of mental illness is invalid?

♦ What is his conclusion about the real nature of these questions?

Thomas Szasz is an American psychiatrist. He began publishing in an uncompromisingly antipsychiatric vein in the late 1950s soon after being made Professor of Psychiatry at Syracuse University in upstate New York. Not surprisingly, he ran into a lot of flack! However, he hung on to his job while at the same time never shifting his basic position. He is now a distinguished Emeritus Professor at Syracuse who continues to publish widely on antipsychiatry themes and to lecture in many parts of the world.

Szasz's objections to the concept of mental illness

Like many other antipsychiatrists, the core of Szasz's objection to the concept of mental illness is that it dehumanizes people. Everyone, Szasz argues, has 'problems of living'. However, we should not see these as illnesses. Why not? Because, essentially, to say that someone is ill is to stop them taking responsibility for dealing with their own problems. (Remember from Session 2, that illness status tends to go with loss of responsibility.)

| **EXERCISE 8** | (5 minutes) |

Think about this for a moment in relation to the map of psychiatry that we looked at in the last session. Where is Szasz locating mental illness?

Remember that as we moved to the left of the map, so the links between mental illness and moral problems became more transparent. In effect, then, Szasz shifts mental illness as a whole right off the edge of the map of mental disorder and into the area of moral (or, more broadly, human) problems.

Mental illness is different from bodily illness

This shift to the left, as we might call it, becomes clearer still if we look at Szasz's method, at how he seeks to undermine the concept of mental illness, to show that mental illness is a myth, that it is not a genuine illness in the sense that bodily illness is genuinely illness. In this, Szasz is in effect pointing to what we could call the right-hand side of our map, taking bodily illness to be the paradigm for all illness. Bodily illness, he says (p. 114), is a deviation from clearly defined factual norms of the 'structural and functional integrity of the human body'. It is a matter of anatomy and physiology. Hence, he suggests, while individual diseases may be defined in different ways, they all involve deviations from these *factual* norms. It is by reference to factual norms, then, that genuine illnesses are defined.

But what about mental illnesses (so-called)—hysteria, depression, schizophrenia even? When we say of someone with depression that they are ill, are we referring, either directly or indirectly, to factual norms of bodily structure and functioning? Surely not. Conditions of these kinds certainly involve deviations from the norm. But the norms concerned, Szasz argues, are 'psychosocial, ethical, and legal' in nature (p. 114). Mental illness, so-called, is thus a concept of a radically different kind from bodily illness, mental illness are, certainly, problems. But they are not *medical* problems. They are, rather, 'problems of living' (e.g. p. 113 and again p. 118).

Szasz' core argument

Szasz's core argument, then, is that all those conditions widely regarded as mental illnesses are, really, defined by moral (or more broadly *evaluative*), rather than by factual (and by implication, *medical*) criteria. In the terms of our map, then, mental disorders are not, merely, closer than bodily illnesses to moral categories. Mental disorders really *are* moral categories. The concept of *mental* illness is thus an illegitimate extension of the concept of bodily illness. Mental illness is a myth.

EXERCISE 9 (20 minutes)

Before going on, spend a few minutes thinking about Szasz's argument. Review his strategy. Revise, if necessary, your original outline of his argument (from problem, to method, to conclusion), and note down briefly its strengths and/or weaknesses from your point of view.

We can summarize the structure of Szasz's argument thus:

1. The *problem*, as understood by Szasz, is the meaning of mental illness: being obscure in meaning, it is problematic in use, merging, in particular, with moral categories (our Feature 4 of the map): the meaning of bodily illness, by contrast, Szasz assumes, as relatively transparent and, correspondingly, the concept is relatively unproblematic in use.

2. Szasz' *method* is to proceed by comparing (the problematic) mental illness with (the unproblematic) bodily illness. He takes examples of bodily illness to be paradigmatic of genuine illness; such examples suggest that genuine illness is defined by (or means) deviation from clear-cut scientific-factual norms of bodily structure and functioning; however, conditions widely regarded as mental illnesses are defined by social-evaluative norms. Hence:

3. Szasz's *conclusion* thus has to be that mental illness, being so radically different in meaning from the paradigmatic bodily illness, is a myth.

Consequences of Szasz's argument

We will look at some of the objections to Szasz's arguments in a moment. It is important to recognize, though, just how fertile his position has been. In his own prolific output, he has explored the consequences of the 'myth of mental illness' in many areas: for particular 'disorders' (e.g. hysteria, schizophrenia, addiction); for its medicolegal implications; for the historical and cultural origins and ramifications of the concept; and so on (see Reading Guide).

A clear and forceful writer, Szasz mounted a strong and direct challenge to the medical model of mental disorder, i.e. to the idea that mental disorders are essentially no different from heart disease, diabetes or GPI (general paralysis of the insane, the tertiary, and before pencillin, final, phase of syphilis).

Szasz and the nature of philosophical problems

Work as fertile as this, whatever the denials of its opponents, is unlikely to be trivial. It may be wrong but it is certainly no mere 'playing with words'. Szasz's work thus illustrates an important general characteristic of philosophical problems. Whether pursued by card-carrying philosophers or not (as noted, Szasz never claims to be a philosopher), the problems of philosophy go to the very basis of our conception of ourselves and of our world.

Problems of this kind are difficult. They are literally at the edge of our powers of penetration, and much philosophical work is thus at best obscure, at worst unproductive. Unlike much scientific research, therefore, philosophy is a high-risk venture, more likely than not to be inconclusive. But when it *does* pay off, it pays off in a big way. (A recurring delusion of philosophers is that they have reached, and can prove that they have reached, the limits of the penetrable. This is one way to understand an element of discontinuity between the earlier and the later Wittgenstein. While in his *Tractatus Logico Philosophicus* (1921) the younger Wittgenstein set out to analyse *the logical form* of the proposition, in his later work he poked fun at the idea that one might have 'absolutely the right concepts'. Indeed he invented hypothetical cases of tribes with different concepts to cast doubt on this.)

We will return to the importance of Szasz's work in Chapter 6 when we look in more detail at the products or outcomes of philosophical work. But we can see already that one important 'pay off' from the ideas he was exploring in the early 1960s, has been what would now be called 'empowerment', an assertion of the *agency* of the patient. His work thus anticipated the whole patient power movement. This has been important practically—patient-centredness in health care, respect for the views of the users of services, and the incorporation of users of services into all stages of the planning and implementation of health care—are nowadays taken for granted in many parts of the world (though sometimes more in word than deed!).

It is important to add that empowerment is especially significant in *mental* health. Psychiatric patients are among those disadvantaged groups who remain notoriously vulnerable to abuse. There are many reasons for this (see later in this chapter and in Part IV). However, the loss of agency implied by taking someone to be ill is a crucially important factor and one that is highlighted by Szasz's work.

Back to the debate about mental illness

The central importance of Szasz's work has been to counter the idea that mental illness is just like bodily illness. In particular, he forced us to take seriously the links between mental illness and moral categories. Szasz also helped to give the whole antipsychiatry movement a high profile by taking a very strong and uncompromising line. It is, however, this strong line that renders his position open to criticism. We return to the counter-arguments of the pro-psychiatrists in Session 4. As to Szasz' position, there are many points, both practical and theoretical, that could be made against him. Here are a few examples (see also Reading Guide).

Practical points

Szasz's extreme position would exclude many from the help they really need. The British social psychiatrist, John Wing, described as 'repellant' (1978, p. 244) those who (like Szasz) would deny treatment to someone with suicidal depression (remember Mr AB in Session 1 of this chapter). Many among the user movement in psychiatry endorse the value even of physical treatments such as drugs, while at the same time insisting on the importance of involving patients themselves in decisions about how and when they are used—Peter Campbell, a writer on user issues in the UK gives a clear and balanced statement of this in his account of his own manic-depressive illness (Campbell, 1996). See also the now classic survey by Rogers *et al.* (1993).

Theoretical points

Szasz's extreme position is vulnerable theoretically in several respects, in particular:

- His characterization of mental illness as defined by social-evaluative norms, seems to exclude all the factual information, including knowledge of brain structure and functioning, currently available and likely to be discovered in the future. Szasz is of course well aware of this. His position is that if a brain basis for schizophrenia is discovered he will regard the condition as being on a par with GPI, i.e. it will then be a *bodily* illness. (For objections to this, see Session 4.)

- His characterization of bodily illness excludes conditions (such as migraine) the bodily causes of which are not known; and it includes conditions (such as extreme physical fitness) that are not illnesses.

- His approach has been attacked as dualistic, driving a false wedge between mind and body, a wedge that psychiatry, in particular, is working to remove.

Szasz and the map of mental disorders

We noted a moment ago that in terms of our map of mental disorders, Szasz's extreme view amounts to locating all mental disorders, however illness-like, off to the left, as moral problems. Another way of putting this is to say that his extreme view emphasizes the differences between mental and bodily illness (in particular the relatively value-laden nature of mental illnesses) at the expense of the similarities.

This is not illegitimate in itself. But as noted earlier, for a satisfactory *philosophical* theory, some account must be given of the features of the map *as a whole*. Hence in order to legitimate his emphasis on the differences between mental disorder and bodily disorder, Szasz must offer some account of why, in other respects, the two kinds of disorder at least *appear* similar. For philosophical purposes, for purposes of getting clearer about the *meaning* of mental disorder, it is not enough merely to draw out and rely on the differences between it and bodily disorder.

So Szasz's antipsychiatry can be characterized as focusing on one part of the map (the value-ladenness of mental disorder) instead of seeking to explain its features as a whole. This is not sufficient philosophically. It *is* important, though. In focusing on this aspect of the map, Szasz has drawn out and emphasized something (variable degrees of value-ladenness) that, as we will see later, is important not only for psychiatry but also, more generally, for medicine as a whole. We will return to the lessons from the debate about mental illness for medicine as a whole at several points in this book.

Antipsychiatries and the map of mental disorders

We have considered Szasz's antipsychiatry in detail as one of the most distinctively *philosophical* attacks on the concept of mental illness, i.e. an attack that goes to the heart of the *meaning* of the concept. Szasz in effect argues that 'mental illness' is an oxymoron—something *cannot* be both an illness and mental, *logically* cannot, because illness *means* 'bodily illness'. The very concept of '*mental* illness', then, is self-contradictory, according to Szasz, in the same way that 'male bitch' is self-contradictory (i.e. because 'bitch' *means* 'female dog').

Other forms of antipsychiatry, and they are many and diverse, are less philosophical, in the sense that they are less concerned explicitly with meanings. Like Szasz's antipsychiatry, though, they can be understood as focusing on parts of the map at the expense of its features as a whole; however, also like Szasz's antipsychiatry, in focusing in this way they have all contributed important new understanding of the diverse forms of mental disorder.

Five forms of antipsychiatry

Some of the main models advanced by antipsychiatrists, mainly in the 1960s and 1070s, can be summarized thus:

1. *The psychological model.* The British psychologist, Hans Eysenck, focusing (in effect) on the behavioural zone of the map, was among those who argued that mental disorders are learned abnormalities of behaviour. The disease model is inappropriate, he claimed, both as a model for investigating aetiology, and as a basis for treatment (e.g. Eysenck, 1968).

2. *The labelling model.* This model has been advanced particularly by sociologists, such as the American Thomas Scheff (1974). It emphasizes the extent to which the features of mental disorder, so called, are, really, no more than a response of the individual to being labelled as deviant. Although not sufficient to explain the onset of mental disorder, labelling processes have been shown to be powerful maintaining factors that may actively inhibit recovery (see, e.g. in the Reading Guide, Rosenhan's (1973) classic study; and recent literature on 'recovery' (Allott *et al.*, 2002)).

3. *Hidden meaning models.* Relevant especially to the psychosis zone of the map, this covers all those versions of antipsychiatry that emphasize the hidden meaningfulness of apparently meaningless (or irrational) behaviour. Thus the Scottish psychiatrist, the late R.D. Laing, in his first book *The Divided Self* ([1960], 1965, with a new preface), gave a detailed analysis of how the apparently meaningless symptoms of someone with schizophrenia could be decoded, once their origins in the patient's contradictory experiences of others were recognized.

4. *Unconscious mind models.* A key feature of the whole psychoanalytic movement is the claim that conscious mental life is a product of unconscious mental activity. Recognizing this, much that is apparently irrational can be made comprehensible in terms of unconscious counterparts of motives, reasons, desires, fantasies, and so forth. The Viennese founder of psychoanalysis was Sigmund Freud (see Part III). His theory was originally inspired by, and remains important especially in relation to, non-psychotic disorders.

5. *Political control models.* The essence of this version of antipsychiatry is that the medical model of insanity is a social or political construction devised (consciously or unconsciously) for the purpose of legitimizing the control of what society deems deviant, dangerous, or otherwise unacceptable. Thus the French philosopher–historian Michel Foucault argued that the medical model was 'invented', or at any rate came to dominance, in the nineteenth century in response to the needs of the industrial revolution, and led to the rise in all industrialized countries of the large asylums (Foucault, 1965). In modern times, as we will see in Part IV, political dissidence has been the basis of attributions of madness in totalitarian regimes; and the boundary between 'madness and morals', or between health care and policing, remains contentious in relation to 'dangerous' conditions such as psychopathy and some sexual disorders.

Highlighting parts of the map

These models are of course not as sharply distinct as this list suggests: labelling, for example, is an important aspect of the learning processes emphasized by psychologists; these in turn play a large part in the effects of the institutionalization of madness resulting from the asylum movement; and practically important ways of understanding these effects have come from the psychoanalytic movement.

None the less, even if not fully distinct, the models do offer well-defined approaches to mental disorder, each of which has proved important to parts of the map. Indeed, their importance, like the importance of Szasz's model, is in part in the extent to which they have become incorporated, alongside the medical model, into current theory and practice. For example,

- psychological treatment methods are now often the treatment of choice for many common non-psychotic disorders (depression and anxiety, for example);
- the power of labelling in reinforcing the features especially of long-term mental illness has been emphasized especially in social psychiatry (see e.g. Wing, 1978).

Schizophrenia may not be, as Laing argued, a sane response to an insane society, but a particular kind of family environment can increase the risk of relapse (Brown *et al.*, 1972; Leff and Vaughn, 1985).

Psychoanalytic and psychotherapeutic ideas, although still far from universally accepted in medicine, have become so well integrated with everyday practice as to be hardly recognizable for what they are. The British psychoanalyst and writer Anthony Storr, in a scholarly reappraisal of Freud's work, brings this out clearly (see Storr, 1989).

Political control models, as noted above, have proved all too tragically prescient with the widespread abuses of psychiatry, most notoriously in the former USSR (Bloch and Reddaway, 1977), but also in many other parts of the world (Chodoff, 1999). We return to the direct links between the latter and Szasz's argument about the concept of mental illness in Part IV.

Empirical evidence that at least some of these models are now present in everyday practice has been produced by the British social scientist, Anthony Colombo, in his work on implicit models of disorder in forensic psychiatry (Colombo, 1997) and in community care (Colombo *et al.*, 2003a). Colombo's work provides a paradigm for combining philosophical and empirical research methods in mental health (Fulford and Colombo, 2004) to good practical effect—see Williams (2004) on training; Heginbotham (2004) on policy, and Williamson (2004) on service delivery.

Antipsychiatry and psychiatry today

The absorption of antipsychiatric themes into mental health practice has led some, especially in psychiatry, to believe that antipsychiatry is dead. That it is not, that antipsychiatry is alive and well, is evident:

◆ in the continued growth in importance of 'patient power' movements;

◆ in the organization of mental health services increasingly along multidisciplinary lines;

◆ in diatribes against psychiatrists from the courts—for example, in the notorious 'Yorkshire Ripper' case (of a man in the UK who murdered several prostitutes in the north of England), the Judge rejected the evidence of both prosecution and defence psychiatrists that the defendant was suffering from schizophrenia;

◆ in 'scandals' about failures of psychiatric care;

◆ in the newspapers; and

◆ in the popularity and continued selling power of antipsychiatry literature.

From the psychiatric side, on the other hand, a strongly biological version of the traditional medical model remains dominant. There is much talk of 'whole person' medicine (see, eg., Cox *et al.*, forthcoming); and of the need for a 'biopsychosocial' model (for an excellent statement of the need for this, see McHugh and Slaveney, 1983, who are two founder members of the American group, the Association for the Advancement of Philosophy and Psychiatry); but the continuing dominance of the medical model is evident, none the less, in the overwhelming priority given to the biological and clinical sciences in research funding, in the syllabus for higher training in psychiatry, and in the papers accepted for academic meetings. The dominance of 'medical' aspects of mental disorder in the implicit models of psychiatrists, as compared with those of social workers and psychiatric nurses for example, has also been demonstrated empirically in Colombo's work (noted above).

In Session 4, we will examine the biological medical model and its role in psychiatry. We will find that like the models of the antipsychiatry movement, the medical model has important strengths. None the less, it also turns out to be a partial view, focusing on one feature of the map of mental disorders at the expense of the rest.

Reflection on the session and self-test questions

As with previous sessions, we are now ready to reflect on the materials in this session. Run over the session briefly and write down the key points that you find significant. Then write brief notes about the following:

1. What was Szasz' essential strategy? On what, precisely, did he focus his arguments?

2. Why exactly did he argue against the medical model in psychiatry? What was he concerned about?

3. What were the three structural elements or stages in his core argument that we identified?

4. What are the strengths of his argument (name two) and its weaknesses (name two)?

5. Name at least three other 'models' of mental disorder reflected in 'antipsychiatric' literature.

6. How, broadly speaking, are different models related to the 'map' of mental disorder introduced in Session 2?

7. Do *you* think antipsychiatry is alive or dead today?

Session 4 The medical model (and beyond)

Until the 1960s, when the debate about mental illness was getting under way, there was little in the way of concern about conceptual problems in medicine. The good and sufficient reason for this was that the problems facing medicine had, to this point, been very largely empirical in nature. The challenge was to understand and find cures for the major diseases—overwhelming infections, cancer, nutritional disorders. That such conditions were indeed *diseases* was not in question; and what was *meant* by calling these conditions diseases seemed all too self-evident.

At about this time, though, concerns began to be raised about the meaning of 'disease' even in physical medicine. These concerns were driven to a large extent by the very success of scientific research. A combination of advances in diagnostic methods and more powerful treatments raised new questions about the distinction between health and disease. Such questions had been the subject of philosophical debate since antiquity. But they became now, for the first time, matters of real *clinical* concern.

R.E. Kendell, philosophy, and pro-psychiatry

Important early work in this area was done by the British chest physician, J.G. Scadding. It is essentially his analysis of the concept of 'disease' (set out fully, for example, in Campbell *et al.*, 1979), which was picked up by British psychiatrists responding to Thomas Szasz and others in the early years of the debate about mental illness. This was notably the case with a newly appointed (at the time) Professor of Psychiatry at Edinburgh University, R.E. Kendell.

EXERCISE 10	(60 minutes)

Read the six extracts from:

Kendell, R.E. (1975). The concept of disease. *British Journal of Psychiatry*, 127: 305–315.

Link with Reading 2.3

Think about Kendell's line of argument comparing it with Szasz' in the last session. Think about the similarities as well as the differences between them in: (1) their characterizations of the problem; (2) their working methods; and (3) their conclusions. In particular, consider why both authors think it important to examine what is meant by bodily illness. And what do they decide 'bodily illness' means?

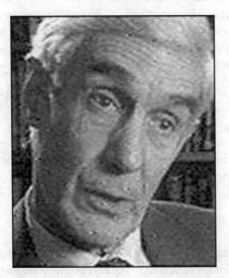

Fig. 2.3 R.E. Kendell

Like Szasz, Kendell was a professor of psychiatry. Also like Szasz, he was concerned directly with the problem of mental illness as a *conceptual* problem. Indeed this paper, which he gave first as his inaugural lecture at Edinburgh, was conceived as a direct response to the challenge of antipsychiatry.

Kendell was very much an establishment figure. After his time as Professor of Psychiatry at Edinburgh University, he became Chief Medical Officer for Scotland. He was then elected President of the Royal College of Psychiatrists in the UK. He was widely read in the philosophy of science and the humanities generally, as well as in medicine. He was one of several psychiatrists working in the UK in the 1970s and 80s, who tackled the conceptual problems of mental health head-on (as well as doing important empirical research). Later in his career, he became a strong supporter of the new philosophy of psychiatry: he gave one of the opening addresses at the millennial international conference in Florence, for example. We return to Kendell's work on psychiatric classification and diagnosis in Part III.

Kendell and Szasz: the same or different?

In this seminal paper, Kendell takes a pro-psychiatry stand which is as uncompromising as Szasz's antipsychiatry stand.

The differences between Kendell and Szasz are clear enough. The most notable difference is of course their contrary conclusions. Szasz had concluded that mental illness is a myth. Kendell concludes that at least some of the conditions widely regarded as mental illnesses are essentially similar to bodily illnesses; hence, mental illness is very far from being a myth. In the terms of our conceptual map of mental illness, then, where Szasz locates mental illnesses right off the map to the left (*as* moral problems), Kendell locates them right off the map to the right, *as* bodily illnesses.

In addition to the differences, though, there are also important *similarities* between Szasz and Kendell. These are more subtle, but also more remarkable. For what they amount to is that Szasz and Kendell, although coming to diametrically opposite conclusions, adopt essentially the same form of argument. Thus, Kendell shares with Szasz *two assumptions about the problem* with which they are concerned, and the same working method, i.e. a common *form of argument*. Thus:

◆ *Shared assumption 1*: *mental illness is the problem*. Kendell and Szasz both assume that it is the concept of mental illness that is 'the problem'. Thus, Kendell (p. 305), notes that the many and varied critics of psychiatry have 'one central argument in common—that what psychiatrists regard as mental illness are not illnesses at all', and he continues 'The purpose of this essay is to examine this proposition'. For Szasz, the assumption that mental illness is the problem, is evident in the very title of his (1960) paper, 'The *Myth* of mental Illness' (emphasis added).

In precisely what sense or senses mental illness is 'the problem' is less clear. Again, however, we can identify at least two shared subassumptions here, (1) that 'mental illness' is more obscure in meaning than 'bodily illness', and (2) that an important respect in which it is more obscure in meaning is that is it more value-laden. Szasz makes this explicit: he argues, as we noted in the last session, that if we look carefully at the concept of mental illness, we see that it is defined by norms that are 'psycho social, ethical and legal' (Szasz, 1960, p. 114). That mental illness is more value-laden is at least implicit in Kendell's paper, for example in his concluding comments (in which he is remarkably close to Szasz) about the unwarranted expansion of psychiatry's concerns from dealing with 'madness' to the 'absurd claims (that) all unhappiness and all undesirable behaviour are manifestations of mental illness' (p. 314).

◆ *Shared assumption 2*: *bodily illness is not a problem*, relatively speaking. Just as both authors take mental illness to be the problem, conceptually speaking, so both take the concept of bodily illness to be at least relatively unproblematic. As with Assumption 1, there are two subassumptions, (1) that bodily illness is relatively transparent in meaning, and (2) that it is relatively transparent because it is defined, straightforwardly, by reference to factual/scientific norms.

This second assumption corresponds with the fact that both authors take examples of bodily illness to be paradigmatic of genuine illness. Both indeed consider some of the same examples (e.g. GPI, or General Paralysis of the Insane, a form of syphilitic brain disease). The underlying message is 'we don't disagree about whether a given condition *is* a bodily illness, hence we must know what we *mean* by bodily illness'.

Kendell does more work on the meaning of bodily illness than Szasz. He reviews the historical development of the concept of disease. Both conclude, however, that whatever the full sense of the term, its core meaning is evident enough. Both, moreover, agree in taking bodily illness to be defined in objective, value-free, scientific terms.

◆ *Common form of argument: to determine the validity of mental illness by comparing it with bodily illness.* Given that Kendell and Szasz both take the meaning of (the paradigmatic) bodily illness to be (relatively) transparent, it is natural that they should both proceed by directly comparing mental illness with bodily illness. This form of argument takes bodily illness to be the template, the true coin against which the less certain coin of mental illness is to be measured.

The key point of disagreement

Most people reading Kendell's (1975) and Szasz's (1960) papers for the first time fail to notice these similarities. This is perhaps because, in a sense, they are just *too* obvious. What stands out is the *differences* between them, their embattled positions at opposite poles of the mental illness debate. We will return in Chapter 4 to the importance for philosophical method of such failures to spot the obvious. For the moment, however, we need to think further about the significance of the *similarities* between Szasz and Kendell as now identified. Where do they take us? Do they matter? In particular, what do they tell us about the debate about mental illness?

EXERCISE 11   (10 minutes)

Take a moment to think about the significance of the points of similarity between Szasz and Kendell. Despite being representatives of opposite poles in the debate about mental illness, they share similar assumptions about: (1) the problem (that the problem is 'mental illness', in particular where it stands between medicine and morals), and (2) the paradigm (that bodily illness is relatively unproblematic and hence the template against which any putative mental illness is to be measured); moreover, (3) both authors adopt the same working method (both compare putative mental illnesses against what they take to be the template of bodily illness).

So, Kendell and Szasz share similar assumptions and a similar method, but they reach opposite conclusions. How come? What is it that they are really disagreeing about? Think about this for yourself and write down your own answer before going on.

The short answer to Exercise 11 is that Kendell and Szasz come to opposite conclusions about mental illness because they

disagree, not, primarily, about the meaning of mental illness, but about the meaning of *bodily illness*.

Thus, Szasz takes bodily illness to be defined by anatomical and physiological norms: whereas, he says, mental illness is defined by norms that are ethical, social, and legal; hence mental illness fails to fit the template of bodily illness; hence, Szasz concludes, mental illness is a myth. Kendell takes bodily illness to be defined rather by reduced life and/or reproductive expectations (these being evolutionarily defined norms of 'biological disadvantage'—we return to biological disadvantage later in this part): he then shows that at least some putative mental illnesses are associated with reduced life and/or reproductive expectations; hence *these* mental illnesses, at least, fit the template of bodily illness; hence, Kendell concludes, mental illness is a reality.

EXERCISE 12   (10 minutes)

Obvious? Again, think about this for a moment. Does it suggest that something odd is going on here? In particular, if this is why, despite similar assumptions and a common form of argument, Kendell and Szasz come to opposite conclusions, does it suggest that their original assumptions may need to be revised?

To repeat: the key point that comes out of comparing and contrasting Kendell's and Szasz's arguments, that what they are *really* disagreeing about is not the meaning of mental illness but the meaning of *bodily illness*, This is the key point because, as we will now see, it is the key to a radical redefinition of the terms of the whole debate.

The debate was about bodily illness not mental illness

Up to this point, the debate has been about mental illness. Mental illness, as we saw, was *the* problem no less for Kendell (the psychiatrist) than for Szasz (the antipsychiatrist). And mental illness has been *the* problem also for the large number of other contributors to the debate.

Now, however, we have found that Szasz and Kendell disagree about mental illness essentially *because they disagree about bodily illness*. The terms of the debate itself thus stand to be radically revised. For the debate has turned out to be a debate, not (primarily) about mental illness at all, but about bodily illness. And this means that both the (implicit) assumptions from which Szasz and Kendell proceeded, and also their working method, have now to be completely revised. We can summarize the revisions thus:

1. the problem is now the meaning of bodily illness (not that of mental illness);

2. 'bodily illness', as well as 'mental illness', is thus very far from being transparent in meaning; and hence

3. the method of direct comparison is not appropriate.

Where do we go from here?

Just *how* we should proceed is the subject of the whole of Chapter 4, on philosophical method. But to anticipate a little, notice that there is a sense in which 'mental illness' could still be said to be genuinely more problematic than 'bodily illness'.

Thus, the meaning of 'bodily illness' has turned out to be at the heart of the debate about mental illness (at least as exemplified by Szasz and Kendell; though the same can be shown to be true of the debate generally, see Fulford, 1989, chapter 1). But the debate *appeared* to be about 'mental illness'. Why? Because the concept of mental illness is more *problematic in use*, i.e. clinically, than that of bodily illness. The concept of bodily illness is of course not *wholly* unproblematic clinically—witness the work of Scadding and others noted above (also, in primary care, that of Helman, 1981). But 'bodily illness' is at least *relatively* unproblematic clinically compared with 'mental illness', notwithstanding the fact that it turns out to be equally difficult to define.

The distinction implied here, between *definition* and the actual *use* of a concept in practice, is the key to a working method in philosophy to which we will turn in Chapter 4. As we will find, this method allows us to build on the foundational work of Szasz and Kendell in the debate about mental illness—or, as we should now say, having so radically revised the terms of that debate, the debate about *bodily* illness!

Reflection on the session and self-test questions

Write down your own reflections on the materials in this session drawing out any points that are particularly significant for you. Then write brief notes about the following:

1. What is the historical link between Kendell's arguments and those of Szasz?

2. From whose work and in what area of medicine (bodily or psychological) did Kendell derive his arguments?

3. How does Kendell's definition of bodily illness (or disease) differ from Szasz's?

4. Identify three similarities between Kendell's and Szasz's arguments.

5. What conclusions can we draw from the similarities and differences between Kendell's and Szasz's arguments for the debate about mental illness?

Conclusions

This chapter has been concerned with the nature of philosophical problems, both in general and as exemplified by our particular subject area, mental health.

In *Session 1*, starting from a practical example (the story of Mr AB), we found that in so far as philosophy and science are distinct, philosophy is concerned with conceptual problems, science with empirical.

In *Session 2*, we came back to a central issue for philosophy and mental health, the meaning of the concept of mental disorder. From a conceptual 'map' of mental disorder we drew out four key features that any philosophical account of the concept must explain: (1) the diversity of the different forms of mental disorder; (2) their different conceptual distance from bodily illness; (3) their differential status as species of illness (evident especially in their status as excusing conditions); and (4) the extent to which, being to a greater or lesser extent close to moral categories, they were more or less value-laden.

It is this fourth feature, the value-ladenness of mental illness, which has driven much of the debate about the concept, as set out in *Sessions 3 and 4*. Taking these together, we found that competing models of mental disorder can be understood as having focused on different parts of the conceptual map while failing to explain its features as a whole. Szasz and Kendell, in particular, representing opposite poles in the debate, focused respectively on the extreme left-hand (moral) and extreme right-hand (medical) boundaries of the map. Szasz took mental illness, because more value-laden than bodily illness, to be a moral concept. Kendell, on the other hand, argued that the value-ladenness of mental illness could be translated into value-free factual norms, and hence that mental illness is essentially no different from bodily illness.

In Chapter 4, we will return to the debate about mental illness. We will find that both sides are, in one sense right, in another wrong; and that this is the clue to a way of understanding the concept of mental disorder which is consistent with, and to this extent explains, all four features of the conceptual map of mental disorder, the Rylean logical geography of the concept, which we have explored in this chapter.

First, though, we need to prepare the ground for this more detailed treatment of the 'problem' of mental disorder by taking a more in-depth look at the features of the wide variety of mental disorders with which we are concerned in mental health.

Reading guide

Introductions to philosophy

A well-balanced introduction is Nigel Warburton's (2004) *Philosophy: the Basics*. Each chapter considers a key area of philosophy, explaining and exploring the basic ideas and themes. Simon Blackburn's (2001) *Think: a Compelling Introduction to Philosophy* is a short introduction with a definite story to tell. More advanced are: Baggini and Fosl's (2003) *The Philosopher's Toolkit*, and Guttenplan *et al.*'s (2003) *Reading Philosophy: Selected Texts with a Method for Beginners*. A light-hearted introduction to some key ideas in philosophy (but not to particular thinkers) is Stephen Law's (2004) *The Philosophy Files*.

Oxford University Press publishes philosophy topics in its 'A very short introductions' series (see www.oup.co.uk/vsi): for example, Tony Hope's (2004) *Medical Ethics: A Very Short Iintroduction*, Martin Davies' (2005) *The Mind*, and Simon Glendinnings' *Derrida* (2005). Lively introductions with cartoon images are published by Ivan Borks, Cambridge, in their 'For Beginners' series; for example John Heaton and Judy Groves' (1994) *Wittgenstein for Beginners*. Routledge has published a series of weightier introductions in its 'Arguments of the Philosophers' series, for example, Peter Caws' (1979) *Sartre*.

Among earlier but still helpful introductions, is Thomas Nagel's (1987) *What Does it All Mean? A Very Short Introduction to Philosophy*, which covers the main themes in modern philosophy for the 'complete beginner'. Slightly more extended is Martin Hollis' *Invitation to Philosophy* (1985, reprinted 1992). Anthony O'Hear's (1985) *What Philosophy Is* gives a more formal account.

Succinct 'lecture notes' covering each of the main areas of modern philosophy (i.e. philosophy of science, philosophy of mind, ethics, etc.) is William James Earle's (1992) *Introduction to Philosophy*. An edited collection with contributions from a wide range of philosophers on each of the main problems of philosophy (free will, mind, and body, etc.; also two chapters on political philosophy) is *Key Themes in Philosophy* edited by A. Phillips Griffiths (1989). A companion volume providing an introduction to classic texts is *Philosophers Ancient and Modern*, edited by Godfrey Vesey (1986). A highly readable introduction to recent French philosophy is Eric Matthews' (1996) *Twentieth Century French Philosophy*.

There are many large dictionaries and encyclopaedias that offer helpful introductions to key topics in philosophy and to individual philosophers. Examples include, *The Oxford Companion to Philosophy*, edited by Honderich (1995), *The Oxford Dictionary of Philosophy*, edited by Blackburn (1994), and *The Cambridge Dictionary of Philosophy*, edited by Robert Audi (1995 second edition, 1999). Edwards and Pap's (1973) *A Modern Introduction to Philosophy* although now somewhat dated, gives key readings from classical as well as contemporary sources. James Rachels' (2005) *Problems from Philosophy* provides an authoritative and fully contemporary introduction. The Blackwell 'Companions' series gives collections of key papers in each main area of philosophy, ethics, aesthetics, political philosophy, logic, philosophy of science, philosophy of mind, etc. Routledge's *Dictionary of Twentieth Century Philosophers* (ed. S. Brown, D. Collinson, and R. Wilkinson; 1996) includes biographies and reading guides to many of the great philosopher-psychologists of the nineteenth and early twentieth centuries. Bryan Magee's (1987) *The Great Philosophers* is the transcripts of a series of television programmes in which contemporary great philosophers talk about the work of earlier great philosophers (e.g. Geoffrey Warnock on Kant and Hubert Dreyfus on Husserl, Heidegger and modern existentialism).

Textbooks of psychiatry

A wide range of introductions to psychiatry is available, of varying lengths and aimed at mental health practitioners with different levels of experience. Among Oxford textbooks, three books of increasing length and detail are: (1) the *Concise Oxford Textbook of Psychiatry* (Gelder, Gath, and Mayou, 1994) primarily for medical students; (2) the *Shorter Oxford Textbook of Psychiatry* (Gelder, Mayou, and Cowen, 2001) giving more detail and aimed at trainees; and (3) the two-volume multi-author *New Oxford Textbook of Psychiatry* (Gelder, Lopez-Ibor, and Andreasen, 2000). The latter is edited by an international team—Michael Gelder (Oxford), Nancy Andreasen (USA), and Juan Lopez-Ibor (Spain)—and includes succinct authoritative chapters by world experts on all the key topics in psychiatry.

A recent introductory text for medical students and psychiatric trainees, covering all the core topics of general psychiatry, but also aiming to make psychiatry 'come alive' with a wealth of quotations, literary extracts, and artwork highlighting the experience of mental illness, is Neel Burton's (forthcoming) 'Psychiatry' (Note: Fulford is Editorial Advisor for this book.)

More specialized, but providing authoritative introductions to key areas are: (1) for old age psychiatry, Jacoby and Oppenheimer's (1996) edited collection *Psychiatry in the Elderly*; (2) for neuropsychiatry, Lishman's (1997) *Organic Psychiatry*; (3) Williams and Kerfoot's (2005) *Child and Adolescent Mental Health Services: Strategy, Planning, Delivery, and Evaluation* (this book is unusual in combining management and practitioner perspectives); Hawton, *et al.*'s (1989) *Cognitive Behavioural Therapy for Psychiatric Problems*; and for forensic psychiatry, there are two core texts in the UK literature, Bluglass and Boden's (1990) *Principles and Practice of Forensic Psychiatry*, and Gunn and Taylor's (1993) *Forensic Psychiatry: Clinical, Legal and Ethical Issues*.

The World Psychiatric Association publishes volumes reflecting different perspectives from around the world in its series on Images in Psychiatry, for example Okasha and Maj's (2001) *Images in Psychiatry: An Arab Perspective*.

The philosophy of psychiatry

Introductions and historical context

The explosion of new work in the interdisciplinary field between philosophy, psychiatry, and abnormal psychology, in the 1990s, is described and set in its historical context in Fulford, Morris, Sadler and Stanghellini's (2003a) introductory chapter to the launch volume to this series, *Nature and Narrative* (Fulford, Morris, Sadler, and Stanghellini, 2003b). Nature and Narrative, together with another volume in the series, Jennifer Radden's (2004) edited *Companion*, both include chapters by many of the recent contributors to the field and between them cover most of the current key topic areas. We note examples from both these sources in later Reading Guides. A succinct account of key topics, linked to the curriculum of the Royal College of Phyciatrists, is Sandy Robertson's (2004) 'Philosophy and History of Psychiatry'. A special issue of the International Review of Psychiatry, edited by Matthew Broome and Paul Bebbington (2004) from the Institute of Psychiatry in London, covers a range of cutting edge topics including developments in psychopathology and psychotherapy since Jaspers (Bolton, 2004), Merleau Ponty's phenomenology and psychiatry (Matthews, 2004), a conceptual framework for studying emotions (Hacker, 2004), the implications of automatism for moral accountability (Levy and Bayne, 2004), Wittgenstein and the limits of empathic understanding (Thornton, 2004), the need for an 'engaged epistemology' for understanding the clinical concept of delusion (Gipps and Fulford, 2004), and an article on reconceiving delusion (Stephens and Graham, 2004).

An early edited collection, based on a series of lectures organized by the Royal Institute of Philosophy in London, is Phillips Griffiths, A. (ed.) (1995) Philosophy, Psychology, & Psychiatry. The introduction and first chapter of this book describe the historical context of the renewal of the cross-disciplinary field (Fulford, 1995a, b). In their Past Improbable, Future Possible, the opening chapter of Nature and Narrative, Fulford et al. (2003a) set these developments in the context of developments in both philosophy and psychiatry in the twentieth century, linking Jaspers' work during psychiatry's first 'biological phase' with modern philosophy of psychiatry as part of psychiatry's second biological phase. As noted in that chapter, although strong traditions of interdisciplinary work between psychiatry and phenomenological and other 'Continental' philosophical traditions, were maintained throughout the twentieth century, philosophical issues in mental health, with the notable exception of studies (mainly critical) of psychoanalysis, were largely ignored by the analytic philosophers of Britain and North America. The potential for work in this area was certainly recognized, notably by Austin (1956/7), to whose 'philosophical fieldwork' we return later in this part, and by the American philosopher, Stephen Toulmin (1980): and there were occasional trail-blazing publications— Jonathan Glover's (1970) 'Responsibility' for example, drew deeply on careful work in different areas of psychopathology. But it was otherwise not until the late 1980s that publications began to appear regularly in the cross-disciplinary field.

Early 'new wave' publications

Early contributors to the current renewal of the field have been concerned with issues in specific areas of psychopathology (Wilkes, 1988; Spitzer et al., 1993; Radden, 1996; Sass, 1994, 1995); but other topics have included concepts of disorder (e.g. Fulford, 1989), the scientific status of psychiatry (e.g. Reznek, 1991), the nature of personal identity (e.g. Glover, 1988), the relationship between psychiatry, philosophy of

mind, and neuroscience (Hundert, 1989), and so forth. Indeed there are few areas of philosophy that have not turned out to have rich interconnections with problems in clinical work or research in psychiatry. The constraints on and potential links between philosophy and practice in mental health are discussed in detail, respectively, in chapters 1 and 12 of Fulford's (1989) Moral Theory and Medical Practice.

Illustrative topics in the cross-over area between psychiatry and the philosophy of mind are brought together in George Graham and G. Lynn Stephens' (1994) edited collection, Philosophical Psychopathology. A corresponding collection with a number of excellent articles broadly in the area of the philosophy of science is Sadler et al.'s (1994) Philosophical Perspectives on Psychiatric Diagnostic Classification.

Journals and book series

The French journal, L'Evolution Psychiatrique, has maintained a long-standing tradition of publications in phenomenology, philosophy, and psychiatry. In English, the journal Philosophy, Psychiatry, & Psychology, which is available on-line as well as in hard copy, publishes peer-reviewed original contributions with commentaries from different disciplinary perspectives, and responses to the commentaries by the authors. The History and Philosophy section of Current Opinion in Psychiatry (also available on-line), gives update review articles. A growing number of publications are appearing in mainline journals in both mental health and in philosophy (for literature search resources, see below).

Among book series, in addition to Oxford University Press' International Perspectives in Philosophy and Psychiatry, to which this book is a contribution, there is a growing international literature, including Disorders in Mind: Philosophical Psychopathology, from MIT Press, edited originally by George Graham and Owen Flanagan, and now by Jennifer Radden and Jeffrey Poland, Gerrit Glas' series in Dutch, the Psychiatry and Philosophy book series from Boom Publishers in Amsterdam, a series from Martin Heinze's group in Germany, the GPWP (Gesellschaft für Philosophie und Wissenschaften der Psyche), and from France a new review published by PSN–Edition in Paris, Psychiatrie, Sciences Humaines et Neurosciences.

Web-based resources

The philosophy of psychiatry

There are a number of web-based resources for the philosophy of psychiatry.

Centrally, the online version of all but the first 2 years of Philosophy, Psychiatry, & Psychology is available on subscription at: http://muse.jhu.edu/journals/philosophy_psychiatry_and_psychology. The contents can be searched online and articles downloaded. Each issue of Philosophy, Psychiatry, & Psychology includes a listing of new publications in the area in its section on *Concurrent Contents: Recent and Classic References at the Interface of Philosophy, Psychology, and Psychiatry*.

Metapsychology offers a list over 2500 reviews of books published in the area and sorted by subject matter at: http://mentalhelp.net/books; and the main site for metapsychology, run By Christian Perring is at: http://www.angelfire.com/ny/metapsychology/

There is a long-standing bulletin board for philosophy of psychiatry announcements also run by Christian Perring at: http://health.groups.yahoo.com/group/philosophyofpsychiatry-announcements

A searchable on-line database of articles and books, developed originally by Paul Sturdee, and extended and now maintained by Richard Gipps, is being set up by the INPP (the International Network for Philosophy and Psychiatry) at www.inpponline.org.

Philosophy

The Philosophers Index is the 'MEDLINE' of philosophy, listing articles and books by subject and author. It is a subscription service and is available through universities and at 'Athens', http://www.athens.ac.uk

There is a free Internet Encyclopedia of Philosophy at: http://www.iep.utm.edu

The Philosophy Research Base contains links to the home pages of academic philosophy departments around the world, plus homepages of many living philosophers: http://www.erraticimpact.com/homepages/home_page_index.htm

The Society for Applied Philosophy provides a focus for philosophical research with a direct bearing on areas of practical concern, including environmental and medical ethics, the social implications of scientific and technological change, philosophical and ethical issues in education, law and economics. http://www.sas.ac.uk/philosophy/sap

Psychology and medicine

Databases, available by subscription through Athens (http://www.athens.ac.uk), include:

- MEDLINE which indexes a large proportion of the leading journals in the medical and health fields from 1965 onwards, and

- PsycInfo which covers psychological literature from 1887 to present day, including journal articles, books, book chapters, technical reports, and dissertations published in over 45 countries.

Online resources include:

- Psychnet, which is run by the American Psychological Association, has a good site map and dedicated search engine for psychology resources on the web. http://www.apa.org/topics/homepage.html

- The Psychology Virtual Library keeps track of online information as part of The World Wide Web Virtual Library. Sites are inspected and evaluated for their adequacy as information sources before they are linked from here. http://www.clas.ufl.edu/users/gthursby/psi/

- Cogprints, which contains archived papers in psychology but also neuroscience, linguistics and philosophy. While coverage is limited it contains some very high quality work. http://cogprints.org

Concepts of disorder: (1) The debate about mental illness

An early but still valuable review of various theories of the nature of mental illness is Anthony Clare's (1979) 'The disease concept in psychiatry' (in *Essentials of Postgraduate Psychiatry*, edited by P. Hill, R. Murray, and A. Thorley). Among classics in the early debate are Laing's *The Divided Self* (1960), Scheff's (1974) and Rosenhan's (1973) work on labelling, and Foucault's (1965) political analysis. Social constructionist models are reviewed in Church (2004). Lewis (1953) gives an early analysis of mental disorder as being distinguished by disturbance of part-functions. Many of the most important classic papers in the debate about mental illness are to be found in the edited collection: *Concepts of Health and Disease*, ed. A.L. Caplan, T. Englehardt, J.J. McCartney (1981). These reviews are brought up to date by Fulford in an entry on 'Mental Illness', for Chadwick, R. (ed.), *The Encyclopedia of Applied Ethics* San Diego, Academic Press (1998); and an article on 'Mental Illness: Definition, Use and Meaning', for Post, S.G. (ed), *Encyclopaedia of Bioethics* (2003); and by Gert and Culver (2004) in *Defining Mental Disorder*.

The Department of Health and Society at Linköping University in Sweden has published a number of books on concepts of disorder and mental health. In addition to Nordenfelt's work (see Chapter 6), examples include Per-Anders Tengland's (1998) *Mental Health: a Philosophical Analysis*, Per Sundström's (1987) *Icons of Disease*, and Tommy Svenson's (1990) *On the Notion of Mental Illness*. Other contributions from a rich Scandinavian literature include Uffe Juul Jensons' (1987) *Practice & Progress*; Henrik Wulff, Stig Andur Pedersen, and Raben Rosenberg's (1986) *Philosophy of Medicine*, and Louhiala and Stenman's (2000) *Philosophy meets Medicine*.

Matthews (1999a) explores the boundary between morals and medicine in *Philosophy, Psychiatry, & Psychology* in his 'Moral Vision and the Idea of Mental Illness', with commentaries by Spitz (1999) and Benn (1999), and a response (Matthews, 1999b). Margree (2002a) opens up a neglected resource for work in this area in her *Normal and Abnormal: Georges Canguilhem and the Question of Mental Pathology*, with a commentary by Gane (2002) and a response (Margree, 2002b).

A detailed analysis of the similarities and differences between anti- and pro-psychiatry theories of the concept of mental illness, together with the arguments leading to the redefinition of the terms of the debate as set out in this chapter, is given in chapter 1 of Fulford's (1989) *Moral Theory and Medical Practice*. The central place of psychotic disorders in the conceptual map of mental disorder is described in chapter 10 of this book. The 'map' of mental disorders in Session 2 was first published in Fulford (1993).

The terms of reference of the debate about mental illness are challenged by Pickering (2003a and b) in his article in *Philosophy, Psychiatry, & Psychology* on the 'Likeness argument and the reality of mental illness', with commentaries by Gipps (2003) Loughlin (2003), Mullen (2003), and Tyreman (2003), and more fully in Pickering (2006). Ian Hacking (1998) explores the influences of cultural factors on the form of mental illness through a richly illustrated historical narrative in his *Mad Travellers*.

Szasz (1987) has drawn together the themes of his work in *Insanity: the Idea and its Consequences*, which includes a full bibliography. A brief but highly readable critique of Szasz' position, including its implicit dualism, is a book by Sir Martin Roth, a former President of the Royal College of Psychiatrists in the UK (and Honorary President of the Philosophy Special Interest Group in the Royal College of Psychiatrists), and Jerome Kroll, a distinguished Professor of Psychiatry in the USA (and a founding member of the American Association for the Advancement of Philosophy and Psychiatry), called, simply, *The Reality of Mental Illness* (1986). A recent collection on Szasz and his critics (with replies by Szasz) is Schaler's (2004) *Szasz Under Fire*; this includes Fulford's (2004) *Values-Based Medicine: Thomas Szasz's Legacy to Twenty-First Century Psychiatry*, which links Szasz' work to recent developments in policy and practice in mental health.

Models of disorder, patient-centred practice and multidisciplinary teams

Although the debate about models of mental disorder is less high profile than it was in the 1960s and 1970s, this is because the issues have now found their way through into policy and practice through developments aimed at, (1) giving the 'user voice' an increasingly central role in all areas of mental health, including research, and (2) reorganizing services around multidisciplinary and multiagency approaches. The importance of both user-centred and multidisciplinary approaches to contemporary service delivery are emphasized, for example, in a national policy document underpinning mental health service provision in England and Wales, the *National Service Framework for Mental Health* (Department of Health, 1999) with direct practical applications in areas such as recovery practice (Allott *et al.*, 2002).

A user-friendly introduction and an integrated approach to the main models of disorder important in clinical work in psychiatry is Tyrer and Steinberg's (2005) *Models for Mental Disorder*. The different perspectives (biological, psychological, and social) important in psychiatry are carefully set out by McHugh and Slaveny (1983) in *The Perspectives of Psychiatry*. The medical model in psychiatry is well reviewed by Macklin (1973) in *The Medical Model in Psychoanalysis and Psychotherapy*.

For a discussion in *Philosophy, Psychiatry, & Psychology* of the applications of Foucault's philosophy to modern user-led developments in service delivery, see Bracken's (1995) *Beyond liberation: Michel Foucault and the Notion of a Critical Psychiatry*, with commentaries by Kendall (1995), Matthews (1995), Heinze (1995), and Kovel (1995). Bracken (2001) and Bracken and Thomas (2001 and 2005) explore the role of post-modern thinking generally for models of service delivery in mental health.

Indications of the practical importance of models of disorder especially in the new circumstances of community care are to be found in, (1) a large literature from patients and patient groups: e.g. Campbell's (1996) *What We Want from Crisis Services*; (2) more systematic studies: e.g. Rogers, Pilgrim, and Lacey's (1993) *Experiencing Psychiatry*; (3) official reports, e.g. the *Report of the Clinical Standards Advisory Group on Schizophrenia* (HMSO, 1995)—this showed that an over-reliance on a consumer-led model could lead to seriously ill patients being neglected; and (4) the ethical and clinical problems posed by community care: e.g. Perkins and Repper's (1998) *Dilemmas in Community Mental Health Practice*. Chapter 11, on *Interprofessional Relations*, of the BMA's (1993) *Medical Ethics Today* is a helpful review of the ethical issues arising in multidisciplinary team working. Fulford, Stanghellini's, and Broome (2004) *What can Philosophy do for Psychiatry?* gives an overview of the role of philosophy in relation to these developments. The *Declaration of Madrid*, the first code of psychiatric ethics to spell out the importance of the 'user' voice in clinical decision-making, was published by the World Psychiatric Association, Geneva (1996).

Anthony Colombo's (1997) *Understanding Mentally Disordered Offenders: a Multi-Agency Perspective* describes an empirical study of the role of different implicit models of disorder in structuring practice. This includes operationalized definitions of each of the key models, medical, social, etc. Anthony Colombo has applied his models methodology to multidisciplinary team working in Colombo *et al.*'s (2003a) 'Evaluating the influence of implicit models of mental disorder on processes of shared decision making within community-based multidisciplinary teams'. This study showed wide differences of implicit models between psychiatrists, social workers, community psychiatric nurses, patients, and carers. An overview of this work is given in *Openmind*, the journal of the UK user advocacy organization, Mind (National Association for Mental Health) (Colombo, *et al.*, 2003b). The philosophical roots of the study in linguistic-analytic philosophy are set out in Fulford and Colombo (2004). The findings from the study and methods developed are included in the training materials for values-based practice described in Chapter 21.

Although biological and other approaches to mental distress and disorder are often presented as being mutually exclusive, among the best of the exponents of different approaches are many who recognize the need for different and complementary models in mental health if the discipline is to serve the diverse needs of individual patients: thus, David Healy's (1990) *The Suspended Revolution*, argues this point from the perspective of psychotherapy, while Nancy Andreasen's (2001) *Brave New Brain* makes the same point from the perspective of the new neurosciences.

References

Allott, P., Loganathan, L., and Fulford, K.W.M. (2002). Discovering hope for recovery. In *Innovation in Community Mental Health: international perspectives*. Special Issue. *Canadian Journal of Community Mental Health*, 21(2): 13–33.

American Psychiatric Association (1994). *Diagnostic and Statistical Manual Of Mental Disorders* (4th edn). Washington, DC: American Psychiatric Association.

Andreasen, N.C. (2001). *Brave New Brain: conquering mental illness in the era of the genome*. Oxford: Oxford University Press.

Aristotle (1980). *Nichomachean Ethics*. Oxford: Oxford University Press.

Audi, R. (ed.) (1995, second edition 1999). *The Cambridge Dictionary of Philosophy*. Cambridge: Cambridge University Press.

Austin, J.L. (1956–7). A plea for excuses. Proceedings of the Aristotelian Society 57: 1–30. Reprinted in White, A.R., ed. (1968). *The Philosophy of Action*. Oxford: Oxford University Press, pp. 19–42.

Baggini, J. and Fosl, P.S. (2003). *The Philosopher's Toolkit*. Oxford: Blackwell.

Bebbington, P.E. and Broome, M.R. (2004). Exploiting the Interface between Philosophy and Psychiatry. *International Review of Psychiatry*, 16, 3:179–183.

Benn, P. (1999). Commentary on Matthew's Moral vision. (1999a). *Philosophy, Psychiatry, & Psychology*, 6(4): 317–320.

Blackburn, S. (1994). *The Oxford Dictionary of Philosophy*. Oxford: Oxford University Press.

Blackburn, S. (2001). *Think: a Compelling Introduction to Philosophy*. Oxford: Oxford Paperbacks.

Bloch, S. and Reddaway, P. (1977). *Russia's Political Hospitals: The Abuse of Psychiatry in the Soviet Union*. London: Victor Gollancz.

Bluglass, R. and Boden, P. (1990). *Principles and Practice of Forensic Psychiatry*. Edinburgh: Churchill Livingstone.

Bolton, D. (2004). Shifts in the philosophical foundations of psychiatry since Jaspers: implications for psychopathology and psychotherapy. *International Review of Psychiatry*, 16, 3: 184–189

Bracken, P.J. (1995). Beyond Liberation: Michael Foucault and the Notion of a Critical Psychiatry. *Philosophy, Psychiatry, & Psychology*, 2/1: 1–14.

Bracken, P. (2001). The radical possibilities of home treatment: postpsychiatry in action. In *Acute Mental Health Care in the Community: intensive home treatment* (ed. N. Brimblecombe). Whurr Publications.

Bracken, P. and Thomas, P. (2001). Postpsychiatry: a new direction for mental health. *British Medical Journal*, 322: 724–727.

Bracken, P. and Thomas, P. (2005). *Postpsychiatry*. Oxford: Oxford University Press.

British Medical Association (1993—new edition in preparation). *Medical Ethics Today: its Practice and Philosophy*. London: British Medical Association.

Brown, G.W., Birley, J.L.T., and Wing. J.K. (1972). The influence of family life on the course of schizophrenia. *Journal of Health and Social Behaviour*, 9: 203–214.

Brown, S., Collinson, D., and Wilkinson, R. (ed.). (1996). *Dictionary of Twentieth Century Philosophers*. London: Routledge.

Burton, N. (forthcoming). *Psychiatry*. Oxford: Blackwells.

Campbell, E.J., Scadding, J.G., and Roberts, R.S. (1979). The concept of disease. *British Medical Journal*, 2: 757–762.

Campbell, P. (1996). What we want from crisis services. In *Speaking Our Minds: an Anthology* (ed. J. Read and J. Reynolds). Basingstoke: The Macmillan Press Ltd for The Open University, pp. 180–183.

Caplan, A.L., Engelhardt, H.J., and McCartney, J.J. (ed.) (1981). *Concepts of Health and Disease*. Reading MA: Addison-Wesley Publishing Co.

Caws, P. (1979). *Sartre*. London: Routledge.

Chodoff, P. (1999). Misuse and abuse of psychiatry: an overview. In *Psychiatric ethics*, (3rd edn). (ed. S. Bloch, P. Chodoff, and S.A. Green). Oxford: Oxford University Press, Chapter 4.

Church, J. (2004). Social constructionist models: making order out of disorder—on the social construction of madness. In *The Philosophy of Psychiatry: a companion* (ed. J. Radden). New York: Oxford University Press, pp. 393–408.

Clare, A. (1979). The disease concept in psychiatry. In *Essentials of Postgraduate Psychiatry* (ed. P. Hill, R. Murray, and A. Thorley). Academic Press, Grune & Stratton, New York.

Colombo, A. (1997). *Understanding Mentally Disordered Offenders: a multi-agency perspective*. Aldershot (England): Ashgate.

Colombo, A., Bendelow, G., Fulford, K.W.M., and Williams, S. (2003a). Evaluating the influence of implicit models of mental disorder on processes of shared decision making within community-based multi-disciplinary teams. *Social Science & Medicine*, 56: 1557–1570.

Colombo, A., Bendelow, G., Fulford, K.W.M., and Williams, S. (2003b). Model behaviour. *Openmind*, 125: 10–12.

Cox., J., Campbell, A.V. and Fulford, K.W.M. (forthcoming) (eds) *Medicine of the Person: Faith, Science and Values in Healthcare Provision*. London: Jessica Kingsley.

Davies, M. (forthcoming). *The Mind*. Oxford: Oxford University Press.

Declaration of Madrid, (1996). Geneva, World Psychiatric Association (reproduced with a brief commentary in the Appendix—Codes of Ethics, 511–531, in Bloch, S., Chodoff P., and Green S.A., (1999). *Psychiatric Ethics* (3rd Edition). Oxford: Oxford University Press.

Department of Health (1999). *National Service Framework for Mental Health—Modern Standards and Service Models*. London: Department of Health.

Earle, W.J. (1992). *Introduction to Philosophy*. New York: McGraw–Hill.

Edwards, P. and Pap, A. (ed.). (1973). *A Modern Introduction to Philosophy*, 3rd edn. New York: The Free Press/London: Collier Macmillan Publishers.

Eysenck, H.J. (1968). Classification and the problems of diagnosis. In *Handbook of Abnormal Psychology*. London: Pitman Medical, Chapter 1.

Foucault, M. (1965). *Madness and Civilization* (trans. R. Savage). New York: Mentor Books.

Fulford, K.W.M. (1989, paperback 1995). *Moral Theory and Medical Practice*. Cambridge: Cambridge University Press.

Fulford, K.W.M. (1993). Value, action, mental illness and the law. In *Action and Value in Criminal Law* (ed. S. Shute, J. Gardner, and J. Horder). Oxford: Oxford University Press, pp. 279–310.

Fulford, K.W.M (1995a). Introduction: Just getting started. pp. 1–3, Introduction to *Philosophy, Psychology, and Psychiatry*, ed. A. Phillips Griffiths. Cambridge: Cambridge University Press, for the Royal Institute of Philosophy.

Fulford, K.W.M (1995b). Mind and Madness: New Directions in the Philosophy of Psychiatry. Chapter 1 in *Philosophy, Psychology and Psychiatry*, Phillips Griffiths, A ed., Cambridge: Cambridge University Press, for the Royal Institute of Philosophy.

Fulford, K.W.M. and Hope, T. (1996). Control and practical experience. In *Informed Consent in Psychiatry—European Perspectives of ethics, law and clinical practice* (ed. H.-G. Koch, S. Reiter-Theil, and H. Helmchen). Report under EU Programme, Biomed 2. Baden-Baden: Nomos Verlagsgesellschaft, pp. 351–379.

Fulford, K.W.M. (1998). Mental illness, Concept of. 5000 word entry for R. Chadwick (ed), *Encylopedia of Applied Ethics*. Vol 3, pp. 213–233. San Diego: Academic Press.

Fulford, K.W.M. (2003). 'Mental Illness: Definition, Use and Meaning', in Post, S.G. (ed). *Encyclopedia of Bioethics*, (3rd edn). New York: Macmillan.

Fulford, K.W.M., Morris, K.J., Sadler, J.Z., and Stanghellini, G. (2003a). Past Improbable, Future Possible: the renaissance in philosophy and psychiatry. Chapter 1 (pp. 1–41) in Fulford, K.W.M., Morris, K.J., Sadler, J.Z., and Stanghellini, G. (eds.) *Nature and Narrative: an Introduction to the New Philosophy of Psychiatry*. Oxford: Oxford University Press.

Fulford, K.W.M., Morris, K.J., Sadler, J.Z., and Stanghellini, G. (ed.) (2003b). *Nature and Narrative: an introduction to the New Philosophy of Psychiatry*. Oxford: Oxford University Press.

Fulford, K.W.M. (2004). Values-Based Medicine: Thomas Szasz's Legacy to Twenty-First Century Psychiatry. Ch 2 in Schaler, J.A (ed) *Szasz Under Fire: The Psychiatric Abolitionist Faces His Critics*, pp. 57–92. Chicago and La Salle, Illinois: Open Court Publishers.

Fulford, K.W.M. and Colombo, A. (2004). Six models of mental disorder: a study combining linguistic-analytic and empirical methods. *Philosophy, Psychiatry, & Psychology*, 11(2): 129–144.

Fulford, K.W.M., Stanghellini, G., and Broome, M. (2004). What can philosophy do for psychiatry? Special Article. *World Psychiatry*, 130–135.

Gane, M. (2002). Normativity and pathology. (Commentary on Margree, 2002a). *Philosophy, Psychiatry, & Psychology*, 9(4): 313–316.

Gelder, M.G., Gath, D., and Mayou, R. (1994). *Concise Oxford Textbook of Psychiatry*. Oxford: Oxford University Press.

Gelder, M.G., Lopez-Ibor, J.J., and Andreasen, N. (ed.). (2000). *New Oxford Textbook of Psychiatry*. Oxford: Oxford University Press.

Gelder, M.E., Mayou, R., and Cowen, P. (2001). *Shorter Oxford Textbook of Psychiatry*, (4th edn). Oxford: Oxford University Press.

Gert, B. and Culver, C.M. (2004). Defining mental disorder. In *The Philosophy of Psychiatry: a Companion* (ed. J. Radden). New York: Oxford University Press, pp. 415–425.

Gipps, R.G.T. (2003). Illnesses and likenesses. (Commentary on Pickering, 2003a). *Philosophy, Psychiatry, & Psychology*, 10(3): 255–260.

Gipps, R.G.T. and Fulford, K.W.M. (2004). Understanding the clinical concept of delusion: from an estranged to an engaged epistemology. *International Review of Psychiatry*, 16, 3: 225–235.

Glendinning, S. (forthcoming) *Derrida*. Oxford: Oxford University Press.

Glover, J. (1970). *Responsibility*. London: Routledge & Kegan Paul.

Glover, J. (1988) *I: The Philosophy and Psychology of Personal Identity*. London: The Penguin Group.

Graham, G. and Stephens, G. Lynn. (1994). *Philosophical Psychopathology*. Cambridge, MA: The MIT Press.

Griffiths, A.P. (ed.). (1985). *Philosophy and Practice*. Cambridge: Cambridge University Press.

Griffiths, A.P. (ed) (1989). *Key Themes in Philosophy*. Cambridge: Cambridge University Press, for the Royal Institute of Philosophy.

Griffiths, A.P. (ed) (1995). *Philosophy, Psychology, and Psychiatry*. Cambridge: Cambridge University Press, for the Royal Institute of Philosophy.

Gunn, J. and Taylor, P.J. (1993). *Forensic Psychiatry: Clinical, Legal and Ethical Issues*. Oxford: Butterworth-Heinemann.

Guttenplan, S., Hornsby, J., and Janaway, C. (2003). *Reading Philosophy: Selected Texts with a Method for Beginners*. Blackwell Publishers.

Hacker, P.M.S. (2004). The conceptual framework for the investigation of emotions. *International Review of Psychiatry*, 16, 3: 199–208

Hacking, I. (1998). *Mad Travelers: Reflections on the Reality of Transient Mental Illnesses*. Charlottesville and London: University Press of Virginia.

Hawton, K., Salkovskis, P.M., Kirk, J., and Clark, D.M. (1989). *Cognitive Behaviour Therapy for Psychiatric Problems: a Practical Guide*, Oxford: Oxford University Press.

Healy, D. (1990). *The Suspended Revolution: Psychiatry and Psychotherapy Re-examined*. London: Faber and Faber.

Heaton, J. and Groves, J. (1994). *Wittgenstein for Beginners*. Cambridge, UK: Icon Books.

Heginbotham, C. (2004). Psychiatric Dasein. *Philosophy, Psychiatry, & Psychology*, 11(2): 147–150.

Heinze, M. (1995). Commentary on 'Moralist or therapist?' (Matthews, 1995). *Philosophy, Psychiatry, & Psychology*, 2/1: 31–32.

Helman, C.G. (1981). Disease versus illness in general practice. *Journal of the Royal College of Practitioners*, 230(3): 548–552.

Hollis, M. (1985, reprinted 1992). *Invitation to Philosophy*. Oxford: Blackwell.

Honderich, T. (ed). (1995). *The Oxford Companion to Philosophy*. Oxford: Oxford University Press.

Hope, T. (2004). *Medical Ethics: a very short introduction*. Oxford: Oxford University Press.

HMSO (1995). *Report of the Clinical Standards Advisory Group on Schizophrenia*, Volume 1, London: HSMO.

Hundert, E.M. (1989). *Philosophy, Psychiatry and Neuroscience*. Oxford: Clarendon Press.

Jacoby, R. and Oppenheimer, C. (1996). *Psychiatry in the Elderly*. Oxford: Oxford University Press.

James, W. (1987) Review of *Grunzuge der Physiologischen Psychologie*, by Wilhelm Wundt (1975). In *Essays, Comments and Reviews*, Cambridge, Mass, Harvard University Press.

Jensen, U.J. (1987). *Practice & Progress: a Theory for the modern Health-care System*. Oxford: Blackwell Scientific Publications.

Kant, I. (1929). *Critique of Pure Reason* (transl. Norman Kemp Smith). London: Methuen.

Kendall, T. (1995). Commentary on 'Beyond liberation. (Bracken, 1995). *Philosophy, Psychiatry, & Psychology*, 2: 15–18.

Kendell, R.E. (1975). The concept of disease. *British Journal of Psychiatry*, 127: 305–315.

Kovel, J. (1995). Commentary on 'Beyond liberation' (Bracken, 1995) and 'Moral therapist?' (Matthews, 1995). *Philosophy, Psychiatry, & Psychology*, 2/1: 33–34.

Laing, R.D. (1960). *The Divided Self*. London: Tavistock.

Law, S. (2004). *The Philosophy Files*. London: Orion Children's.

Leff, J. and Vaughn, C. (ed.). (1985). *Expressed Emotion in Families: its significance for mental illness*. New York: Guildford Press.

Levy, N. and Bayne, T. (2004). Doing without deliberation: Automatism, automaticity, and moral accountability. *International Review of Psychiatry*, 16, 3: 209–215.

Lewis, A.J. (1953). Health as a Social Concept. *British Journal of Sociology*, 4: 109–124.

Lishman, A.W. (1978). (1997 paperback). *Organic Psychiatry*. Oxford: Blackwell Scientific Publications.

Loughlin, M. (2003). Contingency, arbitrariness, and failure. (Commentary on Pickering, 2003a). *Philosophy, Psychiatry, & Psychology*, 10(3): 261–264.

Louhiala, P. and Stenman, S. (ed.). (2000). *Philosophy Meets Medicine*. Helsinki: Helsinki University Press.

Macklin (1973). The medical model in psychoanalysis and psychotherapy. *Comprehensive Psychiatry*, 14: 49–69.

Magee, B. (1987). *The Great Philosophers: an Introduction to Western philosophy*. London: BBC Books.

Margree, V. (2002a). Normal and abnormal: Georges Canguilhem and the question of mental pathology. *Philosophy, Psychiatry, & Psychology*, 9(4): 299–312.

Margree, V. (2002b). Canguilhem and social pathology: a response to the Commentary. *Philosophy, Psychiatry, & Psychology*, 9(4): 317–320.

Matthews, E. (1995). Moralist or therapist? Foucault and the critique of psychiatry. *Philosophy, Psychiatry, & Psychology*, 2/1: 19–30.

Matthews, E. (1996). *Twentieth Century French Philosophy*. Oxford: Oxford University Press.

Matthews, E. (1999a). Moral vision and the idea of mental illness. *Philosophy, Psychiatry, & Psychology*, 6(4): 299–310.

Matthews, E. (1999b). Disordered minds: a response to the commentaries. *Philosophy, Psychiatry, & Psychology*, 6(4): 321–322.

Matthews, E.H. (2004). Merleau-Ponty's body-subject and psychiatry. *International Review of Psychiatry*, 16, 3: 190–198.

McHugh, P.R. and Slavney, P.R. (1983). *The Perspectives of Psychiatry*. Baltimore, MD: The Johns Hopkins University Press.

Mullen, R. (2003). Definition is limited and values inescapable. (Commentary on Pickering, 2003a). *Philosophy, Psychiatry, & Psychology*, 10(3): 265–266.

Nagel, T. (1987). *What Does it All Mean? A Very Short Introduction to Philosophy*. Oxford University Press.

O'Hear, A. (1985). *What Philosophy Is*. Harmondsworth, England: Penguin Books.

Okasha, A. and Maj, M. (ed.). (2001). *Images in Psychiatry: an Arab perspective*. World Psychiatric Association. Egypt: Scientific Book House.

Parsons, T. (1951). *The Social System*. Glencoe, IL: Free Press.

Perkins, R. and Repper, J. (1998). *Dilemmas in Community Mental Health Practice: Choice or Control*. Aberdeen: Radcliffe Medical Press.

Pickering, N. (2003a). The likeness argument and the reality of mental illness. *Philosophy, Psychiatry, & Psychology*, 10(3): 243–254.

Pickering, N. (2003b). The likeness argument: reminders, roles, and reasons for use. (A response to the commentaries). *Philosophy, Psychiatry, & Psychology*, 10(3): 273–276.

Pickering, N. (2006). *The Metaphor of Mental Illness*. Oxford: Oxford University Press.

Putnam, H. (2002). The Empiricist background. Chapter 1 in *The Collapse of the Fact/Value Dichotomy and other Essays*. Cambridge, MA: Harvard University Press.

Quinton, A. (1985). Madness, ch 2 in *Philosophy and Practice* (ed. P.A. Griffiths). Cambridge: Cambridge University Press.

Rachels, J. (2005). *Problems from Philosophy*. Boston: McGraw Hill.

Radden, J. (1996). *Divided Minds and Successive Selves: Ethical Issues in Disorders of Identity and Personality*, Cambridge, Mass: MIT Press.

Radden, J. (2004) (Ed). *The Philosophy of Psychiatry: A Companion*. New York: Oxford University Press.

Reznek, L. (1991). *The Philosophical Defence of Psychiatry*, London, Routledge.

Robertson, S. (2004). Philosophy and History of Psychiatry, chapter 27 pps 551–568, in C. Fear (ed) *Essential Revision notes in Psychiatry for the MRCPsych*. Knutsford, England: Pastest Ltd.

Rogers, A., Pilgrim., D., and Lacey, R. (1993). *Experiencing Psychiatry: user's views of services*. London: The Macmillan Press.

Rosenhan, D. (1973). On being sane in insane places. *Science*, 179: 250–258.

Roth, M. and Kroll, J. (1986). *The Reality of Mental Illness*. Cambridge: Cambridge University Press.

Ryle, G. (1949). *The Concept of Mind*. London: Hutchinson. (London: Penguin, 1963.)

Sadler, J.Z., Wiggins, O.P., Schwartz, M.A. (ed.). (1994). *Philosophical Perspectives on Psychiatric Diagnostic Classification*. Baltimore, MD: Johns Hopkins University Press.

Sass, L.A. (1994). *Madness and Modernism: Insanity in the Light of Modern Art, Literature, and Thought*. Cambridge, MA: Harvard University Press.

Sass, L.A. (1995). *The Paradoxes of Delusion: Wittgenstein, Schreber, and the Schizophrenic Mind*. Cornell: Cornell University Press.

Schaler, J.A (ed.). (2004) *Szasz Under Fire: the Psychiatric Abolitionist Faces his Critics*. Chicago, IL: Open Court Publishers.

Scheff, T. (1974). The labelling theory of mental illness. *American Sociological Review*, 39, 444–452.

Spitz, D. (1999). Commentary on 'How to cut the psychiatric pie: the dilemma of character. (Matthews, 1999a). *Philosophy, Psychiatry, & Psychology*, 6(4): 311–316.

Spitzer, M., Uehlein, F., Schwartz, M. A., and Mundt, C., (1993) eds., *Phenomenology, Language and Schizophrenia*, Springer-Verlag, New York.

Stephens, G.Lynn. and Graham, G. (2004). Reconceiving delusion. *International Review of Psychiatry*, 16, 3: 236–241.

Storr, A. (1989). *Freud*. London: Fontana.

Sundström, P. (1987). *Icons of Disease: A Philosophical Inquiry into the Semantics, Phenomenology and Ontology of the Clinical Conceptions of Disease*. Linköping University, Sweden: Department of Health and Society.

Svensson, T. (1990). *On the Notion of Mental Illness: Problematizing the Medical–Model Conception of Certain Abnormal Behaviour and Mental Afflictions*. Linköping, Sweden: Department of Health and Society.

Szasz, T. (1960). The myth of mental illness. *American Psychologist*, 15: 113–118.

Szasz, T.S., (1987). *Insanity: The Idea and its Consequences*. New York: John Wiley & Sons.

Tengland, P.-A. (1998). *Mental Health: a Philosophical Analysis*. Linköping, Sweden: Department of Health and Society.

Thornton, T. (2004). Wittgenstein and the limits of empathic understanding in psychopathology. *International Review of Psychiatry*, 16, 3: 216–224.

Toulmin, S. (1980). Agent and patient in psychiatry. *International Journal of Law and Psychiatry*, 3: 267–278.

Tyreman, S. (2003). Likening strikes twice: psychiatry, osteopathy, and the likeness argument. (Commentary on Pickering, 2003a). *Philosophy, Psychiatry, & Psychology*, 10(3): 267–272.

Tyrer, P. and Steinberg, D. (2005). *Models for Mental Disorder: Conceptual Models in Psychiatry* (3rd edn). Chichester: John Wiley & Sons Ltd.

Vesey, G. (ed) (1986). *Philosophers Ancient and Modern*. Cambridge: Cambridge University Press.

von Wright, G.H. (1963). *The Varieties of Goodness*. New York: Routledge and Kegan Paul.

Warburton, N. (2004). *Philosophy: the basics (4th edition)*. London: Routledge.

Wilkes, K.V. (1988). *Real People: Personal Identity Without Thought Experiments*. Oxford: Clarendon Press.

Williams, R. (2004). Finding the way forward in professional practice. *Philosophy, Psychiatry, & Psychology*, 11(2): 151–158.

Williams, R. and Kerfoot, M. (eds) (2005). *Child and Adolescent Mental Health Services: Strategy, Planning, Delivery, and Evaluation*. Oxford: Oxford University Press.

Williamson, T. (2004). Can two wrongs make a right? *Philosophy, Psychiatry, & Psychology*, 11(2): 159–164.

Wing, J.K. (1978). *Reasoning about Madness*. Oxford: Oxford University Press.

Wittgenstein, L. (1921). *Tractatus Logico-Philosophicus* (trans. D.F. Pears and B.F. McGuinness). London: Routledge and Kegan Paul.

Wulff, H.R., Pedersen, S.A., and Rosenberg, R. (1986). *Philosophy of Medicine, an Introduction*. Oxford: Blackwell Scientific Publications.

CHAPTER 3

Experiences good and bad: an introduction to psychopathology, classification, and diagnosis for philosophers

Chapter contents

This chapter provides an introduction to psychopathology, classification, and diagnosis in psychiatry for philosophers.

The two aims of this chapter

The chapter has two aims. The first is to give philosophers (or anyone with no background practical experience of mental distress and disorder) a taste of the more formal aspects of psychopathology and the classifications of mental disorder used by professionals working in mental health.

The materials in this chapter, it should be said straight away, are perhaps more characteristic of medical, nursing, and psychological professional work, than, say, social work. The materials, it is true, are the result of over a hundred years of careful observation and development of ideas (covered in detail in Parts II and III). All the same, just as the concept of mental disorder remains subject to widely different interpretations (the various 'models' we explored in Chapter 2), so the classification of these disorders—the particular 'symptoms' identified, the groups and classes and clusters into which they are drawn together—remain much debated. The whole enterprise of classification of mental distress and disorder is indeed challenged by some (see, e.g. Kutchins and Kirk, 1997). As with all the materials in this book, then, this chapter is presented, not as a reflection of a settled or final view, but as a focus for critical engagement and collegial development of ideas.

The second aim of this chapter is to get across the idea that psychopathology and classification in psychiatry are not as easy as many outside the discipline sometimes imagine!

We want to be clear here. The point is not that the discipline is, somehow, arcane or otherwise impenetrable. The point is rather that it is a well-developed area of professional expertise, supported by a wealth of theory, clinical skills, empirical research, and narrative literature. Furthermore, unlike diagnosis and classification in, say, cardiology and renal medicine, psychiatric classification is conceptually as well as empirically difficult. As we noted in Chapter 2, and will develop further later in this part, this conceptual difficulty is at the heart of the engagement between philosophers and practitioners in psychiatry. We will be looking at the historical origins of this engagement in Part II, and at current 'hot topics' later on, in the philosophy of science (Part III), in value theory (Part IV, particularly on the role of values in diagnostic assessment), and in the philosophy of mind (Part V, which explores specific areas of psychopathology). Philosophy, then, has much to contribute here. And the point of this chapter is to encourage philosophers, in engaging with psychiatric classification and diagnosis, to get up to speed with the subject as it really is.

Sources and resources in clinical psychopathology and the aims of this chapter

There is no single source from which a philosopher can get up to speed with classification and diagnosis in psychiatry. Textbooks are written for particular groups of practitioners with particular backgrounds, levels of clinical experience, and training aims.

Diagnostic manuals, similarly, although a helpful source (the DSM has invaluable summary 'boxes', see below), assume a shared 'craft knowledge' and professional expertise. The research literature, as another valuable source, encompasses a number of disciplines (psychological, phenomenological, neuroscientific, etc.), often highly specialized, and necessarily assuming technical expertise and common programme objectives. The growing first-hand narrative literature from users and carers is an especially rich resource, which is becoming increasingly accessible especially through web-based sources.

This chapter includes examples of materials from all these sources set within a framework of the main areas of descriptive psychopathology (symptoms) and categories of disorder (syndromes) recognized particularly by psychiatry and clinical psychology. Clearly, within the scope of this chapter we can claim neither comprehensive coverage nor in-depth treatment of any particular topic. However, we hope that the examples given, taken together with the reading guides here and in later chapters, will provide a clear introduction to *clinical* psychopathology as a basis for well-informed research in the growing discipline of *philosophical* psychopathology.

Structure of the chapter

The chapter is divided into three main sessions:

- *Session 1, diagnosis in medicine and psychiatry*, covers the principles governing diagnosis and classification in psychiatry and medicine (we outlined the *process* of diagnosis in Chapter 2, Session 1).

- *Session 2, descriptive psychopathology*, describes the range of psychiatric symptoms and signs recognized by psychiatry. As the scope of what has become widely known as 'descriptive psychopathology' (Sims, 1988) or, sometimes, 'descriptive phenomenology' (Sims *et al.*, 2000), this will be the largest section of the chapter. It includes brief *Philosophical Annotations* on each of the main areas of symptomatology (anxiety, affect, etc.). These are by way of illustration of philosophical work in psychopathology and are not, of course, exhaustive of this rapidly expanding field. In particular, we have made no attempt to cover the rich resources of Continental phenomenology, which will be the subject of a later book in this series (Parnas *et al.*, forthcoming). A general reading guide to psychopathology, clinical and philosophical, is given at the end of the chapter.

- *Session 3, categories of mental disorder*, outlines the main clinical syndromes included in our current diagnostic classifications of mental disorder, in particular ICD-10 (WHO, 1992) and DSM-IV (APA, 1994). The categories of disorder included in these classifications are built up primarily from the symptoms and signs described in Session 2.

In a brief *Conclusions* we will introduce some of the particular difficulties presented by psychiatric classification and diagnosis and indicate how these connect psychiatry with philosophy. These difficulties are all explored further in other chapters.

Session 1 Diagnosis in medicine and psychiatry

In all branches of medicine, disease classification develops by a kind of natural selection. As medical knowledge advances, so new and clinically more useful categories gradually replace those that have become less useful. In this respect, medicine and psychiatry are no different from other sciences. As Norman Sartorius, at the time Director of the Mental Health section of the WHO, reminded us in the Preface to ICD-10, a classification is no more, and no less, than 'a way of seeing the world at a point in time' (Sartorius, 1992, p. vii). A scientific classification (as we will explore in detail in Part III, chapter 13) thus represents a snapshot of the theory and knowledge base of the science in question at a given stage of its development.

Scientific knowledge in psychiatry has been advancing rapidly in recent years. Psychiatric diagnostic categories are thus correspondingly fluid and this has brought with it a degree of confusion. However, the more widely used classifications are nowadays all broadly similar. DSM-IV and ICD-10 were indeed bound by international treaty to converge as far as possible. They include many of the same overall categories of disorder and they are built up from essentially the same list of basic symptoms and signs. It is mainly in the details of particular category definitions that one classification differs from the next (though as we will see later, particularly in Part IV, chapter 20, some of these differences of detail are conceptually highly significant).

The purposes of diagnosis

In the first exercise in this chapter we consider one of those questions that, so far as doctors are concerned, is generally just taken for granted, namely what purposes are served by medical diagnosis?

Making the purposes of diagnosis explicit helps to explain, first, why diagnostic classifications have developed as they have in bodily medicine, second, why they remain in some respects different in psychiatry, and, third, why philosophy (as well as science) may be important in developing future classifications not only in psychiatry but also in bodily medicine.

EXERCISE 1   (20 minutes)

Write a list of a few medical diagnoses. These could be from your own experience as a doctor or as a patient. Think of minor as well as more serious conditions. Then write down what purposes these diagnoses serve, thinking about this particularly from the perspective of a doctor or other health-care professional.

Here are just a few examples: common cold, migraine, boil, chicken pox, pneumonia, pneumococcal pneumonia, anaemia, iron deficiency anaemia, diabetes mellitus.

Obviously, the list is endless! Each of these diagnoses, however, like any diagnosis in medicine, serves four main purposes. Briefly, these are:

1. *Descriptive*: a diagnostic label provides a summary description of a patient's symptoms, essential for communication, and the key to all other medically relevant decisions about the patient.

2. *Aetiological*: diagnoses, particularly in specialized areas of bodily medicine, are often based on information about aetiology (or causation).

3. *Therapeutic*: knowledge of symptoms and of aetiology is the basis for decisions about treatment and other aspects of clinical management.

4. *Prognostic*: symptoms and aetiology, together with the likely response to treatment, give an estimate of prognosis.

The four main purposes of diagnosis in medicine are served in different ways and to different extents by different kinds of diagnostic category. Thus the diagnosis 'migraine' conveys definite information about a patient's symptoms and their prognosis; however, it suggests only a range of possible treatments, and it tells us little if anything about aetiology. With 'diabetes mellitus', on the other hand, the reverse is the case. This diagnosis conveys definite information about aetiology, it suggests certain specific and effective treatments, and it allows an overall estimate of prognosis; but given the wide variety of possible clinical presentations of this condition, it provides no definite information about the patient's actual symptoms.

We can understand these differences in the terms of what in Chapter 5 we will call differences between strict and ordinary implication. Different kinds of disease category are *defined* in different ways, symptomatically, aetiologically, etc. This is *strict* implication. But they all carry by *ordinary* implication, or contingently, a degree of information relevant to all four purposes of diagnosis.

Differences between diagnosis in bodily medicine and psychiatry

The contested status of psychiatry as part of medicine, as we saw in the last chapter, has its origins in a number of differences between it and general bodily medicine. These are particularly evident in classification and diagnosis.

EXERCISE 2   (20 minutes)

Think about the diagnostic categories you are familiar with in psychiatry, either from your professional or user experience, or by referring back to Figure 2.1 and Box 2.1 in chapter 2. In terms of the four 'purposes' of diagnosis, and their respective representations in the definitions of particular categories, how do the categories of mental disorder differ overall from those in bodily medicine?

A key difference in classification and diagnosis between psychiatry and bodily medicine is that psychiatry's diagnostic categories

Table 3.1 Different kinds of diagnostic category as illustrated by depression

Diagnosis	Symptoms	Aetiology	Treatment	Prognosis
Major or psychotic depression	Severe, often relapsing depression with one or more of: (a) a number of biological symptoms (b) delusions, hallucinations. Sometimes alternating with periods of mania.	Various theories	Physical treatments (drugs, ECT) likely to be effective and may be life-saving (e.g. with suicide risk). Other treatments important but supplementary.	Good, especially with treatment. Likely to relapse but with (often long) periods of normality. When depressed beware high suicide risk.
Minor depression	Usually less severe depression, with neither specific biological symptoms nor delusions or hallucinations. May be chronic, is often relapsing	Various theories	Psychological treatments (e.g. cognitive therapy) often helpful together with counselling, support and social intervention. Physical treatments less likely to be helpful.	Generally good; but sometimes condition is chronic and/or relapsing (merging with personality disorder). Risk of attempted suicide rather than actual suicide.
Depressive personality	Depressive symptoms, usually similar to those of neurotic depression; but continuing largely unchanged throughout adult life	Various theories	Treatment unlikely to change the condition. Management thus concentrates on ameliorating the effects of the condition on the patient's life, and on the lives of those around the patient.	Poor. Likely to remain essentially unchanged.
Adjustment reaction	May include any of the range of depressive symptoms, but these are clearly provoked by loss (e.g. in bereavement) or other psychological trauma.	Experience of loss or other psychological 'trauma' is part of definition.	Counselling, support and social intervention indicated; psychological (and physical) treatments sometimes helpful.	Good. Even if very severe, likely to resolve; but may recur with further stressors.

are more often defined *descriptively*, ie in terms of *symptoms*, rather than aetiologically. Psychiatric diagnostic categories are thus more often like 'migraine' than like 'diabetes mellitus' in the kinds of information that they convey.

Both types of diagnostic category, however, as already noted, also carry important information about aetiology, treatment, and prognosis. This is illustrated by Table 3.1, which shows four important diagnoses of depression. The first three of these differential diagnoses (as a list of this kind is called) are defined primarily by the symptoms present and by their time course. The fourth diagnosis includes a reference to stress as an aetiological factor. However, all four categories carry by ordinary implication information about aetiology, treatment, and prognosis, as well as symptoms. (These categories are described further in Session 3 below, and Table 3.3 and Box 3.1)

The difference between psychiatry and bodily medicine in this respect is of course a difference of degree rather than a difference in kind. This is one reason why the radical antipsychiatry view that mental distress and disorder are *never* pathological, is perhaps not very plausible. As we saw in Chapter 2, though, the fact that there *is* this difference of degree makes the radical pro-psychiatry claim, that mental disorders are *no different* from bodily disorders, equally implausible.

Reasons for the differences: a negative and a positive view

As to why there should be these differences of degree between the diagnostic categories of psychiatry and of bodily medicine, different interpretations are possible. One interpretation, noted in Chapter 2, is that psychiatry is scientifically primitive. Historically, as this somewhat negative line of thought goes, bodily medicine has moved from descriptive categories ('dropsy', the 'staggers', 'fever', etc.) to aetiological categories through a series of remarkable advances in medical science. Psychiatry, then, according to this interpretation, has remained stuck at a descriptive stage, roughly equivalent to pre-seventeenth century general medicine!

A more positive interpretation is that the sciences underpinning psychiatry are just a lot more *difficult* than those underpinning areas such as cardiology and gastroenterology. Psychiatry, then, consistently with this positive interpretation, is in this respect closer to neurology than to cardiology and gastroenterology. For in neurology, too, many of our diagnostic categories, like those in psychiatry, are still primarily descriptive, and for the same reason, namely, that neurological science is peculiarly *difficult* science.

This is not in any way to minimize the importance of the scientific advances made in other areas of medicine. But it *is* firmly to

Box 3.1 **Definition of personality disorder**

1. *Normal.* This shows the regular, moderate mood swings of a normal individual subject to the normal exigencies of an average life.

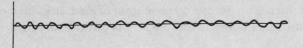

2. *Depressive personality disorder.* Here the subject's mood swings are mainly depressive.

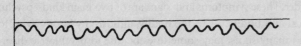

3. *Illness superimposed on a normal personality.* The subject suffers a depressive illness, followed by a manic illness. Note that his symptoms during his first illness are the same as those that subject number 2 suffers most of the time. But for this subject, they represent a change from the norm.

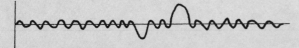

4. *Illness superimposed on an abnormal personality.* Again, the essential difference between illness and personality disorder is a change from the norm for the patient in question, either quantitative (i.e. the first and second blips on the trace) or qualitative (the third, square-shaped blip). Here the personality disorder is cyclothymic, i.e. with excessive mood swings both up and down.

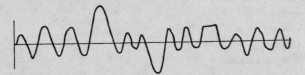

In this diagram, the four longitudinal axes represent the lifetimes of four peopole, from late adolescence through to old age (this being the period over which personality is normally stable). The four horizontal axes represent, for purposes of this example, mood swings – up for happy, down for sad. This axis could represent any other personality trait. (Source: Fulford, 1998).

endorse a positive rather than negative interpretation of the stage of development of psychiatric science. We can spell out this positive rather than negative interpretation in the form of three answers to three questions. Thus,

♦ *Question 1: Why have diagnostic classifications developed as they have in bodily medicine?* Disease classifications in most areas of bodily medicine have moved from a predominantly descriptive to predominantly aetiological basis over the last century or so, because the sciences underpinning them—physiology, bacteriology, and so forth—have developed to the point that an agreed corpus of causal disease theory has reached the threshold of clinically usefulness.

♦ *Question 2: Why do diagnostic classifications remain in some respects different in psychiatry?* Diagnostic classifications remain predominantly descriptive (symptom-based) in psychiatry because progress in the sciences underpinning the discipline has been slower; however, this is because the sciences concerned are a good deal more difficult than those involved in most areas of bodily medicine.

♦ *Question 3: Why may philosophy (as well as science) be important in developing future diagnostic classifications in psychiatry?* Philosophy has a role to play in psychiatric diagnostic classification, because the difficulties in psychiatric science are conceptual (hence in part matters for philosophy) as well as empirical in nature. This is well recognized by many neuroscientists. The American psychiatrist and neuroscientist, for example, Nancy Andreasen, who besides being Editor of the prestigious *American Journal of Psychiatry* has done seminal work both in descriptive psychopathology and in brain imaging, concludes a masterly review of the new neurosciences, concerned as they are with the 'higher' mental functions, of consciousness, personal identity, and so forth, with a ringing endorsement of the importance of the humanities alongside the sciences in psychiatry (Andreasen, 2001).

The positive interpretation in research and practice

A positive rather than negative interpretation of the continuing differences in classification and diagnosis between psychiatry and other medical disciplines is important scientifically. Productive as psychiatry's twentieth century imitation of medical disciplines such as cardiology and renal medicine has been, it can hardly expect to develop fully within a framework of disease theory that is sufficient for these relatively uncomplicated (conceptually speaking) areas of medicine: no more could quantum mechanics have developed within the conceptual framework of nineteenth century mechanical engineering—though of course it could not have developed without it!

We return to the particular conceptual challenges of psychiatric classification and diagnosis below, Conclusions, and in Part III. However, a positive rather than negative interpretation of the stage of development of psychiatric science is perhaps even more important clinically. Much of the difficulty we face in mental health, whether as users or providers of services, whether as psychiatrists, psychologists, nurses, or advocates, arises from the stigmatization of our discipline as being, somehow, an inadequate also-ran to general medicine. Well, it is easier to run up a small hill than a mountain! The scientific mountain of psychiatry is, partly, the empirical challenge of developing methods for investigating the brain. Psychiatry shares this empirical challenge with neurology. However, psychiatric science, in being concerned with the higher functions (of emotion, belief, volition, and so forth) has conceptual challenges as well. These challenges start with the structure of experience and of the disturbed experiences that are the subject matter of descriptive psychopathology.

Reflection on the session and self-test questions

Write down your own reflections on the materials in this session drawing out any points that are particularly significant for you. Then write brief notes about the following:

1. What are the four main purposes of diagnosis in medicine?

2. What is the main difference between the diagnostic categories used in psychiatry and in (most) areas of bodily medicine?

3. Give one positive and one negative interpretation of the differences between diagnostic categories in psychiatry and in bodily medicine.

Session 2   Descriptive psychopathology

In this session, the main psychiatric symptoms and signs recognized by psychiatry will be outlined. As we noted in the last session psychiatric diagnostic categories are mainly like 'migraine'

rather than 'diabetes mellitus', in being defined descriptively rather than aetiologically. In Session 3 we will look at how the symptoms and signs that comprise psychiatry's descriptive psychopathology are aggregated, in various ways, to make up the broad categories of disorder common to most modern psychiatric classifications. A practical scheme giving the steps from symptoms to diagnosis in individual cases is described at the end of that session. Further details of many of psychiatry's diagnostic categories are given in later chapters, in particular in Part V.

The scope of descriptive psychopathology

Descriptive psychopathology covers the symptoms (expressed by the patient) and signs (observed by others) of psychiatric disorder. These symptoms and signs are of two main kinds, psychological and bodily. As to the bodily, almost any bodily symptom, and many signs, may sometimes be due to psychiatric disorder (just as any psychological symptom may sometimes be due to bodily disorder). We will be looking briefly at some of the bodily symptoms important in psychiatry below. But it is on the psychological symptoms that we will be concentrating in this section.

In what follows you may find it helpful to refer to Table 3.2 which gives a checklist of the main psychiatric symptoms and signs.

Table 3.2 Psychiatric symptom check-list

Psychological symptoms

Mood: morbid states of

1. Anxiety
   - generalized (free floating)
   - phobic: specific object, social phobic, agoraphobic
   - panic attacks
2. Affect (sadness/happiness)
   - depression
   - elation (hypomania)
   - mixed
   - diminished

Thought: disorders of

1. Stream
   - slowed
   - accelerated (pressure of thought; flight of ideas;)
2. Connection
   - thought block
   - knight's move
   - positive formal thought disorder (asyndetic thinking, interpenetration of themes, overinclusiveness)
   - negative formal thought disorder ('concrete' thinking)
   - 'word salad' (severe formal thought disorder + neologisms and metonyms)
   - perseveration
3. Possession
   - obsessive-compulsive symptoms
   - thought insertion**/withdrawal**/broadcasting** (schizophrenia)
4. Content
   - delusions,** differentiated by content (paranoid/self-referential; persecutory; grandiose; hypochondriacal; nihilistic; of guilt; of poverty) and origin (primary and secondary)
   - partial delusions*
   - morbid fears
   - overvalued ideas

Perception

1. Hallucinations,** differentiated by mode (auditory, visual, olfactory, gustatory, tactile) and form (simple, complex)
2. Pseudohallucinations*
3. Illusions/distortions

Cognitive function: disturbances of

1. orientation (for time, place, person)
2. attention/concentration
3. memory
   - recent
   - remote
4. IQ (verbal, performance)

Insight: for any symptom, lack of

1. awareness that something is wrong and/or
2. recognition that what is wrong is a symptom of mental illness

Physical symptoms

Any physical symptom may be due to a psychiatric disorder. Important examples include:

1. autonomic symptoms of anxiety (palpitation, tremor, globus, etc.)
2. biological symptoms of depression
3. pain (e.g. in 'masked' depression)
4. disorders of primary sense and voluntary motor systems (in hysteria)
5. disturbances of vegetative functions
   - appetite (loss, anorexia, bulimia); sexual (drive, orgasmic); sleep (increased, decreased)

Psychological signs

Disturbances of appearance, behaviour and speech. Important but mainly as pointing to psychological symptoms; e.g. 1. expressed affect (facial, postural, speech), 2. self-neglect (e.g. in dementia).

* Partial insight; ** psychotic symptoms, ie no insight.

Psychological symptoms

The subdivisions of descriptive psychopathology

As in bodily medicine, accurate diagnosis in psychiatry depends on the details of a patient's symptoms. For example, it is not enough to know that a patient is worried by the thought that he is dirty. You have to decide whether the thought in question is, say, an ordinary preoccupation, an obsession, a delusion, or thought insertion. Each of these has quite different features.

This brings us to the general problem, how to divide up the content of consciousness?

EXERCISE 3	(15 minutes)

Write down your own ideas about how the contents of consciousness might be divided up. Bodily medicine has a (relatively) easy task of dividing the body up into parts and systems—circulatory, gastroenterological, reproductive, etc. What might be the counterparts of these for the mind?

The psychological symptoms of psychiatric disorder are generally divided up by psychiatry for descriptive purposes into disorders of: (1) mood; (2) thought; (3) perception; and (4) cognitive function.

You will probably have had different ideas about the 'parts' of the mind! Different ideas are to be found among authors on psychopathology: delusion, for example, is usually included (as here) among disorders of thinking; however, it is sometimes separated out from disorders of thought as a disorder of belief. So there is work here for philosophy, this being just one of the ways in which psychiatry is conceptually more complex than bodily medicine. In this section, however, our aim is to follow through the categories of mental disorder as currently conceptualized in mainstream psychology and psychiatry.

Disorders of mood

Mood is the prevailing feeling state. In psychiatry, disorders of mood include extreme, or otherwise maladaptive, states of (1) anxiety, and (2) affect (sadness/happiness).

Mood (1): anxiety

EXERCISE 4	(10 minutes)

Think of a situation in which you have been frightened, worried, or just concerned. What did you feel? How did you react, i.e. what if anything did you do? And did you notice any bodily changes?

Anxiety as a symptom

Anxiety is of course a normal response to threat. *Anxiety as a symptom* is a disproportionate or otherwise maladaptive response. Thus, someone who feels anxious with no obvious cause, or who over-reacts to an object or situation, may have anxiety symptoms. But someone whose anxiety is an understandable

response to an imagined threat (e.g. with delusions of persecution), does not: here the anxiety, as such, is proportionate.

Anxiety has three components: subjective (feelings of fear or apprehension); behavioural (avoidance); and bodily (autonomic changes, i.e. changes mediated particularly by the autonomic nervous system, such as palpitation, sweating, shaking, choking and difficulty getting one's breath).

Anxiety as a symptom may be relatively persisting and generalized. This is sometimes called *free-floating anxiety*. Anxiety that is directed or focused, on the other hand, is called *phobic anxiety*.

A phobia is an unreasonable or unfounded fear of an object or situation usually leading to avoidance behaviour. Phobias are of three main kinds: (1) *specific* phobias, i.e. of specific objects or situations, such as fear of thunder or spiders; (2) *social phobias*, in which anxiety is experienced in social situations, such as speaking or eating in public; and (3) *agoraphobia*. Agoraphobic symptoms are diverse but are related mainly to two situations, leaving one's home or other familiar surroundings (sometimes called the 'housebound housewife syndrome'), and being in crowded places (see example below).

A third kind of anxiety symptom is a *panic attack*. Panic attacks are what their name implies, circumscribed (they may last up to a few hours) and usually very intense attacks of anxiety. They are associated with particularly marked autonomic symptoms. These make it especially important to distinguish panic attacks from bodily conditions, such as thyrotoxicosis (overactive thyroid) and some forms of cardiac arrhythmia (disturbance in the rhythm of the heartbeat).

Case 1: the experience of agoraphobic anxiety

Pam Mason describes her experience of agoraphobia as a young woman:

Before long I found the thought of going to Liverpool city centre, only seven miles away, a place I loved more than anywhere else in the world, too hard to imagine. And then Huyton village, a quarter of a mile away, became too far. School was about three hundred yards down the road—somehow I got there during the last few weeks. I got through all my exams, breaking down on the last day, but battling on, doing the papers, getting some good marks, incredibly.

And then I just collapsed. It was a struggle to get as far as the garden gate.

By now I realised I had a form of agoraphobia. I fought. I made myself go out of the house, brief and terrifying as such trips were. Although Mum was fighting her own problems at the time, she offered to go out with me. This meant I could get further from the house and the freedom was as precious to me as it would be to any prisoner travelling under escort. But instead of curing our problems, we had pooled them. I became acutely dependent on her. We acted out the roles of extremely protective mother and sick, frightened toddler. She had to be there all the time now, to hold me and save me when That Feeling came, as it often did, blasting away at my self and all my hope. How could I ever live a normal life when I had this in my head? I read Claire Weekes's books and Open Door newsletters, desperate for a solution, but only terrified myself with other people's symptoms.

Mason (1996, pp. 3–8)

Philosophical annotations

Anxiety is perhaps the commonest psychiatric problem (it is often diagnosed by general practitioners rather than by hospital specialists), and it has a well-understood physiological basis. Yet it has also been a topic of particular interest to philosophers. Anxiety thus provides a unique bridge between medicine and the humanities. The existentialists are the philosophers best known for their distinctive focus on anxiety ('Angst'). Soren Kierkegaard who has sometimes been described as the father of existentialism wrote extensively about anxiety in *The Concept of Anxiety* (1981) and also in *The Sickness Unto Death* (1983). Later Martin Heidegger used an examination of anxiety to reveal the fundamental aspects of our 'being-in-the-world'. According to Heidegger, we are anxious when our natural, fluid engagement with the world is disrupted; in this state the fact that we are not in our essence self-contained but dependent on an engagement with the public world is revealed to us (Heidegger, 1962, see especially part 1, chapter 40). Heidegger's philosophical ideas were then deployed in a psychiatric context by Ludwig Binswanger (1975) and Medard Boss (1963; 1983). Similarly, the existential analyst Irving Yalom (1981) urges that an unacknowledged anxiety about our own death is the source of much psychopathology. For a recent attempt to build bridges between medical and philosophical accounts of anxiety, see the Dutch philosopher and psychiatrist, Gerrit Glas (2003).

Mood (2): affect

The term 'affect' is used in psychiatry to refer to the sadness/happiness aspect of mood. As with anxiety, sadness and happiness are of course normal affects, being responses respectively to loss and to success; and, also similarly, they are pathological if disproportionate or otherwise maladaptive. Depression of mood is a more common symptom than mania and (the less severe) hypomania (pathological elation). Anxiety and depression commonly occur together.

EXERCISE 5   (20 minutes)

Think of a situation in which you have had a disappointment or loss. This might be a major 'life event', such as bereavement, or a more minor loss. How did you react? How did you feel? Were your feelings limited to the loss or disappointment in question or were they generalized to other aspects of your life? As with anxiety (exercise 4 above), think also about what you did, if anything, and any bodily change you noticed.

Then repeat all this for a situation in which you had a particular success.

Depression and elation as symptoms

Depression as a symptom varies in intensity. When it is relatively mild it is like ordinary sadness, except that it is inappropriate to the patient's circumstances. More serious states of depression on the other hand ('major depression'—see below, Session 3) may differ qualitatively from normal. Often the seriously depressed patient does not complain of depressed mood as such, though he or she usually appears extremely sad, unsmiling, and inert. Depression of this kind is associated with motor and psychological slowing (*psychomotor retardation*), though sometimes with the opposite, *agitation*. There may be associated biological symptoms (fixed diurnal variation of mood, together with loss of appetite and weight, and early morning waking) and delusions (see below).

Sometimes depression is masked, i.e. the patient presents with bodily symptoms (such as unexplained pain, tiredness or weight loss) rather than with a complaint of lowered mood.

Hypomania is the counterpart of major rather than of minor depression in that the patient generally does not complain of

Case 2: The experience of depression

The comedian, Spike Milligan describes his depression in an interview with the Irish psychiatrist and broadcaster, Anthony Clare,

Clare: Could you try to describe how you feel when you are depressed? [Just answering this question was a struggle. This man, normally fast and furious with words, had to make a Herculean effort just to make conversation. Responding to questions about how he felt took an almost physical struggle.]
Milligan: There is this terrible emptiness. I just want it to go away, disappear, cover myself up until it goes away. It is like pain yet it is not a physical pain. I cannot describe it. It is like every fibre in your body is screaming for relief yet there is no relief. How can I describe it? I cannot really. I cannot, of course, escape because I have to keep working, which I just about do—though once or twice I have had to stop, had to just hide away and wait till I could summon up the energy just to keep going.

Later in the interview, Clare asks,
Clare: 'But do you retreat? Do you close the door behind you?
Milligan: Yes. The whole world is taken away and all there is, is this black void, this terrible, terrible, empty, aching, black void and the only thing that helps is the psychiatrist coming in with the right tablet. But of course there isn't really a right tablet. It is a little like jacking a car. The psychiatrist can jack up the car but he can't change the tyre. You have to wait. You need tremendous patience. You need the patience. You need the patience of Job.

Milligan and Clare (1993, pp. 16 and 18)

Among other powerful first-hand accounts of depression, see Styron (1991) and Wolpert (1999).

their altered mood state as such (see below, Insight). There is euphoria, self-confidence, pressure of speech and 'flight of ideas' (see below), excessive energy, lack of sleep, heightened sexuality, an infectious jollity (which often gives way to impatience and irritability), an expansive and grandiose manner, and, as the condition worsens, hallucinations and delusions.

Many of the features of both depression and hypomania (full-blown mania is rarely seen, nowadays) can be understood as exaggerations of our normal responses, respectively to loss and to success. These responses include the prevailing moods, of course, sad or happy; but also the tendency of our mood to generalize (we speak of seeing everything through rose-tinted spectacles when happy, for example, and, correspondingly, dark glasses when sad!); the emergence of associated behaviours (withdrawal when sad, engagement when happy); and marked bodily changes (inertia, tiredness, and loss of energy when sad; activity, alertness, and lots of energy when happy).

Case 3: The experience of hypomania

Kay Jamison, a professor of psychiatry at the Johns Hopkins University School of Medicine, includes a number of first-hand accounts of hypomanic symptoms in her study of the relationship between creativity and hypomania. From among poets, her examples include,

1) Euphoric Mood (p. 28). Theodore Roethke . . .
'For no reason I started to feel very good. Suddenly I knew how to enter into the life of everything around me. I knew how it felt to be a tree, a blade of grass, even a rabbit. I didn't sleep much. I just walked around with this wonderful feeling.'
2) Grandiosity (p. 29). Robert Lowell . . .
'The night before I was locked up I ran about the streets of Bloomington Indiana crying out against devils and homosexuals. I believed I could stop cars and paralyze their forces by merely standing in the middle of the high-way with my arms outspread . . . I suspected I was a reincarnation of the Holy Ghost, . . .
3) Pressure of speech and subjective ideomotor pressure (p. 29). John Ruskin . . .
'I roll on like a ball, with this exception, that contrary to the usual laws of motion I have no friction to contend with in my mind, and of course have some difficulty in stopping myself when there is nothing else to stop me . . . I am almost sick and giddy with the quantity of things in my head—trains of thought beginning and branching to infinity, crossing each other, and all tempting and wanting to be worked out'.
Jamison (1996a)

Mixed affective states are sometimes seen, in which features of both depressed and elated mood coexist. These are different again from states of *diminished affect* in which the person's actual *capacity* to feel happy or sad is reduced: examples of this include flattened affect in schizophrenia and 'belle indifference' in hysteria.

Philosophical annotations

Extremes of mood have been associated traditionally with creativity particularly in the arts: both melancholy and euphoria have provided inspiration for poetry, for example (as Jamison's, 1996a book, above, richly illustrates). Quantitative differences between (normal) sadness and (pathological) depression have been a focus of recent work in phenomenology (see, e.g. the German psychiatrist and phenomenologist, Alfred Kraus, 2003). Changes in mood provide particularly sharp tests of 'models' of mental disorder: see, e.g. on depression, the American philosopher, Jennifer Radden's (2003), *Is this Dame Melancholy*, and, another American philosopher, Loretta Kopelman's (1994a) study of 'normal grief'; also Eigen, 2001, on ecstasy. On hypomania, see, Moore *et al.* (1994), for the relationship between pathological elevation of mood and Aristotelian eudaimonia; also the British psychologist, Richard Bentall's (1992) brilliant spoof on the traditional medical model of mental disorder; and replies in the *British Journal of Psychiatry* by Harris (1993), Birley (1993) and Fulford (1993).

Mood is generally thought to be somehow quite distinct from intellectual understanding. But Heidegger, in particular, urged that we should not think of mood as something extrinsic to our reality contact—as something which merely subjectively colours our experience. Rather we are always in some or other mood, and it is in and through these moods that things in the world 'show up' for us in the first place. (See Dreyfus, 1991, chapter 10.)

Disorders of thought

Disturbances of thinking are usually divided into disorders of: (1) stream; (2) connection; (3) possession; and (4) content.

Thought (1): stream

Disorders of the stream of thought

The stream of thought—how fast one thought follows another—may be slowed (as with psychomotor retardation in depression) or accelerated. Acceleration of the stream of thought occurs typically in hypomania and may take the form of pressure of thought (thoughts rushing on one after another) and/or flight of ideas (rapid changes of topic that are none the less still connected up, e.g. through meaning, rhyme, pun, or metaphor).

Case 4: The experience of flight of ideas

The British psychiatrist and psychopathologist, Andrew Sims, gives a short sample of the speech of a woman, aged 45, with hypomanic symptoms: 'They thought I was in the pantry at home . . . Peekaboo . . . there's a magic box. Poor darling Catherine, you know, Catherine the Great, the fire grate, I'm always up the chimney. I want to scream with joy . . . Hallelujah!' Sims (1988, p. 108)

Like the third extract from Kay Jamison's book (above, case example 3), this patient shows pressure of speech. Flight of ideas is shown by her rapid, though still connected, changes of topic.

Sims, 1988, gives a particularly clear and well-illustrated account of the many different ways in which the form of thought may be disturbed. Besides acceleration and retardation, these include: circumstantiality, derailment, fusion, and other disturbances to the flow of thought, thought block (see below), crowding, perseveration, overinclusive and 'concrete' thinking.

Thought (2): connection
Disorders of the connections between thoughts

A variety of *disorders of the connections between thoughts* are seen particularly in people with schizophrenia (though also sometimes in other psychotic disorders, see below, this section, also later in relation to Insight, and Session 3).

Thought block is a simple stopping of the line of thought. It can be a normal phenomenon in states of anxiety, fatigue, and stress. As a psychiatric symptom, it often occurs in an extreme form in schizophrenia when it may be associated with other symptoms of *schizophrenic thought disorder*: e.g. *knight's move* in thought, a shift from one topic to another without any logical connection. A more general *loosening of the associations* between thoughts occurring in schizophrenia is called *asyndetic thinking*. This may be combined with *interpenetration of themes* (two or more topics woven more or less haphazardly into the patient's speech) and with *overinclusiveness* (a tendency to excessive generalization beyond the normal boundaries of a given topic).

In addition to these aspects of thought disorder, people with schizophrenia sometimes produce *neologisms* (invented new words) and *metonyms* (approximately correct, idiosyncratic uses of real words and phrases). The net effect of schizophrenic thought disorder is to leave the listener baffled. In extreme form, the patient's speech may become wholly unintelligible (called *word salad* or *verbigeration*).

Case 5: the experience of thought block

The psychiatrists Julian Leff and Anthony Isaacs, describe a clinical interview with a patient experiencing thought block.

Interviewer: Do you ever find that your thoughts stop dead and leave your mind a complete blank?
Patient: This happens sometimes, yes.
I: What is it like?
P: It's not very good. You're just drifting around like a leaf.
I: Is it just that your thoughts drift off what you were thinking about or do they actually disappear?
P: Your mind just goes more or less blank. You just sort of tick over.
I: Is it as though your thoughts have been taken away or is it just that they've stopped?
P: No, not taken away. It's just as though they've stopped for a little while.

Comment: This patient describes thought block but not thought withdrawal (see below).　Leff and Isaacs (1990)

(Leff and Isaacs' slim volume is full of clear descriptions and vivid clinical examples of all the main areas of descriptive psychopathology.)

Neologisms and metonyms also occur in hypomania. Combined with flight of ideas, this may give a picture not unlike thought disorder in schizophrenia. Note, however, that flight of ideas differs from thought disorder in schizophrenia in that there is always a residual connection of meaning between the thoughts expressed (as described above).

Phenomena similar to those seen in schizophrenic thought disorder may occur in organic states, though usually associated with disturbance of cognitive function (e.g. clouding of consciousness, memory impairment, etc.—see below). In addition, organically impaired patients may show other disturbances of the connections between thoughts such as *concrete thinking*, namely an acquired inability to think in abstract terms (demonstrated for example by overliteral proverb interpretation), and *perseveration*—an inability to switch topics, manifesting as a senseless repetition of the last part of what is said...is said...is said; i.e. like a gramophone getting stuck. Perseveration may be shown in behaviour as well as in speech. Perseveration is a sign particularly of damage to both sides of the frontal lobes of the brain (behind the forehead).

Associationism was the school of psychology/philosophy of mind that stressed the importance of the connections between thoughts. Eugen Bleuler's ([1911]1950) notion of 'schizophrenia' or 'split mind' was developed and set out in associationist terms, the various symptoms being traced back to disorders of association. Thus, formal thought disorder, directly reflecting Bleuler's associationist sympathies, was for him the most basic symptom. (He also talked about dissociation of complexes as well as splitting of the associations, putting himself in both a prototypical psychoanalytic as well as an associationist camp.) The idea that the mind is constructed out of chains of associations, which in a sense was the first mechanistic psychology, was an important influence on European and American psychology/philosophy of mind throughout the nineteenth century.

Thought (3): possession
Disorders of the possession of thought

Disorders of possession of experience are of two very different kinds: (1) obsessive-compulsive, and (2) psychotic; the latter are divided into (a) thought insertion, withdrawal, and broadcasting, and (b) other passivity phenomena.

Obsessive-compulsive symptoms. An obsessional thought is stereotyped in form and comes back repeatedly into the patient's mind. The patient regards the thought as irrational and unpleasant and usually tries to resist it but is largely unable to do so. In this respect it is like a very bad case of getting a tune stuck in your head. More generally, an obsession is any mental content with these features; e.g. ruminations, doubts, images, impulses, series of numbers, repeated words and phrases, and so on. Compulsive acts are the behavioural counterparts of obsessions. Common examples include compulsive hand-washing, tidying, touching, and cleaning.

Case 6: the experience of obsessive-compulsive symptoms

In an article in the *New Scientist*, Zulfikar Abbany describes his own (ultimately successful) attempt to overcome his obsessions and compulsive behaviour related to fear of contamination. In this extract, he describes the effect of builders coming into his flat to carry out essential repairs. On top of the general problems of dust and dirt, one builder had cut himself.

No matter how I scrubbed the pot, it was impossible to convince myself that there was no risk of HIV or hepatitis.

Empty bottles of bleach and disinfectant littered the tiny floor space. The walls of my flat began to cramp my already diminished style. All notions of autonomy, rationality and calm were being squeezed out of me as the walls closed in. Maybe I should try harder. Maybe if I wiped a little more vigorously, fears about disease and intrusion would all go away. It would be like starting again.

That was the theory. In practice, the more I cleaned, the more I felt I had to. If I had used one bottle of bleach on Monday, I would use two—returning to the same spot—on Tuesday. My demand for the stuff was escalating and so was my need for new shops. The local sales assistants, I felt, already viewed me with suspicion.

At the end of June, the builders finally finished. I had made it to the other side, but I was left with a heightened sense of insecurity. Order, and therefore equilibrium, had been restored, but what would it take to throw the fragile status quo off balance again? By now, I had closed down altogether to visitors, and the rigorous 'de-polluting' rituals of handwashing and scrubbing when I came home were horribly time-consuming. I soon tired of going out at all.

I had been avoiding a confrontation with my obsessions and compulsions for a decade. But this time I feared the situation was terminal. I gained strength through that fear—this was the last time it was going to overwhelm me. I set out to find a therapist.   Abbany (2001, pp. 46–49)

Other common themes for obsessive-compulsive symptoms are violence, orderliness, religion and sexuality.

Psychotic disorders of possession of experience: (a) thought insertion, withdrawal, and broadcasting. Obsessional thoughts differ only quantitatively from normal experiences: as just noted, they are similar to a severe case of the experience of getting a tune stuck in one's mind. Obsessional thoughts are 'out of control' (Abbany, 2001, writes of having to 'confront' them) but they remain otherwise one's own thoughts. People with very violent or sexual obsessional thoughts, often describe these as not being their own. However, they mean by this only that they are completely out of character, rather than they are someone else's thoughts.

Thought insertion, withdrawal and broadcasting on the other hand, differ qualitatively from normal. With *thought insertion*, remarkably, the patient actually experiences the thoughts in their head, although thoughts that they are thinking (and in this sense first-personal thoughts), as those of *some other person or agency*, as thoughts *put there by somebody else*. (See also Chapter 29. This symptom, understandably, has been the subject of considerable philosophical interest.) *Thought withdrawal* is the experience of one's thoughts being taken out of one's head. *Thought broadcasting* is an extension of thought withdrawal, in which the patient experiences their thoughts travelling out of their head and being available for other people to inspect.

Case 7: the experiences of thought insertion, withdrawal, and broadcasting

The Canadian psychiatrist, C.S. Mellor, gave a series of case vignette examples of symptoms common in schizophrenia (and other psychotic conditions). His examples include disturbances in the possession of thought. We can pair these (Mellor, 1970) with the definitions in the glossary (Wing *et al.*, 1974) to one of the first standardized instruments for assessing the mental state, the Present State Examination (PSE). Developed by a group at the Institute of Psychiatry, London University, headed by the social psychiatrist, John Wing, the PSE provides an interview schedule and clear definitions allowing reliable identification of all the major symptoms of mental distress and disorder. Thus,

7.1 Thought Insertion. PSE definition (Symptom 55, pp. 160–161) includes... 'The essence of the symptom is that the subject experiences thoughts *which are not his own* intruding into his mind' (emphasis in original).

Example (C.S. Mellor, p. 17, example 6): A 29-year-old housewife said 'I look out of the window and I think the garden looks nice and the grass looks cool, but the thoughts of Eamonn Andrews come into my mind. There are no other thoughts there, only his... He treats my mind like a screen and flashes his thoughts on to it like you flash a picture.'

7.2 Thought Withdrawal. The PSE (Symptom 58, pp. 162–163) treats thought withdrawal as an explanatory delusion for thought block'... The subject says that his thoughts have been removed from his head so that he has no thoughts.' C.S. Mellor (p. 16) describes thought withdrawal as the 'experience (of the patient's thoughts) being withdrawn by some external force'.

Example (C.S. Mellor, pp. 16–17, example 5): A 22-year-old woman said 'I am thinking about my mother, and suddenly my thoughts are sucked out of my mind by a phrenological vacuum extractor, and there is nothing in my mind, it is empty...'

7.3 Thought Broadcasting. PSE definition (Symptom 56, pp. 161–162) includes '...the subject experiences his thoughts actually being shared with others, often with large numbers of people...'.

Example (C.S. Mellor, p. 17, example 7): A 21-year-old student said: 'As I think, my thoughts leave my head on a type of mental ticker-tape. Everyone around has only to pass the tape through their mind and they know my thoughts.'

Psychotic disorders of possession of experience: (b) passivity phenomena. Although often described as 'delusions of control', passivity phenomena are closely related to phenomena like thought insertion, in consisting of experiences of the will being taken over by some other agency: movements, volitions, even feelings are experienced as being out of one's own control and taken over by someone or something else. These are sometimes called 'made phenomena', e.g. made acts, made volitions, made affect.

Case 8: experiences of passivity

C.S. Mellor's brief descriptions and case vignettes illustrate the remarkable range of passivity phenomena (reference above).

8.1 Somatic passivity (p. 16)

The patient is a passive and invariably a reluctant recipient of bodily sensations imposed upon him by some external agency. According to Jaspers the perception is simultaneously experienced as being both a bodily change and externally controlled. It is a single experience and not simply the delusional interpretation of an abnormal bodily sensation.

Example: A 38-year-old man had jumped from a bedroom window, injuring his right knee which was very painful. He described his physical experience as, 'The sun-rays are directed by U.S. army satellite in an intense beam which I can feel entering the centre of my knee and then radiating outwards causing the pain.'

8.2 'Made' feelings (p. 17)

The patient experiences feelings which do not seem to be his own. The feelings are attributed to some external source and are imposed upon him.

Example: A 23-year-old female patient reported, 'I cry, tears roll down my cheeks and I look unhappy, but inside I have a cold anger because they are using me in this way, and it is not me who is unhappy, but they are projecting unhappiness onto my brain. They project upon me laughter, for no reason, and you have no idea how terrible it is to laugh and look happy and know it is not you, but their emotions.'

8.3 'Made' impulses or drives (p. 17)

The impulse to carry out an action is not felt to be one's own, but the actual performance of the act is.

Example: A 26-year-old engineer emptied the contents of a urine bottle over the ward dinner trolley. He said, 'The sudden impulse came over me that I must do it. It was not my feeling, it came into me from the X-ray department, that was why I was sent there for implants yesterday. It was nothing to do with me, they wanted it done. So I picked up the bottle and poured it in. It seemed all I could do.'

8.4 'Made' Volitional Acts (p. 17–18)

The patient experiences his actions as being completely under the control of an external influence.

Example: A 29-year-old shorthand typist described her actions as follows: 'When I reach my hand for the comb it is my hand and arm which move, and my fingers pick up the pen, but I don't control them... I sit there watching them move, and they are quite independent, what they do is nothing to do with me... I am just a puppet who is manipulated by cosmic strings. When the strings are pulled my body moves and I cannot prevent it.'

Philosophical annotations (see also Chapter 29)

The topic of the ownership of thought has been of interest to philosophers at least since Kant, who claimed that an 'I think' accompanies each and every one of my representations, which is to say that I must be able to be aware of all of my representations as being mine in order for me to have experience. The topic of 'immunity to error through misidentification' of the subject, has been taken up in the twentieth century by analytical philosophers such as Shoemaker (1968). Their significance for psychopathology has been examined (among others) by Campbell (1999) and Gallagher (2000, 2003).

The diagnostic significance of these phenomena has long been controversial. Schneider (1959), for example, stressed the pathognomic character of disorders of thought ownership and passivity experiences (made actions etc.) in the diagnosis of schizophrenia. This is reflected in DSM-IV-TR. However, for Schneider the passivity experiences were not criterial for, but merely pathognomic of (highly indicative of, mainly likely to occur in the context of), schizophrenia (See Bentall, 2003, pp. 31–35.) These and other traditional hallmark symptoms of schizophrenia are now known to occur in any of the psychotic disorders.

Thought (4): content

Delusions are the central symptom of psychotic disorders (see below). Psychotic disorders, in turn, as we noted in Chapter 2, and illustrated in the philosophical map of psychiatry (Figure 2.), are a conceptually central kind of mental disorder—it was for just this reason, that Thomas Szasz (1974), the author of 'The Myth of Mental Illness', called schizophrenia, in another book (Szasz, 1976), the 'Sacred Symbol of Psychiatry'.

Yet despite their importance, the proper place of delusions in descriptive psychopathology, remains highly contentious. They are generally included as the most important of the disorders of the content of thought, and then described as abnormal beliefs, of one kind or another. As such, they are closely related to other abnormalities of the content of thinking, e.g. *morbid fears* in anxiety and obsessional states, such as a fear of collapsing or of 'losing control' in public; also, *overvalued ideas*—beliefs of a highly idiosyncratic nature with which the patient is much preoccupied. Overvalued ideas are like delusions in being firmly held (see below); but they are understandable given the patient's particular circumstances and background.

Partial delusions are like delusions except that they are not held with complete conviction. They are ideas with which the patient is much preoccupied while yet not quite believing that they are true.

Delusional mood is a state of perplexity in which the patient senses that something important is going to happen but they are not sure what. With delusional mood, the patient often experiences brief delusion-like ideas that fluctuate in content over short periods of time.

Delusions take various forms (see below) but are usually defined as (1) false beliefs, which (2) are not susceptible to the ordinary processes of reasoning and appeal to evidence, and which (3) are culturally atypical, i.e. out of step with the beliefs conventionally held among people of the same cultural and ethnic background as the person concerned. To be a delusion, a belief must be held with complete conviction (see e.g. the definition in Harré and Lamb, 1987).

The difficulties with clauses (2) and (3) of this standard definition have been widely recognized (see Spitzer, 1990; and for a review of failures of empirical research to demonstrate disturbances of cognitive functioning that are characteristic of delusion, Garety and Freeman, 1999, pp. 113–154 for a valuable review). More radically, as the below examples illustrate, delusions, contrary to clause (1), may be neither false beliefs, nor, even, beliefs at all (at any rate as to matters of fact), but value judgements. With delusion, then, we have, in the terms than we will be adopting in Chapter 4, an excellent example of the use of the concept being far richer and more subtle than received definitions.

Case 9: the varieties of delusional experience

Any theory of the meaning of delusion must explain the wide variety of different logical forms that delusions may take in practice. Examples include,

False Factual Belief
Example: Mr P.D. Age 48. Bank manager [Diagnosis—major depression with hypochondriacal delusions of cancer]

Attended psychiatric clinic with biological symptoms of depression and the delusion that he had HIV infection (repeated tests normal). History of attempted suicide. Refused to believe that he was suffering from depression.
True Factual Belief
Example: Mr O.S. Age 45. Publican [Diagnosis—Othello syndrome or delusions of infidelity]

Attended general practitioner's surgery with his wife who was suffering from depression. On questioning, delivered an angry diatribe about his wife being 'a tart.' Unable to talk about anything else. Offered unlikely evidence (e.g. pattern of cars parked in road). Psychiatric referral confirmed diagnosis even though the doctors concerned knew that Mrs. O. was depressed following the break up of an affair.
Paradoxical
Example: Mr. M.I. Age 40. [Diagnosis—Delusional Disorder with hypochondriacal delusion of mental illness]

Brought to casualty after an overdose. Had tried to kill himself because he believed he was mentally ill. Diagnosis of monosymptomatic hypochondriacal delusional psychosis.
Delusional Value Judgement (Negative)
Example: Mr. E.D. Age 40. Postman [Diagnosis—major depression with delusions of guilt]

Emergency admission with depressed affect, early morning waking and weight loss. Had forgotten to give his children their pocket money, but believed this to be the 'worst sin in the world,' himself 'worthless as a father,' and so on.

NOTE: 1) delusions of guilt may also be factual in form, e.g. the person believes he has caused the HIV epidemic and feels (appropriately) guilty; 2) evaluative delusion with positive rather than negative content are common in hypomania, (see Fulford, 1989, chapter 10).

These examples, which are all based on real cases with biographical details changed, are all described in Fulford (1989, chapter 10). See also, for further examples, Fulford (1991).

Delusions are conventionally divided up, not according to their logical form, but mainly according to their subject matter, i.e. what they are about. The most important kinds are: paranoid, reflecting a distorted relationship between the patient and the world about them, e.g. persecutory, self-referential, and grandiose delusions; hypochondriacal; nihilistic, e.g. that the person has lost all their money; that their body is rotting away, or even that they are actually dead (Cotard syndrome); delusions of guilt; and delusions of impoverishment.

Delusions are also divided up according to their apparent relationship to other pathology. Most delusions are *secondary*, that is they are secondary to some other morbid phenomenon, e.g. delusions of guilt or of impoverishment in depression. Some delusions are *primary*, however, springing into the patient's mind with minimal or no understandable relationship to other aspects of their mental state. A *delusional perception* is a primary delusion sparked by some quite normal percept. Primary delusions are nearly always symptoms of schizophrenia or of some related psychotic condition (but see Chapter 20, which includes an example of a non-pathological delusional perception).

Philosophical annotations

The question of how to define delusion has proved a struggle for philosophers at least since Jaspers (1913, *General Psychopathology*, see especially, Vol. 1 pp. 93–108, 195–198, 409–413). Jaspers (as we describe in Part II) offered a preliminary characterization (which in a related guise is still in general use today) of delusion as false judgement, held with extraordinary conviction, impervious to other experiences and compelling counter-arguments, and with an impossible content—but then went on to urge (p. 93) that this definition 'gives only a superficial and incorrect answer to the problem' of the meaning of delusion. In short, the definition does not explain to us what the distinctive ('internal') irrationality of delusion consists in, but merely documents some standard ('external') features that many (but not all) delusions happen to have. The tendency of definitions of delusion to simply presuppose rather than actually provide an understanding of the distinctive irrationality of delusion has been made clear by Schmidt (1987). Early (modern) discussions of delusion in the philosophical literature include Quinton (1985), Flew (1973), and Glover (1970). Fulford, 1989, chapter 10, and 1996, develops a model of delusion in terms of practical reasoning. The failings of the standard definitions are noted, and an attempt at a more adequate understanding of the character of delusion is attempted, in Gipps and Fulford (2004).

Disorders of perception

A variety of abnormalities of perception may be significant diagnostically but the most important in psychiatry are hallucinations.

Hallucinations in general are perceptions occurring in the absence of a stimulus. These may be normal: for example, hearing a voice calling as you fall asleep (hypnagogic hallucination) or on waking up (hypnopompic hallucination); or the experience during grief of glimpsing the deceased loved one. *True, or psychotic hallucinations*, on the other hand, are hallucinations that the person concerned takes to be real, e.g. a patient hearing voices shouting obscenities at him. *Pseudohallucinations* are similar to true hallucinations except that they lack the full qualities of true perceptions; for example, an auditory hallucination heard in one's head rather than in outside space; or voices coming from the outside world but which the patient regards as possibly not being real.

Hallucinations can affect any sensory modality and come in many forms. Besides *auditory*, as in the above case, they may be *visual, olfactory* (smell), *gustatory* (taste), *tactile* (touch), or *somatic* (bodily or visceral sensations). Then again, they may be well or ill defined in content—*simple* or *complex* hallucinations,

respectively. Voices speaking clearly would be complex hallucinations; simple auditory hallucinations include mutterings, scrapings, slitherings. Similarly, complex visual hallucinations include well-formed images of people, animals, etc., while simple visual hallucinations may take the form of geometric shapes, or brief flashes, or patches of colour.

Illusions differ from hallucinations in being deceptions of the senses, e.g. a stick that looks bent when it is partly immersed in water. Unless very frequent or bizarre, illusions are not generally of pathological significance. Certain distortions of perception may be pathological, however, e.g. micropsia (things looking too small) and hyperacusis (things sounding too loud).

Déjà vu and *jamais vu* experiences, i.e. things seeming excessively familiar or excessively unfamiliar respectively: these are both sometimes significant medically, e.g. in temporal lobe epilepsy. *Derealization* is the experience of things appearing unreal, like a stage set, or as though made of cardboard. *Depersonalization* is a similar experience of one's self or one's body feeling unreal. These are often anxiety-related symptoms but may occur in other psychiatric conditions. *Disturbances of body image*, for example in *anorexia* (in which the patient may perceive her body as being fatter than it is), and *body dysmorphophobia* (in which some part of the body is misperceived as ugly).

There are also a remarkable variety of disturbances of the perception of the body related to neurological lesions (for example, visual neglect, in which a person can see their arm, say, but fails to recognize it as their own).

Philosophical annotations

A standard 'empiricist' or 'non-disjunctivist' line has supposed that perception is to be understood as the having of inner 'sense impressions' or 'representations', which are caused in the right way by the outer objects of which they are impressions or representations. On this view hallucination is to be understood as the occurrence of inner impressions in the absence of the appropriate outer stimuli. Other 'disjunctivist' philosophers of perception, however, have urged that there is no need to think that there is anything 'inner' in common between cases of veridical perception and hallucination. Thus experience is a disjunction of either perceptually taking in a fact or it is a mere appearance (see, e.g. Hyman, 1992, pp. 277–296). Now, however, the challenge is to offer an account of hallucination that does not leave out its sensory element (i.e. doesn't construe it simply in terms of belief—as in an 'intellectualist' account.). An attempt to understand hallucination, not in terms of aberrant inner experiences, but in terms of alterations in the structure of the modalities of experience, can be found in Straus (1958). The failures of 'empiricist' and 'intellectualist' accounts of hallucination, and an alternative (which views hallucination as 'much less the presentation of an illusory object than the spread and, so to speak, running wild of a visual power which has lost any sensory counterpart') can be found in Merleau-Ponty (1996, pp. 334–345).

Disorders of cognitive functioning

Disturbances of cognitive functioning (as the term is used in psychiatry) include: (1) *disorientation* (for time, place, and person); (2) *defects of attention* and *concentration*; (3) impaired *memory* (recent and remote); and (4) *reduced general intelligence* or IQ (for both verbal and non-verbal tasks).

A mild global impairment of cognitive functions is called *clouding of consciousness*. This is the first slip away from full consciousness towards coma. *Delirium* is clouding of consciousness with a high output of verbal and non-verbal behaviour. *Stupor* is a state of consciousness in which the patient is inert and mute but appears none the less to be conscious of his or her surroundings (this may occur, for example, with severe psychomotor retardation in depression, or with lesions in the brain stem).

Dementia as a descriptive term means an acquired impairment of cognitive functioning of a long-term nature, which is usually progressive, and often starts with marked impairment of short-term memory. The term is also used of a group of specific diseases defined partly by particular psychopathological features and partly by particular pathological changes in the brain (see also session 3).

Insight

Insight is not a symptom as such. It is the degree of understanding that a patient has of their symptoms. Understanding is a complex matter involving, among other things, awareness that there is something wrong, and recognition of the nature of what is wrong as illness.

Insight in the former sense may be lacking with any symptom, psychological or bodily. However, insight in the second sense is typically lacking in respect of certain particular psychological symptoms, specifically with delusions, hallucinations and certain kinds of thought disorder (marked with ** in Table 3.2, or with * indicating partial insight). Symptoms of this kind are called psychotic.

The difference between non-psychotic and psychotic symptoms is well illustrated by the difference between obsessions and delusions. As described above, with an obsessional symptom, the patient, although sometimes equivocal about the need for their obsessive-compulsive rituals, ultimately regards them as something wrong with them, and hence as needing therapy. Thus Zulfikar Abbany (2001), in case 6 (p. 41), sought a therapist for his obsessions about contamination and related compulsive behaviours. With a delusion of contamination, however, the patient does not experience their belief that they are contaminated as something (medically) wrong with them. The problem, as they see it, is, simply, that they are contaminated. Similarly with guilt: obsessional guilty thoughts are 'something wrong', for which the person concerned may seek help; but with delusions of guilt, what is wrong, for the person concerned, is that they have done something wrong, and they behave accordingly—going to the police, or, more tragically, committing suicide in remorse and expatiation.

With psychotic symptoms, then, the patient is well aware that something is wrong, but fails to recognize that what is wrong is

that he or she is mentally ill. Conditions in which symptoms of this kind typically occur are called psychotic conditions (see below, session 3, this chapter). Assessment of insight is important diagnostically (Session 3), and to medico-legal issues involving compulsory treatment and legal competence (see Chapter 17).

Philosophical annotations

A useful starting point for current psychiatric thinking on insight is David (1990). See also the various chapters in Amador and David (1998) and Fulford (1992), and the journal article by Lewis (1934).

The philosophical challenge (as with delusion) is to produce a definition of insight that is neither (1) circular, nor (2) narrowly medical. Aubrey Lewis' (1934) account is essentially of the latter (narrowly medical) kind, i.e. he takes it that somebody is lacking in insight they do not see things the way *the psychiatrist does*. This seems to privilege the psychiatrist's understanding of events in an unwarranted way (see Bentall, 2003, pp. 496–497). As to the former (narrowly circular) kind of definition, it is worth noting that insight is a tensed phenomenon: what one recognizes is that one *has been* psychotic. David (1990) empirically, and Fulford (1989, chapter 10) conceptually, seek to establish models of insight that are consistent with the clinical psychopathology of psychotic symptoms.

Julian Hughes, Stephen Louw and Steven Sabat (2006) have brought together an important collection of articles on philosophical and ethical issues raised by dementia.

Bodily symptoms and signs

Among the bodily symptoms and signs of particular importance in psychiatry are the following.

Autonomic symptoms

A variety of autonomic symptoms are associated with anxiety, including palpitation, tremor, sweating, blurring of vision, loose stool, and urinary frequency. Sometimes these may be the presenting symptoms of an anxiety disorder. Certain specific symptoms are recognized, e.g. 'globus hystericus' (psychogenic difficulty swallowing).

Biological symptoms of depression

As noted earlier, with major depression there may be marked 'biological' symptoms such as reduced appetite and extreme weight loss. Depressed patients may sometimes complain of these or of other bodily symptoms (e.g. pain, as below) rather than of lowered mood. As noted above, this is called 'masked depression'.

Pain

Pain is an important presenting symptom in psychiatry as well as in bodily medicine. Besides hypochondriacal conditions, it is common in both anxiety disorders and depression. In anxiety disorders, chest pain, colicky abdominal pain, and headache are common. Headache and facial pains are also common in depression (see, for example, Mr AB's case history, in Chapter 2; and Sullivan, 1995).

Dissociative symptoms

Dissociative symptoms are symptoms usually either of the primary sense and voluntary motor systems or of memory, which turn out to be due to psychological rather than to bodily pathology: examples include paralysis, blindness, and memory loss. Symptoms of this kind are traditionally called *hysterical conversion symptoms*. The term 'dissociative' is sometimes restricted to disorders of memory (memory loss and fugue states), the term 'conversion' then being used for the remainder. The theory reflected in the term 'hysterical conversion' is that an intolerable psychological conflict is 'converted' into a tolerable bodily symptom. The term 'dissociation' reflects the idea that one part of consciousness (such as a painful memory) is split off (or dissociated) from the rest. Both terms are (nowadays) used in mainstream psychiatry descriptively rather than with these aetiological implications.

Vegetative symptoms

Vegetative symptoms include disorders of *appetite*, of *sexual drive*, and of *sleep*. Specific disturbances of appetite include the reduction and loss of appetite of *anorexia* (a persistent active refusal to eat) and *bulimia* (binge eating). The sexual symptoms included under this heading are those involving drive and performance; drive may be reduced (*impotence* in men, *frigidity* in women); difficulties of performance are called 'orgasmic' difficulties, e.g. *premature* and *delayed ejaculation* in men, *vaginismus* in women. Disorders of sleep include insomnia, hypersomnia (excessive sleeping), disorders of *sleep rhythm*, and a variety of specific disorders such as *sleepwalking* and *night terrors* (attacks in which the patient wakes screaming and apparently terrified but with little or no recall the next morning).

Psychological signs

Signs of disorder are as important in psychiatry as they are in bodily medicine. Specifically psychiatric signs are limited to disturbances in the patient's appearance, behaviour, and speech. These may be as important diagnostically as simply listening to what the person concerned says. Important examples include (1) expressed affect (e.g. in depression—unsmiling and immobile face, minimal eye contact, slumped and inert posture, monotonous speech, slowed movements), and (2) dress (e.g. flamboyant in hypomania, idiosyncratic in schizophrenia, neglected in dementia).

Reflection on the session and self-test questions

Write down your own reflections on the materials in this session drawing out any points that are particularly significant for you. Then write brief notes about the following:

1. What are the main groups of psychological symptoms generally recognized in psychiatry?

2. What is the most important (growing) resource for interdisciplinary work between philosophy and mental health in any of these areas of 'psychopathology'?

3. In what specific sense may 'insight' be lost in a person with a psychotic disorder.

4. Give one psychotic and one non-psychotic symptom where both have the same content, for example where the person concerned has a recurring worry that they have done something wrong. By what features would the two different symptoms (psychotic and non-psychotic) be distinguished?

5. Is psychiatry concerned at all with bodily signs and symptoms?

Session 3 Categories of mental disorder

As noted above, the two most widely used classifications of psychiatric disorders are the International Classification of Diseases (the 'ICD') published by the WHO, and the APA's *Diagnostic and Statistical Manual* (the 'DSM'). Both classifications have been developed in a series of editions over a number of years, the current versions being ICD-10 (WHO, 1992) and DSM-IV TR (for Text Revision) (APA, 2000).

The 'basic' classification

Although these classifications differ in detail, they include much the same broad categories of disorder. These are summarized in Table 3.3. An initial division is made between disorders in adults and disorders in children and adolescents. Both are then further subdivided into a variety of main kinds of mental disorder, defined mostly in terms of symptoms (as described above), personality disorders and stress-induced disorders.

Some classifications are organized in part around a number of 'axes'. Thus, the DSM has a multi-axial structure: Axis I covers clinical syndromes, Axis II personality disorders, and Axis III bodily disorders; Axis IV covers the severity of psychosocial stressors, and Axis V the level of adaptive functioning. We will be focusing here on the main categories of disorder (incorporated in Axes I and II in DSM).

Main categories of adult mental disorder

Six main categories of psychiatric disorder are generally recognized in adults.

Organic

Consistently with the predominantly descriptive basis of psychiatric classification, organic *disorders* are defined in terms of organic *symptoms*, i.e. certain specific symptoms that suggest the presence of underlying bodily pathology. (Although you will also find the term 'organic' used to mean that such pathology has actually been demonstrated.) Bodily pathology, in this context, means gross pathology of the kind with which general medicine

Table 3.3 Main categories of psychiatric disorder

Main categories of adult disorder	Organic	Acute (confusional states) Chronic (dementias—primary, secondary) Special syndromes (e.g. frontal lobe syndrome)
	Alcohol/drug related	Addiction states Complications of use/abuse Withdrawal syndromes
	Psychotic disorders other than organic and affective	Schizophrenia (simple, hebephrenic, paranoid, catatonic) Persistent delusional disorder Brief psychotic episode
	Affective disorders (happiness/sadness)	Depression—major ('psychotic'/'biological') Minor ('neurotic') Hypomania Bipolar Schizoaffective
	Anxiety and related disorders	Anxiety disorder (generalized, phobic, panic) Obsessive-compulsive Dissociative (hysteria) Somatoform (e.g. psychogenic pain, hypochondriasis)
	Disorders of vegetative function	Eating (anorexia nervosa, bulimia) Sexual function (orgasmic, drive) Sleeping (insomnia, hypersomnia, sleep terrors, etc.)
Other categories of adult disorder		Personality disorder: very long-term maladaptive personality traits Stress-induced disorders: psychiatric disorder as a reaction to extreme stress; 'psychological trauma'
Child/adolescent disorders		Learning difficulties (or mental retardation): mild, moderate, severe, profound Specific developmental delays: e.g. speech, reading, spelling, arithmetic
		'Pervasive disorders': autism; disintegrative psychosis; schizoid disorders of childhood
		Behavioural disorders: hyperkinetic syndrome; conduct disorder, socialized and unsocialized
		Disorders of physiological functions: e.g. enuresis, encopresis

is concerned, for example degenerative changes (as in dementia), brain tumours and other space-occupying lesions (such as a bleed into the brain), intoxications and infections.

The most important organic symptoms are disturbances in cognitive functioning, especially clouding of consciousness and impaired memory, as described above. However, there are other organic symptoms, for example organic hallucinations are, as it were, good quality hallucinations: they are formed (of people, etc.), often show size distortion (Lilliputian characters are typical), coloured (rather than black and white) and moving; and they are usually worse in the evenings (i.e. when it is getting dark). Organic delusions, by contrast, are poor quality delusions: reflecting the impaired cognitive functioning of organic states, organic delusions are minimally elaborated, not well sustained (they vary in content from one day to the next), and they lack the emotional charge of functional (i.e. non-organic) delusions.

There may also be warning signs of organic aetiological factors in the history, e.g. first onset of a depressive illness or anxiety state in later life in the absence of stressful life events (though the *presence* of stressful life events does not preclude organic factors: for example,

in one study of brain tumours presenting with functional symptoms, 40% of subjects reported a history of stressful events associated with the onset of their symptoms (Minsky, 1933).

The complex relationship between functional symptoms and bodily causes is one reason why, as described in Chapter 2, in psychiatry it is helpful to write a *diagnostic formulation* (setting out separately the descriptively defined differential diagnoses, the aetiology, treatment and prognosis for a given case) rather than relying on brief composite diagnostic labels. It is all too easy to assume that functional symptoms equal functional causes, and indeed vice versa! This complication is further compounded by the fact that organic disorders are generally non-specific, i.e. they point to bodily pathology of *some* kind (space-occupying, cardiovascular, infections, etc.) affecting the brain, but tell us very little about the nature or precise location of the pathology.

Organic disorders, on the other hand, *are* affected by the rate at which the pathology develops. Hence they are subdivided broadly into *acute* and *chronic*. An example of the former would be a 'toxic confusional state' in which there is clouding of consciousness with disorientation, especially for time, progressing to semi-coma and unconsciousness—getting drunk is a familiar example of this! Dementia is the most familiar example of a chronic organic disorder. Here the earliest change is usually a disturbance of memory, especially for recent events. But as with acute organic states, as the condition progresses impairment of all cognitive functions, usually with organic hallucinations and other organic symptoms, is the rule.

The term *secondary dementia* means a dementia caused by some other medical condition (e.g. myxoedema), with the implication that the condition can be arrested or reversed with treatment. Most dementias are primary. A number of specific syndromes are recognized. The most common is the eponymously named Alzheimer's disease (from which the Oxford philosopher, Iris Murdoch, suffered, as portrayed in the film 'Iris' based on the book by her husband, John Bayley, 1999) and cardiovascular dementia.

A limited number of specific organic syndromes are recognized, e.g. frontal lobe syndrome (a syndrome of disinhibition, due usually to damage to the frontal lobes of the brain—see the case history of 'Mrs Lazy' in Chapter 22, and various kinds of memory disorder such as Korsakoff's psychosis (short-term memory loss with confabulation, i.e. spontaneous filling in of lost memories with false memories: this is due to thiamine deficiency, usually secondary to long-term alcohol abuse).

Alcohol/drug-related disorders

This is the only group of psychiatric disorders in which the causal factors are sufficiently well defined to allow an aetiological rather than symptomatic basis for classification. Hence they are generally divided up partly according to the substance involved (alcohol, opioids, cocaine, hallucinogens, etc.), partly by clinical syndrome. The clinical syndromes are of three main kinds, *addiction states*, direct *complications of abuse* (e.g. Korsakoff's syndrome in alcoholism, as above), and *withdrawal syndromes* (most of which, in addition to craving, have features specific to each substance).

Psychotic disorders other than affective and organic

As we saw in Session 2, a psychotic disorder may be thought of as one in which hallucinations and/or delusions and/or certain types of thought disorder typically occur, these being the symptoms that are defined (in part) by the presence of specifically psychotic loss of insight.

In ICD-9 psychotic disorders were classed together as a separate category distinct from all non-psychotic disorders (sometimes called 'neurotic' disorders). In ICD-10 and in DSM-IV, they are included partly in the categories of organic and affective disorders, partly in a residual category for psychotic disorders of other kinds. These latter disorders include *schizophrenia* (defined by certain specific kinds of delusion, hallucination and thought disorder; and subdivided, according to the predominant symptomatology, into simple, hebephrenic, paranoid and catatonic forms—see Chapter 20 for the DSM summary box for the diagnosis of schizophrenia), *delusional disorders* (disorders in which delusions predominate, without specific symptoms of organic, schizophrenic or affective psychoses), and *brief psychotic episodes* (any psychotic disorder of acute onset, limited duration, and without serious sequelae).

The abandonment of a primary division between psychotic and non-psychotic mental disorders was motivated primarily by the difficulty of defining psychotic loss of insight, originally pointed out by Lewis (1934). Yet the concept of loss of insight continues to be widely used in psychiatry: it is important in medico-legal contexts, for example, as we will see in Chapter 17; the term psychosis, furthermore, continues to be used in both everyday medical discourse and in technical journals; and, most remarkably of all, it persists (albeit in an altered form) as a primary division in ICD and DSM, and this notwithstanding the intentions of the authors of these classifications.

Thus, in ICD-10 and DSM-IV the original primary distinction between psychotic and non-psychotic disorders has been replaced with a larger number of primary categories. But most of these new primary categories includes, explicitly or implicitly, a subdivision into psychotic and non-psychotic varieties. Hence, so far as the psychotic-non-psychotic division is concerned, our new classifications have retained the same essential structure as our traditional classifications, albeit turned 'upside down'. 'Insight', then, and 'psychotic', one of us has argued elsewhere (Fulford, 2004), should be understood as one of those high-level concepts (like 'time', see Chapter 4) that we have difficulty defining but which is none the less useful, even essential, for understanding and giving meaning to the world around us (psychotic loss of insight can in fact be partially defined in terms of the phenomenological features of our experience of illness—see Fulford, 1989, chapter 10).

Affective disorders

The most common affective disorders are depressive. Depressive disorders are subdivided into major and minor according partly to the depth of depression, and partly to the presence or absence of associated symptoms. Major depression is associated with biological symptoms as described earlier. It is in major depression also that psychotic symptoms (mainly delusions, sometimes hallucinations) occur. Major depression is for this reason sometimes called psychotic depression. Minor depression is often associated with anxiety symptoms. It is sometimes called neurotic depression. The terms reactive depression and endogenous depression are no longer used because the symptoms of depression have been shown to be the same whether or not there is an obvious external event to which the person concerned is 'reacting' (see e.g. the classic paper by Kiloh and Garside, 1963).

Hypomania (together with its more severe form mania) is the elevated mood counterpart of major depression. It is a psychotic disorder, commonly associated with hallucinations and delusions. There are often biological symptoms (e.g. reduced sleep, increased sexual appetite) and specific forms of thought disorder (e.g. pressure of speech and flight of ideas).

Bipolar affective disorder is a condition in which episodes of major depression and of hypomania alternate (the term is sometimes used of one or the other, e.g. 'bipolar disorder, depressed type'). In schizoaffective disorder schizophrenic and affective symptoms, either depressive or hypomanic, are combined.

Anxiety and related disorders

The disorders in this category are sometimes referred to as 'neurotic disorders'. These disorders cluster together; mixed forms are common; and different forms may occur at different times in the same patient. They are defined by their predominant symptomatology, as described above in session 2. The main categories are anxiety disorders (generalized, phobic, and panic), obsessive-compulsive disorders, dissociative (hysterical) states, and somatoform disorders. The latter includes conditions presenting with bodily symptoms that are not sufficiently explained by bodily pathology and in which there is also positive evidence of psychological disorder (notably other psychological symptoms).

Disorders of vegetative functions

These disorders are defined by the presence of specific vegetative symptoms as described above (session 2). The most important categories are disorders of eating (e.g. anorexia nervosa and bulimia), of sexual function (disorders of drive and of performance), and disorders of sleep (insomnia, hypersomnia, sleep terrors, etc.).

Personality disorder

Personality disorder can be thought of as a maladaptive exaggeration of a personality trait. Symptomatically, a personality disorder may appear very similar to one or other of the categories of mental disorder described above. However, where mental disorder represents a *change* from what is normal for the person concerned, a personality disorder is normally established by late adolescence and continues more or less *unchanged* into old age. Thus, in order to decide whether someone is suffering from a personality disorder or a mental disorder proper, you have to establish the longitudinal pattern of their symptoms. This is illustrated in for depressive personality disorder Box 3.1.

Stress-induced disorder

Stress-related disorders are analogous to physical trauma. Stress is of course an important aetiological factor for both bodily and psychological disorders. However, where a psychiatric condition is very clearly and manifestly a reaction to major stress, the diagnosis is of a stress-induced disorder, e.g. grief reaction, battle fatigue.

The symptoms of stress-induced disorders are very varied. Anxiety and depression are common, as are somatic complaints. But hallucinations, confusion, mania, and many other symptoms also occur.

Stress-induced disorders are generally divided into *acute* and *chronic*. The term 'post-traumatic stress disorder' (PTSD) has

been introduced fairly recently to cover people who experience ongoing distress associated with nightmares, flashbacks, anxiety, depression, and a variety of other symptoms, following major trauma.

Disorders of childhood and adolescence

Many of the disorders of childhood and adolescence are different from those occurring in adults, and they are conventionally classified separately. The main groups of disorder are listed above in Table 3.3. Learning difficulties (previously called mental retardation) and specific developmental delays are separated out as distinct categories. The so-called pervasive disorders correspond approximately with adult psychotic disorders, the emotional disorders of childhood with adult anxiety related (or neurotic) disorders. The remaining groups of disorder include behavioural disorders (e.g. conduct disorder), and disorders of physiological functions (e.g. enuresis and encopresis).

Summary of psychiatric diagnosis: from symptoms to diagnostic categories

Diagnosis in adult psychiatry can be thought of as involving three main stages: (1) clarification of symptoms; (2) exclusion of drug/alcohol-related, personality and stress-induced disorders; and (3) differential diagnosis of remaining disorders according to symptomatology.

1. *Clarification of symptoms.* As it is in bodily medicine, this is the basis of diagnosis in psychiatry. Psychiatry, though, as noted earlier, is like neurology in relying *primarily* on symptoms and signs. This is why the clinical skills of history taking and mental state examination are so crucial.

2. *Exclusion of: (a) drug/alcohol-related problems; (b) personality disorder; and (c) stress-induced disorders.* Excluding drug and alcohol-related disorders depends partly on identifying any organic symptoms that may be present, partly on history, physical examination, and appropriate laboratory tests. Excluding personality disorder depends on establishing the long-term pattern of a patient's symptoms (see above and Box 3.1). Excluding stress-induced disorders involves establishing whether the patient's condition is mainly a direct reaction to some major stress factor. The latter two kinds of category should be used very sparingly and only when they are quite definitely present.

3. *Differential diagnosis of remaining disorders.* This covers all the symptomatically defined categories. Anxiety and related disorders, together with minor depression, are the most common, followed by disorders of appetite and sexual function. Psychotic disorders are the least common but also generally the most serious.

As emphasized above, it is essential to exclude bodily conditions, not only when presenting with obvious organic symptoms, but also with any other psychiatric presentation. Major bodily pathology presenting psychiatrically (such as a brain tumour) is relatively unusual (though all the harder to diagnose for that!). But bodily illness is commonly a *complicating* factor in mental distress and disorder. Unrecognized bodily pathology, for example, is a factor in treatment-resistant depression. Again, common conditions such as anaemia and asymptomatic urinary infections, may reduce the capacity to cope with stressful events. Conversely anxiety and depression may lead to loss of sleep, failure to eat properly and other forms of self-neglect. So the bottom-line message in psychiatry, as it should be in all areas of medicine, is that a balanced 'whole person', mind plus body, approach to diagnosis is essential.

The boundary problem

Finally, it should not be forgotten that many patients presenting psychiatrically, especially in general practice, do not have anything wrong with them as such. They have life problems and difficulties with which they need help. The uncertain boundary between distress and disorder is one reason why classification and diagnosis in psychiatry are conceptually, as well as empirically, difficult.

Reflection on the session and self-test questions

Write down your own reflections on the materials in this session drawing out any points that are particularly significant for you. Then write brief notes about the following:

1. What are the main categories of adult mental disorder?

2. How does personality disorder differ from the main categories of adult mental disorder?

3. How does a stress-induced disorder differ from the main categories of adult mental disorder?

4. What are the main additional categories of disorders of childhood and adolescence?

5. What are the main steps in developing a differential diagnosis in psychiatry?

6. Are all distressing experiences matters for psychiatric diagnosis?

Conclusions: to diagnose or not to diagnose?

In this chapter we have focused particularly on how *psychiatrists* approach the assessment of mental distress and disorder, illustrating, in particular, the rich variety of resources available from such sources as textbooks, diagnostic manuals, psychological 'measures', research studies and narrative literature for cross-disciplinary work in this area.

Uses and misuses of psychiatric diagnosis

The psychiatric approach to diagnostic assessment is not uncontentious, of course. It reflects the 'medical' model, at least to the extent that it assumes much the same principles of diagnosis and classification as are assumed in other medical specialities, such as cardiology and rheumatology. As we saw in Chapter 2, there are competing models of mental distress and disorder—psychological, social etc.—each of which has its own approach to assessment. There are many, furthermore, particularly in the politically-active 'user movement', who reject the very idea of *medical* diagnoses of mental distress and disorder, arguing for the importance of individual understanding over general descriptive categories (Kutchins and Kirk, 1997; see also Reading Guide). Within psychiatry, too, there are other approaches. Leaving aside psychoanalysis, a whole school of twentieth century psychiatry, Adolf Meyer's 'psychobiology of the individual', was based on the belief that psychiatric assessment should take the form of a detailed understanding of an individual's experiences in the context of their particular life history and circumstances. The need for 'idiographic', alongside the currently dominant categorical diagnostic schemas, has been emphasised by recent authors (Mezzich, 2002; Mezzich *et al.*, 1996 and 2003) and is the basis for a psychiatric classification recently adopted in Spanish-speaking South America with the support of the World Psychiatric Association (see also chapter 13).

There is a danger, particularly under the growing managerial and financial pressures on clinical work, of psychiatric diagnostic categories being used in a crudely positivist way. This is a danger to which this chapter, with its necessarily descriptive and schematic format, is at risk of contributing. But such uses of psychiatric diagnosis are *misuses*. Read any authoritative account of psychiatric diagnosis and you will find a strong emphasis, first, on the need to contextualize the process by attending to the meanings of individual experiences as well as to their general form, and, second, on the nature of diagnosis itself being best understood as a form of cautious hypothesis building. Indeed Karl Jaspers, to whose foundational work on psychopathology we return in Part II, emphasized that diagnostic categories should come, if at all, *last* in the assessment of a patient, and then only after a full and in depth exploration of their individual circumstances and experiences (Jaspers, 1997, p. 20).

Difficulties of psychiatric diagnosis and classification

Much (though certainly not all) of the criticism of psychiatric diagnosis, has been criticism of a 'straw man' model of the discipline; and as we noted at the start of this chapter, part of our aim here has been to give a picture of what psychiatric assessment is really about.

All the same, psychiatric diagnosis *is* difficult. It is difficult empirically, of course: we are only at the beginning of developing scientific instruments that are up to the task of investigating the brain. But it is also difficult conceptually. The conceptual difficulties presented by psychiatric diagnosis, compared with diagnosis in bodily medicine, have been treated by those external to the subject as grounds for criticism. But the difficulties are all too evident, in substance if not in name, to those internal to the discipline. This is vividly illustrated by the APA's 'research agenda' for the next edition of the DSM, the DSM-V (Kupfer *et al.*, 2002). We return to this in detail in chapter 13. As we will see, although ostensibly concerned with enriching the 'empirical database' of the new classification (p. xv), the agenda starts with a whole chapter (called issues of 'Basic Nomenclature') on conceptual difficulties, the first of which is, as in this book, the problem of defining mental disorder itself! And many of the other conceptual items on the DSM-V agenda, either in the first or subsequent chapters, are covered by topics in this book, notably in Part III, though also in Part IV and Part V.

A (resistible?) role for philosophers

From the perspective of the traditional medical model it may seem something of a paradox, that as the scientific basis of psychiatry has become more sophisticated, with advances particulary in the neurosciences, conceptual issues in psychiatric diagnostic classification should have become, as in the APA's Research Agenda for DSM-V, more, not less, evident.

Yet this process, of conceptual issues becoming more not less evident with scientific advances, is no paradox. To the contrary, it directly reflects the wider renaissance in philosophy of psychiatry, which, as Fulford *et al.*, (2003) note, directly parallels the flowering of philosophy during psychiatry's first biological phase, with Karl Jaspers' foundational work on psychopathology in the early years of the twentieth century.

If we are to respond appropriately to present challenges, then, at the very least avoiding the mistakes of the past, there may be lessons to be learned from the history of ideas of that period. We examine the philosophical history of psychopathology in the next part of the book. First, though, we return to the debate about mental illness, with detailed considerations of how it illustrates, first the methods employed in philosophical research (Chapters 4 and 5), and then the kinds of outputs or results that philosophy delivers (Chapter 6).

Reading guide

Further reading on each of the main groups of mental disorders is given in the relevant sections of this chapter. We note here only illustrative introductions and overviews.

Concepts of disorder: (2) firsthand and other narrative accounts

As indicated in this chapter, there is a growing and increasingly important literature of firsthand narrative accounts, including websites. The latter can come and go but current examples include, 'Jane's Mental Health Source Page' http://www.chinspirations.com/mhsourcepage/storybook.html and http://serendip.brynmawr.edu/sci_cult/mentalhealth/inside.html#general. An early and still useful edited collection is Bert Kaplan (ed.), (1964) *The Inner World of Mental Illness: a series of first-person accounts of what it was like*. Many examples

are given in Fulford, Dickenson, and Murray's (2002) edited collection, *Healthcare Ethics and Human Values*.

In addition to the examples cited in the chapter, firsthand accounts of the experience of specific conditions include,

1. *Schizophrenia*. Morag Coate (1964) *Beyond All Reason*; Lori Schiller and Amanda Bennett (1996) *The Quiet Room: a journey out of the torment of madness*; Daniel Paul Schreber (2000) *Memoirs of My Nervous Illness*; Barbara O'Brien (1976) *Operators and Things: the inner life of a schizophrenic*; Marguerite Sechehaye's (1996a) *Autobiography of a Schizophrenic Girl: the true story of 'Renee'* (the author is in fact the psychoanalyst who interprets the material).

2. *Manic depression*. Hert and colleagues (2004) *Anything or Nothing: self guide for people with bipolar disorder*; and Kay Redfield Jamison's two books (1994) *Touched with Fire*, and (1996b) *An Unquiet Mind: a memoir of moods and madness*. As noted in the chapter, these include many extracts of firsthand narratives.

3. *Depression and grief*. Personal accounts include: William Styron (1991) *Darkness Visible: a memoir of madness* (an extract of this is given in the chapter); Stuart Sutherland (1998) *Breakdown: a personal crisis and a medical dilemma*; Louis Wolpert's (1999) *Malignant Sadness*. The American philosopher Loretta Kopelman (1994a) explores the distinction between normal and pathological grief in *Normal Grief: Good or bad? Health or disease?* with commentaries by Dominion (1994) and Wise (1994), and a response by Kopelman (1994b). A valuable edited collection is Donna Dickenson and Malcolm Johnson's (1993) *Death, Dying & Bereavement*.

Spirituality and mental health

There is a growing literature on spirituality and mental health with increasingly strong links into policy and practice in the UK. A valuable outline of the issues and initiatives is given in the NIMHE (National Institute for Mental Health in England) policy document 'Inspiring Hope' (Department of Health, 2003). A foundational publication is Swinton's (2001) *Spirituality in Mental Health Care*. Publications illustrating the practical developments in this field include two by the Mental Health Foundation (1999 and 2002), Albert Persaud's (1999) description of the importance of spirituality in cultural contexts, and the report of the *Somerset Spirituality Project Group* (2002). Recent policy guidance is given in the UK Department of Health's (forthcoming) *Meeting the Spiritual and Religious Needs of Patients and Staff*. (See also below, under 'Psychosis and Delusion'.)

Discursive approaches

The power of discursive analysis for exploring personal meanings is shown by Sabat and Harré (1997) in their article on

'The Alzheimer's disease sufferer as a semiotic subject', with commentaries by Hope (1994) and Greenberg (1994). Sabat went on to develop practical tools for improving communication with Alzheimer's disease sufferers in his (2001) *The Experience of Alzheimer's Disease: life through a tangled veil*. Gillett has worked with Harré on discursive approaches (see e.g. Harré, R. and Gillett, G. (1994) *The Discursive Mind*.) and his book, Gillett, G. (1999) *The Mind and its Discontents*. See also in *Nature and Narrative*, Gillett's (2003) *Form and Content: the role of discourse in mental disorder*; and in *Philosophy, Psychiatry, & Psychology*, Gillett's (1994) 'Insight, delusion and belief', with commentaries by David, 1994, Loizzo, 1994, and Davidson, 1994. Harré (1997a) applies a discursive approach to problems in forensic psychiatry in his 'Pathological autobiographies', with commentaries by Adshead (1997) and Norrie (1997) and a response by Harré (1997b).

The importance of narrative is also explored in a special issue of *Philosophy, Psychiatry, & Psychology* (December 2003, issue 10/4) on 'Agency, narrative, and self', edited by Melvyn Woody. Of particular relevance from this issue, in addition to Woody's (2003) 'When narrative fails', are Wells (2003) on 'Discontinuity in personal narrative', which gives a number of firsthand reports, Phillips (2003) on 'Psychopathology and the narrative self', and Thornton's (2003) commentary titled 'Psychopathology and two kinds of narrative account of the self'. (See also Reading guide to Chapter 6.)

An illustration of the value of 'embedded' case histories is Deeley's (1999a) 'Ecological understandings of mental and physical illness', with commentaries by Fabrega (1999), Harré (1999), and Littlewood (1999), and a response by Deeley (1999b). Depression and the role of insight are discussed in Martin's (1999a) 'Depression: illness, insight, and identity', with a commentary by Ghaemi (1999a) and a response by Martin (1999b). The German psychiatrist, Christoph Mundt (a successor to Jaspers as Professor at Heidelberg) gives an important discussion of the diversity of psychopathology in Mundt, 2003.

An exploration of the role of literature in improving understanding of otherwise incomprehensible experiences is Read (2003a) on 'Literature as philosophy of psychopathology: William Faulkner as Wittgenstein', with commentaries by Sass (2003), Coetzee (2003), and a response by Read (2003b).

Psychiatric symptoms

General introductions

In addition to the sources given in the chapter, note: (1) clear descriptions of all the important psychiatric symptoms together with clinical examples, in Leff, J.P. and Isaacs, A.D. (1990) *Psychiatric Examination in Clinical Practice* (3rd edn is 1990 reprinted 1992); (2) case studies in 'cognitive disorders', such as delusions (e.g. Cotard and Fregoli syndromes) and disorders of volition (such as 'alien hand' syndrome), in Halligan

and Marshall's (1996) *Method in Madness: case studies in cognitive neuropsychiatry*, and Campbell's (1992) *Mental Lives: case studies in cognition*; (3) detailed clinical and neurological accounts combined with philosophical analysis in John Cutting's *Principles of Psychopathology* (1997) and *Psychopathology & Modern Philosophy* (1999); and, among modern classics; (4) Sims (1988) *Symptoms in the Mind*. Sims, Mundt, Berner, and Barocka (2000), and Mundt and Spitzer (2001) give excellent detailed overviews.

Psychosis and delusion

Psychotic experiences have received particular attention in *Philosophy, Psychiatry, & Psychology*. Thus, the first article in the first issue of PPP was on thought insertion (by Stephens and Graham, 1994a, with a commentary by Wiggins, 1994); and this was followed by Chadwick (1994, with a commentary by Stephens and Graham, 1994b).

More recently, there has been a double special issue on Schizophrenia (June/September 2001, issues 8/2 and 8/3), edited by the Warwick philosopher, Christoph Hoerl. Hoerl's (2001a) introduction on 'Understanding, explaining and intersubjectivity in schizophrenia', reflects the weaving together of analytic and Continental sources in this double issue. Thus, Eilan (2001) in her 'Meaning, truth and the self', responds both to Campbell's analytic article on 'Rationality, meaning, and the analysis of delusion', and to Parnas and Sass' (2001) more Continental approach in 'Self, solipsism, and schizophrenic delusions'. The issue also illustrates the value of looking in detail at particular symptoms. Thus, Davies *et al.* (2001) give a two-factor account of 'Monothematic delusions', with a commentary by Currie and Jureidini (2001); Roessler (2001) explores delusions of alien control; and Hoerl (2001b) explores 'Thought insertion'. Similarly, in Sass' special issue on 'The phenomenology of schizophrenia' (issue 8/4, December 2001), Gerrans (2002a) explores 'A one-stage explanation of the Cotard delusion', with commentaries by Young and de Pauw (2002) and Phillips (2002), and a response (Gerrans, 2002b). Thought insertion is also the subject of Gibbs (2000a) 'Thought insertion and the inseparability thesis', with a commentary by Stephens (2000) and a response (Gibbs, 2000b).

The border between psychotic illness and spiritual and religious experience is explored in a series of interconnected articles in the December 2002 (9/4) issue of *Philosophy, Psychiatry, & Psychology* with lead articles by Brett (2002a) on 'Psychotic and mystical states of being', and Marzanski and Bratton (2002a) on the importance of theological sources, together with a series of related articles (McGhee, 2002; Jackson and Fulford, 2002: and Sykes, 2002) and cross-commentaries (Brett, 2002b and 2002c; Marzanski and Bratton, 2002b and 2002c). (See also above, 'Spirituality and mental health').

Among particular psychotic phenomena, delusions have attracted an especially rich literature. Thus, in *Philosophy,*

Psychiatry, & Psychology, issue 11/1 (March 2004) was devoted entirely to this topic, with three target articles respectively by Bayne and Pacherie (2004a) on 'Bottom-up or top down?' (This was an article-length response to Campbell's (2001) account of monothematic delusions), Georgacha (2004a) on 'Factualization and plausibility in delusional discourse,' and Klee (2004a) on 'Why some delusions are necessarily inexplicable beliefs'. In this particular issue of *Philosophy, Psychiatry, & Psychology*, commentators were invited to respond to the group of target articles. From the clinical perspective, these included Broome (2004), Ghaemi (2004), and Harper (2004), and from a philosophical perspective, Gerrans (2004), Hohwy (2004), and Sass (2004). The authors of the target articles responded similarly to the group of commentaries (Bayne and Pachererie, 2004b; Georgaca, 2004b; Klee, 2004b).

Max Coltheart and a Martin Davies have been particularly active in this field, see their edited volume in Blackwell's 'Mind and Language' series, on *Pathologies of Belief* (2000). This is reviewed in Christoph Hoerl's Special Issue on Schizophrenia by Atkinson (2001) in 'Pathological beliefs, damaged brains'. James Phillips and James Morley's (2003) 'Imagination and its pathologies' provides a complementary collection from the perspective of Continental Philosophy.

An article that adopts a 'philosophical fieldwork' approach to delusions is Jones (1999a) 'The phenomenology of abnormal belief: a philosophical and psychiatric inquiry', with commentaries by David (1999), Ghaemi (1999b), Stephens (1999), and a response by Jones (1999b).

Psychiatric classifications of mental disorder

The two main international classifications of mental disorders (which are discussed further in Part III, chapter 13)are:

1. Chapter 8 of the World Health Organization's *International Classification of Diseases and Related Health Problems* (the ICD—current edition is ICD-10, World Health Organization, 1992) *The ICD-10 Classification of Mental and Behavioural Disorders: clinical descriptions and diagnostic guidelines.*

2. The American Psychiatric Association's *Diagnostic and Statistical Manual* (the DSM—current edition is DSM-IV, 1994; and note DSM-IV TR, for Text Revision, American Psychiatric Association, 2000).

Most of the larger psychiatric textbooks include sections on classification and diagnosis: for example chapter 1.11, by Dilling (2004), in Gelder, Lopez-Ibor and Andreasen's (2000) *New Oxford Textbook of Psychiatry*. A classic but still valuable publication covering technical and research aspects is Kendell's (1975) *The Role of Diagnosis in Psychiatry*. Christian Perring (2004) gives a philosophically nuanced account of developmental disorders of childhood and adolescence. (See also Reading guide to Chapter 13.)

Philosophy, Psychiatry, & Psychology has included articles exploring specific kinds of mental disorder. For example, a detailed discussion of false memory syndrome is Hamilton's (1998a) 'False memory syndrome and the authority of personal memory-claims: a philosophical perspective', with commentaries by Braude (1998), Eacott (1998), and Lowe (1998), and a response by Hamilton (1998b). The importance of narrative and meaning in intellectual disability (illustrated by bereavement counselling) is explored in Clegg and Landsall-Welfare (2003a) 'Death, disability, and dogma', with commentaries by Colman (2003), Casenave (2003), and Reinders (2003), with a response by the authors (Clegg and Landsall-Welfare, 2003b).

References

Abbany, Z. (2001). Caught in a trap. *New Scientist*, 169 (2283): 46–49.

Adshead, G. (1997) Pathological autobiographies. (Commentary on Harré, 1997) *Philosophy, Psychiatry, & Psychology*, 4(2): 111–114.

Amador, X.F. and David, A.S. (1998). *Insight and Psychosis*. Oxford: Oxford University Press.

American Psychiatric Association (1994). *Diagnostic and Statistical Manual Of Mental Disorders* (4th edn). Washington DC: APA.

American Psychiatric Association (2000). *Diagnostic and Statistical Manual of Mental Disorders*, Fourth Edition, Text Revision. Washington, DC: American Psychiatric Association. [DSM-IV-TR]

Andreasen, N. (2001). *Brave New Brain: conquering mental illness in the era of the genome*. New York: Oxford University Press.

Atkinson, A.P. (2001). Pathological beliefs, damaged brains: a review of Max Coltheart and Martin Davies, Ed., Pathologies of Belief. *Philosophy, Psychiatry, & Psychology*, 8/2(3): 225–230.

Bayley, J. (1999). *Iris and Her Friends: a memoir of memory and desire*. New York: W.W. Norton.

Bayne, T. and Pacherie, E. (2004a). Bottom-up or top-down? Campbells rationalist account of monothematic delusions. *Philosophy, Psychiatry, & Psychology*, 11/1: 1–12.

Bayne, T. and Pacherie, E. (2004b). Experience, belief, and the interpretive Fold. *Philosophy, Psychiatry, & Psychology*, 11/1: 81–86.

Bentall, R.P. (1992). A proposal to classify happiness as a psychiatric disorder. *Journal of Medical Ethics*, 18: 94–98.

Bentall, R.P. (2003). *Madness Explained*. London: Penguin.

Binswanger, L. (1975). *Being in the World*. (trans. J. Needleman). London: Souvenir Press.

Birley, J.L.T. (1993). Invited response to Bentall, R.P. (1993). *British Journal of Psychiatry*, 162: 540–541.

Bleuler, E. (1911). *Dementia Praecox; or the group of schizophrenias*. New York: International Universities Press. (Translated and printed by IUP in 1950.)

Boss, M. (1963 [1957]). *Psychoanalysis and Daseinanalysis*. (Transl by Lefebre, L.). New York: Basic Books.

Boss, M. (1983 [1979]). *Existential Foundations of Medicine and Psychology* (Transl by Conway, S. and Cleaves, A.). New York: Jason Aronson.

Braude, S.E. (1998). False memory syndrome. (Commentary on Hamilton, 1998a) *Philosophy, Psychiatry, & Psychology*, 5(4): 299–304.

Brett, C. (2002a). Psychotic and mystical states of being: connections and distinctions. *Philosophy, Psychiatry, & Psychology*, 9(4): 321–342.

Brett, C. (2002b). Commentary: Spiritual experience and psychopathology: dichotomy or interaction? *Philosophy, Psychiatry, & Psychology*, 9(4): 373–380.

Brett, C. (2002c). Commentary: The application of nondual epistemology to anomalous experience in psychosis. *Philosophy, Psychiatry, & Psychology*, 9(4): 353–358.

Broome, M.R. (2004). The rationality of psychosis and understanding the deluded. (Commentary for Special Issue on Delusion). *Philosophy, Psychiatry, & Psychology*, 11/1: 35–42.

Campbell, J. (1999). Schizophrenia, the space of reasons and thinking as a motor process. *The Monist*, 82: 609–625.

Cambell, J. (2001). Rationality, meaning, and the analysis of delusion. *Philosophy, Psychiatry, & Psychology*, 8/2(3): 89–100.

Campbell, R. (ed.) (1992). *Mental Lives: case studies in cognition*. Oxford: Blackwell Publishers.

Chadwick, R.F. (1994) Kant, Thought Insertion and Mental Unity. *Philosophy, Psychiatry and Psychology*, 1(2): 105–114.

Casenave, G. (2003). Death, disability, and dialogue. (Commentary on Clegg, J. and Lansdall-Welfare, R., 2003a) *Philosophy, Psychiatry, & Psychology*, 10/1: 87–90.

Clegg, J. and Lansdall-Welfare, R. (2003a). Death, disability, and dogma. *Philosophy, Psychiatry, & Psychology*, 10/1: 67–80.

Clegg, J. and Lansdall-Welfare, R. (2003b). Living with contested knowledge and partial authority. (Response to the commentators). *Philosophy, Psychiatry, & Psychology*, 10/1: 99–102.

Coate, M. (1964). *Beyond All Reason*. London: Constable.

Coetzee, J.M. (2003). *Commentary "Fictional Beings"*. Philosophy, Psychiatry, & Psychology, 10/2, 133–134.

Colman, S. (2003). What's in the box then, Mum?—Death, Disability and Dogma. (Commentary on Clegg, J. and Lansdall-Welfare, R., 2003a) *Philosophy, Psychiatry, & Psychology*, 10/1: 81–86.

Coltheart, M. and Davies, M. (eds). (2000). *Pathologies of Belief*. Oxford: Blackwell Publishers.

Currie, G. and Jureidini, J. (2001). Delusion, Rationality, Empathy: A Commentary on Davies *et al.* (2001). *Philosophy, Psychiatry, & Psychology*, 8/2(3): 159–162.

Cutting, J. (1997). *Principles of Psychopathology: two worlds-two minds-two hemispheres*. Oxford: Oxford University Press.

Cutting, J. (1999). *Psychopathology and Modern Philosophy*. England, West Sussex: The Forest Publishing Company.

David, A.S. (1990). Insight and psychosis. *British Journal of Psychiatry*, 156: 798–808.

David, A.S. (1994). Insight, delusion, and belief. (Commentary on Gillett, 1994) *Philosophy, Psychiatry, & Psychology*, 1(4): 237–240.

David, A.S. (1999). On the impossibility of defining delusions. (Commentary on Jones, 1999a) *Philosophy, Psychiatry, & Psychology*, 6/1: 17–20.

Davidson, L. (1994). Insight, delusion, and belief. (Commentary on Gillett, 1994) *Philosophy, Psychiatry, & Psychology*, 1(4): 243–244.

Davies, M. and Coltheart, M. (2000). Introduction: pathologies of belief. In *Pathologies of Belief* (ed. M. Coltheart and M. Davies). Oxford: Blackwell Publishers, Chapter 1.

Davies, M., Coltheart, M., Langdon, R., and Breen, N. (2001). Monothematic delusions: towards a two-factor account. *Philosophy, Psychiatry, & Psychology*, 8/2(3): 133–158.

Deeley, P.Q. (1999a). Ecological understandings of mental and physical illness. *Philosophy, Psychiatry, & Psychology*, 6(2): 109–124.

Deeley, P.Q. (1999b). Response to the Commentaries. *Philosophy, Psychiatry, & Psychology*, 6(2): 135–144.

Department of Health (2003). *Inspiring Hope: recognising the importance of spirituality in a whole person approach to mental health*. National Institute for Mental Health in England. Web: www.nimhe.org.uk. For further information please contact: Peter Gilbert, Project Lead, pgilbert@gilbert88.fsbusiness.co.uk.

Department of Health (forthcoming). *Meeting the Spiritual and Religious Needs of Patients and Staff: Guidance for Staff*. London: HMSO.

Dickenson, D. and Johnson, M. (ed.). (1993). *Death, Dying and Bereavement*. London: Sage Publications in association with The Open University.

Dilling, H. (2000). Classification Chapter 1. 11 in Gelder, M., Lopez-Ibor, J. J. and Andreasen, N. (eds) *New Oxford Textbook of Psychiatry*. Oxford: Oxford University Press.

Dominion, J. (1994). Commentary on normal grief: Good or bad? Health or disease? (Commentary on Kopelman, 1994). *Philosophy, Psychiatry, & Psychology*, 1(4): 221–222.

Dreyfus, H.L. (1991). *Being-in-the-World: A commentary on Heidegger's Being and Time*. Division 1. Cambridge, MA: The MIT Press.

Eacott, M.J. (1998). False memory syndrome. (Commentary on Hamilton, 1998a) *Philosophy, Psychiatry, & Psychology*, 5(4): 305–308.

Eigen, M. (2001) *Ecstasy*. Middletown, CT: Wesleyan University Press.

Eilan, N. (2001). Commentary: Meaning, truth, and the self: A Commentary on Campbell (2001) and Parnas and Sass (2001). *Philosophy, Psychiatry, & Psychology*, 8/2(3): 121–132.

Fabrega Jr. H. (1999). Elegant case history analysis or original contribution? (Commentary on Deeley, 1999a) *Philosophy, Psychiatry, & Psychology*, 6(2): 125–128.

Flew, A. (1973). *Crime or Disease?* New York: Barnes and Noble.

Fulford, K.W.M. (1989, reprinted 1995 and 1999). *Moral Theory and Medical Practice*. Cambridge: Cambridge University Press.

Fulford, K.W.M. (1991). Evaluative delusions: their significance for philosophy and psychiatry. *British Journal of Psychiatry*, 159 (Suppl. 14): 108–112.

Fulford, K.W.M. (1992). Thought insertion and insight: disease and illness paradigms of psychotic disorder. In *Phenomenology, Language, and Schizophrenia* (ed. M. Spitzer, F. Uehlein, F.A., M.A. Schwartz, and C. Mundt). New York: Springer-Verlag.

Fulford, K.W.M. (1993). Invited response to Bentall R. A proposal to classify happiness disease as a psychiatric disorder (*Journal of Medical Ethics*, 1992; 18: 94–98). *British Journal of Psychiatry*, 162: 541–542.

Fulford, K.W.M. (1994 [1988]). Diagnosis, Classification and Phenomenology of Mental Illness. Ch. 1 in Rose, N. (ed) 2nd Edition *Essential Psychiatry*. Oxford: Blackwell Scientific Publications.

Fulford, K.W.M. (1996) Value, illness and action: delusions in the new philosophical psychopathology. In *Philosophical Psychopathology* (ed. G. Graham and G. Lynn Stephens). Cambridge, MA: MIT Press.

Fulford, K. W. M., Morris, K. J., Sadler, J. Z., and Stanghellini, G. (2003). Past Improbable, Future Possible: the renaissance in philosophy and psychiatry. Chapter 1 (pps 1–41) in Fulford, K. W. M., Morris, K. J., Sadler, J. Z., and Stanghellini, G. (eds.) *Nature and Narrative: an Introduction to the New Philosophy of Psychiatry*. Oxford: Oxford University Press.

Fulford, K.W.M. (2004). Insight and delusion: from Jaspers to Kraepelin and back again via Austin. In *Insight and Psychosis* (2nd edn) (ed. X.F. Amador and A.S. David). New York: Oxford University Press.

Fulford, K.W.M., Dickenson, D. and Murray, T.H. (ed.) (2002). *Healthcare Ethics and Human Values: an introductory text with readings and case studies*. Malden, USA and Oxford, UK: Blackwell Publishers.

Gallagher, S. (2000). Self reference and schizophrenia: a cognitive model of immunity to error through misidentification. In *Exploring the Self*. (ed. D. Zahavi). Amsterdam: John Benjamins Publishing Company.

Gallagher, S. (2003). Self-narrative in schizophrenia. In *The Self in Neuroscience and Psychiatry* (ed. T. Kircher and A. David). Cambridge: Cambridge University Press, pp. 336–357.

Garety, P.A. and Freeman, D. (1999). Cognitive approaches to delusions: a critical review of theories and evidence, *British Journal of Clinical Psychology*, 38: 113–154.

Georgaca, E. (2004a). Factualization and plausibility in delusional discourse. *Philosophy, Psychiatry, & Psychology*, 11/1: 13–24.

Georgaca, E. (2004b). Talk and the nature of delusions: defending sociocultural perspectives on mental illness. *Philosophy, Psychiatry, & Psychology*, 11/1: 87–94.

Gerrans, P. (2002a). A one-stage explanation of the Cotard delusion. *Philosophy, Psychiatry, & Psychology*, 9/1: 47–54.

Gerrans, P. (2002b). Multiples paths to delusion. *Philosophy, Psychiatry, & Psychology*, 9/1: 65–72.

Gerrans, P. (2004). Cognitive architecture and the limits of interpretationism. (Commentary for Special Issue on delusion) *Philosophy, Psychiatry, & Psychology*, 11/1: 43–48.

Ghaemi, S.N. (1999a). Depression: insight, illusion, and psychopharmacological Calvinism. (Commentary on Martin, 1999a) *Philosophy, Psychiatry, & Psychology*, 6(4): 287–294.

Ghaemi, S.N. (1999b). An empirical approach to understanding delusions. (Commentary on Jones, 1999a) *Philosophy, Psychiatry, & Psychology*, 6/1: 21–24.

Ghaemi, S.N. (2004). The perils of belief: delusions reexamined. (Commentary for Special Issue on delusion) *Philosophy, Psychiatry, & Psychology*, 11/1: 49–54.

Gibbs, P.J. (2000a). Thought insertion and the inseparability thesis. *Philosophy, Psychiatry, & Psychology*, 7(3): 195–202.

Gibbs, P.J. (2000b). The limits of subjectivity: a response to the Commentary. *Philosophy, Psychiatry, & Psychology*, 7(3): 207–208.

Gillett, G. (1994). Insight, delusion, and belief. *Philosophy, Psychiatry, & Psychology*, 1(4): 227–236.

Gillett, G. (1999). *The Mind and its Discontents*. Oxford: Oxford University Press.

Gillett, G. (2003). Form and content: the role of discourse in mental disorder. In *Nature and Narrative: an introduction to the new philosophy of psychiatry* (ed. K.W.M. Fulford,

K.J. Morris, J.Z. Sadler, and G. Stanghellini). Oxford: Oxford University Press, Chapter 9.

Gipps, R.G.T. and Fulford, K.W.M. (2004). Understanding the clinical concept of delusion: from an estranged to an engaged epistemology. *International Review of Psychiatry*, 16(3): 225–235.

Glas, G. (2003). Anxiety—animal reactions and the embodiment of meaning. In *Nature and Narrative: an introduction to the new philosophy of psychiatry* (ed. K.W.M. Fulford, K.J. Morris, J.Z. Sadler, and G. Stanghellini). Oxford: Oxford University Press, pp. 231–249.

Glover, J. (1970). *Responsibility*. London: Routledge & Kegan Paul.

Greenberg, W.M. (1994). Commentary on Sabat and Harré (1997). The Alzheimer's disease sufferer as semiotic subject. *Philosophy, Psychiatry, & Psychology*, 1(3): 163–164.

Halligan, P.W. and Marshall, J.C. (ed.) (1996). *Method in Madness: case studies in cognitive neuropsychiatry*. Oxford: Psychology Press.

Hamilton, A. (1998a). False memory syndrome and the authority of personal memory-claims: a philosophical perspective. *Philosophy, Psychiatry, & Psychology*, 5(4): 283–298.

Hamilton, A. (1998b). Response to the Commentaries. *Philosophy, Psychiatry, & Psychology*, 5(4): 311–316.

Harper, D.J. (2004). Delusions and discourse: moving beyond the constraints of the modernist paradigm. (Commentary for Special Issue on delusion). *Philosophy, Psychiatry, & Psychology*, 11(1): 55–64.

Harré, R. (1997a). Pathological autobiographies. *Philosophy, Psychiatry, & Psychology*, 4(2): 99–110.

Harré, R. (1997b). Response to the Commentaries. *Philosophy, Psychiatry, & Psychology*, 4(2): 119–120.

Harré, R. (1999). Bringing relations to life. (Commentary on Deeley, 1999a). *Philosophy, Psychiatry, & Psychology*, 6(2): 129–132.

Harré, R. and Lamb, D. (ed.) (1987). *Dictionary of Philosophy and Psychology*. Oxford: Blackwell.

Harré, R. and Gillett, G. (1994) *The discursive mind*. London: Sage.

Harris, J. (1993). Invited response to Bentall, J. (1993). *British Journal of Psychiatry*, 162: 539–541.

Heidegger, M. (1962). *Being and Time*. (Trans. John Macquarrie and Edward Robinson). New York: Harper & Row.

Hert, M. De, Thys, E., Magiels, G., and Wyckaert, S. (2004). *Anything or Nothing: self-guide for people with bipolar disorder*. Antwerp: Janssen-Cilag/Organon.

Hoerl, C. (2001a). Introduction: understanding, explaining, and intersubjectivity in schizophrenia. *Philosophy, Psychiatry, & Psychology*, 8/2(3): 83–88.

Hoerl, C. (2001b). On thought insertion. *Philosophy, Psychiatry, & Psychology*, 8/2(3): 189–200.

Hohwy, J. (2004). Top-down and bottom-up in delusion formation. (Commentary for Special Issue on delusion). *Philosophy, Psychiatry, & Psychology*, 11(1): 65–70.

Hope, T. (1994). Commentary on Sabat and Harré (1997). The Alzheimer's disease sufferer as semiotic subject. *Philosophy, Psychiatry, & Psychology*, 1(3): 161–162.

Hughes, J.C., Louw, S.J., Sabat, S.R. (eds) (2006) *Dementia: Mind, Meaning, and the Person*. Oxford: Oxford University Press.

Hyman, J. (1992). The causal theory of perception. *The Philosophical Quarterly*, 42(168): 277–296.

Jackson, M.C. and Fulford, K.W.M. (2002). Psychosis good and bad: values-based practice and the distinction between pathological and nonpathological forms of psychotic experience. *Philosophy, Psychiatry, & Psychology*, 9(4): 387–394.

Jamison, K.R. (1996a). *Touched With Fire: manic depressive illness and the artistic temperament*. California: Touchstone Books.

Jamison, K.R. (1996b). *An Unquiet Mind: a memoir of moods and madness*. New York: Free Press.

Jaspers, K. ([1913] 1997). *General Psychopathology* (trans. by Hoenig and Hamilton). Baltimore, MD: Johns Hopkins University Press. (1959) *Allgemeine Psychopathologie*. Berlin: Springer, 1959.

Jones, E. (1999a). The phenomenology of abnormal belief: a philosophical and psychiatric inquiry. *Philosophy, Psychiatry, & Psychology*, 6/1: 1–16.

Jones, E. (1999b). Response to the Commentaries. *Philosophy, Psychiatry, & Psychology*, 6/1: 27–28.

Kaplan, B. (ed.) (1964). *The Inner World of Mental Illness: a series of first-person accounts of what it was like*. New York: Harper & Row.

Kendell, R.E. (1975). *The Role of Diagnosis in Psychiatry*. Oxford: Blackwell Scientific Publications.

Kierkegaard, S. (1981). *The Concept of Anxiety*. Princeton: Princeton University Press.

Kierkegaard, S. (1983). *The Sickness Unto Death*. Princeton: Princeton University Press.

Kiloh, L. and Garside, R. (1963). The independence of neurotic depression and endogenous depression. *British Journal of Psychiatry*, 109: 451–463.

Klee, R. (2004a). Why some delusions are necessarily inexplicable beliefs. *Philosophy, Psychiatry, & Psychology*, 11/1: 25–34.

Klee, R. (2004b). Delusional content and the public nature of meaning. *Philosophy, Psychiatry, & Psychology*, 11/1: 95–100.

Kopelman, L. (1994a). Normal Grief: Good or Bad? Health or Disease (with commentaries by Dominion, 1994, and Wise, 1994, and a response by Kopelman, 1994b) *Philosophy, Psychiatry, & Psychology*, 1(4): 209–220.

Kopelman, L. (1994b). Rejoinder (to Commentaries on Kopelman, 1994a). *Philosophy, Psychiatry, & Psychology*, 1(4): 225–226.

Kraus, A. (2003). How can the phenomenological-anthropological approach contribute to diagnosis and classification in psychiatry? In *Nature and Narrative: an introduction to the new philosophy of psychiatry* (ed. K.W.M. Fulford, K.J. Morris, J.Z. Sadler, and G. Stanghellini). Oxford: Oxford University Press, pp. 199–216.

Kupfer, D., First, M., and Regier, D. (ed.) (2002). *A Research Agenda for DSM-V*. Washington, DC: American Psychiatric Association.

Kutchins, H. and Kirk, S.A. (1997). *Making Us Crazy: DSM—the psychiatric bible and the creation of mental disorder*. London: Constable.

Leff, J.P. and Isaacs, A.D. (1990). *Psychiatric Examination in Clinical Practice* (3rd edn). Oxford: Blackwell Scientific Publications.

Lewis, A.J. (1934). On the psychopathology of insight. *British Journal of Medicine and Psychology*, 14: 332–348.

Littlewood, R. (1999). Ecological understandings and cultural context. (Commentary on Deeley, 1999a). *Philosophy, Psychiatry, & Psychology*, 6(2): 133–134.

Loizzo, J. (1994). Insight, delusion, and belief. (Commentary on Gillett, 1994). *Philosophy, Psychiatry, & Psychology*, 1(4): 241–242.

Lowe, E.J. (1998). False memory syndrome. (Commentary on Hamilton, 1998a). *Philosophy, Psychiatry, & Psychology*, 5(4): 309–310.

Martin, M.W. (1999a). Depression: illness, insight, and identity. *Philosophy, Psychiatry, & Psychology*, 6(4): 271–286.

Martin, M.W. (1999b). Response to the Commentary. *Philosophy, Psychiatry, & Psychology*, 6(4): 295–298.

Marzanski, M. and Bratton, M. (2002a). Psychopathological symptoms and religious experience: a critique of Jackson and Fulford. *Philosophy, Psychiatry, & Psychology*, 9(4): 359–372.

Marzanski, M. and Bratton, M. (2002b). Commentary: Minding your language: a response to Caroline Brett and Stephen Sykes. *Philosophy, Psychiatry, & Psychology*, 9(4): 383–386.

Marzanski, M. and Bratton, M. (2002c). Commentary: Mystical states or mystical life? Buddhist, Christian, and Hindu perspectives. *Philosophy, Psychiatry, & Psychology*, 9(4): 349–352.

Mason, P. (1996). Agoraphobia: letting go. In *Speaking Our Minds: an anthology* (ed. J. Read and J. Reynolds). London: Macmillan Press Ltd, for the Open University, pp. 3–8.

McGhee, M. (2002). Mysticism and psychosis: descriptions and distinctions. (Commentary on Brett 2002a). *Philosophy, Psychiatry, & Psychology*, 9(4): 343–348.

Mellor, C.S. (1970). First rank symptoms of schizophrenia. *British Journal of Psychiatry*, 117: 15–23.

Mental Health Foundation (1999). *The Courage to Bare our Souls*. London: Mental Health Foundation.

Mental Health Foundation (2002). *The Somerset Spirituality Project*. London: Mental Health Foundation.

Merleau-Ponty, M. (1996). *Phenomenology of Perception*. London: Routledge.

Mezzich, J. E. (2002). Comprehensive diagnosis: a conceptual basis for future diagnostic systems. *Psychopathology*, Mar–Jun; 35(2–3):162–5.

Mezzich, J.E. Kleinman, A, Fabrega, H. and Parron, D.L. (eds) (1996). *Culture and Psychiatric Diagnosis: A DSM-IV Perspective*. Washington: American Psychiatric Press Inc.

Mezzich, J.E., Berganza, C.E., Von Cranach, M., Jorge, M.R., Kastrup, M.C., Murthy, R.S., Okasha, A., Pull, C., Sartorius, N., Skodol, A., Zaudig, M. (2003). IGDA. 8: Idiographic (personalised) diagnostic formulation. In Essentials of the World Psychiatric Association's International Guidelines for Diagnostic Assessment (IGD), *The British Journal of Psychiatry*, Vol 182/Supplement 45: 55–57.

Milligan, S. and Clare, A. (1993). *Depression and How to Survive It*. London: Arrow.

Minsky, L. (1933). The mental symptoms associated with 58 cases of cerebral tumour. *Journal of Neurology and Psychopathology*, 13: 330–343.

Moore, A., Hope, T., and Fulford, K.W.M. (1994). Mild mania and well-being. *Philosophy, Psychiatry, & Psychology*, 1(3): 165–178.

Mundt, C.H. (2003) Editorial: Common Language and Local Diversities of Psychopathological Concepts—Alternatives or Complements? *Psychopathology*. 36(3): 111–113.

Mundt, C.H. and Spitzer, M. (2001) Psychopathology Today. In: *Contemporary Psychiatry*, Vol. 1 *Foundations of Psychiatry*, (ed. F. Henn, N. Sartorius, H. Helmchen and H. Lauter). Berlin: Springer-Verlag, pp. 1–28.

Norrie, A. (1997). Pathological autobiographies. (Commentary on Harré, 1997). 115–118.

O'Brien, B. (1976). *Operators and Things: the inner life of a schizophrenic*. London: Sphere Books Ltd.

Parnas, J. and Sass, L.A. (2001). Self, solipsism, and schizophrenic delusions. *Philosophy, Psychiatry, & Psychology*, 8/2(3): 101–120.

Parnas, J., Sass, L. and Stanghellini, G. and Fuchs, T. (forthcoming). *The Vulnerable Self: the clinical phenomenology of the schizophrenic and affective spectrum disorders*. Oxford: Oxford University Press.

Perring, C. (2004). Development: disorders of childhood and youth. In *The Philosophy of Psychiatry: A Companion* (ed. J. Radden). New York: Oxford University Press, pp. 147–162.

Persaud, A. (1999). *Respect for Privacy, Dignity and Religious and Cultural Beliefs*. Wiltshire: Wiltshire Health Authority.

Phillips, J. (2002). Arguing from neuroscience in psychiatry. (Commentary on Gerrans, 2002a). *Philosophy, Psychiatry, & Psychology*, 9(1): 61–64.

Phillips, J. (2003). Psychopathology and the narrative self. *Philosophy, Psychiatry, & Psychology*, 10(4): 313–328.

Phillips, J. and Morley, J. (ed.) (2003). *Imagination and Its Pathologies*. Cambridge, MA: MIT Press.

Quinton, A. (1985). Madness. In *Philosophy and Practice* (ed. A.P. Griffiths). Cambridge University Press, Chapter 2.

Radden, J. (2003). Is This Dame Melancholy? Equating Today's Depression and Past Melancholia. *Philosophy, Psychiatry, & Psychology*, 10/1, 37–52.

Read, R. (2003a). Literature as Philosophy of Psychopathology: William Faulkner as Wittgensteinian. *Philosophy, Psychiatry, & Psychology*, 10/2, 115–124.

Read, R. (2003b). "On Delusions of Sense: A Response to Coetzee and Sass". *Philosophy, Psychiatry, & Psychology*, 10/2, 135–142.

Reinders, H. (2003). The ambiguities of meaning: a commentary. (Commentary on Clegg, J. and Lansdall-Welfare, R., 2003a). *Philosophy, Psychiatry, & Psychology*, 10/1: 91–98.

Roessler, J. (2001). Understanding delusions of alien control. *Philosophy, Psychiatry, & Psychology*, 8/2(3): 177–188.

Sabat, S.R. (2001). *The Experience of Alzheimer's Disease: life through a tangled veil*. Oxford: Blackwell Publishers.

Sabat, S.R. and Harré, R. (1997). The Alzheimer's disease sufferer as semiotic subject. *Philosophy, Psychiatry, & Psychology*, 1(3): 145–160.

Sartorius, N. p vii in World Health Organization (1992). *The ICD-10 Classification of Mental and Behavioural Disorders: Clinical Descriptions and Diagnostic Guidelines*. Geneva: World Health Organization.

Sass, L.A. (2003). Commentary "Incomprehensibility and Understanding: On the Interpretation of Severe Mental Illness". *Philosophy, Psychiatry, & Psychology*, 10/2, 125–132.

Sass, L.A. (2004). Some reflections on the (analytic) philosophical approach to delusion. (Commentary for Special Issue on Delusion). *Philosophy, Psychiatry, & Psychology*, 11/1: 71–80.

Schiller, L. and Bennett, A. (1996). *The Quiet Room: a journey out of the torment of madness*. New York: Warner Books.

Schmidt, G. (1987). A review of the German Literature on delusion Between 1914 and 1939. In *The Clinical Roots of the Schizophrenia Concept* (ed. J. Cutting and M. Shepherd). Cambridge: Cambridge University Press, pp. 101–134.

Schneider, K. (1959). *Clinical Psychopathology* (trans. M.W. Hamilton). New York: Grune & Stratton.

Schreber, D.P. (2000). *Memoirs of My Nervous Illness*. New York: New York Review of Books.

Sechehaye, M. (1994). *Autobiography of a Schizophrenic Girl: the true story of 'Renee'*. New York: Penguin.

Shoemaker, S. (1968). Self-reference and self-awareness. *Journal of Philosophy*, 65(19): 555–567.

Sims, A. (1988). *Symptoms in the Mind: an introduction to descriptive psychopathology*. London: Baillière Tindall.

Sims, A., Mundt, C., Berner, P., and Barocka, A. (2000). Descriptive phenomenology. Volume 1, Chapter 1.9, pps 55–70 in *New Oxford Textbook of Psychiatry*. Oxford: Oxford University Press.

Somerset Spirituality Project Group (2002). It would have been good to talk. *Mental Health Today*, October 2002.

Spitzer, M. (1990). On defining delusions. *Comprehensive Psychiatry*, 31(5): 377–397.

Stephens, G.L. (1999). Defining Delusion. (Commentary on Jones, 1999a) *Philosophy, Psychiatry, & Psychology*, 6/1: 25–26.

Stephens, G.L. (2000). Thought insertion and subjectivity. (Commentary on Gibbs, 2000a) *Philosophy, Psychiatry, & Psychology*, 7(3): 203–206.

Stephens, G.L. and Graham, G. (1994a). Self-consciousness, mental agency and the clinical psychopathology of thought-insertion. *Philosophy, Psychiatry and Psychology*, 1(1): 1–10.

Stephens, G.L. and Graham, G. (1994b). Commentary on Chadwick (1994). *Philosophy, Psychiatry and Psychology*, 1(2): 115–116.

Straus, E.W. (1958). Aesthesiology and hallucinations. In *Existence: a new dimension in psychiatry and psychology* (ed. R. May, E. Angel, and H.F. Ellenberger). New York: Basic Books, pp. 139–169.

Styron, W. (1991). *Darkness Visible: a memoir of madness*. London: Jonathan Cape.

Sullivan. M.D. (1995) Key concepts: pain. *Philosophy, Psychiatry. & Psychology*, 2(3): 277–280.

Sutherland, S. (1998). *Breakdown: A personal crisis and a medical dilemma*. Oxford: Oxford University Press.

Swinton, J. (2001). *Spirituality in Mental Health Care: rediscovering a forgotten dimension*. London: Jessica Kingsley Publishers.

Sykes, S. (2002). Commentary: The borderlands of psychiatry and theology. *Philosophy, Psychiatry, & Psychology*, 9(4): 381–382.

Szasz, T. (1974). *The Myth of Mental Illness*. New York: Harper and Row.

Szasz, T.S. (1976) *Schizophrenia: The Sacred Svmbol of Psychiatry*. New York: Basic Books

Thornton, T. (2003). Psychopathology and two kinds of narrative account of the self. *Philosophy, Psychiatry, & Psychology*, 10(4): 361–368.

Wells, L.A. (2003). Discontinuity in personal narrative: some perspectives of patients. *Philosophy, Psychiatry, & Psychology*, 10(4): 297–304.

World Health Organization (1992). ICD-10. *International Classification of Diseases and Related Health Problems* (10th edn). Geneva: World Health Organization.

Wiggins, O.P. (1994). Commentary on Stephens and Graham (1994). *Philosophy, Psychiatry, & Psychology*, 1(1): 11–12.

Wing, J. K., Cooper, J.E., and Sartorius, N. (1974). *Measurement and Classification of Psychiatric Symptoms*. Cambridge: Cambridge University Press.

Wise, T.N. (1994). Normal Grief: Good or Bad? Health or Disease? (Commentary on Kopelman, 1994a) *Philosophy, Psychiatry, & Psychology*, 1(4): 223–224.

Wolpert, L. (1999). *Malignant Sadness*. London: Faber and Faber.

Woody, J.M. (2003). When narrative fails. *Philosophy, Psychiatry, & Psychology*, 10(4): 329–346.

Yalom, I.D. (1981). *Existential Psychotherapy*. New York: Basic Books.

Young, A. and de Pauw, K.W. (2002). One stage is not enough. (Commentary on Gerrans, 2002a). *Philosophy, Psychiatry, & Psychology*, 9/1: 55–60.

CHAPTER 4

Philosophical methods in mental health practice and research

Chapter contents

In Chapter 2 we saw that while the term philosophy covers a broad church, an important strand in Western philosophy has been a concern with concepts, with the framework of ideas— usually of a high level or general kind—by which we organize the world around us. Problems about the concept of mental disorder, correspondingly, turned out to be a particular focus for the new philosophy of psychiatry. In Chapter 3 we filled out the basic 'data' from which philosophical work in this area must start, with an introduction to the wide variety of conditions widely subsumed within the concept of mental disorder.

In this chapter we turn our attention from philosophical problems to philosophical methods. Philosophical methods, like views about what philosophy is, are not only diverse but also themselves the subject of philosophical scrutiny. Hence this chapter, rather than attempting to do justice to the full variety of philosophical methods, will focus on a sample of those that have thus far figured most prominently in the new philosophy of psychiatry.

It happens that these methods have been developed particularly within the two great traditions of twentieth century 'Western' philosophy, called (as we will see, not entirely accurately) Anglo-American analytic philosophy and Continental philosophy. It is important, therefore, before coming directly to these two traditions, to emphasize that there are other great traditions, which in the longer term may prove more fruitful still. Emerging traditions in this regard already include the more meditative and practice-based disciplines of 'Eastern' philosophy–see, for example, the French philosopher, Natalie Depraz', work on schizophrenia (Depraz, 2003); and also the rich resources of classical philosophy, as illustrated by the British philosopher, Christopher Megone's, application of Aristotelian philosophy to concepts of functioning (Megone, 1998, 2000) and the Swedish philosopher, Lennart Nordenfelt's application of Stoic philosophy to cognitive-behavioural psychotherapy (Nordenfelt, 1997). There are also untapped resources in other cultures and language groups. Thus, African philosophy, for example (Gbadegesin, 1991, and Coetzee and Roux, 2002), provides unique insights (inter alia) into the formation and maintenance of personal identity, a deeper understanding of which, as we will see in Part V, is crucial to how we conceptualize (and may come to reconceptualize) a wide variety of mental disorders.

Session 1 Better definitions: philosophy as 'an unusually stubborn effort to think clearly'

You will recall from Chapter 2 William James' characterization of philosophy as a 'an unusually stubborn effort to think clearly'. But how should we go about this? And why does this search have to be 'determined'? Surely we 'know what we are talking about', as we say. And if there are misunderstandings, or if someone uses a word that someone else does not understand, we can just ask them to explain what they mean. 'Define your terms,' as the saying goes. And what are dictionaries for, after all?

In this session we will be digging down a little beneath the surface transparency of language. We will be exploring the scope we have for 'defining our terms' and considering the advantages and disadvantages of definition itself as a way of getting clear about meanings.

As in Chapter 2, we will be starting with an example, though in this case with a non-clinical and (apparently) simple example. Drawing on this example, we will be: (1) looking at the strengths, but also the limitations, of dictionary-type definitions; (2) exploring some of the tensions and trade-offs between different kinds of definition, thinking particularly about the definitions in psychiatric classifications; (3) coming up with a (far from exhaustive) list of seven distinct kinds of definition, reflecting in different ways these tensions and trade-offs; and, finally (4) applying this list to issues in mental health.

How to define 'chair'

So let's start with an everyday, non-clinical, example to look at how we might go about defining our terms.

Starting with an (apparently) simple example, by the way, is itself a feature of (some) philosophical methods. This can be helpful in demonstrating a general point before applying that point to a substantive but more complex case (logic is often taught like this, for example—see Chapter 5). Often, though, what appears to be a simple example turns out to have hidden depths. The meaning of 'bodily disease' in Chapter 2, you will recall, turned out to be considerably more complex than its relatively unproblematic use in practice (compared with the concept of mental disorder) had led everyone to believe. We will find in this chapter that hidden depths are a feature of the meanings of many concepts, non-clinical as well as clinical.

EXERCISE 1	(30 minutes)

How do we search for clear meaning? Think about this with an example in mind (as always, write down your thoughts as you go along). Pick out any everyday object near you: an example would be a chair, but select your own example to work on.

Now, are you clear what 'chair' (or 'door', or 'clock', or 'ceiling', or whatever) means? Write down one or more definitions (if you are working in a group, write your own definitions separately, before comparing notes). Could you define 'chair' for someone who does not speak English? If you did not speak English, or could speak English but had not come across this word before, how would you find out what 'chair' means?

Remember the critical place of *practice* in philosophy. This is especially important in this chapter. If you just read the chapter through in 'passive' mode you will get very little out of it. If you try out the exercises, however, really engaging actively in the argument, you will be starting to develop your own philosophical skills.

How to define 'chair'

For the rest of this session we will be thinking about the concept 'chair'. However, try out the points and follow through the arguments for yourself with whatever object you selected, and preferably with a range of objects, to get a feel for how concepts work and the problems of meaning they raise. From this you will get a better idea of why the search for clear meaning (on this view of philosophy, the philosopher's core activity) has to be in William James' phrase 'particularly determined'.

One common reaction to exercises of this kind is that it all seems a bit dry and, dare one say, trivial. At first sight it seems obvious that everyone (who speaks English) knows what 'chair' means. If you are working in a group, you will probably find that your definitions were along the lines of '...thing to sit on', 'an article of furniture for sitting on', and so forth. There will be variations between definitions even here, of course (an important observation to which we will return). However, they all seem to approximate broadly to the same idea.

Dictionary definitions

So, no philosophical (conceptual) problems here? No 'stubborn' search for clear meaning required from the philosophers? With concepts such as 'chair', the meaning seems clear enough, and if there are differences between us over the details, well, we can always refer to a dictionary.

> **EXERCISE 2** (30 minutes)
>
> Try this for the concepts you are working with. Any reasonable sized dictionary will do. Look up the definition given for your own example. You may find several versions. If so, choose the one nearest to your own definition and write it down. Now look in one or more other dictionaries. Write down the corresponding definitions given in these. Finally, notice any differences between the various definitions you have come up with.
>
> Looking at these definitions, write brief notes on the following questions:
>
> 1. In what ways, if any, do the dictionary definitions differ from each other and from the definitions you brainstormed in exercise 1 of the session?
>
> 2. Why do you think there are these differences even about an everyday and (apparently conceptually uncomplicated) thing like a chair?
>
> 3. Is one or other definition definitely right or wrong?

The *Shorter Oxford English Dictionary* (*SOED*) defines 'chair' as 'A seat for one person; now normally a movable four-legged seat with a rest for the back'. Again, at first glance, this seems reassuringly familiar. Notice, though, that this is a rather more detailed and specific definition than most of our spontaneous definitions will have been: it makes 'chair' a seat for *one person*, for example, thus distinguishing it from, e.g. a settee.

So far so good. But how consistent is this with other 'authorities'? Thus the *Concise Oxford English Dictionary* (*COED*) has it that a chair is a '*separate* seat for one'. So even a dictionary in the same family as the *SOED*, gives a different definition. Hence, turning to a dictionary will not always be enough to resolve differences of view about the meanings even of everyday concepts like 'chair'.

Four kinds of difficulty with defining 'chair'

The difference between the two definitions of 'chair' just noted, one from the *COED* and the other from the *SOED*, illustrates the first of four kinds of difficulty that we run into when we try to define even an apparently simple term such as 'chair', namely that we run straight into a tension between *specifity* and *range* of use.

Difficulty 1: specificity versus range of use

An ideal definition is neither over-inclusive (i.e. it includes too much—thus 'a thing to sit on' includes, e.g. cushion) nor overexclusive (i.e. it excludes too much). However, the attempt to make a definition less inclusive (by making it more specific) always risks it excluding things that in some legitimate understandings of the concept, it should include.

For example, chairs are indeed usually 'separate' (the *COED's* term); however, they need not be (they are not separated in a twin 'baby buggy', for example). There is, certainly, a sense in which any object has to be separable from other objects to be definable at all. But in this sense the *COED's* 'separate seat for one' could be one of the seats in a two-seat settee. And indeed, if the *COED* is right, why are the seats in a theatre not 'chairs'; or in an aeroplane (especially in 'first class' where they may be fully separated)? The *SOED*, avoiding 'separate', introduces the idea that chairs are 'movable'. This explains the theatre and the aeroplane cases up to a point. But the *SOED* says that chairs are 'usually' movable. So, when can a chair be immovable and still a chair? Why are the (relatively) immovable theatre and airline seats not chairs? When, in a word, is a chair not a chair?

Specificity, range of use, and clinical practice

Difficulties of these kinds are thrown up by all definitions. There is always to some extent a tension between specifity and range of use that generates ambiguities and disagreements about the proper sense of the term in question. But does this matter practically?

> **EXERCISE 3** (5 minutes)
>
> Take a few minutes at this stage to think about the practical relevance of the tension between specificity and range of use. Where might this be important in mental health?

We will come across problems of this kind particularly in Part III, when we look at the major psychiatric classifications of mental disorders. Recent attempts to make the definitions in these classifications more specific by using explicit inclusion and exclusion criteria, have resulted in greater reliability (i.e. diagnostic agreement); however, this has been at the expense of certain aspects of validity, notably 'face validity' (i.e. the extent to which a term as defined in the classification corresponds with the way it is understood by patients and practitioners as stakeholders in the classification), and 'construct validity' (i.e. the coherence of the classification with theory—the problem here being that such definitions are disjunctive and classifications based on disjunctive categories are difficult to accommodate in scientific theory and law; see Part III).

A criticism of modern psychiatric classifications has thus been that they fail to capture or correspond with the way mental disorder terms are actually employed. The definition of schizophrenia, for example, in the American classification *The DSM-IV, The Diagnostic and Statistical Manual* (APA, 1994) requires an overall duration for the disorder of more than 6 months (APA, 1994, p. 285, Criterion C). This is to distinguish it from, for example, brief psychotic episodes. However, the WHO's *International Classification of Diseases* (1992) specifies a duration of only 1 month. DSM-IV, to complicate matters further, distinguishes between the duration of individual symptoms (1 month) and of the disorder as a whole (6 months). There are also qualitative as well as quantitative differences. DSM-IV includes a criterion (Criterion B) for schizophrenia that does not appear in ICD-10 at all. (We return to the significance of Criterion B at length in Part IV.)

Authorities vary, therefore, over psychiatric classification. In everyday practice, such very precise definitional points are largely ignored, the diagnostic term being used to cover a relatively wide range of disorders: it is only in research that very specific definitions are required (to allow comparability of results between studies). Note, though, that in the USA, and increasingly in other countries as health-care budgets come under ever-greater pressure, more specific diagnostic categories are demanded clinically.

Difficulty 2: brevity versus depth of understanding

The tension between specifity and range of use leads to a second kind of difficulty with definitions—a tension between on the one hand *brevity*, and, on the other, the *depth of understanding* which can be achieved with a more long-winded treatment.

A brief definition aims to capture the essence of the meaning of a term; however, it has to rely on other terms that may be (and often are—see below) more obscure than the term being defined. A brief definition may therefore actually mask deeper embedded difficulties of meaning. A longer definition, on the other hand, although it can unpack some of these embedded difficulties of meaning, may end up too long-winded to be practically useful.

The idea of *tautology* comes in here. There is a sense in which an accurate definition has to be tautologous (i.e. any definition expresses the same meaning in different terms). In fact some definitions do not rely solely on the meanings of the words they employ and so escape the problem of being tautologous

(see below). In most types of definition, however, their tautologous nature creates a tension between brevity (which is, normally, a function of the degree of precision of the definition in question) and the depth of understanding it offers (which is, normally, a function of the degree of informativeness). To be helpful, therefore, the tautology should be neither so narrow as to be un-illuminating nor so long-winded as to be impractical. (The so-called 'paradox of analysis' is attributed to G.E. Moore; see Langford, 1942.) The problem is this. If one takes philosophical analysis to be an attempt to say what something is (e.g. causation is...; free will is...) then it offers an analysis of a problematic concept P by saying 'P = Q'. But then either 'P' and 'Q' have the same meaning in which case the claim is trivial or they do not in which the identity is false. Either way, Moore argued, it does not seem that philosophy can offer true but non-trivial analysis.

We can see the tension between brevity and depth of understanding being played out in the development of psychiatric classifications. The last edition of the WHO's Classification, the *ICD-9* (WHO, 1978), gave brief synoptic definitions of particular disorders, mostly of not more than four or five lines. *ICD-10* gives much longer descriptions (often a page or two); however, it seeks to preserve the utility of the classification by including summary checklists of key symptoms (e.g. of schizophrenia; WHO, 1992, p. 87). DSM-IV takes this further. DSM-IV gives so much information it can be used as a really helpful stand-alone textbook of psychiatry (at least on diagnostic categories); however, it preserves utility by summarizing the essential diagnostic features of each category in 'boxes' giving key diagnostic criteria.

Difficulty 3: embedded terms and embedded difficulties of meaning

That the tension between brevity and depth of understanding is not special to the definitions of psychiatric terms is evident if we return to the example of 'chair'. Both the *SOED* and the *COED* define chair as a kind of seat and then seek to specify exactly what kind of seat a chair is (as we have seen, in rather different ways). Both definitions are brief, the *COED*'s especially so. 'Seat' includes 'chair', however, so the definition, given the meaning of the embedded term 'seat', seems clear. But is it? Testing this point a little reveals a third kind of difficulty even with such apparently simple definitions as 'chair', namely that they depend on embedded terms the meanings of which, although taken for granted in the definition in question, are in fact very far from transparent.

Thus, suppose that you do not know what 'seat' means. Can you find this out from a dictionary? The *SOED* gives us 'place or thing to sit upon'. But what does 'sit' mean? It is what you do on seats, but this is too narrowly tautological to help. So we look up 'sit'. This means 'of persons, to be or remain in that posture in which the weight of the body rests upon the posteriors...'; and, in turn, 'posteriors' (note the increasingly strained terminology) are 'the hinder parts of the body'.

EXERCISE 4   (5 minutes)

Is this feature of definitions—that as we press them we may unearth hidden difficulties of meaning—hazardous at all? Can you think of any examples, in mental health practice or elsewhere, of a definition giving the *appearance* of clear meaning by relying (explicitly or implicitly) on terms the meanings of which, although taken for granted, are far from transparent?

There is nothing inherently wrong with the embedded nature of definitions. As we have seen, they *have* to be like this. The danger, though, is that the embedded difficulties of meaning are not recognized for what they are. Brief definitions, in particular, useful (indeed essential) as they may be in some contexts, risk masking obscurities of meaning, thus giving the impression of full understanding, where, in reality, understanding is lacking.

Embedded meanings in mental health terms

There are many examples of this in mental health practice, often traceable, ultimately, to difficulties in the meaning of 'mental illness'. We will return to this idea at several points in this book. One example we have already come across (in Chapter 3, on psychopathology) is the standard definitions of 'delusion' as a 'false belief...' (with various further qualifications): in most everyday contexts, we can take the meanings of the terms 'false' and 'belief' to be, if not transparent, at least unproblematic. Hence the apparent transparency of the standard definition of delusion. A moment's reflection, however, shows that neither 'false' nor 'belief' is self-evident in meaning, and, in fact, the standard definition of delusion, as we saw in Chapter 3, turns out to be highly unsatisfactory clinically.

However, it is important to recognize that the definition of 'delusion', and indeed the definitions of other notoriously difficult 'terms of art' in psychiatry, are not alone in depending on the meaning of even trickier embedded terms being taken for granted. This is clearly illustrated by our everyday case of 'chair'. The *SOED* (like the *COED*), you will recall, defined 'chair' as '.... (a kind of) *seat*'; this in turn being defined as 'a place or thing to sit on', and 'sit' being defined as 'of persons, to be or remain, etc.....' Well, we might jib at 'person', the meaning of which is notoriously obscure, at least among philosophers (we return to this in Part V). However, there is difficulty enough further back in the chain of embedded terms, in the definition of the (wholly neglected by philosophers!) term 'seat'. Notice, for example, that in defining 'seat' both dictionaries imply, not merely that seats (whether chairs or not) are sat on, but that they have the *purpose* or *function* of being sat on. The *SOED* has it as a 'place or thing *to* sit upon'; the *COED* is even more explicit, making it a 'thing *used, especially one made, for* sitting on...'. In order, therefore, to understand the meaning of 'chair', we have to understand the meaning of 'seat'; and in order to understand the meaning of

'seat', we have to understand the meaning of 'purpose' and/or 'function'; and with these terms we are swept up into that whole stable of deep philosophical difficulties, in the philosophy of biology, in ethics, in action theory, and so forth, packed into the one word 'teleology'!

So we seem to be getting into deep waters. But just what kind of waters are we in?

EXERCISE 5   (5 minutes)

At this point, take a moment to think about the concepts of 'purpose' and 'function'. Are these radically different from 'chair' or 'seat'? Are they concepts of a qualitatively different kind?

Difficulty 4: from concrete to abstract terms

With the introduction of 'purpose' and 'function', we have fallen back on concepts that are of a radically different kind from our original 'chair' or even 'seat'. To be specific, we have jumped over a divide, from concrete to abstract.

With this divide we come to a fourth kind of difficulty with definitions, namely that as we trace back the embedded terms on which their apparent transparency of meaning depends, these terms become both more general and more abstract. We will come back to the specific difficulties raised by 'purpose' and 'function' at several points in the book. As just noted, they are core concepts not just for mental health but for the whole of biology and the 'human' sciences. As such, they have been subject to endless philosophical dispute and debate, aspects of which we will be covering later in this book. So, if you think you can get clear about their meanings easily, watch this space! This is quite definitely an area where the search for clear meaning has to be determined indeed. And because the meaning of 'chair' depends on the meanings of the terms in which it is defined being taken for granted, the meaning of 'chair', too, turns out to be, as the meaning of 'bodily illness' in Chapter 2 turned out to be, considerably less transparent than it seems.

Concepts are context dependent

We have now looked at four difficulties complicating attempts to define even an apparently straightforward concept such as 'chair': (1) a tension between specificity and range of use; (2) a tension between brevity and depth of understanding; (3) a tendency for definitions to rely on embedded terms the meanings of which may be far from self-evident; and (4) a particular sense in which these embedded terms become less transparent in meaning, namely that they become more general and abstract.

These difficulties are themselves instances of a further feature of concepts, which complicates the search for clear meaning, namely the extent to which meanings themselves are *context dependent*.

The context-dependent nature of concepts is important in mental health. Contrary to the message of the ongoing debate about mental illness (noted in Chapter 2), different classifications, indeed different models of mental disorder itself, are not necessarily competitors. Different models (concepts) may be appropriate for different people and in different contexts. Trading different meanings without falling into confusion is not always easy! But it is important to recognize that context dependence is a feature of concept use in general rather than a 'little local difficulty' for mental health.

Thus, the tensions and difficulties we have looked at—just *how* specific the definition of 'chair' should be, just how *far* the embedded terms should be spelt out, etc.—depend on the context in which a definition is required and the reason *for* which it is required. In the *SOED*, a chair is said to be 'usually [a] moveable four-legged seat with a rest for the back'. So far so good. However, if there were a dispute between, say, the stool-makers union and the chair-makers union, both the number of legs and the presence or absence of a back-rest could become crucial criteria for demarcating their respective territories. Similarly for embedded terms. The *COED* allows a chair to be anything that is used for sitting on (albeit that it is usually 'made for the purpose'). Leaving aside the problem of how to define 'purpose' (critical in philosophy, as noted a moment ago), however, even the term 'made for' could be problematic (what about a 'shooting stick', for example, isn't that 'made for' the purpose of sitting on?).

The context dependence of meaning is evident in other ways. We have assumed so far in this session that in defining 'chair' it was 'chair' as an article of furniture that we were talking about. This assumption was legitimate given the context in which the example was set up, i.e. Exercise 1 above involved picking out an object in the room. However, suppose you had been asked simply, 'define chair'. This would have brought in a range of other, related but distinct, meanings of the term: the *COED* includes (1) seat of authority, e.g. professorship, mayorality; (2) seat of office, e.g. person presiding over a meeting; (3) iron or steel socket holding a railway line in position; and (4) various corresponding verbs.

Different definitions for different purposes

Given all these tension and difficulties with definitions, the question arises, where to stop, where to take the meaning of a term as being sufficiently clear?

This is not pre-fixed. The point at which a definition ceases to be too narrowly tautological to be helpful, the point at which 'other words' illuminate the meaning of the term to be defined, and hence the point at which the definition in question becomes useful, depends on such factors as the given understanding of the person seeking the definition and the uses to which the definition is to be put. In this important sense, everyday definitions (including those we find in dictionaries), and the philosophers' 'search for clear meaning', are both normative in character.

Seven different ways of defining your terms

Dictionaries such as the *COED* and *SOED*, being designed for general reference purposes, offer definitions that, in effect, aim to provide the best overall balance between the various tensions and trade-offs outlined above.

Before finishing this session, it will be worth distinguishing some of the many ways in which, for *particular* purposes and in *particular* contexts, different kinds of definition can be generated. In practice, these are not always clearly distinguished, the different kinds of definition being run together, often without any awareness that this is happening. In the pursuit of clear meaning, however, it can be helpful to recognize different kinds of definition for what they are.

Seven kinds of definition

We will first list seven varieties of definition (the list is not exhaustive!) and then go on to Exercise 6, in which we will look at these in action in different areas of mental health.

1. *Ostensive definition*: pointing out instances, illustrating the meaning of a term by shared experience of actual cases. This is how, directly or indirectly, most descriptive terms are learned. 'Chair', obviously, but also more technical descriptive terms, such as 'mitral heart sound': this sound (a particular noise that the heart makes when one of its values, the mitral valve, is damaged and that a doctor hears through a stethoscope) is described in detail in the medical textbooks; however, could you fully understand what it is without having it pointed out to you and hearing it for yourself?

2. *Conventional definition*: agreement on a meaning by convention. The covention may be more or less explicit. Much of statute law rests on explicitly conventional definitions; a group (with authority) establishes the conventional definitions of 'larceny', 'theft', etc. The Oxford philosopher J.O. Urmson gave the example of 'good apple' as defined by the Ministry of Agriculture (Urmson, 1950).

3. *Persuasive definition*: this is the advertiser's definition. A term is used deliberately to persuade you to attach a given meaning to a concept. A famous book on alcoholism was called *The Disease Concept of Alcoholism* (Jellineck, 1960) in order to persuade people that alcoholism should be understood as a disease.

4. *Declarative definition*: a declarative or formal explanation of the significance of a word or phrase (Oxford English Dictionary (OED), CD-Rom version). For example, the meaning of the word 'gold' must contain a reference to the colour of the element gold, as it is this that supplies the meaning of the predicate 'golden'.

5. *Contextual definition*: definition as revealed by use. A definition that does not provide an equivalent for the expression to be defined, but instead replaces the whole context in which the expression occurs by an equivalent not containing that expression (OED). Thus, in mathematics, an 'incomplete' symbol is one that is defined by its role in a formula or equation—its *use* is thus defined, but in itself it is without

meaning. In practice, many technical and scientific definitions are contextual in this sense—remember the proofs in algebra that start with 'let 'x' stand for . . .'?

6. *Essential definition*: a precise statement of the essential nature of a thing, a statement of form by which anything is defined (OED). Thus, we may define velocity as speed plus direction, or a sentiment as a combination of an idea and an emotion.

7. *Semantic definition*: the action of defining what a word means using only the meanings of other words. Thus the seventeenth century English philosopher John Locke, in his *Essay Concerning Human Understanding* (1690) writes: 'Definition being nothing but making another understand by Words, what idea the Term defin'd stands for' (Bk III, CH.III, §10).

Seven kinds of definition in health care

All seven kinds of definition may be important in health care. Think about this for a moment before going on.

EXERCISE 6   (15 minutes)

Where might distinguishing these seven ways of producing definitions be important in mental health? Make a note of any contexts that occur to you.

The most obvious area in mental health where definitions are important is in the classification of mental disorders. We will be returning to classification and diagnosis later, in Parts III and IV. Psychiatric classification, as we will see, has both descriptive (or factual) and evaluative aspects; hence its appearance in both modules. It can be helpful, however, in understanding how classifications of mental disorders work, to distinguish the different kinds of definition that are woven together in them. As we noted a moment ago, these are not always clearly distinct. However, identifying an element of a particular kind of definition in a mental disorder term, can help us to understand the purpose that term serves practically, what its correct use should be, what would be an incorrect use, and so on. Here are a few examples.

1. *Ostensive definition*. If psychiatry is a branch of medicine, learning the meanings of mental state terms ('phobia', 'obsession', 'delusion') should be like learning the meaning of 'mitral heart sound'. We will see later that learning by shared experience is indeed important here. There is a great deal in the use of classifications that has to be learned 'on the job' and which cannot be conveyed simply by definition in words.

   So far as *ostensive definition* goes, however, there is a difference between something that can be pointed out ('chair', 'mitral heart sound') and something that cannot (i.e. an experience in someone else's mind). At any rate, there *seems* to be a difference. We will need to look very carefully at this later on to get a better grasp of how we come to understand (or may fail to understand) other people's experiences (see especially Part V). Psychiatric classification sometimes takes the form of

a kind of substitute ostensive definition. Instead of trying to define a mental disorder (or symptom) explicitly, examples (or paradigms) are offered that aim to help us 'recognize it when we see it'.

2. *Conventional definition*. This is the basis of all official classification terms, including those used in psychiatry. Recognizing this is the starting point for a whole series of important observations about these classifications: the extent to which they reflect 'natural kinds' (see Part III); how values become (covertly) incorporated into them (see Part IV); and so on.

   A second, and very different, example of conventional definition is what is sometimes called 'operational definition'. This concept, developed originally in the 1920s by the physicist, Bridgman, substitutes for an explicit definition of a term a process (or operation) by which the meaning of the term is realized. Thus Einstein, in one of the thought experiments that led to the theory of relativity, substituted for 'time' the behaviour of precise clocks. Another example would be 'circle'—operationally, this could be defined as the shape marked out by moving in a plane and keeping a fixed distance from a given point.

   The definitions of mental disorders in later editions of both ICD and DSM have sometimes been described as operational, the idea being that they are based on the results of a standardized process of history taking and mental state examination. The use of the term in this context carries overtones of scientific precision and objectivity (an example of persuasive definition!); however, the inclusion and exclusion criteria of these classifications *are* certainly closer to the processes by which diagnoses are made than the synoptic definitions of earlier editions (again, we return to this in Part III).

3. *Persuasive definition*. There is also a good deal of *persuasive definition* in medical classifications. The 'disease concept' of alcoholism (Jellineck, 1960, noted above) was promoted to attract health funds into preventing and treating the condition. Debates during the development of DSM about whether homosexuality or, more recently, 'premenstrual tension', should be included in psychiatric classifications, reflected propaganda (rhetoric!) rather than science—the psychiatric 'advertisers' called the latter 'late luteal phase dysphoric disorder' in order to make it medically and politically acceptable.

4. *Declarative definition*. This is not unlike (indeed it is often a subcategory of) conventional definition. You can think of a declarative definition as a formal enactment of a conventional definition. Thus, the introduction to the DSM includes a definition of 'mental disorder'. The authors of the DSM make clear that they recognize the many difficulties and subtleties involved in defining this term. The ICD, like most textbooks, leaves the meaning of 'mental disorder' implicit (see below, 'contextual definition'). The authors of DSM, however, opted to set out explicitly the definition they chose to adopt and

against which they judged whether a given condition should be included in the classification.

5. *Contextual definition.* This is effectively how the ICD defines 'mental disorder'. Instead of defining the term explicitly, a mental disorder is any condition appearing in the ICD classification. Thus the classification as a whole replaces, and provides an equivalent for, a formal enactment of a conventional definition, without employing the term as such. We will return to the validity of this later. However, it reflects the way many doctors think about diagnosis (i.e. if you don't have a recognized disease then you are not ill!); and it is increasingly how those responsible for health-care budgets operate— insurance companies, for example, may recognize only those conditions that appear on a given list of recognized diseases.

6. *Essential definition.* The DSM includes a summary statement of the precise inclusion and exclusion criteria required for each disorder (i.e. inclusion criteria specify the features that *must* be present for a diagnosis to be made of the disorder; exclusion criteria specify the features that *preclude* that diagnosis). These inclusion and exclusion criteria attempt to capture between them the essential nature of the disorder in question.

Definitions and the illusion of understanding

The slogan 'define your terms', with which we started this session, was traditionally held out as the 'Royal Road' to clear thinking. It is good advice if it is taken as an injunction to be alert to meaning, to think about the meanings of the terms you are using. Meanings are slippery and tricky and often far from transparent: the Oxford moral philosopher R.M. Hare (more on him later) used to say that to be an effective philosopher you have to have good (conceptual) peripheral vision.

You will notice that there is no example in the list above of a semantic definition. In fact, there are elements of semantic definition in all of 1–6, but a *pure* semantic definition (as in a dictionary, for example) tends not to be very helpful in practice precisely because of its tautologous nature. We considered the various features and difficulties raised by this earlier in this session, when we looked at the example of 'chair'.

So, defining your terms *is* important, and it is an activity to which philosophers can contribute. But if this is taken to mean that there is some simple, relatively brief statement waiting for us to capture as the essence of the meaning of a given concept, then this is an illusion.

Ludwig Wittgenstein, the Austrian philosopher whose work (carried out mainly in Cambridge in the inter-war period) did much to expose this illusion, talked of concepts as forming family groups (in his most famous work *Philosophical Investigations*, 1953). This is a helpful image. The concepts we use are evolving, overlapping, variable, and subject to non-rational as well as rational changes; they are not a passive framework within which facts are organized, but engaged in a dynamic interplay with

experience. The search for clear meaning, then, is no mere preliminary defining of terms. It is an open-ended search, requiring all of that 'determination' to which, at the start of this session, William James pointed us.

Reflection on the session and self-test questions

Write down your own reflections on the materials in this session drawing out any points that are particularly significant for you. Then write brief notes about the following:

1. Are dictionaries fully consistent in the definitions they offer of everyday objects like chairs?

2. What are some of the main difficulties with defining everyday objects like chairs? (We noted four.)

3. Are these difficulties confined to defining everyday objects like chairs or do they apply more widely, including in mental health?

4. In how many different ways could you respond to the maxim 'first define your terms'? (We noted seven different kinds of definition.)

5. How many different kinds of definition are important in health care? Give an example of at least one.

6. Having worked through this chapter, how should we understand the maxim 'first define your terms'?

7. What makes a definition meaningful? What makes it useful?

Session 2   Use and definition: J.L. Austin and the Linguistic Analytic (Oxford) move in philosophy

In the last session we found that even an apparently straightforward concept such as 'chair' can be difficult to define adequately. Brief definitions, as in dictionaries, work well up to a point, but only because they are able to take for granted the hidden complexities upon which the full meaning of the word depends. This is not to say that brief definitions as such are unsatisfactory. On the contrary, within a given 'shared discourse' they have genuine explanatory power and can help to sustain clear and consistent language use.

Brief definitions and clinical utility

Brief definitions are important in many areas of the 'shared discourse' of medicine. Hence, as we noted in Session 1, the traditional medical injunction to 'first define your terms'. We will be looking at the value of defining our (medical) terms in later sessions, in particular in relation to psychopathology and classification. A good example of the value of definitions (though also of their hazards, see Part III), is the US–UK Diagnostic Project on Schizophrenia. This showed that reported differences between the US and UK in the prevalence of schizophrenia reflected no more than differences between them in the definitions of schizophrenia being employed (unwittingly) in the two countries (Cooper *et al.*, 1972). Agreeing on a common set of criteria for schizophrenia (an example of conventional definition, see Session 1), has thus improved the consistency of language use in clinical practice and increased the extent to which valid cross-comparisons can be made between research projects.

So, brief definitions, although not necessarily plumbing the full depth of meaning behind a concept, may be helpful. However, the very success of 'defining your terms' in medicine has led to a widespread assumption that clear explicit definition is a *precondition of clinical utility*. That is to say, because *some* difficulties in the uses of our diagnostic concepts have turned out to be due to a lack of clear explicit definitions, it has been assumed that concepts can *only* be useful clinically if their meanings can be set out in this way (Fulford, 2001 and 2003).

From definition to use

The main aim of this session, then, is to undermine the 'first define your terms' assumption by driving a wedge between the definition and use of concepts. We will find that far from use being dependent on definition, there is an important sense in which definition (even in the context of 'scientific' work like the US–UK Diagnostic Project) is dependent on use.

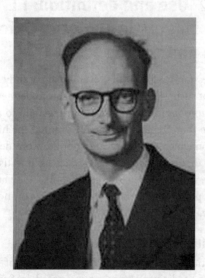

Fig. 4.1 J.L. Austin

This will take us a step towards a better understanding of the debate about mental illness: you will remember from Chapter 2 that this debate started out as a debate about 'mental illness' but ended up as a debate about 'bodily illness', this apparently unproblematic (in use) concept turning out to be highly obscure in meaning. It will also introduce us to a method for tackling some kinds of philosophical problem, a method associated especially with the Oxford philosopher J.L. Austin. Working in the 1940s and 1950s, Austin was among those who emphasized the value of looking at the way a concept is actually used in ordinary language as a guide to its meaning. We will find in later sessions that Austin's work, although not widely fashionable in philosophy at present, is helpful at several points in the search for a deeper understanding not only of the concept of mental illness but also of the conceptual structure of medicine generally.

Use and definition of everyday concepts

We will be reading one of Austin's articles later in this session (Exercise 8). True to his method, though, we will start with a practical exercise.

EXERCISE 7   (30 minutes)

Look around you and list 10 things you see (objects, events, actions, persons, or whatever). Now distribute them in a 2 × 2 table like the one shown in Table 4.1, i.e. according to ease or difficulty of *use*, and ease or difficulty of *definition*.

Take a little time over this. It is not always easy to decide into which box things should go. As you do this, make brief notes on:

1. how often ease/difficulty of use goes with ease/difficulty of *definition* (in other words, if a concept is easy to use, it is likely to be easy to define, and vice versa);

2. just *why* a given concept may be difficult to define and/or use; and

3. overall, which boxes you find most trouble in filling.

Finally, repeat this exercise with terms from medicine and psychiatry (as in Table 4.2 below).

This exercise reinforces the point that definition and use are not correlated. As Table 4.1 illustrates, ease of use may sometimes go with ease of definition (as with 'winner of a race'); and difficult to use may sometimes go with difficult to define (as with 'fine wine'). Equally, though, a concept (like 'time' in Table 4.1) may be easy to use but difficult to define or (like 'genuine Ming vase' in Table 4.1) difficult to use and easy to define. Use and definition thus do not have to go together at all. Contrary to the usual medical view (the 'first define your terms' view), the capacity to use a concept effectively is not dependent on the capacity to provide a clear definition.

Table 4.1 Two-way table of use and definition for everyday concepts

		Definition	
		Easy	Difficult
Use	Easy	Winner (of a race) A 'four' (in cricket)	Time Baroque
	Difficult	Genuine Ming vase Square root of −1	Tort Fine wine

Table 4.2 Two-way table of use and definition for medical concepts

		Definition	
		Easy	Difficult
Use	Easy	Proptosis Aphonia	Delusion Bodily illness
	Difficult	Depressive affect Anaemia	Schizophrenia Mental illness

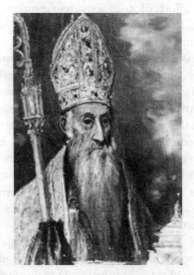

Fig. 4.2 St Augustine

Use and definition of medical concepts

A similar point is made for medical rather than everyday concepts by the table in Table 4.2, which reflects our response to the final part of Exercise 8 above.

Thus, 'proptosis' (bulging eyes) is easy to use and easy to define while 'schizophrenia' is difficult to use and difficult to define (as noted above, schizophrenia is an example of where better definition, provided by the US–UK Diagnostic Project and other research initiatives, led to better use). With other examples, however, ease of use may go with difficulty of definition: 'delusion', like 'time', is a concept that is relatively easy to use clinically (it is a reliably identifiable symptom) yet peculiarly difficult to define (see Chapter 3); and conversely, 'depressive affect' (sadness) is easy to define but often difficult to use (it is not always easy to identify, due to, for example, variation in cultural expression; and it is not reliably differentiated from anxiety).

Again, then, notwithstanding the traditional 'first define your terms', effective use of concepts, in medicine as in everyday non-technical contexts, is not dependent on definition.

Difficulties with concepts

There are many reasons why concepts may be, respectively, difficult to use and/or difficult to define. Recognizing this will be important when we come to consider use and definition in relation to the concepts of bodily illness and mental illness.

For the moment, though, here are just a few examples: difficulties of definition include: (1) complexity of criteria ('baroque', 'schizophrenia'); (2) obscurity of meaning ('time', 'delusion'); and (3) uncertain or inconsistent reference norms ('fine wine', 'tort'). Some of these also apply to difficulty of use, e.g. complexity of criteria for schizophrenia. 'Baroque' and 'time', on the other hand, can be used by and large without difficulty *despite* the extreme difficulties of definition they present. Difficulties of use are more often empirical, involving, for example, fine observational

distinctions ('mitral heart sound'; 'depression', especially its distinction from anxiety), or technical difficulties ('Genuine Ming vase', in Table 4.1 is a concept that is easy to define but difficult to use because the empirical question of whether a particular vase was made in the Ming dynasty is, in practice, difficult to settle).

Both definition and use may present many different kinds of difficulty, then. This is no less true of non-technical areas (concepts taken from around the room, as in Table 4.1) as of technical concepts (medical and psychiatric concepts, as in Table 4.2). In general, though, and coming now to the third question in Exercise 8, we have less trouble in using concepts than defining them. 'Time', one of the examples in Table 4.1, provides an excellent example of this, which we owe to the work of the theologian and philosopher St Augustine.

I know what 'time' is until I think about it

St Augustine was Bishop of Hippo, not far from Carthage in North Africa, in the early decades of the fifth century AD, during the final collapse of the Roman Empire. In Book XI of his *Confessions*, he struggles with the theological paradoxes generated by the notion of an eternal or timeless Creator and a created universe in time. It is only as he comes to think about time that he realizes he does not know what it is. 'So what is . . time?' he asks. 'If no one asks me, I know; if they ask and I try to explain, I do not know' (St Augustine, Confessions, Bk 11, ch. 14, no. 17).

We thought about 'chair' in Session 1 and found that, despite first appearances, even this turned out to be difficult to define. But with 'time' we do not even have a first order stab at a definition to offer. (*Try this for yourself.*) The concept, none the less, is entirely straightforward to use, so much so that it requires an effort of conscious reflection to realize with St Augustine, that in an important sense, we do not (really) know what 'time' means.

Philosophers have sometimes argued that to understand the meaning of a concept is to use it correctly. Thus Wittgenstein (1953), for example, says: 'For a large class of cases—though not for all—in which we employ the word "meaning" it can be defined thus: the meaning of a word is its use in the language.' According to this behaviourist account, we all understand the concept of time. But if so, our understanding is wholly *independent* of the ability to give a clear, explicit definition. Yet it is precisely this ability (to give clear, explicit definitions) that medical science seems to expect in the pronouncement 'first define your terms'.

By and large, then, we are better overall at using concepts than at defining them. This is a hard lesson for most of us to learn, especially in medicine. Yet it makes sense developmentally: we come to understand the meanings of concepts by shared use in a social context rather than by looking them up in dictionaries to find explicit definitions. And once the lesson that we are better at using concepts than defining them *is* learned, it has a number of important consequences for mental health.

I know what 'illness' is until I think about it

One rather general consequence of learning the lesson that we are better at using concepts than at defining them is that it gives us a more positive way of approaching the whole question of the conceptual difficulties raised by mental illness.

Thus, we saw in Chapter 2 that because 'mental illness' is problematic clinically (i.e. in use) while 'bodily illness' is not, the debate about the meaning of 'mental illness' has proceeded on the assumption that 'bodily illness' is relatively easy to define. On this assumption, then, 'bodily illness' has been used as a kind of 'probe' for explaining the meaning of 'mental illness'.

In Chapter 2, we found that this assumption was unwarranted, the debate about mental illness in fact turning on the meaning of '*bodily* illness'. This led us to reframe the debate as a debate about the meaning of 'bodily illness'. We can now reframe the debate more precisely as involving two questions:

1. Why is 'mental illness' problematic *in use*?, and

2. Why is 'bodily illness' relatively *un*problematic in use, *despite* being obscure in meaning?

We will return to the debate about mental illness, and to these two questions, in Chapter 6. The point for now is the effect that reframing the debate in this way has on our attitude to 'mental illness'. So long as difficulties in the use of a concept are equated with lack of a clear explicit definition, psychiatry appears to be merely a muddled or confused version of bodily medicine. This is how it is often portrayed (see Session 3). As the argument proceeds, however, we will find that the conceptual problems associated with the use of

'mental illness', far from being marks of muddle, actually point to aspects of the meaning of 'illness' which are masked by the relatively unproblematic nature of 'bodily illness'. So 'mental illness', not 'bodily illness', will turn out to be the more appropriate 'probe' to the meaning of these difficult concepts.

Use of concepts as a guide to their meaning (philosophical fieldwork)

A first consequence, then, of recognizing the pre-eminence of use over definition is to push back against the negative stereotyping of mental disorder arising from the difficulties associated with it in everyday usage. A second consequence is methodological. This brings us back to Austin. We are, in general, better at using concepts than defining them. Hence, Austin suggested, exploring the use of a concept—'fieldwork in philosophy', as he called it (Austin, 1956/7, p. 25)—may be a better way to get clear about the meaning of that concept than by attempting to define it.

> ### EXERCISE 8   (90 minutes)
>
> Read the two short extracts from:
>
> Austin, J.L. (1968). A plea for excuses. In *The Philosophy of Action* (ed. A.R. White), reprinted. Oxford: Oxford University Press, pp. 19–42 [This is reprinted from original Austin, J.L. (1956/57). A plea for excuses. Proceedings of the Aristotelian Society, 57: 1–30.]
>
> ―――――――――――――――――――――
> Link with Reading 4.1
> ―――――――――――――――――――――
>
> Make brief notes about:
>
> 1. the method of 'doing' philosophy Austin is advocating (and illustrating in the paper as a whole);
>
> 2. what objections there might be to Austin's method; and
>
> 3. the extent to which he claims this to be a panacea for solving philosophical problems.

In this paper, Austin gives a clear statement of his views about philosophical method. He envisages a huge if largely hidden resource of distinctions built up over the lifetime of our culture and embodied in the everyday use that we make of concepts. Actively exploring concept *use*, therefore, rather than the traditional passive reflection on *definition*, is one way to get a clearer understanding of the meanings of the concepts in question.

As we have seen, this approach reflects the fact that our powers of direct introspection on the meanings of our concepts are really quite limited. The Austrian-born Cambridge philosopher, Ludwig Wittgenstein, who preceded but overlapped with Austin, drew an essentially negative conclusion from this. As with any major philosopher there is a whole literature about the possible interpretations of his view (see, e.g. Baker, 2003). For our purposes, though, we can take the nub of his position to be that when philosophers (or other people) try to think directly about the meaning of a concept, they inevitably focus on one or other aspect of its meaning and neglect others. This leads to what are in effect illusions (one-sided or otherwise distorted perceptions) of language. Wittgenstein writes of 'grammatical illusions' (Wittgenstein, 1953, §110), of being 'bewitched' by language. The way to solve philosophical problems, then, according to one interpretation of this passage, is to bring the grammatical illusions to light, to reveal the mistaken assumptions that are the origin of much philosophical theorizing. In effect, Wittgenstein suggested that we should reject all philosophical theory.

'Ordinary', technical, and lay usage

Note by the way, that the term 'ordinary usage', as employed by Wittgenstein, means ordinary as distinct from philosophical usage: it thus includes technical as well as lay usage. A psychiatrist's use of the term 'delusion' in everyday clinical contexts is 'ordinary usage' in this sense. A lay person's use of the term 'delusion' is also 'ordinary usage'. A philosopher, or indeed a psychiatrist or lay person, trying to *define* 'delusion' is involved in philosophical usage (in this 'ordinary language' philosophical sense). Austin, as Warnock indicates in the next reading, distinguishes technical (as in law) and non-technical (lay) usage. But both are equally resources for his 'philosophical fieldwork'.

Modest claims for philosophical fieldwork

For Wittgenstein, then, philosophical problems were no more than pseudo-problems, artefacts of the philosophical enterprise. Austin took a more positive view, regarding ordinary usage as a resource on which philosophers may draw in exploring the meanings of concepts.

A modest methodology

Coming, though, to questions 2 and 3 in Exercise 9, Austin is careful not to overstate the case. Linguistic analysis (as this approach came to be known) is not a panacea. Its critics have often pointed out (*contra* Wittgenstein) that if ordinary usage is taken as a guide to meaning, it may well incorporate all the obscurities and deep metaphysical difficulties that philosophical analysis seeks to explicate. But as G.J. Warnock (another Oxford philosopher, and one of Austin's literary executors) has emphasized (G.J. Warnock, 1989), Austin was quite clear that linguistic analysis is at most one way of getting started with some kinds of philosophical problem.

> ### EXERCISE 9
> (20 minutes)
>
> Read the two extracts from Warnock's philosophical biography of Austin:
>
> Warnock, G.J. (1989). *J.L. Austin*. London: Routledge
>
> ---
>
> Link with Reading 4.2

Warnock's 'oft-quoted passages' from Austin are those given in the last exercise. In what sense does he think the usual interpretation of these passages is the wrong way up?

Also, how many parallels can you spot between law and psychopathology in what Warnock says about Austin's choice of excuses as an appropriate place for 'philosophical fieldwork'?

Warnock's introductory chapter gives a succinct and well balanced account of Austin's 'method'. His bottom line is that this has often been overblown! There is no 'method', in the sense of a fully worked up, detailed approach, beyond the basic point about philosophical fieldwork.

The 'usual interpretation', moreover, is upside down in the sense that, in these passages at least, Austin is not so much advocating a method (in general) as suggesting that *if* one wants to work on excuses (and by implication agency), then this approach (of doing some fieldwork among legal cases) is a good way of getting started. And in this very limited sense, much of what Warnock/Austin says about law (in the second paragraph of this extract), applies to psychopathology. In both, there is 'useful material to hand', and

* '…an immense miscellany of untoward cases'…together with
* '…a good deal of acute analysis …'. Both also…
* …extend the resources of non-technical language since they face '…an immense variety of novel and complicated questions…', and
* there is a pressure of necessity, since, unlike philosophy, '…we have to *decide*'.

The methodological claim, then, of Austin's paper is modest indeed. But, as a modest claim, it is as apposite to philosophy and mental health as to Austin's topic of excuses.

A modest metaphysics

Philosophical fieldwork, on the other hand, does have *some* contribution to make to the traditional 'problems of philosophy'. As a moral philosopher, Austin was interested in the nature of agency and action. These concepts raise, in traditional philosophy, deep problems of causation, free will, determinism, and so forth. Rather than tilting directly at such deep problems, however, Austin seeks to learn something more modest about some of the components of agency and action by looking at a range of cases where actions fail or go wrong. This is his 'plea for excuses'. We *excuse* something we have done by claiming that in some sense it was not fully *our own* action (in an Austinian example, I knocked over the salt, but intended only to pick up the glass: my excuse— 'it was an accident').

Much the same, correspondingly, is true of psychopathology. Here, too, the deep problems of general philosophy lurk just below the surface of the subject. Austin indeed says as much at the end of his paper, pointing to abnormal psychology as a further resource for philosophers interested in studying action (Austin, 1968, p. 42).

A modest contribution to mental health

As a philosophical method, then, philosophical fieldwork, although not an end in itself, still less the only game in town, does have a role to play. As Austin himself (in Reading 4.1) put it, 'Certainly, then, ordinary language is *not* the last word: in principle it can everywhere be supplemented and improved upon and superseded. Only remember, it *is* the *first* word.' (Austin, 1968, p. 27). As the first word, moreover, whatever its limitations as a philosophical method in general, examining ordinary language turns out to be peculiarly appropriate to the kind of conceptual problems which are practically important in medicine and mental health.

EXERCISE 10	(5 minutes)

Before moving to the next part of this session, think for a moment about the claim made at the end of the last paragraph. Write down as many reasons as you can think of why the linguistic analytical method, Austin's 'ordinary use as a guide to meaning', may be helpful in medicine and mental health.

As we have emphasized, the linguistic analytical method is only one way of 'doing philosophy'; it is only one way of pursuing William James' 'stubborn effort to think clearly' (see last session). We will be looking at other important methods before the end of this chapter.

None the less, linguistic analysis *is* important in medicine and psychiatry for several reasons:

1. *The right level of problem*. It is at the Austinian level of ordinary usage that conceptual problems arise in practice. Difficulties, *conceptual* difficulties, in the use of 'mental illness', are not, as such, 'merely' philosophical. They do reflect deeper philosophical difficulties (see Chapter 6). But as difficulties arising in ordinary (as distinct from philosophical) usage, they are difficulties arising at the clinical (and/or research) coal-face.

2. *Useful results*. We do not have to trace these conceptual problems to their metaphysical roots to get clinically useful results. Austin, as we saw, focuses in his paper on everyday excuses rather than attempting a (direct) assault on 'freedom of the will'! Correspondingly, therefore, just as the conceptual problems with which we are concerned in mental health arise at the level of ordinary clinical usage, so any *clarification* of these problems is necessarily at the same clinically relevant level. (We come to a clinical example of this in Chapter 6.)

3. *Well-defined parcels*. The linguistic analytical approach tackles conceptual problems in manageable parcels. General philosophical theorizing often seems excessively open-ended for practitioners whose essential requirement is to take action, to decide and to do. Linguistic analysis, with its focus on actual use, encourages a closer connection with practical utility. (Again, we come to examples of this in Chapter 6.)

4. *Cases and case studies*. The linguistic analytical method is (partly) empirical and often case based. These features of the method 'gel' naturally with the methods with which practitioners are familiar. They also make linguistic analysis a natural partner of all the techniques of empirical research— statistical, methodological, and so on—used in such areas as sociology and anthropology. Austin's critics complained that he operated at an amateur level as a linguist (Fann, 1969). But he died relatively young and who knows how far, given time, he could have developed the method through partnerships with other disciplines. In 'A plea for excuses', he was working in partnership with law; however, psychology, ethnography, comparative linguistics, history, and so on are all natural partners of philosophical linguistic analysis. The method is thus capable of potentially very rich interdisciplinary connections. (See Reading Guide for examples.)

5. *A connection with deep metaphysics*. Although not primarily metaphysical in focus, the method may contribute to the analysis of the traditional problems of philosophy. Austin worked on excuses as a step towards analysing the concept of action as a contribution to the philosophy of action. Thus, although the conceptual problems of mental health arise at the level of ordinary usage, like most problems of this kind they reflect deeper metaphysical difficulties and thus provide at the very least, a resource of examples for general philosophy.

This means that general philosophy as a whole (not just the linguistic analytical method) is relevant to mental health. It also means, conversely, that the problems of mental health are critically relevant to general philosophy. For example, if various kinds of psychopathology may impair responsibility, and if this in turn reflects issues about freedom of the will, philosophy has in principle something to offer mental health. But mental health, conversely, through the rich variety of forms of psychopathology it covers, may have much to offer philosophy. Austin indeed makes exactly this point at the end of his paper, encouraging philosophers to examine abnormal psychology as a rich resource for the philosophy of action. More recently, the Oxford philosopher, Kathleen Wilkes, argued that philosophy of mind as a whole should give up its current reliance on 'thought experiments' and turn instead to the rich resources offered by psychopathology (Wilkes, 1988).

There is thus considerable potential for *two-way* exchange between philosophy and practice by way of the conceptual problems arising in ordinary usage in mental health. Here, perhaps above all, there is in the resources of ordinary (technical as well as lay) usage, '...gold in them thar hills', as Austin put it (Austin, 1968, p. 24).

Who wears the trousers?

But Austin has yet one further point to make, directly relevant to the importance of psychopathology (and hence to reframing our view of the 'problem' of mental illness). This is summed up in his memorable, if politically unreconstructed, aphorism to the effect that in linguistic analysis it is often the negative word that may 'wear the trousers' (Austin, 1968, p. 32).

We can see what he meant by this if we think back to the last session for a moment. Recall how even the concept of 'chair' turned out to have hidden depths of difficulty. Austin's point was that much of the difficulty inherent in the meanings of concepts is effectively hidden by the ease with which we normally use them. It is the facility with which we are able to use even deeply obscure concepts, such as time, that hides their complex meanings behind what Austin called 'the blinding veil of ease and obviousness' (Austin, 1968, p. 23).

Well, there is nothing easy or obvious about the concept of mental illness. We noted above that a first consequence of recognizing the pre-eminence of use over definition is to push back against the negative stereotyping of mental disorder arising from the difficulties associated with the concept in practice. Austin's final point takes this a step further, showing that these difficulties may actually provide a valuable window on the meanings of the medical concepts. The bottom line, then, as we will see in later sessions, is what one of us has called elsewhere, 'mental health first' (Fulford, 2000). The bottom line, just as Austin anticipated, is that the trickiness of the negative concept of mental illness, far from being a mark of muddle, actually points directly to important if all too easily overlooked aspects of the meaning of the apparently more transparent concept of bodily illness.

Reflection on the session and self-test questions

Write down your own reflections on the materials in this session drawing out any points that are particularly significant for you. Then write brief notes about the following:

1. Does ease of 'use' of a term go with transparency of 'definition'? Either way, think of at least one example.

2. What are the implications for the stigmatizing of mental health compared with bodily health, of the fact that the concept of 'mental illness' is not only difficult to define (like the concept of 'bodily illness') but also difficult to use (unlike the concept of 'bodily illness')?

3. What did Austin call the philosophical method that exploits our greater ability to use than to define concepts?

4. What are the strengths and limitations of Austin's method?

5. Which is the more likely to be illuminating about the meaning of 'illness', mental illness or bodily illness?

6. What does 'ordinary usage,' as in Austin's 'philosophical fieldwork' model of how to get started with a philosophical problem, include?

Session 3 Illness and disease: definition and ordinary usage

In the last two sessions we have looked at the work that can be done towards clarifying the meanings of concepts, first by defining them explicitly, then by examining the way they are used.

In this session we return to the debate about mental illness but focusing on the concept of bodily illness. You will recall from Chapter 2, that one outcome of the Szasz/Kendell version of the debate about mental illness was to point the analytical finger at bodily illness. It was the meaning of bodily illness about which Szasz (1960) and Kendell (1975) disagreed, not, as they thought, mental illness. Hence a more careful analysis of bodily illness was called for.

In this session, we consider such an analysis by way of definition. We look at an ingenious attempt by the American philosopher, Christopher Boorse, to define mental illness by way of a more careful definition of the concept of bodily illness. The key to Boorse's approach, as we will see, is to draw a distinction that we have so far ignored, between 'illness' and 'disease'.

Boorse on the distinction between illness and disease

In much of the debate about mental illness, and notably in the papers we examined in Chapter 2 by Thomas Szasz and R.E. Kendell, the terms 'illness' and 'disease' are used interchangeably. In everyday English these terms, although often used as synonyms, can also express the distinction between, broadly speaking, a *patient's experience of illness* and *medical or specialist knowledge of disease*.

The distinction between illness and disease can be analysed in a number of ways (see Fulford, 1989, chapter 2). Christopher Boorse (1975), in an important and widely cited paper, developed a particular technical form of the distinction, specifically targeted at improving our understanding of the concept of mental illness.

EXERCISE 11   (2 hours)

Read the following article:

Boorse, C. (1975). On the distinction between disease and illness. *Philosophy and Public Affairs*, 5: 49–68

Link with Reading 4.3

Make brief notes on:

1. Boorse's view of the problem of mental illness.

2. How he conceives the distinction between illness and disease.

3. The use that he makes of this distinction in attempting to resolve the problem of mental illness.

4. Any strengths and/or weaknesses of Boorse's account, in particular of his central treatment of the concepts of 'illness' and 'disease'.

It is important to think about these points for yourself before going on. The temptation is just to skim Boorse's paper (or not read it at all!), and to jump directly to the account given below. Remember, though, that learning philosophy is not primarily a matter of absorbing facts. It involves learning new skills. Hence, like all skills acquisition, it is critically dependent on practice, with appropriate feedback. You learn philosophy by *doing* it. This is what the exercises in this book aim to achieve: a problem is set up, you do some work on it, and only then get feedback.

Boorse's paper is rich and detailed. It illustrates the power of philosophical work directed towards clearer understanding of the meaning of concepts by direct reflection on their definitions. Here are some notes on the four questions you have been thinking about. Don't take them as 'gospel'. Think about them; compare them with your own notes; see if you agree or disagree with them.

1. *Boorse's view of the problem represented by mental illness.* Like Szasz and Kendell, in Chapter 2, Boorse takes mental illness to be the target problem. He recognizes, though, that the development of a better definition of *bodily* illness is central to making progress in understanding the concept of mental illness.

Also like Szasz and Kendell, he identifies the value-ladenness of mental illness as being central to its problematic nature. In terms of our map of the logical terrain of mental health (see above, Chapter 2), Boorse argues that the real problem with mental illness is its territorial ambitions. Psychiatry, he says, is laying claim to more and more of life's problems. It is the 'medicalisation of morals' that is the danger, as the territory of 'mental disorder' is allowed to extend further and further to the left of the map. The way to put a stop to this, he says, is to establish a value-free science of health (here he is back with both Szasz and Kendell), a science that can tell us unambiguously which conditions are properly within, and which are not within, the territory of medicine.

2. *Boorse's core distinction, between 'illness' and 'disease'.* Recall that both Szasz and Kendell moved fairly quickly to definitions of bodily illness. We noted at the time that a definition of '*disease*' would not necessarily be, as both authors assumed, an appropriate mould or template for deciding the validity of this or that concept of *illness*, mental or otherwise.

Boorse avoids this conflation. Indeed his argument shows that in a critical respect, 'disease' is *not* an appropriate template for 'illness'. He draws attention to an important feature of 'illness' by which, in general, it is distinguished from 'disease', namely that it is more overtly value-laden. As

you will have gathered from his paper, he identifies 'disease' with scientific medical theory, 'illness' with the application of that theory to practice. He defines 'disease', broadly as Kendell (1975) did, in terms of 'biological disadvantage'. Boorse has a more sophisticated analysis of what it is for a function to be impaired (see Reading Guide for a sample of Boorse's other papers). But, like Kendell, he takes survival and reproduction to provide key *factual* criteria (he identifies these as 'apical goals' towards which the functioning of all an organism's parts are directed). 'Illness', on the other hand, is a value concept. It is defined by adding an evaluative element to the concept of disease. An illness is a disease which is 'serious enough to be incapacitating' (p. 4).

Boorse's separation of 'illness' and 'disease' has many advantages:

(a) it is consistent with ordinary use (in as far as they are distinct, we use 'disease' of medical scientific theories, 'illness' of our direct experience of being ill);

(b) it allows for the self-evidently value-laden nature of the experience of illness, whether mental or bodily (to be ill is to be in a bad condition, other things being equal); and

(c) it gives Boorse what he is after, a value-free science of health by which, in principle, the proper scope of medicine can be defined, a science 'continuous with biology and the other basic sciences'.

3. *How Boorse applies this to the demarcation of 'mental illness'.* Boorse (1975) has relatively little to say about the concept of mental illness in this paper: he writes about it in detail in a second paper (Boorse, 1976a). He presages his general line of argument in his first paper (Boorse, 1975), though, when he says that the demarcation between medicine and morals in mental health should be made by reference to scientifically defined norms of mental functioning. Mental diseases, then, are defined in precisely the same way as bodily diseases. Of course, the science of psychology is not as well-developed as that of biology. Hence, he says, we lack norms of mental functioning against which to make the relevant comparisons in many cases. But the principle, at least, is clear; and as psychology and the related brain sciences develop, so the demarcation of genuinely *medical* territory among mental disorders will become clearer in practice.

The relatively value-laden nature of 'mental illness', meanwhile, is legitimate. It reflects the value-laden nature of the concept of illness, which in the case of 'mental illness', lacks, to this point in time, the relevant scientific disease criteria to mark out medicine from morals. 'Mental illness' differs from 'bodily illness' only contingently, then, by the current lack of an adequate science of the mind.

4. *Some strengths of Boorse's argument.* Boorse takes seriously the value-laden nature of the medical concepts while at the same time recognizing the importance of medical science. As an

argument about 'mental illness', therefore, his model represents a significant advance on the polarized pro-psychiatry/antipsychiatry debate. He is able to acknowledge and thus seek an explanation for the value-laden nature of 'mental illness' (rather than simply denying it or seeking to define it away, as Kendell does); at the same time, though, he is able to provide a central place for future scientific advances in understanding mental disorder (which Szasz's position, taken literally, would preclude; though as noted in Chapter 2, Szasz says that when we find a 'lesion' to explain schizophrenia he will accept it as a genuine illness, albeit a bodily illness).

Boorse's value-free definition of disease

Boorse's model is a sophisticated form of what has become widely known as the 'medical' model. In fact, this is a large group of models. (The American philosopher, Ruth Macklin (1973), gives an excellent summary of the varieties of medical models in the literature.) The term, though, serves as a generic for the kind of model of medicine that most doctors more or less explicitly hold. This model assumes that medicine is, at heart, a science; in medicine, facts are accumulated and built into disease theories, which in their fully developed form, are set out in terms of disturbances of well-defined bodily and/or mental functions.

As in Boorse's model, then, the medical model takes the theoretical basis of medicine to be defined by three elements—facts, diseases, and disturbances of function. Many doctors will acknowledge that there is more to medicine that just science. But, as also in Boorse's model, it is science that is at the core: values and the patient's experience of illness are important but peripheral. As specifically *medical* concerns, these are secondary to and dependent on the body of scientific theory by which the proper scope of medicine is defined.

Boorse's model is shown diagrammatically in Figure 4.3. As a model, which is immediately recognizable to the medical mind, it is consistent also with much thinking in psychiatry—in forensic psychiatry, for instance, psychiatrists have sometimes sought to limit their expertise to 'scientific' questions of mental disease, leaving issues of responsibility, with their value-laden overtones, to others.

But is this model correct? You will probably have come up with a number of problems with the model when you were thinking about question 4 of Exercise 11 (above). Many of these are similar to the problems with Kendell's model (both models rely, ultimately, on the same 'biological' criteria). We can also ask, is Boorse's account of 'function' correct? Is his account of the relationship between illness and disease correct (e.g. it explains cases where we can say that someone has a disease but is not ill; however, does it explain cases where we want to say that someone is ill (physically ill) when we do not know whether they have a disease in Boorse's sense? For a discussion of some of these issues, see Fulford, 1989, chapters 2 and 3).

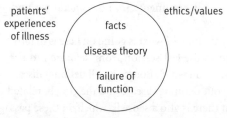

Fig. 4.3 As in Boorse's account, most doctors conceive of medicine as being based on a value-free body of scientific disease theory, which, in its fully developed form, is cast in terms of disturbances of the functioning of bodily and/or mental systems. The patient's experience of illness, their values, and the incapacities (or disturbances of action), which are the key features of the experience of illness, are recognized to be important but they are marginalized.

Boorse's value-laden use of disease

A more critical question, though, is whether Boorse's central claim to have established a value-free definition of disease (and with it a value-free science of health, and with this an unambiguous scientific criterion for demarcating genuine mental illness), is correct.

EXERCISE 12	(10 minutes)

Before going on, go back to Boorse's paper (1975) and re-read from the bottom of p. 56 to, and including, the top half of p. 59. In this passage, he offers two definitions of disease. In each case, think carefully about Boorse's own *use* of words, in particular as they reflect his use of the concept of disease. Is he consistent? If not, what might this tell us about the concept of disease?

This passage is central to Boorse's argument. It summarizes the connection he requires between disease and function and then extends the definition of disease to take account of endemic diseases. He thus offers two definitions of disease both of which are value-free: a disease is (1) a 'deviation from (statistically) normal functioning', and (2) a deviation that is 'mainly due to environmental causes' (see p. 59). Thus far, Boorse is consistent.

The critical shift from definition to use

But now notice this. Immediately after defining disease in these value-free ways, value terms leap back in: four lines after disease has been defined value-free as a 'deviation' from a statistical norm (of functioning), it becomes the value-laden '*deficiency* in functional *efficiency*' (emphasis added); and correspondingly, in the same passage, immediately after the definition of disease has been extended by the value-free 'due to environmental causes', it becomes the value-laden '*hostile* environment' (again, emphasis added).

So, Boorse is inconsistent. 'So what?' you may say. Is this not merely a slip of the pen? Well, hardly, for Boorse is a careful philosopher, and at this point in his paper he is establishing the very core of his argument. So, how *should* we understand this inconsistency?

One way to think of what is going on here is in terms of the shift introduced in the last session from *definition* to *use*. Of course, there is a sense in which Boorse is still defining disease—his whole paper is about defining disease and the closely related concept of illness. But there is also a sense in which, in these passages, having explicitly *defined* the concept of disease he then goes on to *use* it. And it is a crucial observation about his *use* of the concept of disease that, once his eye is off the definitional ball, value terms slip straight back in. What this suggests, given the thrust of Session 2 (that use is a better guide to meaning than definition), is that 'disease', despite its more 'scientific', and less overtly value-laden, appearance compared with 'illness', is after all a value term. Boorse (1997) firmly resists this conclusion. But if even Boorse cannot *use* 'disease' value-free, and even in the context of a paper the whole aim of which is to establish a value-free definition of the term, this suggests, from a linguistic analytic perspective, that an evaluative element really is essential to its meaning. We follow up some of the implications of this in Chapter 6.

Reflection on the session and self-test questions

Write down your own reflections on the materials in this session drawing out any points that are particularly significant for you. Then write brief notes about the following:

1. In so far as they are distinct, how do the terms 'illness' and 'disease' differ in their everyday usage.

2. How does Boorse develop this distinction into a more formal version of the medical-scientific model?

3. In what important ways does Boorse's analysis represent an advance on the Szasz/Kendell debate and earlier work on 'biological dysfunction' analyses of the medical-scientific model?

4. In what respect does Boorse's *definition* of 'disease' differ from his own *use* of the term?

5. What is the significance of the difference between Boorse's use and definition of 'disease' from the perspective of Austin's 'philosophical fieldwork'?

Session 4 Anglo-American and Continental philosophy

So far in this chapter we have concentrated on two ways of exploring the meanings of concepts, directly by careful definition, indirectly by way of their actual uses. As we have seen, both are relevant to many of the conceptual problems arising in day-to-day practice and research in mental health.

We will be looking at some of the products or outcomes of these ways of analysing concepts in Chapter 6. But before going on, we need to set them in context with the main traditions of philosophy and to consider a selection of the many other philosophical perspectives and methods available. As we will see, many of these are important for research and practice in mental health. Indeed, part of the richness of the new philosophy of psychiatry consists in the range of philosophies relevant in principle to mental health, and, vice versa, the range of problems in mental health available as material for philosophical research of different kinds.

With many schools of philosophical work, it is easier to illustrate their approaches than to define them. Hence in what follows we will often be referring you to examples. We will be returning to many of them in detail in later sessions. The idea of this session is just to give you a first impression of the scope and diversity of philosophical approaches relevant to mental health.

We begin the session with a brief overview of two major intellectual orientations by which philosophy was characterized through much of the twentieth century, Anglo-American and Continental.

The split between Anglo-American and Continental philosophy

For much of the twentieth century, Western philosophy has been broadly separated into two main traditions, generally called Anglo-American and Continental. Both traditions include many subdivisions, and the traditions themselves also overlap. However, they may be distinguished roughly thus:

- *Anglo-American philosophy* has been more analytic in orientation, seeking explicit understanding of the meanings of high-level concepts such as agency, mind, person, and so on. The approach, indeed, has been called, simply, analytic philosophy. The distinction between definition and use, as explored in this chapter, is associated particularly with Anglo-American philosophy (through J.L. Austin).

- *Continental philosophy* has generally sought to explore meaning and ethical value through a more intuitive understanding of human experience and expressiveness. Its three main subdivisions are *phenomenology*, *existentialism*, and *hermeneutics* (see below).

Both kinds of philosophy can be thought of as working at the edge of the meaningful. Yet as they split apart, they became increasingly suspicious of each other, essentially because their basic assumptions and methodologies appeared so radically different. Anglo-American philosophy sought explicit clarification of concepts and the structure of reason; Continental philosophy was more implicit, seeking better understanding of the human predicament. Yet in mental health, in which the most radical *failures* of meaning are to be found, the two approaches are entirely complementary. Here, above all, philosophy, in helping us to explore meanings, can draw to excellent effect on both approaches.

The linguistic turn

The origins of the split in philosophy into these two great traditions are complex. One important factor was a development in late nineteenth century philosophy that culminated in the early twentieth century in what came to be called 'the linguistic turn'. Certain influential philosophers during this period gradually became convinced that the key to improving the understanding of philosophical problems lay in the study of language. No one philosopher can be credited with precipitating the linguistic turn; many were involved in what was a gradual process, and it came to maturity only in the 1920s.

So far as the split in philosophy was concerned, the effect of the linguistic turn was indirect. It did not, directly, cause philosophy to split into two subdisciplines; its effect was rather to emphasize the differences between the two traditions in philosophy, each of which had been gradually taking shape for at least a century. The focus on language was then taken up particularly by that strand of philosophy that later came to be called 'Anglo-American'.

The origins of Anglo-American philosophy

The name 'Anglo-American philosophy' reflects the fact that the analytic tradition, which grew out of the linguistic turn, has been most influential in Britain and America. In its origins, however, it is strongly European—the Oxford philosopher of language, Michael Dummett, has suggested that a more appropriate name for this philosophical tradition should be 'Anglo-Austrian', in recognition of its geographical origins (Dummett, 1993).

Thus, four key figures, who established the tradition in the first half of this century, were all either German-speaking or English: Gottlob Frege (working at the University of Jena between 1890 and 1925, his most influential work being *On Sense and Meaning*, 1892); the Cambridge philosopher G.E. Moore (who worked on ethics and the theory of knowledge from around the turn of the century until the 1950s, his best-known work being *Principia Ethica*, 1903); Bertrand Russell, also at Cambridge (especially important being his work on logic and the foundations of mathematics, which culminated in a book co-written with the Cambridge philosopher, A.N. Whitehead, *Principia Mathematica*, 1910); and Ludwig Wittgenstein (we met Wittgenstein earlier; he was Austrian, but worked mainly at Cambridge).

Moore and Russell were most influential during their lifetimes; Wittgenstein has had a continuing influence; Frege was unfashionable for a while (essentially because Russell exposed certain fundamental flaws in his logic of mathematics), but there is currently renewed interest in his work on the relationship between thought and language (see, e.g. Dummett, 1981).

Logical Positivism and the Vienna Circle

The formative years of Anglo-American philosophy were contemporaneous with the birth of the philosophical and scientific movement known as Logical Positivism. In fact, many influential figures were common to both.

As a detailed philosophy, Logical Positivism was developed by a group of philosophers based mainly in Vienna. This 'Vienna Circle', as the group came to be known, included many of the big names of pre-Second World War philosophy—Maurice Schlick, Rudolph Carnap, Herbert Feigl, Kurt Gödel, and Otto Neurath. It was following a visit to this group that the young Oxford philosopher, A.J. Ayer, wrote *Language, Truth and Logic* (first published in 1936), virtually single-handedly introducing Logical Positivism to the English-speaking world. The influence of Logical Positivism declined sharply after the Second World War, but Anglo-American philosophy has continued to maintain a strong interest in the philosophy of the natural sciences (see, for example, Reichenbach, 1951).

With the rise of Nazism in the 1930s, members of the Vienna Circle were forced to relocate, mostly to America. It was partly through this dispersion that analytic philosophy came to be so influential on both sides of the Atlantic. (We return to logical positivism in Part III.)

Three kinds of Continental philosophy

The three main subdivisions of Continental philosophy, as noted above, are *phenomenology*, *existentialism*, and *hermeneutics*. As with Anglo-American philosophy, these are heterogeneous and overlapping (many philosophers in the Continental tradition have worked in more than one area). None the less, the terms mark distinct philosophical approaches, each of which has been important in different ways to philosophy and mental health. We will look briefly at these by way of introduction and then consider each of them in more detail.

Phenomenology and existentialism put people first. *Phenomenology* (as it has been understood since the work of the German philosopher Edmund Husserl in the early twentieth century) is a philosophical method: it seeks in human awareness, and the structure of consciousness, the ways in which we structure and give meaning to experience. Husserl's greatest pupil, Martin Heidegger, moved away from Husserl's later focus on transcendental methodology (i.e. reasoning beyond the limits of experience) and his idealism, preferring instead to develop Husserl's earlier ideas on the nature of lived experience. Heidegger is probably unique in being highly influential on all three main strands of Continental philosophy. The influence of both Husserl and Heidegger is evident in the work of later phenomenologists, including the French philosophers Jean-Paul Sartre and Maurice Merleau-Ponty.

Existentialism, founded by the nineteenth century Danish philosopher Søren Kierkegaard, is a philosophical attitude or position, which in its twentieth century form, has developed largely out of phenomenology. Its defining claim is that existence precedes essence: in other words, there are no 'essences' independent of our individual existences; we create the world as we know it through our actions. In the second quarter of the twentieth century existentialism was developed into a school of philosophical thought by the writings of Heidegger, the German philosopher–psychiatrist Karl Jaspers, and the French philosophers Gabriel Marcel and Jean-Paul Sartre. There is an emphasis in existentialism on the understanding of the individual's subjective view of the world and his/her place in it, and it is in this sense that existentialism is like phenomenology in putting people first.

Hermeneutics is often characterized in such terms as 'it takes as primitive the semiology of discourses'. This rather grandiose phrase just means that it seeks to provide a clearer understanding of language through the interpretation of the meanings of instances of discourse and the texts in which they appear. The German philosopher Hans-Georg Gadamer has done most to shape contemporary philosophical hermeneuticism, drawing on the influence of Martin Heidegger (as above). There is also an Italian school of hermeneutics (which stresses the *techniques* of interpretation rather than the intuitive and existential nature of Gadamer's hermeneutics) of which the most influential figure is Emilio Betti. In addition there is a strong French influence through the work of philosophers such as Jacques Derrida, Michel Foucault, Jacques Lacan, and Paul Ricoeur. Despite its rather formidable image, hermeneutics, like phenomenology and existentialism, also puts people first by placing human expressiveness at the centre of its concerns.

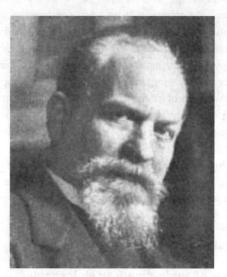

Fig. 4.4 Edmund Husserl

Phenomenology, existentialism, and hermeneutics

We will now look at these philosophies in a little more detail, and especially as they relate to the philosophy and ethics of mental health, starting with phenomenology.

Phenomenology

Although the term 'phenomenology' goes back at least to the eighteenth century German philosopher, Immanual Kant, in its twentieth century form phenomenology is generally attributed to Edmund Husserl with a series of books published in the first half of the twentieth century, in particular *Ideas Pertaining to a Pure Phenomenology and to a Phenomenological Philosophy, First Book* (1931; published in English translation in 1982), *Cartesian Meditations* (1950; English translation in 1960), and, his greatest work, *Logical Investigations* (1900–1; English translation in 1970).

Husserl's ideas (to which we return in detail in Part II) became highly influential, and were later adopted by his pupil, Martin Heidegger, and by Jean-Paul Sartre and Maurice Merleau-Ponty. As with many philosophers working in the Continental tradition, each of these philosophers has also attracted the label 'existentialist'. This is one reason why the distinction between phenomenology and existentialism can sometimes be problematic. One way to think of the difference is this: existentialism is primarily a philosophical *attitude* (broadly, of being aware of and insisting on our powers of self-determination—see later), while phenomenology is best understood as a philosophical *method* for exploring the structure of consciousness. It is thus quite consistent to be *both* a phenomenologist *and* an existentialist.

The best known connection between phenomenology and psychiatry is of course through the work of the founder of modern descriptive psychopathology, the German philosopher–psychiatrist, Karl Jaspers. We return to Jaspers in detail later (in Part II). For an introductory reading in phenomenology in this chapter, however, we are going to look at a passage from Merleau-Ponty's major work, *The Phenomenology of Perception* ([1945], transl. 1962) (see Exercise 13). First, though, a brief introduction to Merleau-Ponty himself and to his philosophical project.

Merleau-Ponty (1908–61) had close ties with Sartre (they collaborated on, and edited, the journal *Les Temps Moderns*), and was in debt to a number of Heideggerian themes, although the roots of his thought were primarily in Husserl's brand of phenomenology combined with key concepts from Gestalt psychology. He anticipates recent work in the philosophy of psychiatry by drawing explicitly on disturbances of consciousness associated with neurological problems (such as aphasia) in developing his themes (see below).

Merleau-Ponty's phenomenological project was to develop a theory of perception. The key to this, he believed, was to undermine of any type of dualism, whether it be the Cartesian *res cogitans (mind)* and *res extentia (matter)*, or the Sartrian being-for-itself (mind) and being-in-itself (matter). In place of dualism, Merleau-Ponty sought to develop a description of our 'pre-reflective' or primordial perceptual *interaction* with the world, what he called our 'being-in-the-world'.

Merleau-Ponty: the phenomenology of perception

Merleau-Ponty sketches out his project in the 'Preface' and 'Introduction' to *The Phenomenology of Perception* (translated into English, 1962, original French edition 1945). He adopts a

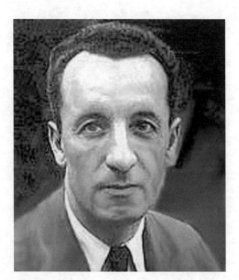

Fig. 4.5 Merleau-Ponty

two-pronged strategy. First, he rejects 'associationist' empirical theories of perception, launching an attack upon the empiricist employment of distinct units of 'sensation', which, he argues, leave us with the problem of how the units are associated and unified (see Introduction, chapter 2). Second, he criticizes 'intellectualist' theories of perception, attacking both the privileging of the transcendental subject (namely, a subject set apart from and monitoring perception—i.e. a subject, somehow, separate from and standing over and above the world), and the conflation of judgement and perception (see Introduction, chapter 3).

Having rejected both empiricism and intellectualism, Merleau-Ponty then draws on elements from both to build up a picture of the lived-experience of the 'Phenomenal Field' (See Introduction, chapter 4). Critical to his argument is that our access to the phenomenal field is given by our *body*. This is the irreducible link to a particular world. The 'lived-body' is thus always already *in* the world prior to any reflection. It cannot be objectified (set *apart* from the world or the individual), and perception must be taken as *embodied* perception that exists only within a specific context or mode of activity.

One way to understand Merleau-Ponty's antidualism—his rejection of both empiricism and intellectualism—is to reflect on our everyday experiences of perception. Try this for yourself. Look at an object, any object near you—a lamp, say. When you reflect on this you might think of the pattern of colours and shapes that can seem to form the basis of an interpretation: that those colours and shapes comprise a lamp. But ordinarily we do not do this. We do not infer the lamp experience from anything more basic. Ordinarily, we do not separate an intellectual

interpretation 'seeing a lamp' from any more basic experience of colours and shapes. We just *see a lamp*.

Merleau-Ponty argues, in effect, that it is the 'seeing a lamp', the pre-reflective experience, which is the basic unit of consciousness. There are no further perceptual 'atoms' from which the perception of the lamp is built up (as the associationists argued); there is no transcendental subject 'judging' that what we see is a lamp (as the intellectualists thought). There is just our lived-experience of meaningful engagement with the world.

Merleau-Ponty on aphasia

So far so good. But how does this help us to understand psychopathology? The following reading is taken from part 1 of *The Phenomenology of Perception*. It comes from chapter 6 ('The body as expression and speech'). Here Merleau-Ponty examines the issue of how speech represents an effort to project one's self towards a world of meaning. He tackles this by looking at the breakdown of speech in aphasia.

EXERCISE 13 (30 minutes)

Read the two short sections from Merleau-Ponty:

Merleau-Ponty, M. (1945/1962). The body as expression and speech. In *The Phenomenology of Perception* (transl. Colin Smith). London: Routledge, pp. 174–177, 184–185

Link with Reading 4.4

Make brief notes on:

1. the approach of 'traditional' theories towards the breakdown of expression, and how they relate to Merleau-Ponty's previous criticisms of empiricism and intellectualism;

2. the relationship between authentic speech, gesture, and the body;

3. the difference between the pre-reflective or existential layers of language and its conceptual layers; and finally

4. how the loss of figure-background horizons and self-transcendence are part of Merleau-Ponty's existential theory of aphasia.

Again, much of what motivates the reading with Exercise 13 is Merleau-Ponty's attack on dualism: he wants to bridge any distinction between language and thought, and to show instead that language is not part of a specific mental realm, rather that words themselves have significance or meaning. Merleau-Ponty rejects the empirical psychologists' approach to the loss of expression in aphasia on the grounds that language is treated as a type of 'verbal image' (p. 176), thereby reducing speech to an inert, third-person phenomenon, that fails to take the function of the word into account. Equally, the intellectualist approach merely attributes the problems of aphasia to a breakdown in thought and the categorial (i.e. rationally ordered) operation of the intellect—language is seen to be an external counterpart to inner thought.

Merleau-Ponty proposes that the word is not some outer layer of thought, rather the recognition of an object is in fact the act of naming it, and thus speaking accomplishes thought. This immediacy of naming and perceptual recognition in language is a glimpse into the primordial-existential layer of language that lies before the categorial level of reflection and objectification. Our access to this primordial level is through the body, indeed the body of speech—the gesture (pp. 184–186). Meaning is gained immediately, through the gestural aspect of speech, and prior to any subsequent intellectual or reflective clarification. In Merleau-Ponty's account of aphasia, then, the *disruption* of expression occurs because of phenomena losing their meaningfulness for the patient.

This example illustrates the power of the modern phenomenological method to afford a richer conceptualization of the processes at work in pathological forms of experience. The link between meaning and psychopathology was important for Karl Jaspers. But as we will see in Part II, Jaspers also used the phenomenological method to develop a detailed classification of the phenomena of consciousness and then of its specific breakdowns in psychopathology.

Modern authors, too, have used phenomenology in both ways, general and specific. As an example of the former, Pat Bracken, a psychiatrist who has worked with the humanitarian organization, Amnesty International, in post-conflict situations, has explored the breakdown of meaning in PTSD (post-traumatic stress disorder); and, drawing on Heidegger's phenomenology, he has developed approaches to management that depend on re-establishing social relationships rather than individual 'counselling' (Bracken, 1998). As to specific uses of phenomenology, there are many current examples from the work of both philosophers and psychiatrists. This work has been given a new urgency by the demands of the new neurosciences, such as brain imaging and behavioural genetics. (See Reading Guide.)

Existentialism

As a philosophical *attitude* rather than a school of thought, existentialism has bred a number of highly individualistic philosophers. The first exponent is generally acknowledged to have been the nineteenth century Danish philosopher Søren Kierkegaard, but as already noted, in its twentieth century form existentialism has developed largely out of phenomenology. It has been adopted by, among others, the German philosophers Martin Heidegger and Karl Jaspers, and also by the French philosophers Gabriel Marcel and Jean-Paul Sartre.

The existential attitude involves the rejection of the primacy of objective knowledge, putting in its place the primacy of *being* (i.e. existence). An individual's experience of his or her situation is the starting point of inquiry. This is the ground of what Sartre called the 'authentic', any concessions to the expectations of others being 'inauthentic'. Existentialist thinkers differ in their view of what resources we have in facing up to the deceptions and depredations of the demands of society. They also differ over the status of the self and whether this is authentic or inauthentic.

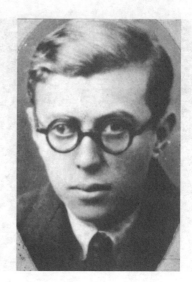

Fig. 4.6 Sartre

Being and nothingness

One of the most influential existentialist thinkers was Jean-Paul Sartre. Like many existentialists, Sartre initially adopted a phenomenological philosophy, his existentialist ideas developing as a response to what he took to be the limitations of his initial position. Sartre's best-known work is *Being and Nothingness*, published originally in 1943. In this he introduces his famous distinction between 'being in-itself' (matter) and 'being for-itself' (mind). In the next exercise, we will be reading the introduction to this work, in which Sartre sets out the issues he will address.

EXERCISE 14   (30 minutes)

Read the opening paragraphs from:

Sartre, J-P. (1956). Introduction, The pursuit of being. I. The phenomenon. In *Being and Nothingness* (trans. Hazel E. Barnes). New York: The Citadel Press, pp. xlv–lxvi

---

Link with Reading 4.5

Do not write anything down, instead reflect upon the ideas in the text as you read it.

Note how carefully Sartre sets up his project, building both on his dissatisfaction with phenomenology, and also on what he sees as its strengths. Note how the idealism of Berkeley is disposed of, as providing insufficient grounds for the existence of consciousness. Finally, note how Sartre sets up the argument for Being-for-itself and Being-in-itself. How do you feel about this? Are you convinced?

Sartre's basic position is that Being is self-revealing and cannot be denied. Whatever one feels about this, there is no doubt that its influence in France in the middle years of the twentieth century was enormous. By the time of his death Sartre had become almost a cultural icon, his ideas inspiring a generation of intellectuals, influencing moral and political thought, and also the expressive arts (through his novels).

Sartre versus Freud

The existentialist concern with the nature of consciousness and its status as the primary ontological category brought it into conflict with the ideas of psychoanalytic theory. In a later chapter of *Being and Nothingness* Sartre offers a damning critique of Freud's ego theory, especially of the censor mechanism. He argues that Freud's mechanism of repression cannot function as it would involve an untenable division of the psyche, and, in any case, once the censor knows of the material to be repressed, the conscious mind must also know it. Sartre's reading of Freud has attracted much criticism, a recent example being by Sebastian Gardner (1993, chapters 2 and 3). We will be returning to Sartre's critique of Freud later in this book.

Hermeneutics

The term 'hermeneutics' originally referred to the techniques of Biblical exegesis. It was first used in its modern sense by the German philologist Freidrich Schleiermacher in the early nineteenth century. Hermeneutic theory and methodology was further developed by the German philosopher Thomas Dilthey in the late nineteenth century; and later still by the German philosopher Martin Heidegger (until just after the publication of *Being and Time* in 1927, after which he no longer described his project as hermeneutical). In more recent times hermeneutics has been dominated by the work of the German philosopher Hans-Georg Gadamer; by the Italian philosopher Emilio Betti; and by French philosophers such as Michel Foucault, Jaques Lacan, Jacques Derrida, and Paul Ricoeur.

In relation to mental health, hermeneutics is directly concerned with one side of the tension (to which we will be returning several times in this book) between causal and meaningful accounts of human experience and behaviour, and the closely related tension between explanation and understanding. It has also been highly influential in the philosophy of psychoanalysis. Put crudely, science in the twentieth century has focused largely on causes and explanations, hermeneutics on meanings and understanding (although of course it has not been alone in this).

An accessible and at the same time seminal example of the application of hermeneutics to psychoanalysis is provided by the French philosopher Paul Ricoeur. In his influential *Freud and Philosophy* (1970), Ricoeur offered an interpretation of Freud's texts which was both original and thought provoking. In the following exercise, we are going to read a passage from this book, in which Ricoeur sets out his view of the methodology of hermeneutics.

EXERCISE 15 (30 minutes)

Read the two extracts from:

Ricoeur, P. (1970). Hermeneutic method and reflective philosophy. In *Freud and Philosophy* (trans. Terry Savage). London: Yale University Press, pp. 37 and 41–42

Link with Reading 4.6

From the start, you will find this very different from the paper by J.L. Austin, which we studied earlier (see Exercise 8). But exactly how does it differ from Austin's work? The difference is not merely of style—there is something fundamentally different about the philosophical presuppositions and methodology of each philosopher. As you read, make short notes on the main characteristics of Ricoeur's philosophical method.

Finally, what is it about Ricoeur's hermeneutics that makes it eminently suitable as a tool for interpreting psychoanalytic texts? Do you think Freud would have recognized himself in this? Does it matter?

We will be returning to Ricoeur's text later in this book (in Chapter 11). The point now is that hermeneutics is concerned with uncovering the hidden meanings behind the explicit story. Freud conceived his project (rightly or wrongly) as part of science, producing generalizations based upon observation of specific instances; in contrast, hermeneutics is concerned with the individual meaning generated in a specific instance of discourse, and also with the methodology by which the meaning can be extracted. By concentrating on the way in which texts can be interpreted at two levels, as having a superficial and a deeper meaning, it is possible to chart the interplay of ideological influences and symbolic forms. As we will find when we return to Ricoeur's text in Part III, he interprets psychoanalysis as a kind of hermeneutics of the mind.

Continental and Anglo-American philosophy: a new partnership

We have looked at examples of how all three main branches of Continental philosophy have produced ideas that are important for mental health. Ricoeur's hermeneutics contains a thorough analysis of Freud's ideas; Merleau-Ponty's phenomenology offers a rich and detailed account of psychopathology (as noted earlier, we return to Karl Jaspers' phenomenology and the origins of descriptive psychopathology in Part II); and existentialism produced its own critique of Freud. It also had an important influence on the early movement in antipsychiatry through the work of such seminal figures as R.D. Laing. We will be returning to each of these later.

In philosophy and mental health, then, the two great traditions, the Continental and the Anglo-American, should be partners, rather than split apart. In the philosophical world generally, there is indeed a growing awareness that Anglo-American and Continental philosophy have many concerns in common. For example, both traditions are increasingly focusing on the nature of the self, and even their methods should be seen as complementary (in that each illuminates aspects of an issue which is neglected by the other).

Thought experiments, the case method, and real people

The complementary nature of these two approaches is also well illustrated by work on the concept of mental illness. We noted the importance of Foucault's work, for example, to the debate about mental illness in Chapter 2. Methodologically, however, perhaps the most exciting development, particularly with mental health research and practice in mind, is the increasing focus on substantive human issues and experience. We have seen that this has been explicitly so with all the main schools of Continental philosophy, but it is now also emerging in some contemporary work in Anglo-American philosophy. Traditionally, Anglo-American philosophy has employed abstract general notions, avoiding the concrete and specific. This allowed it to operate with great rigour, but also gave it a reputation for 'armchair philosophy'.

By the 1970s, however, there was a growing realization among some philosophers that much was to be gained from the consideration of real cases. This found expression in a number of areas, but particularly in the philosophy of mind and in ethics, and coincided with the recognition among practitioners of the need to engage with the philosophical issues (ethical and conceptual) generated by difficult cases. In ethics, one result of this has been a shift from general theory to the consideration of actual cases and the development of a modern version of casuistry (we will return to this in Part IV).

In the philosophy of mind, a strong statement of the requirement for philosophy to return to empirical (as well as conceptual) methods, has been made by the Oxford philosopher, the late Kathleen Wilkes, in her book noted above, *Real People: Philosophy without Thought Experiments* (1988). It is from this book that the last reading in this session is taken.

EXERCISE 16   (15 minutes)

Read the two extracts from:

Wilkes, K. (1988). *Real people: personal identity without thought experiments*. Oxford: Oxford University Press

---

Link with Reading 4.7 (2 extracts: 'Losing touch with reality' and 'A promissory note')

Note what Wilkes says about Kripke's methodology (p. 43)—in what way does J.L. Austin's methodology (examined earlier in this chapter) try to avoid criticism of this kind? What is Wilkes's central message in these last two sections of chapter I of her book?

Wilkes is attacking philosophical methods that rely on thought experiments to the exclusion of the rich variety of material available in the real world of real people. Elsewhere in her book she examines multiple personality disorder in particular. The *general* claim that she and other philosophers (notably another Oxford philosopher, Jonathan Glover, 1988), are making is that psychopathology offers a wide variety of real experiences that are more challenging than anything philosophers can imagine by mere reflection, and yet which, at the same time, are rooted in the real world.

This is the central message in the final two sections of Wilkes's chapter 1. Philosophers are mistaken, she argues, if they believe that by imagining fantastic and impossible thought experiments, they can give greater clarity to the concepts that we use in the real world.

Wilkes agrees with Wittgenstein in saying that the analysis of concepts that have no application in our lives does not thereby give them meaning, and, therefore, they cannot possibly help us to a better understanding of the concepts we find problematic in the real world. We should, instead, look at real life instances where our ordinary concepts seem to be inadequate, and, as Wilkes makes clear later in her text, it is psychopathology that offers possibly the best opportunities of this kind.

This was, after all, precisely Austin's point. Austin was concerned with agency; Wilkes and Glover were concerned with personal identity. But all three are pointing to psychopathology as a resource for philosophy.

Reflection on the session and self-test questions

Write down your own reflections on the materials in this session drawing out any points that are particularly significant for you. Then write brief notes about the following:

1. How does Anglo-American philosophy differ from Continental philosophy (in so far as they are distinct)?

2. What are the three 'schools' of Continental philosophy? Give an exemplar from each whose work is relevant to psychiatry, psychoanalysis and/or psychopathology.

3. Continental and Anglo-American philosophy are beginning to converge—What is the link between them?

4. Are the methods of philosophy and empirical science essentially antagonistic, independent or complementary? (Think about this before reading the Conslusions, below.)

Conclusions: philosophy, science, and mental health

In this chapter, we have reviewed a variety of methods from both Continental and Anglo-American philosophy. We have also noted that these two great traditions are increasingly working together in a complementary way and that this is especially important in relation to mental health.

We have covered a lot of ground in this chapter, but before finishing it will be worth spending a few minutes reviewing the relationship between philosophical methods generally, whether Anglo-American or Continental, and those of science.

Science versus philosophy versus dogmatic religion?

Much philosophy proceeds imaginatively, through the manipulation of thoughts, symbols, meanings, concepts, and so on, 'in the mind'. In this it is sometimes thought to stand in contrast to science, which is taken to proceed by observation of the world. Indeed, 'natural philosophy' (the late medieval term for natural science) could be said to owe its origins to the stand, sometimes taken in the face of great personal danger, by Bacon, Galileo, and others for the primacy of observation over the received authority of religion (Rossi, 2003).

But philosophy, too, had to liberate itself from theology. Indeed, in 'Western' Europe, it emerged as an independent subject only in the seventeenth century: compare, on the one hand, Hobbes's *Leviathan*, published in 1651, the second half of which is biblical exegesis aimed at legitimating the ideas in the first half of the book in order to appease religious sentiment, and, on the other, Locke's views on the role of philosophy in his *Essay Concerning Human Understanding*, published in 1690. Locke felt able, in his 'Epistle to the Reader' at the beginning of his book, to characterize philosophy as being aimed as removing impediments to knowledge (he meant religious superstition, among other things). Locke visualized philosophy as an 'underlabourer' to those who produce real knowledge (he meant, here, natural scientists). Science and philosophy *can* work productively together, and this is, in part, a function of the fact that they produce different, but complementary, sorts of output.

Science and philosophy versus authority

We will be looking in Chapter 6 at some of the ways in which the outputs of science and philosophy differ. As to their methods, though, they are closer than either side is generally prepared to recognize. Thus, the stand of both disciplines is characteristically anti-authoritarian; Socrates was the 'gadfly of Athens'. We will find in Part III that according to at least one influential view (Kuhn, 1962), science as well as philosophy is subject to fashions, to periods of relative stability during which given authorities shape the development of theory. However, both disciplines aim to advance knowledge and understanding primarily through the overthrow of received views rather than by their exegesis.

Parallel experimental methods

Both disciplines, moreover, are experimental, in the broad sense of following through the implications of an idea and seeing whether it remains tenable. Philosophical experimentation is more conceptual, scientific more empirical. But they are both experimental. Nor is the divide between the two kinds of experiment as sharp as is often supposed. Scientific breakthroughs are often made initially by thought experiments—Einstein's crucial insight, leading to the theory of relativity, was generated by thought experiments, such as imagining how to determine whether two widely separated events were simultaneous, or what it would be like to travel on a beam of light. And, of course, philosophy, like science, often proceeds through inspired guesswork or intuitions rather than cold reason alone.

Complementary disciplines

We argued in Chapter 2 that philosophy is more concerned with conceptual, while science is more concerned with empirical, problems. For our purposes, of clarifying the role of philosophy in mental health, this is perhaps a helpful generalization. But neither discipline can proceed indefinitely in isolation from the other.

Reading guide

Concepts of disorder: (3) Austin and other analytic methods

Austin and the concept of mental disorder

G.J. Warnock's biography, *J.L. Austin* (1989), provides a lively and readable overview of Austin's philosophy. The introductory chapter, in particular, offers a well-balanced appraisal of the strengths and weaknesses of linguistic analysis as a philosophical method. The collection, *Symposium on J.L. Austin*, edited by K.T. Fann (1969), includes articles exploring these issues in detail. Austin's papers have been brought together in a collection edited by J.O. Urmson and Geoffrey Warnock (1961, 1989).

The potential importance of linguistic analysis as a bridge between philosophy and mental health is set out in an article by Fulford (1990) 'Philosophy and medicine: the Oxford connection' and in Fulford (2003). For empirical research combining linguistic analytic and empirical methods, see Colombo *et al.* (2003) 'Evaluating the influence of implicit models of mental disorder on processes of shared decision making within community-based multidisciplinary teams', Fulford (2001), and Fulford and Colombo (2004a and 2004b). Linguistic analytic methods are also the basis of new policy and practice developments in mental health (Fulford, Stanghellini and Broome, 2004) including training programmes in working with complex values developed for mental health practitioners, see Woodbridge and Fulford, 2004. Austin's approach influenced Hare, Warnock, Urmson, and others in the 'Oxford School', whose work has directly influenced these practical developments (see also Reading Guide to Chapter 6). As noted in the chapter, a thorough discussion of the importance of philosophers working on real cases, and on the real cases represented by the different forms of mental disorder, is Kathleen Wilkes' (1988) *Real People: philosophy without thought experiments*.

Illness, disease, and disorder

In addition to Christopher Boorse's work, as examined in the chapter, the distinction between disease and illness is discussed further by Barondess, J.A. (1979) 'Disease and illness—a crucial distinction'; and in chapter 2 of Fulford (1989). There are a number of philosophical refutations of the value-free status of disease assumed by the traditional medical model. An early argument to this effect was set out by the English sociologist, Peter Sedgwick (1973), in his 'Illness-mental and otherwise'. A number of American philosophers have made important contributions to this literature, in particular George Agich (1983) 'Disease and illness: a rejection of the value-neutrality thesis'; Loretta Kopelman (1994) 'Normal grief: good or bad? Health or disease?; and Tristram Engelhardt (1975) 'The concepts of health and disease'. A useful discussion of key aspects of this debate is to be found in Sadler and Agich's (1995) critique of Wakefield's analysis in their *Diseases, Functions, Values and Psychiatric Classification*, with a response by Wakefield (1995).

Murphy and Woolfolk (2000a) explore Wakefield's analysis in *The Harmful Dysfunction Analysis of Mental Disorder*, with a commentary by Wakefield (2000), and a response to Wakefield by Murphy and Woolfolk (2000b). Boorse's (1976a) follow-up paper on mental illness, 'What a theory of mental health should be', is in *Journal of Theory and Social Behaviour*. Boorse (1976b) in 'Wright on functions' and 'Health as a theoretical concept' (1977), gives more detailed treatments of the concept of 'function'. Boorse (1997) has developed a detailed update of his work in his 'A rebuttal on health'.

Combining philosophical and empirical methods

An early contribution to the field illustrating the value of analytic philosophy in supporting empirical work is Marshall (1994) 'How should we measure need? Concept and practice in the development of a standardized assessment schedule', with commentaries by Crisp (1994) and Morgan (1994). Marshall's article explores the resources from Oxford analytic philosophy on which he drew in developing a new psychometric measure for assessing need.

Van Staden (2002a and 2002b) draws on Frege's logic of relations in an empirical study of recovery (with commentaries by Falzer and Davidson, 2002, Gillett, 2002, and Suppes, 2002). Similarly, philosophical and empirical techniques are combined in Fulford and Colombo's (2004a) 'Six models of mental disorder', with commentaries by Bendelow (2004, from a social science perspective), Heginbotham (2004, from a policy

perspective), Williams (2004, from a training perspective), and Williamson (2004, from a voluntary sector perspective), and a response by the authors (Fulford and Colombo, 2004b). (All based on Colombo *et al.*, 2003).

Continental philosophy

A highly accessible introduction in English to some of the main schools of recent Continental philosophy is Eric Matthews' *Twentieth Century French Philosophy* (1996).

Merleau-Ponty's phenomenology

Merleau-Ponty's (1945) *Phenomenology of Perception* (trans. Colin Smith, 1962, original French edition 1945) has been in print in English for many years, and is probably his best known work. Less well-known is *The Structure of Behaviour* (1963/5; original French edition 1942). Also of interest is *Signs* (trans. Richard C. McCleary, 1964, original French edition 1960), *The Visible and the Invisible* (ed. Claude Lefort, trans. Alphonso Lingis, 1968, original French edition 1964), and a collection of Merleau-Ponty's papers, *The Primacy of Perception*, edited by James M. Edie (1964) (trans. various).

Of the secondary literature, two useful texts are M. Hammond *et al.* (1991) *Understanding Phenomenology* (chapters 4–9), and M. Langer (1989) *Merleau-Ponty's Phenomenology of Perception: a guide and commentary*. Eric Matthews' (2002) *The Philosophy of Merleau-Ponty* provides an authoritative and accessible introduction.

For a contemporary firsthand analysis of the experience of illness drawing on Merleau-Ponty's phenomenology, see Kay Toombs (1993) *The Meaning of Illness*. As a sufferer from multiple sclerosis, and also an expert in phenomenological philosophy, Toombs offers a uniquely insightful account of the core feature of illness, incapacity.

Additional readings on Merleau-Ponty and concepts of mental disorder are given in the Reading guide to chapter 8 on 'Phenomenology and psychopathology today'.

Existentialism

The existentialist literature is freely available in English translation. Sartre's *Being and Nothingness* has appeared in two versions. One lacks the passages critical of Freud (which were originally published in English translation as a separate volume). The most widely available translation of *Being and Nothingness* is that by Hazel Barnes (see Sartre, 1956) with an introduction by Mary Warnock. This is available with and without the 'Freud' passages. A paper by Sartre (1967) entitled 'Consciousness of self and knowledge of self' appeared in *Readings in Phenomenological Psychology* (ed. N. Lawrence and D. O'Connor). For an example of a detailed application of Sartre's phenomenology to psychopathology, see Morris (2003).

Peter Caws' (1979) *Sartre* gives a clear overview. Mary Warnock's (1970) 'Existentialism' is a readable and comprehensive introduction. A classic title is John MacQuarrie's (1973) *Existentialism*.

Hermeneutics

A well-chosen selection of readings from the hermeneutic literature from the early nineteenth century to the present is provided by Gayle Ormiston and Alan Schrift (ed.) (1990) *The Hermeneutic Tradition*, and (1989) *Transforming the Hermeneutic Context*.

In *Philosophy, Psychiatry, & Psychology*, Phillips (1996) gives an excellent and clear introduction in his Key Concepts article on 'Hermeneutics'. Widdershoven (1999a) explores the relationship between hermeneutics and psychological methods of treatment in his 'Cognitive psychology and hermeneutics', with commentaries by McMillan (1999), Phillips (1999), and Warner (1999), and a response (Widdershoven, 1999b). An early article in *Philosophy, Psychiatry, & Psychology* exploring the relationship between hermeneutic and scientific explanations is Drury (1994) 'Cognitive science and hermeneutic explanation: symbiotic or incompatible frameworks'.

A highly readable introduction to a debate that took place between Michel Foucault and Jacques Derrida on the nature of reason and madness is Roy Boyne's (1990) *Foucault and Derrida: the other side of reason*.

The French psychoanalyst-philosopher Jacques Lacan wrote a number of highly influential works, his best known being Ecrits (1966), available in English as *Ecrits. A Selection* (trans. Alan Sheridan); and *The Four Fundamental Concepts of Psychoanalysis* (The Seminar, Book XI), (ed. Jacques-Alain Miller, trans. Alan Sheridan, 1997/1991). Carlo Strenger's (1991) *Between Hermeneutics and Science*, offers a thought-provoking account of the interplay between the scientific and hermeneutic conceptions of psychoanalysis.

Continental and analytic philosophy: bridging the divide in the philosophy of psychiatry

The complementary roles of analytic and Continental philosophy are particularly evident in descriptive psychopathology. Stimulated by developments in neuroscience, recent work in this area draws equally on phenomenological as well as analytical philosophy; see, for example, several articles in the 1996 *Current Opinion in Psychiatry*, History and Philosophy Section, Vol. 9, September 1996.

The journal, *Philosophy, Psychiatry, & Psychology*, publishes work from both Continental and Anglo-American perspectives. See, for example, Read (2003a) in 'Literature as Philosophy of Psychopathology', with responses by Coetzee (2003) and Sass (2003), and a response by Read (2003b). Similarly, recent edited volumes on philosophy and mental health include chapters by authors from both traditions. In addition to Fulford, Morris, Sadler, and Stanghellini's (2003) *Nature and Narrative*, and Radden's (2004), *The Philosophy of Psychiatry: A Companion*, see for example, Sadler, Wiggins and Schwartz's (1994) *Philosophical Perspectives on Psychiatric Diagnostic Classification* and Graham's and Stephens' (1994) *An Introduction to Philosophical Psychopathology*.

References

Agich, G.J. (1983). Disease and Value: A rejection of the Value-neutrality Thesis. *Theoretical Medicine*, 4, 27–41.

American Psychiatric Association (1994). *Diagnostic and Statistical Manual Of Mental Disorders* (4th edn). APA: Washington DC.

Austin, J.L. (1956–7). A plea for excuses. Proceedings of the Aristotelian Society 57:1–30. Reprinted in White, A.R., ed. (1968) *The Philosophy of Action*. Oxford: Oxford University Press, pps 19–42. (Page numbers in the text are from the 1968 edition)

Ayer, A.J. (1936). *Language, Truth and Logic*. London: Victor Gollancz.

Baker, G. (2003). Wittgenstein's method and psychoanalysis. In *Nature and Narrative: an introduction to the new philosophy of psychiatry* (ed. K.W.M. Fulford, K.J. Morris, J.Z. Sadler, and G. Stanghellini). Oxford: Oxford University Press, Chapter 3.

Barondess, J.A. (1979). Disease and illness – a crucial distinction. *The American Journal of Medicine* 66: 375–376.

Bendelow, G. (2004). Commentary: Sociology and concepts of mental illness. (Commentary on Fulford and Colombo, 2004a) *Philosophy, Psychiatry, & Psychology*, 11(2): 145–146.

Boorse, C. (1975). On the distinction between disease and illness. *Philosophy and Public Affairs*, 5: 49–68.

Boorse, C. (1976a). What a theory of mental health should be. *Journal of Theory and Social Behaviour*, 6: 61–84.

Boorse, C. (1976b). Wright on functions. *Philosophy Review*, 85, 70–86

Boorse, C. (1977) Health as a theoretical concept. *Philosophy of Science*, 44, 542–573.

Boorse, C. (1997). A Rebuttal on Health. Ch 1 in Humber J.M. and Almeder, R.F. eds *What is Disease?* Totowa, New Jersey: Humana Press, pps 1–134.

Boyne, R. (1990). *Foucault and Derrida: the other side of reason*. Unwin Hyman Ltd. Reprinted 1994 and 1996 London/New York: Routledge.

Bracken, P.J. (1998). Hidden Agendas: Deconstructing Post Traumatic Stress Disorder. Chapter 2 in Bracken, P.J. and

Petty, C. (eds) *Rethinking the Trauma of War.* London and New York: Free Association Books, pps 38–59.

Caws, P. (1979). *Sartre.* London: Routledge.

Colombo, A., Bendelow, G., Fulford, K.W.M., and Williams, S. (2003). Evaluating the influence of implicit models of mental disorder on processes of shared decision making within community-based multi-disciplinary teams. *Social Science & Medicine*, 56: 1557–1570

Coetzee, P.H. and Roux, A.P.J. (eds) (2002). *Philosophy from Africa.* 2nd edition. Cape Town, South Africa: Oxford University Press.

Coetzee, J.M. (2003). Fictional beings. (Commentary on Read, 2003a) *Philosophy, Psychiatry, & Psychology*, 10(2): 133–134.

Cooper, J.E., Kendell, R.E., Gurland, B.J., Sharpe, L., Copeland, J.R.M., and Simon, R. (1972). *Psychiatric Diagnosis in New York and London.* Maudsley Monograph No. 20. London: Oxford University Press.

Crisp, R. (1994). How should we measure need? (Commentary on Marshall, 1994) *Philosophy, Psychiatry, & Psychology*, 1(1): 37–38.

Depraz, N. (2003). Putting the *ép.oché* into practice: schizophrenic experience as illustrating the phenomenological exploration of consciousness. In *Nature and Narrative: an introduction to the new philosophy of psychiatry* (ed. K.W.M. Fulford, K.J. Morris, J.Z. Sadler, and G. Stanghellini). Oxford: Oxford University Press, Chapter 12.

Drury, J. (1994). Cognitive science and hermeneutic explanation: symbiotic or incompatible frameworks. *Philosophy, Psychiatry, & Psychology*, 1(1): 41–50.

Dummett, M. (1981). *The Interpretation of Frege's Philosophy.* London: Duckworth.

Dummett, M. (1993). *Origins of Analytical Philosophy.* London: Duckworth.

Edie, J.M. (ed) (1964). *The Primacy of Perception.* (trans. various)

Engelhardt, H.T. Jr. (1975). The concepts of health and disease. In Engelhardt, H.T., Jr. and Spicker, S.F. eds. *Evaluation and explanation in the biological sciences.* Dordrecht, Holland: D. Reidel.

Falzer, P. and Davidson, L. (2002). Commentary: Language, logic, and recovery: a commentary on Van Staden. (Commentary on Van Staden, 2002a) *Philosophy, Psychiatry, & Psychology*, 9(2): 131–136.

Fann, K.T. (1969). (ed) *Symposium on J. L. Austin.* Routledge and Kegan Paul: London.

Frege, G. (1892). *On Sense and Reference* in Translations from the philosophical writings of Gottlob Frege, Peter Geach and Max Black. Oxford: Basil Blackwell, 1960.

Fulford, K.W.M. (1989). *Moral Theory and Medical Practice.* Cambridge: Cambridge University Press.

Fulford, K.W.M. (1990). Philosophy and Medicine: The Oxford Connection. *British Journal of Psychiatry*, 157, pp. 111–115.

Fulford, K.W.M. (2000). Teleology without tears: naturalism, neo-naturalism and evaluationism in the analysis of function statements in biology (and a bet on the twenty-first century). *Philosophy, Psychiatry, and Psychology*, 7(1): 77–94.

Fulford, K.W.M. (2001) Philosophy into Practice: The Case for Ordinary Language Philosophy. Chapter 2, pps 171–208 in Nordenfelt, L., *Health, Science and Ordinary Language.* Amsterdam: Rodopi.

Fulford, K.W.M. (2003). *Mental Illness: definition, use and meaning.* Long entry for Post, S. G. (ed.). *Encyclopedia of Bioethics*, (3rd edn). New York: Macmillan.

Fulford, K. W. M, Morris, K. J., Sadler, J. Z. and Stanghellini, G. (eds.) (2003). *Nature and Narrative: an Introduction to The New Philosophy of Psychiatry.* Launch volume for a new book series. Oxford: Oxford University Press.

Fulford, K.W.M., Stanghellini, G. and Broome, M. (2004). What can philosophy do for psychiatry? Special Article for *World Psychiatry* (WPA), Oct 2004, pps 130–135.

Fulford, K.W.M. and Colombo, A. (2004a). Six models of mental disorder: a study combining linguistic–analytic and empirical methods. *Philosophy, Psychiatry, & Psychology*, 11(2): 129–144.

Fulford, K.W.M. and Colombo. A. (2004b). Professional judgment, critical realism, real people, and, yes, two wrongs can make a right! *Philosophy, Psychiatry, & Psychology*, 11(2): 165–174.

Gardner, S. (1993). *Irrationality and the Philosophy of Psychoanalysis.* Cambridge: Cambridge University Press.

Gbadegesin, S. (1991). *African Philosophy: Traditional Yoruba Philosophy and Contemporary African Realities.* New York and London: Peter Lang.

Gillett, G. (2002). The self as relatum in life and language. (Commentary on Van Staden, 2002a) *Philosophy, Psychiatry, & Psychology*, 9(2): 123–126.

Glover, J. (1988). *I: The Philosophy and Psychology of Personal Identity*, Oxford: Oxford University Press.

Graham, G., and Stephens, G. Lynn., (1994). An Introduction to Philosophical Psychopathology: Its Nature, Scope, and Emergence. pps 1–23 in Graham, G., and Lynn Stephens G., (eds) *Philosophical Psychopathology.* Cambridge, MA: MIT Press.

Hammond, M., Howarth, J. and Keat, R. (eds) (1991). *Understanding Phenomenology.* Oxford, UK and Cambridge, USA: Blackwell.

Hare, R.M. (1952). *The Language of Morals.* Oxford: Oxford University Press.

Heginbotham, C. (2004). Psychiatric Dasein. (Commentary on Fulford and Colombo, 2004a) *Philosophy, Psychiatry, & Psychology*, 11(2): 147–150.

Hobbes (1651, English edn) (1658, Latin edn, Revised). *Leviathan*. London: Andrew Crooke.

Husserl, E. ([1900–1] 1970). *Logical Investigations* (transl. J.N. Findlay). London: Routledge.

Husserl, E. ([1913] 1982). *Ideas Pertaining to a Pure Phenomenology and to a Phenomenological Philosophy, First Book* (transl. in English by F. Kersten). Dordrecht: Kluwer.

Husserl, E. ([1931] 1960). *Cartesian Meditations* (transl. D. Cairns). The Hague: Nijhoff.

Jellineck, E.M. (1960). *The Disease Concept of Alcoholism*. New Haven, CT: College and University Press.

Kendell, R.E. (1975). The concept of disease and its implications for psychiatry. *British Journal of Psychiatry*, 127, p.305–315

Kuhn, T.S. (1962). *The Structure of Scientific Revolutions*, (2nd edn). *International Encyclopedia of Unified Science*, Vol. 2, No. 2. University of Chicago Press.

Kopelman, L.M. (1994). Normal Grief: Good or Bad? Health or Disease? *Philosophy, Psychiatry, & Psychology*, 1(4), 209–220

Lacan, J. (1966). *Ecrits: A Selection*. (trans. Alan Sheridan) London: Tavistock Publications and Routledge, 1977.

Lacan, J. (1977/1991). *The Four Fundamental Concepts of Psychoanalysis* (trans. Alan Sheridan) Harmondsworth: Penguin Books.

Langford, C.H. (1942). *The Notion of Analysis in Moores Philosophy*. In Schilpp, pp. 321–342.

Langer, M. (1989). *Merleau-Ponty's Phenomenology of Perception: a guide and commentary*. Basingstoke: England: Macmillan.

Locke, J. (1690). *Essay Concerning Human Understanding*, Bk III, CH.III, §10.

Macklin, R. (1973). The medical model in psychoanalysis and psychotherapy. *Comprehensive Psychiatry*, 14: 49–69.

MacQuarrie, J. (1973). *Existentialism*. London: Penguin Books.

Marshall, M. (1994). How should we measure need? Concept and practice in the development of a standardized assessment schedule. *Philosophy, Psychiatry, & Psychology*, 1(1): 27–36.

Matthews, E. (1996). *Twentieth Century French Philosophy*. Oxford: Oxford University Press.

Matthews, E. (2002). *The Philosophy of Merleau-Ponty*. Chesham, England: Acumen Publishing Ltd.

McMillan, J. (1999). Cognitive psychology and hermeneutics: two irreconcilable approaches? (Commentary on Widdershoven, 1999a) *Philosophy, Psychiatry, & Psychology*, 6(4): 255–258.

Megone, C. (1998). Aristotle's function argument and the concept of mental illness. *Philosophy, Psychiatry, and Psychology*, 5(3): 187–202.

Megone, C. (2000). Mental illness, human function, and values. *Philosophy, Psychiatry, and Psychology*, 7(1): 45–66.

Merleau-Ponty, M. ([1945] 1962). *The Phenomenology of Perception* (transl. Colin Smith). London: Routledge.

Merleau-Ponty, M. in McCleary, R. C. (trans) *Signs*. (1964 Evanston, Ill: Northwestern University Press; original French edition 1960).

Merleau-Ponty, M. (1963/5). *The Structure of Behaviour*. A. L. Fisher (trans.) Boston, Mass: Beacon Press, 1963 and London: Methuen, 1965.

Merleau-Ponty, M. (1964). *Le Visible et l'invisible* (Paris: Gallimard), edited byt Claude Lefort, English trans. *The Visible and the Invisible*, trans. Alphonso Lingis, (Evanston, Ill: Northwestern University Press, 1968).

Moore, G.E. (1903). *Principia Ethica*. Cambridge: Cambridge University Press. *Ethics*, Home University Library, Thornton Butterworth (1912); Oxford Paperbacks University Series, Oxford University Press (1966).

Morgan, J. (1994). How should we measure need? (Commentary on Marshall, 1994) *Philosophy, Psychiatry, & Psychology*, 1(1): 39–40.

Morris, K. J. (2003). The phenomenology of body dysmorphic disorder: a Sartrean analysis. Chapter 11 in Fulford, K. W. M., Morris, K. J., Sadler, J. Z., and Stanghellini, G. (eds.) *Nature and Narrative: An Introduction to the New Philosophy of Psychiatry*. Oxford: Oxford University Press, 270–274.

Murphy, D. and Woolfolk, R.L. (2000a). The harmful dysfunction analysis of mental disorder. *Philosophy, Psychiatry, & Psychology*, 7(4): 241–252.

Murphy, D. and Woolfolk, R.L. (2000b). Conceptual analysis versus scientific understanding: an assessment of Wakefield's folk psychiatry. *Philosophy, Psychiatry, & Psychology*, 7(4): 271–294.

Nordenfelt, L. (1997). The stoic conception of mental disorder: the case of Cicero. *Philosophy, Psychiatry, and Psychology*, 4(4): 285–292.

Ormiston, G. and Schrift, A. (eds.) (1989). *Transforming the Hermeneutic Context*. New York: State University of New York Press.

Ormiston, G. and Schrift, A. (eds.) (1990). *The Hermeneutic Tradition*. New York: State University of New York Press.

Phillips, J. (1996). Key concepts: hermeneutics. *Philosophy, Psychiatry, & Psychology*, 3(1): 61–70.

Phillips, J. (1999). The hermeneutical critique of cognitive psychology. (Commentary on Widdershoven, 1999a) *Philosophy, Psychiatry, & Psychology*, 6(4): 259–264.

Radden, J. (2004) (Ed) *The Philosophy of Psychiatry: A Companion*. New York: Oxford University Press.

Read, R. (2003a). Literature as philosophy of psychopathology: William Faulkner as Wittgensteinian. *Philosophy, Psychiatry, & Psychology*, 10(2): 115–124.

Read, R. (2003b). On delusions of sense: a response to Coetzee and Sass. *Philosophy, Psychiatry, & Psychology*, 10(2): 135–142.

Reichenbach, H. (1951). *The Rise of Scientific Philosophy*. Berkeley, CA: University of California Press.

Ricoeur, P. (1970). Hermeneutic method and reflective philosophy. In *Freud and Philosophy* (transl. Terry Savage). London: Yale University Press, pp. 37–47.

Rossi, P. (2003). Magic, science, and equality of human wits. In *Nature and Narrative: an introduction to the new philosophy of psychiatry* (ed. K.W.M. Fulford, K.J. Morris, J.Z. Sadler, and G. Stanghellini). Oxford: Oxford University Press, Chapter 17.

Sadler, J.Z., Wiggins, O.P., & Schwartz, M.A. (eds) (1994) *Philosophical Perspectives on Psychiatric Diagnostic Classification*. Baltimore: The Johns Hopkins University Press.

Sadler, J.Z., and Agich, G.J. (1995). Diseases, functions, values and psychiatric classification. *Philosophy, Psychiatry, & Psychology*, 2(3): 219–232.

Sartre, J-P. (1956). 'Introduction', 'The Pursuit of Being', pp. xlv–lxvii from *Being and Nothingness*, trans. by Hazel E. Barnes. New York: The Citadel Press.

Sartre, J-P. (1967). *Consciousness of self and knowledge of self* in *Readings in Phenomenological Psychology* (ed. N. Lawrence and D. O'Connor) (1967)

Sass, L.A. (2003). Incomprehensibility and understanding: on the interpretation of severe mental illness. (Commentary on Read, 2003a). *Philosophy, Psychiatry, & Psychology*, 10(2): 125–132.

Sedgwick, P. (1973). 'Illness - Mental and Otherwise', *The Hastings Center Studies* I (3), 19–40 (Institute of Society, Ethics and Life Sciences, Hastings-on-Hudson, New York).

Van Staden, C.W. (2002a). Linguistic markers of recovery: theoretical underpinnings of first person pronoun usage and semantic positions of patients. *Philosophy, Psychiatry, & Psychology*, 9(2): 105–122.

Van Staden, C.W. (2002b). Language mirrors relational positions in recovery: a response to commentaries by Falzer and Davidson, Gillett, and Suppes. *Philosophy, Psychiatry, & Psychology*, 9(2): 137–140.

St Augustine. *Confessions*, Translated with Introduction and Notes, Henry Chadwick (1991). Oxford: Oxford University Press.

Strenger, C. (1991) *Between Hermeneutics and Science: An Essay on the Epistemology of Psychoanalysis*. Madison, CT: International Universities Press.

Suppes, P. (2002). Linguistic markers of recovery: underpinnings of first person pronoun usage and semantic positions of patients. (Commentary on Van Staden, 2002a). *Philosophy, Psychiatry, & Psychology*, 9(2): 127–130.

Szasz, T.S. (1960) The myth of mental illness. *American Psychologist*, 15: 113–118.

Thornton, T. (2003). Psychopathology and two kinds of narrative account of the self. (Commentary on articles in the Special Issue on agency, narrative, and self). *Philosophy, Psychiatry, & Psychology*, 10(4): 361–368.

Toombs, S. Kay. (1993). *The meaning of illness: a phenomenological account of the different perspectives of physician and patient*. Dordrecht, The Netherlands: Kluwer Academic Publishers.

Urmson, J.O. (1950). On grading. *Mind*, 59: 145–169.

Urmson, J.O. and Warnock, G.J. (eds) (1961, revised 1989). *J.L. Austin: Philosophical Papers*. (Third edition). Oxford: Oxford University Press.

Wakefield, J.C. (1995). Dysfunction as a value-free concept: a reply to Sadler and Agich. *Philosophy, Psychiatry, & Psychology*, 2(3): 233–246.

Wakefield, J.C. (2000). Spandrels, vestigal organs, and such: reply to Murphy and Woolfolk. The harmful dysfunction analysis of mental disorder *Philosophy, Psychiatry, & Psychology*, 7(4): 253–270.

Warner, M. (1999). Theory and practice: negotiating the differences. (Commentary on Widdershoven, 1999a). *Philosophy, Psychiatry, & Psychology*, 6(4): 265–266.

Warnock, M. (1970). *Existentialism*. Oxford: Oxford University Press.

Warnock, G.J. (1989). *J.L. Austin*. London: Routledge.

Whitehead, A.N. and Russell, B. (1910, 1912, 1913). *Principia Mathematica*, 3 vols, Cambridge: Cambridge University Press. (2nd edn), 1925 (Vol. 1) 1927 (Vols 2,3).

Widdershoven, G.A.M. (1999a). Cognitive psychology and hermeneutics: two approaches to meaning and mental disorder. *Philosophy, Psychiatry, & Psychology*, 6(4): 245–254.

Widdershoven, G.A.M. (1999b). Response to the Commentaries. *Philosophy, Psychiatry, & Psychology*, 6(4): 267–270.

Wilkes, K.V. (1988). *Real People: personal identity without thought experiments*. Oxford: Clarendon Press.

Williams, R. (2004). Finding the way forward in professional practice (Commentary on Fulford and

Colombo, 2004a) *Philosophy, Psychiatry, & Psychology*, 11(2): 151–158.

Williamson, T. (2004). Can two wrongs make a right? (Commentary on Fulford and Colombo, 2004a) *Philosophy, Psychiatry, & Psychology*, 11(2): 159–164.

Wittgenstein, L. (1953). *Philosophical Investigations*. Oxford: Blackwell.

World Health Organization (1978). *International Classification of Diseases*, (9th edn). Geneva: WHO.

World Health Organization (1992). *International Classification of Diseases*, (10th edn). Geneva: WHO.

Woodbridge, K., and Fulford, K.W.M. (2004). *Whose Values? A workbook for values-based practice in mental health care*. London: Sainsbury Centre for Mental Health.

CHAPTER 5

Arguments good and bad: an introduction to philosophical logic for practitioners

Chapter contents

Achilles joyfully exclaimed, as he ran the pencil into its sheath. 'And at last we've got to the end of this ideal race-course! Now that you accept A and B and C and D, *of course* you accept Z.'

'Do I?' said the Tortoise innocently. 'Let's make that quite clear. I accept A and B and C and D. Suppose I *still* refuse to accept Z?'

'Then Logic would take you by the throat, and *force* you to do it!' Achilles triumphantly replied.

What The Tortoise Said To Achilles
Lewis Carroll, originally published in *Mind*
(1895, No. 4, pp. 278–280)

We will return to Lewis Carroll's account of the debate between the Tortoise and Achilles about the effectiveness of logic a little later in this chapter. However, Achilles's suggestion that Logic might take one by the throat and force one to a conclusion is a striking expression of the power it holds on our conception of reason and rationality. At the same time, formal logic is often thought to be a subject only for specialists. In this chapter we aim to give an outline of some of the tools available for argument and some of the general issues raised by them.

Two aims of the chapter

Like Chapter 3 (on psychopathology), this chapter has two main aims. The first is the counterpart of the corresponding first aim of Chapter 3, i.e. to give non-philosophers a 'feel' for the work of professional philosophers. Just as medical and psychology students learn the details of psychopathology, so most undergraduates on philosophy degrees include logic; and just as

psychiatrists and clinical psychologists have to be able use current diagnostic classifications, so professional philosophers have to be able to use logic.

The second aim of this chapter is in a sense the opposite of the corresponding aim of Chapter 3. In setting out the details of descriptive psychopathology, we aimed to get across to philosophers that if they want to work in this area, there is a good deal of detail with which they have to be prepared to get up to speed— detail derived not just from professional but also lay (narrative) sources. The message was, psychopathology is not as easy as it may seem!

Here, the message is that logic is not as *difficult* as it may seem. Of course, like most subjects, advanced logic is difficult. However, the basics are relatively easy to grasp. Logic, as you will see, is a set of tools for developing and testing arguments. It helps to frame sound arguments, and to spot arguments that are unsound. So, the second aim of this chapter is to start you thinking in a critical philosophical way as a contribution to the improved 'thinking skills' that are one of main outputs from engagement with philosophy in mental health (Chapter 1). In this chapter, therefore, we provide an introduction to some of the main principles of logic, and the terminology you are likely to come across, together with suggestions for further reading.

How to read this chapter . . .

Unless you are interested in logic for its own sake, there is no need to struggle with the details of this chapter. The intention is not to turn practitioners into 'mini-logicians' (most philosophers do a full course on Logic and Philosophy of Logic in their first degree). It is rather to enable you to become familiar with the terminology of logic, and, in the process, to start to develop your own skills of argument.

. . . and what you should get out of it

1. *Terminology*. By the end of the chapter you should have developed a degree of familiarity with a number of important terms that philosophers pick up by absorption during a first degree (e.g. 'entails', 'paradox', 'syllogism', etc.). All these terms are themselves the subject of detailed philosophical work (we review some of the work on 'implication' later). But for the purposes of this book, you only need to be broadly familiar with them, so that you can 'speak the same language' as philosophers.

2. *Skills of argument*: By the end of the chapter you should also have improved your own skills of argument. As noted above, much of logic is about what makes for a good or bad argument, a valid or fallacious one. These notes aim to outline some of the tools philosophy has come up with to help us here. The importance of an exposure to philosophical logic is not, primarily, to learn the names of this or that fallacy (we list 18 of the more common ones at the end). It is to give you the skills to present good arguments and to spot bad

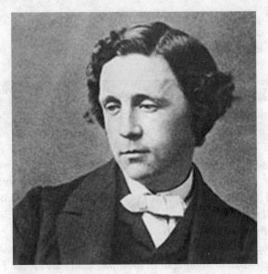

Fig. 5.1 Lewis Carroll

ones. So this is above all an area where *practice* is essential. Don't just read this chapter passively. Try out the exercises for yourself and invent examples of your own. That said, the aim of this chapter is not to teach you the whole of 'undergraduate logic'. That would take more than a chapter and there are many good introductory textbooks on logic for that purpose. The aim is instead to introduce the kind of tools and way of approaching an argument that is at the heart of logic.

3. *Grasp of the broader issues.* By the end of the chapter you should also have a better understanding of the purpose of logical argument, of its strengths and some of its limitations. The *philosophy of* logic is much less settled than the standard logical tools taught to philosophy students (this is not to say that there is no disagreement at the level of logic research), but the central questions about what underpins inference and so on are important for thinking about reasoning and rationality as a whole: surely of central concern to the philosophy of mental health!

Session 1 An introduction to deductive reasoning and formal logic

Why argue deductively?

Argument is one way of attempting to arrive at the truth. There are other ways, such as careful observation and experimentation but even these are usually combined with argument to establish what they show and their impact on our other beliefs. Argument is thus a key element in any general intellectual project that has truth as its goal. This, however, raises a question: How does the proffering of sentences justify or establish the truth a further sentence? Logic is the name of the codification of how sentences can bear on the truth of other sentences in argument.

An argument is described as having two parts: the *premisses* (usually plural) from which we argue to the *conclusion* (usually singular). The point of an argument is to demonstrate the truth of the conclusion, given the truth of the premisses. This is a *semantic* claim. It is a claim about the extent to which the sentences correctly report the state of the world they purport to describe. (Semantics is the name of the formal study of how words and sentences can refer to and be true of features of the world.)

But if the aim of an argument is to demonstrate the truth of one sentence from the truth of others, if the success of the argument is in question it seems that we cannot rely on this semantic relation holding. To know that the truth of the conclusion follows from the truth of the premisses seems to require that we know both the truth of both premisses and conclusion. But it was the purpose of the argument to establish the truth of the conclusion.

This circularity is broken by appeal not to the content or the particular sentences serving as premisses and conclusion but to the relation of the structure of the sentences. The argument can be characterized not just in semantic terms—in terms of the world-involving claim expressed—but syntactic terms, terms having to do with the structure of sentences. The idea behind 2000 years of the study of deductive logic is that the structure of arguments that establish the truth of their conclusions can be articulated.

Deductive logic thus codifies the relationship between structures of sentences. We will discuss, albeit briefly, three ways of codifying this structure:

♦ syllogism,

♦ sentential or propositional logic, and

♦ predicate logic.

Logical validity, truth, and soundness in syllogisms

Valid and invalid inferences

A good starting point is Aristotle, the first person to write a systematic treatise on logic, and thus the inspiration behind of all systems of modern logic. In his *Topics*, written sometime in the fourth century BC, he gives a number of examples of a form of inference, which is known as the *syllogism*. Every syllogism is a sequence of three propositions such that the first two imply the third, the conclusion. Thus:

1. All men are mortal
   Socrates is mortal
   Therefore Socrates is a man

2. All men are mortal
   Socrates is a man
   Therefore Socrates is mortal

EXERCISE 1   (10 minutes)

Think about these two arguments. One is valid; one not—which is which, and why?

These examples are both syllogisms. They each have two premisses, one of which is general (the major premiss), the other of which is particular (the minor premiss), and a conclusion (third line). They illustrate many of the points we need to cover in this brief introduction to philosophical logic.

Syllogism 1 is *invalid*. It illustrates one of the classical fallacies—that of arguing from the *minor term* ('are mortal') in the major premiss to a conclusion about the *major term* ('all men'). Clearly, the premisses could be true and the conclusion false (e.g. Socrates could be a mortal *dog* consistently with the major and minor premisses).

Syllogism 2 is *valid*. In a valid argument, as we shall see, *if* the premisses are true, then the conclusion *must* be true. This illustrates the compulsion of valid arguments—i.e. if it is true that all men are mortal and that Socrates is a man, then it *has* to be true that Socrates is mortal.

There are in fact very many forms of syllogism, only some of which are valid. The *Columbia Electronic Encyclopedia* gives the following brief account:

> There are three basic types of syllogism: hypothetical, disjunctive, and categorical. The hypothetical syllogism, *modus ponens*, has as its first premiss a conditional hypothesis: *If p then q*; it continues: *p, therefore q*. The disjunctive syllogism, *modus tollens*, has as its first premiss a statement of alternatives: *Either p or q*; it continues: *not q, therefore p*. The categorical syllogism comprises three categorical propositions, which must be statements of the form *all x are y, no x is y, some x is y*, or *some x is not y*. A categorical syllogism contains precisely three terms: the major term, which is the predicate of the conclusion; the minor term, the subject of the conclusion; and the middle term, which appears in both premisses but not in the conclusion. Thus: *All philosophers are men* (middle term); *all men are mortal*; therefore, *All philosophers* (minor term) *are mortal* (major term). The premisses containing the major and minor terms are named the major and minor premisses, respectively. Aristotle noted five basic rules governing the validity of categorical syllogisms: The middle term must be distributed at least once (a term is said to be distributed when it refers to all members of the denoted class, as in *all x are y* and *no x is y*); a term distributed in the conclusion must be distributed in the premiss in which it occurs; two negative premisses imply no valid conclusion; if one premiss is negative, then the conclusion must be negative; and two affirmatives imply an affirmative.

One of the preoccupations of medieval scholastic philosophy was with the elucidation of the valid forms. But from the above account it is worth asking: How would one determine whether a form of syllogism was valid? What general method is available?

Fortunately, the syllogism is now recognized as a fairly limited form of argument. What it can achieve can be more perspicuously represented using modern logical systems, of which more later. So, thankfully, there is no need to study the many different forms of syllogism!

But even this initial introduction to logical argument raises the question: What makes an argument a good one? What are the qualities or virtues of an argument?

Validity, truth, and soundness

Validity, truth, and *soundness* are three of the most important concepts in logic and are related notions. Validity and truth are used in loose and informal senses in everyday assessments of statements and arguments. Soundness is confined to philosophical use.

In common-sense understanding, a valid argument is simply a *good* argument. But what exactly makes an argument good?

EXERCISE 2 (10 minutes)

Go back to syllogism (2) again. Is the conclusion true? On what does its truth or falsity depend? If the premisses were false, could the conclusion be true? If the premisses were true could the conclusion be false?

Now read:

What the Tortoise Said To Achilles, by Lewis Carroll. Originally published in *Mind* (1895) No. 4, 278–280

Link with Reading 5.1

In the light of the first questions, of what would one need to be persuaded in order rationally to be persuaded of the conclusion of the argument discussed: (*Z*) The two sides of this Triangle are equal to each other?

The truth of the premisses and the validity of the argument

Now one response to the first question set would be to say that the sentence 'Socrates is mortal' is true because it reports the fact that Socrates is (or was) mortal. However, in this context the right response turns on the nature of the argument offered. The conclusion is supposed to follow from the premisses asserted in the argument. Thus there are two issues to be resolved:

* Are the premisses true?

* Does the conclusion follow from the premisses?

This double dependence of the conclusion on what has been placed before it is summarized by Carroll's Tortoise thus.

> 'Readers of Euclid will grant, I suppose, that *Z* follows logically from *A* and *B*, so that anyone who accepts *A* and *B* is true, *must* accept *Z* as true?'

> 'Undoubtedly! The youngest child in a High School—as soon as High Schools are invented, which will not be till some two thousand years later—will grant *that*.'

> 'And if some reader had *not* yet accepted *A* and *B* as true, he might still accept the *Sequence* as a *valid* one, I suppose?'

> 'No doubt such a reader might exist. He might say "I accept as true the Hypothetical Proposition that, if *A* and *B* be true, *Z* must be true; but I *don't* accept *A* and *B* as true." Such a reader would do wisely in abandoning Euclid, and taking to football.'

> 'And might there not *also* be some reader who would say 'I accept *A* and *B* as true, but I *don't* accept the Hypothetical'?'

> 'Certainly there might. *He*, also, had better take to football.'

> 'And *neither* of these readers,' the Tortoise continued, 'is *as yet* under any logical necessity to accept *Z* as true?'

> 'Quite so,' Achilles assented.

What The Tortoise Said To Achilles, by Lewis Carroll, Originally published in *Mind* (1895, No. 4, pp. 278–280)

Note two important things: First, the validity of an argument is independent of the truth of its premises. Secondly, validity functions so as to preserve truth in an argument. Together, the effect is that if the premises of an argument are true, and the form of the argument is valid, then the conclusion will be true also. If one or more of the premises of an argument is false, however, then even if its form is valid, we cannot conclude anything at all about the truth of its conclusion. Similarly, if an argument has true premises but an invalid form may have either a true or false conclusion, just by chance. This is why an argument that has an invalid form cannot be cited as a piece of reasoning from the premises to the conclusion, in other words the truth of the conclusion does not follow from the truth of the premises.

(We will return to the Tortoise and Achilles in the next section. But for now it is worth noting that the Tortoise's last claim above is not so innocent as it appears.)

What is 'truth'?

What of 'truth'? How do we know when something is *true*? And, by knowing this, do we thereby have an understanding of the *concept* 'truth'? These are difficult questions (see suggestions for further reading at the end of this chapter). Consider, for example, a long-standing approach to the nature of truth called a 'correspondence theory'. One might aim to clarify the notion of truth by saying that a true sentence, e.g. corresponds to a fact. Aside from the choice of 'truth bearer' (are sentences, propositions, or beliefs the sorts of things that are paradigmatically true or false?) whether this approach can work or not depends, however, on whether the right-hand side can offer clarification. In this statement of the correspondence relation we would need to know independently what sort of thing a *fact* is. And there is reason to believe that our best grasp of what a fact is, is that it is what a true sentence states! In other words, no independent clarification is offered.

A more modest approach takes the connection between a true sentence and the fact it states as marking not an explanation but the limits of the concept. Take an example of what is called the T schema (meaning True schema) (or sometimes the disquotational schema) following the work of the Polish-American mathematician-logician Alfred Tarski in the 1940s:

T schema: 'P' is true if and only if P.

P stands for a sentence. The sentence that 'P' stands for on the left is *mentioned* while on the right it is stripped of its quotation marks and *used* to state a worldly fact. The most famous examples is: 'Snow is white' is true if and only if snow is white.

This says that the sentence on the left, 'snow is white' has a particular property under particular circumstances. It is true if it is a fact that snow is white. The sentence is true if snow is white. Which sentence? 'Snow is white.'

The philosopher of language Donald Davidson calls this a 'snow bound triviality'. It is a particular example of the relation that a correspondence theorist hopes to use to explain truth.

A minimalist or deflationist argues, by contrast, that there is no substantial property of truth that 'true' picks out. As a recent commentator Bernard Weiss puts it: 'Minimalists or deflationists about truth argue that our concept of truth is all but captured via (some version of) the disquotational schema, '*P*' is true iff *P*.' (Weiss, 2002, p. 63). (NB 'iff' just means if and only if.) The underlying idea of such an approach is that there is no substantial explanatory property common to truths. Because 'is true' is a predicate there may be 'no harm' in taking truth to be a property (Dodd, 2000, p. 136). However, there is no prospect of a successful philosophical project to show, e.g. that all truths correspond to facts where 'correspondence' and 'fact' have independent analyses.

The most miminal such theory was put forward by Frank Ramsey. His 'redundancy theory' proposed that since 'is true' served simply as a device for disquotation in T schema instances it could be eliminated without loss (Ramsey, 1927). Truth is not, however, eliminable because of the need sometimes to make indirect or compendious assertions, e.g. in cases where what is said is not known, although it is known to be true. We might want to say, e.g. that everything the Pope said was true. Hence Weiss's (2002) comment that truth is 'all but captured' in the disquotational schema. Nevertheless, this need not commit us to thinking that there is anything more to truth than the transparent property expressed in the equivalence between asserting that *P* and asserting that '*P*' is true (for elaboration see Horwich, 1990).

Fortunately, for present purposes there is no need to offer a substantial analysis of truth, even if that were possible. Logic codifies good arguments on the assumption that we already know enough what truth is.

True premisses plus valid form = a sound argument

We are now in a position to consider the notion of *soundness*. Soundness is the property an argument has if it is both valid and its premises true. Recall that a valid form of argument is one which, if its premises are true then it cannot fail to have a true conclusion. The concept of 'soundness' is required because we need some way of referring to such arguments, in virtue of the specific effect of the coincidence of validity and truth. Thus, syllogism (2) is a sound argument. Its premises are true, its form is valid, and therefore it has a true conclusion.

What is far from clear, however, is what property of an argument serves to guarantee this relation (i.e. of the truth of the premiss(s) to the truth of the conclusion). In order to inquire into this, we need to introduce the idea of *logical operators*.

Summary so far

So far, we have used the example of syllogism to exemplify the idea that deductive logic is a codification of argumentative structure. If an argument is of the right syntactic form then it can possess a further semantic property: if the premises are true then so is the conclusion. This is the form of a valid argument. Such an argument never leads from truth to falsity.

But validity is not sufficient for the truth of a conclusion. That requires, in addition, that the premisses actually are true. If they are, and if the argument is valid, then it is also a sound argument. Validity of form plus true premisses equals soundness.

But while scholastic philosophy attempted to codify valid forms of argument through syllogisms there is a simpler, more modern approach—propositional or sentential logic—which in turn leads to modern powerful predicate logic devised by Frege. While we will not discuss predicate logic at any length, we will present a brief sketch shortly.

Propositional logic: the logic of simple connectives

Propositional logic and logical operators

Consider the short argument:

> It is raining and the sun is shining
> Therefore, it is raining

This is a valid argument. If the premiss is true then the conclusion must be true. But why?

In this case the answer is obvious. It turns on the structure of the premiss and conclusion. Consider this argument:

> Brix is the best cat in the world and Wittgenstein is the hardest philosopher
>
> Therefore, Brix is the best cat in the world

It shares the same form as the previous argument. If the one is valid then so is the other and in fact both are because of their shared structure which runs as follows:

> P and Q
> Therefore, P

Simple arguments of this form help highlight the way logical form can underpin validity. Take any two basic sentences represented by P and Q, conjoin them with the word 'and' and that gives a complex sentence that can serve as the premiss of an argument from which the first basic sentence can be derived as a valid conclusion.

The branch of logic that deals with this kind of structure is called Propositional or Sentential logic because it takes as its basic building blocks whole sentences or propositions linked together by some basic logical operators.

Sentences and propositions

The word 'proposition' in philosophy refers to the contents of sentences, what can be shared by sentences with the same meaning in different languages, for example. A proposition is what is expressed and is distinct from the particular form of words in which it is expressed. But this distinction—between proposition and sentence—plays no part in what follows and hence the equivalence here of 'propositional' and 'sentential' logic.

In propositional logic the sentences discussed are restricted to *indicative sentence*. An indicative sentence expresses a proposition about the world, about how things are (or might be in imagination); it indicates things. So, 'All swans are white', and 'All men are mortal', are both indicative. Indicative sentences can be asserted, denied, contended, assumed, supposed, implied, or presupposed. (Indicative sentences contrast with questions and orders, interogative and imperative moods. So 'the door is closed' contrasts with 'Is the door closed?' and 'Close the door!'. Only the first plays a role in propositional logic.)

Thus the basic sentences considered can be true or false.

Logical operators and connectives

The other ingredient of propositional logic is the set of logical connectives or logical operators. A logical operator is a word (or phrase) used either to modify one statement to make a different statement or to join two statements together to form a more complicated statement.. The connectives deployed in propositional logic include 'and', 'or', 'if ... then'. 'Not' is also an operator, although not intuitively a connective (because it 'connects' to only one sentence at a time).

Some but not all connectives in English are 'truth functional'. These are connectives that, when used to form complex sentences from more basic ones, give sentences whose truth depends only on the truth or falsity of the basic sentences. Thus 'and' and 'or' are (more or less) truth functional in English. (More or less because some uses of 'and' in English imply more than just conjunction but rather something like 'because', which is not truth functional.) The truth of the complex sentences 'A & B' and 'A or B' are given by the following rules:

> A & B is true if and only if A is true and B is true.
> A or B is true if and only if A is true or B is true.

These rules can be symbolized in a 'truth table': the notation devised by the Austrian philosopher, who was based in Cambridge for most of his professional life where he was a professor, Ludwig Wittgenstein (1889–1951). Symbolizing 'and' as '&' and 'or' as '∨' so as to emphasize that these are connectives in the language of propositional logic rather than English and using P and Q to stand for sentences the truth tables are as follows.

> P & Q
> T T T
> T F F
> F F T
> F F F
>
> P ∨ Q
> T T T
> T T F
> F T T
> F F F

The tables set out the truth value of the complex sentences ('P & Q' and 'P ∨ Q') for the component truth values of the basic sentences. Because the connectives combine two basic sentences we need to have four rows to capture the permutations of truth and falsity (P is T and F when Q is T and P is T and F when Q is F). the truth of the whole sentence: the conjunctive and the disjunctive is given by the column of T and F in the centre.

In the case of '&', the complex is true only if both P and Q are true. For 'or' or '∨' the composite requires that one or the other is true. (Note that 'because', which is not truth functional, could not be expressed in this form. We will come to if...then shortly.)

The basic connectives are given below. The last pair are if...then, the material implication, symbolized with the horseshoe and if and only if symbolized ≡.

P	Q	−P	−Q	P∨Q	P & Q	P⊃Q	P≡Q
T	T	F	F	T	T	T	T
T	F	F	T	T	F	F	F
F	T	T	F	T	F	T	F
F	F	T	T	F	F	T	T

The basic language of propositional logic is quite powerful. Given the rules for combining basic sentences using connectives, there is no limit to the number of complex sentences that can be formed. There is no limit, for example, simply to conjoining one atomic sentence with others, or even perhaps different tokens of the same sentence type. The resultant complex sentence can then be further conjoined with other atomic or complex sentences. The truth condition of the final result will still be determined by a complex function of the truth conditions of the component atomic sentences and thus derivable from them. But since the process of conjoining sentences can in principle be repeated without limit, a general method of spelling out the truth conditions of arbitrary sentences of the object language will have to be *recursive*. It will have to be repeatedly applicable so that the output of one operation can feed in as the input to the next application until the constituent atomic sentences are reached.

Imagine that a version of propositional logic contains just the following connectives: not, and , or and if...then. One might then define the 'well formed formulae' of that language by a recursive definition as follows:

1. Any letter standing for a sentence or proposition (e.g. A, B, C...) is a well-formed formula, wff.

2. If α (standing for A, B , C or for sentences constructed from them using rules 1–6 etc.) is a wff, then so is '¬α' (i.e. not α)

3. If α and β are wff, then so is '(a & b)'

4. If α and β are wff, then so is '(α ∨ β)'

5. If α and β are wff, then so is '(α ⊃ β)' (i.e. if α then β)

6. Only sentences according to steps 1–6 is a wff.

A grammar like this, in conjunction with the truth tables for the connectives allows the calculation of the truth value of arbitrarily complex sentences in propositional logic from the truth values of its basic sentences.

Arguing with propositional logic

In fact for many arguments in both philosophy and everyday life the structure of the argument used is quite simple. Thus one tool for assessing whether an argument is valid is by relating it to known valid and invalid forms. Here are some common forms:

Modus ponens

> If P then Q
> P
> Therefore Q

This is a valid argument and perhaps the most common argument form actually used.

Modus tollens

> If P then Q
> Not Q
> Therefore, not P

This is a form of argument used in the hypothetico-deductive model of diagnosis. If the patient has syndrome X then he will have such and such symptoms. He does not have those symptoms. Thus he does not have syndrome X.

Affirming the consequent

> If P then Q
> Q
> Therefore, P

This is a common fallacy. It is not valid. If Socrates is a man then he is mortal. He is mortal. Therefore he is a man. But in fact not all mortals are men and he may be a rabbit.

Denying the antecedent

> If P then Q
> Not P
> Therefore, not Q

This is another fallacy. If patient has syndrome X they will have such and such symptoms. They do not have syndrome X. Therefore they do not have such and such symptoms. But in fact those symptoms may come about for different reasons.

Disjunctive syllogism

> Either P or Q
> Not P
> Therefore, Q

This is again a valid argument.

Reductio ad absurdum

One other form of argument is worth particular note less for its general application than for its more colloquial associations: reductio ad absurdum.

The basic idea is that if by assuming P one can derive an absurdity—such as Q and not Q—then one can conclude that not P is true. This follows from the idea that a valid argument cannot lead from true premises to a false conclusion. If the conclusion is false—e.g. if it is a contradiction and could not be true—and if the argument is valid, then at least one of the premisses must be false. In practice it is often a matter of debate in real argument, which the false premiss is. (Logic problems generally allow ways to target a particular premiss perhaps by assuming each in turn is false and deriving a reductio for each.)

A very famous reductio is Pythagoras's proof that the square root of 2 is not a rational number:

1. Assume that $\sqrt{2}$ is a rational number, i.e. a number that can be expressed as a fraction x/y and, further, the faction is expressed in terms that cannot be further reduced, i.e. divided through by common factors. (The terms in the fraction 4/6 by contrast do have a common factor of 2 and thus that fraction can be reduced to 2/3, which is an irreducible fraction.)

2. If $\sqrt{2} = x/y$ then $(x/y)^2 = 2$

3. Thus $x^2/y^2 = 2$ and $x^2 = 2y^2$

4. Therefore x^2 is an even number

5. Thus x is even (because only even numbers have even numbered squares)

6. If x is even then for some z, $x = 2z$

7. Thus $2y^2 = (2z)^2$

8. Thus $2y^2 = 4z^2$

9. Thus $y^2 = 2z^2$

10. As $2z^2$ is even then y^2 is also even and thus y is even.

11. Thus both x and y are even. So x/y is not irreducible, which contradicts the first premiss.

12. Thus $\sqrt{2}$ is not a rational number.

Assessing validity with truth tables

Truth tables

For more complex arguments, propositional logic has another trick up its sleeve. Return to the key idea that complex sentences can be built using more basic sentences and truth functional connectives according to some rules of grammar. The rules of that grammar allow a complex sentence to be broken up into smaller parts but that still leaves rather a complicated final analysis.

There is, however, an elegant way of calculating the truth or falsity of a complex sentence, which depends on its component parts: truth tables, again. The basic idea is that a truth table sets out the truth value of complex sentences in terms of its constituents. However, the basic truth table can be applied to more complex cases than connections applied to just two atomic sentences. By careful application of truth tables recursively to complex combinations the truth value of the complex sentence can be displayed as a function of its parts. This in turn allows for calculating whether one sentence is implied by another.

The method is quite mechanical. One first calculates the truth values of sentences in the premisses in terms of the basic atomic sentences that make them up, and likewise for the conclusion. Recall that the key test for validity is that the conclusion is never false when the premisses are true. Thus one can see whether the argument is valid by checking that, for a combination of atomic sentence truth values, the premisses are never true and the conclusion false.

Most statements will have some combination of T and F in their truth table columns; they are called contingencies. Some statements will have nothing but T; they are called tautologies. There are true whatever the truth values of their component parts. Others will have nothing but F; they are called contradictions. They cannot be true whatever the truth value of their component parts.

Consider the following arguments:

Not (P & Q)

P

Therefore, not Q

And:

(not P or not Q)

Therefore, not (P or Q)

P	Q	Not (P & Q)	(P & Q)	P	Not Q
T	T	F	T	T	F
T	F	**T**	F	**T**	**T**
F	T	**T**	F	**F**	**F**
F	F	**T**	F	**F**	**T**

The table represents the premisses of the first argument: Not (P & Q) and P in the third and fifth columns of Ts and Fs. The conclusion is the final column. Now the test for validity is that true premisses should never lead to false conclusions. Do they? The premisses are only both true in the second row and then the conclusion is true also. So the premisses are never true and the conclusion false. So the argument is valid.

But the next argument is invalid. The premiss is the fourth column and the conclusion the sixth but in the second and third row the premiss is true when the conclusion is false.

P	Q	(not P	or	not Q)	not	(P or Q)
T	T	F	F	F	F	T
T	F	F	**T**	T	**F**	T
F	T	T	**T**	F	**F**	T
F	F	T	**T**	T	**T**	F

The language of predicate logic

The need for predicate logic

While propositional logic is powerful it cannot capture even everything in the first syllogisms described at the start of this chapter: All men are mortal, Socrates is a man, therefore Socrates is mortal. But there is a more powerful logic devised by Gottlob Frege (1848–1925). We will merely introduce the kind of symbolism used and give directions for further reading on the subject.

Predicates and quantifiers

Frege's innovation was to provide a notation to symbolize a structure within whole basic sentences rather than just relying on whole sentences as building blocks for more complex sentences. This analysis could thus deploy some of the resources of propositional logic (although not the mechanical test of validity based on truth tables) but augment them with further tools.

The basic building blocks of Frege's predicate logic are variable terms standing for objects: x, y, z, etc. terms standing for predicates F, G, H and two quantifiers (universal and existential).

Predicates have one or more places. Thus a one place predicate might be 'Rx' and mean that x is red. Or it might have two places and express a relation between two objects. xLy, or Lx,y might mean x loves y. Note that order may be important. Much sadness turns on the fact that xLy does not imply that yLx!

The quantifiers are the universal quantifier and the existential quantifier. The universal quantifier symbolized $\forall(x)$ says 'For all x' or 'For every x'. Thus $\forall(x)$ Rx says that every x is R, which might mean red: every object in the universe is red.

The existential quantifier $\exists(x)$ says that there is at least one x, or there is some x such that (where some might be singular)... Thus $\exists(x)$ Rx says that there is at least one thing that is R or red, in this case.

Quantifiers predicates and variables can be put together to form whole sentences. Note that every variable in a sentence has to be bound by a quantifier for the sentence to be whole and thus capable of truth or falsity. A sentence that has at least one unbound variable is called an 'open sentence', but it does not actually say anything capable of truth or falsity.

The order of quantifiers

Note the difference between the second and third case below. Simplifying the universe discussed to people the following instances might have the following prose interpretations.

$\forall(x)$ $\forall(y)$ xLy says: that for everyone x the following is true: x loves everyone y. In other words, everyone loves everyone including themselves.

$\forall(x)$ $\exists(y)$ xLy says that for every person x there is at least one person y such that x loves that person.

$\exists(x)$ $\forall(y)$ xLy says that there is at least one person x who loves every person y.

$\exists(x)$ $\exists(y)$ xLy says that there is at least one person x such that there is at least one person y and x loves y.

The quantifiers thus allow careful articulation of sentences in which in English are ambiguous. Take a textbook favourite example:

Every nice girl loves a sailor.

This might mean any of:

There is one sailor that every nice girl loves

Every nice girl loves some sailor or other (not necessarily the same one.

Every nice girl loves every sailor.

The difference between these can be expressed using combinations of the two quantifiers.

We will not, however, go further in setting out the logical inferences that this powerful symbolism allows.

Summary of the session

The purpose of this session has been to introduce some of the key terms and tools of modern logic. Deductive logic seeks valid arguments by careful attention to their form or structure. A valid argument cannot lead from true premises to a false conclusion. If the premises are true then so is the conclusion. An argument is sound if its premises are true and it is valid.

While Aristotle discussed forms of syllogism more modern approaches to logic have been developed from the end of the nineteenth century. Propositional logic is the logic of the connectives and, or, if then, not etc. These are truth functional: the truth values of complex sentences made using them dependent only on the truth values of the components. Truth tables allow the definition of connectives and a mechanical test for the validity of arguments.

Predicate logic refines this structure and adds predicates, variables and quantifies to analyse structure within basic sentences.

In the next session we will examine the nature of logical inference: what underpins it?

Reflection on the session and self-test questions

Write down your own reflections on the materials in this session drawing out any points that are particularly significant for you. Then write brief notes about the following:

1. What is the aim of deductive argument?

2. What is meant by 'valid' and 'sound' as applied to arguments?

3. How can the validity of arguments be assessed?

4. What forms of deductive argument or logic are there?

5. What is propositional logic? And what is a truth table?

Session 2   An introduction to the philosophy of logic: what underpins deductive logic?

Deduction and induction

Thus far, we have been considering a form of inference known as *deduction*. The codification of deductive validity in propositional logic suggests that its strength lies in an essential modesty: the conclusions of deductive are somehow contained within the premises. The arguments simply unpack something that was already implicit in the premises. It is this very fact that ensures that true premises cannot lead to false conclusions. By comparison with another kind of argument, however, that can seem very modest indeed. We will argue briefly, however, that deduction still has a clear use. We will then consider more deeply what underpins logical inference, and what precise sense there is in saying that the premisses contain the conclusions.

The other central form of inference is *induction*. Where deductive reasoning relies only on the definitions of the terms in which it is conducted, inductive reasoning relies on the way things are in the world. An oft quoted example is this: 'because the sun has risen in the East for millions of years, therefore it will rise in the East tomorrow'. Inductive reasoning, being in this way experience based, is crucially important to scientific reasoning. In induction, the premisses supply only a part of what appears in the conclusion. That is to say, the induction is *ampliative*, in that it goes further than deductive argument will allow.

Deduction is uninformative, circular, and tautologous

All deductive inference has three major features that distinguish it from inductive inference. These three features are that it is, strictly, *uninformative, circular*, and *tautologous*.

Deductive inference is *uninformative* in a quite straightforward way: in not allowing us to go beyond the information contained in the premisses, it does not offer us any new information about the world.

A *circular* argument argues in a circle. It ends where it started from. But circularity is not necessarily a bad thing. Deductive inference is such a powerful tool of reasoning just because is allows us to check the correctness of a claim, given certain starting assumptions. If it were not the case that this involved a certain amount of circularity (as in syllogism (2) above), then a valid deduction would not be compulsive. Valid deduction is compelling in that we cannot deny that the truth of the conclusion is a logical consequence of the truth of its premisses, in virtue of its form. But it does suggest a constraint on how deduction can play a useful role. Consider:

> All swans are white
> Cygnus is a swan
> Cygnus is white.

Suppose that knowing the truth of the first premiss involved or required checking each swan. Then it seems that the only way to know the truth of the premiss would be to check each and every swan *including Cygnus*. And that seems to make the argument useless. There is no use for the argument given that knowledge of the premiss requires prior knowledge of the conclusion. But, as we will see, there are still uses for such argument.

Tautology

We suggested that the third characteristic of deductive argument was that it is tautological. This can seem surprising. A tautology, on a standard dictionary definition, means something like: saying the same thing twice over. That also does not sound very useful but as we will see it does not undermine the purpose of deductive argument.

In logic a tautology is a defined as a complex statement whose truth is independent of the truth or falsity of its component parts. As a result it does not tell us anything about the world. Consider the statement:

> Either it is Monday or it is not Monday.

That whole sentence is true if either of its parts is true. These are:

> It is Monday
> It is not Monday

Now if it is Monday, the first component is true and so is the whole sentence. But in all other cases, the second component is true and so, again, the whole sentence is true. Thus its truth is independent of the truth or falsity of the components. Furthermore, the fact that it is true tells us nothing about the day of the week.

Valid arguments are, however, related to tautologies in this way. Consider the argument,

> P
> If P then Q
> Therefore, Q

This is valid. This means that if the premisses are true then the conclusion is true (it must be true). This means that a single whole sentence that conjoins the premisses and connects them to the conclusion with the connective if ... then will always be true. So the sentence

> 'If (P and (if P then Q)) then Q'

is always true whatever truth values of P and Q.

Consider now the argument:

> It is Monday, and
> If it is Monday then the weekend is at least four full days away
> Then the weekend is at least four full days away.

This is a valid argument. If the premisses are true then so must the conclusion be. But the argument is clearly related to the following statement:

> If, it is Monday and, if it is Monday then the weekend is at least four full days away, then the weekend is at least four full days away.

This statement is tautological. The structure of the sentence is so formed that whatever day of the week it is, the sentence as a whole is true.

Whenever we can frame a valid argument we can translate it into a tautological statement. It is the validity of the argument that guarantees this.

The role of deductive argument given that it is 'uninformative'

If the conclusions of deductive arguments are strictly uninformative and circular what is the purpose of deductive inference? In scientific inquiry there are at least three positive uses (which in turn motivate examination of logical inference and argument).

1. Scientific theories and hypothesis make *general* claims. Testing such theories, however, relies on the examination of (some of) their consequences in *particular* circumstances. As the general claims cannot be directly tested as a whole it is necessary to *derive* particular consequences for experiment and observation.

2. Deep explanatory theories often postulate unobservable or hidden causes. (These may unify diverse observable phenomena.) As the claims about unobservable causes cannot be directly tested (by definition), testable claims need to be derived from them. Thus there is a positive advantage in the fact that the deductive move from general theory to particular claim involves a loss of information (about the hidden cause).

3. Claims about the world couched in ordinary sentences deploy concepts that have implicitly general consequences. To say that there is a particular chair in a particular corner is to make a particular claim. But it also implies—because of the implicit generality of the concept 'chair'—that there is something substantial, enduring, of mass, etc. in the corner. Drawing deductive conclusions is one way of highlighting the aspects of that content with which we are interested in a particular context.

Consider just the first of these cases. Diagnosis in general practice is often described as following a hypothetico-deductive pattern. Presented with the signs and symptoms, one forms a provisional list of possible diagnoses. Starting with the most likely, one derives an observable deductive consequence. If the symptoms result from such and such underlying cause then that cause would also produce so and so. Is so and so present? Yes or no? This process relies on deduction in a way that escapes the worry about circularity mentioned above.

Can one ever reach a conclusion?

We have so far briefly outlined three ways to codify logical argument: syllogism, propositional and predicate logic. And we have flagged the apparent weakness of deductive argument: that it simply unpacks its premises. But that way of justifying deductive argument faces the following historically significant objection.

EXERCISE 3   (10 minutes)

Look back at the reading with Exercise 2 from *What The Tortoise Said To Achilles* by Lewis Carroll and the continuation that goes with this exercise.

Link with Reading 5.1

How does the Tortoise generate a sceptical challenge against the rational force of logic? What is the significance of his comment: 'Whatever *Logic* is good enough to tell me is worth *writing down*,'? How could the scepticism be defused?

Summary of the problem

The bare bones of the Tortoise's challenge can be thought of like this. The Tortoise asks what the conditions are for being rationally convinced by the argument 'A, B therefore Z' of the truth of the conclusion Z? He suggests that there are two components.

1. Rational belief in the truth of the premises and . . .

2. Rational belief in the validity of the sequent.

The Tortoise accepts (1) but asks to be persuaded of (2). It seems reasonable to suppose that if logic is to be a means of persuasion then there should be the resources to convince him.

But, in fact, the Tortoise suggests that there is a regress. The problem is that rationally believing (2) amounts to accepting that:

   C: If A, B then Z

So the Tortoise must necessarily accept C as well as A, B if he is to be rationally persuaded of Z. Because what logic is good enough to teach is worth writing down he adds this to the list of claims he has to believe alongside the first two premises. Strangely while a moment before he did not believe C he is willing to grant it when asked by Achilles, proving it is written down. It might seem—as it does to Achilles—that this has now solved the problem.

But now the argument seems to have changed to:

   A, B, C therefore Z

and the Tortoise now says that rationally to believe Z he must necessarily accept the new hypothetical:

   D: If A, B, C then Z

Now there is a regress. It appears one has to accept an infinite number of premises before one can be rationally persuaded of Z. Thus one cannot be rationally persuaded. And thus in general, logic cannot rationally persuade!

It is worth pausing at this point. If the Tortoise is correct then logical inference is like Zeno's paradox, as he mentions at the start, but without the solution that the steps involved in getting to the end (the end of the race or the conclusion of the argument) get smaller each time and can be summed. It seems that Carroll wrote this piece because he was genuinely confused.

Diagnosis

In general in philosophy if a sceptical argument is deployed it is wise, if possible, to try to block it before it gets off the ground. In this case the addition of premiss C that codifies the hypothetical involved is what starts the problem off.

Note first that in general, adding extra premises that codify the hypothetical involved to arguments is not a good idea. Consider two cases:

◆ If the argument is valid already then adding the extra hypothetical premiss is unnecessary. If it was valid before then it will be no more valid afterwards.

◆ If the argument was invalid before then adding the premiss will make it valid. But recall that there are two ingredients for rational persuasion: belief that the argument is valid and belief that the premisses are true. The strengthening extra premiss in this case reports that the prior argument is valid. But that is false. So one of the premisses of the new argument is false. The argument is not sound. And thus Z does not follow.

The moral that Carroll should have drawn is this: the Tortoise confuses grasp of rules of inference with acceptance of further premisses. They are distinct. Thus although the Tortoise must accept the rule equivalent to the hypothetical C, this is not a further premiss.

Justification of an argument is a meta-level commentary on that argument, not an extra step in the same argument. The correct way to persuade the Tortoise is not to ask him to accept a further premiss but to show why the argument is valid in the first place, it is to show that it has the correct form.

But a problem remains

The purpose of looking at Carroll's brief article is not, ultimately, to call the force of logic into question but to shed light on how it has that force. It is not a matter of implicitly knowing an infinite number of premisses. Nor is it a matter of external compulsion.

Recall Achilles rather desperate cry: 'Then Logic would take you by the throat, and *force* you to do it!' That is a natural expression of a platonist view. Logic can be pictured as wholly independent of human subjects. But Achilles's hope is in vain. (We will return to Wittgenstein's criticism of platonism in Chapter 25.) Rather, if one has eyes to see it, then one can see that the premisses are indeed sufficient for the truth of the conclusion without the need to pile up further assurance.

That, however, still leaves a question: What is it that underpins the transition from premiss to conclusion? We can ask this not in a sceptical tone but for clarification of the nature and origins of logical force.

In what sense is the conclusion of an argument contained in its premisses?

> **EXERCISE 4**   (10 minutes)
>
> Look at the extract from the following reading:
>
> Prior, A. (1960). The runabout inference-ticket. Analysis 21: 38–39 (Reprinted in Strawson (ed.), *Philosophical Logic*. pp. 217–218)
>
> ———————————————————————
> Link with Reading 5.3
> ———————————————————————
>
> ◆ What is the analytic theory of validity, and how does the connective tonk undermine that picture?

The analytic theory of validity

Prior's target is a family of views about the nature and underpinnings of logic that he calls the 'analytic theory of validity'.

This is the intuitive and attractive view that logical inferences are sustained solely by the definitions of the logical connectives involved. Connectives and inferences are completely mutually defined *de novo*. The inferences fix the meaning of the connectives and the connectives fix the inferences allowed. Neither answer to anything else. Logic is a kind of self-contained game.

Imagine that someone were to ask why the knight in chess can move in the way it can? Now in a modern design of chess set it might be reasonable to ask why 'that piece!' has moved as it has and the correct answer might be that looks notwithstanding it is a knight and thus that is a move it is allowed. But identification of the chess piece is not an issue then there is no very helpful answer to give except to say that knight's are just defined in the game of chess by being permitted that move. That is what makes it a knight and because it is a knight it can move in that way. Moves and pieces are defined together and answer to know uber-chess facts. Chess is not, for example, a representation of a real battle. It does not have to describe anything.

So the analytic theory gives an austere answer to the question of what sustains logical inference: the mutual definition of connectives and inferences.

Tonk's challenge

Tonk is deployed in a kind of *reductio ad absurdum*. Its definition fits the analytic theory of validity. However, it leads to the absurd conclusion that anything may be inferred from anything else. Thus it is absurd and thus so is the analytic theory.

> 'Tonk' is defined thus:
> A implies A tonk B, and A tonk B implies B.
> Thus A implies B for arbitrary A, B.

But from the perspective of the theory, there should be nothing wrong with these rules of inference given the meaning of tonk and the meaning, given the rules. There is no other standard of correctness.

What response should we give to this challenge? We will consider two.

Belnap's context of deducibility response

In a brief paper in the philosophy journal *Analysis*, which specializes in very short pieces, the logician Nuel Belnap (1961–62) offered the following diagnosis. First, he suggested that there could be no such connective as tonk just as there could be no such mathematical operator '?' defined as follows. For any fractions a/b and c/d then,

$$\{a/b \;?\; c/d\} = \{(a + c)/(b + d)\}$$

The problem with the function '?' so defined is that it gives different results, e.g. $\{2/3 \;?\; 4/5\}$ and $\{4/6 \;?\; 4/5\}$. (Calculate the result for both!) But 2/3 equals 4/6 and thus it should not matter which one picks.

Belnap says that this definition contradicts prior assumptions about mathematics (that e.g. 2/3 = 4/6). From this he draws the moral that new mathematical functions have to be defined in a way that is consistent with—or conservative of—prior assumptions.

Likewise, in logic, new connectives should be defined in terms of inferences in such a way that inferences not involving them do not permit inferences that were not possible before. They should preserve the context of deducibility.

The rules governing 'tonk' fail because they allow the inference of statements *not involving tonk*, which were not previously deducible by the rules of deduction. The reason for saying statements *not involving tonk* is this. The inference of the 'contonktive' A tonk B from A does not violate prior assumptions. This was not a statement that had any meaning before tonk was introduced. It is the next stage: deriving B from the contonktive, that was not possible before but which violates logical inference.

This raises the general question, however: What characterizes the context of deducibility? Belnap suggests that all new rules must be conservative extensions of a context of deducibility defined: Gentzen's structural rules.

Gerhard Gentzen

Gerhard Gentzen (1909–45) worked on logic and the foundations of mathematics. His structural rules are very general rules that are supposed to characterize permitted rules of inference. They are fairly intuitive allowing, e.g. the addition of extra premises to already valid arguments (cf. the Tortoise above) and swapping round of premises within arguments. These are the rules:

> *weakening*: from A1,…, An ⇒ C infer A1,…, An, B ⇒ C
>
> *permutation*: from A1,…, Ai, Ai +1 ,…, An ⇒ B infer A1,…, Ai + 1, Ai,…, An ⇒ B
>
> *contraction*: from A1,…, An, An ⇒ B infer A1,…, An, ⇒ B
>
> *transitivity*: from A1,…, Am ⇒ B and C1,…, Cn, B ⇒ D infer A1,…, Am, C1,…, Cn, B ⇒ D

It is outside the scope of this chapter to discuss whether they are successful in characterizing the 'context of deducibility'. But in the context of this chapter—the context of asking what underpins logical inference—they do raise the following problem. They simply repeat, albeit in a more abstract structural way, a list of permitted inferences. And that leaves open the question: What underpins these rules? (Again the question is not being asked in the Tortoises sceptical way. Rather, the question is what in general underpins inferences?) Simply listing more rules does seem to address this question.

Stevenson's vindication through truth tables

In another short paper in the journal *Analysis*, Stevenson (1961) provides a different response to Prior (1960).

He points out that tonk is defined as a kind of permissive game, without any consideration of the injunction that should characterize logic: that truth be preserved in a valid argument. True premises should never lead to a false conclusion. That is the essence of logical validity set out in the previous session. Stevenson suggests that if an inference is called into question—as, e.g. the Tortoise does—it should be *validated* by showing that it follows a rule and then that rule should be *vindicated*.

How should a rule be vindicated? Stevenson argues that this can be done with a truth table. One can spot that something is wrong with tonk because no single truth table can represent how it functions. The introduction of tonk (from A infer A tonk B) looks like 'or' and the elimination (from A tonk B infer B) looks like 'and'. Thus it needs two truth tables.

So a condition of possibility for connective introduction is that they can be represented by a single truth table. This is a sensible response to tonk. But it leaves open the question of whether Stevenson's response undermines the analytic theory of validity—i.e. agrees with Prior—or whether it merely augments it. In other words can we say that inferences and connectives are mutually defined, answer to nothing else, but that the definition has to meet a particular internal consistency constraint: they must be codifiable in a truth table? There is no clear answer to that question.

(Comment on vindication by truth table)

Although Stevenson (1961) provides a sensible criticism of tonk, and it can serve as a necessary test of a potential connective, there remains a general problem with using truth tables to justify rules of inference. This was made clear in a paper by the philosopher Sue Haack (1976). She suggests that typically, at least, the application of the truth table will use (at the meta-level) the very (ground-level) rule to be justified. So as a general method of vindication truth tables only work if one can already presuppose correct rules of inference and that is question-begging.

She gives the following example using Modus Monens and contrasting it with the fallacy of affirming the consequent (symbolized MM in her paper):

> *A1: The justification of Modus Ponens* (using the truth table for if..then.)
>
> Suppose 'A' is true and 'A ⊃ B' is true.
>
> By the truth table for '⊃' if 'A' is true and 'A ⊃ B' is true, then 'B' is true too.
>
> So 'B' must be true too.

This argument has the form:

> A1*
> Suppose C (that 'A' is true and that 'A ⊃ B' is true).
> If C then D (if 'A' is true and 'A ⊃ B' is true, then 'B' is true).
> So D ('B' must be true too).

Now Haack (1976) suggests that this justification is akin to inductive justifications of induction (which will be discussed in Chapter 16).

A2: Justification of induction:

Induction has usually been successful in the past.

Therefore (by induction) induction is usually successful.

This inference assumes the very rule of inference—induction—it is designed to justify. Is this circularity vicious or virtuous? It is hard to tell. But the problem is that counter-induction is also self-justifying. Counter-induction is the principle that what has happened in the past will not happen in the future. It can also justify itself:

A3 Justification of counter-induction:

Counter-induction has usually not been successful in the past.

Therefore (by counter-induction) counter-induction is usually successful.

So if there is a problem with induction—and many philosophers think there is as we will discuss in chapter 16—Haack suggests that there is in deduction as well. Because justifying Modus Ponens—perhaps the key form of inference—using truth tables invokes that very principle. But is there an analogue of counter-induction for deduction? Yes: affirming the consequent (MM in what follows).

Deductive analogue of counter-induction:

Define MM: from A ⊃ B and B infer A

A4 Suppose that 'A ⊃ B' is true and 'B' is true, then 'A ⊃ B' is true ⊃ 'B' is true.

Now by the truth table for '⊃', if 'A' is true, then if 'A ⊃ B' is true, 'B' is true.

Therefore 'A' is true.

To make this a little clearer it has this form:

A4* Suppose D (if 'A ⊃ B' is true, then 'B' is true)

If C, then D (if 'A' is true, then, if 'A ⊃ B' is true, 'B' is true).

So C ('A' is true).

But we will not consider this worry further here.

Analyticity

So something like the analytic theory of validity remains attractive. It is prompted by a response to the Tortoise that you may have arrived at yourself in thinking about his problem. Recall, the Tortoise questions why he should believe the conclusion Z given that he accepts the premises A and B. Recall also what the argument actually was:

(A) Things that are equal to the same are equal to each other.

(B) The two sides of the Triangle are things that are equal to the same.

(Z) The two sides of this Triangle are equal to each other.

Now one response is to say that if the Tortoise accepts A and B then he has *already* accepted Z. Z is already contained with A and B! But what is the sense of 'containment'? Premises are not literally containers.

We will consider this response a little more.

Analytic versus synthetic

The terms *analytic* and *synthetic* were introduced by the eighteenth century Prussian philosopher Immanuel Kant. A statement expresses an *analytic truth*, only if the concept of the predicate is contained within the concept of the subject. For example, 'All husbands are male' is composed of a subject term ('All husbands') and a predicate term ('male'), with a connective ('are') that functions as the logical operator of predication (i.e. 'have the property of 'x'-ness' where 'x' = 'male'). But because the idea of maleness is contained in the idea 'husband', an analysis of the latter necessarily reveals the idea of maleness.

Thus an analytic truth is a truth that depends upon meaning alone. By contrast a synthetic truth depends on meaning (to be the truth it is) but also on how the world is. Thus 'all bachelors are happy' is true in virtue both of what the terms mean but also, given what they do mean, on whether bachelors are, as a matter of fact, happy.

Necessary versus synthetic

There are two other influential distinctions between kinds of truth. The analytic synthetic distinction is a distinction within semantics. It has to do with the relation of truth and meaning. The other two are metaphysical and epistemological.

A truth is necessary if it could not have been false and contingent if it could have been false. A necessary truth is true in all possible worlds. A contingent truth is true only in some possible worlds, worlds most like ours.

A priori versus a posteriori

Arguably, some truths can be known only through experience. Other truths can be known without experience (whether or not they could also be known through experience). This is the epistemological distinction between the a priori—which is knowable prior to experience—and the a posteriori—which can be known only after experience.

EXERCISE 5 (10 minutes)

Consider the following thought experiment. Suppose that you had access to all the truths about the world, the earth, its place in the cosmos, the truths of reason, etc. Imagine that you were to divide the truths up using the three distinctions above: semantic, metaphysical, and epistemological. Would they divide the truths in the same way?

Why might they align?

Many philosophers have thought that the three kinds of truth will divide truths up in the same way: philosophers from Hume—in so far as we can ascribe a semantic thesis to him—to the Logical Positivists of the early twentieth century. Here is an argument why they might:

1. If we can know a truth a priori we can know it without knowing which possible world we inhabit.

2. Thus is must apply in all possible worlds.

3. Further, it must be something we bring to knowledge of the world rather than being given by the world.

4. So it must be analytic.

To find truths which do not fit this alignment we need to think of, e.g. synthetic but a priori truths or a posteriori but necessary truths. And indeed two philosophers have made such claims.

Kant argued that the truths of arithmetic were a prior. But they were not analytic. No amount of thinking about the concept of 7 and plus and 5, for example takes one beyond 7 and plus and 5. It takes a further intuition to get to 12.

More recently, Saul Kripke (1940–) metaphysician and logician has argued that there are a posteriori necessities. If water is H_2O then it is H_2O necessarily. There is no possible world in which there is water but no H_2O. Of course there may be possible worlds in which there is something that looks and tastes like water; however, if it is not H_2O it is not water. Still, it took much empirical work to discover that.

In Part V we will look at Kripke's argument that mental states are not physical states for reasons based on this claim.

Quine's attack

W.V.O. Quine has argued, however, that not only do the distinctions between truths not align, there are no such distinctions. He argued this in a seminal paper: 'Two dogmas of empiricism', which often tops the polls of most influential philosophical paper among analytic philosophers.

The kernal of Quine's argument is that we cannot explain what we mean by analyticity. He claims that there is no distinction between the analytic and synthetic on the grounds that we cannot explain what that distinction amounts to. All attempts at explanation presuppose equally mysterious concepts.

Thus for example, he argues that we cannot define analytic truth by appeal to logical truths. We might have thought that 'all bachelors are unmarried' might be derived from the logical truth 'all unmarried men are unmarried' via substitution of the synonym 'bachelor' for' unmarried man'. But, Quine argues, synonymy is just as dubious as analyticity.

We cannot attempt to explain that term through the notion of definition because most, at least, definitions attempt to capture prior relations of synonymy rather than explaining that notion.

We might have attempted to define synonymy by noting that when one substitutes a synonym for a word in a sentence then its truth or falsity is unaffected. (Of course this is not true if the sentence, e.g. refers to the number of letters in a word.) So one might have assumed one could turn this around and define synonymy as that which leaves the truth of sentences unchanged when substitutions are made. But in fact it needs to be stronger than that. Truths about 'creatures with a heart' will be the same as truths about 'creatures with kidneys' because they are the same creatures, as a matter of fact. But those phrases do not mean the same. But any strengthening of the relation will require using terms

such as 'of necessity' ('the substitution is truth value preserving of necessity'), which Quine asserts, are just as obscure.

Quine concludes that because analyticity can only be explained in terms of a small number of equally opaque concepts, there is no such concept. Why does this follow? Quine does not himself say but one thought is that if there is no way of testing correct understanding, there is nothing determinate to be understood.

Quine's conclusion is radical but influential. There are no analytic truths. What look like analytic truths are simply truths at the centre of our web of beliefs or concepts. We might revise them but to do so would require revising many other concepts and beliefs. Logic too is simply a central part of the structure of our thought but, like any other part of that structure, could be revised in the face of experience.

Analyticity and containment

The problem Quine raises in answering the question of this session though is this: What sense can we give to the idea that logical validity is explained by the idea that the conclusion to a valid argument is contained within the premises? Usually it is not explicitly contained there. So the notion of containment is a kind of metaphor. And analyticity might have 'unpacked' that metaphor. But Quine threatens that idea.

Note also that even in arguments where the symbols used in the conclusions are also in the premises this will not help. Consider the argument:

Not P
Therefore, P

Here 'P' is in both but that does not make it a valid argument.

In fact whether Quine's argument is successful or not is very much a matter of debate. The Oxford philosophers of language H.P. Grice and P.F. Strawson raised a number of objections in a seminal paper (see the further reading). A key point they make is that Quine puts two restrictions on explanations of analyticity:

1. They should not use related expressions.

2. The explanation should be of the same general character as the related expression.

In a piece of English understatement they suggest that such explanations will be 'hard to come by'. What they mean is that the requirements are incompatible and thus, with them in place, it is no surprise that no explanations of analyticity can be given.

More recently, the American philosopher Hilary Putnam (2002) has argued that a distinction can be drawn between distinctions and dichotomies. A dichotomy requires that cases it concerns all fall on one side or another. A distinction, by contrast, does not and can simply be a way of dividing cases for a particular purpose, in a particular context. Putnam argues that there can be a distinction between the analytic and synthetic even if not a dichotomy. (This is also discussed in Chapter 2.)

Thus it remains very much a matter of debate whether the notion of analyticity can really be used to explain the intuitive idea that the premises contain the conclusion. That notion of containment may be best explained by pointing to valid logical inferences. But if so it cannot itself explain the force of logic.

Reflection on the session and self-test questions

Write down your own reflections on the materials in this session drawing out any points that are particularly significant for you. Then write brief notes about the following:

1. In what sense is logic uninformative?

2. Does this undermine deduction?

3. What underpins logical inference?

4. Can truth tables be used to justify inferences?

Session 3 Conclusions: implication and entailment

Formal and informal logic

This chapter has concerned *formal logic*.

Formal logic is concerned with the *form* of arguments, and the focus is upon the abstract structure of the most general kinds of claim. This helps avoid distraction by the *content* of the statements under consideration. The aim is to arrive at a complete, consistent and transparent axiomatic system of logical relations and principles (i.e. a system derived from a few axioms, which, rather as in classical geometry, are an agreed starting-point—one of the problems in logic has always been to agree on which axioms are in this sense basic!). Formal logic is *context-free* in that what makes an argument valid is independent of any specific context, and it is usually presented in the form of symbolic notation (more on this shortly).

Informal logic, on the other hand, eschews recourse to symbolic notation, and does not aim at the elucidation of a perfect logical system, or the derivation of rules of inference from a set of axioms. Its ambitions are modest in that it seeks only to clarify and render more precise the argumentative strategies recognized and accepted as valid in ordinary usage. It is therefore diagnostic in its approach, and deals exclusively with examples of everyday language. As a result, informal logic cannot remove itself from concern with the *content* of the arguments it studies, as an important aspect of its inquiry is into the way in which the *context* (i.e. the setting of the content) of an argument can influence the validity of application of a logical construction or form.

Equivocation

Consider the following hypothetical syllogism:

If I had a high forehead I would be intelligent

If I were an elephant I'd have a high forehead

Therefore, if I were an elephant I'd be intelligent

Now, as it stands, this argument appears valid. Translated in formal logic it looks valid, whether or not its premises are true (so it may not be sound). But informal logic, on the other hand, is concerned with the context of an argument, and, as this example suggests the context of an argument can have an important bearing. Informally we have reason to doubt this argument.

The problem here is one of *equivocation*: it is unclear that the possession of a high forehead in elephants means the same thing as the possession of a high forehead in humans—so even if it were true that being a human and having a high forehead was correlated with intelligence, it is not necessarily true that being an *elephant* and having a high forehead is correlated with intelligence. There is thus equivocation in the use of the relation 'high forehead and intelligence' between the human context and the elephant context. We cannot assume that the relation is the same in both contexts, and that therefore the meaning is the same. And if we cannot assume this, the argument doesn't work—it has committed the *fallacy of equivocation*.

Thus one of the aims of formal logic is to escape this danger. But, as we will see, there is a cost to formal codification.

Ordinary implication and everyday fallacies

Logic is concerned with what follows from what. To argue to a conclusion is to presuppose that there is a relation between the starting-point of the argument and where it ends. This relation, of something (logically) following from something else, is commonly known as *implication*. For example, in syllogism (2), the two premises seem to imply the conclusion:

2. All men are mortal
   Socrates is a man
   Therefore Socrates is mortal

This seemingly straightforward idea (of one thing following logically from another) has been subject to intense scholarly debate concerning its exact properties. The problem has been to try to formalize the relation in logical notation. So far no totally satisfactory account has been produced. But because of the importance of the mechanism of implication for *any* argument, some knowledge of its properties is essential. While such knowledge will not guarantee immunity from error (all humans are prone to faults of reasoning), it will enable one to avoid the more egregious errors, i.e. to be able to recognize the obvious fallacies is to be forewarned!.

At the end of this chapter we give a list of the more common forms of invalid or fallacious argument (see Appendix). We also suggest an exercise that will get you into the spirit of fallacy-spotting. Many of the fallacies cited are well-known, and even have names. It is remarkable, though, how commonly fallacious arguments are used, and to very good (or bad!) effect. So this is one area in which philosophy, by helping to sharpen up our thinking skills, can be useful in practice.

Problems with codifying ordinary informal implication

One problem for codifiying implication stems from the way it is used in everyday reasoning. Consider the statement: 'If I water this seed, then it will germinate'. This is in the form 'If *A* then *B*'. It is an example of an ordinary informal implication, and it does indeed sound as if it might be true.

But note that the inference 'I have watered this seed therefore it will germinate' is not formally valid, because there is no *logical connection* between the statement 'I have watered this seed' and 'therefore it will germinate', which will ensure that germination will indeed follow the watering of the seed. The relation between the watering of a seed and its germination is determined by the properties of the water and the seed, not anything to do with logical form. That seeds germinate following watering is, for example, only *contingently* true and not true if the seeds are also subject to very high levels or heat or radiation in addition to being watered.

Material implication

We have already seen that formal logic in the shape of propositional logic concentrates on truth-functional connectives. This is the case with the account given in the first session of 'if…then' (symbolized by the horseshoe) and which represents 'material implication'

The idea behind this is to try to capture what is meant by 'if…then' in English but in truth-functional terms. And this is what causes problems.

The codification gives conditional argument the minimum possible logical force, so that '*p* ⊃ *q*' simply asserts only that it is not in fact the case that *p* is true and *q* is false. That is what the truth table codifies. It can be summarized as equivalent to 'Not (*p* & not-*q*)', or ~(*p* & ~*q*).

Unfortunately, problems remain. They are known as the *paradoxes of material implication*, and their origin lies in the role of '−' and '⊃' as *truth-functional operators*.

Truth-functional operators

Recall the truth table for 'if…then'(⊃):

p ⊃ *q*
T T T
T F F
F T T
F T F

This truth-table defines the relationship between '*p*', '*q*', and '⊃'. It shows that the material conditional may be true even when there is no connection whatsoever between its antecedent and consequent, e.g. 'If elephants are pink, then the sky is blue' (i.e. the third line down: FTT). In other words, a true conclusion can follow from a false premise, under the rules of material implication.

It thus permits true conclusions to be inferred from irrelevant premises but it also allows us to draw inferences about non-existent objects.

More generally, for any statement *A*, if *A* is false, '*A* ⊃ *B*' is true; and if *A* is true, '*B* ⊃ *A*' is true, no matter what statement *B* is. The paradoxes emerge because it is possible to assert that a conditional that contains a false propositions as either a premiss or as its conclusion, or both, is true. So all the following would be true:

If elephants are pink, then the sky is blue
If elephants are pink, then the sky is not blue
If elephants are not pink, then the sky is not blue

The problem is that capturing the notion of implication in merely truth-functional terms does not capture the relevance of the premiss to the conclusion.

Strict implication

We can sum up the problem thus: as a simple matter of *fact*, it may be true that 'If *A* then *B*' (i.e. it may be true according to its truth table definition), but it does not follow that the inference '*A* therefore *B*' is valid in a more intuitive sense. It may not be true that *B* follows from *A*. Everyday entailment seems not to be a matter merely of the truth and falsity of sentences in premises and conclusions, whereas materal implication is truth functional.

One intuition is to say that, for the inference from *A* to *B* to be valid, is for it to be *impossible* for *B* to be false when *A* is is true. One way of achieving this is to define the relation in terms of *necessary* truth. This is called *strict implication*.

The Oxford philosopher, C.I. Lewis, writing in the 1950s, introduced the notion of strict implication in his system of *modal logic*. Modal logic affords a distinction between ordinary truth and *logically necessary truth*. In strict implication, 'P strictly implies Q' means 'It is logically necessary that P materially implies Q'. This is the reasoning behind it. Consider:

1. If elephants are pink then the sky is not blue.

Clearly (1) is false, because the colour of elephants has no bearing on the sky. Now one can represent (1) as

2. elephants are pink ⊃ the sky is not blue.

But (2) is true because the antecedent is false and thus it is not a good translation of (1). Lewis's is suggested translation is:

3. [] (elephants are pink ⊃ the sky is not blue.)

This says (roughly) that in every possible world where elephants are pink, the sky is not blue. As one can easily imagine a world of pink elephants and a blue sky, (3) is false. Hence, it seems a better of (1).

This avoids the paradoxes of material implication, but entails similar paradoxes of strict implication. Namely, an impossible statement P strictly implies any statement Q, and a necessary statement Q is strictly implied by any statement P. Consider:

4. If elephants are pink then 2 + 2 = 4.

Rendered formally with strict implication, (4) becomes

5. [] (if elephants are pink ⊃ 2 + 2 = 4)

which says (roughly) that in every possible world where elephants are pink, 2 + 2 = 4. Because it's impossible for there to be a world where 2 + 2 fails to equal 4, (5) is true. But surely (4) is false.

Nuel Belnap (1961) offered a very strict and conservative relation analysing premises and conclusion into Boolean 'atoms' and requiring the literal containment of the conclusion-atoms among the premiss-atoms. But their relation eliminates all the paradoxes mentioned so far, but ruthlessly also eliminates much else that seems innocent, in particular, the rule of inference called disjunctive syllogism: P or Q, not-P, therefore Q.

Implication and entailment

The continuing debate about how best to analyse implication in logical terms presents some of the strengths and weaknesses of modern deductive logic.

On the one had it presents a series of powerful tools—which this short introduction can merely point towards—for establishing rigorous argument and for disambiguating ambiguous claims made in everyday English. By articulating forms of argument it can provide the basis of a critique of reasoning that is impartial and independent of particular contents. One cautionary aspect of this is that by looking to the structure of argument one can also highlight fallacies: forms of argument that do not preserve truth. The Appendix lists some of these and learning to identify fallacies as well as valid arguments is a valuable thinking skill.

But on the other hand there is a cost to translating our everyday terms and ideas into the rigorous but minimal language of formal logic. It is particularly striking that one of the most difficult translations is of the central aim of logical argument: implication!

Back to the opening quote

We began this chapter with Achilles's cry that Logic would compel the Tortoise bodily: it would take him by the throat. In fact, while the Tortoise's particular challenge seems to have been based on a misunderstanding, the actual force of logic is more mysterious than we might have thought. But some aspects are very clear. Logical validity is based on the form or structure of arguments and if an argument is valid it cannot lead from truth to falsity. That guarantee comes at a cost: the conclusion to an argument does not contain more information than the premises. A statement of the argument is a tautology: it cannot but be true but that is because it is independent of the world. Nevertheless logical inference plays a vital role in teasing out implicit assumptions or testing hypotheses. But at the same time, if the conclusions of arguments are contained in the premises that is so only for subjects with eyes to see it, subjects able to play the game of logical reasoning. Acquiring that vision is a key thinking skill developed through practice in argument and exercises. The Appendix below outlines some logical fallacies, recognition of which is one aspect of that skill.

Reflection on the session and self-test questions

Write down your own reflections on the materials in this session drawing out any points that are particularly significant for you. Then write brief notes about the following:

1. What is the key strength of formal logic? What is a key limitation?

2. What central paradox is raised by the logical codification of implication and of the connective 'if…then'?

3. What possible solutions have been proposed?

Appendix Some of the more common forms of invalid argument

In the 2500 years during which logic has been studied, a variety of fallacies and invalid forms of argument have been identified. Some of the more common ones are given below.

Spotting fallacies or invalid arguments is a skill like any other, and as with all skills, it is practice that leads to competence. So it is worth getting into the habit of looking for logical errors! The list here is necessarily in a very summary form. There is no single source for reading more about these. Many philosophical dictionaries include at least some of them and a good general account is Walton's (1989) *Informal Logic*, given in the suggestions for Further reading at the end of the chapter. However, there is no need to memorize the list. It is helpful to have an idea what philosophers are talking about when they use the names given below. But the important thing is to develop a sharp eye for misleading or otherwise fallacious arguments (in your own work as well as other people's!)

EXERCISE 6	(30 minutes)

Take any everyday piece of text (this could be a newspaper, a brochure, etc.) or record a discussion programme on the TV/radio:

1. note down any argument you see/hear which seems to you fallacious; then,

2. go through the following list and see if the fallacies can be identified there; finally,

3. return to your text/recording, and see if you can spot any further fallacious arguments.

Ad baculum

The rhetorician's tactic of arousing strong emotions in the audience as a persuasive device. While it might be understandable that strong emotions should be aroused by certain claims or exhortations, *ad baculum* has nothing whatsoever to lend to the logic of an argument, and to claim (even implicitly) that it has is to commit this particular fallacy. A variant is *ad misericordium*, or the appeal to pity.

Ad hominem

To attack the personal reputation of a debating opponent is a well-known recognized manoeuvre in public debate. To do so is almost invariably fallacious, but there is one situation in which it might be valid. This is when the opponent's argument relies on some relevant claim about himself as one of its propositions. In such circumstances, the use of *ad hominem*, if based on relevant and true information about the speaker, can render his own argument worthless. A great favourite of politicians, though not always for the right reasons!

Ad populum

The appeal to popular opinion: another great favourite of politicians and hustlers ('The British people know...'). Invariably fallacious, as the claim that the speaker's point is already accepted by a great number of people can have no bearing on the validity of the argument. And of course, it is always possible that this great number of people, even if they do agree with the speaker, could be equally wrong.

Ad verecundium

The appeal to sapiential authority, expert knowledge, or wise judgement. Prone to notorious problems. The main errors: (1) irrelevance; (2) misattribution; (3) omissions of context; (4) inappropriateness; (5) lack of direct evidence; (6) favouring one authority over another (equally qualified) but dissenting authority; (7) ignoring relevant points of difference among expert authorities.

Ignoratio elenchi

The misconception of refutation—or simply confusing the issue with irrelevant claims. This might be why so many politicians in debate take so long to get to the point. At its clumsiest it consists simply of changing the subject. More sophisticated versions can be more difficult to detect, for example, the introduction of irrelevant or illegitimate qualifiers, e.g. one might assert that 'No *true* Scotsman would put ketchup on a haggis!', but such an invocation would neither disqualify Scotsmen who did so from being Scottish, nor the practice itself from being a legitimate habit of the Scots (although it might be disqualified on other grounds!). It is worth noting that this fallacy is not detected by most kinds of formal logic. *Ignoratio elenchi* can be combined with any of the preceding fallacies.

Petitio principii

The circular argument. In *vicious* circularity the conclusion has already appeared earlier in the argument (sometimes only implicitly); in *virtuous* circularity the claim is that as there is no better argument, this will have to do, but this does not make the

logic any better. J.S. Mill argued that *all* deductive logic is infected with circularity! (1879) and (as noted above, this chapter) there is a sense in which mathematics is too. So what matters is whether the 'circle' is large enough, or sufficiently unobvious, to add anything useful to our understanding of the issues.

Post hoc ergo propter hoc

(Or simply *post hoc*) A complex family of related fallacies, to do with inferring an incorrect causal relation between two events. There are seven variations: (1) inferring a causal connection after just one instance; (2) inferring a causal connection on the basis of just one correlation with previous instances; (3) reversing cause and effect; (4) inferring a direct causal connection between two events that are connected only in that they share a common cause; (5) confusing causation and resemblance; (6) attributing cause to an (apparently) necessary (but not sufficient) condition; (7) ignoring inconvenient counter-instances or confounding data.

Affirming the consequent

This is an invalid inference from a conditional statement. Given 'If p then q', it is a fallacy to argue in reverse that because q then p. It is valid, however, to *deny the consequent*, arguing that, if q is false, p must also be false—this inference is licensed by the conditional, if true.

Denying the antecedent

Another invalid inference from a conditional statement. Given 'If p then q', it is a fallacy to argue that because p is false, q must also be false. It is valid, however, to affirm the antecedent, arguing that, if p then q (this is simply the inference licensed by the true conditional statement).

Equivocation

Relies on *semantic ambiguity* to allow a shift in the meaning or scope of a word between different parts of an argument. Whether it is fatal to the validity of the argument depends on how crucial the shift in meaning is. If the argument hangs on it, then it could be fatal. The danger of equivocation is greatest when *systematic ambiguity* exists (e.g. 'money', 'value'). This is a fallacy that is probably impossible to detect using formal logic.

Amphiboly

Relies on *grammatical ambiguity* to allow a shift between the grammatical status of a word, usually the shift is from an adjective to a verb or vice versa. Probably rare, if it exists at all (some writers claim it is not a true fallacy).

Illegitimate changes in the scope of a key operator

For example, negation or conjunction may range over variable domains in the same argument, but the conclusion relies on the scope of these operators being held constant. Easier to detect in formal logic than in informal logic—in fact, in the latter it can be almost impossible to detect.

Semantic vagueness

Closely related to equivocation, and the two can coexist. The point about semantic vagueness is that, if there is a lack of clarity or precision as to the meaning of key terms, then the same problem will infect any conclusion that is reached.

Inconsistency in a conjunction claimed as true

Where a proposition is actually a conjunction of propositions, the existence of inconsistency among this set will produce one or more contradictions; and, as a contradiction can never be true, the premiss will be false; and if the argument depends on the premiss being true, then the conclusion will be false.

The fallacy of composition

Concerns confusion over the transferability of valid forms of inference over different levels of composition. The reasoning that applies at the micro-level is confused with the reasoning that applies at the macro-level; when the confusion is downwards in scale, the label *fallacy of division* is sometimes used (e.g. macro-economics versus microeconomics).

The fallacy of independence

Assuming in probabilistic calculations that successive outcomes are independent when they are not. It involves a faulty estimation of the conditional probability of each event—for independence to hold, conditional probability must be held constant.

Confusing prior and posterior probabilities

Assuming in probabilistic calculations that outcomes are dependent when they are not. Usually involves a misconception of randomness: randomness is uninfluenced by preceding outcomes, e.g. 'it comes up 'heads' this time, so it must be 'tails' next'.

Secundum quid

Assuming that one has sufficient information to make a generalization. Unfortunately, what is true in a certain respect (or under certain circumstances) may not be true in others. Faulty generalization of this kind is behind many errors of reasoning, but it is probably impossible to produce a heuristic for detecting it at work, because to do so would involve generating a method for revealing whether all the necessary qualifications have been made, and this is highly ambitious. And, of course, it takes only one counter-example to disprove any general claim. This fallacy lies behind many sampling errors in statistical analysis, two of the most serious being insufficient sample size, and sample bias.

Masked man fallacy

Arguing that knowledge of something under one description entails knowledge of it under another description; conversely, arguing that ignorance of something under one description entails ignorance of it under another description. For example, just because I know your identity but do not know the identity of the masked man, does not entail that you are not the masked man.

Quantifier shift fallacy

A fallacy involving a shift in the scope of quantifier terms; e.g. 'every girl loves some boy (or other), therefore there is some (one) boy whom every girl loves'. The shift in scope of the quantifier is possible only because it is ambiguous in ordinary language. In formal logic it is easier to detect. In symbolic form: $(\forall x)\,(\exists y)\,(Fxy)$ therefore $(\exists y)\,(\forall x)\,(Fxy)$.

The socratic fallacy

To argue that knowledge is founded on the ability to define the object(s) of knowledge. This fallacy is committed by the Socrates of the early Plato dialogues. It produces two paradoxes: first, it disqualifies from knowledge many who have every appearance of possessing it (in terms of intuitive ability); second, it disqualifies testing of definitions of the object of knowledge against known instances of that object. This fallacy is behind much of the faulty thinking about concepts of disorder that we covered in Chapters 2–4.

Reading guide

Introductions to logic

◆ Informal logic is more accessible than formal logic and is therefore a useful starting-point. A well established introduction is: Douglas Walton's *Informal Logic* (1989).

◆ The following more recent introductions to informal logic are particularly clear: Warburton, N. (2000) *Thinking from A to Z*, and Baggini, J. and Fosl, P. (2003) *The Philosopher's Toolkit: a compendium of philosophical concepts and methods.*

◆ A very readable introduction to the study of fallacies is Woods, J. & Walton, D. (1982) *Argument: the logic of the fallacies.*

Formal logic

◆ An accessible introduction to formal logic is Guttenplan, S. (1997) *The languages of logic: an introduction to formal logic.*

◆ Less readable but with many exercises is Lemmon, E.J. (1965) *Beginning Logic.*

Philosophy of logic

◆ Two highly readable treatments of the philosophy of logic (sometimes called philosophical logic) are: Haack, S. (1978) *Philosophy of Logics*, and Wolfram, S. (1989) *Philosophical Logic.*

◆ For a more advanced text, there is Simpson, R.L. (1988) *Essentials of Symbolic Logic.*

Truth

◆ An introductory level text on truth is Schmitt, F.F. (1995) *Truth: a primer*.

◆ More advanced is Kirkham, R.L. (1995) *Theories of Truth: a critical introduction*.

◆ For a critique of the very notion of truth, try: Allen, B. (1995) *Truth in Philosophy*.

Logical puzzles

◆ For those who like logical puzzles, there is Sainsbury, R.M. (1988) *Paradoxes*.

References

Allen, B. (1995). *Truth in Philosophy*. London: Harvard University Press.

Baggini, J. and Fosl, P. (2003). *The Philosopher's Toolkit: a compendium of philosophical concepts and methods*. Oxford: Blackwell.

Belnap, N. (1961–62). Tonk, Plonk and Plink. *Analysis*, 22: 130–134.

Dodd J. (2000). An identity theory of truth. London: Macmillan.

Guttenplan, S. (1997). *The Languages of Logic: an introduction to formal logic*. Oxford: Blackwell.

Haack, S. (1976). The justification of deduction. *Mind*. 83: 112–119.

Haack, S. (1978). *Philosophy of Logics*. Cambridge: Cambridge University Press.

Horwich, P. (1990). *Truth*. Oxford: Blackwell.

Kirkham, R.L. (1995). *Theories of Truth: a critical introduction*. London: MIT Press.

Lemmon, E.J. (1965). *Beginning Logic*. London: Van Nostrand Reinhold.

Lewis, C.I. and Langford, C.H. (1932). *Symbolic Logic*. New York: The Century Co.

Mill, J.S. (1879). *System of Logic*. London: Longman.

Prior, A. (1960). The runabout inference-ticket. *Analysis*, 21: 38–39.

Putnam, H. (2002). *The Collapse of the Fact/Value Dichotomy and other Essays*. Cambridge, MA: Harvard University Press.

Ramsey, F. (1927). Facts and propositions. *Proceedings of the Aristotelian Society*, 7 (Suppl.): 153–170.

Sainsbury, R.M. (1988). *Paradoxes*. Cambridge: Cambridge University Press.

Schmitt, F.F. (1995). *Truth: a primer*. Oxford: Westview.

Simpson, R.L. (1988). *Essentials of Symbolic Logic*. London: Routledge.

Stranson, P.F. (ed) (1967). *Philosophic Logic*. Oxford: Oxford University Press.

Stevenson, J. (1961). Roundabout the runabout inference ticket. *Analysis*, 21: 124–128.

Walton, D. (1989). *Informal Logic*. Cambridge: Cambridge University Press.

Warburton, N. (2000). *Thinking from A to Z*. London: Routledge.

Weiss, B. (2002). *Michael Dummett*. Chesham: Acumen.

Wolfram, S. (1989). *Philosophical Logic*. London: Routledge.

Woods, J. and Walton, D. (1982) *Argument: the logic of the fallacies*. New York: McGraw-Hill Ryerson.

CHAPTER 6

Philosophical outputs in mental health practice and research

Chapter contents

Thus far in this part we have considered the kinds of problem characteristically tackled by philosophy (Chapters 2 and 3) and philosophical methods (Chapters 4 and 5). In this chapter we will be thinking about the outputs from philosophical work, about what we should expect to get out of doing philosophy.

It is important to spend some time on this. Views about the value of philosophy (whether indeed it has any discernible worthwhile outputs at all!) are as diverse as views about philosophical problems and philosophical methods. As we will see, they range from the overoptimistic to the overpessimistic. So we need to get a balanced perspective appropriate to the particular contingencies of philosophy and mental health.

It is with this balanced perspective on the outputs from philosophy that we are concerned in Session 1 of this chapter. Our broad conclusion in Session 1 is that philosophy gives us a more complete view of the meanings of the concepts by which we structure and make sense of the world. It is, as a former Professor of Psychiatry at the Institute of Psychiatry in London, Sir Denis Hill, once put it, a 'consciousness raising exercise' (D. Hill, personal communication, 1976). In Sessions 2–4, we then go on to show how philosophy gives us a more complete understanding of the medical concepts than that offered by the traditional medical model: philosophy adds, respectively, values to the facts emphasized in the medical model (Session 2), illness to disease (Session 3), and action to function (Session 4).

The end result, it is important to emphasize, is not to diminish or undermine the importance of science in medicine, as reflected in the traditional medical model. To the contrary, everything that is genuinely scientific about medicine remains intact and is indeed clarified. The end result, rather, is an enriched model in which human and scientific aspects of the discipline—values besides facts, patients' experiences of illness besides medical knowledge of disease, and loss of personal agency besides disturbances of bodily and mental functioning—are fully and equally represented.

Session 1 'I wonder if this headache is mine?'

For many people, philosophy is an arcane discipline, at best self-indulgent, at worst self-deluded. The cartoon in Figure 6.1 sums up the popular image of the philosopher. Most people just have headaches. This philosopher is asking whether his headache is his!

This cartoon appeared in the course book to a programme in philosophy run over 30 years ago by the Open University (a major provider of 'distance learning' programmes in the UK). Intended ironically it none the less illustrates some important points about the value of philosophy.

EXERCISE 1   (15 minutes)

Think carefully about the cartoon in Figure 6.1. Taken as it is from an introductory course in philosophy, it was intended to illustrate the difference between philosophical and non-philosophical questions.

◆ How *practical* is the question this philosopher is asking?

◆ What might you get out of thinking about it?

◆ Could you go to the Medical Research Council (one of the major funders of medical research in the UK) for support to do research on this question? If not, why not?

Write down your own answers to these questions before going on.

The self-evident and the practical

On first inspection, the cartoon is a comment on the pointlessness of philosophical questions, and this is often how it is taken. Whoever needs to ask if the headache they feel is their own! That a headache is one's own headache, surely, is all too painfully self-evident.

Well, we will see especially in Part V, that the 'ownership' of experiences is, on the one hand, one of the deepest and longest running of metaphysical questions, and, on the other, crucially relevant to mental health practice (the symptom of 'thought-insertion', in schizophrenia, described in Chapter 3 provides one of the clearest examples of the remarkable *separation*, in this condition, between first-personal experiences and the sense of ownership of those experiences).

We return to thought insertion in Chapter 30 at the end of Part V. But the point for now, and a key point to take from the Open University's cartoon of the philosopher with a headache, is

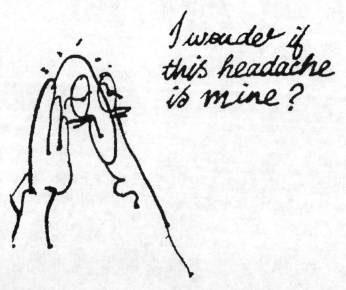

Fig. 6.1

that philosophers, in asking questions that others may think pointless, because self-evident, may often be asking questions that are highly practical when it comes to navigating in the conceptually tricky waters of mental health.

Questions of this kind, however, often do seem entirely pointless to 'practical' people. To the busy doctor, it may seem that they have problems enough without raising questions about the (apparently) self-evident. The Medical Research Council is unlikely to commit its increasingly scarce resources here! Of course, *ethics* has come into its own since the time of the Open University cartoon. A practical 'bioethics' is now widely accepted as being essential to good practice in all aspects of health care. In some ways, though, the success of ethics has increased, rather than decreased, the distance between philosophy and everyday practice.

Ethics, yes! Philosophy, no!

The continuing separation between philosophy and practice, notwithstanding the growth of bioethics, is illustrated by another cartoon, from a more recent publication, shown in Figure 6.2.

This cartoon appeared on the cover of an issue of the *Drugs and Therapeutic Bulletin* in 1996 dedicated to ethical dilemmas. The *Bulletin* is distributed to all medical practitioners in the UK as an update service. That an issue should be devoted to ethics, unthinkable even a few years ago, shows how far the

subject has come. The cover cartoon, however, points a warning finger at 'philosophy'. The suggestion is that there is a difference between asking for a doctor (who could do something practically useful) and asking for a philosopher (who, the cartoon implies, could not.)

And of course in circumstances of this kind, the philosopher, *qua* philosopher, should certainly get smartly out of the way of the first aid crew. For in circumstances of this kind, the problems are indeed primarily empirical rather than conceptual. The problems are the empirical problems of deciding what is wrong and of doing something decisive about it. The problems are not the conceptual problem of deciding whether the condition of the person in the cartoon (lying collapsed on the floor) is properly understood as a medical condition. For precisely this reason, then, because the problem is not a philosophical problem, what is needed when someone has collapsed, is a first aid crew not a philosopher. But what gives the cartoon its point (an ironic point, no doubt) is the implication that philosophers may have *any* role to play in medicine.

The self-evident and the practical

As with all academic subjects, philosophy is not justified primarily by being practically relevant. It may, legitimately, be pursued for its own sake; as may poetry or mathematics, or, indeed,

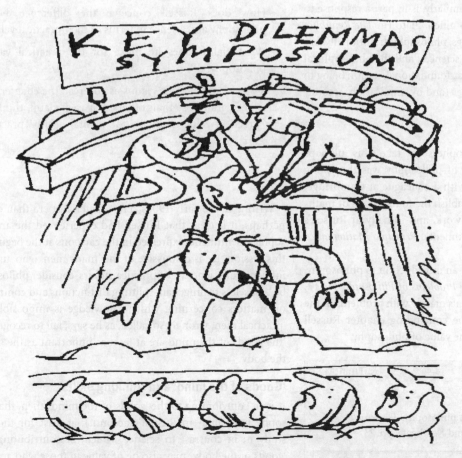

"Is there a philosopher in the house?" Fig. 6.2

biochemistry or economics. Some philosophers, though, the counterparts of those practitioners who assume that philosophy is point*less*, believe that doing philosophy for any reason other than for its own sake is a form of intellectual prostitution.

That you are reading this book—whether as a philosopher or practitioner—suggests that you sense there may be something of value in linking philosophy and practice. We will see in this session that part, at least, of the value of bringing the disciplines together consists *just in questioning the (apparently) self-evident*. We will come to this conclusion, though, by way of the (very divergent) views of philosophers themselves as to what we should expect from philosophy. As we will see, some philosophers have been unduly pessimistic about the value of philosophy, others unduly optimistic. Somewhere in between will be the point of balance.

Philosophers manic . . .

The antipsychiatry movement (Chapter 2) was in part a response to psychiatrists claiming too much, or at any rate to their having had too much claimed for them on their behalf. This was Szasz's concern, you will recall; and it was shared by many of those less inimical to the subject—the starting point for Boorse's work, for example, was a concern about the 'medicalisation' of morals, about more and more of the human condition being assimilated to psychopathological categories.

Antiphilosophical sentiment, similarly, is in part a response to philosophers having claimed too much. Plato (in *The Republic*) wanted to make philosophers kings; philosophy, traditionally, has been acclaimed the queen of the sciences; and the philosophical project has often been conceived as foundational, its aim being to establish the foundations for other (and by implication, secondary or derivative) subjects.

The last great philosopher?

One of the last great philosophers to take this perhaps rather manic view of the value of philosophy was the young Bertrand Russell (Figure 6.3). With a colleague at Cambridge, A.N. Whitehead, he set out to establish the foundations of mathematics in logic. After years of work, and initially at Russell's expense, they published the monumental *Principia Mathematica* (in 1903).

Shortly after this, Russell wrote an introduction to philosophy, aimed at the general reader, *The Problems of Philosophy* (1912, with numerous reprints). This deals mainly with problems in the theory of knowledge, but in the concluding chapter Russell draws together his views about the value of philosophy.

EXERCISE 2   (30 minutes)

Read the extract from:

Russell, B. (1912). The value of philosophy. *The Problems of Philosophy*. London: Williams and Northgate, pp. 237–250

Link with Reading 6.1

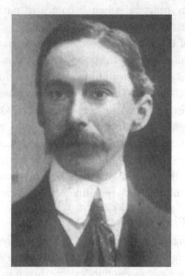

Fig. 6.3 Bertrand Russell

- How does Russell conceive the difference between philosophy and science in terms of their practical value?

- What claims does he make for the practical value of philosophy?

  Make a note of these claims as you read the chapter. Some are more grandiose than others. For each claim, think what its practical value might be for mental health (practice or research).

Writing in the early 1900s, a less materialist era than our own perhaps, it is clear that Russell had experienced the antiphilosophical sentiments expressed in the cartoons at the beginning of this session. He is dismissive of the 'many men' who 'under the influence of science or of practical affairs' consider philosophy to be '... useless trifling, hair-splitting distinctions and controversies on matters concerning which knowledge is impossible'. Such 'practical men', wrongly so called, as he says, fail to recognize that 'the goods of the mind are at least as important as the goods of the body'.

'Goods of the mind' and thinking skills

It is in contributing to the 'goods of the mind', then, that philosophy has value (in Russell's account), at least for those who study it; in contrast to science, which, in contributing to the 'goods of the body', may also be of value to those who are wholly ignorant of it.

Well, there is something in this contrast, of course. But in mental health, the 'goods of the mind'—improved thinking skills, as we indicated in Chapter 1, may be of very real value to others through improved practice. And improved thinking skills certainly seem to have been among the goods that Russell had in mind. Philosophy, he says, provides knowledge of the kind '... which results from a critical examination of the grounds of our convictions, prejudices and beliefs' (p. 239). This last phrase would not look out of place among the aims of an (enlightened) training programme in any area of mental health! We will see later in the book that the lack of just such a critical examination has been an important factor leading to abusive practices in psychiatry (for example, in Part IV).

'Goods of the mind' and 'grand unifying theories'

Russell's other main claim for philosophy, on the other hand, would look distinctly odd among such practical aims. Philosophy, he suggests (also on p. 239) is concerned with '... the kind of knowledge which gives unity and system to the body of the sciences ...'.

To the modern ear this claim has a distinctly grandiose ring. Indeed, although entertained in one form or another by philosophy in many periods of its history, it has been largely abandoned since Russell wrote these words. Philosophers, nowadays, far from being concerned with 'unity and system', perceive themselves as working piecemeal and opportunistically. It is theoretical physics, ironically, which now claims a *Grand Unified Theory* as its goal!

One reason for this is cultural. Ours is not an age of heroes. We are embarrassed by Russell's talk of philosophical contemplation leading to 'greatness of soul', of the 'free intellect' seeing 'as God might see'; of the 'unalloyed desire for truth', a quality of mind 'which, in action, is justice, and in emotion ... universal love'. Perhaps we should not be embarrassed by these phrases. We have an urgent, and most practical, need for idealism, not least in mental health. But as claims for philosophy, these would cut little ice with a modern psychiatric training committee or research panel.

A second reason for the abandonment of philosophy's loftier ambitions is its (apparent) failure to make progress. This is foreshadowed by Russell. It must be admitted, he acknowledges, that compared with science, mathematics, or even economics, philosophy is long on questions and short on answers. This is partly because when a subject matures to the point where definite answers become possible, it stops being philosophy—astronomy, physics, and, most recently, psychology, have been lost to philosophy (J.L. Austin talked of them being 'kicked upstairs'). But this has still left the big questions at the heart of philosophy's agenda as open as ever: the nature of consciousness, good and evil, free will, the purpose of life, the possibility of knowledge....

A third reason comes from within philosophy itself, namely proof positive that foundations, at least as traditionally conceived, are not to be had, that, to the contrary, uncertainty goes all the way down. Two figures stand out head and shoulders above other twentieth century philosophers in the discovery of this radical uncertainty. The first is Ludwig Wittgenstein, the

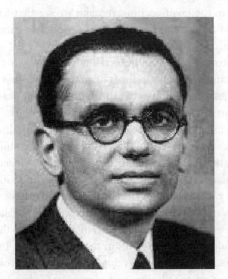

Fig. 6.4 Kurt Gödel

Austrian-born Cambridge philosopher, to whose work we return in a moment. The second is the Austrian philosopher and logician, Kurt Gödel (Figure 6.4). The nub of Gödel's extraordinary insights is that there are no foundations to be had even for mathematics, let alone philosophy. Contrary to Russell and Whitehead's claims, Gödel showed that any mathematical system sufficiently complete to allow the basic procedures of addition, subtraction, multiplication, and division, must contain statements that are fully meaningful within the system, yet the truth or falsehood of which can be determined only by going up a level to a more complex system. But then there will be 'Gödel-undecidable' statements at this next level up; and so on, *ad infinitum*.

Radical uncertainty: a win–win situation?

Gödel's work, being in philosophical logic, is not well known outside philosophy. But the discovery of radical uncertainty is a win–win result for both philosophy and mental health.

In philosophy, it shows that, contrary to the common perception, philosophy really does make progress—not the progress it expected, perhaps, but progress none the less. After centuries of working towards foundations, philosophy itself has shown that it has been chasing a rainbow. But this means that philosophy has turned out to be falsifiable, much as science—in the model of another great philosopher of the twentieth century, Karl Popper—is falsifiable (we return to Popper's work in Part III). And more than this, philosophy has turned out to be falsifiable through the careful accumulation of argument and counterargument. Gödel was Russell's bane: he showed that Whitehead and Russell's *Principia Mathematica* (1910) was fatally flawed; and

Russell in turn was the bane of the great nineteenth century German philosopher of mathematics Göttlob Frege. Put this sequence in the positive, however, and we see that Russell and Whitehead built on Frege's work, and Gödel in turn built on Russell and Whitehead's work.

The discovery of radical uncertainty is also a 'win' for mental health because it goes to the heart of what one of us has called the 'pathologies of certainty' by which the subject was plagued throughout the twentieth century (Fulford, 2000). Time and again, the most adverse developments in mental health over this period have been driven, not by lack of knowledge, still less by ill intention, but by false certainties, by the all-too-sincere conviction of this group or that, often of particular individuals, that they have *the* answer—psychoanalysis, social psychiatry, anti-psychiatry, and, latterly, biological psychiatry, have all fallen prey to becoming overblown. We will return in a moment to the positive side of philosophy's contribution to mental health, but this, at least, is crucial—it helps us develop a mind set that, avoiding false certainties, is open, reflective, and responsive to change.

...and philosophers depressive

Russell was well aware of the value of uncertainty and of the importance of philosophy in helping to avoid false certainties. Russell (1912) indeed sees this as central: 'The value of philosophy', he writes on p. 242, 'is, in fact, to be sought largely in its very uncertainty'. And it is uncertainty of the kind Russell had in mind, which is crucial to mental health: in everyday clinical work, it is the 'arrogant dogmatism' (Russell's phrase) of the practitioner unreflectingly convinced that his or her approach is best, which is at the heart of much abusive practice (we look at this in detail in Part IV); and in research, 'confining ourselves to definitely ascertainable knowledge' although good for one's CV, and attractive to funding agencies, undoubtedly stifles 'that speculative interest' which is the mainspring of innovation.

It is perhaps natural, none the less, that with his monumental *Principia Mathematica* so quickly overtaken by Gödel, Russell should have adopted a far less grandiose vision of the role of philosophy in his later work. Certainly he was not alone among twentieth century philosophers, faced with the apparent failure of their project, and unfavourable comparisons with science, in swinging from their long historical high to a distinctly depressive low. The extremes of this depressive reaction are illustrated by the following readings.

EXERCISE 3   (10 minutes)

Read the brief extracts from:

  Wittgenstein, L. (1921). *Tractatus Logico-Philosophicus* (trans. by D.F. Pears and B.F. McGuinness). London: Routledge and Kegan Paul, last page

---

Link with Reading 6.2

Russell, B. (1962). *An Inquiry into Meaning and Truth*. London: Penguin Books, p. 23

Link with Reading 6.3

Williams, B. (1985). *Ethics and the Limits of Philosophy*. London: Fontana Press/Collins, p. 23

Link with Reading 6.4

Think about how their respective views about the characteristic outcomes of philosophy stand up to the work we have done already in this part on the concept of mental illness.

Wittgenstein's essential point, in the first of these three readings, seems to be that the value of philosophy is to self-destruct. This extract comes right at the end of his first book (and the only one to be published in his lifetime), the *Tractatus Logico-Philosophicus* (1921). His pithy, aphoristic style, makes him very difficult to read. It can seem that there is no 'story-line'. In fact, this somewhat negative view of philosophy is a mark of continuity between the younger Wittgenstein and the later Wittgenstein, the author of the *Philosophical Investigations* (1953). It is in the later work that he makes explicit the view that philosophical problems are merely 'grammatical illusions', products of a 'bewitchment of our intelligence by means of language'. In effect, then, philosophical problems are artefacts of philosophy itself, to be *dissolved* (rather than solved) by taking us back to a clear (rather than philosophically befuddled) view of ordinary, non-philosophical, language use (remember this distinction, between ordinary and philosophical usage, introduced in Chapter 4). (On a recent interpretation of the *Tractatus Logico-Philosophicus* nearly every paragraph of that work is a sophisticated *reductio ad absurdum*; Crary and Read, 2000. The eventual conclusion of an intelligent reader is that although it seems to make sense, the *Tractatus* is really, strictly, a piece of nonsense. It does not advance meaningful philosophical claims.)

The outcome, though, the result, once we have this clear view, is the end of philosophy! Wittgenstein indeed thought for a while that he had finished (off) philosophy, that there was nothing left to do once this point had been recognized. Having climbed the rungs of the ladder, as he puts it in the extract you have just read, he did indeed push the ladder away. He went off for 10 years and worked as a gardener in a monastery.

Grammatical illusions and mental health

Wittgenstein was hugely influential on philosophy in the second half of the twentieth century and we will see later that there are important truths in his conception of philosophical problems. But does his negative conclusion—that philosophical problems are, merely, illusions—stand up to our experience *in mental health*?

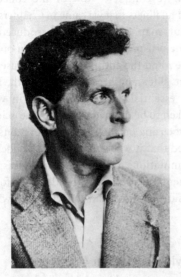

Fig. 6.5 Wittgenstein

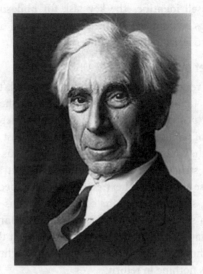

Fig. 6.6 Russell

The debate about mental illness sprang up entirely outside philosophy, after all. So much so, that most of its most active participants were not philosophers—Szasz and Kendell, although drawing on philosophical ideas, were not philosophers. The debate, and the related debate about concepts of illness, disease, and so forth, arose not among philosophers but *within* ordinary usage. Those involved may, perhaps, have been under the influence of 'grammatical illusions': Szasz could be taken as saying that the concept of mental illness is one big grammatical illusion. All the same, the conceptual problems posed by the medical concepts, far from being artefacts of philosophical usage, are products of practical issues of the deepest urgency. And to the extent that philosophy can help with these issues, its outputs, correspondingly, will be practically relevant. Practical problems *in*, practical solutions *out*!

This is the relevant point also in reply to the extracts from Russell and Williams. Russell's picture of philosophers giving us a 'complicated structure' in place of what we take to be self-evident (that one has two eyes), comes in the introduction to one of his books on epistemology, or the study of knowledge. His ironic comment, that 'as to the value of this, he did not feel competent to judge', may be right for practically unimportant questions (about whether one has two eyes). But had he been concerned with practically *important* questions, his 'complicated structure' would have been correspondingly important practically. And how dramatically different in tone and temper are his claims for philosophy in 1962 compared with the claims he felt able to make as a young man 50 years earlier, in 1912.

The mob and the moderates

Bernard Williams, a former White's Professor of Moral Philosopher at Oxford, has at times been positively dismissive of philosophy, at least of the analytic kind. Like many non-philosophers, he thinks the abstractions teased out by philosophers are powerless against the real world . . . in his evocative image, the Professor's arguments will be impotent when the mob 'break down the door, trample his spectacles, take him away'.

In relation to mental health, though, our reaction must be that if arguments fail, what have we left? It is after all the 'mob' that is our enemy. Of course arguments will fail against the fanatic. But aside from countering plain prejudice, it is critical to good practice in mental health that we recognize the subtleties, uncertainties, and complexities of the situations with which we are dealing day-to-day. In a later section we will look at the history of abusive practice in psychiatry. As already noted, we will find that a crucial factor in this, whether institutionalized as in the former Soviet Union, or sporadic, has been, not deliberate malpractice but the enthusiasms of those who are convinced that they have 'the answer'.

And this, after all, is Russell's point, in the extract from his 1912 book (Exercise 2), over again. At that stage in his philosophical development, as against the later extract, he was still confident of the value of philosophy, not in providing 'answers' but as a foil against false answers, against prejudice, against narrowness of view, against dogmatism. It is to this view, too, that he comes in his *History of Western Philosophy* (first published in 1946). This remarkable overview of philosophy, from its earliest beginnings up to the early twentieth century, places each major figure in their historical and social context. And in his introductory overview (p. 14), Russell identifies the key task for philosophy, in our generation, as helping us to cut the umbilical cord of blind conviction and to learn to live with uncertainty.

Gadflies get swatted

This is not a recipe for popularity, it should be said. The work we have done so far on the concept of mental illness, shows that neither extreme position, neither the manic nor the depressive view of the value of philosophy, is likely to be right, at least in respect of mental health. We have already come up with a Russellian more complicated structure (his phrase in the 1962 extract). So this will not please either kind of extremist! Moreover, because a more complicated structure *is* more complicated, it is not readily reduced to a slogan. There is no 'sound-bite' around which to rally. So it may seem that philosophy, to the extent that its value consists in showing us that the answers we thought we had are wrong, offers nothing in return.

Socrates, the 'gadfly' of Athens, paid the price for this. He was one of the manic philosophers. Where Wittgenstein, Russell, and Williams, in the above three extracts at least, are all depressives, adopting excessively pessimistic views of the value of philosophy, Socrates (as reported by Plato in *The Republic*) thought philosophy so important he would have made philosophers kings. In fact, so irritated were the Athenians by his capacity to show that everything they took to be self-evident was wrong, they ended up executing him. His arguments at his trial certainly had all the naïveté Bernard Williams so vividly portrays. Call that a defence! But it is a good example of what happens when the Bernard Williams' mob *do* break in.

A more complete view

So far in this session, we have seen that philosophy is not the end of its own story, as Wittgenstein thought; it offers us a Russellian longer story; and *contra* Williams, in mental health at least, the recognition that there is a 'longer story', even if ultimately no defence against the mob, is in itself a contribution to good practice—it puts discursive argument in the path of dogma, reflection in the place of prejudice and presupposition.

In the remainder of this chapter, we will be looking in more detail at the 'longer story' itself, at the kind of story it is, and at its main elements. This will take us from the negative side of the role of philosophy in mental health, to its positive side.

EXERCISE 4   (25 minutes)

Think about the account of philosophy's role given here, i.e. as giving us a more complete view, in relation to the work we have done in earlier chapters on the concepts of bodily illness and mental illness. Are the conclusions we reached there consistent with this account? Write brief notes on your conclusions before going on.

Two incomplete views in Chapter 2

It was to a more complete view of the concepts of bodily illness and mental illness that we came in Chapters 2 and 4. Thus, in terms of our 'map' of psychiatry introduced in chapter 2, Kendell and the pro-psychiatrists focused on one side, the *fact* side, while Szasz and the antipsychiatrists focused on the other side, the *value* side. The arguments of both, however, were driven by an essentially 'medical' model in which genuine diseases are taken to be defined by 'value-free' scientific criteria. Hence Szasz, focusing on the value connotations of mental illness, concluded that it was a myth; while Kendell, focusing on its factual connotations, concluded that at least some mental disorders are genuine diseases. Both sides, therefore, were working with one-sided views of the concepts with which they were concerned.

A one-sided view in Chapter 4

Boorse, in chapter 4, working primarily by careful definition, took a first step towards giving us a more complete view by introducing the distinction between illness and disease. However, his approach was still governed by a one-sided (or perhaps lopsided) view, to the extent that he sought to define disease, which he took to be the theoretical core of all things genuinely medical, in terms of the fact-side only.

So the whole debate, to this point, was dominated by one or other incomplete view, by the illusion that one or other side is, as it were, definitionally pre-eminent.

Coming to a more complete view

In the remainder of this chapter we will be coming to a more complete view of the medical concepts: in Session 2 by adding values to the facts of the medical model; in Session 3 by adding the patients' experiences of *illness* to specialist knowledge of disease; and in Session 4 by adding an analysis of the experience of illness in terms of incapacity, or a particular kind of *failure of action*, to the analysis of disease in terms of failure of function.

As already emphasized, this will amount, not to abandoning the medical model, but to seeing its elements (facts, disease, failure of function) as parts, important parts to be sure, but still only parts, of the conceptual structure of health care. The traditional medical model as a whole, then, will, according to this line of argument, turn out to be a Wittgensteinian illusion or incomplete view.

The power of the medical model

First, though, to pave the way for this, we will end this session by looking at just why the (Wittgensteinian) illusion of a value-free concept of disease should have been (and remains) so powerful and pervasive.

EXERCISE 5 (30 minutes)

Think carefully about the 'medical' model in mental health. List as many examples of its continued influence as you can think of (if you are working in a group, this is best done in pairs, brainstorming a list for each pair and then combining your findings as a group).

Now make brief notes on three questions:

1. Why is this model so powerful and pervasive?

2. What are its strengths?

3. What would we lose if we gave up the idea that the medical concepts are value-free?

Once the 'medical' model is recognized for what it is—not a mistaken view, but a one-sided view—it is evident everywhere we look in mental health. The dominance of 'biological' psychiatry, in so far as it is conceived exclusively, is the 'medical' model writ large. But mechanistic interpretations of social and psychological psychiatry are one-sided in the same way.

The pre-eminence of the medical model is a natural consequence of the importance of science in medicine. Science has given us major advances in our understanding of the causes and treatments of illness. Hence it is natural that we should have come to focus on the factual element in the structure of medicine, that we should have taken disease concepts, and disease concepts developed in terms of disturbed functioning, to be, in some exclusive, or (as in Boorse's model) central way, its *defining* feature.

Science plus

The more complete view, as introduced here, does nothing to undermine the importance of science in medicine. It suggests, only, that other elements are important also.

We have said this several times now and we make no apology for repeating it. It is crucially important to see from the start that what is involved here is not an overthrow of science. If this were the result of philosophical work in health care, it really would be a case of killing the goose that lays the golden eggs. Yet philosophy is still too often seen (and perhaps at times presents itself) as the enemy of science. This is sometimes true even of the new philosophical discipline of bioethics. But as we will see in Part IV, even in relation to values, the results of philosophical work in medicine are not to substitute for the illusion of a value-free (medical) model, an equally illusory fact-free model! (We will see in Part III, on the philosophy of science, that many would argue that science itself is far from value-free.)

Both kinds of element, then, fact *and* value, disease *and* illness, function *and* action, are important. Both are already there in the conceptual structure of health care and it is the task of philosophy, in giving us a more complete view, to make them explicit. This is the sense in which, in an earlier reading in this session, Wittgenstein said that philosophy 'leaves everything as it is'

(Wittgenstein, 1953). But this is not the end of philosophy. In health care at least, making *both* kinds of element explicit is an important move, an Austinian 'first step', towards using *both* more effectively.

Reflection on the session and self-test questions

Write down your own reflections on the materials in this session drawing out any points that are particularly significant for you. Then write brief notes about the following:

1. Is it good or bad practice to be concerned with apparently self-evident questions?

2. Some philosophers have been unduly optimistic about the contribution that their subject can make to practical disciplines: give one example of such a philosopher.

3. Whose work in particular burst the bubble of philosophy's traditional grand claims?

4. Other philosophers have been unduly pessimistic about the returns from philosophy for practical disciplines: give one example of such a philosopher.

5. How should we understand the practical pay-off from philosophy according to the view developed in this chapter?

Session 2 Adding value to fact

In Chapter 4, we found that even Christopher Boorse, having defined 'disease' in value-free terms, was unable to sustain its use in a consistently value-free way. This suggested that there is an essential evaluative element in the meaning of 'disease'. In other words, however carefully Boorse (or anyone else) stipulates a purely descriptive or factual definition of 'disease', the term simply cannot do the work that is required of it in ordinary (i.e. technical as well as lay) usage if it is shorn of its evaluative meaning.

If this is true of 'disease', then, the most 'scientific' of the core medical concepts (and hence marked out by Boorse as the concept around which medical theory is to be built), it seems likely that despite (scientific) appearances, the medical concepts through and through are value concepts.

In this session, we follow up this idea by looking at some of the properties shared by all value terms in ordinary usage and applying these to the medical concepts. This will give us a quite different way of understanding the concept of 'bodily illness', and, hence, of interpreting the debate about 'mental illness'. We will come to some of the many practical implications of this later in the book (especially in Part IV).

Agreeing and disagreeing about values

In the 1950s and 1960s, a number of philosophers, working mainly in Oxford and influenced by Austin, began to explore the properties of value terms in ordinary usage. We will be drawing on their findings in this session. They were not concerned with the medical concepts, still less with the debate about mental illness. But their observations are highly pertinent none the less.

To get into the spirit of their work, and to provide us with a basis from which to come back to the debate about mental illness, try the following brief exercise.

EXERCISE 6   (20 minutes)

Make two lists of objects, events, sensations, or any other category of things that may be evaluated as good or bad:

1. The first list should be of things about which most people *agree*, evaluatively speaking (i.e. if one person thinks something is a good example of its kind, most other people will, and vice versa).

2. The second list should be of things about which people characteristically *disagree* (i.e. if one person thinks something is a good example of its kind, the next person may well think that it is a bad one, and so on).

An example for the first list would be eating apples—most people agree that a good eating apple is crisp, sweet, and clean-skinned. An example for the second list would be pictures—people tend to disagree about what makes a good picture.

If you are working in a group, try this in pairs. Once you have got two lists (of, say, half a dozen items each), consider what it is exactly that you are agreeing about for list 1 and disagreeing about for list 2. Write down your conclusions.

This can be a surprisingly difficult exercise, especially working on your own. Before we think directly about the two lists, it will be worth looking at why this should be.

Two reasons why this exercise is difficult

One reason why this exercise is difficult is because values are built so deeply into the way that we think about the world, we take them for granted. This will be an important observation later, especially in Part IV, when we examine the values that govern practice in mental health and the extent to which they have remained largely covert.

A second reason for the difficulty of this exercise is that it is set up, deliberately, in a very open way. A natural reaction, on starting to think about agreement or disagreement on questions of value, is to say '*value for what?*'. Again, this is an important observation. There are different kinds of value—aesthetic (beauty, ugliness), prudential (sensible, foolish), moral (good, wicked); there are different kinds of value-norm (personal, social, legal); and within all these, many values depend on the particular context (what's sauce for the goose is not always sauce for the gander).

Analytic moral philosophy has been concerned with the *general* logical properties of value terms, of whatever kind and in whatever context, and it is on these that we will be drawing in this session. But the differentiation *between* values of different kinds will also be important to us later on, in particular when we come to consider the various symptoms by which particular kinds of mental disorder are defined (i.e. psychopathology).

R.M. Hare on descriptive and evaluative meaning

So, values are often implicit; and there are values of different kinds. None the less, if you managed the two lists, you will have recognized that there are some things about which, at least in a given context, people characteristically agree (like good eating apples), and other things about which they characteristically disagree (like good pictures). There are not two distinct categories here, of course, more a spectrum from agreement to disagreement.

We will see in this session that this spectrum is crucial to our understanding of the medical concepts. To get to that point, however, we need to look first at the second part of Exercise 6, at what lies behind agreement and/or disagreement over questions of value, what it is that we are agreeing or disagreeing about.

This was one of the questions studied by philosophers working in the linguistic analytical tradition. A particularly clear and well worked out approach to the question was developed by a former White's Professor of Moral Philosophy in Oxford, R.M. Hare (Figure 6.7), in his first book, *The Language of Morals* (1952). The

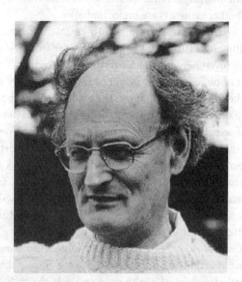

Fig. 6.7 R.M. Hare

nub of Hare's argument on this point comes in his chapter 7, on 'Description and evaluation'. In the next exercise we read two key sections from this chapter.

EXERCISE 7   (30 minutes)

Read sections 7.1 and 7.2 from:

Hare, R.M. (1952). Description and evaluation. Chapter 7, in *The Language of Morals*. Oxford: Oxford University Press, pp. 111–117

Link with Reading 6.5

In these sections Hare distinguishes descriptive and evaluative meanings. Make a note of the similarities he identifies between them; and of any differences.

- What meanings are normally carried by the value term 'good', according to Hare?

- What is the logical connection that he identifies between the two kinds of meaning in this case?

In these two sections Hare introduces the distinction between descriptive and evaluative meanings by way of examples of descriptive and evaluative expressions: e.g. 'This strawberry is sweet' (descriptive), 'This is a good strawberry' (evaluative).

Evaluative expressions convey descriptive information

The first part of his argument can be summarized thus:

- These two kinds of expression, descriptive and evaluative, share many similarities. In particular, both may convey information.

- In the case of an evaluative expression, its information content is contained in the descriptive part of its meaning.

- This descriptive part of the meaning of an evaluative expression is carried by the criteria for the value judgement it expresses.

Thus, the evaluative expression 'This is a good strawberry' conveys the descriptive information 'This strawberry is sweet' because and to the extent that for most people sweetness is a criterion of goodness in strawberries.

Evaluative expressions also commend

This, however, also points up a key *difference* between the two kinds of expression. The *primary* function of 'This strawberry is sweet' is to convey information; whereas 'This is a good strawberry' conveys information only *secondarily*. Moreover, 'This is a good strawberry' conveys the specific information 'This strawberry is sweet' *only* to the extent that sweetness happens to be a widely shared criterion of goodness in strawberries. This, then, is only a *contingent*, not a necessary, part of the meaning of 'good strawberry'. The primary meaning of 'good', according to Hare's account, is to *commend*. (See above, Chapter 5,

introduction to logic, for the distinction between contingent and necessary.)

Value judgements have descriptive criteria

We can sum up the connection between the descriptive and evaluative meanings of an evaluative expression, as defined by Hare, thus:

An evaluative *expression* (e.g. 'This is a good strawberry') expresses a value *judgement* (e.g. 'I commend this strawberry') the criteria for which are *descriptions* of the object of the evaluation (e.g. 'This strawberry is sweet').

Back to Exercise 6

We now have all the conceptual tools we need to deal with the second part of Exercise 6.

EXERCISE 8   (10 minutes)

Go back to Exercise 6 and think about the reasons you wrote down for agreeing or disagreeing on questions of value. In terms of Hare's analysis of the descriptive and evaluative meanings of evaluative expressions, what is it that you are agreeing or disagreeing about?

On Hare's account, agreement or disagreement over questions of value is likely to be agreement or disagreement over the *descriptive* criteria for the value judgements in question. When we make a value judgement, we do so by reference to criteria. But the criteria are not in themselves evaluative. They are, as we have seen, *descriptions of the things evaluated*. And when we agree or disagree over questions of value, we are agreeing or disagreeing over these descriptive criteria.

Good apples and good pictures

How far is this account true of your own lists? It certainly seems to be true of apples and pictures. The descriptive criteria for goodness in (eating) apples are more or less consistent, at least given everyday situations: as we noted a moment ago, for someone buying apples from a grocer, say, a good (eating) apple is clean-skinned, sweet, and crisp. Even this assumes an everyday context, of course, hence the parenthetical 'eating'.

A good eating apple is not *necessarily* like this, of course. It is open to someone to prefer sharp rather than sweet apples, for example. A *cooking* apple should *not* be sweet. A *cider* apple should be rotten! But in a given context, it just is the case that most people more or less agree about the criteria for good eating apples. Whereas, by contrast, people tend to *disagree* about the criteria for good pictures—hospital committees have broken up over this question, and even the 'experts' often disagree violently!

'Good apple' describes; 'good picture' does not?

Thus far, then, we have seen that the criteria for the value judgements expressed by value terms are descriptive, that agreement on questions of value is (often) agreement on the descriptive criteria for the value judgement in question, and that disagreement is (often) disagreement on the descriptive criteria.

These observations, however, have the consequence that the two kinds of value term (the agreement kind, as in 'good apple', and the disagreement kind, as in 'good picture') end up looking quite different in ordinary usage. We will see in a moment that this is a crucially important consequence for our understanding of the debate about mental illness. First, we will look at how Hare sets this out in a further extract from his chapter 'Description and evaluation'.

EXERCISE 9   (20 minutes)

Read section 7.5 from:

> Hare, R.M. (1952). Description and evaluation. Chapter 7 in *The Language of Morals*. Oxford: Oxford University Press, pp. 121–126

Link with Reading 6.6

Again think about your two lists. Hare notes that value terms expressing value judgements over which people *agree*, appear different from those expressing value judgements over which people *disagree*.

In what way do the two kinds of value term appear different, according to Hare?

Hare's point here is that where the descriptive criteria for a value judgement are widely agreed upon, *the descriptions in question can become attached by association to the meaning of the value term in question*. Hence, if the descriptive criteria are widely *agreed*, the corresponding value term comes to look like a *descriptive* term, whereas if the descriptive criteria are *not* widely agreed upon, the corresponding value term remains clearly *evaluative* in meaning.

Hare illustrates this with the difference between 'good egg' and 'good poem'. It is also shown clearly by our examples of 'good apple' and 'good picture'. As noted above, 'good (eating) apple' normally implies a clean-skinned, sweet, and crisp apple. Hence, although 'good apple' is a value term, it has come to look like a descriptive term (describing the apple to which it refers as 'clean-skinned, sweet, and crisp'). In everyday contexts this is taken for granted. If you are out shopping, as above, and the grocer gives you anything else in your pound of apples, you have grounds for complaint. You don't need to spell this out. Whereas with pictures, you do. The descriptive criteria for 'good picture' are not widely agreed, and there is no corresponding stable descriptive meaning that can become attached to 'good picture'.

A brief overview of Hare's account

Before returning to the debate about mental illness (immediately below), we will briefly summarize Hare's observations about the properties of value terms in ordinary usage.

Value terms express (explicitly or implicitly) value judgements. A value judgement, Hare suggests, has two components:

- a *prescriptive*, action-guiding or commending component, and
- a *descriptive* component, representing the criteria adopted.

His emphasis on the prescriptive component has led to his account being called *prescriptivism*. Thus, the value term 'good apple' expresses the value judgement that the apple in question is good. The descriptive component of this is, in the case of eating apples, likely to include 'crisp, sweet, etc.'; but in addition to this descriptive meaning, the value judgement includes the prescriptive or action-guiding meaning 'eat it', or such like.

Hare also makes value-judgements *universalizable*. This is a property that marks out value judgements from other prescriptions, such as orders or instructions. The latter are one-offs. Value judgements are universalizable in the sense that if you judge something good, then you imply the same judgement of all (relevantly) similar things under (relevantly) similar conditions. This is important for ethics, but not here.

The exact extent to which descriptive meaning can become attached to a value term is a matter of philosophical dispute: 'non-descriptivists', such as Hare, consider that there will always remain a gap, even if very small, between description and evaluation; descriptivists such as another Oxford philosopher, G.J. Warnock, consider that the gap can close altogether. We return to this in the next session, when we re-examine the possibilities for a medical model of mental illness in the light of descriptivism. The point for now, though, is one on which both sides are agreed, namely that in cases such as 'good apple', a value term can come to look like a descriptive, or factual, term; while in cases such as 'good picture', its appearance remains clearly evaluative.

Back to the debate about mental illness

The above observations, about the shifts in appearance of value terms in ordinary usage, have a clear *prima facie* relevance to the debate about 'mental illness'. The point of departure for this debate, as we saw in Chapter 2, was the overtly evaluative connotations of 'mental illness' compared with the factual or descriptive connotations of 'bodily illness'. And we have now seen that value terms, similarly, may sometimes have overtly evaluative connotations (as in 'good picture') and sometimes overtly descriptive (as in 'good apple').

Good apple and good picture; bodily illness and mental illness

The correlation between the two kinds of case could be merely superficial of course. They could look similar but for quite different reasons. But it is also possible that 'illness', if a value term, varies in appearance between its uses in respect of mental and bodily conditions, much as 'good', as a value term varies in appearance between its uses in respect of pictures and apples. Before we consider this possibility, try one further exercise.

EXERCISE 10   (10 minutes)

Write down two lists, one of increasingly painful situations (i.e. involving bodily pain), one of increasingly frightening or anxiety-producing situations. Now rate each of the situations on both lists according to whether they are welcome or unwelcome in their own right, i.e. something to take pleasure in or avoid in themselves, as distinct from being necessary for some other end.

If you are working in a group, make the value ratings individually for yourselves and then compare the results. If you are working on your own, make the ratings for yourself and then try to imagine someone who might take pleasure in either a painful or frightening situation, respectively, that you would avoid (or vice versa).

Most groups doing this exercise find that they agree on the pain list but not on the anxiety list. Correspondingly, for those working individually, most people find it is harder to think of people who would evaluate pain positively (for its own sake) than to think of people who would evaluate anxiety positively—some people enjoy horror films, some enjoy hang-gliding, some even bungee-jumping!

The key point is that there is considerable and legitimate variation between people in their evaluations of anxiety experiences; whereas for pain experiences, anything other than the mildest of brief pain is for nearly everyone at best a necessary evil. There *could* be differences of evaluation even of pain, but to envisage this we have to depart further and further from the everyday. There is nothing abnormal (non-everyday) about a good afternoon's hang-gliding; but what would we think of someone who enjoyed a good afternoon's pain? A masochist, or perhaps a saint?

This second exercise, then, has in effect added pain and anxiety to our initial two lists, of things that people respectively agree and disagree about evaluatively. But pain and anxiety are symptoms, respectively, of mental illness and bodily illness. Hence, if 'illness' is a value term, then simply because people tend to agree in their evaluations of pain but to disagree in their evaluations of anxiety, 'illness' used of bodily conditions (at least of pain, as in a 'heart attack', for example) will have relatively marked descriptive connotations compared with its use of mental conditions (at least of anxiety). If, then, illness is a value term, *for this reason alone, 'bodily illness' will have to have more marked descriptive connotations than 'mental illness'.*

No special pleading

We have now got right back to the debate about 'mental illness' in Chapter 2, specifically to the more value-laden connotations of 'mental illness' compared with 'bodily illness'. We have come a long way round to get back to this starting point in order to make clear that whatever follows depends, not on anything special to medicine, still less to mental health, but only on, 1) a general logical property of value terms, taken together with, 2) an important characteristic of human beings.

1 The required logical property of value terms is the variation in the strength of their descriptive connotations with the degree of agreement on the descriptive criteria for the value judgements they express.

2 The required human characteristic is our widely varying evaluations of the aspects of human experience and behaviour with which psychiatry is concerned—anxiety, as we saw in Exercise 10, but also, more generally, affect, belief, desire, motivation, sexuality, and so forth. These, as areas of human experience and behaviour with which psychiatry is concerned, are also all areas of human experience and behaviour over which our values differ widely and legitimately.

That there is no special pleading involved here is shown diagrammatically in Figure 6.8. The top half of this figure shows the parallels between everyday evaluations and the value-ladenness or otherwise of the term 'illness' in different contexts: 'good' used of things such as apples carries mainly factual connotations, while used of pictures it carries evaluative connotations; correspondingly 'illness' used of things such as pain carries mainly factual connotations, while used of things such as anxiety it carries evaluative connotations. The bottom half of the figure indicates that (if 'illness' is a value term) *precisely the same explanation* operates in the case of 'illness' as in the case of 'good'. People differ in their evaluations of some things (e.g. pictures and anxiety) more than others (e.g. apples and pain). Where they agree, the value terms in question come to carry factual connotations by simple association with the factual criteria for the value judgements the terms in question express.

Differences of values, it is worth noting, are important. They reflect our very individuality as human beings. It is our individuality as human beings, then, which is expressed in the more value-laden nature of 'mental illness'.

A watershed of understanding

The point we have now reached represents a watershed in our understanding of the medical concepts. For if the model represented in Figure 6.8 is right, it gives us an entirely different way of understanding the debate about 'mental illness'. Traditionally, 'bodily illness' was assumed to be a scientific term, if not value-free then capable of being so defined; and 'mental illness' had

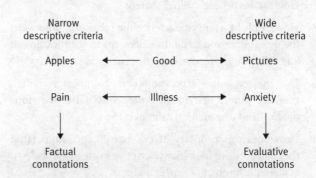

Fig. 6.8 Diagrammatic representation of the parallels between 'good' and 'illness' as value terms.

then either to be *capable* of a corresponding value-free definition (as Kendell supposed, and, in a more complex argument, Boorse), or it had to be shown to be *incapable* of value-free definition, and hence not genuinely illness (as Szasz concluded).

The work of Hare, Urmson, and Warnock on the way value terms work in ordinary usage has now given us a picture that is in several respects the reverse of the traditional view. Instead of 'bodily illness' being value-free, it is now understood to have mainly factual connotations *just because it is a value term*. Like 'good apple', the criteria for the value judgement expressed by 'bodily illness' are relatively uncontentious, but it is no less of a value term for that. Moreover, on this scenario, the more marked evaluative connotations of 'mental illness' reflect *legitimate disagreement* over the criteria for the value judgements it expresses. Hence, attempting to force 'mental illness' into the mould of 'bodily illness', far from being a legitimate way of proceeding, could be positively dangerous. For it would only be possible to make 'mental illness' look like 'bodily illness' by suppressing the legitimate differences of values between people that are the basis of the more marked evaluative connotations of 'mental illness'.

'Mental illness', on this model, is more complicated and contentious than 'bodily illness'. In this respect the antipsychiatrists are right—'mental illness' is *not* just like 'bodily illness'; and so long as people have different values, it never will be. But 'mental illness' is not, thereby, invalid. On the contrary, 'mental illness', in being evaluatively more problematic, and hence more overtly value-laden, reveals the true nature of 'illness' as a value term, a nature that is hidden by the covertly evaluative concept of 'bodily illness'. We will examine the practical importance of this for bodily medicine as well as psychiatry later in this book (in Part IV). But it is a prime example of Austin's 'negative concept wearing the trousers'.

Reflection on the session and self-test questions

Write down your own reflections on the materials in this session drawing out any points that are particularly significant for you. Then write brief notes about the following:

1. How far are people's values shared?

2. How did R.M. Hare characterize the relationship between the descriptive and evaluative elements in the meaning of an evaluative expression (e.g. 'this is a good strawberry')?

3. How may *evaluative* expressions come to appear as though they are purely *descriptive* expressions? Give one non-medical and one medical example.

4. How does this property of evaluative expressions (that they can come to look like descriptive expressions) help to explain the 'problem of mental illness'.

5. What is added by this session to the traditional medical-scientific model?

Session 3 Adding illness to disease

The model of the medical concepts set out in the last session, although certainly more complete than the standard medical model (it offered a *clearer* view, as Wittgenstein would have said), none the less remains in an important respect *in*complete. One way to see this is in terms of the map, or logical geography, of mental disorders introduced in Chapter 2.

Medical and other values

If you refer back to this map, you will recall that it showed a variety of different forms of mental illness merging with bodily illness on one side and moral categories on the other. M*ere* fact (or psychopathology) and *mere* value, are not sufficient to explain the feature of the map, therefore. What is also required is some means of differentiating *medical* value from other *kinds* of value: illness from immorality, disease from delinquency, ugliness, and so forth.

There is more to mental illness than (negative) value simpliciter

This further differentiation is important in principle. It is also important in practice: many of the trickiest conceptual problems in mental health practice arise not from differences over values *per se*, as from difficulties about the particular *kind* of value involved. 'Mad or bad?' is the standard form of this problem in forensic psychiatry. But what about more everyday cases?

EXERCISE 11	(30 minutes)

Go back to the cases we examined in the first session in Chapter 2. Are the problems considered there sufficiently characterized as problems about people's values? In Mr AB's case, for example, was there significant disagreement about whether or not he was in a *bad* condition? If not, what was the disagreement really about?

Mr AB's case, as a case of involuntary psychiatric treatment, is an example of the non-forensic equivalent of 'mad or bad?'. There is unlikely to have been disagreement about whether he was in a bad condition as such. As we will see later (when we retain to Mr AB in Part IV), there *is* disagreement about whether he should be treated under the Mental Health Act (roughly a 50:50 split). But the disagreement here was about whether his bad condition is a bad condition of the kind that is appropriately regarded as mental *illness* (and hence appropriately treated by doctors under the Mental Health Act). The issue, then, was in effect, 'mad or, just, *sad*?'.

Little help from moral philosophy

Surprisingly little work has been done by philosophers on the differentiation between different kinds of value—moral, aesthetic, prudential, medical, etc. Most moral theory is concerned with the properties of value terms in general. The differentia, though, are critical for mental health. The demarcation problem (which was Boorse's problem) consists in just this. Ugliness, wickedness, illness, etc., are all negative value terms. Recognizing this has important implications. But the differentiation between them as different *kinds* of negative value term (mad or bad, mad or sad, etc.) is central to the conceptual problems presented by mental health.

More help from the medical model?

In this session and the next we start to fill out our picture of the conceptual structure of medicine by sketching in the elements of an account of the particular kind of negative value judgement expressed by illness. This will in effect pick up on the line of argument we started to explore in Chapter 4 in relation to Boorse's work on the distinction between illness and disease. Boorse, you will recall, was concerned with the demarcation problem, namely with where the boundary between medicine and morals should be drawn. He tackled this by distinguishing between illness (broadly, what the patient experiences) and disease (broadly, scientific medical knowledge of the disturbances of bodily structure and functioning that cause illness), and he argued that we could distinguish medical from moral values by reference to the latter. However, Boorse's approach to the demarcation problem, we suggested, failed to the extent that it depended on disease being defined value-free while his own *use* of the concept remained value laden.

In the remainder of this session we consider two ways of attempting to preserve a traditional medical model, i.e. a model in which (as in Boorse's theory) values have a place but remain secondary to facts. The failure of both these approaches will reinforce the essential (and indeed primary) importance of values, and of the particular kind of value expressed by illness, in the conceptual structure of medicine and psychiatry. This in turn will lead us, in the final session of the chapter, to a positive characterization of the concept of illness as a particular kind of disturbance of action or of agency. What all this will amount to, as we anticipated in the first session of this chapter, is an enlarged or more complete picture of the conceptual structure of medicine and psychiatry, thus providing a framework for much of the material we will be covering in the rest of the book.

A medical model by logical reduction of illness to disease?

The two ways of attempting to preserve a medical model while retaining a place for values in the medical concepts, are both reductive: one involves a *logical* reduction, the other a *causal* reduction.

The logical reductive route is via moral descriptivism. This is the theory, advanced by authors such as the Oxford philosophers Phillippa Foot and G.J. Warnock, that at least some value judgements are *entailed* by certain matters of fact. This is a strong claim. It means that, given certain matters of fact, particular value judgements follow by *definition*. (We covered entailment in Chapter 3.)

EXERCISE 12 (45 minutes)

Read the two extracts from:

Foot, P. (1967). Moral beliefs. Chapter VI in Foot, P. (ed) *Theories of Ethics*. Oxford: Oxford University Press, pp. 83–84, 85–86

Link with Reading 6.7

Refer back to the section of the Introduction to Logic concerned with the difference between ordinary and strict implication. In the light of this, what do you think of Foot's arguments in 'Moral beliefs'? What is the relevance for the medical model of her view of the logical relationship (the relationship of meaning) between facts and values?

Foot's argument is to the effect that there are cases in which to reject a particular evaluation (of good or bad) seems not merely to be perverse but to show a failure of understanding of the very meaning of good and bad. G.J. Warnock develops a similar argument in his *The Object of Morality* (1971). If these (descriptivist) authors are right, cases of the kind they discuss would be the equivalent of the example of strict implication in the *Introduction to Logic*, 'bitch is a female dog'. Hence values, in cases of this kind, would be reducible (logically) to facts. An expression of value correspondingly could be restated without loss of meaning in terms only of statements of fact.

Can we have our cake and eat it?

Moral descriptivism, making values (sometimes) reducible to matters of fact alone, is a highly attractive theory for the traditional medical model. For it effectively allows us to have our cake and eat it, evaluatively speaking. On the one hand, if the *medical* value terms (disease, dysfunction, and so on) can be reduced to purely factual terms, then this (logical) reduction would satisfy Boorse's requirement (in Chapter 4) for a value-free science of health. On the other hand, though, because these facts entail the relevant negative value judgements, the medical value terms can continue to be used (as Boorse himself continues to use them, remember) with evaluative connotations.

Hare, however, whose work we drew on earlier, offers some powerful arguments against the reduction of values to facts, even in the *prima facie* plausible cases offered by Warnock and Foot.

EXERCISE 13 (30 minutes)

Read the two extracts from:

Hare, R.M. (1972) Descriptivism, ch 5 in *Essays on the Moral Concepts*. London: The Macmillan Press (Extracts, pp. 70–73, 97–100.)

Link with Reading 6.8

These two extracts are both short. But think carefully about them, again with the ideas introduced in Chapter 3 (introduction to logic) in mind, before going on. Hare mounts two main arguments against descriptivism, one in each extract. What are they? Do you agree with him?

In the first extract (pp. 70–73), Hare suggests that the plausibility of descriptivism consists in the fact that the descriptive terms in the cases discussed by Foot (and Warnock) are so widely, perhaps universally, adopted as criteria for the value judgements in question. But this is a contingent fact about human beings, a fact of psychology, not a necessary requirement of logic. We can see this by applying what Mary Warnock, in *Ethics Since 1900* (1978) calls the test of non-contradiction: it would *not* be self-contradictory, in the case of ethics, to acknowledge the descriptions but deny the evaluation; while it really *would* be self-contradictory to acknowledge that an animal is a bitch but deny that it is a female dog. But as Hare points out in this extract the examples given by descriptivists, such as Warnock (G.J.) and Foot, do not pass this test. The force of descriptivism is, rather, contingent. The force of descriptivism derives from the fact, which is a fact of psychology not logic, that over some things (things of the kind on which descriptivists draw) our values are largely shared. Hare, in this extract, anticipating later descriptivists on the medical concepts (like Kendell, in Chapter 2), gives by way of example the biological needs of survival and reproduction ('procreation', p. 72). There is a strong compulsion to say of something that contributes to our survival and/or reproductive potential, that (other things being equal) it is a good thing. But this trades on the merely contingent fact of our psychology that over situations of the kind in question our values are very widely shared. It would be psychologically odd, to the point perhaps of being disingenuous, to admit the facts but deny the values in such cases. But it would not be self-contradictory.

Hare's argument in the second extract (pp. 97–100) is more complex but amounts to the same end result. The plausibility of the descriptivist's case, he argues, consists in the fact that the supposed descriptions are not, actually, value free. 'Harm' appears to be a matter of fact, in the sense that it only makes sense to call certain things or states of affairs harmful. But this is because 'harm' is connected logically to 'interests', which in turn is connected logically to 'desiring' and 'wanting', neither of which can be defined value-free. So 'harm', despite its factual or descriptive appearance, itself contains a hidden element of evaluative meaning, a hidden evaluative premiss. (For the relevance of this point to philosophical work on the concepts of function and 'dysfunction', see Session 4, below, and Fulford, 2000.)

The debate about mental illness and the 'is-ought' debate

In both cases, then, Hare argues, despite appearances, values cannot be reduced to facts; or, equivalently, no set of descriptions of a situation will in themselves entail a value judgement.

In taking this position, Hare is the latest in a long line of philosophers who have argued that there is an unbridgeable logical gap between description and evaluation. This 'is-ought' gap, as it is sometimes called, was first explicitly pointed out by David Hume (in his *Treatise of Human Nature*, (1739/40) III, I, i, final paragraph). But the debate between reductionists (like Warnock and Foot) and non-reductionists (like Hume and Hare)

has produced a large literature on the logical links between description and evaluation.

Most philosophers nowadays accept the Hume/Hare line. They argue, however, that the gap between fact and value is not very important in practice. Be that as it may, in mental health at least, we will find that this is far from the case. Disentangling description from evaluation, and recognizing values for what they are, turns out to be crucially important, for example in relation to the abuse of psychiatry (see later).

But there is, anyway, a decisive argument against the *general* effectiveness of descriptivism as a device for preserving the medical model, at least in mental health. In so far as it is plausible at all, descriptivism depends on (more or less universal) agreement in the criteria for a value judgement. This is what made Foot's (and Warnock's) examples persuasive—everyone, surely, agrees that it would be absurd to claim that clasping and unclasping your hands, etc. (as in Foot's example) is a good thing. Agreement on factual criteria of this kind, as we saw in Session 2, is characteristic of 'bodily illness' (or at any rate 'disease'); however, as we also saw in that session, mental illness differs from bodily illness *just in that the criteria for the value judgement expressed by mental illness are not widely agreed upon.*

In relation to mental illness, then, the conditions for a descriptivist reduction of values to facts are not satisfied. Hence, even if the descriptivist's reduction were valid in principle, it would not work when (from the perspective of the traditional medical model) it is most needed, in mental health.

A medical model by causal reduction of illness to disease?

Although less radical than the logical reduction offered by moral descriptivism, the causal reduction of illness to disease is by far the more familiar, at least among doctors.

EXERCISE 14	(10 minutes)

Spend a few minutes thinking about what happens when you go to see your doctor feeling unwell; for example, unusually tired, or with a sore throat. How does your doctor deal with this, typically? What does he or she do? What kind of thing does he or she say to you by way of a diagnostic conclusion?

In terms of the demarcation problem, this scenario amounts to going to your doctor in a bad condition and wanting to know 'if there is anything (medically) wrong?'. The doctor asks a few questions, does a 'physical' examination, may take a few tests; and then comes up with a diagnosis. 'Yes, you are anaemic' or 'you have a "strep" sore throat', etc.; or, 'No, there's nothing wrong. You are just tired'/'have been overworking', etc. The line of reasoning implied in this process is that if a known disease (anaemia, streptococcal infection) is causing your bad condition, then your condition is an illness; if not, it is not. In other words, if the *cause* of your bad condition (e.g. feeling tired) is a *disease* (e.g. anaemia), then your bad condition is an *illness*; if not, it is not (i.e. No, there's nothing (medically) wrong. You're just tired).

Diagnosis by causes

We return to the diagnostic process in detail in Parts III and IV. The point for now is that, consistently with the medical model, diagnosis of this kind (by reference to causes) in effect seeks to differentiate between medical and non-medical negatively evaluated conditions, by tracing the *cause* of a symptom to some underlying bodily abnormality (such as low blood haemoglobin or the presence of specific bacteria in the throat).

This is a common line of reasoning in other areas of medicine when issues of responsibility come up. In forensic psychiatry, for example, the courts are always impressed by such 'physical' findings as abnormal EEG's (patterns of electrical activity in the brain); this is taken to imply (1) that the person concerned 'could not help' what he or she did, and (2) that a 'physical' finding means that they are ill (again, hence not responsible).

Causes and responsibility

The model of mind and brain implicit in diagnosis of this kind, is also one that is widespread in the biological sciences, and indeed in everyday thinking.

EXERCISE 15   (10 minutes)

Think about the issues raised by the quest for a gene for homosexuality. There has been much published on this issue. You might want to look up on the Web a summary of one such book: *The Sexual Brain* by Simon LeVay (MIT, 1994), which MIT describes as follows: 'Written with clarity, directness, and humor, *The Sexual Brain* examines the biological roots of human sexual behavior. It puts forward the compelling case that the diversity of human sexual feelings and behavior can best be understood in terms of the development, structure, and function of the brain circuits that produce them.'

This book was reviewed by John Diamond in the *Sunday Times* (15 July 1993) in a short review called 'Born to be Gay?', which we discuss below. If you have access to this review you can use it to think about the following issues: what model of the relationship between mind and brain is implied here? What answer to the problem of differentiating medicine from morals (the Boorse demarcation problem), does this suggest? If you do not have access to the review, think about these questions in general.

Work on the brain 'abnormalities' underpinning homosexuality suggests the same model of mind and brain as 'diagnosis by causes'. The abnormality, described in Simon LeVay's book and summarized in the *Sunday Times* review by John Diamond, in the anterior hypothalamus, is taken, somehow, to show that being gay is not freely chosen but determined by the individual's brain. At the top of the fourth column of the *Sunday Times* review this is made explicit. LeVay, the researcher, is said to claim that this finding '... proves that gays are ... no more able to choose their sexual

orientation than blacks ... are able to pick a skin colour'. Well, perhaps so, but if this is the case, then, (1) the same must be true of heterosexuals, and (2) there is nothing in this to make the brain abnormality (in the statistical sense) into a disease. Yet, as we have just seen, these are both corollaries that are regularly drawn, albeit usually implicitly, in medical and legal contexts.

It is important to add that 'diagnosis by causes' is legitimate up to a point. It is legitimate to the extent that it depends on the relevant causal conditions *already being defined as diseases*. By the same token, though, it is wholly illegitimate to extend it to areas where this is not the case, where the point at issue is whether the condition in question is a disease at all.

Two kinds of differential diagnosis

To see this, it is helpful to recognize that there are, really, two different types of diagnosis:

- *Type 1* seeks to allocate a diseased condition to a particular category *within* an established classification of diseases (we can call this 'disease diagnosis').

- *Type 2* seeks to determine whether a condition is properly included in a classification of diseases at all (we can call this 'illness diagnosis').

In medical contexts, these two kinds of differential diagnosis are often conflated. The situation is complicated. But one way to see that these really are distinct types of diagnosis, albeit often run together, is by considering conditions for which the causes are not yet known. The diagnosis of migraine, for example, depends on the features of the condition itself (one-sided headache, etc.). Various risk factors for migraine are recognized (stress, chocolate, etc.) but its underlying causes, at a (medically) acceptable physiological level at least, are not understood. None the less, migraine is firmly within the established classification of diseases. Hence, it cannot be in the classification, it cannot be 'on the list', by virtue of our knowledge of any underlying causal process.

We return in Session 4 of this chapter to just what it is about 'symptomatically defined' conditions such as migraine that gets them on the list of diseases. This is important for psychiatry, most mental disorders being, like most neurological disorders, defined symptomatically. But the key point for now is that causation, although one basis for differential diagnosis of type 1 (disease diagnosis) cannot be the basis for differential diagnosis of type 2 (illness diagnosis).

Some practical sequelae

The practical problems caused by conflating these two types of diagnosis are particularly prominent in psychological medicine but also occur in bodily medicine. There can be few doctors who believe that we have already identified all existing diseases, still less that new diseases will not continue to arise. Yet all too commonly, a patient who feels *ill* is told there is 'nothing medically wrong' simply because their condition cannot be allocated to a known *disease* (conflating the two types of diagnosis).

This is a common experience in all areas of medicine. But in forensic psychiatry, as we saw above, there is a strong tendency to equate the *mere* discovery of a cause with the presence of disease. Yet health, no less than disease, must be caused. So at the very least, it is a *disease*-as-cause that is relevant to the attribution of responsibility in law.

Illness defines disease

The essence of the objection of principle to the standard diagnostic process amounts to the idea that it puts the cart before the horse. Far from diseases-as-causes marking out negatively evaluated conditions as illnesses, it is illnesses (patients' negatively evaluated experiences) that mark out causal conditions *as* diseases. This is shown schematically in the diagram. The direction of causation (from disease to illness) is the opposite of the flow of meaning (from illness to disease).

Asymptomatic diseases

Once a bodily state has been identified as a cause of illness, however, and hence as a disease, it can then be used diagnostically; and this is what legitimizes (up to a point) the standard diagnostic process. This is true, in particular, of asymptomatic diseases, i.e. where a person is said to have a disease even when they are not aware of anything wrong. Causes, as Ayer (1976) put it, are 'connections of tendency'. Hence discovering a 'shadow on the lung', say, picked up on a routine chest X-ray, may lead to the person concerned legitimately being said to have a disease, because the condition in their lungs is one that has a causal 'connection of tendency' with people becoming ill. But what legitimizes this, is that the causal connection, between conditions of this kind in lungs and people being ill, has already been identified.

It is, then, even in the case of asymptomatic diseases, the experience of illness by which, ultimately, a bodily condition is marked out *as* a disease. But the enormous extent to which such bodily conditions have been marked out as causes of illness, especially in the last hundred years, has led to the illusion that diagnosis *as a whole* is nothing more than recognizing already identified diseases. This can indeed give us short cuts to diagnosis (a blood test, or X-ray, etc.). But the short cuts depend on a long (logical) route having already been mapped out.

So far as causal reduction is concerned, then, far from preserving a medical model answer to the demarcation problem, it shows

that the medical model actually depends on a prior, and essentially non-medical model, answer. The 'disease' answer depends on a prior 'illness' answer. It is illness, not disease, which drives the logic of diagnosis, whatever logical short cuts are available once the prior process of discovery of diseases-as-causes has gone through.

So what is illness?

The failure of causal reduction reinforces the need for an account of illness which is not dependent on that of disease. As we have seen, part of what is involved here is a negative value judgement. But this is not sufficient. In the next session, we outline a more complete account of the concept of illness, and how it gives us a clearer picture of the conceptual structure of medicine.

Reflection on the session and self-test questions

Write down your own reflections on the materials in this session drawing out any points that are particularly significant for you. Then write brief notes about the following:

1. Is adding 'values to facts' sufficient for a more complete picture of the conceptual structure of medicine? If not, why not?

2. What philosophical account of the relationship between descriptive and evaluative meaning might be used to reduce the evaluative element in the meanings of the medical concepts to a descriptive element?

3. What is the difference between the causal and logical relationship between illness and disease?

4. Does disease define illness, or illness disease? If the latter, how do we account for asymptomatic diseases?

5. What does a non-descriptivist account of the relationship between illness and disease add to the traditional medical model?

Session 4 Adding action to function

If illness is not defined by disease, as the medical model requires, how is it to be characterized? How, generally, do we come to think of an experience *as* an illness?

This question has been studied as much by sociologists as by philosophers. It is indeed one of those questions that admits equally of empirical and of conceptual answers. In reviewing some of these answers in this session, we will be adding a further element to our more complete picture of the conceptual structure of medicine; a picture around which, as we will suggest in the conclusions to this chapter, many of the topics at the interface between philosophy and mental health can be assembled.

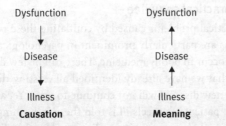

Fig. 6.9 The different directions of the causal and logical connections between the experience of illness and dysfunctional states as diseases (based on chapter 4 of Fulford's *Moral Theory and Medical Practice*, 1989).

A logical geography of illness
The experience of illness

Before we get to this more complete picture, however, we need to look at the features of our everyday use of the concept of illness. Philosophically, this will involve a further exercise in philosophical fieldwork. So, rather than starting with a reading, we will begin with a practical exercise.

EXERCISE 16   (60 minutes)

This exercise comes in two parts, a practical exercise and then a reading. They should take about 30 minutes each. Please do both!

1. Think about moving and not moving. Move your hand, to put down a book, say. Now rest your hand on the table. Or, stand up and walk around the room; then, sit still in your chair. Now imagine that you go to perform any of these actions (including those that involve keeping still) and find that you can't. Would you think there is something wrong with you? Would you think you were ill? Write down (a) as many aspects of the experience of failing to move or keep still that you can think of which, for you, would be likely to increase and/or decrease the likelihood of thinking that you are ill; and (b) any alternative accounts of your experience that you can think of, i.e. ways in which you might think of it other than as something (medically) wrong with you.

2. Now read the four brief extracts from:

Locker, D. (1981). The construction of illness. Chapter 5 in *Symptoms and Illness*. London: Tavistock Publications, pp. 95–96, 96–97, 100, 101

Link with Reading 6.9

David Locker did important empirical work on the features of experiences by which they are marked out as illnesses. As you read the extract, particularly the way the interviewees talked about their experiences, see how far this connects with your own responses in the first part of the exercise.

The point of this exercise is to start us thinking about the features of an experience that identify it as an experience of *illness*. As we should expect (from the fact that we are in general better at using concepts than at defining them, see Chapter 4), this is a surprisingly difficult thing to do. As David Locker notes elsewhere (in the introduction to his book), even sociologists have largely taken for granted that the meaning of 'illness' is self-evident.

This extract illustrates a number of important points. First, illness is related to but not the same as disease, or underlying disorder. This comes out also in cross-cultural work (see especially Fabrega's work in the Reading Guide). Second, as we should expect, elements of the concept of disease are very much mixed up with the experience of illness (e.g. p. 96 of this extract, Locker

notes that illness, as in the interview at the bottom of the preceding p. 95, is perceived as ' . . . the product of some underlying disorder'). Third, though, the experience of illness has a number of important features in its own right. We can summarize these features thus:

◆ *Feature 1—negative evaluation*: the experience (of failing to move or keep still) is *negatively* evaluated. We should expect this from everything we have done so far on the concepts of illness and disease; and this is a theme that runs right through Locker's interviews. They are all about 'problems', 'disorders', and so on.

◆ *Feature 2—intensity and duration*: the experience must have a certain *intensity and duration*. Again, this is implicit in Locker's interviews and is likely to have been clear from your own responses to part 1 of Exercise 16. Thus, in the case of movement/keeping still, a very brief difficulty in initiating action, one immediately rectified, is not experienced as illness. You might think that you had been clumsy, perhaps, or inattentive. These would be reasonable alternative accounts of such experiences. But a failure to move or to keep still has to be of a certain intensity and/or duration before you start thinking there is something wrong, before you 'call the doctor'.

◆ *Feature 3—not 'done or happens to' me:* the experience must not be obviously due to some *obstruction*. If I fail to walk around the room because someone trips me up, the experience is not of illness. In Locker's interviews, this is implicit at several points, and fully explicit, for example, at the bottom of p. 101, where a mother describes her daughter having hurt her leg: 'that's not an illness. . . .', she says.

In general, anything that we experience as being *done or as happening to* us is not, in this experiential sense, illness. Things being done or happening *to* me, to revert to part 1 of the exercise, are further alternative explanations for a failure to move or to keep still, even where such failures are intense (I fall heavily) or sustained (I keep falling over because people keep tripping me up).

◆ *Feature 4—not 'done by' me*: the experience must not be of me *doing something*. If I simply keep my hand still, or sit firmly in my chair, that is not paralysis. It is, simply, me keeping still. So long as a movement, or keeping still, remains under my control it is not experienced as illness.

Thus, in Locker's study, the experience of illness is sharply distinct from what he calls 'motivated behaviour'. The lady referred to illustrates this point very well. She could not do what she would ordinarily have done (go to her son's school concert): she felt so sick, she had to lie down. There is a sense, then, in which her behaviour (lying down) was something she did; but as Locker puts it, it was, really, imposed on her by her subjective state. (Hence, it is also not something that is done or happens to her, in the sense of feature 3 above, because there is no external agent.)

Illness and failures of 'ordinary doing'

In chapter 7 of his *Moral Theory and Medical Practice*, Fulford (1989) argues that these features of the experience of illness can be drawn together if we think of the experience of illness as involving, at least in the first instance, a failure of a particular kind of action.

EXERCISE 17   (45 minutes)

Read the extract from chapter 7 in:

Fulford, K.W.M. (1989). Illness and action. In *Moral Theory and Medical Practice*. Cambridge: Cambridge University Press, pp. 115–119

Link with Reading 6.10

Concentrate for the moment on the analysis offered of 'illness'. There is a good deal elsewhere in the chapter about the relationship between 'function' and 'action', and we will return to this later in this session. But what do you make of the analysis offered of illness? In particular, note:

1. how Fulford derives the features of the experience of illness from the notion of 'action failure', and

2. of the many different kinds of action of which people are capable, the particular kind of action (failure) that he argues is relevant to the experience of illness.

In this extract, Fulford argues that the primary experience of illness (at least as instantiated by movement and/or keeping still), can be analysed as a failure of 'ordinary doing' in the perceived absence of obstruction and/or opposition. The term 'ordinary doing' is borrowed from Austin. It means those things that are done, not reflexly, but usually without thinking too hard about them. As illustrated in the extract, then, ordinary doings, in Austin's sense, are actions we normally just get on and do, but which, if we reflect on them, are none the less seen to be intentional.

The details of this part of Fulford's analysis of the medical concepts are complicated, but the main points of his derivation of the features of illness can be summarized thus:

- Feature 1 (negative evaluation) follows directly from the fact that actions involve intentions that entail positive evaluations (hence *failures* of action entail the *negative* evaluation entailed by 'illness'). Spelling this out a bit, to act intentionally is to act for a reason (or intentionally, on purpose); this implies that your intention, your object, is one which, for you, is desired, wanted or in some other way positively evaluated; hence the *failure* of this is, correspondingly, a *negatively* evaluated experience.

- Feature 2 (intensity and duration) derives from the way that ordinary, everyday actions are defined by reference to norms or expectations of our capacities. We expect to be a bit slow or clumsy. The norms involved here are individual as well as group specific—an athlete failing to run a 4-minute mile might think there was something wrong with him, whereas you or I, perhaps, would not. Illness experiences thus fall outside the range of normal expectations as set by individual and collective norms.

- Feature 3 (not done or happens to); this too derives from ordinary actions. Our experience of performing actions is derived in contrast to being pushed or pulled by the world. Hence being obstructed is experienced as action being prevented rather than as a *failure* of action.

- Feature 4 (not done by). That illness is not something we do, is simply the action-failure theory made explicit.

Illness as a kind of 'action failure' corresponds with the idea that illness entails incapacity—the inability, rather than refusal, to do things. Talcott Parsons, in his classical sociological studies of deviance (Parsons, 1951), made this a central feature of illness: illness is something for which we are not responsible; it is therefore an excuse. (We noted this as a feature of the conceptual map of psychiatry in Chapter 2.)

The phenomenology of illness

Our understanding of the experience of illness is a good example of the way in which the explicit analyses offered, typically, by Anglo-American philosophy, are complemented by the more intuitive appreciation that we get from Continental Philosophy (see Chapter 4). This is well illustrated by the work of the American philosopher and phenomenologist Kay Toombs.

EXERCISE 18   (45 minutes)

Read the four extracts from:

Toombs, K. (1993). The body. Chapter 3 in *The Meaning of Illness: a phenomenological account of the different perspectives of physician and patient*. Dordrecht, The Netherlands: Kluwer Academic, pp. 62–63, 63, 66–67, and 70–71

Link with Reading 6.11

Make notes as you go along on the features of the experience of illness as Kay Toombs draws them out through her work in phenomenological description. In particular, note how she uses descriptions of the lived body to illuminate the experience of illness.

In this chapter, Kay Toombs is concerned with the experience of bodily illness. She starts with an account of the lived body as this has been developed in the phenomenological literature. Essentially, the lived body is our prereflective mode of being, in particular our continuing (and normally taken for granted) potential for action, which arises from our open relationship with the world. Hence, the essential characteristic of the experience of illness is a closing down or diminution of this open relationship, with a consequent restriction of our potential for action.

Kay Toombs introduces this idea initially on pp. 62–63. A particularly clear example is given on p. 67 in relation to our experience of space (this being a component of our relationship with the world upon which our taken-for-granted potential for action critically depends, but of which we are normally unaware, i.e. it is prereflective).

There are obvious parallels between this phenomenological account of illness and that derived above linguistic analytically; the phenomenological 'taken for granted potential for action' is very close to Austin's 'ordinary doing'; the phenomenological 'restriction of action' is very close to Fulford's 'failure of ordinary doing'. The two kinds of account, then, are indeed not in conflict but complementary.

Two objections

The importance of 'action failure' (failure of 'ordinary doing' in the perceived absence of obstruction and/or opposition) as being at least a feature of the experience of illness, is thus supported both by empirical evidence (your own practical experience; and the social scientific literature) and by philosophical analysis (linguistic and phenomenological).

At this point, however, two objections to an 'action failure' account of the experience of illness may have occurred to you: (1) that 'action failure' may seem little different from the 'failure of function' (or 'incapacity') emphasized by writers such as Boorse—so are we back with the same disease model by another name?, and (2) that this account may work for movement (tics, chorea, etc.) and keeping still (paralysis), but most illness experiences involve sensations (fear, pain, dizziness, etc.). Indeed in bodily medicine, sensations (fear, pain, dizziness, etc.) and perceptions (blindness, etc.) are more common than disturbances of movement; and in psychiatry, illness experiences involve a whole range of other phenomena—emotions, desires, motivations, etc. So, the question is, is an action-failure account of the experience of illness generalizable?

Objection 1: action and function

Taking these two objections in turn will fill out the action failure account of illness. The first objection, then, is that there may seem little difference between 'action failure' and 'failure of function'. This is covered in detail in Fulford (1989, chapter 7). We read a section from that chapter in Exercise 17 above and will be looking at a further brief extract below (Exercise 20). First, though, a good way to get clear about this is with a further practical exercise.

EXERCISE 19	(10 minutes)
Carry out any of the simple actions you tried at the start of this session; for example, putting down a book. Now, under what circumstances would you naturally think of this as your hand/arm functioning rather than as an action of yours? Write down one or more suggestions before going on.	

This exercise brings out a number of points (covered in Fulford, 1989, chapter 7) about the relationship between function and action. It shows, in particular, that they are not sharply

distinct, that, indeed, for some things we do they are two sides of the same coin. Which side of the coin we use then depends on the context. Putting down a book—one of Austin's 'ordinary doings'—is an *action* in the context of human beings relating to each other as agents. But once we focus on the parts or systems of which people are composed (arms, hands, etc.), it becomes natural to talk of *functions*. This would be true, for example, of a neurologist carrying out an examination of someone's arm.

Failure of action and failure of function

So, people (as agents) perform actions; bits and parts of people function. And this difference maps neatly on to the distinction between the patient's experience of illness and the doctor's knowledge of disease. This is spelled out in the next reading.

EXERCISE 20	(10 minutes)

Read the extract from:

Fulford, K.W.M. (1989). Illness and action. Chapter 7 in *Moral Theory and Medical Practice*. Cambridge: Cambridge University Press, pp. 126–127

Link with Reading 6.12

♦ Note the way in which, on this account, action failure is the natural way to analyse illness, where failure of function is the natural way to analyse disease.

As the reading in the above exercise indicates, differences in the uses of 'action' and 'function' correspond with differences in the uses of 'illness' and 'disease'. The most important of these is that actions are typically predicated of people while functions are typically predicated of organs, limbs, systems, or other parts of people. This is also true of illness and disease. Insofar as these are distinct, it is people who fall ill, the parts of people (livers, cardiovascular systems, etc.) which become diseased.

There is a spectrum here, of course, in which, as Fulford notes, ordinary doings, relatively simple actions, fall about mid-way. The more complex an activity, the more voluntary, the more it is something that a *person* does, then the stronger is the use of 'action'; conversely, the simpler an activity, the less voluntary, the more it is something that a *part* of a person does (a nerve, a blood cell, etc.), then the stronger becomes the use of 'function'. And the kinds of action-failure by which illness is characterized (i.e. the 'ordinary doings') fall in that part of the spectrum where action and function are equivocal. And this directly corresponds with the equivocal nature of illness and disease.

As Figure 6.10 indicates, then, the direct correspondence of these two equivocations (the equivocation between function and action corresponding with that between dysfunction and illness), strongly supports the wider claim that where dysfunction, and hence disease, are naturally analysed in terms of 'functional doing', the experience of illness is naturally analysed in terms of

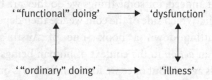

Fig. 6.10 The relationship between action and function, illness and dysfunction. Source: Fulford, K.W.M. (1989). Illness and action. In *Moral Theory and Medical Practice*. Cambridge: Cambridge University Press, p. 127.

failure of the particular kind of action that Fulford, following Austin, characterizes as 'ordinary doing'.

Objection 2: movement and pain

So much for objection 1. What about objection 2, that illness experiences often involve sensations such as pain, rather than movement, or indeed emotions, beliefs, etc. as in mental health, and hence are not so obviously linked with action failure as this account might suggest. The question, then, is how far is this account generalizable from movement-as-illness to other kinds of illness experience?

EXERCISE 21   (30 minutes)

Some authors (e.g. including Boorse, 1975) have sought to define illness in terms of either incapacity or pain. Do we need another kind of illness? Or is 'action failure' generalizable to things other than movement? Try running through the four features of illnesses (noted above) for (1) pain, and (2) memory. Are these assimilable to action-failure?

Like movements, not all pains are experienced as illness, and, at a first level at least, pain-*as*-illness appears to be very similar to movement-*as*-illness.

Thus, pain-as-illness is *negatively evaluated*. However, negatively evaluated experiences of pain are not necessarily experienced as illness (pain, although usually negatively evaluated, is not *necessarily* so; for an excellent discussion of this, see Hare [1964]1972). Hence, even granted that an illness experience (of pain) is a negatively evaluated experience of pain, there must be other features of the experience as well. These features, as for movement-as-illness, include a certain *intensity and duration* (a very brief, mild pain is unlikely to be experienced as illness); moreover, and again analogously with movement-as-illness, pain-as-illness is distinguishable both from '*done or happens to*' experiences, i.e. from pain that is manifestly either inflicted by others or due to some other external cause, and, pain that is being '*done by*' someone, i.e. is self-inflicted. Thus, pain-as-illness is distinct both from my hand held in the flame by others, and from me holding it there.

Movement, sensations, and the machinery of action

There are thus *prima facie* parallels between pain-as-illness and movement-as-illness. But this still leaves the basic objection, that pain, unlike movement, just does not 'look like' an action. So, if the experience of illness is, somehow, derived from action-failure

(of a particular, 'ordinary doing', kind), how does pain become experienced as a symptom? The next exercise focuses on this question.

EXERCISE 22   (15 minutes)

This is a two-stage exercise.

1. Start by thinking about whether there is any sense in which pain is involved with action. There is a crucial step here, crucial to our understanding of the concept of mental illness.

Link with Reading 6.13
---

2. After thinking about this for yourself, read the further extract from:

   Fulford, K.W.M. (1989). Illness and action. Chapter 7 in *Moral Theory and Medical Practice*. Cambridge: Cambridge University Press, pp. 135–136

As this reading brings out, there is clearly a sense in which movement and pain are quite different *viz-à-viz* action. Movement is executive. There is more to action than movement, as we saw a moment ago (there is intention, motivation, perception, etc.). But without movement, actions could not be performed. From the vibrating of vocal cords to the striding of legs, it is by movements that actions are executed. Pain, on the other hand, along with other sensations, is on the receiving rather than output side. It is among the sensory mechanisms by which actions are generated; in particular, it prompts withdrawal from potentially harmful situations.

Pain, therefore, is integral to what Fulford, using Austin's phrase, calls the *machinery of action*. We will return shortly to Austin on the 'machinery of action' in the last reading in this chapter (see Exercise 23). But the point for now is to see that pain, no less than movement, is part of the machinery of action. It is a different part from movement, to be sure. But it is a part of the machinery, none the less. Hence, like movement-as-illness, pain-as-illness is eligible in principle for an action-failure analysis. Specifically, as Fulford goes on to argue, to the extent that pain prompts withdrawal, then, pain-as-illness is parallel to movement-as-illness in that *it can be understood as pain from which one is unable to withdraw in the perceived absence of obstruction and/or opposition.*

Back to the map of mental illness

This way of understanding the experience of illness, as (or as derived from) a particular kind of failure of action, can be extended to the full range of illness experiences, mental as well as bodily, by considering these as involving different parts of the machinery of action.

That this 'machinery' is in principle rich enough (conceptually speaking) to encompass the full variety of illness experiences is evident from the next reading, a brief extract from Austin's *A Plea for Excuses* on this topic.

EXERCISE 23 (20 minutes)

Read the extract from:

Austin, J.L. (1956–7). A plea for excuses. *Proceedings of the Aristotelian Society*, 57: 1–30. [Reprinted in White, A.R. (ed.) (1968). *The Philosophy of Action*. Oxford: Oxford University Press, pp. 19–42.] (Page numbers from reprint.)

Link with Reading 6.14

As you read through this long paragraph, 1) list any of the distinct parts of the 'machinery of action' mentioned by Austin, and 2) try to think what particular areas of psychopathology would correspond with (to extend Austin's metaphor) *failures* of each of these. (You may want to refer back to chapter 3 here.)

In the first part of this (very long) paragraph, Austin notes, among other parts of his 'machinery of action', attention (reduced in distractability in hypomania, for example), guarding against likely dangers (overactive in obsessional disorders), and 'judgement or tact' (again reduced in hypomania; also in 'frontal lobe syndrome').

Austin's purpose, here, is to illuminate excuses, i.e. as relying on ways in which our actions can 'go wrong'. All these, he says, are 'executive'. But there are also 'intelligence and planning', 'decision and resolve', and, a part of the machinery he distinguishes from all these, 'appreciation'. 'We can know the facts', he says, 'and yet look at them mistakenly or perversely, or ... even be under a total misconception'. Here, he says, with failures of appreciation, 'troubles and excuses abound' (p. 34).

Austin's special mention of 'appreciation' turns out to be particularly relevant for understanding a key feature of the 'map' of mental disorder. You will recall from Chapter 2 that psychotic disorders, defined centrally by delusions, are the central case of mental illness as an excuse. Yet exactly why this should be so is far from clear: delusions, as we saw in Chapter 3, are not characteristically marked by any failure of the cognitive functions, such as memory and intelligence. Austin, although of course not concerned here with delusion as an excuse, gives us, in the concept of appreciation, as a part of the machinery of action distinct from knowledge, memory, intelligence and such like, a basis for explaining (or at any rate exploring) the distinct status of delusion as an excuse.

Thus, Fulford (1989, chapter 10), argues that the psychopathological features of delusion suggest that it should be understood as a failure of practical reasoning (i.e. the reasoning characteristic of whole persons as distinct from the particular cognitive part-functions of memory, IQ etc.); and in a widely used assessment measure of decision-making capacity, the MacCAT-T, developed by the psychiatrist Paul Appelbaum and the psychologist Thomas Grisso in the States, the loss of insight by which delusion is characterized is measured on a scale distinct from understanding and reasoning. And this distinct scale, in a neat coincidence with Austin's terminology, Grisso and Appelbaum actually call 'appreciation' (Grisso and Appelbaum, 1998).

Many meanings of illness

Not only movement and pain, then, but a wide range of other sensations (and lack of sensations) can be analysed similarly, as can the far more diverse phenomena by which mental illness is constituted. Some of these phenomena are more like movement (thought, for example, and memory, as in the second part of Exercise 16); others are more like pain (anxiety, sadness, and so forth); none are *quite* the same, though, and some (like delusion) are altogether different.

Illness, then, the patient's actual experience, can be analysed in terms of a particular kind of action failure. The *similarities* between different kinds of illness experience, including those between mental and bodily illness, derive, on this analysis, from their common origins (conceptual origins) in action-failure; while the *differences* between them derive from differences in the way the phenomena concerned are built into the machinery of action.

This account, it is important to add, is not exclusive of function-based analyses of disease. As we have seen, action and function, failure of action and failure of function, are complementary. But if the indications we can take from Austin's (brief) account of the machinery of action are right, when it comes to understanding the diverse phenomena by which *mental* illness (include delusion) is constituted, action-failure, as well as function-failure, is essential.

Reflection on the session and self-test questions

Write down your own reflections on the materials in this session drawing out any points that are particularly significant for you. Then write brief notes about the following:

1. What are the features of the actual experience of illness? (We suggested four key features.)

2. Among the different kinds of actions (or things that a person does), which kind of action is particularly associated with early experiences of illness?

3. What objections might there be to analysing the experience of illness in terms of a particular kind of failure of action? We noted two objections.

4. How can an analysis of the experience of illness in terms of disturbance of agency be connected with an analysis of disease in terms of disturbance of functioning?

5. How can an analysis of the experience of illness in terms of a particular kind of disturbance of agency be generalized from movement (and loss of movement) to other kinds of illness experience?

6. What does an analysis of the experience of illness as a particular kind of disturbance of agency add to the traditional medical model?

Conclusions: a full-field model and a two-way exchange

In this chapter we have looked at the outputs of philosophical work, at what we get out of doing philosophy. The broad conclusion has been that philosophy gives us a more complete picture (Wittgenstein's 'clearer view') of the meanings of the concepts in a given area of discourse.

A full-field model

The more complete picture of the medical concepts to which we have come, and its relationship to the traditional medical model, is shown diagrammatically in figure 6.11

As the top half of this figure illustrates, a full-field model adds to, rather than subtracts from, the traditional medical model. It incorporates the medical model elements of fact, disease, and failure of functioning, but adds to these the elements of value, illness, and failure of action. This is why it is a 'full-field' model, incorporating both the traditional 'right field' of the medical model, and the 'left field' of illness experience, rather than suggesting that either field should exclude the other.

The inclusive (fact+value, etc) rather than exclusive nature of a full-field model is worth emphasizing. Too often science and the humanities are thought to be, somehow, antithetical in medicine. One could be forgiven for thinking this given the way in which

scientifically minded doctors and ethicists often appear to be at loggerheads! But a full-field model incorporates everything that is genuinely scientific in medicine alongside and on an equal basis with everything that is genuinely humanistic.

Many methods

We have drawn in this chapter, as in earlier sections, particularly on Austinian 'fieldwork' as one method for building up this more complete picture, this clearer view, of our concepts. As we have seen, this is a powerful method. But as Austin himself emphasized, it is only one way of getting started with some kinds of philosophical problem. We noted in the last chapter the way in which Continental and Anglo-American methods are entirely complementary in coming to a more complete view of the 'logical geography' of illness. The bottom half of figure 6.11 illustrates the wide range of other philosophical disciplines that are relevant in this respect. Nor should philosophy as a whole be thought of as working in isolation. To the contrary, it is a natural partner of empirical and other research methods—thus we drew on empirical sociological work in session 3, for example.

A two-way exchange

We will find many examples in this book of the ways in which, either directly, through giving us a clearer picture of the medical concepts, or indirectly, by drawing on more general philosophical topics, the clearer view offered by philosophy can contribute to good clinical work and research in mental health.

It is important, though, finally, to remind ourselves that, as we learned from Austin, Wilkes and others in Chapter 4, the 'outputs' of this clearer view, what we 'get out of it', is not a one-way flow from philosophy to practice. Just as important is the flow back from practice to philosophy.

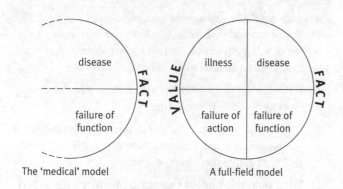

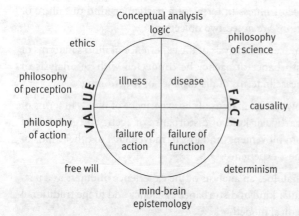

Fig. 6.11 The full-field view and its philosophical context.

Reading guide

Concepts of disorder: (4) Values and philosophical value theory

Hare's (1952) *The Language of Morals*, his first book, remains an excellent introduction to his approach. It was followed in 1963 by *Freedom and Reason* Hare, 1963a, and later in 1981 by *Moral Thinking: levels, methods and point*. He wrote extensively on descriptive and evaluative meaning, see for example, his article 'Descriptivism', first published in 1963 in *Proceedings of the British Academy* (Hare, 1963b); reprinted in Hare, R.M. (1972) *Essays on the Moral Concepts*. G.J. Warnock's (1971) version of descriptivism, which opposes Hare's prescriptivism, is set out in his *The Object of Morality*. Two accounts which defend the reduction of evaluative aspects of classification to the factual (naturalized) aspects are C.R. Pigden's (1993) 'Naturalism' in Peter Singer's, *A Companion to Ethics*; and

John Searle's contentious 'How to derive "ought" from "is" ', in Phillippa Foot's (1967), *Theories of Ethics*.

A useful brief introduction to the main philosophical views on the logical properties of value terms, and an excellent summary of the debates between descriptivist and non-descriptivist positions, is given in Geoffrey Warnock's (1967) *Contemporary Moral Philosophy*. As noted in chapter 2, the American philosopher, Hilary Putnam has recently (2002) set out an 'entanglement' view of the relationship between fact and value in his collection of essays, *The Collapse of the Fact/Value Dichotomy and other Essays*. Chapters 2–4 of Fulford's *Moral Theory and Medical Practice* (1989) explore the implications of this debate for our understanding of the concepts of illness and disease (as mixed fact-value concepts) in medicine and psychiatry. The applications of the debate specifically between non-descriptivist and descriptivist positions to the debate about mental illness, are set out in chapters 3 and 6 (corresponding to the first and second of the Hare extracts in this chapter of this book). A more complete treatment of a descriptivist version of the medical model is to be found in Fulford's (1995) chapter on 'Psychiatric ethics' in Almond's *Introducing Applied Ethics*.

The nature of the causal reduction is a large topic in its own right in the philosophy of science—see Reading Guides in Part III. For a discussion of causal reduction and its relevance to concepts of illness and disease, see Thornton, T. (2004) 'Reductionism/Antireductionism' in Radden's. (Ed) (2004) *The Philosophy of Psychiatry: a companion*. The complex relationship between illness and disease, including the way in which the ordinary usage of these terms is driven by their properties as value terms, is set out in chapters 2 and 4 of Fulford's *Moral Theory and Medical Practice*.

We will be returning to the relationship between facts (as in Hare's descriptive criteria) and values, both in their own right and as this is relevant to practical issues in mental health, at several points later in the book (in particular in Part IV).

The experience of illness: sociological studies

In addition to David Locker's work as noted in the chapter, important sociological studies of illness behaviour and experience include Talcott Parsons' (1951) classic account of deviance and the way society uses the sick role to maintain stability; Robert Dingwall's (1976) study of illness in terms of social action; David Mechanic's (1981) 'The social dimension' work on the way in which illness behaviour is related to effective problem-solving (including delivery of health care); and work by labelling theorists, some of it offering radical critiques of mental illness (e.g. Pearson, 1975, *The Deviant Imagination*).

Early work on the cross-cultural aspects of the experience of illness includes Fabrega (1972) 'The study of disease in relation

to culture'. Recent work, building on these early studies, includes Fitzpatrick et al's (1984) *The Experience of Illness*, Michael Calnan (1987) *Health and Illness: the lay perspective*; and Wendy Stainton Rogers (1992) *Explaining Illness*. A valuable edited collection is Marx and Johnson's (1991) *The Illness Experience: Dimensions of Suffering*.

Values, agency, and illness

An account of the relationship between agency and values concerned with the concept of health, and hence with a different focus from that outlined in the chapter, has been developed by the Swedish philosopher, Lennart Nordenfelt (1987) in his *On the Nature of Health: an action-theoretic account of health*. This explores in detail the conceptual links between health, the 'vital goals' of the individual, and their biological and social origins. Nordenfelt's account fills in the social dimension of health. Although developed originally for bodily illness, Nordenfelt has extended his analysis to mental health in his *Talking about Health* (1997) and *Health, Science, and Ordinary Language* (2001).

The argument linking the experience of illness to loss of agency is developed in chapter 7 of Fulford's (1989) *Moral Theory and Medical Practice* and is extended to mental illness generally in chapter 8. (This includes the discussion of 'memory-as-illness', see Exercise 16.) The psychiatrist, Jeremy Holmes, and the philosopher, Richard Lindley (1989), have explored the relationship between values, agency and illness in psychotherapy in their *The Values of Psychotherapy*. The South African psychiatrist, Werdie Van Staden, has examined the relationship between recovery and agency in a linguistic-analytic study of first personal pronoun use in psychotherapy (Van Staden, 2002a; Van Staden and Fulford, 2004). Martins' *et al*. (2000) *Delusion According to the Speech Acts Theory*.

Two articles in the debate between Fulford and Nordenfelt have been published in the *Journal of Theoretical Medicine*—see especially, Fulford's (1993) 'Praxis makes perfect: illness as a bridge between biological concepts of disease and social conceptions of health'; also Fulford and Nordenfelt's contributions to Nordenfelt (2001) 'Health, science and ordinary language', respectively Nordenfelt's (2001) 'Toward a critical assessment of the reverse theories of health and illness' (pp. 75–112), and Fulford's (2001) 'Philosophy into practice: the case for ordinary language philosophy' (pp. 171–208) in Nordenfelt (2001).

Agency has been explored by a number of authors in *Philosophy, Psychiatry, & Psychology*. The first paper in the first issue of *Philosophy, Psychiatry, & Psychology* was on agency, Peter Binns' (1994) 'Affect, agency, engagement: conceptions of the person in philosophy, neuropsychiatry, and psychotherapy', with a response by Peter Caws (1994). Other papers on agency include, Campbell (2000a) 'Diagnosing agency', with a commentary by Loizzo (2000) 'Guarding patient agency', and a response by Campbell (2000b) on 'Naturalizing agency'. A Special Issue of *Philosophy, Psychiatry, & Psychology*, guest edited by Melvin Woody, explores themes around 'Agency, narrative and self' (2003, issue 10/4). This issue was made up of an introduction by Sadler and Fulford (2003), and four target articles: Wells' (2003) 'Discontinuity in personal narrative: some perspectives of patients'; Kennett and Matthews (2003) on 'The unity and disunity of agency'; Phillips (2003) 'Psychopathology and the narrative self'; and Woody (2003) 'When narrative fails'. Commentaries on the set of four papers were provided by Glas (2003) on 'Loss of the self', Hardcastle (2003) on 'Emotions', Radden (2003) on 'Learning from disunity', Thornton (2003) on 'Two kinds of narrative accounts of the self', Weiner (2003) on volition, and Woodbridge (2003) on 'The forgotten self' (which covers the implications for training).

A novel analysis of the links between recovery and restoration of agency is Van Staden (2002a) on 'Linguistic markers of recovery: theoretical underpinnings of first person pronoun usage and semantic positions of patients', with commentaries by Gillett (2002), Suppes (2002), and Falzer and Davidson (2002), and a response by Van Staden (2002b). Van Staden's paper explores the philosophical underpinnings in Frege's logic of relations of the empirical work reported in Van Staden and Fulford (2004).

(See also Reading guide, Chapter 26.)

References

Austin, J.L. (1956–7). A plea for excuses. *Proceedings of the Aristotelian Society*, 57: 1–30. [Reprinted in White, A.R. (ed.) (1968). *The Philosophy of Action*. Oxford: Oxford University Press, pp. 19–42.]

Ayer, A.J. (1976). *The Central Questions of Philosophy*. London: Penguin.

Binns, P. (1994). Affect, agency, engagement: conceptions of the person in philosophy, neuropsychiatry, and psychotherapy', with a response by Peter Caws (1994).

Boorse, C. (1975). On the distinction between disease and illness. *Philosophy and Public Affairs*, 5: 49–68.

Calnan, M. (1987). *Health and Illness: the lay perspective*. London: Routledge.

Campbell, P.G. (2000a). Diagnosing agency. *Philosophy, Psychiatry, & Psychology*, 7(2): 107–120.

Campbell, P.G. (2000b). Naturalizing agency: a response to the Commentary. *Philosophy, Psychiatry, & Psychology*, 7(2): 123–124.

Caws, P. (1994) *Commentary on Binns, P. (1994) "Affect Agency, and Engagement"*. Philosophy, Psychiatry, and Psychology, 1/1, 25–26.

Christodoulou, G.N. (1977). The syndrome of Capgras. *British Journal of Psychiatry*, 130: 556–64.

Crary, A. and Read, R. (eds) (2000). *The New Wittgenstein*. London: Routledge.

Diamond, J. (1993). Born to be gay? *The Sunday Times*, 15 July.

Dingwall, R. (1976). *Aspects of Illness*. London: Martin Robertson.

Eigen, M. (2001). *Ecstasy*. Middletown, CT: Wesleyan University Press.

Fabrega, H., (1972), The study of disease in relation to culture. *Behavioural Science*, 17: 183–203.

Falzer, P. and Davidson, L. (2002). Language, logic, and recovery: a commentary on Van Staden. (Commentary on Van Staden, 2002a). *Philosophy, Psychiatry, & Psychology*, 9(2): 131–136.

Fitzpatrick, R., Hinton, J., Newman, S., Scrambler, G., and Thompson, J. (1984). *The Experience of Illness*. London: Tavistock Publications.

Foot, P. (ed.) (1967). Moral beliefs. Chapter VI in Foot, P. (ed) *Theories of Ethics*. Oxford: Oxford University Press, pp. 83–92.

Fulford, K.W.M. (1989). *Moral Theory and Medical Practice*. Cambridge: Cambridge University Press.

Fulford, K.W.M. (1993). Praxis makes perfect: illness as a bridge between biological concepts of disease and social conceptions of health. *Theoretical Medicine*, 14: 321–324.

Fulford, K.W.M. (1995). Psychiatric ethics. In *Introducing Applied Ethics* (ed. B. Almond). Oxford: Blackwell.

Fulford, K.W.M. (2000). Teleology without Tears: Naturalism, Neo-Naturalism and Evaluationism in the Analysis of Function Statements in Biology (and a Bet on the Twenty-first Century). *Philosophy, Psychiatry, & Psychology* 7/1: 77–94.

Fulford, K.W.M. (2001). Philosophy into practice: the case for ordinary language philosophy. Part 2. In *Health, Science and Ordinary Language* (ed. L. Nordenfelt). Amsterdam: Rodopi, pp. 171–208.

Gillett, G. (2002). The self as relatum in life and language. (Commentary on Van Staden, 2002a). *Philosophy, Psychiatry, & Psychology*, 9(2): 123–126.

Glas, G. (2003). Idem, ipse, and loss of the self (Commentary on Wells, 2003, Kennett and Matthews, 2003, Phillips, 2003 and Wooding, 2003). *Philosophy, Psychiatry, & Psychology*, 10(4): 347–352.

Grisso, T. and Appelbaum, P.S. (1998). *Assessing Competence to Consent to Treatment: a guide for clinicians and other health professionals*. New York: Oxford University Press.

Hardcastle, V.G. (2003). Emotions and narrative selves. (Commentary on Wells, 2003, Kennett and Matthews, 2003, Phillips, 2003 and Wooding, 2003). *Philosophy, Psychiatry, & Psychology*, 10(4): 353–356.

Hare, R.M. (1952). *The Language of Morals*. Oxford: Oxford University Press.

Hare, R.M. (1963a) *Freedom and Reason*. Oxford: Oxford University Press.

Hare, R.M. (1963b). Descriptivism. *Proceedings of the British Academy*, 49: 115–134. (Reprinted in Hare, R.M., 1972, ch 5 in *Essays on the Moral Concepts*. London: Macmillan.)

Hare, R.M. (1964). Pain and evil. *Aristotelian Society Supplement*, XXXVIII. (Reprinted as Chapter 6, *Essays on the Moral Concepts*, 1972, London: The Macmillan Press.)

Hare, R.M. (1972). *Essays on the Moral Concepts*. London: The Macmillan Press.

Hare, R.M. (1981). *Moral Thinking: levels, methods and point*. Oxford: Oxford University Press.

Holmes, J. and Lindley, R. (1989). *The Values of Psychotherapy*. Oxford: Oxford University Press.

Hume, D. (1739/40). *Treatise of Human Nature*. III, I, i, final paragraph.

Kennett, J. and Matthews, S. (2003). The unity and disunity of agency. *Philosophy, Psychiatry, & Psychology*, 10(4): 305–312.

LeVay, S. (1993) *The Sexual Brain*. Cambridge: MIT Press.

Locker, D. (1981). The construction of illness. Chapter 5 in *Symptoms and Illness*. London: Tavistock Publications.

Loizzo, J. (2000). Guarding patient agency. (Commentary on Campbell, 2000a). *Philosophy, Psychiatry, & Psychology*, 7(2): 121–122.

Martins, F., Costa, A. and Porto, K. (2000). Delusion according to the theory of speech acts. *Psicol. Reflex. Crit.*, vol. 13, p. 189–198.

Marx, M.J. and Johnson, J.L. (1991). *The Illness Experience: Dimensions of Suffering*. Newbury Park, London: Sage Publications.

Mechanic, D. (1981). The social dimension. In *Psychiatric Ethics*, (1st edn) (ed. S. Bloch and P. Chodoff). Oxford: Oxford University Press, pp. 46–59.

Nordenfelt, L. (1987). *On the Nature of Health: an action-theoretic account of health*. Dordrecht: D. Reidel Publishing Co.

Nordenfelt, L. (1997). *Talking about Health: A Philosophical Dialogue*. Amsterdam: Rodopi.

Nordenfelt, L. (2001). *Health, Science, and Ordinary Language*. Amsterdam: Rodopi.

Nordenfelt, L. (2001). Toward a critical assessment of the reverse theories of health and illness. Part I. *Health, Science and Ordinary Language*, pp. 75–112.

Parsons, T. (1951). *The Social System*. Glencoe, IL: Free Press.

Pearson, G. (1975). *The Deviant Imagination*. London: Macmillan Press.

Phillips, J. (2003). Psychopathology and the narrative self. *Philosophy, Psychiatry, & Psychology*, 10(4): 313–328.

Pigden, C.R. (1993). Naturalism. In *A Companion to Ethics* (ed. P. Singer). Oxford: Blackwell.

Plato. (2003). *The Republic*. Harmondsworth, England: Penguin Books Limited.

Putnam, H. (2002). *The Collapse of the Fact/Value Dichotomy and other Essays*. Cambridge, MA: Harvard University Press.

Radden, J. (2003). Learning from disunity. (Commentary on Wells, 2003, Kennett and Matthews, 2003, Phillips, 2003, and Wooding, 2003). *Philosophy, Psychiatry, & Psychology*, 10(4): 357–360.

Radden, J. (2004). (Ed) *The Philosophy of Psychiatry: A Companion*. New York: Oxford University Press.

Russell, B. (1912). The value of philosophy. In *The Problems of Philosophy*. London: Williams and Northgate, pp. 237–250.

Russell, B. (1946). *History of Western Philosophy*. London: George Allen and Unwin.

Russell, B. (1962). *An Inquiry into Meaning and Truth*. London: Penguin Books.

Sadler, J.Z. and Fulford, K.W.M. (2003). Agency, narrative, and self: a philosophical case conference. *Philosophy, Psychiatry, & Psychology*, 10(4): 295–296.

Searle, J. (1967). How to derive 'ought' from 'is'. In *Theories of Ethics* (ed. P. Foot). Oxford: Oxford University Press.

Stainton Rogers, W. (1992). *Explaining Illness*. Milton Keynes: Open University Press.

Suppes, P. (2002). Linguistic markers of recovery: underpinnings of first person pronoun usage and semantic positions of patients. (Commentary on Van Staden, 2002a). *Philosophy, Psychiatry, & Psychology*, 9(2): 127–130.

Thornton, T. (2003). Psychopathology and two kinds of narrative account of the self. (Commentary on Wells, 2003, Kennett and Matthews, 2003, Phillips, 2003 and Wooding, 2003). *Philosophy, Psychiatry, & Psychology*, 10(4): 361–368.

Thornton, T. (2004). Reductionism/antireductionism. In The *Philosophy of Psychiatry: a companion* (ed. J. Radden). New York: Oxford University Press, pp. 191–204.

Toombs, K. (1993). The body. In *The Meaning of Illness: a phenomenological account of the different perspectives of physician and patient*. Dordrecht: Kluwer Academic, pp. 51–71.

Van Staden, C.W. (2002a) Linguistic markers of recovery: theoretical underpinnings of first person pronoun usage and semantic positions of patients. *Philosophy, Psychiatry, & Psychology*, 9(2): 105–122.

Van Staden, C.W. (2002b). Language mirrors relational positions in recovery: a response to commentaries by Falzer and Davidson, Gillett, and Suppes. *Philosophy, Psychiatry, & Psychology*, 9(2): 137–140.

Van Staden, C.W. and Fulford, K.W.M. (2004). Changes in semantic uses of first person pronouns as possible linguistic markers of recovery in psychotherapy. *Australian and New Zealand Journal of Psychiatry*, 38(4): 226–232.

Warnock, G.J. (1967). *Contemporary Moral Philosophy*. London: Methuen.

Warnock, G.J. (1971). *The Object of Morality*. London: Methuen.

Warnock, M. (1978). *Ethics Since 1900* (3rd edn). Oxford: Oxford University Press.

Weiner, S. (2003). Unity of agency and volition: some personal reflections. (Commentary on Wells, 2003, Kennett and Matthews, 2003, Phillips, 2003 and Wooding, 2003). *Philosophy, Psychiatry, & Psychology*, 10(4): 369–372.

Wells, L.A. (2003). Discontinuity in personal narrative: some perspectives of patients. *Philosophy, Psychiatry, & Psychology*, 10(4): 297–304.

Whitehead, A.N. and Russell, B. (1910, 1912, 1913) *Principia Mathematica*, 3 vols, Cambridge: Cambridge University Press. (2nd edn), 1925 (Vol. 1), 1927 (Vols 2, 3).

Williams, B. (1985). *Ethics and the Limits of Philosophy*. London: Fontana Press/Collins.

Wittgenstein, L. (1921). *Tractatus Logico-Philosophicus* (trans. D.F. Pears and B.F. McGuinness). London: Routledge and Kegan Paul.

Wittgenstein, L. (1953). *Philosophical Investigations*. Oxford: Blackwell, §124.

Woodbridge, K. (2003). The forgotten self: training mental health and social care workers to work with service users. (Commentary on Wells, 2003, Kennett and Matthews, 2003, Phillips, 2003 and Wooding, 2003). *Philosophy, Psychiatry, & Psychology*, 10(4): 373–378.

Woody, J.M. (2003). When narrative fails. *Philosophy, Psychiatry, & Psychology*, 10(4): 329–346.

PART II

A philosophical history of psychopathology

Part contents

Introduction to Part II

In Part I of this book, we explored current ideas about mental disorder, the variety and subtlety of descriptive psychopathology (in Chapter 3), and the range of often competing ways in which the concept of mental disorder itself has been understood (Chapters 2, 4, and 6).

In this part we will be looking at the historical origins of these ideas. We will be asking such questions as: how have we come to recognize the variety and subtlety of psychopathological concepts? Where have our categories of disorder come from? Who decided which phenomena are 'symptoms'? And why? Are current classifications the last word on the subject?

Reinventing psychopathology

Questions of this kind have been given a new urgency as we enter a new century with dramatic developments in the neurosciences. A classification in any science is a snapshot of the current state of theory: from respiratory medicine to quantum theory, nature is divided up in accordance with prevailing assumptions and theories.

Critics of psychiatry often point to its relatively unstable classifications of disorder as a mark of scientific immaturity. However, such instability is a mark equally of an actively evolving science. And the neurosciences are nothing if not actively evolving! Brain imaging techniques, psychopharmacology, behavioural genetics, and artificial intelligence, are opening up the possibility of new ways of classifying and theorizing about the nature of psychopathology. We return to psychiatric clarification, and to the challenges of the new neurosciences, in detail in Part III.

A second mark of an actively evolving science is close engagement with philosophy. As Fulford et al., (2003) note, the conceptual challenges of the new neurosciences are one of the reasons behind the late twentieth century renaissance in philosophy of psychiatry. This is why, as Fulford et al., (2003) put it, the decade of the brain turned out to be also the decade of the mind. Similar close encounters between empirical science and philosophy are evident in other actively evolving sciences, notably in theoretical physics and in psychology.

History as a guide

At times of rapid change, history may be a helpful guide. This is true generally in mental health: many of the failings of community care could have been avoided if we had taken the lessons of history—William Parry-Jones' *The Trade in Lunacy* (1972), for example, to which we return in Chapter 7, showed how the initially well-intentioned reforms of the eighteenth and nineteenth centuries degenerated into abusive practices, partly through under-resourcing.

In the history specifically of psychopathology, we have a particularly compelling guide, for there are important respects in which the state of the discipline now, at the turn of the twenty-first century, was paralleled by its state a hundred years ago at the turn of the twentieth century (Fulford et al., 2003). Then, as now, the brain sciences were in a period of rapid advance: the localization of functions, such as speech and movement, in specific cerebral areas, the invention of differential staining methods in neuropathology, and the discovery of specific disease entities (such as neurosyphilis and Alzheimer's disease), had much the same 'gee-whiz' impact as modern brain imaging; then, as now, there were competing paradigms (the soon-to-be-born psychoanalysis, as a psychological theory, for example, paralleling our modern cognitive psychologies); and then, as now, there were wide-ranging debates about the classification of psychopathology.

A number of major figures in the history of psychopathology emerged from this period—the German psychiatrist, Emil Kraepelin, and, from Switzerland, Eugen Bleuler, for example, who defined 'schizophrenia'. It was also during this period that the great German philosopher-psychiatrist, Karl Jaspers, on whose foundational work in philosophical psychopathology we will be focusing in this part, published the first edition of his *Allgemeine Psychopathologie (General Psychopathology,* 1913/1963).

The storyline of Part II

The histories of particular symptoms and syndromes have been widely studied (see Chapter 7, Exercise 1 and the Reading Guide). In this part, though, it is with the history of the underpinning conceptual structure of psychopathology that we will be mainly concerned, this being the set of ideas by which, through most of the twentieth century, psychiatrists have organized and tried to give meaning to psychopathology.

It is above all to Karl Jaspers that we owe this structure as it has come down to us today. This is why it is with Jaspers, and with the philosophical influences on his psychopathology, that we will be

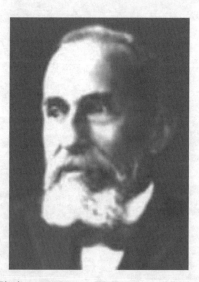

Fig. II.1 Eugen Bleuler

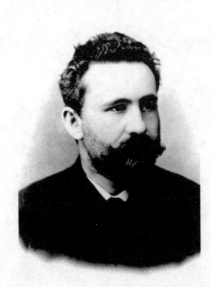

Fig. II.2 Emil Kraepelin

mainly concerned in this Part of the book. We will start, in Chapter 7, by placing Jaspers' work in context with an overview of shifting ideas about mental distress and disorder over the last two and a half millennia. As we will see, a key theme of Part I is reflected in this two and a half thousand year history, namely the tension between moral (as in Szasz' work, for example) and scientific (as in Kendell's reply to Szasz) interpretations. It is this theme, too, as we will also see, that runs through Jaspers' work, though now translated into the need for meaningful as well as causal accounts of psychopathology. We take an overview of Jaspers, of his biography and of his key theoretical ideas, in Chapter 8. We then look in detail at two key philosophical influences on Jaspers, respectively, phenomenology in Chapter 9, and, in Chapter 10, the *Methodenstreit*, a nineteenth century debate about method in the human sciences.

Jaspers and psychopathology today

By the end of this part, we will find that Jaspers' work, important as it has been, was incomplete. The conceptual framework for psychopathology that he built up is still, perhaps, the most coherent available. But there remain within it, as a reflection of Jaspers' thinking, unresolved tensions. This is no criticism of Jaspers, however. For the tensions are essentially those that, in Part I, we found between moral (Szaszian) and medical (Kendellian) models of mental disorder. These tensions, in turn, we will find in Chapter 7, run though the last two and a half thousand years of the history of ideas about mental disorder. They persist, still, in different forms, in the philosophy of science (Part III) and in ethics (Part IV). And they persist, above all, in the philosophy of mind (Part V), in continuing debates about the relationship between (human) reasons and (scientific) causes.

The incompleteness of Jaspers' psychopathology, then, his failure fully to reconcile meanings with causes in our understanding of mental disorder, far from being a matter for criticism, is a direct reflection of a deep feature of psychopathology itself. Twentieth century psychiatry, as we have seen, and as we will examine further in Part III, The Philosophy of Science, made giant strides in improving the reliability of its psychopathological and diagnostic concepts, progress that indeed laid the foundations for the new neurosciences. This progress, though, was made possible by focusing on the scientific (descriptive and causal) side of psychopathology at the expense of its human (meaningful and rational) side. We will see later in this part that a strong phenomenological tradition was maintained through the twentieth century, particularly in Continental Europe. Mainstream psychiatry, however, in many parts of the world, moved increasingly away from meanings and towards causes.

It is, however, a final vindication of Jasper's insistence on the need for *both* meanings *and* causes in psychopathology, that, with the renaissance of philosophy of psychiatry in the late twentieth century, a renaissance directly driven in part by the new neurosciences, we find ourselves back where we started, with Jaspers' twin-track psychopathology, a psychopathology, not rejecting science, but seeking to incorporate alongside our increasingly powerful scientific insights into the causes of experience and behaviour, the personal meanings that make psychiatry as a medical discipline a genuinely human science.

References

Fulford, K. W. M., Morris, K. J., Sadler, J. Z., and Stanghellini, G. (ed.) (2003). Past improbable, future possible: the renaissance in philosophy and psychiatry. In *Nature and Narrative: an introduction to the new philosophy of psychiatry*. Oxford: Oxford University Press, pp. 1–41.

Jaspers, K. ([1913] 1963/1997). *Allgemeine Psychopathologie* (4th edn). Berlin: Springer-Verlag; *General Psychopathology* (trans. J. Hoenig and M.W. Hamilton). Chicago: University of Chicago Press. New edition with a Foreword by Paul R. McHugh (1997) Baltimore: The Johns Hopkins University Press.

Parry-Jones, W. (1972). *The Trade in Lunacy*. London: Routledge and Kegan Paul.

CHAPTER 7

A brief history of mental disorder

Chapter contents

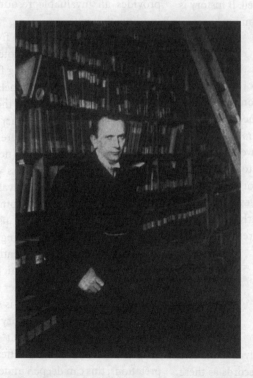

Fig. II.3 Jaspers as a young man in the library of the Department of Psychiatry in the University of Heidelberg.

There are many in psychiatry, and in other mental health disciplines, who see the history of early twentieth century psychiatry, not as a guide to the paradigm shifts we now face, but as a record of psychiatry's paradigms finally reaching a settled state. Those responsible, in particular, for the development of our modern classifications of mental disorders, the ICD and DSM, have often appeared to take this view of our history.

We touched on these classifications at various points in Part I and we will be returning to them in more detail in Part III. As we will see, they have played a vital role in the descriptive groundwork necessary for the application of modern neuroscience to mental disorders, and hence for the changes of paradigm which this is likely to catalyse. However, the architects of these classifications have too often seen themselves not so much as catalysts as crystallizers. They have seen their role as settling once and for all the theoretical tools for shaping our diagnostic concepts. Future researchers, according to this view, will provide new data: but how we organize the data, what indeed counts as data, they take to be largely settled.

This could be right. The history of science itself, though, makes it unlikely, for predictions of the 'end of history' in science have always been falsified, and not least in that hardest of hard sciences, physics. At the end of the nineteenth century, many physicists believed their theoretical paradigms were largely settled—yet within 20 years, they had relativity theory and quantum mechanics! Whether psychiatry will produce its Einstein or Heisenberg, whether we have a twenty-first century Karl Jaspers perhaps already working on his or her PhD, only time will tell. If history is any guide, she or he will have trouble with the examiners!

This chapter and this part of the book

In this chapter, then, we will be taking a whistle-stop tour through a two and a half thousand year history of ideas about mental disorder. This will be by way of preparation for a closer study of Karl Jaspers' work in Chapter 8, and of the main philosophical sources of his psychopathology in Chapters 9 and 10. To understand Jaspers' work on psychopathology, however, we need to understand the problem he was tackling: and to understand Jaspers' problem, we need to understand its historical context. This is why this chapter will be taken up with a few basic facts about the history of psychiatry, focusing particularly on the way mental disorders have been understood at different historical periods.

Session 1 Introduction and overview

Facts and fictions

'Facts' in history, even 'basic facts', are notoriously elusive. The historical record is always incomplete; and such records as there are always have to be interpreted. The difficulties of interpretation, moreover, are compounded for the history of *ideas* by the problems of translation: from one language to another; from one culture to another. And to all these difficulties, when it comes to the history of ideas in *psychiatry*, we have to add the fact that the relevant ideas—rationality, reason, responsibility, and so forth—are themselves complex and difficult to understand.

Few have made a greater individual contribution to assembling the facts, such as they are, of the development of our psychopathological concepts than the Cambridge historian and psychiatrist, German Berrios. As a philosopher as well as historian, few have been as aware as Berrios of the methodological and conceptual pitfalls of work in this area. In our first reading, Berrios sets out some of these issues.

EXERCISE 1   (30 minutes)

Read the extract from:

Berrios, G.E. (1996). Matters historical. *The History of Mental Symptoms. Descriptive psychopathology since the nineteenth century.* Cambridge: Cambridge University Press, p. 7

Link with Reading 7.1

◆ Note the different ways in which some of the founders of modern psychiatry used historical sources.

Together with a companion volume, *History of Clinical Psychiatry: the origin and history of psychiatric disorders* (co-edited with Roy Porter, 1995), Berrios' *The History of Mental Symptoms* provides an invaluable resource for work on the history of psychopathology.

In the introductory section from which the extract linked with Exercise 1 is taken, Berrios notes the wide variety of approaches to psychiatric history, ranging from Haslam, who was interested in 'historical semantics', to Pinel, who regarded history as a record of past failures against which the triumph of 'the modern' should be contrasted. These and other approaches are complementary, illuminating practice in different ways. Yet history, like science, has been 'post-modernised' (not Berrios' term!). In place of the 'Whiggish' march-of-progress view, we now have a more cautious, piecemeal, and perspectival model. Traditionally, the history of medicine has seen itself somewhat like a science, discovering the truth. Current history of psychiatry is understood more on the model of a sculptor, carving out a story. Which model we opt for in the history of psychopathology, Berrios goes on to argue, should be determined by which is 'more suitable to [our] own beliefs and the symptom under study' (p. 11).

If Berrios is right, then, it is small wonder that the history of psychiatry, let alone the history of the concept of mental illness, has been given widely different 'spins' by different authors. This is not in itself a bad thing. If different authors have different interpretations, this can deepen understanding. If the historical record is explained in different ways, this can increase the resources for philosophical and other studies. We will be looking at some aspects of all this later in this session. But it is, none the less, important to be aware of the 'spins'. If history is a guide, historians may guide us in different directions!

The rest of this chapter

With these caveats, we will start with an outline of how psychiatry has developed. This will help us to locate Karl Jaspers in the history of the subject. As we will see, his seminal work on psychopathology in the early years of the twentieth century, rides on the back of

a history, spanning two and a half millennia, of attempts to make sense of madness.

One 'spin' on this history, as a history of ideas, is that it reflects a continuing tension, oscillating sometimes one way and sometimes the other, between moral and natural conceptions of mental disorder. This is illustrated diagrammatically in Figure 7.1. As this shows, the modern debate, outlined in Chapters 2, 4, and 6, between antipsychiatry (moral) and psychiatry (natural), including

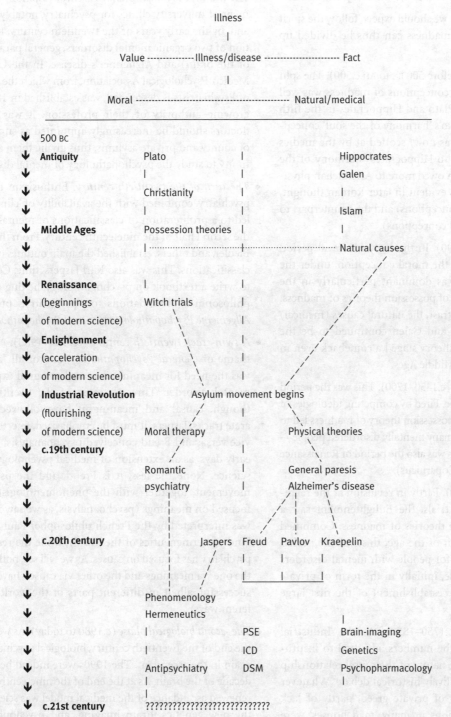

Fig. 7.1 Flow diagram of a conceptual history of mental disorder.

their different 'takes' on the roles of facts and values in the definitions of psychopathological concepts, is but the latest manifestation of this historical tension. Our understanding of mental disorder (or madness) has oscillated between the two extremes over at least two and a half millennia.

We will start with an overview of this history of moral and medical interpretations before considering each of its stages in a little more detail.

A history of mental disorder in twenty minutes

Ideas about mental disorder, as we should expect, follow the spirit of the times. The history of madness can thus be divided up broadly by historical periods.

- *The Classical Period* (from before 500 BC to AD c.500). The split between moral and natural conceptions of madness was well established by the time of Plato and Hippocrates in the fifth and fourth centuries BC. Plato's 'harmony of the soul' conception of mental health was (as now) scoffed at by the medics of the day, who subscribed to Hippocrates' 'harmony of the humours' conception (which owed more to Aristotelian physiology). A similar division is evident in later Roman thought, between the Stoics (moral conceptions) and the counterpart to Hippocrates, Galen (medical conceptions).

- *The Middle Ages* (c.500–1500). In the early Medieval period (also called the Dark Ages) the moral conception, under the influence of Christianity, was dominant particularly in the Western Empire, in the form of possession theories of madness. In Islamic countries, by contrast, the natural causes (medical) conception of Hippocrates and Galen continued to be the dominant theory; and this theory staged a comeback even in western Europe in the later Middle Ages.

- *Renaissance and Reformation* (c.1450–1700). This was the period of the 'witch panics' in Europe. Fired by competing ideologies of Catholic and Protestant, the possession theory of madness led to the torture and execution of many mentally disordered people—and note the paradox that this was also the period of Renaissance science (e.g. Bacon, Galileo, Copernicus).

- *Enlightenment* (c.1700–1800). Partly in revulsion at the religious excesses of the witch trials, the Enlightenment saw a reassertion of natural cause theories of madness. Combined with the humanitarian spirit of the age, this was the period when provision of 'asylum' for people with mental disorders first became widely available, initially in the form of private 'mad houses', later with the establishment of the first large public asylums.

- *The Great Confinement* (c.1750–1850). As the Industrial Revolution gathered pace, the numbers admitted to institutional care rose sharply. The nature of the causal relationship here remains the subject of lively historical debate. Whatever the case, for reasons partly of private greed, partly of lack of public resources, conditions in many 'mad houses' were

appalling. And the fate of those committed was compounded by 'medical' theories that favoured restraint and other punitive treatments, such as ducking and spinning. It was against such abuses that the great reformers at the turn of the nineteenth century (Pinel and Esquirol in France; Samuel Tuke and John Connolly in England) sought to establish more humane regimes based on what came to be called 'moral therapies'.

- *The first biological phase* (c.1850–1910). The nineteenth century, though, was also the century of scientific medical advance; it saw the first localizations of cerebral function, the establishment of university clinics for psychiatry, notably in Germany, and, by the early years of the twentieth century, the identification of two organic mental disorders, general paralysis (syphilis of the brain) and Alzheimer's disease. In the UK, the Royal Medico-Psychological Association, from which the Royal College of Psychiatrists is descended, was established in 1841. With the growing authority of their profession, it was natural that doctors should be increasingly appointed as superintendents of county and private asylums, thus giving them ample opportunity to study the psychopathology of mental disorders.

- *The turn of the twentieth century*. Enthusiasm for biological psychiatry, combined with the availability of 'clinical material', led to a proliferation of classifications of mental disorders in the second half of the nineteenth century. From this, Kraepelin, Bleuler, and others, established the main outlines of our current classifications. This was also Karl Jaspers' time. Commissioned to write a textbook on psychopathology, he dug deep into the philosophical foundations of psychiatry, producing his *Allgemeine Psychopathologie* (*General Psychopathology*) in 1913.

- *A twin-track twentieth century* (c.1900–1980). An important theme of *General Psychopathology*, and of all Jaspers' work, was the need for meaningful as well as causal explanations of mental disorder. Through most of the twentieth century, though, 'causal' and 'meaningful' have followed largely separate tracks. Jaspers, it must be emphasized, rejected Freud, and vice versa; and Freud conceived psychoanalysis, at least in its early days, as an extension of medical psychology and neuroscience. None the less, it is Freud, and the psychoanalytic movement, together with the phenomenologists, who have focused on meanings (psychoanalysis, as we saw in Chapter 4, was interpreted by the French philosopher Paul Ricoeur, as a kind of hermeneutics of the mind), while the rest of medical psychiatry has focused on causes. As we will see, both approaches, the one via meanings and the other via causes, have been hugely successful, albeit in different parts of the world and in different ways.

- *The second biological phase* (c.1980 to today): As we approached the end of the twentieth century, biological psychiatry was once again in the ascendant. The 1990s were indeed heralded as the decade of the brain. As at the end of the nineteenth century, this renewed ascendance of the medical model was science driven—the new genetics, brain imaging, and psychopharmacology were the inspirations for late twentieth century biological psychiatry, just as neuroanatomy, differential histological stains and germ theory were the inspirations for late nineteenth century biological psychiatry.

Such is the 'march' of history, then! But what will follow? What will future histories of psychiatry add retrospectively. For besides intriguing similarities, there are also important differences between the state of psychiatry now and its state at the end of the nineteenth century. We will return to these later. But a key difference is the state of our classifications of mental disorders. At the end of the nineteenth century there was 'diagnostic anarchy'; at the end of the twentieth century we have, at least within medicine, a broadly agreed outline of a classification of mental disorders to serve as the descriptive springboard for the causal theories promised by the new neurosciences.

As already noted, it is to Jaspers (among others) that we owe the psychopathological theories on which these classifications are based. We will return to Jaspers' psychopathology in Chapter 8. First, though, in the remainder of this chapter, we will take a more detailed look at some of the key stages in the development of psychiatry.

Reflection on the session and self-test questions

Write down your own reflections on the materials in this session drawing out any points that are particularly significant for you. Then write brief notes about the following:

1. How far back does the concept of mental illness (broadly understood) go?

2. What is the historical relationship between medical-scientific and moral-humanistic models of 'madness'?

Session 2 The main historical periods

The Classical period

The Greeks had a word for it

Most histories of 'madness' start with the Greeks. Interpreting how such a complex notion was understood over 2000 years ago, raises all the key problems noted above of historical analysis of ideas! But 'madness' was certainly recognized in one form or other in Classical times, it was subject to competing causal theories (including a link with disease), and it had many of its present-day moral and legal connotations.

The American philosopher and psychologist, Daniel Robinson, to whose remarkable history of the insanity defence we return below (Robinson, 1996), points (slightly tongue in cheek) to the earliest record of a successful defence on grounds of madness in Homer's epic poem, the *Iliad*. The warring parties in the Trojan wars having fought each other to a standstill, King Agamemnon

seeks to excuse his original provocative actions, 'It was not I that did it' he says, 'Zeus and Fate, the erinys that walk in darkness struck me mad when we were assembled on the day that I took from Achilles the prize that had been awarded him . . .'. Similarly, in Book IV of the Odyssey, Helen excuses her original abandonment of hearth and home as 'the madness that Aphrodite bestowed when she led me here' (pp. 8–9).

It is with Plato, though, a few centuries later, and at the height of Classical Greek culture, that we find one of the first recognizably modern accounts of mental health. Our next reading is taken from a classic paper on Plato's conception of mental disorder by the Oxford philosopher, Anthony (A.J.P.) Kenny.

EXERCISE 2   (60 minutes)

Read the opening passage from:

Kenny, A.J.P. (1969). Mental health in Plato's *Republic*. *Proceedings of the British Academy* (3.12.1969), pages 229–253

Link with Reading 7.2

Note the strikingly confident assertion with which Kenny opens his article, that 'The concept of mental health was Plato's invention'; however:

1. In which of Plato's books does Kenny identify the first non-metaphysical use of the concept of mental health?

2. What competing' models' were there in Classical Greece?

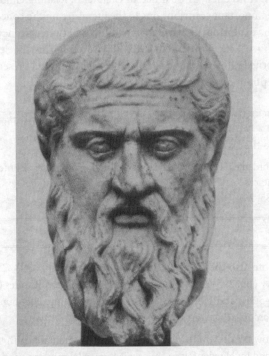

Fig. 7.2 Plato

Like Robinson, Kenny notes many early examples of the use of medical metaphors; but it is with the Plato of *The Republic*, he suggests, that we find for the first time a genuine theory of madness as a sickness or disease of the mind. In the rest of this article, Kenny goes on to describe how the standard 'medical' model of the time (i.e. of Hippocrates and, in later Roman medicine, of Galen) was of a balance or harmony of the elements of the constitution (Kenny notes the Galenic 'wet, hot, dry, cold, sour and sweet', p. 231). Plato, he suggests, applied this model to 'disorders of the soul' (p. 231), identifying, with some variation, three constituents of the soul, reason, appetite, and temper. Reason, aided by temper, rules appetite. There are shades of Freud here, as Kenny notes (p. 238 et seq.). By the start of section V, though, Kenny is clear that Plato, although developing what appears to be a *moral* concept of mental health, is intent on assimilating the moral to a *medical* model. He (Kenny) deplores this attempted assimilation, identifying a similar move underpinning modern attitudes to mental disorder (notably in the Mental Health Act, 1959, the legislation in force at the time in the UK governing issues such as involuntary treatment). Reacting against the assimilation of morals to medicine, as many others have done, Kenny identifies with an overtly medical model: 'In the paradigmatic cases of mental illness (e.g. schizophrenia)', he says, 'organic causes are known or suspected'. Hippocrates and Galen would have approved!

Roman stoicism

Some of the difficulties of translating Classical conceptions into a modern context are illustrated by a debate in *Philosophy, Psychiatry and Psychology* around an article by the Swedish philosopher, Lennart Nordenfelt, on Stoic conceptions of mental health. Nordenfelt, as we noted in Chapter 6, Reading Guide, has made important contributions to the literature on the concept of health, exploring in particular the links between agency and health (see, e.g. Nordenfelt, 1987). However, in this article he is concerned rather with the parallels between Stoic and present day conceptions of mental health.

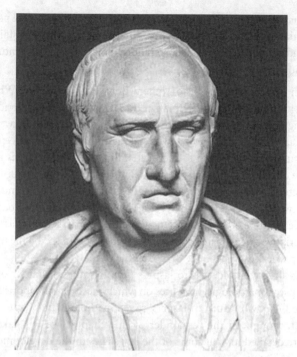

Fig. 7.3 Cicero

In the passage preceding this extract, Nordenfelt describes (p. 286) how Stoic philosophy was 'material, deterministic but at the same time teleological', i.e. in the sense that the course of the world is guided by '*Logos* or *God*...for the good of human beings'. We should thus 'meet every event with a sense of security or independence'. This 'apatheia' is the basis of what Nordenfelt claims is a Stoic theory of mental health (p. 286). This theory, as he spells out in this extract, can be identified as being developed into a Stoic classification of mental disorders not entirely unlike our modern classifications. He emphasizes that the analogy should not be pushed too far: 'apatheia' itself, at the heart of Stoic philosophy, has no obvious parallel in modern mental health; and we should certainly not want to go as far as Cicero in regarding extremes of emotion as necessarily disordered! But as to the practical implications of the theory, as to what it implies for how we should *achieve* mental health, there are clear parallels, he concludes later in the paper, with modern cognitive-behavioural approaches. Again, the analogy should not be pressed too far. But the 'nub' of Nordenfelt's paper is the essentially modern point that values, 'ideas about the good and virtuous man', are inextricably intertwined with ideas about mental health (p. 290).

The commentators on Nordenfelt's challenging claims represented a range of very different views. At one extreme, Rosamund Rhodes (1997), a Classical scholar and bioethicist working at The Mount Sinai Hospital, New York, argued for a reading of Stoic philosophy different from Nordenfelt's. At the other extreme, Ivy Blackburn (1997), also a Classical scholar but now a Professor of Clinical Psychology, largely endorsed Nordenfelt's reading, in particular what she called the 'fudge' of mental health and virtue. Stan Leavy (1997), a physician, took from all this, the necessity, the *human* necessity, of retaining some notion of radical freedom, of the reality of choice. Emilio Mordini (1997), a psychiatrist and psychoanalyst (and a Classical scholar) working in Rome, also largely endorsed Nordenfelt's reading; but, locating Stoic philosophy firmly in its cultural and historical context, he noted the extent to which modern philosophy and neuroscience are undermining the traditional separation of reason and emotion.

Reactions to the paper and the ensuing discussion varied widely! Of course, there can be no final answer as to whether Nordenfelt is right or not. In the first place, scholars of equal eminence may 'read' the Stoics differently (Rhodes, for example, clearly read them differently from Nordenfelt and Blackburn). But these different readings are in different ways enlightening. These papers thus illustrate the richness of resources offered by Classical attempts to understand mental distress and disorder. We may end up either for or against a particular point of view, or in some more complex mixture of points for and against, or with a distinct view of our own. The message, though, is in what we learn from the debate itself.

The Middle Ages and beyond

Medieval madness

In the early Middle Ages, as we noted above, attitudes to the insane were very different in the Islamic and (Western) Christian worlds. The Islamic world, influenced by the medical and physiological works of Hippocrates and Galen, continued to regard madness as largely a product of brain disease. In the Christian world, although there were many who subscribed to 'brain' theories, the dominant aetiological theory was of possession by demons. It was this theory that, in the late Middle Ages, as the Church sought increasingly desperately to eradicate heresy, led to the mentally ill sometimes being tried as witches.

The gradual dominance of Christian (moral) conceptions of madness over late Roman (natural causes) theories is graphically charted by Daniel Robinson in his *Wild Beasts and Idle Humours* (from which we quoted above).

EXERCISE 4 (20 minutes)

Read the extract from:

Robinson, D. (1996). Immortal souls, mortal cities. Chapter 2 in *Wild Beasts and Idle Humours: the insanity defense from antiquity to the present*. Cambridge, MA: Harvard University Press, pp. 55–56

Link with Reading 7.4

Robinson summarizes in this section how Christian notions of sin and possession came to overlay and largely displace Classical natural-causes notions of mental disorder. However,

witch trials were not to become widespread until a later period.

♦ Why do you think this was?

♦ Why the delay?

On a separate point, do you see any particular advantages for the history of ideas in studying legal history?

Robinson's book is a scholarly but highly readable history of the insanity defence. He notes in the 'Introduction' (p. 2) that a legal history of insanity has the great advantage for the 'history of ideas' that the law does not have the luxury of idle speculation, but has to dispose of real cases. The history of legal insanity thus provides a valuable 'probe' to the *zeitgeist* on mental disorders of different periods. There is a nice link here, then, with J. L. Austin's comments on the merits of legal cases as a resource for ordinary language philosophy (see especially Chapter 4).

In the section of his book from which this extract is taken, Robinson describes how, despite the rise of Christian ideology, the Middle Ages were not a time of particular persecution of the 'mad'. True, like physical diseases, madness was believed at this time to be often the result of possession. But this was not in itself a matter for persecution. The seeds of later persecution were there, of course; but in the Middle Ages, at least in western Europe, the prevailing ideology was too secure to fear deviance. As we will see shortly it was only with the Reformation that it became increasingly necessary to persecute 'heretics'.

In the late Medieval period, there was a strong revival of Aristotelian naturalistic doctrines. St Thomas Aquinas, for example, seems to have regarded at least many forms of insanity as natural in origin; he recognized different kinds of mental disorder (distinguishing congenital and non-congenital forms, for example); and appears to have regarded the insane as irrational and hence as lacking the capacity for sin. The law, similarly, while seeking to protect society, provided for the insane to be released into the care of their family once they were no longer considered dangerous. There was also a degree of institutional care: a notable example was the hospice established by the Priory of St Mary of Bethlehem in 1403 specifically for the insane. It started with six male patients, and remains with us today in the form of the Maudsley and Bethlem Hospitals in South London. (The original name 'Bethlehem' was shortened to 'Bethlem' from which the corruption 'Bedlam' is derived.) In this period, then, while demon-possession remained a popular 'folk' theory, the official doctrines of Church and State were largely humanistic.

Satan and Renaissance science

The Renaissance period right through to the end of the eighteenth century, was marked by a tension between scientific and satanic explanations of mental disorder. It is important to note the paradox that, even as natural science was becoming ever more successful, demonology, witch-hunts, and the torture and execution of many mentally ill people as witches, reached epidemic proportions.

The cultural environment that fostered the witch trials was the long-running battle between Catholic and Protestant. The Reformation forced the Catholic Church into ever more frenzied attempts to root out heresy. The Counter-Reformation prompted the Protestants to equally frenzied attempts to demonstrate that God was with them. Witches were an easy target for both; and people with severe mental illness, whose psychopathology of course often included delusions of guilt, of satanic possession, and so on, were a ready source of 'witches'. But natural science and medicine were often partners in the witch trials, offering 'expert' evidence, including specific signs such as a third nipple and pain-insensitive areas.

The next reading (see Exercise 5), which is from a major 'text-book' for witch-prickers of the day, the notorious *Malleus Maleficarum* (Kramer and Sprenger, 1996), shows just how easy it was for science to end up as a partner to religion in this way.

EXERCISE 5   (45 minutes)

Read the three extracts from:

Kramer, H and Sprenger, J. (1996). Malleus Maleficarum (The Witch Hammer). Published as *Malleus Maleficarum: the Classic Study of Witchcraft*, translated with an introduction, bibliography, and notes, by Montague Summers. London: Bracken Books, pp. 211, 213, and 227

Link with Reading 7.5

Heinrich Kramer and James Sprenger were two Dominican monks working as Inquisitors in northern Germany in the late fifteenth century. Their book is a detailed and scholarly work, adamant in its opposition to witchcraft, but spelling out meticulous rules of procedure aimed at avoiding the innocent being falsely convicted.

♦ How successful do you think Kramer and Sprenger were in this, however?

♦ As you read the extracts, identify the 'proofs' they offer of witchcraft, and note any modern parallels to the procedures they advocate.

Published with a preface in the form of a Papal Bull from Innocent VIII (1484), the *Malleus Maleficarum* rapidly became the most widely read and respected authority on witchcraft. It is impressive in its detailed treatment of every aspect of the identification, prosecution, and disposal of suspects.

From our perspective, the 'proofs' it offers may seem naïve. But if you believe in witchcraft, then the 'proofs' are little different in form from those offered in modern contexts. Thus, in the first extract (p. 211) they set out what in a modern textbook of medicine we would call the 'history of the presenting complaint'. In the second extract (p. 213), they note that a 'diagnosis' (not their word) should be based on: (1) the bad reputation of the accused;

(2) evidence of the 'fact'; and (3) the words of witnesses. Well, as to (1), it is still true that we say 'give a dog a bad name...', and 'no smoke without fire'. As to (2), evidence of the fact is a Humean 'constant conjunction' theory of causality—the accused touched a child, and it fell sick; the accused was seen looking at her neighbour's cows, and the milk yield fell; she was in the field when the tempest blew up, etc. And as to (3), about witnesses, while Kramer and Sprenger are clear about the danger of false witness, if sufficient 'good men and true' give evidence, then it must be so—an early, and still persisting emphasis on operationalism in psychopathological diagnosis.

There are even objective signs of witchcraft. On p. 227, for example, in the third extract, we find precise details of how to elicit the physical sign of 'inability to shed tears'. The sign of inability to shed tears, moreover, is, in the terms of modern scientific classifications, both reliable (shown by 'worthy men of old and our own experience') and has construct validity (it is caused by the Devil's preventing penitential tears). Of course, as skilled examiners we must beware of malingering (she may smear her face with spittle) and false positives (she may deceive us with her witchery into seeing tears). But these risks can be minimized by repeated examination in different ways (p. 213, also pp. 230–231), and, later in this section, by taking sensible precautions such as avoiding her glance (p. 228), and by following correct procedure (not allowing her to return to her room after she has been apprehended, p. 215). All very 'modern', then, the last in particular strongly reminiscent of 'child abuse' procedures. And if we doubt the effectiveness of all these diagnostic procedures, well Kramer and Sprenger go on to offer us ample supporting case histories (e.g. p. 229).

Values and science

The point of drawing these parallels is not to suggest that demonology is on a par with biology. Many have claimed that *all* knowledge is relative: as we will see in Part III, as a modern form of radical scepticism, this (self-defeating) assertion has been highly influential in some quarters in recent philosophy of science. But the point for us, here, is that science itself, far from guaranteeing objectivity, may give authority to current bias and prejudice.

EXERCISE 6   (20 minutes)

♦ Does all this remind you of anything in the recent history of the abuse of psychiatry?

♦ Can you think of an example of a situation in which a similar conjunction of ideology and science led to grossly abusive uses of medical psychiatry?

As you think about this, read a final extract from the *Malleus Maleficarum*:

Kramer, H and Sprenger, J. (1996). Malleus Maleficarum (The Witch Hammer). Published as Malleus Maleficarum: *the*

Classic Study of Witchcraft, translated with an introduction, bibliography, and notes, by Montague Summers. London: Bracken Books, pp. 1–3

Link with Reading 7.6

In this extract (pp. 1–3) of the *Malleus Maleficarum*, Kramer and Sprenger set out the theoretical foundations on which their treatment of witchcraft is built. The 'bias and prejudice' is clear. They recite alternative theories, current at the time, notably that 'there is no such thing as magic, that it only exists in the imagination…', but they roundly reject such theories as heretical: they are, they say, contrary to 'the authority of the Holy Scripture', and 'the true faith'. Of course, they continue, it is true that magic is sometimes 'merely in the imagination'. But given the overwhelming authority of the Scripture, the Saints, the Canons, and so on, 'those who suppose that *all* the effects of witchcraft are mere illusion and imagination are very greatly deceived' (p. 3, emphasis added).

The driving force, then, behind everything that follows in the *Malleus Maleficarum*, is dogmatic religious ideology. The witch trials of this period thus had the same ingredients as, in recent history, the institutionalized abuse of psychiatry in the final years of the former USSR. We return to this in Part IV (Chapter 18). There are many differences, of course. But in both cases, as we will see, the dominant power group (the communists in the USSR, the Catholics or Protestants in Reformation Europe) needed some way of reinforcing their own value system and beliefs. In both cases, they sought the authority of science to support their persecution of dissenters (in Reformation Europe, medical experts 'proved' that dissenters were witches; in the Soviet Union, they 'proved' that dissenters were insane). In both cases, then, science was harnessed to a value system that made a virtue of suppressing dissent.

We should not be too ready to scoff at Kramer and Sprenger, however. As we will see in Chapter 11, recent work in the history and philosophy of science has shown the extent to which science remains authority led, in its overall theories, and in the extent to which aberrant experimental results are interpreted to fit those theories. There is not an argument for radical scepticism. As the Italian historian and philosopher of science, Paolo Rossi, has argued, the achievements of the Renaissance, '… logical rigour, experimental control, the public character of results and methods…' were hard won at the time and, even today, have to be continually defended (Rossi, 2003, p. 263). Science as such is no sinecure against bias and the *vox populae*!

The Great Confinement

By the end of the seventeenth century, naturalistic theories of madness had once again become the dominant paradigm, science had largely triumphed over Satan, and a more humanistic

approach to the care of people with mental disorders began to emerge. Sporadic public provision had been available since the Middle Ages. But parishes were now made responsible for their mentally disordered members. They responded to this by 'boarding' them out. A large number of private 'madhouses' were thus established, marking the start of what Michel Foucault (1989) called 'the great confinement'. Foucault based his view of the history of this period on the Hôpital Général in Paris. But large public asylums only became widespread in the UK during the nineteenth century, notably after the Lunatics Act of 1845 made it compulsory for every county to establish such institutions. All the same, it is true that there was a progressive shift from 'community care' to confinement; and that the number of people confined rose dramatically through the eighteenth and into the nineteenth centuries.

Many 'madhouses', private and public, sought to offer some form of treatment within a humane environment. Most had either retained physicians or physician-superintendents. Treatment, however, usually took the form of restraint, often with shackles or straightjackets, combined with punitive procedures such as ducking. There were, moreover, many unscrupulous profiteers in the 'trade in madness', a trade made the more profitable by the fact that resources rapidly became wholly inadequate to the rising tide of new admissions. There were also, however, many who stood for a more humanitarian approach. By the end of the century, a Quaker, William Tuke, had established The Retreat at York in England, offering 'moral therapy' based on a homely environment; and in Paris, Phillipe Pinel, and his pupil Jean Etienne Dominique Esquirol, had 'thrown away the chains' of the patients in the Salpêtrière and Bicêtre Hospitals.

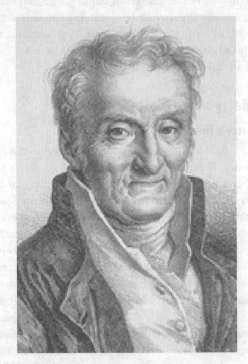

Fig. 7.4 Philippe Pinel

It is difficult to get a balanced view of the treatment of those with mental disorders over this period. The common perception is famously reflected in the contemporary painting by the eighteenth century Dutch—English painter (and cartoonist), Hogarth, called, simply, 'Bedlam'. Modern scholarship has shown, however, that, although abuses were common enough, conditions in private institutions were more often humane by the standards of the day; and the public asylum movement was launched in a spirit of genuine therapeutic optimism. Such misportrayals of 'madness' are common today. Hogarth's picture is an eighteenth century counterpart of Ken Kesey's famous book (and later a film) *One Flew over the Cuckoo's Nest* (1963)!

Complementary approaches to the social history of madness over this period, relevant to contemporary psychiatry, are illustrated by Roy Porter's, *A Social History of Madness* (1987), and William Parry-Jones's *The Trade in Lunacy* (1972). Roy Porter was Professor of History of Medicine at the Wellcome Institute in London. William Parry-Jones was a psychiatrist who won the Year Prize at Cambridge for an MD in the history of medicine on which his book is based. Both explore madness in the eighteenth century. Porter employs much narrative material from accounts of contemporary 'survivors'. Parry-Jones draws particularly on detailed historical analyses of contemporary statistical and other records. Both, in different ways, give us a picture that is far from the 'Hogarthian Bedlam'. Yet both have important messages from the period for modern psychiatry: the dangers of 'graft' and false confinement; the difficult yet crucial balance between care and control; the importance of adequate checks and balances external to the interests of professionals, however well intentioned; the failure of reforms if they are inadequately resourced, and so on.

By the middle of the nineteenth century, then, large numbers of mentally ill patients had been confined mainly under the supervision of medical superintendents. With scientific medical knowledge advancing rapidly, the stage was thus set for the emergence of a recognizably medical psychiatry.

Psychiatry's two biological phases

Psychiatry's first biological phase

Although 'medical' theories of insanity had been around since Hippocrates, it is only in the second half of the nineteenth century, and notably in Germany, that modern causal theories start to appear. There had been important work in descriptive psychopathology in France in the first half of the century. However, the father of biological psychiatry is generally identified as William Griesinger, who, in the 1860s from his position as Professor of Psychiatry at the University of Berlin, coined the uncompromising aphorism that 'Mental illness is cerebral illness' ('Geisteskrankheiten sind Gehirnkrankheiten'—quoted by Jaspers *Allgemeine Psychopathology*, p. 382; *General Psychopathologie*, p. 459).

This was a period of optimistic expansion. Pioneers were opening university clinics of psychiatry in Germany for the first time and appointing professors. The race was on to find the brain abnormalities that lay at the basis of the major psychoses. There were many successes, although more in the field of neurology than psychiatry. Thus, Carl Wernicke, working in Vienna and Berlin, demonstrated an association between patients who could not understand speech and an abnormality in the posterior temporal lobe of the brain. This is still called Wernicke's area. In France, Paul Broca found an association between patients who could understand what was said to them but could not express themselves, and an abnormality in the posterior frontal lobe. This is still called Broca's area.

Next to Griesinger, Theodor Meynert, Professor of Psychiatry in Vienna, was perhaps the most famous representative of psychiatry's first biological phase. Meynert was to be a tutor to Sigmund Freud (he was also a chronic alcoholic). Meynert has no lasting findings to his credit but he did establish the importance of neuro-histology for research into the major psychoses. Meanwhile, in the 1880s, Paul Flechsig, in Leipzig, was creating a map of brain areas responsible for different psychological functions, and Eduard Hitzig, in Halle, was demonstrating that the brain responds to electrical stimulation.

The 'action', then, in the late nineteenth century, was mainly in neurology, which at the time was not sharply distinct from psychiatry. Two disorders, however, were to emerge from this period that are of particular importance for psychiatry—Alzheimer's disease and general paralysis.

Mental illness and brain disorder

We owe the identification of these two disorders to Alois Alzheimer and Franz Nissl. They were great friends. Alzheimer was working in Frankfurt and Nissl in Heidelberg (where he was to become Jaspers' professor). Nissl had developed stains that allowed nerve cell structures to be seen. Together, Alzheimer and Nissl worked on brain histology. Alzheimer described the brain changes in the disease, mostly of senility, which has come to bear his name, and, together, they described the brain changes in general paralysis, a disease that had been rife since the major wars in Europe.

There had been enormous speculation about the cause of general paralysis and whether it had its origins in earlier syphilitic infection. Henry Maudsley, who was later to give his name to the modern descendant of the 'Bedlam' hospital (the Maudsley and Bethlem Hospital in London), believed it was not syphilitic, but events were to prove him wrong. Alzheimer and Nissl showed that general paralysis had a different brain histology to Alzheimer's disease. Then in 1906, Wasserman invented the test that bears his name and showed that patients suffering from general paralysis tested positive for syphilis. Finally, in 1913 Noguchi and Moore demonstrated the existence of *Treponema pallidum* (the bacillus responsible for syphilis) in brain tissue. This was a world-changing event. For the first time, a specific psychiatric disease had been shown to have a specific neuropathological cause. The search for the specific brain causes of the major psychoses was reinvigorated and continues to this day, though with, as yet, little more to show!

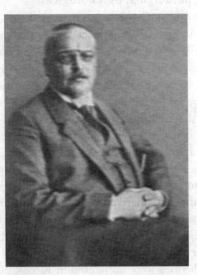

Fig. 7.5 Alois Alzheimer

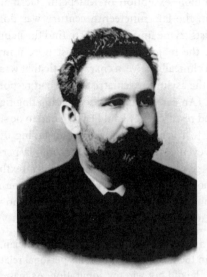

Fig. 7.6 Emil Kraepelin

It is important for our understanding of contemporary psychiatry to note that even in psychiatry's first biological phase, 'moral' theories of madness continued to be influential. This was notably so even in Germany, with the 'Romantic Psychiatry' movement. Recent scholarship, moreover, has shown the extent to which Griesinger himself, the 'father' of biological psychiatry, had a sophisticated understanding of the complexities involved in a genuinely biological psychiatry.

This is vividly illustrated by the philosopher and German scholar Katherine Arens' article in *Philosophy, Psychiatry, & Psychology* on *Wilhelm Griesinger* (1996, 147–164), and the commentary by North American philosopher and psychologist, Aaron Mishara (1996, pp. 165–168). Arens' article gives a sense of the excitement of the dramatic 'new wave' of biological thinking in German psychiatry in the second half of the nineteenth century. It is also an example of how careful scholarship, equipped with philosophical and historical skills, can help us to understand the work of key historical figures in a way which is highly relevant to contemporary problems. It is crucial, in giving balance to the current biological approach to psychiatry, to recognize that its own heroes were acutely aware of the limitations, as well as the strengths, of a brain-based approach to mental disorder. Mishara effectively underscores this point by relating Griesinger's thinking directly to the currently renewed interest in hermeneutics and the importance of phenomenology as a partner to neuroscience in the new biology of psychiatry.

Kraepelin and psychiatric classification

Consistently with the proliferation of theories of the causes of mental disorder in the second half of the nineteenth century, there was a proliferation of classifications. As R.E. Kendell put it in his *The Role*

of Diagnosis in Psychiatry (1975), this was a period when every professor of psychiatry had his own system. It was Emil Kraepelin, a gifted physician and scientist, who, through a series of editions of his *Lehrbuch* (textbook (1915)), started to bring order out of chaos.

Kraepelin arrived in Heidelberg in 1890 and set about collecting around him a formidable range of the major figures in neuropsychiatry of the time, including his friend Nissl (in 1895). Kraepelin had earlier studied brain histology under Paul Flechsig in Leipzig. But he had an eye problem and had difficulty with microscopes. Not surprisingly, perhaps, he got on badly with Flechsig and left. (There is a story that he was sacked.) His career was rescued by the eminent experimental psychologist, Wilhelm Wundt, founder of the first psychological laboratory and the first journal of experimental psychology. Wundt was attempting to build an experimental psychology on the paradigm of the natural sciences—an experimental introspectionism—and Kraepelin was to carry over what he had learned from Wundt into psychiatry.

It was in part because of his problems with microscopes that Kraepelin focussed on clinical research. He kept meticulous records (in the form of cards) on the symptomatology and clinical course of his patients. It was this careful clinical work that came to fruition in his *Lehrbuch*. In the face of the neuroresearch around him, Kraepelin made major advances in the clinical description of psychiatric disorders. His work was not without its problems. Many of the cases he had diagnosed clinically as general paralysis proved not to have syphilis. But he gave us the basis of the psychiatric classification that is still in use today—in particular, the distinction between dementia praecox and manic depressive illness. (The term 'dementia praecox' was changed to 'schizophrenia' by Eugen Bleuler in 1912.)

Patients, brains, and persons

With the notable exception of Kraepelin, German academic psychiatry in the late nineteenth century was dominated by brain scientists trying unsuccessfully to find the neuropathological basis of the major psychoses. Most were uninterested in patients and clinically naïve, a characteristic that was very much resented by the asylum psychiatrists who had responsibility for the patients. (An early round in the ongoing dog fight between clinicians and researchers!) Paul Flechsig had to be sent away on a sabbatical to learn psychiatry prior to taking up his chair. Franz Nissl, even at the time he had become Jaspers' professor in Heidelberg, was said to carry Kraepelin's textbook in his white coat pocket for quick reference on ward rounds! One of Meynert's junior physicians, Arnold Schitzler (who was later to become a playwright), wrote of him:

> He was a great scholar, a splendid diagnostician, but as a physician in the narrower sense, in his personal relations with patients, … he did not win my admiration. As masterful as he may have been in the face of disease, in front of the sick person his behaviour often seemed to me cool, uncertain, if not indeed anxious. Quoted in Shorter (1997, p. 77)

Karl Jaspers and biological psychiatry

It was in this atmosphere of reliance on brain science, that Karl Jaspers began his work. He started as a junior psychiatrist in Nissl's department in Heidelberg in 1908. This was a time of therapeutic pessimism. Despite the rapid advances in neuropathology, very little in the way of treatment was available. All the clinician could do was await spontaneous improvement or not. In 1911, Jaspers was commissioned by Nissl to write a textbook of psychopathology. The first edition of *Allgemeine Psychopathologie* (*General Psychopathology*) appeared in 1913. Jaspers intended this as a methodological and philosophical overview of the subject, examining the nature and possibility of knowledge in psychiatry. Jaspers recognized the importance of natural scientific techniques in psychopathology. He was well aware of Kraepelin's system of classification, of the neuropathological advances in Alzheimer's disease, and of the recently demonstrated syphilitic aetiology of general paralysis. However, he considered that the passion for brain research had gone too far: 'These anatomical constructions, however, became quite fantastic (e.g. Meynert, Wernicke) and have rightly been called "Brain Mythologies" (Jaspers, [1913] 1963/1997 *General Psychopathology*, p. 18)'.

As we will see in more detail in Chapter 8, Jaspers thus came to emphasize the need for meaningful as well as causal explanations in psychiatry. In medical psychiatry, it is the 'causal' side of his work that has been most influential as his psychopathology has come to form the basis of modern 'scientific' approaches to psychiatric diagnosis. But in the meantime, even as Jaspers was developing his psychopathology, competitors to biological psychiatry were already emerging.

Competing paradigms: psychological

By the late 1920s, psychiatry's first biological phase was drawing to a close, not least because of the poverty of findings. The neuropathological causes of the major psychoses had not been found. The field, therefore, was clear for alternative theories.

One such theory, building on earlier associationist psychologies, was based on the Russian psychologist, Ivan P. Pavlov's, concept of the conditioned reflex. Pavlov, as is well known, developed a detailed 'learning theory' based on the observation (familiar to animal trainers) that dogs could be conditioned to salivate to the sound of a bell ringing by associating it with food. (Salivating to the food is an unconditioned reflex, salivating to the bell is the conditioned reflex.) Among other important findings, Pavlov showed that neurotic behaviour could be induced in his dogs if they were exposed to incompatible stimuli (e.g. pain and food), or to inconsistent conditioning.

Pavlov's theories were influential in Russia; other forms of 'learning theory' were developed later in the century (notably by J.B. Watson and B.F. Skinner in the USA); and learning theory approaches (though not specifically Pavlovian approaches) to treating some forms of mental disorder have become highly influential and important in modern psychiatry and clinical psychology (see, e.g. Hawton *et al.*, 1989). Over much of this century, though, even more influential has been psychoanalysis, developed originally by the Austrian neurologist, Sigmund Freud.

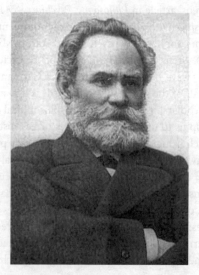

Fig. 7.7 Ivan Pavlov

Freud and the psychoanalytic movement

Freud, although trained as a neuroscientist, was impressed by the therapeutic power of suggestion, notably in Charcot's work on hysteria at the Salpêtrière in Paris; and by Pierre Janet's demonstration of the recovery of lost traumatic memories. This inspired his central (clinical) insight that aberrant experience and behaviour could be an expression of conflicting mental contents (wishes, desires, beliefs, etc.) of which we are unaware (i.e. they are unconscious). Psychoanalysis split early on into a number of movements, Jungian, Adlerian, etc. This has not been to the credit of psychoanalysis, or, indeed, to psychiatry. In the public image, and perhaps in reality, conflicting, rather than competing, paradigms have been characteristic of twentieth century psychiatry.

Psychoanalysis became (and has remained) highly influential in France. But it was in the USA that it reached its zenith. Paradoxically, a major factor in the promotion of psychoanalysis was the rise to power of the Nazis in Germany in the 1930s. The antisemitism of the regime forced the emigration of Freud and his disciples, almost all of whom were Jewish—Freud to London and most of the rest to the USA. Even before this, psychoanalysis had found favour with the private practice/office-based psychiatry of the time in the USA. Many psychoanalysts, including Jung, Ferenzi, Jones, and Freud himself, had visited the USA to give lectures. The first psychoanalytic society was founded by Henry Brill in New York in 1911. The German psychoanalysts moving to the USA included some very 'big names'—Franz Alexander to Chicago, Sando Rado to New York, and Otto

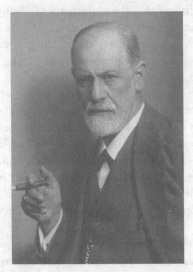

Fig. 7.8 Sigmund Freud

Fenichel to Los Angeles. The influx created some notable linguistic problems. In a lecture at the Menninger Clinic, Fenichel wanted to talk about 'penis envy', but was having problems with the translation. Fenichel tried 'penis envoy' and another émigré suggested 'penis ivy' (reported by Shorter, 1997, p. 167).

Psychoanalysis has had a rather chequered relationship with medicine. In the UK, the two disciplines have developed rather separately. In the States, at least until recently, they were closely related. By 1938, the American Psychoanalytic Association dictated that all candidates for a training analysis must have completed at least 1 year of residency in psychiatry. By the early 1940s, American psychiatry was firmly tied to psychoanalysis and vice versa. Psychoanalysis in the USA boomed until the early 1980s, since when it has gone into steep decline with the rise of a new phase of biological psychiatry. Current views on the status of psychoanalysis are sharply divided. As we will see in Chapter 11, many doubt its scientific credentials. Jaspers, for one, firmly rejected it. He considered psychoanalysis to be a perversion of his method of understanding (*Verstehen*): 'In this way within the confines of psychopathology there grew a methodological comprehension of something which had always been present, but which was fading out of existence and which appeared in striking reverse, "through the looking-glass" as it were in Freud's psychoanalysis—a misunderstanding of itself.' (Jaspers, [1913] 1997, *General Psychopathology*, p. 302).

The second biological phase

The first biological phase was founded on brain pathology, reflecting Griesinger's aphorism 'mental illnesses are brain illnesses'. The second biological phase, although now building on genetics and brain-imaging techniques, started with psychopharmacology and the move from neuroanatomy to neurochemistry as the likely locus of abnormality in the major psychoses.

Modern psychopharmacology of the major psychoses began in the 1950s with the development of such drugs as lithium for hypomania, chlorpromazine for schizophrenia and imipramine for depression. We now know some of the actions of these drugs in the brain. The inference is usually drawn that if a drug acts on a particular system then there must have been something wrong with that system to make the patient ill. Take schizophrenia. The drugs that are effective in schizophrenia all block the neurotransmitter dopamine (a neurotransmitter is a chemical that transmits signals between nerve cells). Therefore, many conclude, there must be an overactivity of brain dopamine in schizophrenia. As an inference, of course, this is not strictly justified. (We looked at inferences of different kinds in Chapter 5.) Moreover, despite considerable effort, the requisite overactivity has not been identified. But as a *hypothesis*, the dopamine theory is entirely reasonable. And it has been the power of the new drugs to alter experience and behaviour, which has kick-started the new wave of biological psychiatry as we head into the twenty-first century.

Reflection on the session and self-test questions

Write down your own reflections on the materials in this session drawing out any points that are particularly significant for you. Then write brief notes about the following:

1. Who represented moral and natural conceptions of madness, respectively, in classical Greek and Roman thought?

2. In which cultures were moral and natural conceptions of madness, respectively, dominant in the early Mediaeval period?

3. With what attitudes to madness were the Renaissance and Reformation associated?

4. How did things change in the Enlightenment?

5. What was the Great Confinement? When did it happen?

6. What was Karl Jaspers' work as a philosopher-psychiatrist a response to?

7. How is Jaspers' work similar to recent developments in the philosophy of psychiatry?

Conclusions: possible futures

The lesson(s) of history

In this chapter, we have looked at a variety of readings, which, although broadly in the area of the history of psychiatry, are very different in nature, form, and style. Each of these illuminates, in different ways, our understanding of psychiatry, and in particular of the theoretical and practical difficulties surrounding the concept of mental illness. But is there an overall direction, an overall trend in this history, pointing us unequivocally to a particular future?

EXERCISE 7   (30 minutes)

In this final exercise, we look at two 'overviews' of the history of psychiatry:

1. A brief extract from the epilogue to a now classic study:

   Zilboorg, G. and Henry, G.W. (1941). The second psychiatric revolution. In *A History of Medical Psychology*. London: George Allen and Unwin, (Extract p. 522–523.)

2. A brief extract from the concluding pages of:

   Shorter, E. (1997). *A History of Psychiatry: from the era of the asylum to the age of prozac.* New York: John Wiley and Sons. (Extract p. 325.)

Link with Readings 7.7 and 7.8

♦ What do you see as the main differences between these two overviews of the history of psychiatry?

Note: the 'Brill' referred to in the first reading is A.A. Brill, one of Freud's pupils who introduced psychoanalysis to America.

These two readings represent two very different overviews of the history of psychiatry. With Zilboorg and Henry, writing in the 1940s, when psychoanalysis was 'all the rage', at least in America and France, Freud was perceived as having rescued a genuinely human psychiatry from the one-sided brain-based approaches of the turn of the twentieth century. By the 1990s, however, Shorter sees the psychoanalytic movement as little more than a distraction from the serious business of biological psychiatry.

Both perspectives are illuminating. Zilboorg and Henry help us to see, especially in the current wave of anti-Freudianism, the clinical importance of the psychoanalytic movement. Shorter gives us marvellous insights into the subversion of biological psychiatry by greed and graft! Neither book, moreover, is naïve as to the perspectives of history: Zilboorg and Henry anticipate that attitudes to Freud may change; Shorter explicitly acknowledges the difficulties of historical interpretation. But both are *basically* convinced that their overview is right. Shorter adopts an engaging contrast between postmodern historians of psychiatry and himself: '*they*' (the postmodernists) are 'revisionists', *he* is a 'neoapologist'! (p. ix).

So, as noted in the introduction to this part of the book, we need to be cautious in projecting forward from history. History does have lessons for us, as we have seen. But, to adapt a familiar aphorism, history never *quite* repeats itself. There are always differences as well as similarities between historical periods, and the differences can be important.

Biologies old and new

One difference between the first biological phase and the second, is the importance, today, of psychological and social methods of treatment alongside physical. *Clinical* psychiatry is nowadays openly eclectic: it is the 'biopsychosocial' approach which is *de rigeur* (McHugh and Slavney, 1983).

A second difference is the importance of descriptive psychopathology. Like general medicine, developments in the neurosciences relevant to psychiatry are building on careful clinical observation of the actual phenomena of mental disorders. As we have seen, we owe the broad outlines of our classification of mental disorders to the careful work of Kraepelin and others at the turn of the twentieth century. But the descriptive psychopathology from which modern descendants of these classifications are constructed, we owe mainly to Karl Jaspers. It is to a more detailed study of Jaspers, then, and the conceptual structure of his descriptive psychopathology, that we turn in the next chapter, chapter 8.

A third difference, and one to which we owe the very existence of this book, is the extent of developments in the philosophy of psychiatry. In psychiatry's first biological phase, as we will see, Karl Jaspers, as a philosopher and psychiatrist, was a central but somewhat isolated figure. In psychiatry's second biological phase, by contrast, as Fulford *et al.* (2003) describe, a whole discipline of philosophy and psychiatry has sprung up around the world. The 1990s was indeed the decade of the brain. But it was also the decade of the mind (Fulford *et al.*, 2003). Exploring, therefore, as we will in the remaining chapters of this part, the details of Jaspers' psychopathology (chapter 8), and its intellectual origins respectively in phenomenology (chapter 9) and the *methodenstreit* (chapter 10), will help to define the new challenges for psychopathology today, a psychopathology that is informed, equally, by the empirical findings of the new neurosciences and by the conceptual insights of the new philosophy of psychiatry.

Reading guide

The history of psychiatry and psychopathology

Although until recently relatively neglected by historians of medicine, the history of psychiatry is now an actively developing discipline.

Outlines of the history of psychiatry will be found in most larger psychiatric textbooks. W.F. Bynam's (1983) chapter, for example, 'Psychiatry in its historical context', offers a highly readable detailed overview. A classic text is G. Zilboorg and G.W. Henry (1941) *A History of Medical Psychology*. Recent years have seen an abundance of new histories. Some of these, like E. Shorter's (1997) *A History of Psychiatry* have a particular story to tell.

Excellent introductions to the histories of all the main areas of psychopathology, are G.E. Berrios' (1996) *The History of Mental Symptoms*, and G.E. Berrios and R. Porter (ed.) (1995) *A History of Clinical Psychiatry*. Beer's (1996) *The Dichotomies* charts the shift in our understanding of psychosis from mental disorder to disease concept.

Perhaps the most acute historian of twentieth century psychiatry is the French historian and psychiatrist, George Lanteri-Laura (eg 1998). The history of British psychiatry has been surveyed in Richard Hunter and Ida McAlpine's (1963) *Three Hundred Years of Psychiatry: 1535–1860*; and Berrios and Freeman's (ed.) (1991) *150 Years of British Psychiatry: 1841–1991*.

The American psychiatrist and historian, Jerome Kroll (1995), has explored the issues raised by historical work on concepts of disorder in a review article in *Philosophy, Psychiatry, & Psychology* on 'The historiography of the history of psychiatry'. See also his historical work on spiritual experience and psychosis (Kroll and DeGanck, 1986, and Kroll and Bachrach, 2005).

History of the concept of mental disorder

Daniel Robinson's (1996) *Wild Beasts and Idle Humours*, from which the reading for Exercise 4 in this chapter was taken, is particularly helpful as a *conceptual* history of psychiatry because of its focus on the 'insanity defence'. A remarkable *tour-de-force* of two and a half millennia of psychiatric history, each chapter combines encyclopaedic scholarship with a lively style to bring to life the ways in which mental distress and disorder were understood at each of the main periods of the history of psychiatry. Paul Hoff's (2005) article (in German) explores the tendency of psychiatry at different periods to fall back on one or another dominant model.

Eighteenth and nineteenth centuries

The history of psychiatry in the eighteenth and nineteenth centuries, has been one of the battlegrounds of the psychiatry/antipsychiatry debate. As we saw in Part I, the French psychologist-philosopher, Michel Foucault (1989), in his *Madness and Civilisation*, argued that the concept of 'mental illness' emerged in parallel with the Great Confinement of the late eighteenth and nineteenth centuries, as a response to the needs of the work-ethic of the Industrial Revolution. Roy Porter (1987; whose richly detailed *A Social History of Madness*, we looked at in this chapter) is among those who, although in the past identified with antipsychiatry, has offered a more balanced understanding of this period: see, for example, his (1985) *The Anatomy of Madness* (2 vols) jointly authored with one of the 'hard men' of psychiatric science, Michael Shepherd. The article by Katherine Arens (1996) in *Philosophy, Psychiatry, & Psychology* on 'Wilhelm Griesinger: psychiatry between philosophy and praxis', and the commentary by Aaron Mishara (1996) suggest, similarly, that we may need to reappraise the received views about the 'birth of biological psychiatry' in the second half of the nineteenth century. As we also saw in this chapter, the historian-psychiatrist, William Parry-Jones' (1972) *The Trade in Lunacy* is a model of careful and scholarly research in this difficult area. But that the battle continues is illustrated by an exchange in *The History of Psychiatry*, between the psychiatrist-historian John Crammer and one of the historical gad-flies of psychiatry, Andrew Scull (see Crammer, 1994, and Scull, 1995).

Other periods

Other periods have also attracted recent research. We looked at Lennart Nordenfelt's (1997a) work on the Stoics in this chapter, in his 'The stoic conception of mental disorder: the case of Cicero', with commentaries by Blackburn (1997), Leavy (1997), Mordini (1997), and Rhodes (1997); and Nordenfelt's response (1997b); and the earlier work of A.J.P. Kenny (1969) 'Mental health in Plato's Republic'. A further example is the New Zealand philosopher, Andrew Moore's, study of Aristotelian 'eudaimonia' and the concept of hypomanic mood disorder in Moore *et al.*'s (1994) 'Mild mania and well-being'; with commentaries by L. Nordenfelt, 1994 and D. Seedhouse, 1994. Recently renewed interest in the importance of classical work for ethics, for example in Bernard Williams' (1985) *Ethics and the Limits of Philosophy*, and Michael Stocker's (1997) 'Aristotelian akrasia and psychoanalytic regression' (with a commentary by P.G. Sturdee, 1997); and the paper by the philosopher, Chris Megone (1998) 'Aristotle's function argument' (with commentaries by Szasz (1998), Hobbs (1998) and Fulford (1998) and a response (Megone, 1998b), and a further special issue of *Philosophy, Psychiatry, & Psychology* on 'Aristotle, function and mental disorder' (Sadler and Fulford, 2000a and 2000b), with contributions by Szasz (2000), Wakefield (2000), Megone (2000), Thornton (2000), and Fulford (2000), all show the classical period to be a potentially fertile field for cross-disciplinary work between history, philosophy, and psychiatry.

An important focus of work on mediaeval conceptions of madness has been the relationship between spiritual experience and psychopathology: the American historian and psychiatrist, Jerome Kroll's. Kroll has also contributed importantly to the philosophical debate, see in particular, Roth, M. and Kroll, G. (1986) *The Reality of Mental Illness*, written as a direct reply to Thomas Szasz's claim that mental illness is a myth.

Coming right up to date, we will see in later chapters (for example, in Chapter 13 on psychiatric classification), that the modern history of psychiatry has important lessons for the development not only of policy and practice but of the research base of the discipline. A recent translation, for example, by Sula Wolff (2000) of a study of abnormal happiness by one of the founders of modern descriptive psychopathology, William Mayer-Gross, has, as the two commentators on the translation by Dominic Beer (2000) and Sir Martin Roth (2000) showed, potentially important implications for the direction of current research into the understanding and classification of disorders of mood.

References

Arens, K. (1996). Wilhelm Griesinger: psychiatry between philosophy and praxis. (Commentary by Aaron Mishara, 1996) *Philosophy, Psychiatry, & Psychology*, 3(1): 147–164.

Beer, M.D. (1996). The dichotomies: psychosis/neurosis and functional/organic: a historical perspective. *History of Psychiatry*, vii, 231–255.

Beer, M.D. (2000). The Nature, Causes, and Types of Ecstasy. (Commentary on Wolff, 2000). *Philosophy, Psychiatry, & Psychology*, 7(4): 311–316.

Berrios, G.E. (1996). *The History of Mental Symptoms. Descriptive psychopathology since the nineteenth century.* Cambridge: Cambridge University Press, pp. 7–11.

Berrios, G.E. and Freeman, H. (ed.). (1991) *150 Years of British Psychiatry: 1841–1991.* London: Gaskell.

Berrios, G.E. and R. Porter (ed.) (1995). *A History of Clinical Psychiatry: the origin and history of psychiatric disorders.* London: Athlone Press.

Blackburn. I.-M. (1997). Commentary: The stoic conception of mental disorder. *Philosophy, Psychiatry, & Psychology*, 4(4): 293–294.

Bynam, W.F. (1983). Psychiatry in its historical context. In *Handbook of Psychiatry*, VI. 5 (ed. M. Shepherd and O.L. Zangwill). Cambridge: Cambridge University Press.

Crammer, J.L. (1994). English asylums and English doctors: Where Scull is wrong. *History of Psychiatry*, 5: 103–115.

Foucault, M. (1989). *Madness and Civilisation*. London: Routledge.

Fulford, K.W.M. (1998). Commentary: Aristotle's function argument and the concept of mental illness. *Philosophy, Psychiatry, & Psychology*, 5(3): 215–220.

Fulford, K.W.M. (2000). Teleology without tears: naturalism, neo-naturalism, and evaluationism in the analysis of function statements in biology (and a bet on the twenty-first century). *Philosophy, Psychiatry, & Psychology*, 7(1): 77–94.

Fulford, K.W.M., Morris, K.J., Sadler, J.Z., and Stanghellini, G. (ed.) (2003). Past improbable, future possible: the renaissance in philosophy and psychiatry. In *Nature and Narrative: an introduction to the new philosophy of psychiatry*. Oxford: Oxford University Press, pp. 1–41.

Hawton, K., Salkovskis, P.M., Kirk, J. and Clark, D.M. (1989). *Cognitive Behaviour Therapy for Psychiatric Problems: a Practical Guide*, Oxford, England: Oxford University Press.

Hobbs, A. (1998). Commentary: Aristotle's function argument and the concept of mental illness. *Philosophy, Psychiatry, & Psychology*, 5(3): 209–214.

Hoff, P. (2005). Die psychopathologische Perspektive. In *Ethische Aspekte der Forschung in Psychiatrie und Psychotherapie* (ed. M. Bormuth and U. Wiesing). Cologne: Deutscher Aerzte–Verlag, pp. 71–79.

Hunter, R. and McAlpine, I. (1963). *Three Hundred Years of Psychiatry: 1535–1860.* London: Oxford University Press.

Jaspers, K. ([1913] 1963/1997). *Allgemeine Psychopathologie* (4th edn). Berlin: Springer-Verlag. *General Psychopathology* (transl. of 4th German edition J. Hoenig and M.W. Hamilton). Manchester: Manchester University Press. Republished by Johns Hopkins University Press, 1997.

Kendell, R.E. (1975). *The Role of Diagnosis in Psychiatry.* Oxford: Blackwell Scientific Publications.

Kenny, A.J.P. (1969). Mental health in Plato's Republic. *Proceedings of the Aristotelian Society* (3 December, 1969), 229–253.

Kesey, K. (1963). *One Flew over the Cuckoo's Nest.* New York: Penguin.

Kraepelin, E. (1902) *Clinical Psychiatry: a text-book for students and physicians.* New York: Macmillan. Translation by A. Ross of the 6th edition of Emil Kraepelin's Lehrbuch der Psychiatrie.

Kramer, H. and Sprenger, J. (1996). *Malleus Maleficarum.* London: Bracken Books.

Kroll, J. (1995). Essay review: the histriography of the history of psychiatry. *Philosophy, Psychiatry, & Psychology*, 2(3): 267–276.

Kroll, J. and DeGank, R. (1986). The adolescence of a thirteenth century visionary nun. *Psychological Medicine*, 16: 745–756.

Kroll, J. and Bachrach, B. (2005). *The Mystic Mind: The Psychology of Medieval Mystics and Ascetics.* London, Routledge.

Lanteri-Laura, G. (1998) *Essai sur les paradigms de la psychiatrie moderne*. Paris: Editions du temps.

Leavy, S.A. (1997). Commentary: The stoic conception of mental disorder. *Philosophy, Psychiatry, & Psychology*, 4(4): 295–296.

McHugh, P. R. and Slavney, P. R. (1983). *The Perspectives of Psychiatry*. Baltimore, USA: The Johns Hopkins University Press.

Megone, C. (1998a). Aristotle's function argument and the concept of mental illness. (Commentaries by Szasz (1998), Hobbs (1998) and Fulford (1998) and a response (Megone, 1998b). *Philosophy, Psychiatry, & Psychology*, 5(3): 187–202.

Megone, C. (1998b). Response to the Commentaries. *Philosophy, Psychiatry, & Psychology*, 5(3): 221–224.

Megone, C. (2000). Mental illness, human function, and values. *Philosophy, Psychiatry, & Psychology*, 7/1: 45–66.

Mishara, A.L. (1996). Commentary: William Griesinger. *Philosophy, Psychiatry, & Psychology*, 3(3): 165–168.

Moore, A., Hope, T., and Fulford, K.W.M. (1994). Mild mania and well-being. (Commentaries by Nordenfelt, pp. 179–184, and Seedhouse, pp. l86–192) *Philosophy, Psychiatry, & Psychology*, 1/3: 165–178.

Mordini, E. (1997). Commentary: The stoic conception of mental disorder. *Philosophy, Psychiatry, & Psychology*, 4(4): 297–302.

Nordenfelt, L. (1987). *Nature of Health: an action-theoretic approach*. Dordrecht: D. Reidel and Co.

Nordenfelt, L. (1994) Mild Mania and Theory of Health. (Commentary on Moore *et al.*, 1994). *Philosophy, Psychiatry, & Psychology*, 1/3: 179–184.

Nordenfelt, L. (1997a). The stoic conception of mental disorder: the case of Cicero. *Philosophy, Psychiatry, & Psychology*, 4(4): 285–291.

Nordenfelt, L. (1997b). Response to the commentaries. *Philosophy, Psychiatry, & Psychology*, 4(4): 305–306.

Parry-Jones, W. (1972). *The Trade in Lunacy*. London: Routledge and Kegan Paul.

Porter, R. (1987). From fools to outsiders. In *A Social History of Madness*. London: Weidenfeld and Nicolson.

Porter, R. and Shepherd, M. (1985). *The Anatomy of Madness*, (2 vols). London: Tavistock.

Rhodes, R. (1997). Commentary: The stoic conception of mental disorder. *Philosophy, Psychiatry, & Psychology*, 4(4): 303–304.

Robinson, D. (1996). *Wild Beasts and Idle Humours: the insanity defense from antiquity to the present*. Cambridge, MA: Harvard University Press.

Rossi, P. (2003). Magic, science, and equality of human wits. In *Nature and Narrative: an introduction to the new philosophy of psychiatry* (ed. K.W.M. Fulford, K.J. Morris, J.Z. Sadler, and G. Stanghellini). Oxford: Oxford University Press, Chapter 17.

Roth, M. and Kroll, G. (1986). *The Reality of Mental Illness*. Cambridge: Cambridge University Press.

Roth, M. (2000). Ecstasy and abnormal happiness: the two main syndromes defined by Mayer-Gross. (Commentary by Wolff, 2000). *Philosophy, Psychiatry, & Psychology*, 7(4): 317–322.

Sadler, J.Z. and Fulford, K.W.M. (2000a). Editors' Introduction. *Philosophy, Psychiatry, & Psychology*, 7/1: 1–2.

Sadler, J.Z. and Fulford, K.W.M. (2000b). *Aristotle, Function and Mental Disorder* (with contributions by Szasz, 2000, Wakefield, 2000, Megone, 2000, Thornton, 2000, and Fulford, 2000). *Philosophy, Psychiatry, & Psychology*, 7/1:

Scull, A. (1995). Psychiatrists and the historical facts. Part two: re-writing the history of asylumdom, *History of Psychiatry*, 6: 387–394.

Seedhouse, D. (1994) The Trouble with Well-Being: A Response to mild mania and well-being. *Philosophy, Psychiatry, & Psychology*, 1/3: 185–192.

Shorter, E. (1997). *A History of Psychiatry: from the era of the asylum to the age of prozac*. New York: John Wiley and Sons.

Stocker, M. (1997). Aristotelian *Akrasia* and psychoanalytic regression. (Commentary by P.G. Sturdee, pp. 243–246) *Philosophy, Psychiatry, & Psychology*, 4/3: 231–242.

Sturdee, P.G. (1997). Aristotelian Akrasia and Psychoanalytic Regression. (Commentary on Stocker, 1997). *Philosophy, Psychiatry, & Psychology*, 4/3: 243–246.

Szasz, T. (1998). Commentary: Aristotle's function argument and the concept of mental illness. *Philosophy, Psychiatry, & Psychology*, 5(3): 203–208.

Szasz, T. (2000). Second Commentary: Aristotle's function argument. *Philosophy, Psychiatry, & Psychology*, 7/1: 3–16.

Thornton, T. (2000). Mental illness and reductionism: can functions be naturalized? *Philosophy, Psychiatry, & Psychology*, 7/1: 67–76.

Wakefield, J.C. (2000). Aristotle as sociobiologist: the function of a human being argument, black box essentialism, and the concept of mental disorder. *Philosophy, Psychiatry, & Psychology*, 7/1: 17–44.

Williams, B. (1985). *Ethics and the Limits of Philosophy*. London: Fontana.

Wolff, S. (2000). The phenomenology of abnormal emotions of happiness: a translation from the German of William Mayer-Gross doctoral thesis. *Philosophy, Psychiatry, & Psychology*, 7(4): 295–310.

Zilboorg, G. and Henry, G.W. (1941). The second psychiatric revolution. In *A History of Medical Psychology*. London: George Allen and Unwin, pp. 479–510.

CHAPTER 8

Karl Jaspers and General Psychopathology

Chapter contents

In this chapter we turn from the broad history of psychopathology to one of its most important exponents in the twentieth century, Karl Jaspers. Jaspers set out his psychopathology in the first edition of his monumental *Allgemeine Psychopathologie* or *General Psychopathology*, published in 1913. We will be looking at a short passage from *Allgemeine Psychopathologie* towards the end of the chapter.

We will be focusing, however, on two papers that Jaspers published at about the same time as *Allgemeine Psychopathologie*; one (Jaspers, 1913a) on the importance of meanings as well as causes in psychopathology, an idea that Jaspers in turn derived from the 'Methodenstreit' (a nineteenth century debate in Germany on methods in the natural and human sciences), the other (Jaspers, 1912) on the distinctive role of phenomenology as a methodology for psychopathology. Taken together, these two papers will give us important insights into some of the key guiding ideas behind Jaspers' *Allgemeine Psychopathologie*. The topics with which the two papers deal will be taken up in more detail later, phenomenology in Chapters 9 and the *Methodenstreit* in Chapter 10.

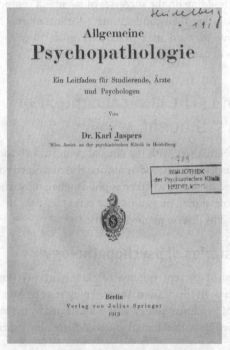

Fig. 8.1 'Jaspers' Allgemeine Psychopathologie, first edition, courtesy of Thomas Fuchs and the librarian, Psychiatry Department, Heidelberg University.

Active engagement not passive review

Psychopathology—how we describe and understand mental distress and disorder—is at the heart not only of clinical work and research in mental health but also of the conceptual issues at the intersection between practice and philosophy. Practitioners learn psychopathology as a 'received system'. But as we have seen, recent developments in mental health—including advances in the neurosciences, the move to community care, and the growing importance of the 'user's voice'—are forcing us to rethink how we conceptualize mental distress and disorder, and, hence,

psychopathology. And it is these developments, too, which, as Fulford *et al.*, (2003) argue, have inspired renewed interest in cross-disciplinary work between philosophers and those with practical experience of mental distress and disorder.

In exploring Jaspers' work and the history of ideas behind modern psychopathology, therefore, we will be actively engaged in a contemporary research programme rather than undertaking a merely historical review. Jaspers' work has many important lessons for us today. It is important to understand why our received system is as it is. But it is equally important to understand the problems, conceptual as well as empirical, with which Jaspers and others were struggling in a period, like our own, of dramatic advances in the neurosciences and of wide-ranging cultural change. In responding to these problems, Jaspers proposed a richer psychopathology than the system in wide use in psychiatry today: Jaspers, as we will see, hoped to create a twin-track psychopathology, incorporating meanings as well as causes, and based on phenomenological as well as empirical research methods. Our current system of descriptive psychopathology, however, outlined in Chapter 3, is the counterpart mainly of the 'causal' side of Jaspers' psychopathology. In arguing the need for meanings as well as causes in psychopathology, therefore, and for phenomenological as well as empirical methods, we can understand Jaspers as seeking to base psychopathology, in the terminology of Chapter 6, on a more complete view of the conceptual structure of the subject.

An unfinished agenda

There are many respects in which Jaspers' psychopathology, although indeed representing a more complete view than that provided by modern descriptive psychopathology, is very far from being the last word on the subject. We will be considering some of the inconsistencies and other respects in which Jaspers' psychopathology is incomplete in this and the next two chapters.

We should not, however, expect complete success in a venture of this kind. The problems with which Jaspers was struggling—the relationship between meanings and causes, the development of phenomenological and other methods for the study of subjectivity, and wider issues of the relationship between the natural and the human sciences—are among, or are closely related to, some of the deepest problems of philosophy. This is why there are such close and natural points of contact between philosophy and practice in this area. We will indeed be following up some of these points of contact in later parts of the book, in two chapters on reasons and causes, for example, one in Part III (the Philosophy of science) and one in Part V (the Philosophy of mind). But with problems as difficult as these, what we should expect is not complete success (no 'theory of everything'); rather, as we outlined in Chapter 6, we should hope for modest advances in understanding, partial insights with which we can move forward in a practically useful, but none the less provisional, way.

Modern descriptive pscychopathology, then, is perhaps best understood in its historical context in this way, as a modest advance in understanding, a partial insight to which Jaspers, along with Kraepelin, Bleuler, and many others contributed, and with which in the twentieth century we have indeed been able to move forward in a practically useful way: the greatly improved reliability and transparency of current psychiatric terminology underpin late twentieth century developments in therapy (psychological as well as pharmacological) and in the neurosciences (as in brain imaging, behavioural genetics, and psychopharmacology).

The danger, though, is that we forget the provisional nature of our current psychopathology and come instead to believe that it is complete. This danger is the greater at the present time because of the evident successes of the new neurosciences. As in Jaspers' time, a vigorous biological psychiatry is ever at risk of becoming trapped in the ideological blind alley of 'biologism'. The danger, though, of believing that our current psychopathology is complete, if increased by our evident successes, is at the same time greatly reduced by our equally evident failures. That the antipsychiatry movement should have got so energetically underway in the 1960s, just as psychiatry was once again beginning to make real progress as a medical science, came as something of a shock and a disappointment to the psychiatrists of the time. And as we noted in Chapter 2, the antipsychiatry movement, far from diminishing in subsequent decades as advances in medical psychiatry have accelerated, has become increasingly absorbed into the mainstream: first, with the expansion of non-medical interventions (psychological and social), then with the move from institutional to community and home-based service provision, and now, at the start of the twenty-first century, with the growing importance of the 'user voice' in all aspects of mental health, including research.

There are no doubt many and complex historical factors behind the success of antipsychiatry, so construed. But a key factor has been resistance—in different ways and from different quarters—to a merely causal-scientific understanding of mental distress and disorder. However powerful the heuristic of current descriptive psychopathology has been, it has alienated, as we saw in Part I, many of those with whom as users and carers psychiatry is centrally concerned. Modern textbooks of psychiatry, we emphasized in Chapter 3, stress the importance of understanding the individual as well as their psychopathology. But judged by the continued criticisms from those on the receiving end, all too often we fail in this. A poor workman, as they say, blames his tools. Perhaps, then, we should just try harder with the existing tools of diagnostic assessment. But perhaps we need to change or at any rate add to the tool bag. Perhaps we need to add to the tools of descriptive psychopathology, powerful as these have been up to a point in working with the causal aspects of psychopathology, tools designed to be equally powerful in dealing with the 'meaningful' aspects of psychopathology.

A return to Jaspers' agenda

There is a *prima facie* case, then, for a return to Jaspers' agenda of developing a psychopathology that encompasses meanings as well as causes and draws on phenomenological as well as empirical methods. Jaspers, as we will describe later in this chapter, after his extraordinary output around 1912 and 1913, appears to have largely given up on psychopathology. True, he regularly revised *Allgemeine Psychopathologie*. But for much of his life he was better known outside Germany for his work in philosophy. We have assets that Jaspers lacked, however: we have new resources, derived from the neurosciences as well as from philosophy (both Continental and analytic), new allies, in the wide variety of new clinical disciplines on which service provision is increasingly based, a new internationalism in mental health, providing a richness of cultural and intellectual perspectives, and, a crucial difference this, a user movement that is in the process of becoming increasingly engaged, no longer in trench warfare against the establishment (important as this has been), but in the design and delivery of services and of research.

In returning to Jaspers' agenda, then, in actively re-engaging with the problems he faced, we do so with a realistic prospect of making further modest advances in understanding, advances which, in building on the successes of twentieth century psychopathology rather than condemning it for its failures, could help us to move forward in a practically useful way to meet the challenges of twenty-first century mental health.

Session 1 The clinical context of Jaspers' thought

We will begin, then, with the clinical context, with the problem faced by Jaspers, and indeed by anyone else concerned with mental distress and disorder (whether as philosopher, researcher, mental health professional, or as a user or carer), of how to order and understand its diverse manifestations.

Seven stories of psychopathology

We looked at current systems of classifying psychopathology in Chapter 3. In this session, we are going start by looking at 'the problem of psychopathology' as it is illustrated by the experiences of seven people with different kinds of distressing experiences.

EXERCISE 1   (25 minutes)

As you read through the following case histories, we will be asking you to think about specific questions in relation to each. These questions will add up to the general question of *how the experiences of the people concerned could be organized schematically*.

This is a question, partly about general organizing principles, partly about specific categories and subcategories. These are not sharply distinct, of course, but any classification involves both (classification will be covered in detail in Part III on the 'Philosophy of science and mental health practice'). We will be looking at Jaspers' answers to this question in this session, but, as ever, it is important to *think about it for yourself* before going on.

Note: two of these case histories are based on notable cases from the past. The remainder are based on the experiences of real people (though with anonymized and amalgamated case histories to protect confidentiality).

Case 1

Ms HG aged 19, diagnosis: hebephrenic schizophrenia

HG shows very childish behaviour. She giggles endlessly to herself. She picks up simple objects and laughs hysterically. She tears innocent notices off the walls. When drinking, she dribbles down her chin and chest. She talks to the television. She is often incontinent, apparently without awareness or concern. She walks backwards down corridors. In the cafeteria she goes for 'seconds' and then returns to a different seat. The ward floor has a damaged tile now replaced with a tile of a completely different colour. She stands endlessly on this 'magic circle' talking to herself. She will give no account or explanation of her unusual behaviour. She does not interact with other patients or staff or with her family.

Questions to think about

- What do you make of HG's behaviour? Is it meaningful or meaningless? Does it serve any purpose and if so what purpose?

- HG is a Hindu Gujerati of very low social class and very limited education. In India she would be an Untouchable. Does her cultural background make any difference and if so what?

Case 2

Mr AM aged 52, diagnosis: post-traumatic stress disorder

AM had been a taxi driver, driving some 30 000 miles per year. In 25 years he had had neither an accident nor an endorsement. He was sitting in his son's car in his drive working on the wing under the dashboard. Another car failed to take the bend, hit a low wall, took off and landed on top of Mr AM's car. He was not physically injured but he developed a severe generalized anxiety state and a phobic avoidance of traffic situations.

He now cannot drive the 5 miles into the next village without severe anxiety. He dreams about road accidents, although usually not his own accident. He rehearses his own and other road accidents endlessly and painfully in his imagination. In response to any extraneous road noise or to road situations on TV he sees dreadful crashes. He finds these 'visions' very compelling and frightening. They are very real to him, in more than one sense modality, and he cannot banish them from his awareness even though he is well aware that they are not really happening. They occur in his 'inner vision' but, nevertheless, they torment him.

Questions to think about

- How would you describe his 'inner visions'?

- Are they perceptions and if not, then what?

Case 3

Mr ST aged 60, diagnosis: obsessive-compulsive disorder secondary to a depressive illness

ST has been depressed for some 6 months with low mood, fleeting suicidal thoughts, ideas of hopelessness and uselessness, poor appetite and sleep, and no energy.

He identifies strongly with the various people he sees when watching television or reading the newspaper. He thinks that he is John Major (the British Prime Minster at the time), that he is the Dunblane killer, that he is responsible for the genocide in Rwanda. He knows none of this is true but he finds the experience very compelling and distressing to the extent that he cannot bear to be in the same room as a television or newspaper in case he catches a glance of them. He knows the experience is 'crazy' but he cannot distance himself from it.

Questions to think about

- How would you describe his avoidance of television and newspapers?

- In what ways do his experiences differ from those of case 2, Mr AM?

Case 4

Ms BC, aged 32, diagnosis: paranoid schizophrenia

BC believes that she is under surveillance by a hi-tech bugging device. The bug is listening to her mundane, everyday conversation and relaying it to the group responsible. She hears her conversations being repeated at work and on public transport, which further convinces her of the surveillance. The surveillance is some sort of malign joke.

She spent £300 having her house 'swept' for bugs. Nothing was found. She concluded that this was because the bugs were actually next door, listening through the wall. She was refused access to carry out a 'sweep' next door. She concluded that the neighbours must be part of the plot. She could not interest the police in her difficulties so she took a course in detection, passed the examination and is now an accredited private detective. On one occasion, however, having smashed the window of her supposed persecutor, she was admitted to hospital under a section of the Mental Health Act, 1983. Within 3 weeks on medication the surveillance had completely disappeared.

Questions to think about

- One explanation for the disappearance of the surveillance was that BC had been ill and had been cured by the medication. Her own explanation for the disappearance of the surveillance, however, was that by getting her admitted to hospital, 'they' had made her appear 'mad', were now satisfied with their handiwork and had moved on to torment someone else! Is there any way of proving which is right?

- How would you describe the differences between BC's experiences and those of both case 2, Mr AM, and case 3, Mr ST?

- BC is a sophisticated Punjabi Muslim. Does her cultural background make any difference and if so what?

Case 5

Mr WE, aged 33, diagnosis: paranoid schizophrenia

WE asked his doctor: 'Do we have the technology to put thoughts into peoples' minds?' The doctor replied that we do not. WE said he agreed but that all the same 'they are doing it to me'. There were thoughts in his mind that he was convinced were not his own thoughts. He had great difficulty describing the nature of these alien thoughts. He gave two descriptions. First, the alien thought has a different 'feel' (he flipped his wrist). Second, the alien thought is like watching a dull, mundane and predictable B-movie on TV when suddenly a rhinoceros intrudes and you think 'What is that rhinoceros doing there?'

Questions to think about

◆ What difference would there have to be in the thoughts going through your own mind before you no longer recognized them as being your own thoughts and experienced them as someone else 'using your mind' for their thinking?

◆ How might *you* describe such alien thoughts if they happened to you?

Case 6

Ms FH, aged 60, diagnosis: schizoaffective disorder

FH was a recluse who only went out to collect rubbish, which she took to her priest for the church jumble sale. She lit her house by candles and would not allow the solidified wax to be moved because it had set into some meaningful pattern. She spent most of her time talking quietly to herself, but suddenly developed a manic episode in which she became elated and enthusiastic. She hardly slept and wrote the following passage. It is extracted from a piece of some 5000 words. She does not use punctuation! It is her spelling—the conceptual shifts and clang associations illustrate what in descriptive psychopathology is called 'flight of ideas'.

Read the passage with some rhythm:

When it's night time in Italy it's Wednesday over here how does a frog sit down to have its why does a fly how does a moth sit down to have its tea I like a nice cup of tea for to start the day you see and after I have sent the breakfast in my idea of him hymn is either a fourth or a fifth cup of tea and when it's getting late almost anything can wait but by golly there'll be folly if they ever touch my tea we all came into the world with nothing and we can't kiss going out and about and if there's about a bit well let's all snap out of it there was the empties and there was the fulls as a fitch is a fish and a ditch is a dish glass like a cup and saucer well my mother said I never should play with gypsies in the wood irrespective of a cook shop and if I do the mass will say naughty girl to disobey but auntie went to Colwyn Bay and so did the rest of people just to see what it was like being an angel without wings rings things looked black at the other side of the great divide divine divinity call it what you will but I thought I had written at least three parts of universe simply because there was a magic carpet attached to it but a set of false teeth on Coney Island was more than a man can stand.

Questions to think about

◆ If you had come across this piece, not as a 'case' but in, say, an *avant garde* literary magazine, what would you have made of it?

◆ How many literary forms (e.g. alliteration) can you identify?

Case 7

Mr MG, aged 42, diagnosis: hebephrenic schizophrenia

MG lived in a squalid flat painted dark green. He had a long history of illicit drug use, mostly 'whiz' (amphetamine). He lived in total isolation from the world. In 8 months in hospital there was not a single visitor or enquiry for him. He says his parents are living on Mars.

The following is a transcript from his speech. He can go on in this vein indefinitely and he never repeats himself. The previous example from Ms FH was written, this example is spoken. Note that in Ms FH's case her shifts of topic, neologisms and so on, always remain linked up in some way (by rhyme, association, etc.), whereas in this extract meaningful links are to all appearances lost. The conceptual jumps illustrated in this passage are called 'knight's move' thinking, implying that within three or four conceptual 'moves' the patient's thinking can be anywhere, as with the knight on the chess board. As described in Chapter 3, this is a feature of 'schizophrenic thought disorder', characterized by loss or loosening of the normal associative links in our thinking.

Just vocal vapour, like a vyrax landroidal sutra. Have they got a special group of people who take an engineering efficiency out of the responsibility of the professionals at the DHSS? My doctrines are very powerful in ball-point hand writing and the silence transmissions that I hear come from somebody somewhere suffering from psychosis. I've got a mental verbal auditory lock on my ears as if one is pressing my . . . Oh I don't know what you call it, my muscle back into normality with a gap in my teeth not, er, er, invokes, invokes diseases, corporalogy, hybrid takes, insects, and it makes you . . . somebody is manipulating me. I don't want you to deal with the fact that I don't know a Turkish drug addict when he sleeps in a box, you know . . . I am sure we can get from planet to planet by mesmeric Father Christmas' children and, if you like, the giant. Dr Johnson's a giant. I am like 'em. I'm a trichlorinectic pilot.

Questions to think about

◆ How does Mr MG's speech differ from Ms FH's writing?

◆ What can be made of his speech? What is he saying and why? Does it mean anything at all? (Notice the novel words or neologisms, e.g. 'vocal vapour . . . vyrax landroidal sutra . . . silence transmissions . . . mental verbal auditory lock . . . corporalogy . . . hybrid takes'.)

Jaspers' four key distinctions

Our responses to these stories

This (deliberately) diverse sample of case histories is at first glance bewildering. The cases are bewildering partly because they *are* diverse. But they are also bewildering because they are in various ways unfamiliar: they are like, yet unlike, everyday experiences (*is* Ms FH's text poetry?); some are understandable, others not (or not obviously so—what *is* Mr MG's 'vocal vapour'?); some we can empathize with, others we cannot (what *would* it feel like to have, like Mr WE, a *first*-personal experience of *other* people's thoughts?).

Karl Jaspers' reaction to these cases

Karl Jaspers, to go straight to his answer to the general questions posed in Exercise 1 above, sought to make the experiences of mental distress and disorder less bewildering by structuring our thinking about it using a number of powerful organizing principles.

Jaspers' key distinctions were:

1. Meaningful and causal connections
2. Understanding and explanation
3. Objective and subjective phenomena
4. Form and content

Our response and Jaspers' reaction

Why and how did Jaspers come to adopt these particular organizing principles? To answer this question, we will want to get a picture of 'Jaspers the man'—of how he came to be a philosopher as well as a psychiatrist, and the main influences on his work. First, though, spend a few minutes thinking for yourself how you would apply these principles to our seven cases.

EXERCISE 2	(10 minutes)

Run briefly through the seven cases described above thinking how Jaspers' four key distinctions might help you to organize the diverse phenomena they illustrate.

Obviously, you will be relying here on your personal understanding of Jaspers' terms and this will vary according to your particular background and experience. We will be aiming to get a deeper understanding of how Jaspers himself used these terms, and hence broadly how they are still used in psychopathology, by the end of the chapter. But you will be helped in this if you try them out for yourself before going on.

Here are a few examples of how Jaspers' organizing principles, understood in a common sense way, could be applied to our case studies. You may have thought of others:

1. *Meaningful*: Ms BC (case 4) has her house swept for bugs because she thinks she is under surveillance. We may not agree with her as to the fact of the matter but we have no difficulty *understanding* why she does this, i.e. there is a *meaningful* connection between her behaviour and her beliefs.

   Causal: Mr MG's (case 7) complex and bewildering speech, by contrast, is not *meaningful* in that we have no idea what he is trying to tell us. We cannot use his speech to *understand* his inner mental state. We are therefore left trying to *explain* his speech in terms of underlying *causal* links alone. One might

hypothesize, for example, that his history of heavy illicit drug use is a *cause*, or contributory *cause*, of his mental disorder.

2. *Understandable*: Mr AM's (case 2) avoidance of traffic situations is *understandable* given that the accident he was involved in was a traffic accident.

   Explainable: yet one also might say that there is no general causal *explanatory* link between traffic accidents and stress disorders, as not everyone who is involved in a traffic accident inevitably becomes mentally disturbed.

3. *Objective*: Ms HG's (case 1) childish, silly and in other ways unusual behaviour, and Ms BC's (case 4) elaborate delusional system, are *objective* in the sense that they are matters of observation (though of course, there are judgements involved in applying such terms as 'childish' and 'delusional').

   Subjective: what Ms HG (case 1) is experiencing, i.e. what it would be like to see the world through her eyes, is *subjective*.

4. *Form*: the *form* of all Mr ST's (case 3) thoughts is the same. They are compelling, known (by him) to be untrue, resisted, but unsuccessfully. Similarly, although Ms FH's (case 6) writing and Mr MG's (case 7) speech appear superficially similar, there is an important difference of *form* between them (Ms FH's retains while Mr MG's has lost apparent *meaningful* connections).

   Content: although identical in *form*, the *content* of Mr ST's thoughts differ. He is successively John Major, the Dunblane killer, and responsible for the Rwanda massacres. Note, however, that he does not really believe he is any of these. In this respect, the *form* of his (obsessive-compulsive) thought is different from that of delusions, which, as in Ms BC's (case 4) belief that she was being 'bugged', are firmly and fully believed to be true. In this respect, delusions are similar in *form* to experiences which in other respects are different in form: 'thought insertion', as in Mr WE's (case 5) experience of alien thoughts, although often classified with delusional beliefs, and sharing the same kind of psychotic 'loss of insight' (see Chapter 3), has the character of a direct experience.

The received and the obvious

All this may seem, at one level, fairly obvious. This is because it makes explicit many of the common sense ways we think about everyday experiences and behaviours. Psychopathology, then, grows out of 'folk-psychology', out of our everyday ways of describing human experience and behaviour. We drew on everyday experiences in Chapter 3 in learning about psychopathology.

Psychopathology, however, differs from everyday experiences and behaviours just in being, to a greater or lesser extent, and in one or more ways, *non*-everyday. A 'science' of psychopathology, then, while it may start from the common sense ways in which we understand everyday experiences and behaviours, must go beyond them if it is to be helpful to us, either clinically or as a basis for other sciences, not least the *neuro*sciences. One way in which it might do this is to ask what principles a *science* of experience would be based on, and how it would compare with the explanatory power of the sciences of the material world, such as physics.

Jaspers and the problem of psychopathology

As we will see, it was precisely this question that was occupying philosophers, psychologists, and psychiatrists at the time Jaspers started work on his psychopathology. The *Methodenstreit* or *Methodological Controversy* was concerned precisely with the question of whether all sciences must model themselves on the natural sciences; and Edmund Husserl's phenomenology, published in his *Logical Investigations* (brought out in 1900—more on Husserl in Chapter 9), promised to be a new rigorous science of psychological experience. But this was also a time of great strides forward in knowledge of the brain and the *neuro*pathological bases of some mental disorders. Indeed, then as now, as we noted earlier, there were high hopes that *all* mental disorders would soon be explained in terms of brain diseases.

Jaspers, then, at this critical time in the development of his psychopathology, and hence for the subsequent evolution of psychopathology in psychiatry, was poised between the (then as now) 'official doctrine' of a biological psychiatry modelling itself on the natural sciences, and what he perceived as the need for a new paradigm if the scientific method itself was to be applied fruitfully to grasp the reality of each individual case and the content of mental life.

So how did Jaspers come to perceive the 'problem of psychopathology' in this way? How did he come to be standing over and against the official line in psychiatry? Why did this bright up-and-coming psychiatrist become a philosopher? Just who was Karl Jaspers?

Reflection on the session and self-test questions

Write down your own reflections on the materials in this session drawing out any points that are particularly significant for you. Then write brief notes about the following:

1. How uniform/diverse are the categories of experiences and behaviours that may be associated with mental distress and disorder?

2. What four key distinctions did Jaspers employ in attempting to categorize these experiences and behaviours?

Session 2   Karl Jaspers the man

Origins

Jaspers was born in 1883, the son of a banker and local councillor. He was chronically ill throughout his childhood and was thus unable to engage in boyish pursuits. He began studying law at university, found it too dry and switched to medicine. His illness was finally diagnosed while he was a medical student. He had bronchiectasis (a chronic cavitating lung infection) with secondary heart failure. In those pre-antibiotic days, the prognosis was death from pneumonia in his late twenties or early thirties at the latest. Jaspers none the less graduated as a doctor in 1908 and began working as an assistant in the department of psychiatry in the University of Heidelberg. In the same year, Kraepelin's influential *Textbook* (*Lehrbuch*) of psychiatry was in its 8th edition. Because of his illness, however, Jaspers did not have a 'proper' job. He did some research, wrote reports, and filled in for absent colleagues. He avoided much human contact: a common cold could be fatal. He continued like this throughout his life, being regarded, as a result, as somewhat distant and aloof.

In the event, he lived to be 86! But his relative isolation as a young man meant that he read widely, studying not only medicine but psychology and philosophy. As we will see, it was the depth of his philosophical understanding that equipped him to make his unique contributions to psychiatry.

Early influences

Jaspers and biological psychiatry

Jaspers' professor in the Heidelberg Department of Psychiatry was Franz Nissl. Nissl was a neurohistologist, who, as we noted in the last chapter, has an important place in the history of medicine as the discoverer of a dye that allowed the structure of nerve cells to be clearly seen for the first time. Using this technique, he had shown that the neurohistological changes in general paralysis were different to the changes described by his friend Alois Alzheimer in dementia. General paralysis was a degenerative dementia that had swept Europe after the wars of the late nineteenth century. It was shortly to prove to be a form of neurosyphylis. These were paradigm-shaking discoveries, therefore, and the young Jaspers was impressed with Nissl as a scientist. When it came to *clinical* work, though, Jaspers was considerably less impressed.

The action in psychiatry at the turn of the twentieth century in Germany had moved out of the large institutions into university clinics. There was considerable resentment among the institutional psychiatrists that their discipline had been taken over by academic neuroscientists whose knowledge of clinical psychiatry was scanty, and who they perceived as being under the spell of a crudely natural scientific model, epitomized by the German psychiatrist, Wilhelm Griesinger's, famous aphorism 'Mental illnesses are brain illnesses' ('Geisteskrankheiten sind Gehirnkrankheiten')—quoted by Jaspers (*Allgemeine Psychopathologie*, p. 382; *General Psychopathology*, p. 459). In fact, Griesinger's *Mental Pathology and Therapeutics* (1867, trans. 1882), argued that mental illness should be interpreted as a product of an individual's response to both biological and cultural factors. (As noted in chapter 7, the philosopher and German scholar, Katherine Arens has given a balanced treatment of Griesinger's contribution to scientific psychopathology in her 'Wilhelm Griesinger: psychiatry between philosophy and praxis', 1996; with a commentary by Aaron Mishara, 1996.)

At all events, researchers at the time, such as Griesinger, Alzheimer, Nissl, Carl Meynert, and Theodor Wernicke, were in hot pursuit of the neuropathological changes by which they believed the major psychoses could be characterized. And, given their success with general paralysis, hopes were understandably very high. Jaspers shared these hopes. But he believed the paradigm had been pushed too far. 'These anatomical constructions' he wrote, as we noted earlier (in chapter 7), 'became quite fantastic (e.g. Meynert, Wernicke) and have rightly been called 'Brain Mythologies' (*Hirnmythologien*).' (*Allgemeine Psychopathologie*, p. 16; *General Psychopathology*, p. 18).

Jaspers and the 'Methodenstreit'

Jaspers' reservations about what he perceived as the excessively natural scientific approach to psychiatry were no mere whim of a relative outsider. They were driven by his understanding of the philosophical debates in psychology in the late nineteenth century, the so-called the *Methodenstreit*. As noted earlier, this was concerned with whether the human sciences (the *Geisteswissenschaften*) should try to emulate their far more successful cousins, the natural sciences (*Naturwissenschaften*), or whether they should go their own methodological way. The positivists—including such eminent figures as John Stuart Mill (in England), Auguste Comte, and Emile Durkheim (in France)—argued that the human sciences were no different from the natural sciences. Others argued that the human or cultural sciences were different from the natural sciences either in terms of the nature of their subject matter (ontology) or their methodology (epistemology) or both. The latter, in Germany, included Wilhelm Windelband, Heinrich Rickert, Wilhelm Dilthey, and crucially for Jaspers, the German philosopher and sociologist, Max Weber.

Jaspers meets Weber

Jaspers met Max Weber in 1909. He was invited to join Weber's elite intellectual circle, which met on Sunday afternoons, and he quickly became one of Weber's three key intellectual antagonists, one of Weber's 'real interlocutors, to whom Weber listened and with whom he had a genuine exchange of ideas' (Loewenstein, 1965, p. 95). For Jaspers, Weber was the 'Galileo of the human sciences' (quoted in Ehrlich *et al.*, 1986, p. 478).

Weber, as just noted, was one of those who believed that the human sciences involved a distinctive approach. However, his view of sociology, his own discipline, was that it was a hybrid subject, living partly within the natural and partly within the human sciences.

General psychopathology

Jaspers' position in the *Methodenstreit* was similar to that of Weber—he wanted to keep a foot in both camps. Jaspers regarded psychopathology very much as Weber regarded sociology—as having a peculiar position among the sciences in that it lives both within the natural sciences, pursuing abnormalities of brain functioning, and also within the human sciences, pursuing the experiences, aims, intentions, and subjective meanings of individual people. Of course, at a time when psychiatry was dominated by the 'brain mythologists', Jaspers' major aim was to bring psychiatry back within the ambit of the human sciences. He wanted to

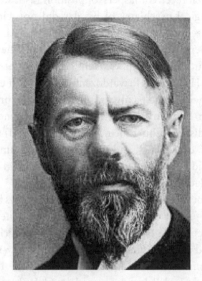

Fig. 8.2 Max Weber

balance things up. In Weber's work, therefore, who in turn had drawn on the work of Dilthey, Windelband, and Rickert, he saw things falling into place, and much of Weber's social theory—interpretation/understanding, *Evidenz*, ideal types, etc.—was to find its way into his psychopathology. Sometime later he wrote:

> My article of 1912 and this present book (1913) were greeted as something radically new, although all I had done was to link psychiatric reality with the traditional humanities. Looking back now, it seems astonishing that these had been so forgotten and grown so alien to psychiatry. In this way within the confines of psychopathology there grew a methodical comprehension of something which had always been present, but which was fading out of existence and which appeared in striking reverse, 'through the looking glass' as it were, in Freud's psychoanalysis—a misunderstanding of itself. The way was clear for scientific consciousness to lay hold on human reality and on man's mental estate, his psychoses included, but there was an immediate need to differentiate the *various modes of understanding*, clarify them and embody them in all *the factual content* available to us.
>
> *Allgemeine Psychopathologie*, p. 251; *General Psychopathology*, p. 302 (emphases in original)

The period 1909–13 was a time of high output for Jaspers. He wrote papers on homesickness, hallucinations, pathological jealousy, phenomenology, and, as noted earlier, the need for both 'causal' (i.e. natural scientific) and 'meaningful' (i.e. human scientific) connections in psychic life. We will be looking at his seminal paper on the latter topic in a moment. But the culmination of this burst of output was that, in 1911, he was commissioned by the publisher, Springer, to write a textbook of psychopathology. It was thus that his *General Psychopathology* (*Allgemeine Psychopathologie*) appeared in its first edition in 1913.

Beyond the (psychiatric and philosophical) pale?

It was not well received! Jaspers' opposition (as it was perceived) to the biological psychiatry of his day did not win him many friends. Indeed, in 1913, Nissl was unable to find an academic post for Jaspers. He offered to set him up with Alzheimer or with Kraepelin but, for personal reasons, Jaspers wanted to stay in Heidelberg. He became Privatdozent (lecturer) in experimental psychology within the faculty of philosophy. His professor here was the neo-Kantian, Wilhelm Windelband. Windelband was famous for distinguishing the nomothetic (natural) sciences that seek general, causal laws, and the idiographic (human) sciences that seek valid, individual descriptions. Windelband died in 1915 and was replaced a year later by Heinrich Rickert.

Relations between Jaspers and Rickert were always bad and they deteriorated further when Weber died a few years later, on 14 June 1920, in the epidemic of encephalitis lethargica, which was sweeping the world after the First World War. On 17 July 1920, Jaspers gave a commemorative address to the student body of the University of Heidelberg. Jaspers claimed Weber as 'a philosopher...perhaps the only one in our time'. After this, Rickert rounded on Jaspers for the 'absurdity' of describing Weber as a 'philosopher'. Rickert also claimed Weber as his pupil and he denigrated Weber's likely future influence. Jaspers was outraged:

> Now the disaster had occurred. I became angry and went so far as to say: 'If you think that you and your philosophy will be known at all in the future, then it will only be because you appear as a footnote in one of Max Weber's works, an author to whom Weber has expressed his thanks for some logical insight'
>
> Jaspers (1957, p. 33.)

Jaspers notes: 'from then on Rickert was my enemy' (Jaspers, 1957, p. 33). This was certainly the case (although as we will see in Chapter 10, Jaspers was influenced by Rickert's philosophy through Weber). In 1921, when Jaspers applied for the second chair in philosophy in Heidelberg he was strenuously opposed by Rickert who advanced his own candidates. In the event, Jaspers was successful. Rickert was indeed Jaspers' 'enemy'. He was scathing about Jaspers' abilities. Jaspers was more charitable, never commenting either on Rickert's disabling agoraphobia or on his later involvement with the Third Reich.

After general psychopathology

The retreat to philosophy

The decade of the 1920s was a quiet period for Jaspers. He published little so that people came to believe that, having achieved his chair, he was resting. In fact, he was preparing his main philosophical work, *Philosophie* (*Philosophy*), published in 1932. The work was in three volumes and it followed Kant's critique of metaphysics very closely. Each of the three volumes took one of Kant's metaphysical topics—the world as a whole, the soul, and God—transformed them into Jaspers' terminology—world orientation, Existenz, and transcendence—and investigated the possibility of metaphysical thinking in the twentieth century.

The Heidegger connection

It was also around 1920 that Jaspers first became friendly with and began working with Martin Heidegger. Heidegger was preparing his most important work, *Being and Time* (*Sein und Zeit*) for its publication in 1927. Heidegger wrote a lengthy review of Jaspers' second book, *Psychologie der Weltanschauungen* (1919) (*The Psychology of World Views*). The review was found in Jaspers' papers after his death. He was to admit that he had never read it. In 1933, Heidegger became Rector of the University of Freiburg under the Third Reich. Jaspers was shocked by his friend's actions and he broke off contact with him. Heidegger's Rectorship was to be short-lived but he never renounced the Third Reich. (For further details, see Ott, 1993.)

Jaspers was removed from administrative functions in the University in 1934. In 1936, he published his *Nietzsche: Einführung in das Verständnis seines Philosophierens* (Jaspers, 1936). Nietzsche had been adopted by the Third Reich as their philosopher. The 'will to power' and the 'superman' had an obvious attractiveness for Hitler's own philosophy. Jaspers bravely showed that Nietzsche could not be used in this way. By 1938, he was forbidden to teach or do research. Unlike many intellectuals, Jaspers did not emigrate. During the Second World War he applied for leave to go to Switzerland. This was granted but his Jewish wife, Gertrud, must remain in Germany. Jaspers elected to stay with her. During the war years, Jaspers had set himself the task of revising his *General Psychopathology* for its fourth edition. The fourth edition was greatly expanded. It became not only a psychopathology of what it is to be human but also a philosophy of what it is to be human.

By 1942, Jaspers and his wife were in hiding with a suicide pact should either be taken. The Americans liberated Heidelberg on 1 April 1945. A few days later, he was handed a note to the effect that his and his wife's deportation to the camps was planned for 14 April. He escaped death by a whisker.

After the war, Jaspers was appointed to the American-led interim government. He was not happy there and his health remained precarious. He took an appointment in the University of Basle in Switzerland where he was to remain until his retirement. Jaspers' interests moved away from academic philosophy to a preoccupation with what he saw as the dangers of being overridden by communist totalitarianism or annihilated in a nuclear war. His writings began to reflect this dual danger. In 1968, still living in Basle, he suffered several strokes and he died in February 1969.

The philosophical basis of psychopathology

In the remainder of this chapter, we will look more closely at Jaspers' thinking by concentrating on the two broad influences on his work: the *Methodenstreit* and phenomenology, as reflected respectively in his two papers, 'Causal and "meaningful" connections between life history and psychosis in schizophrenia' (1913b) and 'The phenomenological approach in psychopathology' (1912). This will allow us to consider in more detail the four key distinctions, introduced above, which Jaspers used in the analysis of mental phenomena. Of these distinctions, Jaspers can be understood as taking the first two primarily from the *Methodenstreit*, the third and fourth primarily from phenomenology. Thus, we have, very broadly, two pairs of distinctions underpinning his psychopathology. From the *Methodenstreit* we get:

1. Meaningful and causal

2. Understanding and explanation.

   From phenomenology we get:

3. Objective and subjective

4. Form and content.

As already noted, we will be considering phenomenology in detail, particularly as introduced by Husserl, in Chapter 9, and the *Methodenstreit* in Chapter 10.

Reflection on the session and self-test questions

Write down your own reflections on the materials in this session drawing out any points that are particularly significant for you. Then write brief notes about the following:

1. When and where did Jaspers work?

2. What was the name of his most famous book? When was the first edition published? What is its significance for psychiatry today?

3. For what was Jaspers better known over much of his life?

Session 3 Causal and meaningful connections

We will look first of all at Jaspers' (1913b) paper 'Causal and "meaningful" connections between life history and psychosis in schizophrenia'. This paper sums up the core of Jaspers' beliefs about the nature of psychopathology in terms of two of the key distinctions we noted above, that between meaningful and causal, and that between explanation and understanding. Building on the one hand on his work with Max Weber on the *Methodenstreit*, and on the other on his recognition of the successes of the brain sciences of his day, Jaspers argues that psychopathology is both a biological natural science seeking general explanations of mental disorders in terms of their neuropathological causes, but also a human science seeking to 'understand' (*verstehen*) the individual patient's experiences.

EXERCISE 3	(75 minutes)

Read the long extract from:

Jaspers, K. ([1913b] 1974). Causal and 'meaningful' connections between life history and psychosis (Kausale und verständliche Zusammenhänge zwischen Schicksal und Psychose bei der Dementia praecox). Translated with an introduction and postscript by J. Hoenig. In *Themes and Variations in European*

Psychiatry (ed. S.R. Hirsch and M. Shepherd). Bristol: Wright, pp. 80–93.

Link with Reading 8.1

How does Jaspers characterize the key differences between understanding (*Verstehen*) and explanation (*Erklären*) in psychopathology. Make a list of the ways Jaspers contrasts them—do we ordinarily think of understanding and explanation as being so distinct? You may want to think about what we mean by 'explaining something' or 'understanding something'. Note too the way that the distinction between causal and meaningful connections mirrors the distinction between explanation and understanding. How would Jaspers apply these to our seven case-histories?

Note: this is just a first reading of Jaspers' paper aimed at introducing some of his key ideas. We will be returning to the details of these ideas and to the influence of the *Methodenstreit* on Jaspers in Chapter 10.

Causes/explanations; and meanings/understanding

Understanding and meaning in Jaspers' psychopathology

The distinction that Jaspers develops between causes/explanations on the one hand and meanings/understanding on the other hand, is complicated by his terminology and the difficulties of translation from the German. The word he uses for 'meaningful' is '*verständlich*', more literally translated as 'understandable'. The importance of this is that it ties his work into the 'understanding' or *Verstehen* tradition of the developing human sciences (*Geisteswissenschaften*), and, thus, into the methodological controversy or *Methodenstreit* of the late nineteenth and early twentieth century.

'Understanding' (*Verstehen*) for Jaspers is the route to other people's inner mental states. It underpins the ability to 'read' their motives and subjective meanings from their actions and speech. For Jaspers, 'understanding' acts both as a technical term grounding psychopathology as a human science and also a non-technical or lay term referring to the ability to read the everyday motives of the people around one.

We return to understanding later in this chapter, in Session 4, when we consider its relationship to empathy and to Jaspers' use of the distinction between objective and subjective symptoms.

Static understanding and genetic understanding

Jaspers goes on to distinguish two main categories of understanding: (1) our understanding of someone's mental states considered individually—this is his 'static understanding' (*statische Verstehen*), and (2) our understanding of how one state may follow on from another—this is his 'genetic understanding' (*genetische Verstehen*).

Thus, on p. 82 we find,

◆ *Static understanding*: 'we present vividly to ourselves separately and describe in detail psychic states experienced'

◆ *Genetic understanding*: 'we understand how psychic events can emerge out of other psychic material'.

EXERCISE 4

Now refer back to the case studies in Session 1 of this chapter.

1. Try applying Jaspers' distinction between 'static understanding' and 'genetic understanding' to them. Pick out at least one example of each.

2. Are there phenomena that defy understanding? In Jaspers' terms, are such phenomena 'un-understandable' or could they still be explained?

Static understanding and the 'un-understandable'

In case 3, Mr ST, his tormenting images of 'being John Major' or 'being the Dunblane killer' can be understood by extension from the more mundane experience of being unable to get a catchy tune or a worrying notion out of one's head. In both instances we know it is inappropriate, but it gets, as we say, 'stuck in our minds'. Similarly, in case 4, Ms BC, most people would 'understand' the feeling of being under surveillance, of being watched, recorded, and reported on. In both cases, then, the patient's experience is understandable as a more extreme version of everyday experiences.

With case 5, Mr WE, and the symptom of thought insertion, we come by contrast, to experiences that are qualitatively different from everyday experiences. The experience of thinking a thought while at the same time experiencing it as someone else's thought is well outside most people's experience. Such experiences thus provide one example of what Jaspers might mean for an experience to be 'un-understandable'. Try, again, to think what it would be like genuinely to take a thought passing before the mind's eye to be someone else's thought. While it may at first sight seem to be an unusual but comprehensible error, there is something close to self-contradiction about the very idea of *me* thinking someone *else*'s thoughts. (See also chapters 3 and 28 for further discussion and examples of thought insertion.)

Genetic understanding

In case 3, beginning from the experience of being under surveillance, Ms BC builds a complex and to some extent self-fulfilling delusional system, which explains both the events themselves and sets them in a wider context of meaningful relations. We understand the 'emergence of one psychic event from another' on the basis of grasping the ideas, which Ms BC has used as her starting assumptions, and include the belief that she is being watched. Thus the development of a complex and internally consistent delusional system can be predicated on the initial (subjective) experience of being watched. Once we have accepted the initial propositions upon which Ms BC's delusional beliefs are based, everything hangs together 'understandably'.

The demand for understanding carries with it a further demand for explanation in terms of how the phenomena themselves are caused. In some cases, the lack of a suitable way of understanding someone leaves only the demand for explanation.

Explanation

We can see this with some of our other case histories. In case 1, Ms HG's behaviour on the ward seems wholly strange. Or, in case 7, Mr MG's speech does not appear to mean anything. We cannot 'get our heads around' Ms HG's behaviour or what Mr MG is saying at all. It seems impossible to know what motive or meaning underpins them. Accordingly, Jaspers describes such phenomena as 'un-understandable' (*unverständlich*). They are not a topic for either static or genetic understanding and, because of this, we must try to 'explain' (*erklären*) them as if they were the meaningless subject matter of the natural sciences—that is, we try to construct a causal account of their production.

The contrast between the demand for understanding in the human sciences and the demand for causal explanation in the natural sciences is a central feature of the *Methodenstreit*. We will be returning to this in Chapter 10 and to related debates about reasons and causes in current philosophy of science in Part III and in the philosophy of mind and in Part V.

Reflection on the session and self-test questions

Write down your own reflections on the materials in this session drawing out any points that are particularly significant for you. Then write brief notes about the following:

1. By what philosophical debate in the nineteenth century was Jaspers particularly influenced?

2. Jaspers wrote two key papers in response to the challenge of the 'biological psychiatry' of his day. What were they about?

3. How are these two papers related to his *Allgemeine Psychopathologie*?

Session 4 Phenomenology

The second of Jaspers' papers that we are going to read from his period of high output, is his 'The phenomenological approach in psychopathology', published in 1912.

'The phenomenological approach in psychiatry' contains a detailed account of Jaspers' use of the distinction between objective and subjective as derived from phenomenology. As just noted, we will be returning to this in Chapter 9 when we consider Jaspers' phenomenological method in more detail. But for now we are concerned with the distinctions he introduces to psychopathology from phenomenology and how he uses these to set out the basic phenomenological structure of psychopathology. In the next reading, we will be thinking particularly about the distinction between objective and subjective. We pick up on the final of Jaspers' four distinctions between form and content later, with a reading from *Allgemeine Psychopathologie*.

EXERCISE 5   (75 minutes)

Read the following paper:

Jaspers, K. (1968 [1912]). The phenomenological approach in psychopathology. *British Journal of Psychiatry*, 114: 1313–1323 (anonymous translation of 'Die Phänomenologische Forschungsrichtung in der Psychopathologie', 1912, *Zeitschrift fur die gesante Neurologie und Psychiatrie*, 9: 391–408)

Link with Reading 8.2

In this paper, Jaspers develops the third of the key distinctions noted earlier, between objective and subjective. As you read his paper, look carefully at how he draws this distinction, particularly on pp. 1313–1316. Is his use of the objective/subjective distinction identical with its contemporary use? What does he mean by 'phenomenology'? Also, (1) note any connections he draws with the other distinctions on which he relies, and (2) consider how you would apply his objective/subjective distinction to our seven case histories.

As with the first of Jaspers' two key papers, on causal and meaningful connections, we will be returning to this paper and to the influences on Jaspers from phenomenology in more detail later in this part, in this case in Chapter 9.

Objective and subjective

The distinction between objective and subjective is one of those everyday distinctions that has been much debated by philosophers. In Jaspers' work, objective symptoms include those that are publicly observable and often quantitatively measurable performances. The analogy with the observation and measurement of a machine drawn by Jaspers is clear:

It is not the feeling of fatigue but 'objective fatigue' which is being investigated. All such concepts as fatiguability, the power of recovery, learning ability, practice, the effects of rest periods, etc., refer to performances that can be measured objectively, and it does not matter whether one is dealing here with a machine, a live but mindless organism, or a human being endowed with a mind.
(p. 1314)

In this regard, then, Jaspers' use of the objective/subjective distinction is reminiscent of its contemporary use: in medicine we distinguish symptoms from signs according to whether we have to depend on reports by the patient of how they are feeling (symptoms) or can be observed (signs). But this is not exactly Jaspers' use of the distinction, for he also includes a very different sort of phenomenon under the term 'objective symptoms'. This is clear right from the start of the article on p. 1313. Look at this again, noting especially the passage we have now emphasized in

the following extracts (in italics):

Objective symptoms include all concrete events that can be perceived by the senses, e.g. reflexes, registerable movements, an individuals' physiognomy, his motor activity, verbal expression, written productions, actions and general conduct, etc.; all measurable performances, such as the patient's capacity to work, his ability to learn, the extent of his memory, and so forth, also belong here. *It is also usual to include under objective symptoms such features as delusional ideas, falsifications of memory, etc., in other words the rational contents of what the patient tells us. These, it is true, are not perceived by the senses, but only understood; nevertheless, this 'understanding' is achieved through rational thought, without the help of any empathy into the patient's psyche.*

Objective symptoms can all be directly and convincingly demonstrated to anyone capable of sense-perception and logical thought; ...
(p. 1313, emphasis added)

The term 'objective' thus covers not only what we would now call behavioural variables, such as how long it takes somebody to say or write something, but also *what is being said*, or in Jaspers' words 'the rational contents of what the patient tells us'. The 'rational contents' of the patient's words is clearly not perceived by the senses in the same way as the physical marks of the words they might write on paper or the sound patterns of their voice.

Subjectivity, understanding, and empathy

It is at this point that we find a key connection with another of Jaspers' distinctions (see point 1 in Exercise 5). For it is clear that in some sense 'understanding' is required to grasp symptoms that are 'objective', i.e. in Jaspers' sense of having rational content. 'Understanding' in this sense is what we came across above in relation to the distinction between understanding and explanation. There is, however, another and different sense of 'understanding', as Jaspers uses the term, i.e. a sense of 'understanding' that requires 'empathy' with the *subjective* side of symptoms. We may think of this subjective side as *what it is like* to have a certain sort of experience. 'Empathy' is Jaspers' term for our grasp of this subjective side of mental states, or what Jaspers calls 'subjective symptoms'. Jaspers argues that these subjective symptoms

... cannot be perceived by the sense organs, but have to be grasped by transferring oneself, so to say, into the other individual's psyche; that is, by empathy. They can only become an inner reality for the observer by his participating in the other person's experiences, not by any intellectual effort. Subjective symptoms include all those emotions and inner processes, such as fear, sorrow, joy, which we feel we can grasp immediately from their physical concomitants.
(p. 1313)

Empathy

Note the way in which Jaspers characterizes 'empathy', or an imaginative 'living along' with the patient's mental state, as an activity that is quite distinct from, and even seems not to require, 'logical thought'. Jaspers will use this idea to develop a stronger notion of 'understanding' than that found above in relation to 'objective symptoms'—these latter can be grasped by 'anyone capable of sense-perception and *logical thought*' (emphasis added).

At this stage it is worth asking yourself whether for Jaspers there is an inherent deficiency in 'logical thought', which means that we cannot use it to form a complete 'understanding' of the patient? Or is it that 'empathy' just offers us a distinctly different kind of insight into the patient's mind? Jaspers writes, for instance: '[The psychiatrist] can share the patient's experiences—always provided this happens spontaneously without his having to take thought over it' (p. 1315). This might strike you as an unusual conception of empathy. As we shall see later, Jaspers' notion of 'understanding' owes much to the work of Wilhelm Dilthey. Dilthey's philosophical approach is often characterized as 'life-philosophy', in that he regards (human) life as something that cannot be comprehended within traditional logical and rational ways of thinking.

Phenomenological seeing

We can now turn to how Jaspers characterizes 'phenomenology'. We will be looking at some of the different meanings of this term in Chapter 9, but in this paper Jaspers uses it in connection with his distinct notion of empathy. Jaspers argues that the psychiatrist, in his role as phenomenologist, must help others in the field to 'see' the subjective symptoms he describes.

> In the same way [as the histologist] the phenomenologist can indicate features and characteristics, and show how they can be distinguished and confusion avoided, all with a view to describing the qualitatively separate psychic data. But he must make sure that those to whom he addresses himself do not simply *think* along with him, but that they *see* along with him in contact and conversation with patients and through their own observations. This 'seeing' is not done through the senses, but through the understanding.' ('Dieses Sehen ist keines sinnliches, sondern ein verstehendes.'). (p. 1316, emphases in the original)

The notion of a phenomenological 'seeing', not mediated by the senses but by direct understanding, may not make much sense to you at this stage. Ordinarily, one tends to think of 'understanding' as a more advanced form of cognitive ability, compared with 'seeing'. It is important to remember, however, that Jaspers wishes to construct notions of understanding and empathy that are distinct from 'logical thought'. Jaspers is thus using the term 'seeing' in connection with 'understanding' in order to emphasize that the latter constitutes a mode of comprehension *distinct* from thinking. Again, this may strike you as strange; we ordinarily think of understanding as a *form of thought*. These ideas will become clearer when we look more closely at Husserl's notion of phenomenology in Chapter 9. Husserl uses the term 'seeing' similarly, in a broad sense, to include whatever we grasp and comprehend in an immediate way without the need for logical thought.

Form and content

The final key distinction we need to look at is 'form' and 'content'. In modern psychopathology (as in Chapter 3) we think of form

and content as distinguishing types of symptom and their subject matter. Thus a *delusion* of guilt has the same content but a different form from an *obsession* of guilt. Conversely, a delusion of *impoverishment* (e.g. that one has been made bankrupt) has the same form but a different content from a delusion of *guilt*.

Multiple form and content distinctions

This version of the form–content distinction is generally attributed to Jaspers but it has a complex history. The terms 'form' and 'content' have been used—and are still used—in a multiplicity of different ways by different philosophers. In order to understand Jaspers' use of the terms, we therefore have to consider which philosophical sources Jaspers might have been drawing on. There is a continuing debate about precisely which philosophers had most influence on Jaspers. We return to this in Chapter 9, in particular to the extent of the influence of Edmund Husserl's phenomenology on Jaspers' phenomenological method. But one philosopher, at least, who is directly acknowledged by the later Jaspers, is Immanuel Kant. In Jaspers' work on Kant (1957), he writes: 'Kant is the nodal point in modern philosophy...Kant is absolutely indispensable. Without him there is no critical basis for philosophy' (1962, pp. 380–381).

In relation to Jaspers' early work, and *General Psychopathology* in particular, it is likely that he drew together, in a complex way, ideas and approaches taken from phenomenology, Weber, the Neo-Kantianism of Windelband and Rickert, the 'life-philosophy' of Dilthey, as well as from his own reading of Kant. But Kant, at least, is important to him, so we will look first at Kant's use of the form–content distinction.

Kant's form and content distinction

A distinction between form and content is central to Kant's theory of knowledge. This sought to draw together features of both empiricism and rationalism. The empiricists thought that knowledge was exclusively the product of incoming sensory experience; rationalists, however, pointed to types of knowledge, for example mathematics and geometry, whose results have a degree of certainty that does not seem consistent with the idea that they have a purely experiential basis. The rationalists thought that at least some beliefs and principles must be innate in our minds and not derived from sensory experience.

Kant attempted to reconcile these two approaches, seeking to do justice to the insights of both. Briefly, Kant argued that knowledge is a product of incoming sensory input as the *content* of what he calls 'intuition', which is also ordered or given *form* by necessary principles or concepts. This is captured in a famous slogan: 'Thoughts without content are empty, intuitions without concepts are blind' (Kant, [1781] 1929, A51/B75). Without an experiential input thought would fail to have meaning or substance. But without the structure provided by concepts the rational significance of thoughts would be missing. Indeed, the suggestion here is that experience itself, as well as subsequent judgement made because of it, is in some sense conceptualized.

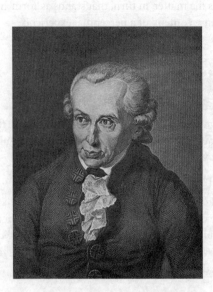

Fig. 8.3 Kant

Kant distinguished three types of necessary and *a priori* (i.e. not derived from experience) principle:

- the Forms of Pure Intuition (principles relating to space and time—for example, the way there is a spatial point between any two other spatial points, or a temporal moment between any two other temporal moments);

- the Categories of Pure Understanding (relating to notions such as 'substance', 'property', 'causality'—for example, the way that our experience is of *objects* with *properties*);

- the Ideas of Pure Reason (relating to the coherence of experience and the systematicity of knowledge—for example, the way that we expect there to be order in and systematic relations between our observations of the world).

Together these can be thought of as the '*formal*' aspects of any and all knowledge and experience. For example, referring to the pure forms of intuition (formal principles of spatial and temporal order), Kant writes in the *Critique of Pure Reason* ([1781] 1929, A20 (first edition), B34 (second edition); parenthesis and emphases added):

> That in the appearance which corresponds to sensation I term its matter [i.e. *content*] but that which so determines the manifold of appearance that it allows of being ordered in certain relations, I term the *form* of the appearance. [. . .] While the matter of all appearance is given to us *a posteriori* only, its form must lie ready for the sensations *a priori* in the mind, and so must allow of being considered apart from all sensation.

Kant's theory of knowledge and experience is thus marked by the use of a contrast between form and content. Essentially he is

arguing that certain very formal structures and forms of ordering are necessary aspects of all objective knowledge and experience. For example, the experience of a green door and a brown carpet are clearly different experiences—but they differ (in Kant's use of the term) only in 'content'. One can think of their 'formal' structure being the same: in each case we are concerned with a type of *object* and a type of *property* (Kant uses the terms 'substance' and 'accident'), and these are pure categories of the understanding.

Jaspers' form and content distinction

Kant's form–content distinction is difficult and abstract, and we will be returning to it later, in Chapter 9, on phenomenology. For now, though, we will pick this up from a section of *General Psychopathology* where Jaspers discusses it explicitly.

EXERCISE 6 (30 minutes)

Read the extract from:

Jaspers, K. ([1913a]1942). *General Psychopathology*, Vol. 1. (trans. by J. Hoenig and Marian W. Hamilton). Baltimore: Johns Hopkins University Press, pp. 58–59.

Link with Reading 8.3 here

- Do you think Jaspers is employing *Kant's* distinction between form and content?

In this section of *General Psychopathology*, Jaspers writes, for example, of 'hypochondriacal *contents*, whether provided by voices, compulsive ideas, overvalued ideas or delusional ideas . . .' (p. 59, emphasis added). Thus, the patient may hear a voice telling him *that he is ill* (auditory hallucination); he may have a persistent and intrusive thought *that he is ill* even though he resists the intrusion and knows it to be false (an obsessional idea); he may have had a long-standing preoccupation with bodily ill-health (an overvalued idea); he may have concluded *that he is ill* in the setting of the pessimism and despair of a severe depression (a secondary delusion or delusion-like idea); or he may have come to hold the belief that he is ill with great conviction and despite reassurance but *without relevant prior changes* in his mental state (a primary delusion). All these phenomena have the same 'content', hypochondriasis, but are present in consciousness in different 'forms'—auditory hallucination, obsessional idea, overvalued idea, delusion-like idea, primary delusion.

That a similar use of the form–content distinction is to be found in modern psychopathology is evident from the examples we gave earlier in this chapter from our seven case histories. Here are a few more: in case 2, Mr AM, the content is dreadful and fatal road accidents; the form is a pseudohallucination (See chapter 3, under 'Disorders of Perception'). In case 3, Mr ST, the content, at different times, is John Major, the Dunblane killer, the Rwanda genocide; the form is a compulsive or obsessional thought. In case 4, Ms BC, the content is 'high-tech' surveillance; the form is a primary delusion, delusion-like ideas, and the development of an elaborate delusional system. In case 5, Mr WE, the content is thoughts in his mind that do not belong to him; the form is thought insertion, a variety of 'made' or passivity experience. In case 6, Ms FH, the content is clever assonance, alliteration and clang associations; the form is that of thought disorder—in this case flight of ideas. In case 7, Mr MG, the content is bizarre, unintelligible prose; the form is that of thought disorder—in this case knight's move thinking.

Useful and powerful as this version of the distinction between content and form in psychic experience is, however, and whatever debt Jaspers may or may not have had to Kant, it is not as such to be found in Kant's approach. We have come across Jaspers' notion of 'content' before—it is what Jaspers called 'rational content' above in discussing the notion of 'objective symptoms' in his phenomenology paper. Remember that Jaspers writing in that paper (p. 1313) claims that, 'It is also usual to include under objective symptoms such features as delusional ideas, falsifications of memory, etc., in other words the *rational contents* of what the patient tells us.' (Emphasis added.)

This version of the form–content distinction in Jaspers' work derives not from Kant but from Husserl's phenomenology. We will be returning to this in Chapter 9, on phenomenology, but we will take a first look at it here.

Husserl's form and content distinction

In the passage you have just read (in Exercise 6) it is clear that Jaspers is using a form–content distinction that is different from that found in Kant. We might call Kant's distinction the distinction between 'sensory content' and 'objective form'; for Kant, these work together so that our experience is an experience of a particular empirical object, for example, a green door. Taken together, however, sensory content and objective form can in turn become the 'content' of a further sort of form. This new form–content distinction would be concerned with the way that the form of our experience of something can itself vary, while that 'something' remains the same. For example, the 'content' of our experience may be 'the door is green', but the 'form' may be one of anger, pleasure, etc. I may be angry *that the door is green* or pleased *that the door is green*. Or more generally, as Jaspers writes: 'Perceptions, ideas, judgments, feelings, drives, self-awareness, are all forms of psychic phenomena; they denote the particular mode of existence in which content is presented to us' (pp. 58–59).

This version of the distinction between form and content is found in Husserl's *Logical Investigations* (again, we return to this work in Chapter 9). Jaspers is right to point out that the terms 'form' and 'content' are widely used in discussions of knowledge, but it is important to be able to distinguish different form–content distinctions! Husserl indeed introduces different terms for the different distinctions. In the above examples, Husserl would call the *anger* or *pleasure* the 'quality' of a psychic phenomenon, while

what they have in common (*that the door is green*) he calls the 'matter'. It is the matter, in turn, that stands as 'form' in relation to the basic 'sense content' of a perceptual experience.

Reflection on the session and self-test questions

Write down your own reflections on the materials in this session drawing out any points that are particularly significant for you. Then write brief notes about the following:

1. What two distinctions does Jaspers derive from phenomenology in developing his psychopathology?

2. What conceptual distinction derived from Jaspers' work is particularly evident in modern descriptive psychopathology? What, in turn, are the philosophical origins of this distinction in Jaspers' work?

Conclusions: the seven stories and Jaspers' four key distinctions

The distinctions we have discussed in this chapter are subtle and have been the object of extensive philosophical debate. You should not be surprised, therefore, if you feel that they are difficult to grasp! Our aim in this chapter, as we have noted several times, is to give you an overview of how they fit into Jaspers' thought, and we will be covering them again in more detail in the next two chapters.

Before finishing, though, it will be worth returning once more to our starting point, to Jaspers' use of these distinctions to frame a psychopathology that is capable of structuring and ordering experiences as diverse as those illustrated by our original seven cases. Just how successful is this?

EXERCISE 7   (40 minutes)

As in Exercise 2 near the start of this chapter, run through the case histories given above with Jaspers' four key distinctions in mind. Look for other examples of how the four distinctions may be applied and ask yourself whether your understanding of these terms has been modified. Finally, how successful do you think Jaspers' distinctions are as a way of structuring psychopathology?

As before, there is room for disagreement over precisely how Jaspers' key distinctions should be applied in a given case, but here are a few examples.

1. *Meaningful*: Ms BC (case 4) takes a course as a private detective *because* she could not get the police to take an interest.

   Causal: one might think that Mr ST's insomnia and lack of energy (in case 3) have a neurophysiological *cause*.

2. *Understandable*: but Mr ST's avoidance of television and radio is *understandable* given his tendency to identify himself with the people he sees.

   Explainable: the onset of Ms FH's manic episodes (case 6) might be *explained* in terms of neurochemical changes in the brain.

3. *Objective*: Mr MG's (case 7) belief that his parents are living on Mars, is *objective* in Jaspers' sense.

   Subjective: What it *feels like* for Mr WE (case 5) when he is having an 'alien thought' is *subjective*.

4. *Form*: Mr AM (case 2) has numerous experiences that take the *form* of 'visions'.

   Content: the *content* of Mr AM's experiences, on the other hand, are always the same—they are about dreadful car crashes.

Sorting out psychopathology?

With selected examples such as these, Jaspers' distinctions do seem to provide order and structure. But if we press the distinctions a little harder things suddenly seem much less clear cut. Thus, *what* is the nature of Mr AM's visions of dreadful car crashes? *Why* does Mr ST get recurrent thoughts that he is John Major or the Dunblane killer? Can you understand these strange phenomena? What about Ms BC's novel explanation of the ending of the surveillance against her. It is very discrepant with our own explanation, but who is correct and how might we demonstrate the correct view? Again, where has Mr MG got the idea that people can put thoughts into his mind? As we asked before, what would a thought in your mind have to be like before you failed to recognize it as belonging to you? Or what of Ms FH's striking and poetic piece, full of alliteration, assonance, rhyme, rhythm, humour, and intriguing associations. Is she trying to tell us something. If so what? Finally, can you understand Mr MG's claim that he is 'a trichlorinectic pilot' and 'Dr Johnson a giant'. Is this purposeful, meaningful speech or just the speech centre running aberrantly, out of control?

The challenge of psychopathology today

We began this chapter with the 'challenge of psychopathology'—to describe, define, differentiate, conceptualize, and classify the diverse and sometimes very unusual phenomena of psychiatric disorder. Jaspers' psychopathology is widely acknowledged as the basis of modern descriptive psychopathology. As we have seen, it has substantial philosophical foundations, drawn from the philosophical currents of his day. In the next two chapters we look further at the two main influences on Jaspers' work, phenomenology and the *Methodenstreit*. Our aim in this will be to gain a deeper understanding of Jaspers' psychopathology and how it drew on the philosophy of the time. By identifying and clarifying the 'history of ideas' behind Jaspers' work in psychiatry's first biological phase, we will be better equipped to take up the challenge of psychopathology today, the challenge of developing a psychopathology that, continuing Jaspers' foundationed work

at the start of the twentieth century in psychiatry's first biological phase, builds on the rich resources equally of modern philosophy and of the neurosciences in psychiatry's second biological phase.

Reading guide

Karl Jaspers

Jaspers' *Allgemeine Psychopathologie* has recently (1997) been retranslated and published in two volumes by the Johns Hopkins University Press, as Jaspers, K. (1997) *General Psychopathology*. Translated from the German by J. Henry and Marian W. Hamilton with a new foreword by Paul R. Mc Hugh. Baltimore and London: The John Hopkins University Press.

In addition to *Allgemeine Psychopathologie*, and papers respectively on phenomenology and on causes/meanings as discussed in this chapter (and in more detail, respectively, in Chapters 9 and 10) key works by Jaspers include:

- Jaspers, K. (1962) *Kant: Leben, Werk, Wirkung*; translated as *Kant*, Vol. II of *The Great Philosophers*, trans. by R. Mannheim.

- Jaspers, K. [1920]. *Max Weber*. (Reprinted in *Rechenschaft und Ausblick*, 1951.)

- Jaspers, K. [1932] *Philosophie*, trans. as *Philosophy* (trans. by E.B. Ashton, 1969).

- Ehrlich, E., Ehrlich, L., and Pepper, G.B. (1986) *Karl Jaspers: Basic Philosophical Writings*.

- Jaspers, K. [1912]. *Zeitschrift fur die Gesamte Neurologie und Psychiatrie* (*The Phenomenological Approach in Psychopathology*, published in translation, 1968, on the initiative of J.N. Curran).

Jaspers: secondary publications

The historical continuities and discontinuities between Jaspers' time and our own, between psychiatry's first and second biological phases, and between its corresponding first and second philosophical phases, are the subject of Fulford *et al.*'s (2003) *Past Improbable, Future Possible*.

Berrios (1992) provides a critical analysis of the relationship between phenomenology, psychopathology and Jaspers work. Other secondary publications specifically on Jaspers and his work, include: Hoenig (1965) 'Karl Jaspers and psychopathology'; Schlipp (1981) *The Philosophy of Karl Jaspers*; Shepherd (1990) *Karl Jaspers: general psychopathology, conceptual issues in psychological medicine*; Schmitt (1986) 'Karl Jaspers' influence on psychiatry'.

Two useful sources on the relationship between Jaspers and Weber are Dreijmanis (1989) *Karl Jaspers on Max Weber*, and

Loewenstein (1965) *Max Weber's Political Ideas in the Perspective of our Time*.

(See also Reading Guide Chapter 9).

Phenomenology and psychopathology today

Building on the foundational work of Eugene Minkowski (eg 1927 and 1968), and his mentor, Henry Bergson (eg 1927), and others, modern exemplars of the phenomenological tradition in psychiatry include such seminal figures as Henry Ey (eg 1954) in France, Kimura Bin (eg 1992) in Japan, and Wolfgang Blankenburg (eg 1971) in Germany. An early modern collection highlighting the links between phenomenology and neuroscience is Spitzer *et al.* (1993). Bracken (1999a) provides a succinct review and his *Trauma: Culture, Meaning and Philosophy* (Bracken, 2002) draws on Heideggerian phenomenology in an explanation of the experience of trauma. *Nature and Narrative* includes many exemplars of modern phenomenological work in psychopathology: Kraus (2003) on classification, Morris (2003) on body dysmorphophobia, Musalek (2003) on delusions, Widdershoven and Widdershoven-Heerding (2003) on dementia, and Heinimaa, 2003, on incomprehensibility. Also in this series, see Phillips, J. (2004), Chapter 12 in Radden, J. (ed.) (2004), on explanation and understanding, and Schwartz, M.A. and Wiggins, O.P. (2004), Chapter 24 in Radden, J. (ed.) (2004), on phenomenological and hermeneutic methods: also Stanghellini's (2004) study of the phenomenology of schizophrenia *Deanimated bodies and disembodied spirits*; and the forthcoming textbook by Parnas, Sass, Stanghellini, and Fuchs, *The Vulnerable Self: the clinical phenomenology of the schizophrenic and affective spectrum disorders*.

Another philosopher working within the phenomenological tradition, Maurice Merleau-Ponty (1908–61), who was influenced by both Husserl and Sartre, has inspired new work in the philosophy of psychiatry, on the concept of mental disorder (Matthews, 2003), and specific areas of psychopathology— see, for example, work by Philpott, drawing on his own experience of dyslexia, in his 1998a paper in *Philosophy, Psychiatry, & Psychology* on 'A phenomenology of dyslexia', with commentaries by Komesaroff and Wiltshire (1998), Rippon (1998), and Widdershoven (1998), and a response by Philpott (1998b). Pringuey and Kohl's (2001) edited collection is illustrative of modern French phenomenology.

Other examples of what Petitot, Varela, Pachoud, and Roy (2000) have called 'naturalized phenomenology', include: Varela, Thompson, and Rosch (1992), Gallagher and Cole (1995), and Gallagher (1996) on body schema; Davis (1997) on positive features of dyslexia; and Parnas and Zahavi (2000) on the self. A contrasting cognitive approach is illustrated by a special issue of *The Monist* (1999) edited by Joelle Proust.

In *Philosophy, Psychiatry, & Psychology*, the Swedish philosopher, Frederik Svenaeus (1999a) has explored the phenomenology of alexithymia, with commentaries by Bracken (1999b), Philpott (1999), Sturdee (1999), Nissim-Sabat (1999), and a response by Svenaeus, (1999b); the Dutch philosopher, Guy Widdershoven (1999a), has applied hermeneutic concepts to issues of meaning and causation in cognitive psychology, with commentaries by McMillan (1999), Phillips (1999) and Warner (1999), and a response (Widdershoven, 1999b); the Canadian psychiatrists Mona Gupta and L.R. Kay (2002a) have explored the impact of phenomenology on North American psychiatry, with commentaries by Morley (2002) and McMillan (2002), and a response (Gupta and Kay, 2002b); and the Italian philosopher and psychiatrist, Giovanni Stanghellini has described work on the phenomenology of schizophrenia (2001a) with a commentary by the North American philosopher and psychologist, Louis Sass (2001a).

Sass (2001b) has also edited a Special Issue of *Philosophy, Psychiatry, & Psychology* on three classic approaches to the phenomenology of schizophrenia (Issue 8(4): December 2001). This includes new translations with commentaries of works, respectively, by Eugene Minkowski (Minkowski and Targowla, 2001: commentaries by Urfer, 2001; Naudin and Azorin, 2001; Stanghellini, 2001b; Pachoud, 2001), by the German psychiatrist and phenomenologist, W. Blankenburg (2001; commentaries by Mishara, 2001; Fuchs, 2001; Wiggins *et al.*, 2001), and by the Japanese phenomenologist and psychiatrist, Kimura Bin (2001: with commentaries by Cutting, 2001; Zahavi, 2001; Phillips, 2001). Louis Sass and the Danish philosopher, Joseph Parnas provided an 'overview and future directions' (2001).

References

Arens, K. (1996). Wilhelm Griesinger: psychiatry between philosophy and praxis. *Philosophy, Psychiatry, and Psychology*, 3(3): 147–164.

Bergson, H. (1927) *Essai sur les données immédiates de la conscience*. Presses Universitaire de France, Paris.

Berrios, G.E. (1992). Phenomenology, Psychopathology and Jaspers: a Conceptual History. *History of Psychiatry*, 3: 303–28.

Bin, K. (1992) *Essais de psychopathologie phénoménologique*. Presse Universitaire de France: Paris.

Bin, K. (2001). Cogito and I: a bio-logical approach. *Philosophy, Psychiatry, & Psychology*, 8(4): 331–336.

Blankenburg, W. (1971) *Der Verlust der Natuerlichen Selbstverstaendlichkeit. Ein Beitrag zur Psychopathologie Symptomarmner Schizophrenien*. Enke, Stuttgart.

Blankenburg, W. (2001). First steps toward a psychopathology of common sense. *Philosophy, Psychiatry, & Psychology*, 8(4): 303–316.

Bracken, P. (1999a). Phenomenology and psychiatry. *Current Opinion in Psychiatry*, 12: 593–596.

Bracken, P. (1999b). The importance of Heidegger for psychiatry. (Commentary on Svenaeus, 1999). *Philosophy, Psychiatry, & Psychology*, 6(2): 83–86.

Bracken, P. (2002) *Trauma: Culture, Meaning and Philosophy.* London: Whurr Publishers.

Cutting, J. (2001). On Kimuras Ecrits de psychopathologie phénomenologique. (Commentary on Bin, 2001). *Philosophy, Psychiatry, & Psychology*, 8(4): 337–338.

Davis, R. (1997). *The Gift of Dyslexia*. London: Souvenir.

Dreijmanis, J. (1989). *Karl Jaspers on Max Weber*. New York: Paragon House.

Ehrlich, E., Ehrlich, L., and Pepper, G.B. (ed.) (1986). *Karl Jaspers: basic philosophical writings.* Athens, OH: Ohio University Press.

Ey, H. (1954) *Etudes Psychiatriques*. Desclee de Brouwer: Paris.

Fuchs, T. (2001). The Tacit dimension. (Commentary on Blankenburg, 2001.) *Philosophy, Psychiatry, & Psychology*, 8(4): 323–326.

Fulford, K.W.M., Morris, K.J., Sadler, J.Z., and Stanghellini, G. (2003). Past improbable, future possible: the renaissance in philosophy and psychiatry. In *Nature and Narrative: an introduction to the new philosophy of psychiatry* (ed. K.W.M. Fulford, K.J. Morris, J.Z.S. Sadler, and G. Stanghellini). Oxford: Oxford University Press, pp. 1–41.

Gallagher, S. (1996). Body schema and intentionality. In *The Body and The Self* (ed. N. Eilen). Cambridge, MA: MIT Press.

Gallagher, S. and Cole, J. (1995). Body schema and body image in a deafferented subject. *Journal of Mind and Behaviour*, 16: 365–390.

Griesinger, W. ([1867] 1882). *Mental Pathology and Therapeutics* (trans. C.L. Robertson and J. Rutherford) New York: William Wood and Co.

Gupta, M. and Kay, L.R. (2002a). The impact of phenomenology on North American psychiatric assessment. *Philosophy, Psychiatry, & Psychology*, 9(1): 73–86.

Gupta, M. and Kay, L.R. (2002b). Phenomenological methods in psychiatry: a necessary first step. (Response to the commentaries). *Philosophy, Psychiatry, & Psychology*, 9(1): 93–96.

Heidegger, M. (1962). *Being and Time* (trans. J. Macquarrie and E. Robinson). Oxford: Blackwell.

Heinimaa, M. (2003). Incomprehensibility. In *Nature and Narrative: an introduction to the new philosophy of psychiatry* (ed. K.W.M. Fulford, K.J. Morris, J.Z.S. Sadler, and G. Stanghellini). Oxford: Oxford University Press, Chapter 14.

Hoenig, J. (1965). Karl Jaspers and psychopathology. *Philosophy and Phenomenological Research*, 26: 216–229.

Jaspers, K. ([1912] 1968). The Phenomenological Approach in Psychopathology. *Zeitschrift fur die Gesamte Neurologie und Psychiatrie*, 9, 391–408. Published in translation, (1968) (on the initiative of J.N. Curran), *British Journal of Psychiatry*, 114: 1313–1323.

Jaspers, K. ([1913a] 1963/1997). *Allgemeine Psychopathologie* (4th edn). Berlin: Springer-Verlag; (1942. *General Psychopathology* (trans. of 4th German edition J. Hoenig and M.W. Hamilton). Manchester: Manchester University Press.) *Note*: new edition, with foreword by Paul R. McHugh, 1997, Baltimore: The John Hopkins University Press.

Jaspers, K. ([1913b] 1974). Causal and 'meaningful' connections between life history and psychosis (Kausale und verständliche Zusammenhänge zwischen Schicksal und Psychose bei der Dementia praecox). Translated with an introduction and postscript by J. Hoenig. In *Themes and Variations in European Psychiatry* (ed. S.R. Hirsch and M. Shepherd). Bristol: Wright, pp. 80–93.

Jaspers, K. (1919). *Psychologie der Weltanschauungen* (*The Psychology of World Views*).

Jaspers, K. (1936). *Nietzsche: Einführung in das Verständnis seines Philosophierens* (*Nietzsche: An Introduction to the Understanding of His Philosophical Activity*) (trans. C.F. Wallruff and F.J. Schmitz). Baltimore, MD: Johns Hopkins University Press.

Jaspers, K. ([1920] 1951). *Max Weber*. Reprinted in *Rechenschaft und Ausblick*. Munich: Piper.

Jaspers, K. (1957). Philosophical autobiography. In *The Philosophy of Karl Jaspers* (ed. P. Schilpp). LaSalle, IL: Open Court.

Jaspers, K. (1962). *Kant: Leben, Werk, Wirkung*. Munich: Piper. (Trans. as *Kant*, Vol. II of *The Great Philosophers*, trans. by R. Mannheim. New York: Harcourt, Brace and World.).

Jaspers, K. ([1932] 1969). *Philosophie*. Translated as *Philosophy* (trans. by E.B. Ashton). Chicago, IL: University of Chicago Press.

Kant, I. ([1781] 1929). *Critique of Pure Reason* (trans. N. Kemp Smith). London: Macmillan.

Komesaroff, P.A. and Wiltshire, J. (1998). Commentary: A phenomenology of dyslexia. *Philosophy, Psychiatry, & Psychology*, 5(1): 21–24.

Kraepelin, E. (1915). *Psychiatry Textbook* (*Lehrbuch*), (8th edn). Leipzig: Thieme.

Kraus, D. (2003). How can the phenomenological-anthropological approach contribute to diagnosis and classification in psychiatry? In *Nature and Narrative: an introduction to the new philosophy of psychiatry* (ed.

K.W.M. Fulford, K.J. Morris, J.Z.S. Sadler, and G. Stanghellini). Oxford: Oxford University Press, Chapter 13.

Loewenstein, K. (1965). *Max Weber's Political Ideas in the Perspective of Our Time*. Amherst, MA: University of Massachusetts Press.

Matthews, E. (2003). How can a mind be sick? In *Nature and Narrative: an introduction to the new philosophy of psychiatry* (ed. K.W.M. Fulford, K.J. Morris, J.Z.S. Sadler, and G. Stanghellini). Oxford: Oxford University Press, Chapter 4.

McMillan, J. (1999). Commentary: Cognitive psychology and hermeneutics: two irreconcilable approaches? *Philosophy, Psychiatry, & Psychology*, 6(4): 255–258.

McMillan, J. (2002). Jaspers and defining phenomenology. (Commentary on Gupta and Kay, 2001). *Philosophy, Psychiatry, & Psychology*, 9(1): 91–92.

Minkowski, E. (1927) *La Schizophrenie. Psychopathologie des Schizoides et des Schizophrenes*. Payot: Paris.

Minkowski, E. (1968) *Le Temps Vecu*. Presse Universitaire de France: Paris.

Minkowski, E. and Targowla, R. (2001). A contribution to the study of autism: the interrogative attitude. *Philosophy, Psychiatry, & Psychology*, 8(4): 271–278.

Mishara, A. (1996). William Griesinger. (Commentary on Arens, 1996). *Philosophy, Psychiatry, and Psychology*, 3(3): 165–168.

Mishara, A.L. (2001). On Wolfgang Blankenburg, common sense, and schizophrenia. (Commentary on Blankenburg, 2001). *Philosophy, Psychiatry, & Psychology*, 8(4): 317–322.

Morley, J. (2002). Phenomenological and biological psychiatry: complementary or mutual? (Commentary on Gupta and Kay, 2001). *Philosophy, Psychiatry, & Psychology*, 9(1): 87–90.

Morris, K. J. (2003). The phenomenology of body dysmorphic disorder: a Sartrean analysis. Chapter 11 in Fulford, K.W.M., Morris, K.J., Sadler, J. Z., and Stanghellini, G. (eds.) *Nature and Narrative: An Introduction to the New Philosophy of Psychiatry*. Oxford: Oxford University Press, 270–274.

Musalek, M. (2003). Meanings and causes of delusions. Chapter 10 in Fulford, K.W.M., Morris, K.J., Sadler, J.Z., and Stanghellini, G. (eds.) *Nature and Narrative: An Introduction to the New Philosophy of Psychiatry*. Oxford: Oxford University Press.

Naudin, J. and Azorin, J.-M. (2001). Schizophrenia and the void. (Commentary on Minkowski and Targowla, 2001). *Philosophy, Psychiatry, & Psychology*, 8(4): 291–294.

Nissim-Sabat, M. (1999). Phenomenology and mental disorders: Heidegger or Husserl? (Commentary on Svenaeus, 1999). *Philosophy, Psychiatry, & Psychology*, 6(2): 101–104.

Ott, H. (1993). *Martin Heidegger: a political life* (trans. by A. Blunden). London: Fontana Press.

Pachoud, B. (2001). Reading Minkowski with Husserl. (Commentary on Minkowski and Targowla, 2001). *Philosophy, Psychiatry, & Psychology*, 8(4): 299–302.

Parnas, J. and Zahavi, D. (2000). The link: philosophy–psychopathology–phenomenology. In *Exploring The Self* (ed. D. Zahavi). Amsterdam: Benjamins, pp. 1–16.

Parnas, J., Sass, L., Stanghellini, G., and Fuchs, T. (forthcoming). *The Vulnerable Self: the clinical phenomenology of the schizophrenic and affective spectrum disorders*. Oxford: Oxford University Press.

Petitot, J., Varela, F., Pachoud, B., and Roy, J.-M. (ed.) (2000). *Naturalizing Phenomenology: issues in contemporary phenomenology and cognitive science*. Cambridge: Cambridge University Press.

Phillips, J. (1999). The hermeneutical critique of cognitive psychology. (Commentary on Widdershoven, 1999a). *Philosophy, Psychiatry, & Psychology*, 6(4): 259–264.

Phillips, J. (2001). Kimura Bin on schizophrenia. (Commentary on Bin, 2001). *Philosophy, Psychiatry, & Psychology*, 8(4): 343–346.

Phillips, J. (2004). Understanding/explanation. In *The Philosophy of Psychiatry: a companion* (ed. J. Radden). New York: Oxford University Press, pp. 180–190.

Philpott, M.J. (1998a). A phenomenology of dyslexia: the lived-body, ambiguity, and the breakdown of expression. *Philosophy, Psychiatry, & Psychology*, 5(1): 1–20.

Philpott, M.J. (1998b). Response to the Commentaries. *Philosophy, Psychiatry, & Psychology*, 5/1, 33–36.

Philpott, M.J. (1999). The how and why of phenomenology. (Commentary on Svenaeus, 1999). *Philosophy, Psychiatry, & Psychology*, 6(2): 87–94.

Pringuey, D. and Kohl, F.S. (ed.) (2001) *Phenomenology of human identity and schizophrenia*. Collection Pheno sous la direction de Georges Charbonneau. France: Association Le Cercle Herméneutique, Société dAnthropologie Phénologique et dHerméneutique Générale.

Proust, J. (ed.) (1999). Special Issue of *The Monist*.

Radden, J. (ed.) (2004). *The Philosophy of Psychiatry: a companion*. New York: Oxford University Press, pp. 180–190, 351–363.

Rippon, G. (1998). A phenomenology of dyslexia. (Commentary on Philpott, 1998a). *Philosophy, Psychiatry, & Psychology*, 5/1: 25–28.

Sass, L.A. (2001a). Commentary: Pathogenesis, common sense, and the cultural framework (Commentary on Stanghellini, 2001a). *Philosophy, Psychiatry, & Psychology*, 8/2/3: 219–224.

Sass, L.A. (2001b). Self and world in schizophrenia: three classic approaches. *Philosophy, Psychiatry, & Psychology*, 8(4): 251–270.

Sass, L.A. and Parnas, J. (2001). Phenomenology of self-disturbances in schizophrenia: some research findings and directions. *Philosophy, Psychiatry, & Psychology*, 8(4): 347–356.

Schlipp, P.A. (1981). *The Philosophy of Karl Jaspers*. LaSalle, IL: Open Court.

Schmitt, W. (1986). Karl Jasper influence on psychiatry. *Journal of the British Society for Phenomenology*, 17: 36–51.

Schwartz, M.A. and Wiggins, O.P. (2004). *Phenomenological and Hermeneutic Models: understanding and interpretation in psychiatry*. Ch. 24 in Radden, J. (ed.) The Philosophy of Psychiatry: A Companion, pp. 351–363. New York: Oxford University Press.

Shepherd, M. (1990). *Karl Jaspers: general psychopathology, conceptual issues in psychological medicine*. London: Tavistock.

Spitzer, M., Uehlein, F., Schwartz, M.A., and Mundt, C. (ed.) (1993). *Phenomenology Language and Schizophrenia*. New York: Springer-Verlag.

Stanghellini, G. (2001a). Psychopathology of common sense. *Philosophy, Psychiatry, & Psychology*, 8/2/3: 201–218.

Stanghellini, G. (2001b). A dialectical conception of autism. (Commentary on Minkowski and Targowla, 2001). *Philosophy, Psychiatry, & Psychology*, 8(4): 295–298.

Stanghellini, G. (2004). *Deanimated bodies and disembodied spirits. Essays on the psychopathology of common sense*. Oxford: Oxford University Press.

Sturdee, P.G. (1999). There has to be a pattern. (Commentary on Svenaeus, 1999). *Philosophy, Psychiatry, & Psychology*, 6(2): 95–100.

Svenaeus, F. (1999a). Alexithymia: a phenomenological approach. *Philosophy, Psychiatry, & Psychology*, 6(2): 71–82.

Svenaeus, F. (1999b). Response to the Commentaries. *Philosophy, Psychiatry, & Psychology*, 6(2): 105–108.

Urfer, A. (2001). Phenomenology and psychopathology of schizophrenia: the views of Eugene Minkowski. *Philosophy, Psychiatry, & Psychology*, 8(4): 279–290.

Varela, F.J., Thompson, E.T., and Rosch, E. (1992). *The Embodied Mind: cognitive science and human experience*. Cambridge, MA: MIT Press.

Warner, M. (1999). Theory and practice: negotiating the differences. (Commentary on Widdershoven, 1999a). *Philosophy, Psychiatry, & Psychology*, 6(4): 265–266.

Widdershoven, G.A.M. (1998). A phenomenology of dyslexia. (Commentary on Philpott, 1998a). *Philosophy, Psychiatry, & Psychology*, 5(1): 29–32.

Widdershoven, G.A.M. (1999a). Cognitive psychology and hermeneutics: two approaches to meaning and mental disorder. *Philosophy, Psychiatry, & Psychology*, 6(4): 245–254.

Widdershoven, G.A.M. (1999b). Response to the Commentaries. *Philosophy, Psychiatry, & Psychology*, 6(4): 267–270.

Widdershoven, G.A.M. and Widdershoven-Heerding, I (2003). *Understanding Dementia: a Hermeneutic Perspective*. Ch 6 in K.W.M. Fulford, K.J. Morris, J.Z. Sadler and G. Stanghellini (eds) Nature and Narrative: an introduction to the new philosophy of psychiatry. Oxford: Oxford University Press.

Wiggins, O.P., Schwartz, M.A., and Naudin, J. (2001). Husserlian comments on Blankenburgs psychopathology of common sense. (Commentary on Blankenburg, 2001). *Philosophy, Psychiatry, & Psychology*, 8(4): 327–330.

Zahavi, D. (2001). Schizophrenia and self-awareness. (Commentary on Bin, 2001). *Philosophy, Psychiatry, & Psychology*, 8(4): 339–342.

CHAPTER 9

Phenomenology and psychopathology

Chapter contents

Introduction

This is the first of two chapters in which we will be looking in detail at the philosophical basis of the work of Karl Jaspers, the philosophical father of modern psychopathology. As we saw in Chapter 8, Jaspers envisaged his psychopathology as being founded on phenomenology. In this chapter, therefore, we will look more closely at phenomenology itself, and, in particular, the way it developed in the work of Edmund Husserl. In Chapter 10, we will move on to the second main philosophical influence on Jaspers' psychopathology, the *Methodenstreit*, and how Jaspers used this to formulate an approach to psychopathology, which draws on aspects of both the natural and human sciences.

Husserl and Jaspers

The purpose of this chapter, then, is to introduce Husserl's work and to assess how, and to what extent, Jaspers was influenced by him. One of Jaspers' early articles, which we introduced in Chapter 8, is indeed called 'The phenomenological approach in psychopathology', but there has been recent debate over whether Jaspers' notion of phenomenology is anything like Husserl's! Husserl's project is a fascinating one in its own right. It is important, therefore, to gain a sense of what Husserl was doing before trying to decide whether Jaspers was doing the same.

Husserl and many others

There is, however, a further reason why a study of Husserl's work is important—even if it turns out, as we shall see, that Jaspers' notion of phenomenology bears little resemblance to Husserl's. Husserl's phenomenology is commonly regarded as setting in motion the distinctive tradition of twentieth century philosophy

usually known as Continental philosophy (introduced above, Chapter 4). This tradition is made up of a highly heterogeneous set of philosophical approaches, all of which, to a greater or lesser extent, have their roots in a critical engagement with Husserl. Some of the more well known philosophers who fall within this tradition are Martin Heidegger, Hans-Georg Gadamer, Emmanuel Levinas, Jean-Paul Sartre, Paul Ricoeur, and Jacques Derrida. Their work has become a rich source for those seeking a philosophical understanding of mental health and illness in the context of a broad and inclusive approach to human life.

We introduced a number of these philosophers in Part I (especially in Chapter 4). We conclude this chapter with a brief look at a further important figure from this tradition, Martin Heidegger. Additional reading on modern phenomenology, including a number of contributions to this book series, is given in the Reading guide to this chapter.

Session 1 Jaspers' phenomenological approach to psychopathology

In Chapter 8, we looked at the later of Jaspers' two articles, 'Causal and "meaningful" connections' (published in 1913), before turning to his earlier article on 'The phenomenological approach in psychopathology' (published in 1912). The reason for approaching Jaspers' work in reverse order was that the later article, in treating the difference between understanding a mental disorder and giving a causal explanation of it, allowed us to come to an initial grasp of the peculiar nature of psychopathology as a discipline with links to both the human sciences (such as history, where one seeks to understand the thoughts and actions of, say, Napoleon) and the natural sciences (where one seeks to formulate causal laws governing the emergence of observed effects).

Mental states and psychopathology

This 'peculiar nature', however, is of course not restricted to psychopathology but is a feature of psyche, or mental states, as a whole. Phenomenology, as developed by Husserl, is concerned with identifying and characterizing exactly what the peculiar nature of mental states consists in.

The term 'phenomenology', as we will see in this chapter, has been and continues to be used with many different meanings. This has led to much confusion, not least, as we will argue in this chapter, for Jaspers himself. Jaspers often uses the term phenomenology, much as it is widely used today, to mean a method for carefully describing and cataloguing particular mental states. But for Husserl, at least, phenomenology was a more fundamental activity: it was an analysis of the basic conceptual framework within which talk of mental states, including such distinctions as that between meanings and causes, is possible at all.

It is this basic conceptual framework, we will argue, rather than phenomenology as a method, that Jaspers owes to Husserl. It is also through critiques of the framework proposed by Husserl,

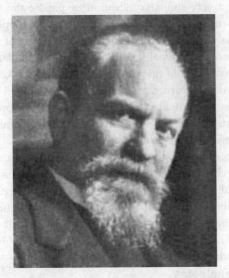

Fig. 9.1 Edmund Husserl

that, as we noted above, later philosophers, in the Continental tradition, have enriched our understanding of psychopathology.

Mental states and Husserl's phenomenology

As a first step, then, in understanding this basic conceptual framework, we will look at the problem with which Husserl himself was concerned, the nature of mental states.

Husserl's problem: what is a mental state?

Consider the following two statements.

- John is depressed because of the death of his friend,
- John is depressed because of a neurochemical imbalance in his brain.

The first statement, in the term of Chapter 8, cites a 'meaningful connection'—one might say that being depressed on account of the death of a friend is 'understandable'; whereas the second statement cites a 'causal connection' between the state of depression and brain chemistry, a connection that has been established through lengthy scientific investigations.

In both, we are talking about a type of conscious mental state or a form of experience. John, we said, 'is depressed'. Are we clear, however, about what these terms, 'mental state' and 'experience' mean? They are terms we can easily take for granted—we use them in everyday life as well as in clinical contexts—but are we really clear about what a mental state is, what the essential aspects of it are, whether there are fundamentally different types of mental state, or whether all mental states have structures in common?

For example, under the broad title of 'mental state' one might list 'belief' and 'perception' as two very different types of mental state—and one might then count 'delusion' and 'hallucination' as abnormal forms of these. While the empirical scientist may be interested in surveying the commonest forms of delusion, from a philosophical perspective we seek to understand what a belief is and how it is related to other fundamental types of mental state. Jaspers was interested in the question of the difference between a causal account of a mental state and an understanding of it, but this presupposes a grasp of the very thing we are considering in these two different ways—what a mental state is! This latter question is not an empirical matter, but a conceptual matter—one is seeking clarification of the everyday and seemingly self-evident concepts we use in talking about other people. This type of conceptual investigation was what Husserl, in his early work, called 'phenomenology'—an investigation of mental phenomena aimed at clarifying the very idea of 'mental phenomena'.

Husserl's project: to clarify the concept of a mental state

Husserl was well aware that his more empirically minded colleagues might regard his project as rather trivial—rather than going out and making an empirical survey of the commonest types of mental state

and their abnormalities, Husserl proposed merely to sit down and analyse what we mean by a mental state in the first place!

Throughout his life, however, Husserl regarded phenomenology as playing a vitally important role in relation to scientific research—the clarification of the basic conceptual schemes within which scientific research is undertaken; and in his early work the conceptual scheme he was interested in is that which we use to talk about other people—their 'mental states'. If someone were to regard such an investigation as concerning itself with mere trivialities, then Husserl would agree, but add that this makes the investigation simply more pressing:

> It ill befits the philosopher, the dedicated representative of purely theoretical interests, to let himself be guided by considerations of practical use. He must surely know that it is precisely behind the obvious that the hardest problems lie hidden, that this is so much so, in fact, that philosophy may be paradoxically, but not unprofoundly, called the science of the trivial. In the present case at least what seems at first quite trivial, reveals itself, on closer examination, as the source of deep-lying, widely ramifying problems.   (Husserl [1900–01] 1970a p. 528)

Husserl and Austin: clarifying concepts basic to science

There are many resonances here with the characterization of the role of philosophy we took from J.L. Austin and others in the Anglo-American tradition of analytic philosophy, developed early in Chapters 2, 4, and 6. But it might otherwise strike you as quite strange that a philosopher should describe philosophy as the 'science of the trivial'. Husserl was concerned throughout his life with a view of philosophy as a process of clarifying the concepts that we normally use without thinking about them, including the concepts that are taken for granted as the basic concepts in a particular science.

This is a very similar conception of philosophy to that of Austin, then. Both philosophers believed that philosophy's role is that of analysing and clarifying our understanding of seemingly trivial concepts—'trivial' because they are so fundamental to our everyday ways of thinking that we normally take them for granted. As you learn more about Husserl, you will see other similarities: in particular, their common emphasis on the need not to just 'play games' with words, but to 'look and see' how concepts are used in concrete practices.

In Husserl and Austin, then, we see the extent to which the distinction between 'analytic' philosophy and 'continental' philosophy breaks down: the father of modern Continental philosophy and a leading figure of British analytic philosophy would seem to be following quite similar paths!

Jaspers' view of Husserl's early and later phenomenologies

The text by Husserl from which the above extract was taken, *Logical Investigations*, although Husserl's second major work, is definitive of what is now known as his 'early' phenomenology. Published in two volumes, in 1900 and 1901, *Logical Investigations* is a huge (over 800 pages in the English translation) and densely written text. We will be looking at it more closely below.

Husserl's first major work was the *Philosophy of Arithmetic*. This is similar in a number of respects to *Logical Investigations* and is the work in which Husserl first sets out his notion of phenomenology. The *Logical Investigations*, on the other hand, is the work that had most influence on Jaspers. Indeed, it appears that Jaspers only ever read two texts by Husserl; the second being Husserl's short piece entitled 'Philosophy as rigorous science' which was published in 1911.

By 1911, with the publication of 'Philosophy as rigorous science', Husserl had moved to a very different notion of phenomenology. This new account of phenomenology, Husserl's 'later phenomenology', is widely distinguished from his earlier work as 'transcendental phenomenology'. Hussel's transcendental phenomenology is sketched out initially in 'Philosophy as rigorous science' and then developed in a programmatic text of 1913 that he took to replace *Logical Investigations* as definitive of phenomenology. This text has the rather unwieldy title 'Ideas pertaining to a Pure Phenomenology and to a Phenomenological Philosophy, first book: General Introduction to a Pure Phenomenology'. The title is universally shortened to *Ideas I*, for obvious reasons! We shall look briefly at Husserl's notion of a transcendental phenomenology below.

As far as is known Jaspers never read Hussel's *Ideas I*. Indeed, having read the 1911 text 'Philosophy as rigorous science', Jaspers concluded that Husserl was no longer pursuing a form of philosophy with which he had any sympathy. It was, then, the earlier phenomenology of *Logical Investigations* that Jaspers regarded as more useful for his own work.

There is a further complication, though, of which we have to take account if we are to properly assess the extent to which Husserl's work forms a foundation for Jaspers' psychopathology. This complication relates to what Jaspers means when he uses the terms 'phenomenology' or 'phenomenological approach'. We shall see that Jaspers' idea of phenomenology is different in important ways even from Husserl's early notion, while at the same time, he draws ideas from Husserl that he does not explicitly acknowledge as phenomenological ideas. What this means is that in assessing the role of Husserl's phenomenology on Jaspers' thinking, we are going to have to look deeper than simply at what Jaspers means when he explicitly uses the term.

Five questions about Jaspers' phenomenology

One way to explore the influence of Husserl's work on Jaspers is through a careful reading of Jaspers' article 'The phenomenological approach in psychopathology'.

EXERCISE 1 (60 minutes)

As part of this exercise, please re-read Jaspers' article, which we first looked at in Chapter 8 (Exercise 5).

Jaspers, K. (1968). The phenomenological approach in psychopathology. *British Journal of Psychiatry*, 114: 1313–1323 (anonymous translation of 'Die Phänomenologische Forschungsrichtung in der Psychopathologie', 1912, Zeitschrift fur die gesante Neurologie und Psychiatrie, 9: 391–408)

Link with Reading 9.1 (This is same as Reading 8.2—Chapter 8/Exercise 5)

A key part of understanding what Jaspers means by 'phenomenology' is to grasp what he means by the 'subjective symptoms' of a patient's disorder. It is 'subjective symptoms' that are the concern of phenomenology for Jaspers. *Before* re-reading the article, therefore, note down what sorts of thing you think would fall under the category of 'subjective symptom'. Then, having read it, answer the following questions:

1. How does Jaspers characterize the nature of 'subjective symptoms'?
2. What does Jaspers mean by 'empathy'?
3. What is the place of phenomenology, for Jaspers, within psychopathology as a whole?
4. What is the task of phenomenology in Jaspers' view?
5. What does Jaspers identify as the 'boundaries of phenomenology'?

Question 1: the nature of subjective symptoms

On the face of it, one might guess that the term 'subjective symptom' would refer to the thoughts, ideas, feelings, attitudes, etc. that we think of as making up a patient's 'state of mind'. However, as you may have noticed at the very beginning of Jaspers' article, things are not so simple! We are going to take the answer to the first question in this exercise rather slowly—indeed, you might think the following paragraphs are rather hair-splitting! However, if we are to grasp what Jaspers means by phenomenology, everything depends on first being as clear as we can about what the 'subjective symptoms' are, with which phenomenology is (on Jaspers' view) concerned.

Subjective and objective symptoms

The best way of approaching what Jaspers means by 'subjective symptoms' is to look at how he sets them apart from 'objective symptoms'. We might think of 'objective' symptoms as the external manifestations of a patient's disorder—things that are, in various senses, publicly on view. Jaspers includes 'all concrete events that can be perceived by the senses', and 'measurable performances', but also, notably, a patient's utterances, written expressions, and ideas.

Jaspers' use of the term 'objective' is thus rather broad; one might, for example, think of the sounds produced or the physical markings made on paper as 'objective' in a strict sense, and clearly the meaningfulness of an utterance is not objective in this sense. Nor is a delusional idea 'objective' in the same way as a facial tic—yet Jaspers counts 'the rational contents of what the patient tells us', i.e. what particular idea is being talked about, what its content is, as 'objective'. Jaspers acknowledges that his notion of objective symptoms includes things that 'are not perceived by the senses, but only understood...through rational thought'—but the problem is that Jaspers tells us that 'subjective symptoms', too, are things that cannot be perceived by the senses. Further, in our initial guess at what might fall under 'subjective symptoms'— thoughts, ideas, beliefs—we included things that precisely are 'not perceived by the senses, but only understood', and are thus 'objective symptoms' for Jaspers! What then does he mean by 'subjective symptoms'?

Things are not helped by what Jaspers goes on to say in the second paragraph of the article. There he says that subjective symptoms 'are all those psychic experiences and phenomena which patients describe to us'—yet if we ask a patient to describe his or her mental state, are we not given 'objective symptoms', in other words, things we 'understand' through 'rational thought'? Given the breadth of what Jaspers counts as an objective symptom, it can begin to seem quite mysterious what precisely a 'subjective symptom' is!

The clue to what Jaspers means by 'subjective symptom' comes in his reference to 'empathy' in the first paragraph. As we have seen, there are objective symptoms that are not purely physical manifestations, and require 'understanding', but our grasp of these symptoms 'is achieved through rational thought, without the help of any empathy into the patient's psyche'. 'Empathy' is again mentioned in the second paragraph, where we find Jaspers directly stating that 'subjective symptoms' are what are given to us through empathy with the patient:

> Subjective symptoms cannot be perceived by the sense-organs, but have to be grasped by transferring oneself, so to say, into the other individual's psyche; that is, by empathy. They can only become an inner reality for the observer by his participating in the other person's experiences, not by any intellectual effort.
>
> (p. 1313)

It seemed, at first, that we were going to be told what 'subjective symptoms' are by setting them off from objective symptoms, but now it seems that to have a grasp of 'objective symptoms' one needs to know what Jaspers means by 'empathy' (as 'objective symptoms' include those that can be understood without empathy). Yet the only grasp we have on the notion of empathy is that it gives us access to 'subjective symptoms'. Before we can properly answer our first question, then, we will need an answer to our second: what does Jaspers mean by 'empathy'?

Question 2: Jaspers' notion of empathy

If phenomenology, for Jaspers, is concerned with 'subjective symptoms', then the notion of 'empathy' must be an essential aspect of it, as it is empathy that gives us access to 'subjective symptoms'. We need, therefore, to come to an initial understanding of 'empathy' if we are to grasp Jaspers' notion of phenomenology. (The idea of empathy will be taken up again in the next section, as Wilhelm Dilthey, one of the key protagonists in the *Methodenstreit*, took empathy to be an essential part of what distinguishes the method of the human sciences from that of the natural sciences.)

Jaspers gives an initial indication of what he means by 'empathy' in the above quotation: it involves 'transferring oneself, so to say, into the other individual's psyche'. The qualification, 'so to say', is all important here—as clearly one cannot literally transfer oneself into another's psyche! Obviously 'transferring oneself' is a metaphor. But the question is: what aspect of 'transferring oneself' in a literal sense is Jaspers drawing on to illuminate the matter? One suggestion might be that when one literally 'transfers oneself', one moves to a different place and thus sees the world from a different viewpoint. If this is what Jaspers is referring to, then empathy is a process of trying to think how the world seems from the patient's perspective. But this is clearly not what Jaspers means. Finding out about how the world seems from the patient's perspective is to find out what their thoughts, beliefs, ideas, attitudes, feelings, etc., about the world are and these are 'objective symptoms' for Jaspers. Empathy is not a process of trying to think how the patient views the world, as Jaspers is explicit that it does not involve 'any intellectual effort' (literally, 'any thinking', *Denken*). Rather, Jaspers says it involves 'participating in the other person's experiences'. But again this must be a metaphor, as it is difficult to see how one can any more literally participate in someone else's experiences than one can participate in someone else's sneezing!

Many of the expressions Jaspers uses to characterize empathy are similarly metaphorical, and one must be careful not to just leave them unexamined, as if their meaning were unquestionably clear. On p. 1315, for example, Jaspers states that the psychiatrist can 'share' the patient's experience; psychiatrists should seek to 'actualise these phenomena for themselves' (p. 1316), it involves a 'seeing', which is not done through the senses, but through the understanding' (*ibid.*). Perhaps even 'understanding' is metaphorical here—some 'objective symptoms' require 'understanding... achieved through rational thought', so empathy must be a form of understanding achieved without rational thought, and it is certainly difficult to know what this might mean.

Empathy as 'Knowing what it's like'

Just what, then, does Jaspers mean by empathy? While we will consider this question again in Chapter 10, it is important to come to an initial view, because of the place of empathy in Jaspers' understanding of phenomenology. Later in the first section of the article, Jaspers complains that a purely objective psychology leads 'quite systematically to the elimination of everything that can be called mental or psychic' (p. 1314). In order to illustrate what he means, Jaspers refers to the assessment of a patient's fatigue through measurable performances: 'It is not the feeling of fatigue but "objective fatigue" which is being investigated' (*ibid.*). This suggests that what does not fall within the category of 'objective symptoms' is what it's like to be fatigued. One could then extend this idea to other types of objective symptom, for example:

- *The thought that one's liver has been removed* would be an objective symptom that a patient might manifest—but this would be different from knowing *what it's like to think that one's liver has been removed.*

- *The belief that one's home is being bugged by Russian spies* would be an objective symptom—but this would be different from knowing *what it's like to believe that one's home is being bugged by Russian spies.*

- *The feeling of depression* would be an objective symptom—but this would be different from *knowing what it's like to feel depressed.*

It would seem, therefore, that for Jaspers empathy is a process of coming to know, in a personal and direct sense, what it is like to undergo the type of experience that the patient is going through. Towards the end of the article Jaspers himself says that phenomenology, using empathy, 'views psychic events "as from within"' (p. 1322), and the suggestion is confirmed—to an extent—by the following statement from Jaspers:

> [The psychiatrist] can share the patient's experiences—always provided this happens spontaneously without his having to take thought over it. In this way he can gain an essentially personal, indefinable and direct understanding, which, however, remains for him a matter of pure experience, not of explicit knowledge.
>
> (p. 1315)

The last part of this statement is quite striking—what empathy gives us remains 'a matter of pure experience, not of explicit *knowledge*'. Thus it is perhaps not strictly accurate to say, as we did above, that empathy is a process of coming to *know* what it's like to undergo a certain type of experience. Coming to *know* something about the patient's type of experience is what happens when one correctly grasps an *objective* symptom, for Jaspers; it would thus be better to say that in empathy one simply lives through—in one's imagination presumably—the same type of experience as that which the patient is living through.

The incommunicability of empathy

Jaspers himself says, in the above quotation, that in this way the psychiatrist comes to 'an essentially personal, indefinable and direct understanding'—but even this cannot be quite right. To possess an 'understanding' of an experience is surely for that experience to be the object of some sort of rational reflection directed to it. In other words, it would involve reflecting upon it, rather than living through it as a 'pure experience'. It is a consequence, of course, of this notion of empathy that what empathy gives you is simply incommunicable—one cannot communicate to anyone else what it's like to undergo a certain type of experience, as this is something that can only be lived through (either imaginatively or in reality). Jaspers seems to acknowledge this when he writes: '[The phenomenologist] must make sure that those to whom he addresses himself do not simply *think* along with him, but that they *see* along with him (p. 1316)'.

The contrast between 'thinking' and 'seeing' is presumably meant to capture the immediacy of living through an experience—an immediacy that is lost when our grasp of it is 'mediated' by concepts—which is what happens when we attempt to communicate it to others.

The question is, of course, what possible use is empathy, in psychopathology, if what it gives us cannot be communicated to anyone else? If I cannot, in principle, communicate the results of empathy to another psychopathologist, then it could be that his exercise in empathy results in something quite different, and we would never know! More seriously, if one cannot, in principle, communicate the results of empathy to another, then it would seem that the notion of empathy becomes a free spinning cog within the science of psychopathology—in other words, it does no real work. The philosopher Ludwig Wittgenstein used similar arguments against theories that give an explanatory role to incommunicable inner mental states, and concluded 'that a nothing would serve just as well as a something about which nothing could be said' (*Philosophical Investigations* # 304)!

We will be looking more closely at Wittgenstein's work in Part V. For the moment it is enough to see that Jaspers' notions of empathy and incommunicable 'subjective phenomena' put him in rather a difficult position. On the one hand he is convinced of the essential role played by empathy in psychopathology:

> Only so do we acquire a fruitful critical faculty which will set itself against the framing of theoretical constructions as much as against the barren deadly denial of any possibility of progress. Whoever has no eyes to see cannot practise histology; whoever is unwilling or incapable of actualising psychic events and representing them vividly cannot acquire an understanding of phenomenology.
>
> (pp. 1316–1317)

And on the other hand he has to acknowledge that, in trying to imaginatively live through a type of experience, one has to rely on things that *can* be communicated, for example statements made by a patient: in other words, things that fall under the category of 'objective symptoms'. Thus rather than subjective symptoms providing any basis for our understanding of objective symptoms, Jaspers has to admit that it is objective symptoms that provide any sort of basis for our imaginative re-creation of subjective symptoms:

> The more numerous and specific these indirect hints become, the more well-defined and characteristic do the phenomena studied appear. Indeed, this personal effort to represent psychic phenomena to oneself under the guidance of these purely external hints is the condition under which alone we can speak of any kind of psychological work at all.
>
> (p. 1316)

One is left wondering why anyone would bother with this 'personal effort' (i.e. of empathy), and how it contributes to 'psychological work', given that: (1) its results could not be communicated to anyone; (2) no one would know if they had performed it in the same way as anyone else; and (3) no one would know if you had attempted it all!

The role of empathy in psychiatry

There is another initial conclusion one might draw at this point. Given that the idea of 'empathy' with a patient does, intuitively, sound like a good and beneficial psychotherapeutic practice, one might conclude that Jaspers has simply given a wrong analysis of it—rather than thinking that the notion itself is wrongheaded. Whether this is the right conclusion to draw, however, is a question that will have to wait until Chapter 10, when we look more closely at the idea that empathy plays a key role in the methodology of the human sciences as a whole. All we can conclude at present is that there is something deeply problematic with Jaspers' notion of empathy as part of a 'phenomenological approach to psychopathology'.

One might be tempted to conclude, further, that Husserl's influence on Jaspers was not altogether a positive thing—but this would be too hasty. One should not conclude that the notion of empathy is central to Husserl's conception of phenomenology, on the basis of its being central for Jaspers. We shall see below that Husserl's phenomenology differs from Jaspers' quite radically on this point. Before turning to consider Husserl's work, however, it will be helpful to look at what else Jaspers says about phenomenology, in order to be able to form a more balanced assessment of Husserl's influence. In other words, we need to put on one side our reservations about the role of empathy in a 'phenomenological approach', and look at what Jaspers says about the place of phenomenology in psychopathology, its particular aims, and how it differs from other types of psychology. It could be that here we do indeed find evidence of Husserl's influence.

Question 3: Jaspers' view of the place of phenomenology in psychopathology

This question is easier to answer. Psychopathology is made up of 'objective psychology' and 'subjective psychology', and phenomenology is a part of the latter.

From the very beginning of the article, Jaspers is concerned to defend the existence of a 'subjective psychology' alongside 'objective psychology'. The explosion of interest in experimental psychology towards the end of the nineteenth century had led to the proliferation of purely quantitative measures of mental ability, for example, experiments designed to test how many items on a list can be remembered in different conditions, or at different ages. This tendency, Jaspers argues, is in danger of producing a 'psychology without a psyche':

> All such concepts as fatigability, the power of recovery, learning ability, practice, the effects of rest periods, etc., refer to performances that can be measured objectively, and it does not matter whether one is dealing here with a machine, a live but mindless organism, or a human being endowed with a mind.   (p. 1314)

It is in the face of the predominance of such 'objective psychology' that Jaspers wishes to defend and develop the idea of a 'subjective psychology', a psychology that retains 'psychic life as its object of study' (p. 1314). Given Jaspers' description of objective psychology above, his complaint that it is a 'psychology without a psyche' looks well founded. It is worth remembering, however, that Jaspers' notion of an 'objective symptom' (i.e. what is studied by objective psychology) is much broader than the above description suggests. The 'rational content' of a person's ideas also counts as an objective symptom for Jaspers—and yet we do not think of this class of objective symptoms as applying indifferently to a machine, a 'mindless organism', and a human being. You would not think of your computer as believing that the sun is shining, even though *believing that the sun is shining* is an objective symptom for Jaspers. He is attempting to strengthen his case for a 'subjective psychology' by presenting an overly narrow view of objective psychology.

Phenomenology as static understanding

For most of the article one might be forgiven for thinking that 'phenomenology' is just another name for subjective psychology; it is only towards the end that we find that it is only a limited part of it. It turns out that subjective psychology is made up of two different ways of understanding mental states, which Jaspers calls 'static understanding' and 'genetic understanding' respectively. In Jaspers' view phenomenology only consists of the former.

> 'Genetic understanding' [is] the understanding of the meaningful connections between one psychic experience and another, the 'emergence of the psychic from the psychic'. Now phenomenology itself has nothing to do with this 'genetic understanding' and must be treated as something entirely separate.   (p. 1322)

While in 'genetic understanding' we are concerned with the meaningful connection between one mental state and another, phenomenology, for Jaspers, is concerned with mental states taken in isolation. A trivial example of a meaningful connection would be that between a belief that one had won the lottery and a state of happiness about having won the lottery; phenomenology, in Jaspers view, would be concerned with each of these mental states—a belief and a state of happiness—taken in isolation.

Jaspers' view of phenomenology and Husserl's

Before we go into Husserl's work in more detail below, it is worth signalling again at this point that Jaspers' conception of phenomenology differs quite considerably from Husserl's. First of all, Husserl always considered his phenomenology as a type of fundamental philosophical investigation, a 'theory of knowledge', or more precisely an analysis of what it means to be a 'knowing subject'. That is, Husserl was concerned to provide an analysis of what it means to be a subject that is capable of scientific knowledge of the world. Phenomenology, therefore, is neither on a par with, nor a part of, other types of scientific investigation, but rather is conceived as a *foundation* for them: a foundation in the sense of clarifying what it means to be capable of scientific investigation in the first place. We will come back to this idea below.

Secondly, Husserl by no means limits phenomenology to the study of mental states taken in isolation, but is deeply concerned with the connections between mental states: both in the way that one (higher order) type of mental state may depend on the contemporaneous existence of another (more basic) type of mental state, and in the way that mental states may be sequentially connected. We shall see, however, that Husserl limits phenomenology to a much narrower notion of 'meaningful connection' between mental states. Simplifying greatly, one might say that Husserl is interested in 'rational connections' where 'rational' signifies a much stronger form of 'meaningful connection'. For example, the emergence of a state of happiness on the basis of a belief that one had won the lottery, would not strictly be a rational connection for Husserl. One is not rationally obliged to become happy on learning that one has won the lottery, and perhaps there are people for whom winning the lottery would not be a reason for happiness at all (though we don't know any!).

In relation to these two points, and in relation to the notion of empathy, we shall see just how little there is in common between Husserl's conception of phenomenology and Jaspers when we look at Husserl's work below. Again, however, in order to come to a balanced assessment we must look further at what Jaspers says about phenomenology. In particular, we have not yet really considered what Jaspers thinks the *aim* of phenomenology is. What does it do, and what does Jaspers think it's for?

Question 4: Jaspers' view of the aim of phenomenology

The aim of phenomenology is stated near the beginning of Jaspers article, on p. 1314: its aim is to inject some sort of initial order into the 'manifold diversity of psychic phenomena'. What is a little confusing is that Jaspers first provides a statement of the aims of subjective psychology as a whole (which, you remember, turns out to be made up of phenomenology and 'genetic understanding'):

> What then are the precise aims of this much-abused subjective psychology? [. . .] It asks itself—speaking quite generally—what does mental experience depend on, what are its consequences, and what relationships can be discerned in it? The answers to these questions are its special aims. (p. 1314)

This is not itself a terribly clear statement, but it helps us to realize that the statement cannot refer to subjective psychology as a whole, but only to 'genetic understanding', despite what Jaspers says. Jaspers does not distinguish phenomenology and genetic understanding until later, and the description does not fit phenomenology at all, this being the study of mental states taken in isolation. Rather, phenomenology's aims are preparatory to those of 'genetic understanding', which constitutes 'real inquiry':

> So before real inquiry can begin it is necessary to identify the specific psychic phenomena which are to be its subject, and

form a clear picture of the resemblances and differences between them and other phenomena with which they must not be confused. This preliminary work of representing, defining, and classifying psychic phenomena, pursued as an independent activity, constitutes phenomenology. (*Ibid.*)

The aim of phenomenology in psychopathology is thus to describe and name the rich diversity of pathological mental states, and to group them in suitable classifications—a taxonomy, one might say, of mental disorder. Jaspers clearly contrasts phenomenology with other psychological approaches that might seek to reduce our appreciation of this rich diversity, by attempting to explain the diverse range in terms of a small number of principles.

> For while the ideal of phenomenology is an infinity of irreducible psychic qualities, classified and ordered to permit of their survey, there exists another, opposite ideal, that of the fewest possible ultimate elements, as in chemistry. [. . .] Phenomenology, on the other hand, rejects the ideal of the fewest possible elements; on the contrary it has no wish to restrict the infinite variety of psychic phenomena, only, as far as possible (for the task is, of course, boundless) to try to make them more lucid, precise and individually recognisable at any time. (p. 1321)

Jaspers' view of the aims of phenomenology and Husserl's

Again, it will be useful at this stage to provide a brief indication of whether the aim that Jaspers attributes to phenomenology bears any resemblance to what Husserl envisages as its aim. On the face of it, as we shall see further below, their views are diametrically opposed. Husserl was precisely concerned in setting out the ultimate elements involved in any mental state—he argued that our everyday rich vocabulary for talking about mental states can be clarified by identifying the essential aspects of our very notion of a mental state. We must be careful not to misunderstand Husserl here, and we will look more closely at this point below. It is not, for example, that Husserl wishes to deny that there are irreducible qualitative differences between mental states, such as happiness, anxiety, worry, fear, hopefulness, anger, etc., but only that in talking about mental states in this way we are referring to a single aspect of mental states, which Husserl calls the 'quality' of a mental state. This aspect of mental states is quite different from another regard in which we talk about them—we are often concerned with the 'content' of a mental state, i.e. *what* someone is happy about, *what* someone is worried about, etc. This aspect of a mental state is what Husserl calls its 'matter'.

To a large extent, then, Husserl abstracts from the rich diversity of mental life, in order to provide a more *formal* description of what belongs to the very idea of mental life, or more precisely, of the mental states or experiences, which we take mental life to consist of. When Husserl does give a detailed description of a specific types of mental state, it is because he takes these to be essential to the very idea of ourselves as capable of knowledge of the world. He talks in detail, for example, about the difference and relation between a belief that such and such is the case, and the perception that such and such is the case. In other words, he is concerned with basic 'knowledge situations', for example, first merely thinking that one has £10 in one's pocket, and then seeing that this is indeed so.

Jaspers, on the other hand, is clearly reacting against this aim of Husserl's phenomenology. Indeed, he over-reacts in that he often emphasizes the irreducible qualitative differences between types of mental states, without being able to see the connection between them:

> Now in the present state of phenomenology, it would seem that there exist numerous groups of phenomena between which no relationship can be perceived. Sense-perceptions and ideas, hallucinations and delusions, seem to be phenomena separated by a gulf rather than united by transitions. Such totally unrelated phenomena can only be placed under separate headings and cannot be organised into any particular pattern within the psychic life.   (p. 1320)

Husserl might respond in two ways: first, given that the 'phenomena' we are picking out all belong to 'psychic life' one might expect them to share formal features in common that belong to the very idea of a mental state. Secondly, might there not be important connections between say a perception and an idea, or a hallucination and a delusion. If one hallucinates an elephant chasing after you, the relation between this and a delusory belief that one is being chased by an elephant, is certainly not a 'gulf'!

Are their views really so opposed?

On the face of it, Husserl's view of the aim of phenomenology is diametrically opposed to that of Jaspers. It is difficult to see how one could suggest any positive influence by Husserl on this point. Indeed, in giving his view of the aim of phenomenology, Jaspers seems to acknowledge that there is another view of phenomenology (i.e. Husserl's) that is quite different:

> As one procedure among others, phenomenology brings to light psychic qualities that appear as constituents of what is being studied. This breaking down of complex structures into constituents is only one way of proceeding; but those who adopt the point of view already described, which is valid only in relation to the origination of psychic phenomena, speak as if it were the only way. They would, for example, explain perception by analysing it into the elements of sensation, spatial perception and intentional act, whereas true phenomenology would first compare perception with imagery, which is composed of the same elements, and come to the conclusion that perception must be characterised as an irreducible psychic quality.   (p. 1321)

This is a very revealing statement, and it is worth noting several points. First, we see Jaspers' concern to regard perception as 'an irreducible psychic quality', playing down the fact that it has elements in common with 'imagery'. Secondly, he contrasts 'true phenomenology' with a brief description of an analysis that is very similar to the approach Jaspers himself takes in other papers, for example his two papers on 'false perceptions'. In the footnote to p. 1314 of the present article, he describes these two papers as

conducting 'systematic phenomenological investigations'—whereas in the above quotation this type of phenomenological investigation is held to be not 'true phenomenology'.

Why does Jaspers refuse to recognize Husserl's more analytic approach as 'true phenomenology'? One reason is that, as we saw above, phenomenology for Jaspers is merely a form of descriptive taxonomy of mental states. There is a second reason, however, which is hinted at in the above quotation—he argues that the approach which is concerned to identify common elements in diverse types of mental state 'is only valid in relation to the origination of psychic phenomena'. What Jaspers means is that an approach that aims at 'analysis into ultimate elements' is a procedure of use only in the natural sciences. Indeed, he explicitly states: 'This ideal takes its cue from the natural sciences, and certainly has a meaning in relation to the origin of psychic qualities.' (ibid.)

In other words, Jaspers regards Husserl's approach of identifying common aspects shared by all mental states as the first step towards a natural scientific explanation of mental states, and their diversity, in terms of a few general principles: 'Just as the infinite variety of colours can be traced to purely quantitative differences in wave-length, so one could wish to explain the origins of psychic qualities and perhaps establish different classifications on this basis.' (ibid.)

It is an aim of natural sciences, clearly, to put forward explanations that are able to account for a diverse range of phenomena in terms of a small number of explanatory principles. Yet, as we shall see below, Husserl in his attempt to analyse mental states into their common elements, was by no means trying to 'explain' them in terms of some simple underlying mechanism, or reduce qualitative differences to merely quantitative ones. Husserl envisages phenomenology as a purely 'descriptive' undertaking—but part of its aim is also to bring clarity to our understanding of mental states by bringing to light the formal structures they have in common. Husserl's phenomenology strives for the simplification of the rich diversity of mental states, but its aim is not 'explanation', but 'clarification' or 'elucidation'. The simplification phenomenology aims for is not that of positing a simple underlying mechanism, but rather is closer to the type of simplification one achieves through 'formalization'. Just as in mathematics we abstract from the rich diversity of things we might choose to count, so in Husserl's phenomenology we abstract from the rich diversity of mental states in order to focus on the formal structures implicit in mental states as such.

It seems then, that while both Jaspers and Husserl regarded phenomenology as a purely descriptive undertaking, Jaspers misunderstood the nature of the type of description Husserl was aiming at, with the result that he did not regard the sort of phenomenological analysis that Husserl would give as 'true phenomenology'. The basic idea, however, that phenomenology is a descriptive and not an explanatory undertaking, still suggests an influence of Husserl on Jaspers, and so we now need to look at what Jaspers says about this 'limitation' of phenomenology more closely.

Question 5: Jaspers' view of the limitations of phenomenology

At the end of the article, Jaspers has a section titled 'The boundaries of phenomenology', the aim of which is to make clear what phenomenology 'does not intend to pursue, and with what phenomenology should not be confused' (p. 1322). You might have picked up on the following points:

1. *Phenomenology is a descriptive and not an explanatory undertaking.* Jaspers makes this point in several different ways: phenomenology does not concern itself 'with any factors that may be thought to underlie psychic events', 'phenomenology can gain nothing from theory', and it 'has nothing to do with the [causal] genesis of psychic phenomena'.

2. *Phenomenology must be kept separate from 'genetic understanding'.* We looked at this point above; Jaspers' term 'genetic understanding' refers to the way that the emergence of one mental state from another may be a 'meaningful connection'. The term should not be confused with 'genetic' in the more modern sense or with a study of the causal 'genesis' of a mental state.

3. *Phenomenology concerns the forms of mental experience, not the particular contents.* You might easily have missed this one, as Jaspers only mentions it in passing at the end of the section while summarizing the above two points!

We have considered the second limitation already, and how it represents a quite different view of what phenomenology looks at, compared with Husserl. The first limitation is going to be our main focus, but it is worth thinking briefly about the third point first.

On the face of it, this again represents a huge departure from Husserl's conception of phenomenology, in that Husserl was predominantly concerned to do justice to the 'content' of mental states—the way that they are about things and events, whether imaginary or real. Having said this, however, Husserl's phenomenology, as a formal analysis of mental states, is not concerned with the particular things people know or believe, or with questions of which beliefs are more common and are more rare. Jaspers is suggesting that phenomenology, as part of psychopathology, is not concerned with providing a taxonomy of, say, all the different things that figure in the context of people's delusions, and Husserl would agree that this is not phenomenology's job.

There is, however, a further more subtle point that needs to be made here. In denying that phenomenology is concerned with the 'contents of the personal experience of the individual' (p. 1323), Jaspers is drawing on a distinction between 'form' and 'content', which he takes to apply to all mental states. Husserl uses the more precise terms 'quality' and 'matter' to name two aspects common to all mental states, but Jaspers is clearly following Husserl in his assumption that one can identify elements common to every mental state. This of course conflicts with Jaspers' expressed conviction that 'true phenomenology' should not attempt to identify ultimate elements that are common to all mental states. It would seem that Jaspers *uses* Husserl's conception of phenomenology (as a conceptual analysis of what belongs to the very idea of a mental state) while at the same time denying that this is 'true phenomenology'. You can begin to see that pinning down Husserl's influence on Jaspers' 'phenomenology' is a rather tricky business, and why, as we shall see below, there has been such disagreement about it!

Jaspers' view of phenomenology as purely descriptive

Returning, then, to point 1 above, a key limitation (though not in a negative sense) of phenomenology for Jaspers, is that it does not, and should not, pursue explanations of the emergence and existence of conscious mental states. This is linked closely in Jaspers' thinking with the limitation to static understanding (point 2). Thus he writes: 'Though its practice is a prerequisite for any causal investigation, [phenomenology] leaves genetic issues aside, and they can neither refute nor further its findings' (p. 1322).

However, the limitation to descriptive rather than explanatory accounts of mental states is also spelled out in its own right. In practising phenomenology, Jaspers argued the psychopathologist must constantly be on guard against allowing his descriptions of mental life to become infected by the conceptual schemes of *explanatory theories* of consciousness. Jaspers cites Wernicke as someone who brings 'theoretical constructions of physiological and pathological cerebral processes' into a phenomenological approach to conscious life: 'Thus Wernicke, who in fact did make important discoveries, distorted them by interpretations in terms of "connective fibres", "sejunctions" and the like. These sort of constructs constantly prevent phenomenological investigations from reaching their proper goal.' (*ibid*).

What Jaspers is suggesting is that in our conscious mental lives we have thoughts, perceptions, beliefs, etc., about objects and events, but in having these experiences we are precisely not aware of the neurophysiological processes that make them possible. Reference to these processes should not, therefore, figure in a pure descriptive account of our conscious lives. The phenomenologist should approach mental phenomena without presupposing any particular theory of their causal origin or of the neurophysiological processes that occur in having a given experience. This point leads us to a related idea: the need for a phenomenological approach to be presuppositionless. Jaspers draws this idea from Husserl, for whom the presuppositionlessness of phenomenology was of paramount importance, so it is worth taking a closer look at what Jaspers says about it.

Jaspers' view of the presuppositionlessness of phenomenology

Jaspers notes the need for the phenomenologist to avoid presupposing any particular explanatory theory in describing conscious life, earlier in the paper.

We should picture only what is really present in the patient's consciousness; anything that has not really presented itself to his consciousness is outside our consideration. We must set aside all outmoded theories, psychological constructs or materialist mythologies of cerebral processes; we must turn our attention only to that which we can understand as having real existence, and which we can differentiate and describe. This, as experience has shown, is in itself a very difficult task. This particular freedom from preconception which phenomenology demands is not something one possesses from the beginning, but something that is laboriously acquired after prolonged and critical work and much effort—often fruitless—in framing constructs and mythologies.   (p. 1316)

There are a number of points we can make about this passage. First, what does Jaspers mean by a 'materialist mythology of cerebral processes'? He is not clear on this point, but we can assume he means the citing of general and experimentally unjustified neurological theories to explain the existence of a particular mental state or a sequence of mental states. We must remember that in Jaspers' day the science of neurophysiology was in its infancy, and there certainly was not the technology available to investigate neurological changes in the brain during a particular conscious experience. In the next section we will look at what Jaspers thought of the possibility of giving a neurophysiological explanation of mental disorders in general—as this will be part of understanding how Jaspers tries to accommodate both natural scientific and human scientific approaches within psychiatry.

'Theory-laden' observation

Note, too, how Jaspers regards the avoidance of theoretical notions drawn from causal accounts of mental disorder as something that is hard work, and only acquired after fruitlessly trying to give such accounts. One might say that after an education in various neurological theories of mental dysfunction, the psychopathologist's very observations become 'theory-laden', such that it takes a new effort to free oneself from theoretical presuppositions in one's descriptions.

In Part III, we will be looking much more closely at the notion of 'theory-laden observation', and the argument that—contra Jaspers—observation is always, and inescapably, theory-laden. In a passage that follows on from the above quotation, Jaspers likens psychopathologists to children, who first draw things as they imagine them to be, not as they later see them to be in an 'unprejudiced' way. Jaspers in this way suggests that it is through the putting aside of theoretical approaches to mental disorder that one learns to see them 'as they really are'. One could, however, use Jaspers' analogy to make the opposite point: that children first draw things as they see them, and only later learn how to draw them 'as they really are', when they are educated into a more 'theory-laden' view of the world! It is by no means obvious, then, that theoretical presuppositions have the distorting effect that Jaspers imagines, but again this is an issue that we will return to in Part III.

There is a further issue we can raise about Jaspers' demand that phenomenology be presuppositionless—and that is to ask: why,

exactly? This may seem like a rather trivial question surely it's obvious why one should seek to avoid theoretical presuppositions, if one can. However, being clear about why Jaspers demands presuppositionlessness will help us distinguish it from other notions of presuppositionless—that which figures in DSM-IV, and also Husserl's notion of presuppositionlessness.

Jaspers demands presuppositionlessness because phenomenology, for Jaspers, is a purely descriptive taxonomy of mental states. Phenomenology thus demands a presuppositionless approach in the same way as any other form of taxonomy, that is, in the interests of scientific accuracy and objectivity in one's observations. Imagine, for example, an entomologist, who in studying millipedes, simply rested content with the presupposition that they all possess a thousand legs. One would certainly demand in this case that he 'set aside all outmoded theories' and 'acquire an unprejudiced direct grasp of [them] as they really are'. In other words, Jaspers' demand for presuppositionlessness is in the service of common sense notions of empirical accuracy.

Presuppositionlessness in classifications of mental disorder

We can contrast this with another view of the avoidance of theoretical presuppositions—the one that figures in psychopathological diagnostic manuals, where there is an emphasis on providing 'atheoretical' descriptions. The following justification for this approach comes from the introduction of DSM-III-R:

> The major justification for the generally atheoretical approach taken in DSM-III and DSM-III-R with regard to aetiology is that the inclusion of aetiological theories would be an obstacle to use of the manual by clinicians of various theoretical orientations, since it would not be possible to present all reasonable aetiological theories for each disorder. For example, Phobic Disorders are believed by many to represent a displacement of anxiety resulting from the breakdown of defence mechanisms that keep internal conflicts out of consciousness. Others explain phobias on the basis of learned avoidance responses to conditioned anxiety. Still others believe that certain phobias result from a dysregulation of basic biological systems mediating separation anxiety. In any case, clinicians and researchers can agree on the identification of mental disorders on the basis of their clinical manifestations without agreeing on how the disturbances come about.
>
>   American Psychiatric Association (1987, p. xxiii)

Here the justification for presuppositionlessness is quite different—and one that is sometimes mistakenly attributed to Jaspers—namely that it should be free from theories of aetiology (or causation). In fact, as we will see in Part III, its origin was the contribution of the American philosopher of science, Carl Hempel, to a WHO symposium on classification, convened under the chairmanship of the British psychiatrist, Irwin Stengel, and incorporated in Stengel's subsequent report and recommendations to the WHO on the future of psychiatric classification). This report led to the publication first of ICD-8 and ICD-9, as symptom rather than aetiology based classifications; and DSM-III extended the approach with the introduction of clear inclusion and exclusion criteria.

The aim of presuppositionlessness, then, in Jaspers' model is the production of good and accurate descriptions. The aim in the ICD and DSM is to avoid getting drawn into the plurality of theoretical explanations that, in the current state of our scientific knowledge, can be given of the aetiology of any particular symptom. The demand to produce good, accurate descriptions of symptoms as the basis of any classification of mental disorder is, Hempel pointed out, a requirement of any taxonomy. The 'atheoretical' approach taken by the later editions of DSM, however, although often characterized as a 'phenomenological approach', is different from Jaspers' notion, in its aims and justification.

Presuppositionlessness in Husserl's phenomenology

It is worth also noting at this point how Jaspers' notion of presuppositionlessness differs from Husserl's. And again the difference relates primarily to the question of why one should seek to avoid introducing theoretical presuppositions into phenomenology.

There are two related reasons why Husserl places a great emphasis on the need for phenomenology to be descriptive in the sense of avoiding theoretical presuppositions. The first relates to Husserl's view of phenomenology as a theory of knowledge, or as we said above, more precisely, a theory of what it means to be a 'knowing subject'. The purpose of phenomenology for Husserl is to give an account of what is involved in the very idea of being a subject that can arrive at knowledge of, and formulate scientific theories about, the world. He, therefore, regarded it as a form of circular argument to appeal to scientific theories about human consciousness in an account of what it means to be able to formulate scientific theories in the first place. Such an attempt to use scientific knowledge to explain our ability to arrive at scientific knowledge is known as 'naturalized epistemology' ('epistemology' being the philosophical term for theory of knowledge). One of Husserl's lifelong obsessions, from the period of *Logical Investigations* onwards, was the question of how to avoid aspects of naturalized epistemology creeping into one's reflections on knowledge. To this end, as we shall see below, Husserl demands that phenomenology, as a type of theory of knowledge, must avoid drawing on any scientific, explanatory theories of consciousness.

The second, and related reason why Husserl demanded that phenomenology should not make use of scientific theories, was that he was concerned to analyse the notion of a 'knowing subject *as such*'. That is, Husserl wished to give an account of what it means to be an entity capable of knowledge of the world irrespective of whether that entity be a human, an alien sulphur-based life form living in another part of the galaxy, or a silicon-based supercomputer that might be developed in years to come. In other words, Husserl wishes to give an account of our very notion of knowing subjectivity, irrespective of who or what they are. Phenomenology for Husserl is a form of conceptual study, and thus it is a mistake to try and draw on the findings of empirical science in one's analysis. The later would always be limited in

their validity to the particular type of organism being studied, whereas the findings of a phenomenological analysis are to hold universally.

Jaspers' and Husserl's views of phenomenology as purely descriptive

It seems, then, that even on the issue of the descriptive and presuppositionless nature of phenomenology, there are clear differences between Jaspers and Husserl. For Jaspers, the phenomenologist must avoid theoretical presuppositions, because phenomenology is a purely descriptive taxonomy of mental states. For Husserl, the phenomenologist must avoid theoretical presuppositions, because phenomenology is a conceptual analysis of what it means to be a subject capable of formulating theories at all.

Throughout our close reading of Jaspers' article 'The phenomenological approach in psychopathology', aspects of Husserl's conception of phenomenology have been introduced. It should be clear to you that the question of Husserl's influence on Jaspers, and the question of the proximity or otherwise of their notions of phenomenology, are not going to have easy 'yes' or 'no' answers! We will look below at some of the views that have been taken on these questions, but first it is time to look more closely at Husserl's own notion of phenomenology.

Reflection on the session and self-test questions

Write down your own reflections on the materials in this session drawing out any points that are particularly significant for you. Then write brief notes about the following:

1. What is the difference between subjective and objective symptoms according to Jaspers?

2. What is empathy?

3. What is the connection between phenomenology and subjective psychology?

4. What is the aim of phenomenology, according to Jaspers?

5. What role does Jaspers accord to phenomenology?

Session 2 The background to Husserl's phenomenology

A review of what you have learned about Husserl so far

In this session, we are going to take a look at the philosophical background to Husserl's project of phenomenology. To an extent this will mean exploring Husserl's early work in mathematics. But don't let this put you off! Before beginning our consideration of Husserl's work, however, it would be a good idea to review what you have learned about Husserl's philosophy so far.

Look back over the previous session, and make brief notes about what has been said about Husserl's work, in the sections which have contrasted it with Jaspers' view of phenomenology.

Here is a quick checklist of what we have learnt about Husserl's phenomenology thus far:

- Husserl's work involves a clarification or elucidation of what is meant by a 'mental state', rather than a taxonomy of the rich and varied types of mental state one might come across.

- Husserl viewed philosophy as a process of clarifying the seemingly trivial concepts we often use without thinking, or the concepts that are taken for granted as basic in a particular science.

- Husserl's thinking went through a number of distinct phases of development.

- Phenomenology for Husserl is not on a par with empirical sciences, but is a form of philosophical theory of knowledge or epistemology, or more precisely an analysis of what it means to be a 'knowing subject'.

- Phenomenology is just as concerned with relations between mental states, as with mental states considered in isolation, but the relations at issue are those that are 'rational', rather than those that are merely 'meaningful'. (Remember that feeling happy when you win the lottery is meaningful but not rational, in Husserl's sense.)

- Husserl's approach to mental life is 'descriptive', in that it aims at clarification and elucidation of the idea of a knowing subject, rather than an *explanation* of it in causal terms.

- Thus, in Husserl's view, one must avoid introducing presuppositions from explanatory theories of mind—phenomenology rejects any form of naturalized epistemology.

You may have surprised yourself by just how much you learned about Husserl's work without realizing it! In this session and the next we are going to look at Husserl's project more closely, and, perhaps more importantly, to get a feel of what Husserl was trying to do and why he was doing it. You might be reassured to know, however, that the points we drew out through comparison with Jaspers already give us, in a nutshell, the broad contours of Husserl's thinking. All we shall be doing is expanding them and weaving them into a coherent whole. As you work through this session on the background to Husserl's thinking, keep the above points in mind, and then we will come back to them in detail in the next session.

Husserl: early work in mathematics

Husserl's early work and the background to phenomenology

Husserl's most important work for our purposes has already been mentioned: it is *Logical Investigations*, volume 1, published in 1900, and volume 2, in 1901. It is this work which first launches Husserl's project of phenomenology. Rather than simply jumping into a discussion of this text, however, it will be helpful to consider the background to it in Husserl's earlier work.

Husserl's original training was in mathematics, and this at a time when new and important developments were taking place in the subject. His first major work, 'Philosophy as rigorous science' (1911), was part of a broad movement at the time concerned with the 'foundations' of mathematics, and a brief consideration of the issues that were in the air will help set the scene for the development of phenomenology.

Husserl's early studies in mathematics were under the tutelage of Weierstrass—a German mathematician whose name is probably unfamiliar to you, but whose work is still recognized by mathematicians today as being of fundamental significance. Weierstrass was concerned with calculus and with the problematic status of some of the key concepts used in it. Calculus is a branch of mathematics concerned, for example, with how one would calculate the acceleration of a body at a given point. It is a vital tool in many natural sciences, as well as a key branch of pure mathematics. The problem was that the traditional proofs of methods used in calculus made reference to shadowy 'infinitesimally small' quantities. For example, in calculating the acceleration of a body at a certain point, one needs, it seems, to consider the distance it travels in an infinitesimally small period of time—a period of time so small that, in fact, no time has passed at all!—as one wants its velocity at a given *point*. It seemed, then, that the foundations of this all important mathematical theory rested on a rather dubious slight of hand. Weierstrass was the first to show how calculus could be put on a firmer basis by drawing on the theory of 'real numbers'.

More mathematical background

To understand Husserl's work we need to look into its mathematical background a little further. The term 'real numbers' can best be explained by introducing two further terms: 'rational numbers' and 'irrational numbers'. Rational numbers are all those numbers that can be expressed as fractions, e.g. 1/2, 1/3, 8/5, etc.; irrational numbers are those numbers that can never be expressed as fractions, for example, the square root of 2—one can always calculate fractions either side of it, but no single fraction hits the mark exactly. 'Real numbers', then, are just the rational together with the irrationals.

A further breakthrough in mathematics was made around the same time. A mathematician called Dedekind finally produced a way of showing how an irrational number could be defined in terms of rational numbers. This was an important breakthrough, because, as we have seen, rational numbers in turn are defined in terms of two natural numbers (making a fraction), and the numbers are simply the numbers we are all familiar with that we use for counting things. In a short space of time, therefore, the theory of calculus, whose foundations were for so long rather shaky, had suddenly been shown to be derivable from the simplest and most secure branch of mathematics—everyday numbers and arithmetic. The question naturally arose, however, of whether natural numbers and arithmetic could be derived from even more basic foundations—and it is at this point in the story that Husserl enters the picture, along with one of the most famous logicians of modern times, Gottlob Frege.

Husserl's 'Philosophy of Arithmetic'

Gottlob Frege (1848–1925) was a German mathematician, logician, and philosopher who worked at the University of Jena. He is credited with putting logic on its modern footing through the construction of a formal system called 'predicate calculus'.

Frege tried to show that even natural numbers and arithmetic could be defined in terms of more basic notions: purely logical notions. If Frege could succeed in this, he would have shown that even the higher reaches of mathematics have their roots in logic and the basic principles of what makes for a valid argument. It would be quite an achievement and Frege (1980), in fact, produced a popular and very readable outline of his project, *The Foundations of Arithmetic*, which is worth looking at if you are interested in the issue. He then went on to write a technical proof of his theory, showing how numbers themselves could be defined purely logically. But just after Frege finished this huge work, a flaw was identified in his proof by the young Bertrand Russell, a flaw that has become known as Russell's paradox. Husserl, however, was unhappy with Frege's approach even before this problem was brought to light, and his early work, *Philosophy of Arithmetic*, is highly critical of Frege's project.

Husserl's objections to Frege's ambitious project are rather technical and we do not need to go into them here. What is important for our purposes is that Husserl concluded that numbers could not be defined in terms of anything more basic—our number

concepts are themselves basic and irreducible. He argued further, however, that a different form of clarification and foundation of our number concepts could be given: a *psychological*, as opposed to logical, foundation. Husserl's line was essentially this: even though we cannot define our number concepts in terms of anything more basic, what we can do is show how they are connected to our abilities to count and to perceive groups of things as groups. For example, to see a pair of objects is not to see one object and then to see another, rather we have to see them 'together'. Yet in seeing them together we do not see them as one thing, rather we see them as two. Husserl thus argued that our basic number concepts—even though they are basic notions—can be clarified by an analysis of the psychological abilities involved in perceiving groups of objects.

Husserl and the problem of psychologism

Husserl's work, *Philosophy of Arithmetic*, is a long and technical mathematical work, though it does contain a number of insights into what we would now call 'Gestalt psychology'—the theory that stresses the importance of the ability to perceive wholes, groups, and patterns. Weierstrass had recommended to Husserl that he should study with the philosopher Franz Brentano, as a way of balancing his mathematical training with a firm grasp of current thinking in psychology. Brentano's key work, *Psychology from an Empirical Standpoint*, had appeared in 1874, and we will come back to him below, as his influence is very much evident in the phenomenology of *Logical Investigations*. The key concept of Brentano's psychology is that of 'intentionality': mental states, he argued, differ from physical states in that the former possess 'intentionality'—they are 'of' or 'about' things. We will be looking at this notion in detail below. It is centrally important because it is at the heart of the psychological analysis of the perception of groups that Husserl gives in the *Philosophy of Arithmetic*, as well as of the phenomenological analysis of mental states generally, which he gives in *Logical Investigations*.

How then do the psychological analyses of the *Philosophy of Arithmetic* differ from the 'phenomenological' analyses of *Logical Investigations*? On the face of it, one might think there has only been a change in subject matter: the early work giving an analysis of mathematical abilities using Brentano's intentional psychology, the later work looking at our more basic logical abilities. In fact, the question of just how close the two works are is a matter of some debate. It depends very much on how one interprets Husserl's project in the earlier work, knowing what we do about *Logical Investigations*, because in many places the *Philosophy of Arithmetic* is unclear and ambiguous.

The main bone of contention concerns a philosophical standpoint known as 'psychologism', and whether Husserl held this position in his early work (what the term means will be explained below). What we do know is that by the time of *Logical Investigations* Husserl comes to reject psychologism completely: the whole of the first volume is taken up with its refutation; an understanding of the issue of psychologism is vital to a proper understanding of Husserl's phenomenology. It is widely held that Husserl's early

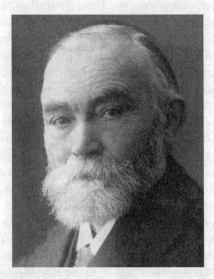

Fig. 9.2 Gottlob Frege

work is a form of psychologism, and this view derives almost entirely from a scathing review that Frege wrote of Husserl's book. Frege was a life-long opponent of psychologism, and his review is widely regarded as having forced Husserl to change his ideas. Frege's review is now, however, itself regarded as unfair and rather uncharitable: picking on the points of unclarity and ambiguity to make it appear to support an extreme form of psychologism. Certainly the review had some impact on Husserl: otherwise he would not have thought it necessary to introduce his next work with a 200-page refutation of psychologism to make sure nobody misunderstood him this time!

To psychologize or not to psychologize?

So what then is psychologism? While there are a number of different forms of psychologism, the basic idea is that logical and/or mathematical truths ultimately have a psychological basis. One way to think about psychologism as a philosophical movement is to keep in mind what you read above about the interest in the foundations of mathematics at the end of the nineteenth century, and then combine this with the fact that huge advances were being made in experimental psychology at the time. That is, in the context of a debate about the foundations of mathematics, it seemed natural to many philosophers to argue that its foundations should be sought in an account of the workings of the human mind or brain. Another, and related, reason why psychologism became widespread at this time, was that mainstream philosophy itself was generally empiricist in orientation.

Empiricism is a philosophical theory about knowledge, which argues that all aspects of knowledge derive from experience. Empiricism became popular in Germany in the nineteenth century as a reaction against the metaphysical excesses of German Idealism. In an extreme form of empiricism one might argue that mathematical truths, such as $2 + 2 = 4$, are generalizations derived from experience—that is, whenever in the past you have put any two objects together with any other two objects, you have ended up with four objects. Frege (1980) commented rather caustically, in *The Foundations of Arithmetic*, that if the truth of $2 + 2 = 4$ depended on being able to put two objects together with two other objects, then it was a good job that not all objects were nailed down, otherwise it wouldn't be true!

In fact, one would be hard pushed to find anyone who seriously held such an odd view of mathematics as having an empirical basis in observations about the world. But psychologism *is* a related position. It holds that logical or mathematical truths are empirical in that there are psychological laws concerning how human minds or brains function. One famous exponent of this view is J.S. Mill. We will come back to Mill in the next section also, as not only did he argue that logic, as a part of psychology, was a form of natural science, but also that the human sciences must seek to base their findings on natural science too. In *Logical Investigations*, Husserl cites the following passage from Mill:

Logic is not a science separate from and co-ordinate with psychology. To the extent that it is a science at all, it is a part or branch of psychology, distinguished from it on the one hand as the part is from the whole, and on the other hand as the art is from the science. It owes all its theoretical basis to psychology, and includes as much of that science as is necessary to establish the rules of the art.

(J.S. Mill *An examination of Sir William Hamilton's philosophy*, quoted by Husserl, [1900–01] 1970a, p. 90)

It is this type of view that Husserl seeks to refute in the first volume of *Logical Investigations*, and that Frege, a life-long opponent of such views, accuses Husserl of holding in the *Philosophy of Arithmetic* (Husserl 1970b). Husserl certainly never explicitly stated such a view in his early work, though many of his remarks are unclear, and generally he did not come to a clear view about the relation between mathematical concepts and psychological concepts. It would also be odd if Frege's review had had the impact on Husserl generally attributed to it, since Husserl was already familiar with Frege's antipsychologism from *The Foundations of Arithmetic*. What is more likely is that Frege's review prompted Husserl to come to a clear view on what the relationship is between logic/mathematics as such, and a psychological analysis of our logical and mathematical *abilities*, and just what sort of 'clarification' a *psychological* analysis can provide.

You may, however, be wondering at this point just what is so wrong with psychologism. It is to this question that we now turn, and this will bring us closer to an understanding of the nature of Husserl's phenomenology in *Logical Investigations*.

What is wrong with psychologism

As noted above the whole of volume 1 of *Logical Investigations*, entitled 'Prolegomena to Pure Logic', is taken up with an analysis and refutation of psychologism. Husserl starts by drawing attention to a number of differences between how we usually think of logical or mathematical laws, and how they would be if psychologism were true, thus suggesting that psychologism does not provide a very suitable analysis of their nature. We think of logical laws, he argues, as having a certainty that outstrips that of even the most well-founded empirical laws of nature. If logical laws were empirical generalizations about how our minds work, then they would only be as certain as the empirical evidence in their favour, but this is simply not how we think of them. The Law of Non-Contradiction (which states that a statement and its negation cannot both be true) would appear to have a degree of self-evidence that no empirical law could have.

Secondly, Husserl cites a further point often made at the time against psychologism, namely that logic, but not psychology, is normative. That is to say, logical laws tell us how one *ought* to think, not how we *do* think. If during a psychological survey, 5% of people were found to hold contradictory beliefs, one would not conclude that the Law of Non-Contradiction holds only in 95% of cases, but rather that people holding two contradictory beliefs *ought* rationally to give up one of them.

The normative character of logic

Many opponents of psychologism held that it was enough to cite the normative character of logic in order to refute psychologism, but Husserl was, in fact, not convinced. Husserl argued, against this traditional antipsychologistic view, that logic was not fundamentally a normative discipline, and for two reasons. First, if logic were a normative discipline giving the rules one ought to follow while thinking, then alongside the Law of Non-Contradiction one would expect to find rules such as: don't listen to loud, distracting music while thinking; make sure you've had enough sleep before thinking etc. Logic as traditionally conceived (and to which we had an introduction in Chapter 5) simply doesn't concern itself with such psychological rules for thinking well.

Husserl's second argument against the ultimately normative character of logic builds on this first argument. Every normative discipline, he argues, is 'founded' on a non-normative or purely 'theoretical' discipline. Husserl doesn't mean that normative principles can be derived from a non-normative science—one cannot derive an 'ought' from an 'is' (see Chapter 4)—but rather that every normative discipline makes reference in its evaluations to a realm of objects and states-of-affairs, which are the subject matter of particular non-normative sciences.

An example will help clarify what Husserl means. Nutrition, as a normative discipline, posits rules about what one *ought* to eat to stay healthy; its value judgements make reference, however, to studies of the effect of certain chemicals or their absence on the human body, and thus are founded (in Husserl's sense) on the findings of biology and physiology. What, then, is the theoretical science upon which logic as a normative discipline is founded? Those who cite the normative character of logic against psychologism tend to leave this question unanswered. If logic is a normative science about how one ought to think, then one might be tempted to think that its value judgements ultimately concern processes ordinarily studied in psychology. Yet, whereas the findings of biology and physiology have relevance for nutrition as a normative discipline, the findings of empirical psychology simply have no relevance to logic. Husserl thus argues that it is not enough to cite the normative character of logic, unless one can make clear what non-normative, theoretical science it is founded on, if this is not psychology.

Relativism and the 'absurdity' of psychologism

Husserl's main arguments against psychologism, however, have a different focus. Basically, Husserl argues that psychologism entails that logical laws are relative to the psychological functioning of human beings as a particular species. This further entails that truth is relative to particular species, and thus it is conceivable that psychologism, as a theory put forward as true by us, could be both true and false (that is, from the same premises, someone from a different species may validly argue, with their logic, to

contradictory conclusions). Psychologism is thus a theory whose truth undermines its own status as true, and this self-conflicting nature of psychologism is what Husserl calls its 'absurdity'. Husserl's argument here is rather dense. It is set out in detail, along with a number of related arguments against psychologism, in chapter 7 of Husserl's *Logical Investigations*, volume 1, a chapter titled 'Psychologism as sceptical relativism'.

For our present purposes we do not need to look in detail at Husserl's 'absurdity' argument against psychologism, but it will be worth looking at a brief example. Consider, then, this famous syllogism:

1. All men are mortal
2. Socrates is a man
3. Socrates is mortal

Now psychologism has to explain why it is we feel obliged to hold the third statement to be true, if we accept the first two. Different types of psychologism would give different answers depending on the type of psychological theory. In general, such explanations will argue that there are psychological laws that govern human thought processes such that if one thinks the first belief, followed by the second, one is caused to think the third. We can imagine, then, as Husserl pointed out, other creatures governed by different psychological laws such that thinking the first two statements causes them to think 'Socrates is not mortal'. If psychologism were correct, this conclusion would be 'true for them' and their 'logic', while 'Socrates is mortal' would be 'true for us' and our 'logic'. In this way, one can see how psychologism entails that truth becomes relative—one cannot talk about truth *per se*, but only 'truth for species x', 'truth for species y', etc. Husserl ends chapter 7 with a tirade against such views:

> One need only try to think out what [psychologism] implies: that there might be peculiar beings, logical supermen, as it were, for whom *our logical principles do not hold*, but rather quite different principles, so that every truth for us is a falsehood for them. For them it is the case that the mental phenomena they are experiencing are not experienced by them. That we and they exist may be true for us, but is false for them, etc. We everyday logicians would say: Such beings are mad, they talk of truth, yet destroy its laws [...]. Yes and No, truth and error, existence and non-existence, lose all their distinctness in their thought.
>
> *Logical Investigations* (pp. 165–166)

The diagnosis of where psychologism goes wrong

Chapter 7 of *Logical Investigations* also introduces elements of Husserl's 'diagnosis' of the problem of psychologism and his proposed 'cure': that is, what the fundamental mistake being made by supporters of psychologism is, and what needs to be put in its place.

> If someone wished to argue from the fact that a true judgement, like any judgement, must spring from the constitution of the judging subject in virtue of appropriate natural laws, we should warn him not to confuse the 'judgement', *qua* content of the

judgement, i.e. as an ideal unity, with the individual, real act of judgement. It is the former that we mean when we speak of the judgement $2 \times 2 = 4$, which is the same whoever passes it. One should likewise not confuse the true judgement, as the correct judgement in accordance with truth, with the *truth* of this judgement or with the true content of judgement. My act of judging that $2 \times 2 = 4$ is no doubt causally determined, but this is not true of the truth $2 \times 2 = 4$.

Logical Investigations (pp. 141–142)

This passage repays careful study. Husserl is arguing that the supporters of psychologism are confusing two senses of the term 'judgement': first, in the sense of the real mental process, or 'act of judgement' that goes on in a particular individual, and then 'judgement' in the sense of *what is being judged*—in Husserl's example, *that* $2 \times 2 = 4$. If two people are both thinking that $2 \times 2 = 4$, then here we have two distinct *acts* of judgement, going on in two different people, but the 'content' of their judgements is identically the same, the judgement or proposition that $2 \times 2 = 4$. Our former example,

1. All men are mortal

2. Socrates is a man

3. Socrates is mortal,

can be thought of in two ways: either as a temporal sequence of real beliefs going on in someone's mind, or as a set of three propositions, between which certain relations hold. If Husserl's diagnosis of psychologism is the confusion of these two, then his 'cure' is to argue that logic is not a study of real, psychological acts of judgement or belief, but a study of relations between propositions. You may have noticed in the above quotation that Husserl calls the content of judgements an '*ideal*' unity. We do not talk of judgement contents or propositions as existing in particular places, or at particular times, which is the way we think of the occurrence of *real* acts of judgement; and Husserl uses the term 'ideal' to mean this atemporal and non-spatial way of being, which we use in our talk of judgement-contents. Husserl's 'cure', to repeat, is the argument that logical laws simply do not refer to real psychological events and their relations, but to relations between propositions:

If the relativist says that there could be beings not bound by these principles [the principles of contradiction and excluded middle]—this assertion is easily seen as equivalent to the relativistic formula stated above. He *either* means that there could be propositions or truths, in the judgements of such beings, which do not conform to these principles, *or* he thinks that the course of judgement of such beings is not *psychologically* regulated by these principles. If he means the latter, his doctrine is not at all peculiar, since we ourselves are such beings.

Logical Investigations (p. 141)

If the supporter of psychologism says there may be beings not bound by the laws of logic, then Husserl is arguing that this either applies to judgement-contents, or propositions, in which case relativism is the consequence, or that it applies to psychological acts of judging, in which case, the supporter is saying nothing more than that there are creatures that sometimes think illogically—i.e. creatures like us!

Psychology as the new 'queen of the sciences'

The entirety of volume 1 of *Logical Investigations*, then, 'Prolegomena to Pure Logic', is concerned with arguing that psychology has nothing to do with logic, and with offering a refutation, diagnosis and cure for the view that logical laws are a type of psychological law.

Husserl, like Frege, felt particularly strongly about this because psychology, at this time, was making a takeover bid for philosophy. Towards the end of the nineteenth century in Germany, many chairs of philosophy in German universities had been awarded to experimental psychologists. At that time most universities did not have separate departments of psychology. In some circles, the recent advances in experimental psychology were taken as a sign that the new science of psychology would come to replace moribund philosophy as the 'queen of the sciences'. Psychology seemed to some to offer a new way of solving the fundamental problems that were traditionally the preserve of philosophy. Franz Brentano, whom we came across above as an influence on Husserl, was one who saw psychology as the 'science of the future':

Let me point out merely in passing that psychology contains the roots of aesthetics, which, in a more advanced stage of development, will undoubtedly sharpen the eye of the artist and assure his progress. Likewise, suffice it to say that the important art of logic, a single improvement in which brings about a thousand advances in science, also has psychology as its source. In addition, psychology has the task of becoming the scientific basis for a theory of education, both of the individual and of society. Along with aesthetics and logic, ethics and politics also stem from the field of psychology. And so psychology appears to be the fundamental condition of human progress in precisely those things which, above all, constitute human dignity.

Brentano ([1874] 1995, p. 21)

It was in this context of the perceived encroachment of psychology into philosophy departments and into the traditional problems of philosophy, that Husserl launched his attack. Essentially, he was arguing for the limitations of empirical psychology—and this, not in relation to questions of aesthetics, ethics, or politics, but in relation to a more fundamental field: logic as the study of reasoning itself.

The confusion caused by volume 2 of *Logical Investigations*

In this context of worries about psychology's encroachment on philosophy, it is not surprising that philosophers at the time welcomed Husserl's sustained attack on psychologism with open arms! Volume 1 of *Logical Investigations* was published in 1900, with volume 2 promised for the next year, and many waited eagerly for it. Perhaps many expected a further development of the sort of formal logical concerns to which Husserl turns at the end of volume 1. But they were in for a surprise! In the next exercise, you are going to read what they read (with dismay!) on opening volume 2, Husserl's introduction to the six 'logical investigations', which constitute the second volume. Part of the reason for looking so closely at the problem of psychologism above was to allow you to 'empathise' with the confusion, consternation, and bewilderment that the early readers of *Logical Investigations* experienced. Having argued in volume 1 for the sharp opposition between logic and psychology, volume 2 suddenly argues that one in fact needs a form of psychology to supplement pure logic. This form of psychology, which Husserl describes as a 'descriptive psychology', is what Husserl calls 'phenomenology'. Some readers at the time must have simply assumed Husserl had gone mad: volume 1 had precisely argued for the *irrelevance* of an empirical, descriptive psychology of how people think, to logic.

In a later introduction to *Logical Investigations* (which Husserl wrote, but never used, for the new edition published in 1913), Husserl talks about the cold reception that volume 2 was given. Part of what he was trying to achieve in volume 1, he says, was to create in people a sense of dissatisfaction with the tension between the purely logical and the psychological. He wanted people to think: well, yes, psychology is irrelevant for logic, but surely logic must have something to do with the way people think. It was this sense of dissatisfaction with the gulf between logic and psychology that Husserl sought to build on in volume 2. The strategy failed. In his own words:

> Quite a few, unfortunately even the majority, of the critics of the book proceed, however, in a different manner. On the basis of a cursory glance at it, they write off the second volume. This happens, for opposite reasons, on the part of both groups: the psychologists take the investigations in question *eo ipso* as psychology, but as a scholastically adulterated form because there is everywhere in them talk of the ideal, of the a priori. But the idealists [the Neo-Kantians] find their expectations of transcendental constructions from above disappointed; instead of such constructions there is everywhere talk of lived-experiences, acts, intentions, fulfilments, and the like—in other words, for them too, talk of the psychological. Time and again they speak of a 'relapse into psychologism'. They find absolutely nothing wrong with the fact that the very same author, who in the first volume displays an acuteness of judgement which they praise highly, would in the second volume seek his salvation in open and outright childish contradictions.
>
> Introduction to *Logical Investigations* (pp. 22–23)

The confusion on the part of his readers was forgivable, though. Husserl's first major work had sought to draw on psychology to provide a 'clarification' of numbers and arithmetic, and had been attacked by Frege, a staunch opponent of psychologism. In the *Philosophy of Arithmetic*, Husserl had indeed used ideas in that earlier work from Franz Brentano, who appeared to strongly support psychologism. And here, again, in the second volume of *Logical Investigations*, Husserl was once more using Brentano's

intentional psychology. Husserl, in volume 1, seemed to have renounced his earlier psychologism, and now it appeared that he had changed his mind again! Just what was going on?

Reflection on the session and self-test questions

Write down your own reflections on the materials in this session drawing out any points that are particularly significant for you. Then write brief notes about the following:

1. With what was Husserl's early work mainly concerned?

2. What is the connection between Husserl's work on logic and 'psychologism'?

3. What is Husserl's key argument for distinguishing logic and arithmetic from psychology and thus against attempting to reduce the former to the latter?

4. Did he succeed in persuading his critics that his theory was not psychologistic?

Session 3 Husserl's conception of phenomenology

Husserl's introduction of phenomenology

In this session we come square on to Husserl's conception of phenomenology as introduced in the second volume of *Logical Investigations*. We will be looking in a moment at the introduction to volume 2. Before doing so, there are a couple of preliminary points worth making. First, the translation you will be reading is the translation of the second edition of *Logical Investigations*, published in 1913. This is important because, as we mentioned above, by 1913 Husserl had radically changed his notion of phenomenology, and the new edition was revised by Husserl from his new standpoint. Depending on one's view of the development of Husserl's thinking, the revisions are simply clarifications, bringing out what was already there, or they are an attempt by Husserl to project back his new ideas into his first account of phenomenology. The answer is probably somewhere in the middle.

There is a change made by Husserl to the new edition at one point, which is particularly striking. Fortunately, the translation of the second edition also gives the text of the first edition at that point. The change occurs in §6 of the Introduction (pp. 260–263): in the first version, Husserl states that 'phenomenology is descriptive psychology', while in the second edition, he writes 'phenomenology is not descriptive psychology'! As early as 1903 Husserl felt that calling phenomenology 'descriptive psychology' was causing a widespread misunderstanding of what he was doing, and clearly the issue bears directly on the relation of Jaspers' work to Husserl's. For Jaspers, remember, phenomenology very much *is* descriptive psychology.

The second preliminary point is simply to warn you that reading Husserl is not easy! Husserl has a writing style that rivals Kant's for its density and difficulty. The result is that one has to work quite hard even to grasp what he means by 'phenomenology' and a 'phenomenological analysis'—not a good idea if one is seeking to launch a fundamentally new approach to the analysis of mental life! Indeed Husserl adds to the confusion by starting off his 'Introduction' by flagging yet another new approach. His analysis of mental life, he says, is going to start not by talking vaguely of 'mental experiences', 'ideas', 'representations', or other traditional psychological terms of the time, but rather with an analysis of *language* ability.

The centrality of language in Husserl's phenomenology

The way to read the Introduction, then, is to hold on to the idea that phenomenology, for the early Husserl, is a type of analysis of the mental states involved in possessing knowledge in a form that can be communicated in language. As *analysis* of our linguistic and cognitive abilities, that is to say, Husserl's intention is that phenomenology will unravel the complexities involved in our everyday, and normally taken for granted, ability to talk about things. Phenomenology is going to ask, for example, about the relation between the following seemingly trivial things:

◆ The proposition that the sun is shining

◆ Saying that the sun is shining

◆ Thinking that the sun is shining

◆ Perceiving that the sun is shining

◆ Perceiving the following series of small black printed marks on the piece of paper in front of you...

    THE SUN IS SHINING

If this list strikes you as rather trivial and hair-splitting, you would not be alone. In part, it was the extraordinary detail that Husserl dug out of our everyday linguistic and cognitive performances, that led to the charge of 'scholasticism' to which Husserl referred above. You need to remember, though, 'that it is precisely behind the obvious that the hardest problems lie hidden', and that the types of ability Husserl will be looking at seem trivial precisely because they are so fundamental to our sense of ourselves, and the sort of beings we are.

Seven questions about Husserl's phenomenology

The crunch question though is, exactly what *type* of analysis it is, which phenomenology attempts to give. In order to grasp what is distinctive about phenomenological analysis, as conceived by Husserl, you need to look out for the places where he contrasts it with an empirical, psychological approach to mental life on one side, and links it up with a purely logical analysis of language on the other.

EXERCISE 3   (60 minutes)

Read:

Husserl, E. ([1900–01] 1970a). 'Introduction' to Logical Investigations Volume II *Logical Investigations*, 2 Volumes, (translated by J.N. Findlay), London: Routledge and Kegan Paul, Volume I pp. 248–266

Link with Reading 9.2

Don't worry if there are parts you can't understand at all!—Husserl introduces technicalities, especially in §§4–5, which we don't have to worry about here. Before you start, though, look through the following list of questions. Then as you read, make brief notes for yourself about what Husserl says.

1. Is phenomenology an empirical science or a 'pure' and 'a priori' discipline?

2. What does phenomenology seek to do for pure logic?

3. Why is a phenomenological approach to mental life so difficult?

4. In what sense is phenomenology a 'descriptive' discipline?

5. What sort of 'theory of knowledge' is phenomenology?

6. In what way is a phenomenological analysis 'free from presuppositions'?

7. Why does Husserl say at the end that the worth of a phenomenological analysis does not even depend on there being 'such things as men'?

Question 1: phenomenology as a 'pure' or 'a priori' discipline

In §1 Husserl uses the term 'pure' to describe both logic and phenomenology. The idea is that each of these disciplines is not an empirical study; they do not seek empirical or experimental evidence for their results. Phenomenology is concerned with 'the experiences of thinking and knowing', but in a quite different way to that of empirical or experimental psychology. Phenomenology is concerned with them 'in the pure generality of their essence, not experiences empirically perceived and treated as real facts, as experiences of human or animal experients' (p. 249). This statement is, in fact, an addition made in the 1913 edition, but what it says certainly characterizes phenomenology as Husserl thought of it in the first edition. Phenomenology is an analysis of the very notions of thinking and knowing, not an empirical study of the real psychological events we identify in human beings as instances of thinking and knowing.

Husserl immediately signals a connection between pure phenomenology and empirical psychology, however:

[Pure phenomenology] analyses and describes in their essential generality—in the specific guise of a phenomenology of thought and knowledge—the experiences of presentation, judgement and knowledge, experiences which, treated as classes of real events in the natural context of zoological reality, receive a scientific probing at the hands of empirical psychology. (*ibid.*)

While empirical psychology studies the mental processes of particular individuals or particular species, phenomenology is concerned with the very idea of such mental processes conceived in 'essential generality', that is, irrespective of their real instantiation in any particular sort of entity. In §6 (though again as part of the 1913 addition) Husserl compares phenomenology with other 'pure' disciplines, such as arithmetic and geometry. In the same way as arithmetic and geometry can play a vital role in empirical sciences and technologies, so phenomenology's findings can have relevance for empirical psychology: 'Our essential insights into perceptions, volitions and other forms of experience will naturally hold also of the corresponding empirical states of animal organisms, as geometrical insights hold of spatial figures in nature.' (p. 262).

Question 2: phenomenology's relation to logic

Aside from having relevance for empirical psychology, in clarifying the very conceptual scheme within which the study of 'mental states' is undertaken, Husserl regards phenomenology as having key relevance for logic. Essentially, Husserl's idea is that formal logic, with its concern to analyse the parts of propositions and relations between propositions, is in danger of simply becoming an esoteric study lacking any relevance to real life. Phenomenology seeks to provide a clarification of the place of logic in everyday life by using it in the analysis of what it means to possess logical, rational abilities, and the place of these abilities in the idea of being a 'knowing subject'. Husserl expresses this idea in two passages which are rather misleading, but which repay careful consideration, precisely because of the misunderstanding they can (and did!) give rise to. At the bottom of p. 249, Husserl writes: 'Phenomenology on the other hand, lays bare the "sources" from which the basic concepts and ideal laws of *pure* logic "flow", and back to which they must once more be traced, so as to give them all the "clearness and distinctness" needed for an understanding and epistemological critique of pure logic.' (p. 249–250)

On the face of it, except for the scare quotes around 'sources' and 'flow', which indicate that we should not take these words at face value, there could not be a clearer expression of psychologism! Supporters of psychologism precisely argued that logic concerns psychological processes, and that its laws are ultimately psychological laws. It prompts one to ask, as Husserl does rhetorically in §6, 'what then was the point of the whole battle against psychologism?'

One might have expected Husserl to be a little more careful, after his experience of being savagely criticized by Frege for saying the same sort of thing about the concepts of arithmetic! What Husserl is trying to say—none too clearly—is that there is a clarity in our understanding of logic which comes by seeing how it is connected to a pure, a priori analysis of what it means to be an entity capable of logical thought. Unless we relate logic back to subjectivity in this non-psychologistic way, then the rejection of psychologism is apt to make logic seem like a free-floating, esoteric discipline. What phenomenology tries to do is bring logic back down to earth, re-connect it with the idea of a cognitive agent, yet not in the sense that logic *derives* from subjective experiences.

Yet in §2 Husserl seems to say that logical concepts originate in intuitions about our mental states. Again, on the face of it, this is a form of psychologism: not only would logical concepts be psychological concepts, but they are formed through empirical introspection upon our own real mental lives in each case. Here is the passage:

Logical concepts, as valid thought-unities, must have their origin in intuition: they must arise out of an ideational abstraction founded on certain experiences, and must admit of indefinite reconfirmation, and of recognition of their self-identity, on the reperformance of such abstraction. Otherwise put: we can absolutely not rest content with 'mere words', [. . .] we must go back to the 'things themselves' (p. 252; translation modified)

'Back to the things themselves' is one of phenomenology's most famous watchwords, yet in the context in which it is introduced, it supports psychologism: to clarify logical concepts, we must go back to subjective, psychological experiences! Yet Husserl is not saying that 'logical concepts' *do* have their origin in intuition, but that they 'must'. Why? In order that one can bring a new 'epistemological clarity' to logic. Again the idea is that logical concepts must be related back to essential types of psychological act, not that they are themselves empirical concepts.

We can understand this better if we consider Husserl's term 'ideational abstraction'. What he has in mind is the sort of procedure used by someone doing geometry. Someone draws a circle in the process of a geometrical proof, but they are not concerned with just this particular circle, they are concerned with *the circle per se*, as a geometrical form. Husserl would say that while perceiving the drawn circle, they are performing an 'ideational abstraction' upon it: they are regarding it as a mere instance of a universal type. If we reflect on our own mental lives, phenomenology demands that we do the same thing: merely use our empirically real mental lives as a useful aid towards formulating an analysis of the *essential types* of mental act that we regard our own mental lives as instantiating, through performing an 'ideational abstraction' upon them.

Question 3: the difficulty of a phenomenological analysis

We mentioned the watchword of phenomenology above, 'back to the things themselves'. Connected to this is the emphasis Husserl puts on the place of 'intuition', and we have already seen that Husserl by no means has simple empirical observation in mind. On the face of it, what Husserl has in mind is the idea that one must not be content with constructing idle, free-floating ideas of what mental life involves, but we *must look and see!*

Yet even this seemingly trivial advice can give rise to misunderstandings. In §3 Husserl talks about the difficulty of doing a phenomenological analysis: in everyday life we deal with things and situations without reflecting on the mental acts we are having at the time; in seeing a chair, for example, it is the chair that is the object of our attention, not the mental act of perceiving it. Phenomenology is, however, the study of the essential types of mental act involved in the perception and recognition of a chair, and Husserl acknowledges that this change in the focus of our attention is difficult. The way Husserl describes this difficulty can make it seem that phenomenology is difficult because it is a form of introspection, and this is difficult because we more often focus on objects and situations in the world and not on our mental states: 'The source of all such difficulties lies in the unnatural direction of intuition and thought which phenomenological analysis requires. Instead of becoming lost in the performance of acts built intricately on one another, [...] we must rather practice "reflection", i.e. make these acts themselves, and their immanent meaning-content, our object.' (pp. 254–255)

The idea that phenomenology is a method of 'introspection' or 'reflection' (note again the scare quotes!) can suggest that Husserl envisages that, with practice, we can achieve a transparent access to our own mental states. While difficult, ultimately all we need do is introspect, and describe what we see. One might call this a 'Cartesian' view of the mind, as Descartes thought that we have a (transparent) grasp of our mental contents ('ideas'), which we can never attain for things out in the world.

Even a passing familiarity with the tortuous arguments of Husserl's *Logical Investigations* is enough to show, however, that phenomenology is not a matter of mere reflection or introspection! There are two passages in the Introduction that give us a better picture of the complexities involved. In the first Husserl points out that in characterizing mental states one must use language suited to talking about objects in the world: 'it is, in fact, impossible to describe referential acts without recurring in our expressions to the things to which such acts refer' (p. 256; translation modified). This suggests that a description of myself or another as 'perceiving a chair' is not a straightforward matter of introspection upon my mental life, or empathy with another's, but depends precisely on a prior ability to use the term 'chair' correctly for objects in the world.

In the course of six Logical Investigations, we find lengthy discussions on the nature of universals (Investigation II), part–whole relations (Investigation III), and logical grammar (Investigation IV). Husserl draws on all these to clarify our understanding of our cognitive and logical abilities, first broached in Investigation I— again, indicating how far phenomenology is from a simple introspective discipline. What we in fact find is described by Husserl himself as a 'zigzag' movement: 'We search, as it were, in zigzag fashion, a metaphor all the more apt since the close interdependence of our various epistemological concepts leads us

back again and again to our original analysis, here the new confirms the old, and the old the new.' (p. 261)

It is clear, then, that we should not think of phenomenology as presupposing a Cartesian, transparent access to our own mental states, such that all we need do is 'reflect' on ourselves and describe what we see. Why then does Husserl constantly stress the importance of 'intuition'? The answer is that while phenomenology seeks to be an analysis of what belongs a priori to the notion of a 'knowing subject', in terms of the essential types of mental state involved in our logical and cognitive abilities, we must constantly check to see that the analysis does indeed make sense of how we think of ourselves. Husserl is concerned that phenomenological analysis should not become a mere flight of conceptual imagination, but rather that the essential types of mental acts posited in the analysis can all the time be found instantiated in ourselves.

Question 4: phenomenology as a descriptive discipline

We can already see that phenomenology is not a descriptive discipline in the usual sense we think of 'descriptive'. It is not concerned with the simple recording of the empirical observations or introspections we make of ourselves; it is not a descriptive taxonomy of mental life, but an a priori conceptual analysis of what it means to be a knowing subject, of which we take ourselves to be an instance. One might argue that phenomenology is no more a descriptive study of mental life, than geometry is a descriptive study of the shapes of different objects we happen to find lying around our homes.

What then led Husserl to call phenomenology 'descriptive psychology'? Given that Husserl envisages that the conceptual scheme of essential types of mental acts, posited in a phenomenological analysis, can also be of use in empirical psychology, it seems likely that Husserl used the description to give a flavour of what a phenomenological analysis is going to look like. Even in the first edition, though, Husserl has reservations about using the term 'descriptive psychology':

> Since it is epistemologically of unique importance that we should separate the purely descriptive examination of the knowledge-experience, disembarrassed of all theoretical psychological interests, from the truly psychological researches directed to empirical explanation and origins, it will be good if we rather speak of 'phenomenology' than of 'descriptive psychology'. It also recommends itself for the further reason that the expression 'descriptive psychology', as it occurs in the talk of many scientists, means the sphere of scientific psychological investigation, which is marked off by a methodological preference for inner experience and by an abstraction from all psychophysical explanation.   (p. 263)

At the end of this passage, Husserl is basically saying that the term 'descriptive psychology' already has a well established use in relation to a particular form of empirical investigation. Indeed, in the next section we will come across the term used by the philosopher and historian, Wilhelm Dilthey, whose work was a great influence on Jaspers. It was thus quite a risk to use the term for an essentially distinct approach to mental life, and Husserl paid heavily for it, in terms of the misunderstandings to which it gave rise.

There is a sense in which the term 'descriptive' is quite apt for phenomenology, so long as we think about the term in the right way. Ordinarily, we think of description as 'empirical description', i.e. the reporting of observations, as opposed to the formulation of an empirical explanation. This is the sense of 'descriptive' in Dilthey's idea of a 'descriptive psychology'.

We can also think of 'descriptive' in the sense of unpacking and clarifying what is implicit or unclear in our ways of thinking; 'descriptive' in this sense is used by the English philosopher Peter Strawson, in his idea of a 'descriptive metaphysics' (Strawson, 1964). In such an approach one must be careful not to draw on ideas that are themselves founded on the very ways of thinking one is seeking to examine. In particular, in this context, one needs to be careful not to draw on explanatory theories of mental life, when one is precisely trying to clarify the idea of the very type of mental life that would make theory formation possible. Husserl hints at this in the above passage, where he states that it is 'epistemologically of unique importance' that one hold off from any ideas drawn from an 'empirical explanation' of mental life. It is, however, the following section, §7, which makes clear this restriction on phenomenology, on the basis of the nature of phenomenology as 'epistemology' or 'theory of knowledge'.

Question 5: phenomenology as a theory of knowledge

§7 refers back to the last chapter of volume 1 of *Logical Investigations*, the 'Prolegomena to Pure Logic'. In that chapter Husserl had developed the idea of pure logic as culminating in the formal study of *theories* as sets of interrelated propositions: logic as a formal theory of what a *theory* is. Phenomenology's task is to relate this abstract study back to a concrete understanding of the essential types of mental act possessed by a subject that can formulate theories:

> This theory of theories goes together with, and is illuminated by, a formal theory of knowledge which precedes all empirical theory, which precedes, therefore, all explanatory knowledge of the real, all physical science on the one hand, and all psychology on the other, and of course all metaphysics. Its aim is not to *explain* knowledge in the psychological or psychophysical sense as a *factual* occurrence in objective nature, but to *shed light* on the *Idea* of knowledge in its constitutive elements and laws.   (p. 265)

This is a very important passage for our understanding of phenomenology. In it phenomenology is described as a 'formal theory of knowledge' that seeks to 'illuminate' or 'shed light' on the Idea of knowledge, as analysed in pure logic as a theory of theories. The terms 'illuminate' and 'shed light' both translate the German term '*aufklären*', which Husserl contrasts with explanation, or '*erklären*'. Husserl's term 'descriptive' for phenomenology thus needs to be understood not as part of the opposition 'empirical description vs. empirical explanation', but in terms of the opposition 'explanation vs. clarification'.

Question 6: phenomenology's presuppositionlessness

The idea that phenomenology must hold back from drawing on any explanatory theories of mental life, is also part of what Husserl means by the 'presuppositionlessness' of phenomenology. This is also discussed in §7: phenomenology is neither an explanatory theory, nor presupposes any explanatory theory. Husserl gives another useful characterization of what sort of theory phenomenology then is: 'The "theory" that it aspires to, is no more than a thinking over, a coming to an evident understanding of, thinking and knowing as such, in their pure generic essence.' (p. 263)

And, as we have seen, this 'thinking over' and 'coming to an evident understanding of' are by no means achieved through simple introspection; it involves a complex zigzag process, drawing on a number of different types of investigation, and on the findings of an analysis of the logical structure of theories. By bearing this in mind, we can also avoid a rather misleading connotation of the idea of a 'presuppositionless' approach to mental life. This connotation can suggest precisely that in phenomenology one simply introspects and describes what one sees without any presuppositions. It is rather the case that formal logic, together with, for example, investigations of formal grammar and formal ontology (which is what Husserl later calls part–whole theory), are presupposed and drawn on to help make explicit what is involved in the idea of knowledge and of being a knowing subject.

What is going on here can be made clearer by drawing on an idea from Husserl's later work, which is only implicitly present in *Logical Investigations*. In his later work, Husserl introduces the idea of 'bracketing' our everyday beliefs and theories. The notion of 'bracketing' does not merely mean that we are to avoid drawing on them, but rather that while they are 'bracketed' our everyday beliefs and theories, *with all their presuppositions*, are precisely to become the objects of study. In the later work, phenomenology becomes a far more general approach to uncovering, making explicit, and clarifying the hidden depths of presuppositions in our everyday 'natural attitude'. In the same way, we can think of the phenomenology of *Logical Investigations* as a more limited investigation aimed at uncovering, making explicit, and clarifying what is involved in the very idea of one sort of entity: ourselves, as knowing subjects.

Question 7: phenomenology does not presuppose the existence of human beings

There is a further and related connotation to Husserl's idea of the presuppositionlessness of phenomenology that we need to consider. We can think about it in this way: it would be odd to imagine that one could undertake a descriptive taxonomy of caterpillars, if none actually existed, yet phenomenology as a 'descriptive psychology' does not presuppose that there is anything with mental states! Husserl makes this point at the very end of the Introduction:

> It can easily be seen that the sense and the epistemological worth of the following analyses does not depend on the fact that there really are languages, and that men really make use of them in their mutual dealings, or that there really are such things as men and a nature, and that they do not merely exist in imagined, possible fashion. (p. 266)

Again, we need to remember that phenomenology, for Husserl, is an a priori, conceptual analysis of the idea of being a certain sort of subject, irrespective of the physical manifestation of such entities. We might think of it as making clear what is implicit in our everyday sense of ourselves, and also what would be implicit in the recognition of a Martian or gaseous extraterrestrial as being a 'knowing subject', i.e. something that we take to possess beliefs and knowledge about the external world. Husserl returns to this point at the very end of *Logical Investigations*, in a passage that underlines the generosity of spirit implicit in the rather formal approach to subjectivity found in phenomenology. It is worth citing this passage, even though it makes reference to a number of concepts that Husserl has analysed in the course of the book, which we cannot go into here.

> An understanding governed by other than the pure-logical laws would be an understanding without understanding. If we define understanding, as opposed to sensibility, as the capacity for categorial acts, also, perhaps, as a capacity for expression and meaning directed according to such acts, and made 'right' by them, then the general laws rooted in the specific nature of these acts belong to the definitory essence of understanding. Other beings may gaze upon other 'worlds', they may also be endowed with 'faculties' other than ours, but, if they are minded creatures at all, possessing some sort of intentional experiences [...] then such creatures have both sensibility and understanding, and are 'subject' to the pertinent laws. (p. 828)

Phenomenology is concerned to make explicit what is involved in the very ideas of 'understanding' and what one might call 'mindedness', such that if we take another entity, a Martian say, as possessing knowledge and beliefs about the world, then the phenomenological analysis will fit them too. From out of the undeniable formality and complexity of Husserl's phenomenology, a commitment shines through: not to allow contingent aspects of our physical constitution—being carbon-based organisms of a certain species, having two eyes and two legs, having blue eyes and blond hair—to encroach upon what properly makes up our sense of who and what we are. This only makes it all the more poignant that in the last years of his life, in 1930s Germany, Husserl suffered under a regime that labelled who and what he was purely in terms of his being Jewish.

Five key concepts in Husserl's *Logical Investigations*

With a background in place of what the nature of Husserl's phenomenology is, we can turn to the some of the key concepts

which figure in *Logical Investigations*—'intentionality', 'quality', 'matter', 'fullness', and the distinction between 'objectifying acts' and 'founding acts'. Although somewhat obscure as terms, Husserl's concepts actually capture rather intuitive aspects of how we think about mental states.

Intentionality and mental acts

Husserl's first key concept aims at drawing a distinction between two forms of experience that make up our mental lives. We think of certain experiences as being *about* or *of* things; for example, thoughts and perceptions. In having a thought, we are thinking *about* or *of* something; a perception is always a perception *of* something. A mental state such as pain, is not about anything in the same way—a pain is just a pain. Husserl distinguished these two types of experience by using the term 'intentional' for the former and 'non-intentional' for the latter. Husserl is here following Brentano, who had introduced the notion of intentionality as a defining characteristic of mental phenomena. Husserl differs from Brentano not only in allowing for non-intentional mental experiences, but also in the clarity of his analysis of the idea. Brentano's sole explication of the term in his major work *Psychology from an Empirical Standpoint* ([1874] 1995) is the following rather obscure passage:

> Every mental phenomena is characterised by what the Scholastics of the Middle Ages called the intentional (or mental) inexistence of an object, and what we might call, though not wholly unambiguously, reference to a content, direction toward an object (which is not to be understood here as meaning a thing), or immanent objectivity. Every mental phenomena includes something as object within itself, although they do not all do so in the same way. In presentation something is presented, in judgement, something is affirmed or denied, in love loved, in hate hated, in desire desired, and so on. (p. 88)

We do not have to worry here, however, about the details of the way Husserl criticizes, in Investigation V, the infelicities in Brentano's account. All we need to be clear about is that, used in this technical sense, 'intentional' does not mean anything like 'done on purpose'. It means purely the 'of-ness' or 'about-ness' of certain mental states, i.e. the way one might say, they are aimed at or directed to particular other things. Husserl introduces the term 'act' or 'mental act' as a short-form for 'intentional experience'.

The quality and the matter of mental acts

'Quality' and 'matter' are terms that Husserl uses to denote two aspects necessarily possessed by any mental act. Matter is the specific 'content' of a mental act, its being about the specific thing it is about; quality is more the 'attitude' one takes to what it is the mental act is of. We can make this clear though a few simple examples:

Quality is what the following mental acts have in common:

Being afraid of spiders
Being afraid that one has left the gas on

Whereas the following differ in quality but have the same matter:

Being afraid *that one has left the gas on*
Hoping *that one has left the gas on*

The fullness of a mental act

'Fullness' is Husserl's term for the third aspect necessarily possessed by a mental act; it is the extent to which a mental act is infused by sensory data. For Husserl, what primarily distinguishes the mental act of merely thinking of a friend, from the mental act of perceiving him in his bodily presence in front of one, is the different extent to which sense-data are woven into the experience. Mere thought of one's friend has a zero degree of sensory content, while a perception of one's friend is infused by visual sensory experiences.

Conceived of in isolation from their part in an intentional experience, sensory data are not of or about anything—they are non-intentional experiences such as pain. It is only when they become part of an encompassing intentional act that they become the visual experience *of* anything, for example, one's friend.

Husserl thinks of this in terms of the matter of an act informing the way that sensory content is 'apprehended'. For example, on a dark and murky night, the very same sensory content may at one moment be taken as giving one the visual experience of a person, and then after closer examination, as the visual experience of tree stump. These two experiences differ not in quality or in sensory content, but in their matter: one is *of a person*, the other is *of a tree stump*.

Husserl gives another example, which it is useful to cite, because it will later illuminate the relation of Husserl's early work both to Jaspers' phenomenology and to Husserl's own later conception of phenomenology.

> Whatever the origin of the experienced contents now present in consciousness, we can think that the same sensory contents should be present with a differing apprehension, i.e. that the same contents should serve to ground perceptions of different objects. Apprehension itself can never be reduced to an influx of new sensations; it is an act-character, a mode of consciousness, of 'mindedness'. We call the experiencing of sensations in this conscious manner the perception of the object in question. [...] I see a thing, e.g. this box, but I do not see my sensations. I always see *one and the same box*, however *it* may be turned and tilted. I have always the *same* 'content of consciousness'—if I care to call the perceived object a 'content of consciousness'. But each turn yields a *new* 'content of consciousness', if I call experienced contents 'contents of consciousness', in a much more appropriate use of words. Very different contents are therefore experienced, though the same object is perceived. The experienced content, generally speaking, is not the perceived object. We must note, further, that the object's real being or non-being is irrelevant to the true essence of the perceptual experience, and to its essence as a perceiving of an object as appearing thus and so, and as thus and so thought of.   (pp. 565–566)

There are a lot of ideas here, but for now we need only take note of two. First, there is the way that by distinguishing between the matter and sensory content of an act, Husserl tries to do justice to the way that perceiving a three-dimensional object can involve very different visual experiences, yet bound into a single mental state, which we would describe as the perception of one and the same object. Secondly, note that being able to distinguish sensory content as part of a mental act does not mean that we are explicitly aware of it when we 'live through' the mental act, so to speak. The object of the intentional experience is the object we are perceiving not the sensory content woven into the intentional mental state.

Objectifying acts and founded acts

In the context of a long discussion of Brentano in Investigation V, Husserl makes the claim that every mental act is either an objectifying act or founded on an objectifying act. What Husserl is getting at here, is the way that we can regard certain complex forms of mental state as having simpler mental acts as components. For example, instead of analysing the mental state of being happy that the sun is shining as a unitary state having a certain quality ('being happy') and matter ('that the sun is shining'), we can think of it as having, as a component, the self-standing mental act of believing that the sun is shining. We can say that the more complex happy mental state is 'founded on' this simpler mental act, in the sense that the former requires the latter for its existence. Husserl's name for these basic mental acts, which serve as a basis for all other attitudes we might take towards things, is 'objectifying acts'. Without going into the technicalities, the term 'objectifying act' is rather broader than 'belief', and is best thought of as the basic mental act involved in simply 'having something in mind'.

This is not to say, however, that in having the more complex mental state of happiness about something, we experience a distinction between what is given in the objectifying act and our attitude towards it. Husserl's analysis precisely tries to take account of what he calls the 'phenomenological unity' of a given experience: 'A sad event, likewise, is not merely seen in its thing-like content and context, in the respects which make it an event: it seems clothed and coloured with sadness.' (p. 574)

Here again we see how inadequate it is to think of phenomenology as simply involving an introspection of our mental states. The distinction Husserl draws between objectifying and founded acts is simply not one that we are aware of in the course of our mental lives. Rather, Husserl is attempting to give an analysis of such complex states as being happy and sad about things, which will show in a convincing way how such states figure in a broader conception of ourselves and our cognitive and logical abilities.

Husserl's later transcendental phenomenology (the attempt to get out of the box)

Before we end this session on Husserl's phenomenology, it would be worthwhile briefly considering his later conception of phenomenology, as found in the two works referred to above: 'Philosophy as a rigorous science' (1911) and *Ideas I* (1913). Rather than going into any detail—as Jaspers was clear that Husserl's later phenomenology was no longer helpful for his purposes—we shall look more at what Husserl thought was wrong with his own earlier conception of phenomenology.

If you look back at the long quotation from *Logical Investigations* above under 'The fullness of a mental act', you will see two things. First, that 'the origin of the experienced contents now present in consciousness' is not relevant to a phenomenological analysis, and second, that 'the object's real being or non-being is irrelevant to the true essence of the perceptual experience'. The picture this gives us of a knowing subject is that of a self-enclosed mental realm, with sensory-content that carries no information about its causal origin, or whether indeed the object we take ourselves to be perceiving exists or not. As a theory of knowledge, Husserl's early phenomenology ends up appearing to deny that we can ever have any knowledge of the external world at all!

Husserl's later diagnosis of what has gone wrong with the analysis is telling. He concludes that he has not been careful enough in 'bracketing' out naturalistic presuppositions in his analysis of subjectivity. What are these presuppositions that have crept in? Well, the knowing subject has been approached as a type of entity existing in the midst of other entities, such as tables and chairs—and it is this natural, everyday conception of ourselves that must now be 'bracketed', for the later Husserl, when we undertake a phenomenological analysis. When we bracket this naturalistic framework, we are no longer thinking of ourselves as an empirical subject, but as a 'transcendental subject'. In this 'transcendental attitude' we conceive of ourselves as a realm of absolute subjectivity, itself 'constituting' the objects that, in the 'natural attitude' we thought of as having independent existence.

Even from this rather brief description of 'transcendental phenomenology', one can see that it will be rather less useful for an empirical psychopathologist, such as Jaspers. If you want to find out more about Husserl's later work, however, and its relation to his earlier phenomenology, you should consult some of the works in the Reading guide at the end of this chapter.

Reflection on the session and self-test questions

Write down your own reflections on the materials in this session drawing out any points that are particularly significant for you. Then write brief notes about the following:

1. How does Husserl's view of phenomenology relate it (in his view) to logic and arithmetic?

2. By what method was phenomenological analysis meant to proceed?

3. What is the object of study of phenomenology, according to Husserl?

4. What does 'bracketing' mean? In modern phenomenology; and in Husserl's work?

5. What is the key aspect of the mind according to Husserl?

Session 4 Assessment of Husserl's influence on Jaspers

We have seen that both Jaspers' and Husserl's phenomenologies are complex and many-faceted. Assessing Husserl's influence on Jaspers, therefore, is itself a complex task. Such an assessment will depend on one's reading and interpretation of the work of both. It will also depend on what one regards as the most important characteristic of Husserl's phenomenology and whether that characteristic is, or is not, reflected in Jaspers' work. All the same, given our examination of Jaspers and Husserl above, it would seem that any assessment of Husserl's influence on Jaspers will need to take account of the following points.

Five differences between Husserl's phenomenology and Jaspers'

1. *The empirical or non-empirical nature of phenomenology.* Phenomenology for Jaspers is clearly an empirical discipline, a part of psychopathology, and more generally of psychology. Its aim is to yield a descriptive taxonomy of mental states. For Husserl, phenomenology is an a priori, conceptual study, quite distinct from empirical psychology, though its results, in terms of the conceptual scheme it yields, may be of use to the psychologist.

2. *The role of introspection and empathy.* For Jaspers, a phenomenological approach involves an empathetic re-living of a mental state by the phenomenologist, in order that he or she may grasp 'what it's like', in a way that cannot be communicated. Husserl, on the other hand, presupposes no transparent access to our own mental states in formulating an account of their essential nature; rather logic and other formal disciplines are used to shed light on what it means to possess logical and cognitive abilities.

3. *Phenomenology as 'static understanding'.* Jaspers thinks of 'phenomenology' as having a narrower range than Husserl envisages. For Jaspers phenomenology is merely 'static understanding', as opposed to 'genetic understanding', which concerns relations between mental states. Phenomenology for Husserl is equally concerned with relations between mental states, but in a more limited regard: connections that are 'rational' in a stronger sense, e.g. the relation between the wish that *p* and the perception that *p*. The notion of 'understanding' does not figure in Husserl's thinking in the same way as it does in Jaspers'. Husserl is more concerned with a priori rational relations between mental states, and not with what relations between belief states are 'understandable' or 'comprehensible', in a weaker sense. We must look elsewhere for the source of Jaspers' concern with 'understanding' and 'empathy', and we will be looking at this in Chapter 10.

4. *Phenomenology as a descriptive, rather than explanatory, undertaking.* For Jaspers, phenomenology should avoid drawing

on explanations of mental life, because it is to be purely a descriptive taxonomy. Phenomenology is descriptive for Husserl because it cannot, without circularity, invoke concepts drawn from explanatory sciences in its clarification of what it means to be an entity capable of engaging in an explanatory science.

5. *Phenomenology as presuppositionless.* Jaspers stresses the presuppositionlessness of phenomenology in virtue of the methodological requirement for a descriptive taxonomy to be undertaken honestly and accurately. For Husserl, the presuppositionlessness of phenomenology is in virtue of its status as a theory of knowledge. Further, as an a priori, conceptual analysis, phenomenology does not even presuppose the real existence of anything possessing mental states; rather it seeks to uncover, make explicit, and clarify the very 'presuppositions' implicit in the idea of a 'knowing subject'.

Signs of influence of Husserl on Jaspers

On each of the above five points, there would appear to be quite major differences between Jaspers' conception of phenomenology and Husserl's. We should not be too hasty in concluding, however, that there is, in fact, no influence by Husserl on Jaspers. This is because there are signs that Jaspers sought to draw on Husserl's phenomenology in the very way Husserl envisaged that an empirical psychologist could. The following passage comes from Jaspers' 1911 paper, 'The analysis of false perceptions':

> We give a second example from Husserl: 'I see a thing, e.g. this box, but I do not see my sensations. I always see one and the same box, however it may be turned and tilted.' The experience of the sensation changes, new sensations always appear in consciousness. It remains the same intending—the box as its object—the same act. We have in the total experience of perception the to-and-fro of the tilting box, changing parts, sensations, and the constant and invariable 'intending' of the box.
>
> Jaspers ([1911] 1963a, p. 197)

Here we see Jaspers directly drawing on Husserl's analysis of perception in terms of the way the matter of an intentional act can remain constant, while its sensory-content changes. In this article, Jaspers uses the concepts that Husserl had developed in the course of an a priori analysis of the knowing subject, in order to understand better the nature of a particular psychopathological symptom. Just as Husserl envisaged, his phenomenological analyses are being used to supply what we called at the start of this chapter, the basic conceptual framework for empirical psychological investigations. This use of Husserl's phenomenology is also much in evidence in Jaspers' major text, *General Psychopathology*. What tends to confuse the situation with regard to an assessment of Husserl's influence, is that Jaspers does not use the term 'phenomenology' for the basic conceptual scheme he takes from Husserl. Rather, as we have seen above, he uses the term 'phenomenology' for a type of psychological investigation

that he regards as an essential component of empirical psychology and psychopathology.

You can easily see, therefore, how one might come to two diametrically opposed conclusions about Husserl's influence on Jaspers. If one focuses on what Jaspers means by 'phenomenology' when he uses the term, one would have to conclude that there is little influence from Husserl: for Jaspers uses the term phenomenology to mean something quite different from Husserl. If, however, one focuses instead on the basic conceptual scheme that informs Jaspers' psychological investigations, one would conclude, to the contrary, that there is clear evidence of Husserl's influence. A brief survey of the current literature on the Husserl–Jaspers question shows that commentators have indeed tended to take up these diametrically opposed positions.

The debate continues

The question of Husserl's influence or lack of influence on Jaspers, has been explored by Osborne P. Wiggins and Michael Schwartz (a philosopher and psychiatrist respectively, working in America), by Manfred Spitzer (a German philosopher and psychiatrist) and by Chris Walker and G.E. Berrios (both psychiatrists working in England), as listed in the Reading guide. Wiggins and Schwartz, and Spitzer, argue that Husserl was indeed a major influence, while Walker and Berrios argue that there is no substantive presence of Husserl's thinking in Jaspers' work.

We cannot do justice here to the detailed way in which each of these authors defends their position. However, in terms of the material presented in this chapter, we can understand their respective positions broadly as follows:

◆ Wiggins and Schwartz (1995) downplay the differences we have noted above, and they do this by emphasizing the role of 'intuition' in Husserl's phenomenology. This allows them to understand Husserl's views of the descriptive and presuppositionless nature of phenomenology in a way that fits far better with what Jaspers says. That is, by emphasizing the way that Husserl demands that we go beyond merely playing with concepts, and directly 'look' at what is going on, Husserl's approach seems very similar to what Jaspers demands for an accurate descriptive taxonomy of mental states.

◆ Walker does much to balance this interpretation, by stressing the purely conceptual (or 'eidetic', to use a term from the later Husserl) nature of phenomenology. He convincingly argues that the clearly eidetic approach of Husserl's later phenomenology—which Jaspers rejected—was already implicit in Husserl's earlier work. He draws the conclusion that Jaspers misunderstood the nature of Husserl's early work, and thus that it had no real influence on him. We have seen, however, that a purely conceptual analysis can be of use to an empirical science, that Husserl envisaged that his phenomenology could be of use in this way, and that Jaspers did indeed use Husserl's phenomenology in this way.

Walker goes on to argue that it is Kant, rather than Husserl, who provides the philosophical force behind Jaspers' psychopathology, and in Chapter 10 we will be looking at the influence of 'Neo-Kantian' thinking more closely.

♦ Berrios, who is a historian as well as psychiatrist (we drew on his work in Chapter 7), does a great service in demonstrating how prevalent the idea was of a descriptive taxonomy of mental states, independent of Husserl's approach, at the time Jaspers was working as a young man in Heidelberg. He goes so far as to suggest that Jaspers cited Husserl's *Phenomenology* merely 'to legitimate his own youthful ideas on psychopathological description' (p. 317). As we saw above, Dilthey for example, also argued for the need for a 'descriptive psychology'.

What Berrios perhaps underplays is the way that even a purely 'descriptive' approach moves within a certain general conceptual framework, and that the key notion of 'intentionality' does not figure, for example, in the 'descriptive psychology' of Dilthey. It was Husserl who, more than anyone, strove to clarify the conceptual scheme in which we talk of *mental states*, and thus one might indeed be able to find evidence of a distinctive influence from Husserl on Jaspers.

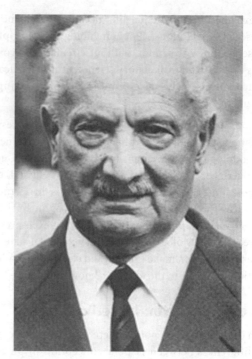

Fig. 9.3 Heidegger

Reflection on the session and self-test questions

Write down your own reflections on the materials in this session drawing out any points that are particularly significant for you. Then write brief notes about the following:

1. Is there a clear answer to the degree of influence of Husserl on Jaspers?

2. Are there differences in the accounts of phenomenology given by Jaspers and Husserl? If so, give an example.

Session 5 Conclusions: the contemporary relevance of the phenomenological tradition in psychiatry

As indicated at the start of this chapter, Husserl's importance for psychopathology and psychiatry is very far from being limited to any influence he may have had, directly or indirectly, on Karl Jaspers. Husserl's phenomenology, as we noted, generated a rich tradition of phenomenological work in the twentieth century, much of it inspired by critical engagement with the master!

A number of major figures from this tradition have had important influences on psychiatry. We noted some of these in Chapter 4—Sartre and Merleau-Ponty, for example. Clearly we cannot do justice, here, to a century of phenomenological psychiatry

and to the work of the many important contemporary figures in the field. We give illustrative references in the Reading guides at chapter 4. A number of books in this series explore phenomenological approaches: *The Vulnerable self*, by Joseph Parnas, Louis Sass, Giovanni Stanghellini, and Thomas Fuchs provides a detailed introduction to contemporary phenomenology and psychiatry; and the sister volume to this book, Jennifer Radden's *Companion*, includes a number of chapters by important contemporary phenomenologists.

By way of illustration, however, we will conclude this chapter with a brief excursion into the contemporary relevance of one of Husserl's most famous pupils, the German philosopher, Martin Heidegger. Heidegger became notorious for his support for the Nazi party (see, e.g., Sheehan, 1988; Farias, 1989). But his phenomenology is important as an illustration of the relevance of phenomenology not just for psychopathology, classification, and diagnosis, but also in generating new approaches to treatment.

Heidegger and Husserl's problem

Heidegger, who worked in Heidelberg before and during the Second World War, was deeply influenced by Husserl, particularly the Husserl of *Logical Investigations*. Like Jaspers, however, Heidegger was unhappy with Husserl's move to a 'transcendental phenomenology'. The work that put Heidegger on the philosophical map was *Being and Time*, first published in 1927. Though dense, and difficult to read, this work caused huge excitement at the time. The book was part of a much larger philosophical project, the first stage of which involved fundamentally questioning our sense of who and what we are. Heidegger was convinced that Husserl's phenomenological analysis of what it means to be a 'knowing subject' was deeply, if largely implicitly, informed by a traditional Cartesian framework.

We saw above how Husserl himself came to be unhappy with the analysis of *Logical Investigations* because it seemed to leave the subject strangely cut off from his or her world, never really in contact with it at all. Husserl sought to avoid this problem by moving to an approach in which one no longer regards oneself as an entity in the world at all, but rather as a 'transcendental ego', the ground of the very existence of the world.

Heidegger and the analysis of Dasein

Heidegger's diagnosis of what had gone wrong was different. The mistake was not in regarding oneself as an entity *per se*, but rather in the Cartesian view of that entity as essentially constituted by a subjective realm cut off from the world outside it. Whereas Husserl sought to analyse what it means to be a 'knowing subject', Heidegger even thought that the very term 'subject' is best avoided, because of its deeply entrenched Cartesian connotations. Instead, Heidegger uses the less 'theory-laden' term 'Dasein' (which is used in everyday German for 'existing' or 'being', and literally means 'being there') as the name for the sort of entity 'we' are. 'We' is in scare quotes here because, following Husserl, Heidegger is not giving an empirical analysis of what it means to be an entity of the empirical species 'human being'. Rather, Heidegger is concerned to give an analysis of what it means to be open to the world in the way we take ourselves to be everyday, and would equally apply to any other entity we take to be like us in this way. *Being and Time* thus involves what Heidegger calls the 'Analysis of Dasein'.

Heidegger argues that traditional views of ourselves, which also inform Husserl's analyses, are marked by certain 'atomistic' ways of thinking. This happens in regard to two 'dimensions' of life, so to speak. First of all, in a vertical dimension, we think of subjectivity as an independent and self-standing realm, with the world outside it; then secondly, we think of mental life as a discrete, 'atomised' series of mental acts or experiences. Heidegger's aim is to re-think life or Dasein in a way free of these theoretical presuppositions, and also to explain why these artificial ways of thinking (as he considers them) come so naturally to us.

You can get a feel for Heidegger's approach in the following brief extract from *Being and Time*, which outlines what he takes to be the proper starting point for a description of Dasein's engagement with the world, which stresses its practical rather than its theoretical nature.

EXERCISE 4   (15 minutes)

Read the short extract from:

Heidegger, M. (1962). *Being and Time* (trans. John Macquarrie and Edward Robinson). Oxford: Basil Blackwell, pp. 95–99

Link with Reading 9.3

◆ What is the role of equipment in Heidegger's account of Dasein's understanding of the world?

One of Heidegger's key innovations in overcoming these two atomistic conceptions is to focus on our involvement in practices by which we use everyday items of 'equipment'—chairs, tables, pens, pencils, hammers, etc. That is, traditionally one might think of mental life as consisting of a series of discrete 'ideas', 'representations', or 'acts' that correspond in some way to items in the world outside. Heidegger, however, suggests that we think of ourselves more in terms of our concrete ability to become involved in ongoing practices, in which such items as chairs and tables take on significance for us.

Heidegger's impact on psychotherapy

This is only the briefest indication of Heidegger's project—for additional reading, see the introductory books on Heidegger in the Reading guide. Heidegger's work has proved a rich source, however, for psychiatrists and psychotherapists unhappy with existing conceptual frameworks for understanding human beings.

One of the first therapists to take up Heidegger's approach was Ludwig Binswanger, who introduced a distinctive type of 'existential psychotherapy' that he called 'daseinsanalysis'. Heidegger's thinking also entered the clinical domain through the work of Medard Boss. Boss, who had trained as a psychiatrist and psychoanalyst, became fascinated with *Being and Time* during the Second World War. After the war Boss wrote to Heidegger and they struck up a close friendship that was to last until Heidegger's death in 1976. Throughout the 1960s Heidegger would often visit Boss's home in Zollikon, Switzerland and hold seminar discussions with Boss's students. Transcripts of these seminars, together with Boss's notes from his conversations with Heidegger were published in 1987 as the *Zollikoner Seminare*. In the introduction, Boss tells us that Heidegger's hope was that his work might 'escape the confines of a philosopher's study and become of benefit to wider circles, in particular to a large number of suffering human beings' (p. 7).

Recent phenomenological strands

In the Reading Guide to this chapter, we include examples from the very rich literature in modern phenomenology and psychopathology. A useful review, which brings the 'phenomenological' approach up to the end of the twentieth century, is a paper by the philosopher and psychiatrist, Patrick Bracken (1999).

In this paper Bracken outlines a number of developments in contemporary thinking about psychiatry. His suggestion—very much in line with the theme of this chapter—is that contemporary psychiatry can learn from the technical uses of the term 'phenomenology'. As Bracken points out, the current use of this term at least in Anglo-American psychiatry is simply as a listing of clearly described symptoms without presupposing any particular aetiological theory. But as we have seen, the term has a rich and complex philosophical history. Bracken suggests that contemporary psychiatry should take note of and could usefully draw on that philosophical history.

Bracken argues further that a key moment in phenomenology for psychiatry was Heidegger's move away from Husserl to the engaged view of Dasein he set out in *Being and Time* as involving everyday practical activities that we normally take completely for granted. Bracken suggests that the Cartesian elements within Husserl's picture would dovetail with contemporary cognitivism in philosophy and the neurosciences, and, hence, that if there are a priori arguments in favour of Heidegger and against Husserl, these might translate into arguments against cognitivism.

Whether Bracken is right in his general claim remains an open question. We have found in this chapter that simply describing Husserl's position as Cartesian is an oversimplification. But as we will see in Part V, when we consider cognitivism in detail (see especially Chapter 24), Bracken is not alone in pointing to the need for 'understanding' and 'meaning' to move outside the skull, as it were, to escape from the narrow confines of the intrapersonal space of cognitivism into an extended interpersonal space of social exchanges (see, for example, the work of Rom Harre, Grant Gillett and Steven Sabat in Part V). And Bracken, taking his Heideggerian phenomenology right through into practice, has developed a distinctively Heidegerian analysis of post-traumatic stress disorder which, combined with his clinical work in Africa, has become the basis of a policy statement by Amnesty International.

Important, therefore, as the links between phenomenology and the new neurosciences may eventually turn out to be, Bracken's work, in drawing on Heidegger's analysis of Dasein to develop new policies and treatment approaches in some of the most challenging areas of clinical practice, provides a clear signal of the continuing relevance of phenomenology for psychiatry today.

Reflection on the session and self-test questions

Write down your own reflections on the materials in this session drawing out any points that are particularly significant for you. Then write brief notes about the following:

1. Besides Jaspers, what other phenomenologist has particularly influenced psychiatry, and in what area?

2. What term does Heidegger use in reference to subjects in *Being and Time*?

3. What does his term mean literally and why does he use it?

4. In what parts of the world did phenomenology particularly develop in the twentieth century?

Reading guide

Husserl

Husserl wrote an overview of his project in the *Logical Investigations* from the perspective of his later position. This has been published in English as:

◆ Edmund Husserl (1977). 'The task and the significance of the *Logical Investigations*' (trans. by J.N. Findlay) in *Readings on Edmund Husserl's 'Logical Investigations'* (ed. J.N. Mohanty). The Hague: Martinus Nijhoff, pp. 197–215.

A useful (though still difficult!) overview of transcendental phenomenology in English is given by Husserl in an article he wrote for the *Encyclopaedia Britannica*:

◆ Edmund Husserl [1927]. 'Phenomenology', Edmund Husserl's Article for the *Encyclopaedia Britannica*, revised translation by Richard E. Palmer, in Husserl, *Husserl: Shorter Works*. Indiana: University of Notre Dame Press (1981), pp. 21–35; reprinted from (1971) *Journal of the British Society for Phenomenology* 2: 77–90.

Among excellent commentaries on Husserl's philosophy, note: Bernet, Kern, and Marbach's (1993) *An Introduction to Husserlian Phenomenology* (this covers each period of Husserl's thinking with great clarity) and de Boer's (1978) *The Development of Husserl's Thought* (trans. by Theodore Plantinga) on Husserl's early work on mathematics up to the point where he develops transcendental phenomenology.

The Husserl–Jaspers question

The Cambridge psychiatrist and historian, G.E. Berrios, whose foundational work on the history of psychiatry and psychopathology we noted in Chapter 7, has written critically of many of the widely held views about the relationship between phenomenology, Jaspers and psychopathology today. See Berrios (1993) 'Phenomenology and psychopathology: was there ever a relationship?', and (1992) 'Phenomenology, psychopathology and Jaspers: a conceptual history'.

The debate in *Philosophy, Psychiatry, & Psychology* exploring contrary views on the importance of Husserl's influence on Jaspers, includes four papers by the British psychiatrist Chris Walker, with a reply in two parts by the American philosopher, Osborne Wiggins, and the psychiatrist (and founder President of the American Association for the Advancement of Philosophy and Psychiatry), Michael Schwartz.

Chris Walker sets out his detailed case in four papers: 'Karl Jaspers and Edmund Husserl—I: The perceived convergence' (1994a); 'II: The divergence' (1994b); 'III: Jaspers as a Kantian phenomenologist' (1995a; with a commentary by Ruth Chadwick, 1995); and 'IV: Phenomenology as empathic understanding' (1995b).

Wiggins and Schwartz reply to Walker in a first paper in *Philosophy, Psychiatry, & Psychology* and set out their own views directly in a later paper:

- Wiggins and Schwartz (1995). 'Chris Walker's interpretation of Karl Jaspers' phenomenology: a critique', with a commentary by Fulwiler and Folstein (1995).
- Wiggins and Schwartz (1997). 'Edmund Husserl's influence on Karl Jaspers' phenomenology', with a commentary by Handin and Azarin (1997).

The original statement of their position is given in: Wiggins *et al.* (1992) 'Phenomenological/descriptive psychiatry: Husserl and Jaspers', in Spitzer, *et al.* (ed.), *Phenomenology, Language and Schizophrenia*.

Heidegger

Heidegger's *Being and Time* is generally acknowledged to be one of the most difficult philosophical texts of modern times! You may, therefore, want to start by reading one of the lecture courses Heidegger gave at the time, which provide more accessible introductions to his project. The lecture course *History of the Concept of Time*, in particular, has a lengthy discussion of Husserl's phenomenology. See: *The Basic Problems of Phenomenology*, trans. by A. Hofstadter (1982) (a 1927 lecture course), and *History of the Concept of Time: Prolegomena*, trans. by T. Kisiel (1985) (a 1925 lecture course).

Heidegger's Zollikon seminars are not available in translation as a whole, however, the following is a translation of a number of extracts: 'On adequate understanding of daseins-analysis: excerpts from Martin Heidegger's Zollikon teaching', translated by Michael Eldred (1988).

Two of the best short introductions to Heidegger's work are: Mulhall (1996) *The Routledge Philosophy Guidebook to Heidegger and 'Being and Time'*, and Polt (1999) *Heidegger: an introduction*.

The Heideggerian tradition in psychiatry

Two key publications marking the translation of Heidegger's philosophy into psychotherapy are: Biswanger (1963) *Being-in-the-World*, and Boss (1963) *Psychoanalysis and Daseinsanalysis*.

The Irish psychiatrist and philosopher, Patrick Bracken, has drawn on Heideggerian phenomenology in developing new approaches to the management of severe trauma in society that retain a strong cultural rather than individual identity (see, Bracken *et al.*, 1997; Bracken and Peay, 1998; Bracken, 2001; Bracken, forthcoming). For an ingenious extension of the concept of *Dasein* to current issues of user and carer empowerment within multidisciplinary (hence multimodel, see Part I) services, see Heginbotham (2004) in *Psychiatric Dasein*.

References

American Psychiatric Association (1987). *Diagnostic and Statistical Manual of Mental Disorders*, (3rd edn), revised (DSM-III-R). Washington DC: American Psychiatric Association.

Bernet, R., Kern, I., and Marbach, E. (1993). *An Introduction to Husserlian Phenomenology*. Evanston: Northwestern University Press.

Berrios, G.E. (1992). Phenomenology, psychopathology and Jaspers: a conceptual history. *History of Psychiatry*, 3: 303–327.

Berrios, G.E. (1993). Phenomenology and psychopathology: Was there ever a relationship? *Comprehensive Psychiatry*, 34: 213–220.

Binswanger, L. (1963). *Being-in-the-World*. New York: Basic Books.

Boss, M. (1963). *Psychoanalysis and Daseinsanalysis*. New York: Basic Books.

Bracken, P.J. (1999). Phenomenology and psychiatry. *Current Opinion in Psychiatry*, 12: 593–596.

Bracken, P. (2001). Post modernity and post traumatic stress disorder. *Social Science and Medicine*, 53: 733–743.

Bracken, P. (2002). *Trauma: Culture, Meaning and Philosophy*. London: Whurr Publishers.

Bracken, P. and Petty, C. (ed.) (1998). *Rethinking the Trauma of War*. London: Free Association Books.

Bracken, P., Giller, J., and Summerfield, D. (1997). Rethinking mental health. work with survivors of wartime violence and refugees. *Journal of Refugee Studies*, 10: 431–442

Brentano, F. ([1874] 1995). *Psychology from an Empirical Standpoint* (trans. Antos C. Rancurello, D.B. Terrell, and Linda L. McAlister). London: Routledge.

Chadwick, R.F. (1995). Commentary: Karl Jaspers and Edmund Husserl—III. *Philosophy, Psychiatry, & Psychology*, 2: 83–84.

de Boer, T. (1978). *The Development of Husserl's Thought* (trans. by Theodore Plantinga). The Hague: Martinus Nijhoff.

Farias, V. (1989). *Heidegger and Nazism*. Philadelphia Temple University Press.

Frege, G. (1980). *Foundations of Arithmetic* (trans. J.L. Austin). Oxford: Blackwell.

Fulwiler, C. and Folstein, M.F. (1995). Commentary: Chris Walkers (1995). Interpretation of Karl Jaspers phenomenology. *Philosophy, Psychiatry, & Psychology*, 2(4): 345–347.

Heginbotham, C. (2004). Psychiatric Dasein. *Philosophy, Psychiatry, & Psychology*, 11(2): 147–150.

Heidegger, M. (1962). *Being and Time* (trans. John Macquarrie and Edward Robinson). Oxford: Basil Blackwell.

Heidegger, M. (1985). *History of the Concept of Time: Prolegomena* (trans. by T. Kisiel). Bloomington, IN: Indiana University Press.

Heidegger, M. (1982). *The Basic Problems of Phenomenology* (trans. by A. Hofstadter). Bloomington, IN: Indiana University Press.

Heidegger, M. (1987). *Zollikoner Seminare: Protokolle—Gespräche—Briefe* (ed. M. Boss). Frankfurt am Main: Klostermann.

Heidegger, M. (1988). On adequate understanding of daseinsanalysis: excerpts from Martin Heidegger's zollikon teaching (trans. by Michael Eldred). *Humanistic Psychologist*, 16: 75–98.

Hempel, C.C. (1994). Fundamentals of taxonomy.

Husserl, E. (1927). Phenomenology. Edmund Husserl's Article for the *Encyclopaedia Britannica* (revised translation by Richard E. Palmer). In *Husserl: Shorter Works*. Indiana: University of Notre Dame Press (1981), pp. 21–35. (Reprinted from (1971). *Journal of the British Society for Phenomenology*, 2: 77–90.

Husserl, E. ([1900–01] 1970a). *Logical Investigations* (trans. by J.N. Findlay), 2 vols. London: Routledge and Kegan Paul.

Husserl, E. (1970b). *Philosophie der Arithmetik* (ed. L. Eley). The Hague: Martinus Nijhoff.

Husserl, E. (1975). *Introduction to the Logical Investigations* (trans. P.J. Bossert and C.H. Peters) (ed. E. Fink). The Hague: Martinus Nijhoff.

Husserl, E. (1977). The task and the significance of the *Logical Investigations* (trans. by J.N.Findlay). In *Readings on Edmund Husserl's 'Logical Investigations'* (ed. J.N. Mohanty). The Hague: Martinus Nijhoff, pp. 197–215.

Husserl, E. (1981). Philosophy as a rigorous science. In *Husserl: Shorter Works* (trans. by Quentin Lauer). Indiana: University of Notre Dame Press, pp. 166–197. (Also in Husserl, E. (1965) *Phenomenology and the Crisis of Philosophy*. New York: Harper & Row, pp. 71–147.)

Husserl, E. (1982). *Ideas Pertaining to a Pure Phenomenology and to a Phenomenological Philosophy, First Book: general introduction to a pure phenomenology* (trans. F. Kersten). Dordrecht: Kluwer.

Jaspers, K. ([1911] 1963a). Zur Analyse der Trugwahrnehmungen' (The Analysis of False Perceptions). In *Gesammelte Schriften zur Psychopathologie*. Berlin: Springer-Verlag, pp. 191–251.

Jaspers, K. ([1913b] 1974). Causal and 'meaningful' connections between life history and psychosis (Kausale und verständliche Zusammenhänge zwischen Schicksal und Psychose bei der Dementia praecox) (trans. J. Hoenig). In *Themes and Variations in European Psychiatry* (ed. S.R. Hirsch and M. Shepherd). Bristol: Wright.

Jaspers, K. (1963b). *General Psychopathology* (trans. J. Hoenig and M.W. Hamilton). Chicago: University of Chicago Press.

Jaspers, K. [1912]. The phenomenological approach in psychopathology (trans. of 'Die phänomenologische Forschungsrichtung in der Psychopathologie); reprinted in *Gesammelte Schriften zur Pschopathologie* (*Collected Writings in Psychopathology*), pp. 314–328; anonymously translated in *British Journal of Psychiatry*, 1968; 114: 1313–1323.

Mulhall, S. (1996). *The Routledge Philosophy Guidebook to Heidegger and 'Being and Time'*. London: Routledge.

Naudin, J. and Azorin, J.-M. (1997). Commentary on Wiggins and Schwartz, 1997, Edmund Husserls influence on Karl Jaspers's phenomenology. *Philosophy, Psychiatry, & Psychology*, 4: 37–40.

Parnas, J., Sass, L., Stanghellini, G. and Fuchs, T. *The Vulnerable Self: the clinical phenomenology of the schizophrenic and affective spectrum disorders*. Oxford: Oxford University Press.

Polt, R. (1999). *Heidegger: an introduction*. London: University of London Press.

Radden, J. (Ed) (2004) *The Philosophy of Psychiatry*. New York: Oxford University Press.

Sheehan, T. (1988). Heidegger and the Nazis. *New York Review of Books*, June 16.

Strawson, (1964). Individuals. London: Routledge.

Walker, C. (1994a). Karl Jaspers and Edmund Husserl—I: The perceived convergence. *Philosophy, Psychiatry and Psychology*, 1: 117–134.

Walker, C. (1994b). Karl Jaspers and Edmund Husserl—II: The divergence. *Philosophy, Psychiatry and Psychology*, 1: 245–265.

Walker, C. (1995a). Karl Jaspers and Edmund Husserl—III: Jaspers as a Kantian phenomenologist. *Philosophy, Psychiatry, & Psychology*, 2: 65–82.

Walker, C. (1995b). Karl Jaspers and Edmund Husserl—IV: Phenomenology as empathic understanding. *Philosophy, Psychiatry and Psychology*, 2: 247–266.

Wiggins, O.P. and Schwartz, M.A. (1995). Chris Walkers Interpretation of Karl Jaspers phenomenology: a critique. *Philosophy, Psychiatry, & Psychology*, 2(4): 319–344.

Wiggins, O.P. and Schwartz, M.A. (1997). Edmund Husserl's influence on Karl Jasperss phenomenology. *Philosophy, Psychiatry, & Psychology*, 4: 15–36.

Wiggins, O.P., Schwartz, M.A., and Spitzer, M. (1992). Phenomenological/descriptive psychiatry: Husserl and Jaspers. In *Phenomenology, Language and Schizophrenia* (ed. Spitzer, M. *et al.*). New York: Springer-Verlag, p. 67.

Wittgenstein, L. (1953). *Philosophical Investigations* (trans. G.E.M. Anscombe). Oxford: Blackwell.

CHAPTER 10

Psychopathology and the 'Methodenstreit'

Chapter contents

Introduction

This is the second of two chapters concerned with the philosophical basis of the work of Karl Jaspers. In Chapter 9 we considered the influence of Edmund Husserl's phenomenology, and concluded that there were aspects of Jaspers' approach to psychopathology that were not 'phenomenological' in Husserl's sense. These included the notions of 'empathy' and 'imaginative re-living', as parts of the psychopathologist's methodology, and 'understanding' (as opposed to 'explanation') as a key aim of the psychopathologist's investigations.

In order to gain a clearer sense of what Jaspers meant by these terms, we need to look at how they were used in a philosophical debate that was being carried on at the time: the debate over the nature and status of the 'human sciences'. This debate was concerned, in particular, with whether the method and aims of the human sciences, such as history, political science, and comparative religious studies, are the same as those of the natural sciences. Hence it has become known as the *Methodenstreit*, literally translated as the 'methodological debate'. This debate, which ran primarily in Germany and drew heavily on Kantian philosophy, had as we shall see, a considerable influence on Jaspers. By looking more closely at the debate itself, therefore, we will be in a better position to understand and assess Jaspers' work on the philosophical foundations of descriptive psychopathology.

Who's who

In this chapter, after an initial exploration of the key distinction between understanding and explaining, we will examine the influences of the *Methodenstreit* on Jaspers particularly through the work of three of the big names in nineteenth century German scholarship, Dilthey, Weber, and Rickert.

- ◆ Wilhelm Dilthey, one of the chief protagonists in the *Methodenstreit*, was a historian and philosopher. He asserted the independent status of the human sciences, citing 'empathy' and 'imaginative re-living' as their distinctive methods, and 'understanding' as their distinctive aim.

- ◆ Max Weber, by contrast, was a sociologist—we looked briefly at Jaspers' close friendship with him in Chapter 8. In this chapter we will be focusing on the aspects of Weber's work which influenced Jaspers, particularly Weber's concept of 'ideal types'.

- ◆ Heinrich Rickert, a leading figure in the philosophical movement known as the South-west German school of Neo-Kantianism, had a considerable influence on Weber. Rickert sought to analyse the distinctive method and aims of history in terms of the place of values in its investigations, and thus to defend the methodological autonomy of the human or 'cultural' sciences.

The *Methodenstreit* today

Dilthey and the South-west German School of Neo-Kantianism were both deeply influenced by Kant, but they regarded his

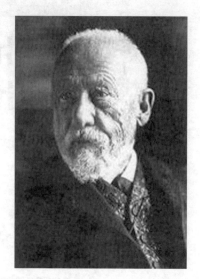

Fig. 10.1 Wilhelm Dilthey

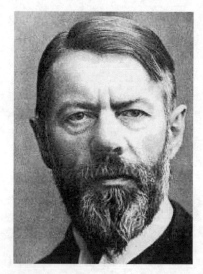

Fig. 10.2 Max Weber

theory of knowledge as having significant limitations, particularly in regard to an account of *historical* knowledge. History is often taken as a paradigm example of a human science, and, in an attempt to make sense of the thoughts, intentions, beliefs, and desires of figures whose way of thinking may be quite different

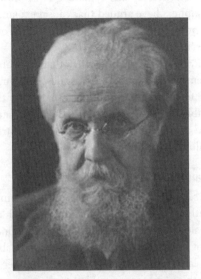

Fig. 10.3 Heinrich Rickert

to their own, the work of historians would seem to resemble in some respects that of practitioners in relation to their patients.

Psychiatry, however, as we have seen, if it is in some respects like history, and thus has connections with (in the terms of the *Methodenstreit*) a paradigmatic *human* science, also draws directly on such disciplines as neurophysiology and neuropharmacology, and thus has connections with paradigmatic *natural* sciences. Psychiatry, then, is at the heart of the *Methodenstreit*. We will conclude this chapter, therefore, with an overview of four unresolved tensions in the way Jaspers conceived of the relation between these two sides of psychiatry. This will lead into a closer examination of the nature of psychiatry as a science in Part III.

Session 1 Understanding, explanation, and the *Methodenstreit*

In the previous chapter, we noted that Jaspers characterized phenomenology as being concerned only with what he called 'static understanding', i.e. the description and classification of mental states taken in isolation.

From 'static' to 'genetic' understanding

In this chapter we are going to be primarily concerned with what Jaspers says about the *connections* between mental states, and in particular the idea of a 'meaningful' connection as opposed to a 'causal' connection. To grasp the meaningful connection between two mental states is to possess what Jaspers calls, in contrast to static understanding, 'genetic understanding'. It is with genetic understanding, then, in Jaspers' terms, that we will be concerned

in focusing on his 1913 paper (introduced in chapter 8), 'Causal and "meaningful" connections between life history and psychosis'. (The German title is 'Kausale und verständliche Zusammenhänge zwischen Schicksal und Psychose bei der Dementia praecox (Schizophrenie)'.) Before coming directly to this, however, we need to start with some terminological issues.

Terms of art and everyday terms

Jaspers' terms of art

In Jaspers' terminology, as we saw in the previous chapter, 'static understanding' together with 'genetic understanding', make up 'subjective psychology', as opposed to 'objective psychology'. However, in the context of discussing the two different types of connection one might seek to find between mental states, Jaspers tends to use slightly different terminology. Rather than 'genetic understanding', Jaspers simply uses the term 'understanding' ('*Verstehen*'), and speaks of '*verstehende psychologie*', translated as 'meaningful psychology'. This type of psychology is then not so much compared with 'objective psychology' as a whole, but rather with that part of it that attempts to formulate *causal explanations* of mental phenomena. What we will be looking at in this session is the distinction that Jaspers formulates in terms of the difference between 'understanding' and 'explanation'.

The reason for starting with these terminological observations is twofold. First, the rather specific way in which Jaspers distinguishes between understanding and explanation does not exactly match colloquial usage. We need to be aware, therefore, that Jaspers is using these as 'terms of art'. This in turn will help us see the extent to which Jaspers is influenced in this by the philosophical context in which his thinking took shape. In particular, the use of the terms 'understanding' and 'explanation' with quite distinct meanings owes much to the *Methodenstreit*: 'understanding' was held to be the aim of human sciences, while 'explanation' was the aim of the natural sciences.

The second reason for starting with terminology is to allow us to sharpen our sense of what these terms mean before going on to look at Jaspers' paper. By taking an initial look at what we mean by 'coming to an understanding' and 'giving an explanation', we will be better placed to assess what *Jaspers* thinks is involved.

'Explaining' and 'understanding'

In everyday life, there are many different forms of what we would describe as an 'explanation'. In Chapter 9, for example, we drew attention to two different sorts of conclusion one might reach in a clinical context:

◆ John is depressed because of the death of his friend.

◆ John is depressed because of a neurochemical imbalance in his brain.

Each of these, in a different way, gives an '*explanation*' of why John is depressed; one might also say that in each case we are being told something, on the basis of which we can '*understand*'

John's state of depression. In everyday usage we do not draw a sharp distinction in our use of the terms 'understanding' and 'explanation', yet we can clearly see that the above statements offer quite different forms of explanation or understanding. Only the second statement is offering us a lawlike 'causal account' of John's depression.

The giving of a causal account of a certain event or phenomena is something we do everyday, of course, but it is also regarded as the chief aim of natural science. We speak of a scientist 'coming to an *understanding*' of why a china vase breaks when it is dropped but a rubber ball does not, and here we think of this *understanding* as consisting in the formulation of a causal story relating to the behaviour of their microscopic constituents.

This type of explanation or understanding seems quite different to the type in which we are told of someone's reasons or motives for acting in a certain way. We might, for example, *explain* why someone is running down the high street in a suit and tie, by saying that he does not wish to miss his bus. Here we would not think of ourselves as giving a causal account of the behaviour of a certain object, but rather as making his behaviour comprehensible in a different way, a way that has to do with his intentions (to catch the bus), beliefs (that the bus is about to leave), and so on.

On the face of it then, while not distinguishing between the terms 'understanding' and 'explanation', we have a clear sense of there being different forms of what we think of as understanding or explaining. Jaspers, following the lead of protagonists in the *Methodenstreit*, uses 'explanation' solely for the giving of a causal account, while 'understanding' is used for an account that concerns the 'meaning' of an action or event. Though we have an intuitive grasp of a difference between these two forms of comprehending the world, it will be useful to think briefly about the extent to which we grasp what is involved in each considered separately.

Giving a causal explanation

In a causal account, we normally think of there being a certain necessity in a sequence of events: we speak of one event 'making' another event happen. We also think of there being a degree of universality, if our causal account is correct; that is, we think that if event A causes event B, then we can expect that, all other things being equal, events of the first type are always followed by events of the second type. As a result, we expect a causal explanation of a particular occurrence to make reference to a general *law* (sometimes called a 'law of nature') connecting an occurrence of that type to an antecedent event of a certain type.

In Chapter 15 (Part III), we will look much more closely at some of the difficulties surrounding the notion of a causal connection. We will be considering, for example, whether it is possible to explain the notion of 'causation' in terms of more basic ideas. Thus, the eighteenth century British philosopher, David Hume, argued that an observation of one thing '*making*' another thing happen is an illusion: our idea of causation, Hume argued,

derives merely from the more basic idea of there having been a 'constant conjunction' of one type of event following another. Other philosophers have argued that causal explanations reflect and rely on nothing more than the formulation of generalizations, such as 'if A then B'.

It turns out, as we will see in Part III, that there are in fact profound problems with attempts such as these to reduce the notion of causation to something more basic; however, this leaves us only being able to say that we correctly give a causal account when we *find* causal connections—and this can strike us as not particularly illuminating!

Coming to an understanding

Jaspers often seems to suggest that our ability to 'comprehend' the world is neatly divided into 'understanding' and 'explanation'. We will see below that he proposes that where we find a sequence of events 'not understandable' or 'ununderstandable', we must there posit a causal connection. There are a number of questions we can ask at this point, however. First of all, is it true that there is just one thing we think of as constituting 'understanding'? Are there more simple types of understanding from which our more complex ways of coming to an understanding are derived? And, paralleling our thoughts about causal explanation, is our notion of what is 'understandable' reducible to more basic ideas?

The very title of Jaspers' paper (in English), 'Causal and "meaningful" connexions between life history and psychosis', suggests that understanding is our ability to grasp a 'meaningful' connection, and thus that 'meaningfulness' is the more basic notion from which our idea of understanding derives. In fact, the term translated 'meaningful' (*verständliche*) in the title, and the term translated 'meaning' as in the phrase 'psychology of meaning' (*verstehende Psychologie*), both derive from the term for understanding (*Verstehen*). Literally then, Jaspers is suggesting that what we become aware of in understanding is an *understandable* connection—and again, this does not appear particularly illuminating!

It is worth noting in passing that we have no better idea how to define (causal) explanation than (human) understanding. Our tendency, perhaps, particularly given the successes of the natural sciences, is to think that while understanding, in the sense now outlined, is rather mysterious, causal explanation is by contrast relatively straightforward. This tendency is part of what is involved in the stigmatizing attitudes towards mental health generated by the naive medical model that we considered in Part I. We also saw in Part I, however, that with higher level concepts we are often better at using than defining them—remember the concept of 'time' in Chapter 4! The concept of causation, as used in the natural sciences, is like time in this respect: apart from extreme cases, like quantum mechanics, the concept of causation is not a problem in practice—scientists of course face deep difficulties working out the causes of things but these are empirical difficulties rather than difficulties arising from the meaning of the concept itself. Yet, like time, and indeed the concept of bodily illness, our ease of use of such concepts is, as we put it in Chapter 4, despite (rather than in virtue of) the availability of clear explicit definitions.

The question, then, paralleling our question about causation, is whether what we become aware of in 'coming to an understanding' can be thought of in more basic terms. A related question, and one which (given the relative ease of use of the concept of causation) it is tempting for those trained in the natural sciences to ask, is whether what we think of as 'coming to an understanding' can itself be reduced to the apparently more transparent terms of causal explanation. We will see in Part V that this is a hot topic in philosophy today: and a key issue in the *Methodenstreit* was precisely the question of whether understanding is simply a disguised form of causal explanation.

The start of the *Methodenstreit*

One of the clearest statements of the view that understanding, as aimed at by the human sciences, should be no different from the causal explanations aimed at by natural sciences, comes from the philosopher John Stuart Mill. The son of another philosopher, James Mill, John Stuart Mill did influential work on logic and epistemology as well as in political philosophy. He was also a Member of Parliament from 1865 to 1868, and a firm advocate of women's suffrage.

The book in which Mill expounds his views on the natural and human sciences is *A System of Logic*, originally published in 1843. This book had a huge impact in Germany when it was translated,

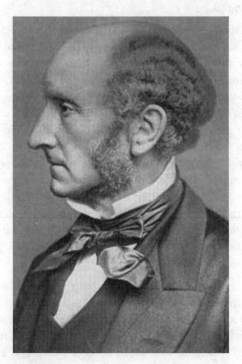

Fig. 10.4 John Stuart Mill

and indeed it can be considered as sparking off the whole *Methodenstreit*!

In the next reading we look at an extract from *A System of Logic* in which Mill gives a robust formulation of what he saw as the deficiencies of the human sciences (then called 'moral sciences') in comparison with the natural sciences.

EXERCISE 1   (30 minutes)

Read the short extract from:

> Mill, J.S. (1974). That there is, or may be, a science of human nature. In *Collected Works of John Stuart Mill*, Vol. VIII: *A System of Logic (Books IV–VI and Appendices)*, (ed. J.M. Robson). Book VI, Chapter III, §1–2, pp. 844–847. (Extracts: p844, p845, pp846–7)

Link with Reading 10.1

Look in particular at (1) the way that Mill characterizes the backward state of the science of human nature, and (2) his claim that the results of investigations in these sciences will ultimately have much the same character as the results of natural scientific investigations.

A unitary conception of science

In the text from which these extracts are taken, Mill claims that there are no substantive differences between the methods or aims of the human sciences and those of the natural sciences. Just as the latter draw general laws from a series of observations, so do the former (though they can only aim at probabilistic laws). In each case, the results can be used to predict the future behaviour of the phenomena studied. It was this view that thinkers such as Dilthey, Rickert, and Weber sought to counter, by arguing for the independent status of the methods and aims of the human sciences. The *Methodenstreit* ran up to the end of the nineteenth century and into the first decade of the twentieth century.

The debate emerged again several decades later, however, in a new context. This time the debate was triggered by the views of a philosophical movement known as Logical Positivism, and their idea of a 'Unified conception of science' ('*Einheitswissenschaft*'). Two of the key protagonists in this new form of the debate were C.G. Hempel and W.H. Dray (see the Reading Guide). Hempel argued that human sciences such as history were underpinned by explanations based on laws. Dray argued instead that it depended on finding reasons or meaningful connections between events that resisted assimiliation even to probabilistic laws. More recently still, the behaviourism found in psychology in the 1960s and since can be seen as an expression of Mill's hard line. Coming right up to date, contemporary attempts to show how reasons can be encoded in brain states, which are themselves governed by neurological laws, are in line with Mill's aim. We will return to the distinction between reasons and causes at a methodological level in Chapter 15 and the attempt to construe reasons as brain states throughout Part V.

The *Methodenstreit* and understanding

As a way of preparing ourselves to look at the debate in the form it took when Jaspers was writing, it will be useful to think a little more about what it is we grasp when we 'understand' something. The translation of '*verständliche*' in the title of Jaspers' paper as '*meaningful*' is, of course, no accident—the 'meaning' or 'sense' of something would seem to be precisely what we are seeking to grasp in 'coming to an understanding'. But we should be careful not to overlook the fact that these are multifaceted concepts. There are very different ways in which we may think of things as having or lacking meaning or sense, or being understandable or not understandable.

We will see by the end of this chapter that one of the unresolved tensions in Jaspers' work, and indeed in psychopathology today, arises from a failure to distinguish different senses of understanding when we move from everyday to technical usage.

EXERCISE 2   (15 minutes)

Note down for yourself as many examples as you can of the different sorts of thing we take to be 'understandable' and to 'have meaning', or to be 'not understandable' and to 'lack meaning'—in other words, the different senses in which we take ourselves to possess 'understanding' or to have 'grasped the meaning' of something.

Varieties of understanding

Here a few examples of the variety of different phenomena we take ourselves to 'understand'. There are of course many others that you may have thought of!

- We think of certain sequences of words or utterances as understandable; this sentence would be one example. Whereas 'certain or think we sequences utterances understandable of words of as' would strike us a lacking any meaning! Husserl, in fact, calls this type of lack of meaning 'nonsense'.

- Husserl distinguishes nonsense (so defined) from 'absurdity'— that is, where words or utterances seem to form a grammatical sequence, but what is being said still does not 'make sense'. For example, 'the square root of two dissolves in water'.

- We also think of ourselves as understanding sequences of sentences, and as not understanding when we can no longer 'see' the 'connection'. For example, 'I'm going to the shops. Grass is green. I have two brothers.' Taken individually, we understand each of the sentences, but we 'fail to understand' what connection they have to each other.

- A further sense in which we may understand a sequence of sentences is where the first one is a reason for asserting the final one. The famous syllogism 'All men are mortal. Socrates is a man. Socrates is mortal' would be an example. If the final sentence had been 'Socrates is not mortal' we might say that we 'fail to understand' how anyone could come to that conclusion.

- Another example would be: 'It is raining. I want to keep dry. I will take my umbrella'. Here the final statement by no means follows from the first two with the strictly (deductive) rationality of the first, yet intuitively we think of the final statement as being 'understandable' on the basis of the other two.

- One might say, then, that in both cases the first two sentences are 'reasons' for taking an umbrella. But clearly not just any old statements would be regarded as 'reasons' here. Why are we apt to think of the first two statements as 'reasons'? It may be that our grasp of what a 'reason' is, is itself derivative from our grasp of the way certain statements make other statements 'understandable'.

- We also, of course, speak of understanding in relation to non-verbal forms of behaviour. If we saw someone crawling aimlessly around in a patch of grass, this would probably strike us as a not very meaningful piece of behaviour; we do not understand what he is doing. Someone then says, 'he is looking for his contact lens, and suddenly, as a result of these words, his behaviour becomes 'understandable'.

- Another way of looking at this same example is to think of the man's behaviour as 'making sense' in the light of the beliefs and motives that are ascribed to him: he believes he has lost his contact lens in the patch of grass, and wants to find it. A motive is provided here by a wishing or wanting, on the basis of which, together with the relevant beliefs, a given behaviour becomes meaningful.

- What, though, makes us think of a certain mental act of wishing or wanting as providing a 'motive'? Thinking that he wants to buy a newspaper, for example, would not make the man's behaviour understandable! It may seem as though it is motives that we are seeking to grasp when we 'understand someone'; but our very grasp of what a motive is, seems to derive from a prior grasp of how the connection between certain forms of mental state and certain actions can be meaningful or *understandable*. In other words, 'understanding' of other people in terms of their 'motives' may be a derivative form of understanding—derivative, that is, upon our ability to first grasp the 'meaningful connection' between such statements as: 'He believes he has lost his contact lens in that patch of grass. He wishes to find the contact lens. He is crawling around the grass on his hands and knees.'

- There is another, related use of the term 'understanding', which is worth mentioning as we will find Jaspers drawing attention to it. This is when we say 'I understand' as a way of signalling our *approval* of an action or decision on the basis of the meaningful connection that someone cites between it and their beliefs. Someone may cite beliefs they held, which turned out to be false, but which they took as good reasons for a certain action, and by saying 'I understand' we convey that we would have done the same on the basis of those beliefs.

You can probably think of many more ways in which we use notions such as 'understanding', 'making sense of something', and 'grasping the meaning', as well as notions of what is, or is not, 'understandable' or 'meaningful'. The purpose of these examples is to bring this variety to light, and also to make us wary of thinking that the notion of understanding is reducible to 'simpler' ideas such as those of 'motives' and 'reasons'.

Reflection on the session and self-test questions

Write down your own reflections on the materials in this session drawing out any points that are particularly significant for you. Then write brief notes about the following:

1. What are the differences between understanding and explanation? Is there a clear distinction between the everyday use of 'understand' and 'explain'?

2. Does everybody agree that there is a distinction?

3. Can explanation and understanding be analysed into more basic terms?

Session 2 Understanding and explanation in Jaspers' psychopathology

Having sharpened our intuitions about 'understanding' and 'explanation', we can now turn to Jaspers' paper on 'Causal and "meaningful" connections' and on the way psychopathology is required to draw on both.

You had a first look at this paper in Chapter 8. We now need to return to it in preparation for being able to see how Jaspers was influenced by the *Methodenstreit*. Many of the ideas he introduces in this paper are also discussed in his major work *General Psychopathology*. In the next reading we will identify some of these ideas. We will then consider them in more detail by reference to Jaspers' discussions in *General Psychopathology* and to the views of the philosophers he himself draws on from the *Methodenstreit*, notably Dilthey, Weber, and Rickert. In this way, we will also be using Jaspers' paper as the basis for an exploration of the *Methodenstreit* itself.

The influences on Jaspers

As a start, it is worth looking at the quotation cited by the translator, J. Hoenig, in his introductory paragraphs to Jaspers' paper. This quotation comes from the long footnote on pp. 301–302 of *General Psychopathology*, where Jaspers talks about the need for the notion of understanding to be reintroduced in psychopathology, as well as about the authors that have influenced him. In the

quotation given by Hoenig, Jaspers says: 'The work of Max Weber was mostly responsible for my deliberate use of understanding as a method which would be in keeping with our great cultural traditions. I was also influenced by [Weber's] *Roscher and Knies*... My ideas were then carried forward by Dilthey ("Ideas Towards a Descriptive and Analytic Psychology" ...) and by Simmel[1] (*Problems in the Philosophy of History*).' (p. 301–302)

In the discussion of Jaspers' paper that follows we will see that there are certain tensions in his view of understanding that stem from his combining ideas from the two rather different philosophies of Weber and Dilthey. Weber, and his teacher Rickert, considered their work to be very much a rejection of Dilthey's approach! It is notable in this respect that in the above extract, Jaspers fails to acknowledge any debt to Rickert. This is perhaps not surprising given that Jaspers and Rickert, as we saw in Chapter 8, became enemies. Yet the result was that Jaspers failed to incorporate in his thinking a key aspect of Weber's account of understanding derived from Rickert's work on values. This failure, we will suggest in our conclusions, could be important for psychopathology.[2]

EXERCISE 3 (60 minutes)

Re-read the paper:

Jaspers, K. ([1913] 1974). Causal and 'meaningful' connections between life history and psychosis (Kausale und verständliche Zusammenhänge zwischen Schicksal und Psychose bei der Dementia praecox). Translated with an introduction and postscript by J. Hoenig. In *Themes and Variations in European Psychiatry* (ed. S.R. Hirsch and M. Shepherd). Bristol: Wright, pp. 80–93

Link with Reading 10.2
(This is same as 8.1—Chapter 8/Exercise 3)

Before you start reading, look through the nine questions listed below—they will help guide your reading. As you read through the paper, write down brief answers to these questions.

Although this is something of a marathon exercise, you can think of the nine questions as being concerned, broadly, with three topics: understanding and its close cognates (questions 1–4), meaningful connections (5–8), and the place of values (question 9).

---

[1] (Georg Simmel (1858–1918) was a German philosopher and sociologist. Famous in Germany as a charismatic lecturer, his courses ranged from logic and the history of philosophy to ethics, social psychology, and sociology. He published *Problems in the Philosophy of History* and *Introduction to the Science of Ethics* as well as major works on sociology.

[2] The terms normative and evaluative are used sometimes as synonyms and sometimes with different meanings. In one fairly widespread use in philosophy, evaluative is a subclass of normative. Normative implies rule following where the rules in question are human in origin (e.g. the rules of a game) as distinct from natural laws. Evaluative, according to this way of marking the distinction, is used only where the rules in question are about judgements of good and bad (aesthetic, moral, prudential, epistemic, etc.). The use of normative in this 'human rule following' sense is illustrated by Peter Winch's account of the difference between social and natural sciences in Part III (Chapter 15).

We have asked you to think about all nine questions together because, as you will see, the answers to them are closely interconnected. In particular, the somewhat different philosophies of Dilthey, Weber, and (indirectly) Rickert, run as three strands through Jaspers' thinking on all nine topics. The result, as we noted above, is a number of unresolved tensions in Jaspers' account of psychopathology. We summarize these tensions and indicate their continuing importance for psychiatry today in the concluding session in this chapter.

So, our nine questions are:

Understanding and its close cognates

1. How does Jaspers use 'inner' and 'outer' sense to distinguish understanding and explanation?

2. What is the difference between 'rational understanding' and 'empathic understanding'?

3. What does Jaspers mean by the 'evidence of genetic understanding'?

4. How does understanding relate to interpretation?

Meaningful connections

5. What appears to be Jaspers' paradigm example of a meaningful connection?

6. What does Jaspers mean by an 'ideally typical' connection?

7. What does Jaspers mean by saying that there are limits to understanding, i.e. to seeing meaningful connections, and what does he mean by 'as if' understanding?

8. Does Jaspers think it is possible to give a causal account of a meaningful connection?

The place of values

9. Does Jaspers think that understanding always involves value judgements?

Understanding and its close cognates

Our first four questions, then, are broadly concerned with what Jaspers means by 'understanding' and how it is related in his thinking to a number of closely related concepts, explanations (question 1), empathy (question 2), genetic understanding (question 3), and interpretation (question 4).

Question 1: 'inner' and 'outer' sense

This first question is perhaps one of the more straightforward of the set. In the first section of the paper, Jaspers suggests that there is a certain analogy between understanding and causal explanation. The analogy is that 'causal thinking' concerns the way we link up the sensory data we receive from our sense organs, and 'show how they hang together by explanations', while psychological understanding concerns what is given to us in 'inner sense'. By this latter phrase,

Jaspers means the 'vivid representation of psychic data' (p. 82), which we arrive at through empathy with another person. Empathy, as part of phenomenology in the sense we looked at in Chapter 9, plays an analogous role to the way our sense organs supply the data for causal thinking, i.e. by supplying data that we then *understand*.

We will see below that this approach to the distinction between understanding and explaining owes much to the early work of Wilhelm Dilthey. In a well known phrase from his essay 'Ideas towards a descriptive and analytic psychology', which we will be looking at below, Dilthey said: 'Nature we explain, psychic life we understand'. This does not tell us what 'explanation' or 'understanding' consist of, only that they apply to different things: explanation applies to sense data from our sense organs, understanding to our own 'inner world' or the re-living, in empathy, of another's inner life. Jaspers uses a suggestive phrase in section 3, where he compares 'psychology of meaning' (*verstehende Psychologie*) with 'performance psychology' (a form of 'objective psychology'). He writes that performance psychology 'does not try to feel itself in any way into the psyche' (p. 83), the implication being that this is what 'understanding' consists of.

The influence of Dilthey

In order to help clarify Jaspers' view here, the next exercise asks you to read an extract from Dilthey's essay 'Ideas towards a descriptive and analytic psychology' (1894). Dilthey's aim in this article was to argue that human sciences, such as history, need to draw on the findings of psychology—but a 'descriptive' psychology rather than an 'explanatory' psychology. In his view, explanatory psychology attempts to use the methods of the natural sciences in its study of the human mind, and this approach needs to be supplemented with a descriptive psychology that is concerned with *understanding* the 'psychic nexus'. You will see that Dilthey characterizes the difference in terms of the nature of our 'inner experience' of our own mental lives.

EXERCISE 4

Read the two extracts from:

Dilthey, W. (1977). Ideas concerning a descriptive and analytic psychology. In *Descriptive Psychology and Historical Understanding* (trans. R.M. Zaner and K.L. Heiges). The Hague: Martinus Nijhoff, pp. 21–120 (Extracts: pp27–28, 52–55)

Link with Reading 10.3

◆ Note in particular how Dilthey characterizes the difference between understanding and explanation in terms of what is given to us from the 'inside' or 'outside' of consciousness respectively.

This essay by Dilthey comes from the middle period of his work, and in it we can also find ideas that were to become more prominent in his later work. In particular, on p. 55, Dilthey mentions that what is peculiar about what is given in 'inner experience' is what we might call its 'holism'. That is, an individual lived experience takes on significance in the light of 'the coherent whole which is livingly given to us'. This emphasis on the relation between a part and the whole is at the heart of Dilthey's interest in hermeneutics, which we will come back to below.

The rejection of Dilthey's approach

The first section of Jaspers' paper (1974) clearly seems to draw on the work of Dilthey in its appeal to the distinction between 'inner' and 'outer' sense. In fact, however, this line of thinking drawn from Dilthey conflicts with another approach to the notion of understanding, which is also present in Jaspers' paper. This other line of thinking becomes apparent when Jaspers suddenly announces at the start of section 6:

> The suggestive assumption that the psychic is the area of meaningful understanding and the physical that of causal explanation is wrong. There is no real event, be it of physical or of psychic nature, which is not in principle accessible to causal explanation. [...] In fact there is no single event known to us which, in this sense, cannot be understood as well as explained. (p. 86)

This line of thought—that there are not two separate realms of reality, one of which is the field of causal thinking and the other the field of understanding—derives primarily from Jaspers' friend, the sociologist Max Weber. Weber in turn takes the approach from his early teacher, Heinrich Rickert, who was a leading figure in what we noted earlier has become known as the 'South-west German School of Neo-Kantianism'.

Neo-Kantianism was a diverse movement in philosophy at the time. This particular school of Neo-Kantianism was a key force in the *Methodenstreit*, arguing for the distinctive and irreducible nature of the human sciences. For Dilthey, 'understanding' was a key aspect of what made the human sciences distinctive, but Rickert objected to the Cartesian thinking that underpinned Dilthey's distinction. We can see the same Cartesian approach in Jaspers' first line of thought—that understanding and explanation apply to two distinct realms of reality, the mental and the physical. It turns out, of course, that Jaspers' first way of introducing the distinction between understanding and explanation is merely a 'suggestive assumption', which he then goes on to say 'is wrong'. However, even in *General Psychopathology*, we find some distinctively Cartesian ideas: 'The understanding of meaning demands other methods than those of the natural sciences. What is meaningful has quite different modes of being from the objects of those sciences.' (*General Psychopathology*, p. 355).

The idea that that which is meaningful or understandable has a 'quite different mode of being' is very suggestive of Descartes. In Descartes' dualism, as we will see in Part V, there are two fundamentally different types of substance or being, mental substance and physical substance.

'Human sciences' and 'cultural sciences'

The term Dilthey uses for 'human sciences' is '*Geisteswissenschaften*', made up of the two words '*Geist*', meaning 'mind' or 'spirit', and

'*Wissenschaft*', meaning 'science'. Rickert objected to this label for sciences such as history, comparative literature, political science, etc., precisely because he felt it suggested a basically Cartesian grounding for their methodologies. Rickert's preferred term was '*Kulturwissenschaften*' ('cultural sciences'), where the term 'culture' indicates an objective social phenomenon rather than a subjective mental world. Rickert argued, against Dilthey, that the natural and human sciences were not sufficiently distinguished in terms of their subject matter, i.e. the natural sciences studying nature while the human sciences study the human mind or spirit (*Geist*). The following quotation comes from Rickert's major work *The Limits of Concept Formation in Natural Science* (1902):

> Despite the necessary connection between history and mental life, whoever wants to understand both the *logical* and the *substantive* differences between natural science and history will not succeed by *beginning* with the mental and the concept of 'human science'. We no longer need to show that in this way, the logical oppositions of method are more obscured than clarified. Even if we construe the concept of 'mind' so narrowly that only volitional and valuing beings fall under it, we must always emphasize that like any other reality, they can also be subsumed under the concepts of natural science or treated in a generalizing fashion. From a logical standpoint, therefore, wherever the understanding of the nature of *historical* science is at stake, the term human science remains as vacuous as ever. (p. 128)

This passage shows a debt to Rickert's teacher Wilhelm Windelband (1848–1915) part of the so-called Heidelberg School of Neo-Kantian philosophy and the first to distinguish between ideographic (based on particular individuals) and nomothetic (based on laws) understanding and explanation. Following his teacher, then, Rickert argues in this passage that one must look for the difference between natural sciences and so-called 'human sciences' not in their *subject matter* but in the *methods*. In the above quotation, Rickert emphasizes that any 'reality', whether mental or physical, 'human' or 'natural', can be studied using the methods of the natural sciences; what is distinctive about 'human' or cultural sciences is the distinctive method and aims they bring to a study of the same reality.

On the face of it, it seems that Jaspers was merely using the Dilthean approach to introduce the distinction between understanding and explanation, and that his real position is closer to the Rickert–Weber line. However, this is not the whole story, since as we shall see below the Rickert–Weber line is also quite opposed to the idea that empathy plays an important role in understanding, an idea which Jaspers took from Dilthey. With this complication in mind, we now need to look more closely at Jaspers' idea of 'empathic understanding'.

Question 2: 'rational understanding' and 'empathic understanding'

In Chapter 9 we noted that in his phenomenology paper, Jaspers distinguishes between subjective and objective psychology; he regards subjective psychology as being made up of phenomenology (which he limits to 'static understanding') and 'genetic under-standing'; and he includes among the 'objective symptoms' of concern to objective psychology, the 'rational contents' of someone's utterances or written expressions.

In section 2 of the present paper, however, Jaspers argues that genetic understanding (which in his phenomenology paper is part of subjective psychology) is divided into 'rational under-standing' and 'empathic understanding'. In other words, the sense of 'genetic understanding' slips depending on whether Jaspers takes it to characterize any understanding of transitions between mental states or whether he restricts it to empathic understand-ing of the subjective aspects of such transitions. In the latter case it does not apply to rational understanding. Rational understand-ing concerns the logical sequence of thought-contents, such as when one proposition follows logically from others. This approach to understanding the sequence of someone's utterances 'is only an *aid* to psychology' (p. 83)—it is not itself a psychological matter. (This perhaps indicates an influence of Husserl's anti-psychologism, which we looked at in Chapter 9.)

Rational understanding thus needs to be distinguished from 'empathic understanding': 'empathic understanding *is* psycho-logy itself' (*ibid.*). Jaspers gives the following characterization of this form of understanding: 'But if we understand the content of the thoughts as they have arisen out of the moods, wishes, and fears of the person who thought them, we understand the con-nections psychologically or empathically'. (*ibid.*)

We should note that Jaspers uses the term 'understand' to charac-terize what is distinctive about empathic understanding, which may strike you as not very illuminating! This may, however, be a sign that the notion of understanding is a basic notion, which cannot itself be understood in terms of anything simpler. Jaspers' use of the term 'empathic' does, though, give us a clue as to what it is that he takes to be 'understandable'—mental states as re-lived imaginatively in empathy. The idea seems to be that when we reflect on our vivid imaginings of another's mental life, certain connections between the imagined mental states strike us as 'understandable' or 'meaningful' (*verständlich*).

The influence of Dilthey

This view of understanding as requiring the imaginative re-enactment of the mental states that we take another person to have, again, owes much to Dilthey, rather than to the Rickert–Weber approach. The depth of Jaspers' debt to Dilthey is evident in Dilthey's work (1976), 'The construction of the historical world in the human sciences', in *Selected Writings* (see Reading guide), where he emphasizes the importance of empathy, of the need to 're-live' or 're-experience' in one's imagination the mental life of another, by 'transposing' oneself into their situation (e.g. pp. 226–228). Again, the context is a discussion of what is distinctive about the science of history, but we need to remember that the work of the historian, in attempting to under-stand the mental life and actions of historical figures, parallels in

many respects the aims of a 'psychology of meaning'. Thus, for Dilthey, the 'state of mind involved in the task of understanding, we call empathy' (p. 226). Jaspers, however, makes a distinction between 'rational understanding' and 'empathic understanding', as we saw above, which does not figure in Dilthey's view of understanding.

In order to clarify why Jaspers makes this distinction, we need to go back to his distinction between subjective and objective symptoms. Remember that for Jaspers, the 'rational contents' of thought, and their rational connections, are objective phenom-ena, suggesting that they are, in some way, public matters, not hidden, so to speak, in the depths of the human psyche. What we grasp in 'empathic understanding', on the other hand, appears to be something irreducibly subjective—we only have access to it through the imaginative re-living of someone's mental life in our own minds. In other words, if we are no longer concerned with strictly logical connections between thoughts, then any other form of 'meaningful connection' between them is something that can only be found in our own subjective mental realm.

This is an extension of the Cartesian approach to what is understandable, as found in Dilthey, and it directly conflicts with the Rickert–Weber line. For Weber, in particular, as we shall see, these weaker, non-logical, forms of meaningful connection are just as objective as the strictly logical type: and we will find this line of thought also represented in Jaspers' paper. To put things in a rather oversimplified form: for Weber, a connection is not meaningful because we can empathize with it, rather we can empathize with it because it is meaningful.

Weber's rejection of empathy

Weber regarded Dilthey's emphasis on empathy as a bit of a red herring, in terms of pinning down what understanding consists in, in the human sciences. In the next reading we consider an extract from a work by Weber, *Roscher and Knies*, which, as we saw above, is cited by Jaspers as an influence on him. Here Weber rejects the idea that understanding derives from an imaginative re-living of the experiences that we take another person to be going through in a given situation. For Weber, understanding does not involve the re-living of another's mental life, but rather the *making of evaluations*, in the sense of setting out the objective norms and values that 'govern' the thinking and acting of a per-son in a given situation. Weber talks, for example, of the 'axiolog-ical relations' of an object—literally, the value of an object, or the normative significance attaching to an event, in a given context. The term translated 'axiological relation' (*Wertbeziehung*) is usu-ally translated 'value relevance' or 'value connection', and we will come back to this notion below in relation to the work of Weber's teacher, Heinrich Rickert. You should also note that Weber has a very broad notion of 'causal explanation', which in this context includes the norms and regulations that 'make' people act in a certain way.

EXERCISE 5 (60 minutes)

Read the extract from:

Weber, M. (1975). *Roscher and Knies: the logical problems of historical economics* (trans. Guy Oakes). New York: The Free Press (Extracts: pp. 179–183, 184–186)

Link with Reading 10.4

Don't worry if you cannot follow everything that Weber is saying—it is rather unclear in parts! What is important to note, however, is the way Weber seeks to replace the centrality of 'empathy' with a notion of 'evaluation'.

Weber's main objection to making the notion of empathy central to what is involved in understanding, is that there is no guarantee that our imaginative re-living of someone's mental state will bear any resemblance to what the person actually experienced.

He further argues that the idea of re-living someone else's 'experiences' is too indeterminate—what we seek to grasp, in understanding someone, is the content of their judgements, in particular their 'value judgements'. Weber understands 'value judgement' in a broad sense, covering not only someone's judgement of whether something is good or bad, but more generally their acknowledgements of the 'meaning' or 'value' which an object or event possesses in a given situation. Weber's conclusion is that '. . . "meaning" interpretable human conduct ("action") is identifiable by reference to "valuations" and "meanings"' (p. 185), rather than by reference to our own empathic re-living of experiences. We will come back to this idea below, when we look at the place of Weber's notion of an 'ideal type' in Jaspers' view of understanding.

Question 3: the 'evidence' of genetic understanding

When you looked at Jaspers' notion of the 'evidence of genetic understanding', you should have picked up on the fact that the term 'evidence' is not being used in the sense in which a detective may seek 'evidence'. The detective seeks to draw inferences from, and arrive at conclusions on the basis of, certain objects or facts which are 'signs' of criminal activity. What Jaspers is suggesting is that this is precisely not what happens in 'understanding'—understanding is not something we arrive at by an inference from objective signs, rather our grasp of what is meaningful or understandable is immediate and direct. There is a certain 'self-evidence' to what is meaningful—the meaningfulness of a connection is simply 'evident' to us. A footprint may be a sign for the detective of where a burglar entered a building, but the footprint itself is not signified by something else, it is simply there. In the same way, Jaspers is suggesting, we must take meaningful connections as given and evident: 'To accept this type of evidence is a precondition of the psychology of meaning, in exactly the same way as acceptance of perceptual reality and causality are preconditions of the natural sciences.' (p. 84)

We must take ourselves as able to 'see' meaningful connections—Husserl argued similarly in relation to logical relations between propositions: a logical deduction has an evidence to it that we must accept and not try to reductively explain in terms, for example, of the causal laws governing a sequence of mental states.

The idea that a meaningful connection is simply something we 'see', would seem to confer a certain objectivity on the existence of meaningful connections. In other words, a connection is meaningful not because we can experience a certain empathy with it, rather what we call empathy would depend on our prior seeing of a meaningful connection. In section 4, on 'the evidence of genetic understanding', we indeed find this idea, which conflicts somewhat with the emphasis on empathy that Jaspers took from Dilthey: 'All psychology of meaning is based on such evidential experiences which we have in relation to quite impersonal, detached, meaningful connections. Such evidence is gained *while* we gather experience in our contact with human personalities but is not gained *through* such experiences and is *never* inductively proved by repetitions of such experiences.' (p. 84)

Here a meaningful connection is 'quite impersonal' and 'detached'—it is being described in the way Jaspers usually thinks of objective phenomena. For Jaspers, we neither infer a meaningful connection from some other form of experience, nor do we arrive at such conclusions by induction. Induction is the name given to the process by which we arrive at a law-like generalization on the basis of a limited number of experimental observations. In Part III, we will be looking much more closely at the so-called 'problem of induction' (the problem of whether we are ever justified in drawing general conclusions from limited observations)—but here Jaspers takes it to be a distinctive feature of forming causal explanations. The contrast with understanding then becomes even clearer: the *meaningful* connection between the wish to keep dry and the taking of an umbrella is not established by the observations of how often the mental state of wishing to keep dry is followed by the person taking an umbrella with them!

Question 4: understanding and interpretation

In section 5 of the paper, Jaspers turns to the question of the relation between understanding and interpretation. At first sight there appears to be a conflict between this section and what Jaspers has told us about understanding so far. He writes: 'All understanding of individual actual events therefore remains more or less an interpretation which can reach a high level of completeness only in rare cases.' (p. 85)

Whereas previously Jaspers describes understanding as consisting in an immediate and direct grasp of meaningful connections, it now appears that understanding is something we construct only on the basis of observing events. It may seem that here we have another inconsistency in Jaspers' approach due to the different lines of thought on which he draws: the emphasis on the 'seeing' of meaning derives from Husserl, whereas an emphasis on the way that coming to an understanding may require a laborious process of interpretation, derives from Dilthey. As a historian, Dilthey was well aware that the understanding of, for example, a historical figure was no easy matter, and required the historian to draw together insights from letters, official documents, memoirs, etc. This Dilthean aspect to Jaspers' notion of understanding is further underlined in *General Psychopathology*, where Jaspers refers to an idea on which Dilthey worked extensively: the idea of a 'hermeneutic circle' (translated in *General Psychopathology*, though, as 'hermeneutic round'). It is worth quoting this passage from *General Psychopathology* in its entirety:

> We understand the content of a particular thought or the flinching of the body in fear of a blow. But such isolated understanding is meagre and unspecific. Moreover, the whole nature of the individual pervades even the most isolated outpost of his being, giving it objective context and the complexity of psychic motivation. Understanding therefore will push on from the isolated particular to the whole and it is only in the light of the whole that the isolated particular reveals its wealth of concrete implications. What is meaningful cannot in fact be isolated: there is no end, therefore, to the collection of our objective facts which provide the starting-point for all understanding. Any one particular starting-point may gain an entirely new meaning through addition of fresh meaningful facts. We achieve understanding within a *circular movement from the particular facts to the whole* that includes them and *back again from the whole* thus reached to the particular significant facts. The circle continually expands itself and tests and changes itself meaningfully in all its parts. A final 'terra firma' is never reached. There is only the whole as it is attained at any time, which bears itself along in the mutual opposition of its parts.   Jaspers [1913] 1997 (pp. 356–357)

Dilthey and hermeneutics

We need not worry about trying to make sense of everything Jaspers says here. It is worth, however, comparing it with a passage from Dilthey's essay 'The development of hermeneutics' (1900). 'Hermeneutics' is the name given to the study of methods of interpretation, and the principles used in arriving at an interpretation. In the following passage Dilthey is talking about the interpretation of a text, but the difficulty he identifies is, as he says, a 'general difficulty of all interpretation':

> Here we encounter the general difficulty of all interpretation. The whole of a work must be understood from individual words and their combination but full understanding of an individual part presupposes understanding of the whole. This circle is repeated in the relation of an individual work to the mentality and development of its author, and it recurs again in the relation of such an individual work to its literary genre. [. . .] Theoretically we are here at the limits of all interpretation; it can only fulfil its task to a degree; so all understanding always remains relative and can never be completed. *Individuum est ineffabile* [The individual is ineffable].   (p. 259)

For Jaspers and Dilthey, interpretation is something that never comes to a final conclusion—there is always the possibility of one's grasp of the whole throwing new light on a particular part, which in turn adds to our understanding of the whole, which in turn throws new light on a part, and so on. Jaspers follows Dilthey further in tending to *identify* understanding with interpretation; for Dilthey interpretation, as a distinct scholarly activity, is simply an extension of everyday understanding: 'All interpretation of literary works is merely the methodological development of the process of understanding, which extends over the whole of life and relates to any kind of speech or writing.' ('The development of hermeneutics', in *Selected Writings*, p. 258)

The evidence versus incompleteness of understanding

However, when Jaspers says of understanding that a 'final "terra firma" is never reached', this would seem to be in direct conflict with what he has previously said about the straightforward *evidence* of what we grasp as understandable. Further, the reference to 'the collection of our objective facts which provide the *starting-point* for all understanding' in the above quotation from *General Psychopathology* would seem to conflict with what Jaspers says about the *immediacy* of our grasp of what is understandable. In section 5 of the paper, Jaspers suggests that the 'application' of our grasp of a meaningful connection 'to a particular case' can be wrong—suggesting the constant possibility of a gap between the objective facts and the understanding arrived at from this starting-point.

It may be, however, that the inconsistency is not as great as it first seems. To start with, it is not clear what Jaspers means by the 'objective facts' on which an interpretation rests, in the above passage. If by 'objective facts' one understands that which is described by physics, and if this is taken as the starting-point for understanding, then clearly all understanding is a hypothetical interpretation based on these objective phenomena. On this view of understanding we are essentially in the position of a 'cosmic exile' (to use a phrase introduced by the philosopher W.V.O. Quine, 1960, p. 275). That is, all we have to go on, in trying to interpret what is happening or being said in a given situation, are observations of the physical movements and changes of objects. However, we need to remember that Jaspers' notion of what is 'objective' is much wider than merely what would figure in a physical description: it includes the 'rational contents' of utterances and written expressions, for example.

Reconciling Jaspers' views of understanding

It may be the case, therefore, that the 'objective facts which provide the *starting point* for *all understanding*', are things of which we *already* possess an *understanding* in the sense of an immediate, direct grasp of their meaning. In the above passage, Jaspers does indeed speak of 'meaningful facts' and 'significant facts'. It could be that when Jaspers writes that 'all understanding' is based on 'objective facts', what he really means is that certain higher types of understanding (such as in the hermeneutic circle of interpretation) are based on other more fundamental types (such as in the immediate grasp of meaning).

The second way in which the inconsistency may be dissolved, is to look more closely at what Jaspers says about 'the whole' in the light of which particular facts are interpreted. Certainly our grasp of the meaning of a certain word or gesture depends on an awareness of the context in which it occurs. In one context, somebody waving their hand is correctly understood as a greeting, while in another context as an appeal for help. Again, this might suggest that there is never a direct grasp of meaning, and that understanding is only ever an *inferring* of meaning from the wider context, thus always open to future revision. It may, however, be possible to reconcile Jaspers' emphasis on the immediacy of our grasp of meaning with this emphasis on its 'contextuality'. One might argue, for example, that for simple cases of understanding, the necessary context is that of our upbringing in certain practices and 'forms of life', and it is precisely this that *allows* us to 'see' the meaning of words, gestures, and actions. In other words, it is by becoming immersed in a context constituted by language and cultural traditions and practices, that we learn to 'see' meaningful facts in the first place: meaningful facts that would not be apparent to a 'cosmic exile'. These are issues we shall come back to in Part III; for the present we need simply to see that there is not necessarily a conflict between the immediacy of our grasp of meaning and the way that actions or words only take on determinate meaning in a given context.

The final way in which one might try to reconcile the idea of an immediate grasp of meaning with what Jaspers says about interpretation, is to suggest that in talking about interpretation Jaspers means the ascription of *motives* to people. To return to our example of the umbrella: the meaningful connection between wanting to keep dry and taking an umbrella is understandable in an immediate and direct way, but it may not be the correct 'understanding' of why someone took an umbrella in a particular case. 'Understanding' here refers to the linking of an action to the motive for that action—and it may be that someone takes his umbrella in order to show it off to a friend. Of course, the simplest, though not infallible, way of ascertaining whether we have understood someone's motives correctly is to ask them. Understanding in this sense depends, as indicated above, on our grasp of the meaningfulness of the connection between a certain stated desire or wish and an action. This again suggests that when Jaspers says that 'all understanding... remains more or less an interpretation', Jaspers does not mean *all understanding*, but rather a higher type that in turn depends on more fundamental forms of understanding.

Meaningful connections

Question 5: Jaspers' paradigm example of a meaningful connection

Part of the answer to why Jaspers appears to say such inconsistent things about understanding is that he has a quite unusual paradigm example of finding a meaningful connection. This only becomes clear as the article progresses, and we find Jaspers referring

repeatedly to Nietzsche and his thesis about the genesis of Christian morality. Nietzsche is mentioned in sections 4 and 5, and in section 11 Jaspers writes: 'Entirely unique and the greatest of all subjective psychologists is Nietzsche' (p. 90). Whether one agrees with Nietzsche's analysis or not, one would have to admit that it is by no means a 'fundamental' type of understanding. Jaspers introduces Nietzsche's thesis, developed at length in his book *On the Genealogy of Morals*, in the context of the evidence of genetic understanding:

> The basis from which this evidence is derived is demonstrated, for example, when Nietzsche convincingly makes us understand how, out of the awareness of weakness, wretchedness, and suffering, moral principles, moral demands, and a religion of deliverance can arise because the psyche, via this roundabout way, wants to satisfy its will to power in spite of its weakness; we experience immediate evidence which we cannot reduce further nor base on any kind of other evidence.   (p. 84)

This is itself a strange statement: while on the one hand arguing for the evidence of Nietzsche's account, Jaspers refers also to Nietzsche's highly metaphysical, and by no means obvious, theory of the 'will to power' to explain the connection. In section 5 Jaspers again uses the example, this time to illustrate how we might not be sure that an evident meaningful connection applies in a particular case:

> When Nietzsche tries to apply the connection (which in itself is meaningful and convincing) between awareness of weakness and morality to the actual particular historical events of the origin of Christianity, it is possible that such an application to a particular case can be wrong in spite of the correctness of the general (ideal-typical) understanding of that connection.   (p. 85)

The problem with Jaspers' choice of Nietzsche

The choice of such a distinctive type of understanding as a paradigm case is problematic to the extent that it can mislead us over the nature of other forms of understanding. Jaspers also relates Nietzsche's analysis to Weber's notion of 'ideal types', which we will look at below. There are not many commentators who would regard Nietzsche's analysis as a particularly representative example of an ideal-typical understanding, though! One needs to appreciate that Nietzsche's analysis is an attempt to simplify a complex cultural phenomenon by using a theory that accounts for people's motivations within a simple model of power relations. This makes it surprising that Jaspers should champion Nietzsche's account while simultaneously criticizing Freud for over simplifying matters: 'An error in the Freudian teaching consists in the increasing simplification of his understanding which is connected with the transformation of meaningful connections into general theories. Theories tend to simplification. Understanding finds infinite variety and complexity.' (p. 92)

In this statement, Jaspers is no longer thinking about understanding in the Nietzschean model; he has switched back to thinking of understanding in terms of the evident meaningful connections we grasp in everyday life, in their irreducible multiplicity. This is quite different to the notion of understanding in the sense of an encompassing model of cultural life, or in the sense of the meaningful connections that 'have been discovered through the intuition of exceptional persons' (p. 90).

Question 6: ideally typical connections

While recognizing that Nietzsche's work is perhaps not a central example of what we mean by understanding, nor a type of understanding that is common in a clinical context, it is still worth considering the notion of 'ideal type' understanding. The notion comes from Weber, and this is what Jaspers says about it: 'Meaningful connections are ideally typical connections. They are self-evident (not arrived at by induction) and do not lead to theories; they remain only a kind of model by which particular real events can be assessed and recognised as being more or less understandable.' (p. 85)

There has been much debate about Weber's notion of an ideal type, and also about their place in psychopathology (see the work by Wiggins and Schwartz in the Reading guide for details. The above quotation does not help very much). It tells us that ideal types are 'models', which are of help in assessing the understandability of particular real events, but it is unclear what is meant by a 'model' here. Natural scientists often speak of, and construct, 'models' of certain natural phenomena: a computer simulation of the weather, for example, running a particular 'mathematical model'. Commentators on Jaspers, such as Wiggins and Schwartz, take an ideal type to be a type of diagnostic tool— it is a grouping of symptoms that are often found together, and can be given a convenient name, though it is not necessary for a patient to display all of the symptoms in the group in order to be diagnosed as having the named syndrome. While this is undoubtedly a useful way of thinking of diagnostic classifications, it is not necessarily what Jaspers means by an ideal type.

In *General Psychopathology*, Jaspers distinguishes an ideal type from what he calls an 'average type'. It is worth quoting the passage at length:

> How are types arrived at? We create them through thoughtful contemplation whereby we develop the construct of a coherent whole. We make a distinction between the average type and the ideal type. Average types are created, for instance, when we establish certain measurable properties in a group of individuals (height, weight, powers of registration, fatiguability, etc.) and calculate the mean. If we gather together the results for all these properties this will give us the average type for this group. Ideal types are created when we proceed from given presuppositions and develop the consequences either through causal constructions or the exercise of psychological understanding; that is, we envisage a whole on the occasion of our experiences, but do not actually experience it. To establish the average type we need a great number of cases; but for the development of an ideal type we only need to be stimulated by the experience of one or two individuals. It follows from the very nature of ideal types that they carry no significance as a classification of what really is, but provide an instrument all the same which helps us to assess real, individual cases. In so far as they correspond to the ideal type,

we can comprehend them. [...] In addition ideal types enable us to give order and meaning to psychic states and developments *in concreto*, not through disjointed enumeration of them but by revealing the ideally typical connections in so far as they really exist.   (pp. 560–561)

This passage tells us a number of things: first that ideal types are not constructed on the basis of what properties or symptoms are seen to often go together; they are of no significance for empirical classifications; they are used to form a meaningful whole, rather than giving a 'disjointed enumeration' of 'psychic states and developments'. To understand Jaspers more fully here, we need to look at what Weber meant by an 'ideal type', and how he understood their usefulness.

Weber's notion of ideal types

In his work *Roscher and Knies*, Weber characterizes an ideal type as 'a teleological scheme of rational action' (p. 191). What he means is that an ideal type is a conceptual scheme that sets out the aims, goals, and ends that are valued in a particular context, together with the rules, regulations, and norms that govern what counts as proper or correct behaviour in pursuit of them. There are other complications to Weber's notion of an ideal type, which we do not need to worry about here. What is important to grasp is the way that an ideal type sets out the normative or rule-governed framework that informs the actions and behaviour of the members of a society. This model of the framework is called an *ideal* type, because it gives a picture of how the agents would behave if they acted in accordance with the values and norms in force—which, of course, they do not always do! The following exercise will ask you to read an extract from one of Weber's 1907 essays, where he discusses ideal types in relation to the idea of rule-following.

EXERCISE 6   (30 minutes)

Read the extract from:

Weber, M. (1989). The concept of 'following a rule'. In *Max Weber: selections in translation* (ed. W.G. Runciman) (trans. E. Matthews). Cambridge: Cambridge University Press, pp. 99–110 (Extract p99)

Link with Reading 10.5

◆ Note carefully how Weber distinguishes various senses of 'rule' and 'law', particularly the distinction between a natural law and a normative rule.

Note in this extract how Weber makes a fundamental distinction between 'laws of nature' and a rule in the sense of 'a "norm" against which present, past or future events can be "measured" in the sense of a value judgement' (p. 99). He then goes on to distinguish various types of rule, broadening our conception beyond that of merely 'regulative' rules governing behaviour (such as legal rules), to rules that constitute certain forms of behaviour in a more fundamental sense (think of the rules that constitute the game of football). The philosopher John Searle characterizes the difference between regulative and constitutive rules as follows:

> We might say that regulative rules regulate antecedently or independently existing forms of behaviour; for example, many rules of etiquette regulate inter-personal relationships which exist independently of the rules. But constitutive rules do not merely regulate, they create or define new forms of behaviour. The rules of football or chess, for example, do not merely regulate playing football or chess, but as it were they create the very possibility of playing such games. The activities of playing football or chess are constituted by acting in accordance with (at least a large subset of) the appropriate rules.
>
> Searle (1969, pp. 33–34)

An ideal type as a normative model

As a first approximation, we can think of Weber's notion of an ideal type as the making explicit of the constitutive and regulative rules that inform a certain social context; it tries to map out the prevailing aims and goals valued in a given situation, and thus to make clear what would be considered as good reasons in a certain situation for certain types of behaviour. We can thus think of an ideal type as a model of the meaningful context in which people 'live' in a given situation, that is the framework of rules that people draw on in their own understanding of themselves, their actions, and their reasons for acting. In constructing his technique of ideal types, Weber drew heavily on the philosophy of the South-west German School of Neo-Kantianism, which emphasized the irreducible 'normative' dimension of meaning and rationality. We can therefore think of an ideal type as a 'normative model' rather than a causal model, such as used in the natural sciences. A normative model gives the framework of 'norms' that people draw on in their self-understanding, in a given situation.

The legal framework of a society at a given time is perhaps the most obvious example of the norms that might figure in the ideal type of a certain historical situation. One such law may be the law against murder. The fact that this law is not always followed, does not make it any less of a law (compare this with a causal law!). Connected with the law against murder would be other regulations governing procedures that are brought into play if the law is contravened. Yet the fact that murders take place and these procedures are not followed (for example, the murder goes undetected), does not mean that the regulations are not 'in force' in that situation.

An ideal type is a mapping of the normative framework in a much broader sense than just the institutionalized legal framework, yet the same principles apply: it is a type of model that takes account of the fact that not everyone acts rationally or in accord with other normative rules. It is thus quite different in nature to an 'average type' or a statistically frequent diagnostic grouping of symptoms, even though in these cases also it is not expected that each individual's behaviour conforms exactly to the average, or shows all the symptoms associated with a particular diagnosis.

Jaspers and ideal-typical understanding

In his 'Causal and "meaningful" connections' paper, Jaspers emphasizes particularly the irrelevance of statistical surveys of behaviour for the construction of an ideal type (remember that the number of murders does not change the status of the law as a norm in force in a particular society). One of Jaspers' examples gives a good illustration of the way that what is seen as a meaningful connection both cannot be inferred from statistical information, and also can change from period to period. He writes, 'The meaningful connection between autumn weather and suicide is in no way confirmed by the suicide curve which is highest in spring, but that does not mean that this meaningful connection is wrong.' (p. 85)

Jaspers is suggesting that at the time he wrote, and in his cultural world, autumn carries rather depressing connotations. We can think of this in terms of there being a 'meaningful connection' in force such that its being autumn is accepted as a reason for feeling melancholic. Yet in other times and other cultures—indeed, perhaps for many in our own culture—autumn carries no such connotations, i.e. there is no such meaningful connection in force.

While Jaspers himself says that ideal types 'carry no significance as a classification of what really is', the notion does throw important light on how we think about 'understanding'. In particular, Jaspers' reference to Weber's theory again signals a move away from a simple 'empathic' model of understanding. A connection is not meaningful because we can subjectively empathize with it in our own psychic life, rather a connection is constituted as meaningful by the 'objective' and normative framework of meaning in which we live.

Question 7: the limits of understanding

When Jaspers writes that 'there is no single event known to us which, in this sense, cannot be understood as well as explained' (p. 86), one might be forgiven for thinking that any event is in principle capable of being either understood or causally explained. This was very much the view of Rickert, who argued as we saw above that understanding and causal explanation do not apply to two distinct realms of reality (the mental and the physical, respectively), but that they represented two distinct approaches to one and the same reality. For Rickert, the difference between a human scientific approach and a natural scientific approach lie in the difference in the aims and logical structure of how we choose to conceive of a given event. And as we also saw above, Jaspers clearly draws on Rickert's thinking (through Weber). But now we come across a difference: 'Whereas with the method of causal explanation in principle we nowhere encounter barriers, but can gain new ground in all directions and without limitation, with understanding we encounter limitations everywhere.' (p. 86)

Jaspers is thus saying that any event that we understand as involving a meaningful connection, can in principle be investigated causally, though not every event can be understood in the first place.

'As if' understanding

What Jaspers means becomes clearer if we consider his idea of 'as if' understanding: something he particularly finds in some of Freud's explanations of psychic life. 'As if' understanding, for Jaspers, results from the attempt to extend understanding beyond its proper limits, such that one cites a *meaningful* connection where properly one should cite a *causal* connection. We need to be careful, however, about just what Jaspers means by the 'limits' to understanding: given enough ingenuity, there is no event that cannot be understood, it is rather that certain events are more *properly* conceived of as causal connections.

This becomes clearer when we look at Jaspers' example of an event that, in the past, was understood meaningfully, but that we now regard as not appropriately understood in this way: '...In a mythological age men thought they could understand Donar in thunder and lightning' (pp. 86–87). Clearly, today, someone who accounted for thunder and lightning by understanding it as the intentional action of a divine agent, would be thought of as living in the past. Weber indeed talks of the 'disenchantment' of nature in the modern age: by which he means the way in which the finding of purposes and intentional actions behind natural events slowly became unacceptable.

What then marks out a certain attempt to understand an event as 'unacceptable' or as an instance of extending understanding beyond its 'proper' limits? It cannot be that understanding is inappropriate in the case of events that *can* be given a causal explanation—as Jaspers acknowledges that every event is susceptible to causal explanation. Jaspers seems certain, though, that it is possible to identify inappropriate uses of understanding, and indeed he finds such in Freud's work: 'The confusion of meaningful connections with causal connections is the basis of the incorrect Freudian postulate that every aspect and event in psychic life can be understood (is meaningfully determined). However, it is only the postulate of unlimited causality, not the postulate of unlimited meaningfulness, which is justifiable.' (p. 91)

Jaspers gives no indication of how one tells, in general, whether an attempt to understand is appropriate or not—and maybe it is not possible to give general guidelines for this. In certain cases, such as the taking of an umbrella, or a clap of thunder, it seems clear when understanding or causal explanation is appropriate, but in other cases the question of which approach is more appropriate in the context, may be an issue for discussion and debate.

Development or process?

The issue of whether a sequence of events is more properly understood or causally explained is at the heart of psychopathology for Jaspers. In *General Psychopathology*, the 'basic problem' is 'personality development or process?':

> The investigation of the basic biological events and the meaningful development of the life-history culminates in a differentiation of two kinds of individual life: *the unified development of a personality* (based on a normal biological course through the

age-epochs and any contingent phases) and the *disruption* of a life which is *broken* in two and falls apart because at a time a *process* has intervened in the biological happenings and irreversibly and incurably altered the psychic life by interrupting the course of biological events. (p. 702)

By 'process', Jaspers means a biological or neurological dysfunction that we cite as explaining a mental illness. We might loosely speak of a neurological dysfunction as 'disrupting' someone's mental life, or a life 'broken in two', but clearly what we mean by this is a complex issue. In part it will depend on our assessment of 'normal' biological development. In part also it involves our failure to see the sequence of someone's thoughts and behaviour as amenable to understanding: that is, as not subject to a 'proper' use of understanding. But again, it is difficult to imagine how one could lay down general principles about when we 'see' and do not 'see' a meaningful connection—except that we are more likely not to see one where we possess a detailed account of the causal mechanism linking events. That is, while one might accept in principle that every event can be subject to a causal account, the question of whether a concrete causal account is available in a particular case is an important criterion in deciding whether or not it is appropriate to understand the event meaningfully.

In general we can see Jaspers' discussion of meaningful and causal connections as torn between two competing motives. On the one hand, Jaspers wished to re-establish the place of understanding in a discipline that was increasingly viewing mental disorder in biological and natural scientific terms; on the other hand, he wished to make clear that understanding has 'limits', so that the possibility of fruitful research into the biological or neurological basis of certain disorders is not discounted. The question of where understanding ends and causal explanation begins becomes more appropriate is presented as rather cut and dried, in order to balance these two motives; but in practice, the answer will be much more difficult, and very much up for debate.

Question 8: a causal account of meaningful connections?

We have seen that Jaspers regards psychopathology as unusual in drawing on the methods and aims of both the natural sciences and the human sciences. He says, for example, that 'in almost all psychological investigations, understanding and explanation go hand in hand. This combination of methods is indispensable for psychology' (p. 86). In answering the previous question (about the limits of understanding) we saw how a clinician may turn to a causal explanation when attempts to understand someone's mental life fail. There is a further question we can ask, however, and that is whether this *combination of methods* is indispensable for philosophical reasons, or for merely pragmatic reasons.

To put this another way: are there aspects of what it means to understand someone that are simply irreducible to a causal account, or is it merely that there are *practical* obstacles to giving a full causal account of a meaningful connection, even though *in theory* it would be possible? Certainly in Jaspers' day the technology was simply not available to undertake detailed neurological investigations of the kind (like brain scanning) available today. So could it be that one speaks of a 'meaningful connection' between mental states simply as a short-hand for speaking about a causal connection that we are not yet in a position to explain fully? In other words, the 'combination of methods' may be 'indispensable for psychology' for merely *practical* reasons, rather for any reason of *principle*: and indeed a causal account could perhaps ultimately be given in cases where we now 'make do' with describing a meaningful connection.

'Folk psychology' as a primitive explanatory theory

This question, of whether we speak about 'understanding' someone's mental life merely as a substitute for a causal explanation that we are not yet in a position to give, is a central issue in contemporary philosophy of mind. We should not be surprised by this. Rapid advances in the neurosciences in the late twentieth century, like the corresponding advances in Jaspers' time, once more seem to hold out the prospect of a complete causal account of human experience and behaviour. This has given rise to a very influential contemporary philosophical position called 'physicalism'. This is the view, roughly, that everything that is explicable is explicable ultimately in physical terms. (See Gillett and Loewer, 2001.) Many, then, not least in philosophy, have argued that causes will increasingly displace meanings in the human sciences as they have in the natural sciences.

We return to this debate in detail in Part V, especially Chapter 23. As we will see, our everyday (meaningful) ways of understanding people's experiences and behaviours are often referred to in modern philosophy of mind as 'folk psychology'. Although not intended pejoratively, the implication is clear: just as the causal stories of modern physics have increasingly made the 'folk physics' of pre-scientific imagination redundant, so advances in the neurosciences will increasingly make meanings and understanding redundant in the human sciences. The question, then, with which we will be concerned in Part V, is whether folk psychology is ultimately a primitive form of explanatory theory that now needs to be updated in the light of modern neurological investigations. For the present we will simply lay the ground for this more detailed discussion by showing that there appears to be a tension in Jaspers' mind over what the answer is. It is clear that he thinks we need both—both causal and meaningful amounts of psychopathology. But it is not clear whether he thinks it is *in principle* impossible to give a causal explanation of a meaningful connection, or whether there are merely contingent reasons why such an explanation could never be given in *practice*.

The reducibility or irreducibility of meaningful connections

Jaspers' view of the 'reducibility' or 'irreducibility', in principle, of meaningful connections to causal connections can be found in section 6:

> It is not absurd to think that it might one day be possible to have some rules which could causally explain the sequence of meaningfully connected thought processes without paying heed to the meaningful connections between them. In such cases the meaning of the connection would be just as irrelevant and accidental for the causal explanation as, in another case, is the lack of meaning. It is therefore in principle not at all absurd to try to understand as well as to explain one and the same real psychic event. These two established connections, however, are of entirely different origin and have entirely different kinds of validity. [. . .] In fact there is no single event known to us which, in this sense, cannot be understood as well as explained. To find such an event is an infinitely remote problem.   (*ibid.*)

It is worth looking at this passage carefully! At the beginning Jaspers suggests that it is 'possible' that 'one day' we will be able to give a causal account of thought processes that we at present understand in a meaningful way. Again, we can think of analogies with physics: great 'significance' used to be attributed to a solar eclipse, but now, when we can give a causal explanation of it, the 'meaning' of the event is 'irrelevant and accidental'. Are mental events like this? Will we, one day, regard the attribution of 'meaning' to a sequence of brain states as a primitive and pre-scientific way of thinking? Jaspers would seem to suggest that it is not absurd to think so—in other words, Jaspers here suggests the *reducibility in principle* of meaningful connections to causal connections.

Yet Jaspers also says that understanding and explaining 'have entirely different kinds of validity'—i.e. that understanding is not merely a primitive or shorthand form replaceable by a more adequate causal account. This would suggest the *irreducibility in principle* of meaningful connections to causal connections.

The final two sentences suggest yet another possibility: that the giving of a full causal account of a particular meaningful connection 'is an infinitely remote problem'. That is, while possible in principle, there is an *irreducibility in practice* of meaningful connections to causal connections. Is it possible, then, to make sense of what Jaspers means here? Can we reconcile Jaspers' different views of the relation between meaningful connections and causal connections?

A reconciliation of Jaspers' views?

A possible clue to reconciling Jaspers' views of the reducibility or irreducibility of meaningful connections to causal connections comes toward the end of the same paragraph from which the above quotation comes. Jaspers writes that 'in no case do the understanding and explanation, coming as they do from different sides, converge on one and the same real aspect of the complex psychic event under study' (p. 86). At first sight it is difficult to know precisely what Jaspers means here. One interpretation might be that Jaspers is claiming that while one might be able to give a causal explanation of the relation between two states that are picked out initially as standing in a meaningful connection, it is not possible to give a causal account of their relation *qua* (in respect of its being a) meaningful connection.

Here is an analogous case: imagine swapping five 2p pieces for a 10p piece. There are all sorts of physical relation one could describe between the 2ps and the 10p—for example, the relation between their weights. However, what one could never describe in physical language is the 'meaningful connection' between five 2p pieces and a 10p piece—i.e. that they carry the same monetary value. In other words, one can give an physical account of the relation between the items picked out as '2p pieces' and '10p pieces', but it is not possible to give a physical account of their relation *qua* monetary relation.

This would be a more subtle form of the 'irreducibility in principle' thesis—one that acknowledges that a causal explanation of the states picked out as standing in a meaningful connection may be possible. We return to this idea in Chapter 23 in the sophisticated form (called 'anomalous monism') developed by the American philosopher Donald Davidson.

The continuity between understanding and explanation

There is evidence against this interpretation of Jaspers, however. In the above quotation, he uses the image of understanding and explanation coming 'from different sides'. It is difficult to know what precisely he means by this. Interestingly, Jaspers does use a similar image in a related context in *General Psychopathology*. However, whereas in the above quotation from his paper on 'Causal and "meaningful" connections', the image is used to suggest the irreducibility of meanings to causes, here, in *General Psychopathology*, the image suggests precisely the *reducibility of* meaning to causes! The passage in fact is concerned with the connection between mind and brain (or 'psyche' and 'soma'), though the link to the present context should be obvious: mind is what we seek to understand, the brain is investigated causally. This is the passage:

> Investigation of somatic function, including the most complex cortical activity, is bound up with investigation of psychic function, and the unity of soma and psyche seems indisputable. Yet we must remember that neither line of enquiry encounters the other so directly that we can speak of some specific psychic event as directly associated with some specific somatic event or of an actual parallelism. The situation is analogous with the exploration of an unknown continent from opposite directions, where the explorers never meet because of impenetrable country that intervenes. We only know the end links in the chain of causation from soma to psyche and vice versa and from both these terminal points we endeavour to advance.   *General Psychopathology* (p. 4)

Here Jaspers likens the relation between the understanding of mental states and the causal explanation of brain states to 'the exploration of an unknown continent from opposite directions'. In the analogy the explorers never meet because of obstacles in practice—in principle they could meet, if they were better

equipped or their technology improved. Analogously, then, it seems that understanding is reducible to causal explanation in principle: it is only practical difficulties and technological limitations that prevent us from arriving at a meaningful connection (i.e. one side of the continent) by undertaking a causal investigation (i.e. starting at the other side). This would suggest that there is a fundamental continuity between the understanding approach and the explanation approach. Given enough technical know-how, the one will merge with the other.

It would seem that Jaspers wavered between the ideas of *irreducibility in principle* and *irreducibility in practice*, and given the relatively primitive state of neurology at the time, it is likely that he felt the question could be deferred. As noted above, however, with enormous advances in the technology required to investigate the causal functioning of the brain, the question is now once again more pressing: are there aspects of what it means to understand someone which are irreducible in principle to the giving of a causal account?

The place of values

Question 9: understanding, normativity, and value judgements

One reason for thinking that there is an irreducibility in principle of understanding to causal explanation would be that understanding necessarily involves value judgements or at any rate has an inescapable normative (i.e. human rule following) dimension of some kind.

Since the time of the Scottish philosopher, David Hume, it is commonly held that normative statements cannot be reduced to, nor derived from, statements of fact. As we saw in Part I, this idea is often expressed in terms of the 'is-ought' distinction: statements of what *ought* to be the case cannot be derived from statements purely about what *is* the case. In section 10 of his article, Jaspers suggests that understanding 'inevitably' involves a value judgement, and it is worth looking closely at what he says for two reasons. First of all, it may throw light on Jaspers' view of the reducibility or not of understanding to causal explanation. Secondly, it may help us understand the place of value judgements within psychiatry—an issue we considered in some detail in Part I, and to which we return particularly in respect of psychiatric diagnosis in Part IV. Thus, Jaspers writes,

> It is a fact that when dealing with meaningful connections as such we inevitably tend to value positively or negatively, while everything meaningless we merely value, if we do so at all, only in relation to something else. Thus the emergence of moral demands from resentment we may value as something despicable, whereas we value memory merely as a tool. In the *science* of psychology, however, we must strictly refrain from any such value judgement. Our task is merely to grasp the meaningful connections as such and to recognize them.   (p. 89)

(*Note*: The translation is rather misleading here. A more literal translation of the first sentence would be 'It is a fact that we value all genetically understood connections in themselves positively or negatively, while everything ununderstandable . . .'.)

Jaspers' view of the need to avoid value judgements

Jaspers' view then, in this passage, is that, as a matter of course, we tend to place a positive or negative value on that which we understand, and purely in virtue of our understanding of it (not merely in virtue of its being good or bad as a means to something else). However, this evaluative aspect of understanding is not an essential part of it: in the 'science of psychology' we must seek to avoid making any value judgements.

On the face of it, therefore, there is no essentially normative, or value-laden, aspect to understanding, according to Jaspers, such that this could be cited as a reason for the irreducibility of understanding to causal explanation. Further, and contrary to what we concluded in Part I, Jaspers seems to suggest that a scientific psychiatry should be value-free (or at least that any normative considerations are merely extraneous additions). Jaspers gives the following explanation of why we tend to confuse (in his view) understanding *per se* with a 'valuation' (*Wertung*) of what we understand: 'Since everyone likes to be judged favourably they usually only feel themselves properly "understood" if the result is such a favourable valuation [*Wertung*]. Hence common usage takes the word "understand" frequently to be identical with "favourably judged" '. (p. 90)

But is this right? An example may help make clear that the issue is not as clear-cut as Jaspers seems to be suggesting. When we think about the meaningful connection between someone's motives and their actions, we may conclude that we can see the *reason* for their action. In identifying a belief or motive as the *reason* for acting in a certain way, we imply that there is a *rational* connection between the belief or motive and the action. This in turn implies that it would have been *right* for any *rational agent* to have acted the same way, given those beliefs or motives.

For example, if someone wishes to catch a train and believes that the station is a mile to the north then it is rational for them to head north because by doing that they will, with luck, be able to catch a train. In order to explain their action—their purposeful striding out in a northerly direction—we can cite their desire to catch a train and their beliefs and the relative direction of the station. Note that this sort of explanation does not depend on doing further psychological experiment or market research. We do not need to know, for example, that this is what 90% of people questioned in the past have done. Instead we can understand the point or purpose of the action by placing it in the context of the subject's belief and desire. In that context, the action is the *right* thing to do. Thus the explanation is *normative*. It depends, in part, on citing the outcome valued by the subject. But the pattern of beliefs, values, and actions is itself a pattern that seems rational or right to the person offering the explanation. Of course there remains a further question of value: whether heading to the station to catch a train in order to commit a crime in a distant city is morally the right thing to do.

Thus even putting aside any considerations of the morality of an action, there seems to be a normative dimension to our judgements of the very rationality of an action in the light of given motives. If we decide that someone ought (rationally) not to have acted in a certain way, that person may indeed feel themselves not 'properly understood'; but rightly so, if there are considerations that we did not take into account that show the action to have indeed been the *right* thing to do (rationally).

It seems, then, that there *is* an inescapable normative dimension to the type of understanding where we recognize a 'rational' connection between a motive and an action—to call it 'rational' implies that any other rational agent *ought* to have done the same. Jaspers would, therefore, appear to be wrong in suggesting that it is only 'common usage' that links 'understanding' and 'favourably judged'. There would seem to be a conceptual connection between them when we are talking about rational meaningful connections.

Of course, not all types of understanding are concerned with rational connections: a particularly strong form of meaningful connection. Could it be, then, that there are types of meaningful connection, and thus types of understanding, which have no essential connection to value judgements? As we saw above, there are a great many ways in which we use the notion of understanding—we would need to look at them one by one. However, if we take Weber's notion of ideal types as a good model of what understanding involves in the sophisticated sense in which human sciences seek to understand people and events, then it again appears that a normative dimension is inescapable. Indeed, we saw above that what is distinctive about an ideal type is that it specifies the *normative* framework within which we act on, and formulate, motives.

A tension in Jaspers' mind

As with the relationship between causal and meaningful connections above, there is a tension in Jaspers' own thinking on the relationship between understanding and evaluation. While in the article he clearly states that we must refrain from making value judgements, and goes on to suggest that the linking of understanding and evaluation is mistaken, his position in *General Psychopathology* is quite different. Here he states that there is an *inescapable* link between understanding and evaluation, and that there is indeed a good reason why people identify understanding with judgements of value—the reason being that understanding actually *implies* judgements of value! It is worth quoting the passage from *General Psychopathology* to see the contrast:

> Meaningful human activity is in itself an expression of values, and everything understandable carries for us an immediate positive or negative colouring; everything understandable has a constituent potentiality of worth. [. . .] In understanding a concrete case we inevitably appear to make an appraisal, and to fail in scientific understanding, because with human beings every meaningful connection as such is immediately judged negatively or positively. This is due to the fact that the understandable as

such implies some evaluation. To understand correctly is to appraise; to appraise correctly is finally to understand.   (p. 310)

So what are we to make of this? On the one hand Jaspers says we must avoid making value judgements in understanding people, on the other he says that understanding is unavoidably linked to the making of value judgements!

Jaspers and Weber's demand for 'freedom from value judgements'

Two answers are possible here. The first is that the value judgements Jaspers is talking about in the article are really *moral* judgements. In the example he gives, 'the emergence of moral demands from resentment' (Nietzsche's thesis), Jaspers may be referring to our tendency to judge such an occurrence as *morally* repugnant. It would indeed seem possible to understand a person or event without coming to a *moral* evaluation, and this may be what Jaspers is suggesting.

The second answer, connected to the first, is that when Jaspers asserts, in the article, that understanding must be free of value judgements, he does not properly distinguish between different types of value judgement. That is, there may be unavoidable normative aspects to the notion of understanding, quite apart from any moral considerations, and it may be these that Jaspers acknowledges in the passage from *General Psychopathology*.

We can get a deeper understanding of what is going on here by considering the background to Jaspers' approach in the (contrasting) work, respectively, of Weber and Rickert. In the article, Jaspers is following Weber to a large extent, in his emphasis on the need for a science, even one that involves understanding, to be 'value-free'. Weber is well known for insisting on 'freedom from value judgements' (*Werturteilsfreiheit*) in social sciences—and there is debate on this issue right up to the present day (see Dirk Käsler's book in the Reading Guide for further details). A clear statement comes from a 1917 essay by Weber, but the ideas he expresses are also present in his earlier work. The essay title is translated as 'The meaning of "ethical neutrality" in sociology and economics', though the translation is again a little misleading: Weber is talking about 'freedom from values' (*Wertfreiheit*), not simply 'ethical neutrality'. Weber writes, for example:

> What is really at issue is the intrinsically simple demand that the investigator and teacher should keep unconditionally separate the establishment of empirical facts (including the 'value-oriented' [*wertenden*] conduct of the empirical individual whom he is investigating) and *his* own practical valuational [*wertende*], i.e. evaluational stance [*beurteilende…'bewertende' Stellungnahme*] toward these facts as satisfactory or unsatisfactory (including among these facts valuations [*Wertungen*] made by the empirical persons who are the objects of investigation).
> Weber ([1917] 1949 p. 11)

On the face of it, it would appear that Jaspers agrees with Weber: value judgements must play no part in our scientific understanding of people. The term both Weber and Jaspers predominantly use is '*Wertungen*' (from '*Wert*', 'value')—scientific understanding must be free of 'valuations'.

Weber and the 'value-philosophy' of Rickert

We need to look deeper into this issue, however. As we noted earlier, one of the major influences on Weber was the philosophy of the South-west German School of Neo-Kantianism, in particular the work of Rickert. The philosophy of this school is often called 'value-philosophy', because of the emphasis those involved placed on values in scientific investigations. In the value-philosophy of Rickert one finds a distinction between *Wertungen* ('valuations') and *Beurteilungen* ('evaluations'). An 'evaluation' in Rickert's sense is an expression of the 'value relevance' (*Wertbeziehung*) of an object or event, that is, the normative significance attaching to it in the light of a norm or rule. The following passage comes from Rickert's *The Limits of Concept Formation in Natural Science*:

> It is simply not the business of historical science to offer positive or negative *valuations*: in other words, to assert that the individual realities they represent are either good or bad, valuable or antagonistic to value. For in that case, how is history to arrive at *generally* valid value judgements? It is rather the case that we have to scrupulously distinguish what we mean by the 'relevance' of an individual to a value from the direct positive or negative *valuation* of this individual. Indeed, if our view were conceived as if we held that rendering positive or negative *value judgements* is a task of historical *science*, and thus that history is a *valuing* science, this would be the *most reprehensible of all misunderstandings*. On the contrary, we must regard the dissociation of every 'practical' positive or negative value judgement from the *purely theoretical relevance* of objects to values as an essential criterion of the *specific* historical conception. Indeed, insofar as the value perspective is decisive for history, this concept of the 'value relevance'—in opposition to 'valuation'—is actually *the* essential criterion for history as a pure science.   Rickert [1902] 1986 (p. 91)

Rickert argues that the historian, for example, must avoid giving his own *valuations* of an event (i.e. whether it was from the historian's own point of view a good or bad thing), but cannot avoid the *evaluations* that are part and parcel of understanding something as an historical or cultural happening. The evaluation (in Rickert's sense) of a historical event is the act of placing it into a pattern that reveals its point and purpose—and thus what about it was valued by the historical agents who brought it about—but the pattern itself is a rational pattern. It is the pattern of what is the appropriate, right thing to do in the context of an agent's beliefs and desires. An historian might, for example, attempt to understand the actions of Hitler's deputies before and during the Second World War by characterizing the peculiar culture of leadership Hitler developed. This could underpin an account of the way in which decisions were made and implemented in accordance with the rules of 'proper' behaviour and of ways to impress the leader. Individual acts could then be seen to make sense in that context. But none of this need be taken to be implicit or explicit support (or, for that matter, condemnation) of that regime.

While Weber is well known for his insistence on 'freedom from value judgements', this can tend to obscure the place of values, and 'evaluations' (in Rickert's technical sense), in his analysis of what is involved in understanding. The following quotation comes from Weber's 1904 essay ' "Objectivity" in social science and social policy'. It is worth quoting at length, because of the clarity with which Weber expresses the idea that the type of understanding undertaken by human or social sciences cannot do without an investigation of the 'value relevance' (or what Rickert would call the evaluation) of, for example, the actions, words, and behaviour of the people studied.

> The concept of culture is a *value-concept*. Empirical reality becomes 'culture' to us because and insofar as we relate it to value ideas. It includes those segments and only those segments of reality which have become significant to us because of this value-relevance. Only a small portion of existing concrete reality is coloured by our value-conditioned interest and it alone is significant to us. It is significant because it reveals relationships which are important to us due to their connection with our values. Only because and to the extent that this is the case is it worthwhile for us to know it in its individual features. We cannot discover, however, what is meaningful to us by means of a 'presuppositionless' investigation of empirical data. Rather perception of its meaningfulness to us is the presupposition of its becoming an *object* of investigation. (p. 76)

> The transcendental presupposition of every *cultural science* lies not in our finding a certain 'culture' or any 'culture' in general to be *valuable* but rather in the fact that we are *cultural beings*, endowed with the capacity and the will to take a deliberate attitude towards the world and to lend it *significance*. Whatever this significance may be, it will lead us to evaluate [*beurteilen*] certain phenomena of human existence in its light and to respond to them as being (positively or negatively) meaningful. Whatever may be the content of this attitude—these phenomena have cultural significance for us and on this significance alone rests its scientific interest. Thus when we speak here of the conditioning of cultural knowledge through *value* ideas [*Wertideen*] (following the terminology of modern logic), it is done in the hope that we will not be subject to crude misunderstandings such as the opinion that cultural significance should be attributed only to *valuable* phenomena. (p. 81)

There are several important ideas here that underline the distinction between (in Rickert–Weber terminology) 'valuation' (actually making value judgements) and 'evaluation' (studying value and other normative judgements as objects of inquiry that help to make sense of human actions and events). The passage as a whole indeed spells out the point that while Weber does indeed insist that the human sciences do not and should not consist in making value judgements about the things people say and do (Weber's 'freedom from value judgements'), he nonetheless also insists that understanding the meaning of what someone says or does includes evaluation, i.e. understanding the values and other norms that are a (necessary) part of the meaning of what they say or do.

First, he emphasizes that an investigation of the meaningfulness of human phenomena cannot expect to start from a 'presuppositionless' investigation of empirical data. We expressed this above in terms of Quine's (1960) notion of the 'cosmic exile': the cosmic exile, setting out to study human behaviour, has access only to the 'value-free' findings of a physical investigation of the movements of and other changes in his objects of study. Weber stresses that an investigation of the meaningfulness of human phenomena cannot start from this 'exiled' perspective; it must rather presuppose that a direct 'perception' of meaningfulness is possible. This is what Weber means by a 'transcendental presupposition' of a cultural science. It is a condition of the very possibility of a cultural (or human) science that social scientists do not attempt to be cosmic exiles, but can instead directly perceive meanings in what people say and do.'

The second important point is the role of values and evaluations as part of what it means to perceive the meaningfulness of a human phenomenon. When we seek to understand the 'significance' of actions, utterances, or behaviour, this significance derives from our evaluation of them in connection to norms and rules, that is, our evaluation of their 'value-relevance'. Thus it is our norms that are used to make sense of others' actions. This contrasts with the idea that we test experimentally the idea that people who want to go to the station and believe it is to the north go there. Rather we know this to be right a priori and we thus impose this standard on them to read their actions. So in one sense it is an imposition of values, i.e. in the sense of the right thing to do. But it is not the morally or aesthetically right thing to do. Rather, it is the *correct* thing to do if they want to get what they want. We cannot, however, flesh out a general third person theory of the correct thing to do in all circumstances. We put ourselves in their place and reason it out.

One must be careful not to be misled, then, by Weber's well-known insistence on 'freedom from value judgements'. Given Jaspers' clear debt to Weber (for example, in connection with the idea of an 'ideal type'), it may be that Jaspers' own insistence on the need to avoid 'value judgements' in understanding might itself reflect a misunderstanding of Weber on this point. Another way of putting this would be to say that Jaspers overlooked the distinction made by Rickert between valuations and evaluations, and focused too much on Weber's insistence that we should avoid the former.

Understanding and 'evaluation'

Rickert's own theory of the nature of *Beurteilungen* ('evaluations') and *Wertbeziehung* ('value-relevance') is complex, and we need not go into it here. What is being suggested, however, is that while rejecting the place of *Wertungen* ('valuations') in understanding, Jaspers fails to acknowledge that there may be other forms of 'evaluation' that are essentially constitutive of it. For Rickert, it was this constitutive aspect of evaluation that fundamentally distinguished the investigations of the 'cultural sciences' from the natural sciences. A natural-scientific form of investigation disregards the 'value relevance' of an object or event, and regards it merely as an instance of a general type, irrespective of its cultural context, and thus indistinguishable from any other instance of that type. In a set of lectures entitled *Science and History*, Rickert (1962) puts this point as follows:

> We see now why it was important earlier to emphasize the fact that the criterion of *value* is what distinguishes cultural events from nature, as regards their scientific treatment. It is *only* in such terms that the individual content of what we may now perhaps call the 'concepts of culture' become comprehensible, not as a separate kind of reality, but as divergent from the general content of the concepts of nature. Accordingly, in order to bring out the distinctive character of this difference even more clearly, we must describe the individualising procedure of the historical sciences as one *oriented to values*, in contrast to that of the natural sciences, whose investigations are directed toward the discovery of laws or the formation of general concepts without regard to cultural values or the relationship in which the objects of nature stand to them.   (p. 87)

While Rickert is here focusing again on history, we can extend the point he is making to cover what is distinctive about the nature of understanding found in human sciences generally. That is, what is distinctive about understanding, in contrast to causal explanation, is the presence in understanding, and the absence in causal explanation, of normative, or as Rickert would say evaluative, considerations.

As the above quotation from *The Limits of Concept Formation in Natural Science* (1902) suggests, if we can distinguish these normative considerations from the making of overt valuations, then there is no reason to think of human sciences as being any less 'scientific' due to their not being 'value-free'. In other words, a properly scientific investigation of the meaningfulness of human actions and behaviour cannot disregard the 'value' attaching to them, as their 'value relevance' is, in a broad sense, precisely what constitutes their meaningfulness. 'A human science has to include the study of values because it is by values that the meanings that are the distinctive objects of study of a human science are in part constituted. But provided the "human scientist" (the historian or whatever) avoids making value judgements of their objects of study their work is no less scientific than that of a natural scientist.' Indeed the actions studied in a human science can only be recognized as the actions they are by fitting them into a rational pattern. The giving of rings, for example, may be partly constitutive of a marriage, because of the rituals and intentions involved. But in other circumstances it may be part of the division of the spoils of war or theft. Fitting actions into a broader context is not like fitting them into a system of laws of nature but rather into a pattern that reveals their purposes.

It is perhaps worth signalling, by the way, that we will be arguing in Part IV (Chapter 21), consistently with the 'fact + value' conclusions of Part I, that as a practical discipline psychiatric diagnosis differs from Rickert's account of a human science, in that it involves, in Weber–Rickert terminology, valuations (i.e. actual value judgements) as well as evaluations (i.e. understanding in terms of relevant value norms).

Thus, anthropologists studying mental distress and disorder can limit themselves to *evaluation*, i.e. to studying values without making value judgements, exactly as Rickert suggests; and such studies can certainly inform diagnostic practice (that which otherwise appears meaningless may become understandable once the relevant values are made clear). But in *making* a diagnosis in a particular case, there are (we will argue) also elements of *valuation*, i.e. value judgements. Diagnostic value judgements are implicit, we will argue, in such concepts as rationality and capacity, and explicit in the judgements involved in applying diagnostic criteria such as the DSM's Criterion B for schizophrenia. So *evaluations* (based on our own understanding as well as on the findings of the human sciences) may inform, but they cannot replace, the *valuations* that are part of diagnosis. As we will see in Chapter 21, this is true in principle of diagnosis in all areas of medicine. But it is important practically when, as in psychiatry, the relevant values are divergent rather than shared and hence may be contested.

Moving towards a conclusion

We have now come to the end of our consideration of the nine questions that guided our reading of Jaspers' article on 'Causal and "meaningful" connections'. We have seen how Jaspers draws considerably on the work of those involved in the *Methodenstreit*, in his conception of psychopathology as being concerned with connections of both kinds. We have also seen how Jaspers' tendency to combine ideas from different protagonists in the *Methodenstreit* leads to certain tensions in his account of understanding. In the concluding session to this part we will bring together the different threads of our analysis in terms of these tensions in Jaspers' thinking, and look briefly at what general conclusions we can draw about the nature of psychiatry and its philosophical foundations.

Reflection on the session and self-test questions

Write down your own reflections on the materials in this session drawing out any points that are particularly significant for you. Then write brief notes about the following:

1. What did Jaspers take, respectively, from the work of Dilthey, Rickert, and Weber?

2. How did the various influences on Jaspers affect his use of terms such as 'empathy', 'understanding', and 'ideal type'?

3. What is the connection between 'ideal types', normativity, and Jaspers' use of the term 'meaningful'?

4. What notable tension is present in Jaspers' thought about the relationship between meanings and causes?

5. Have the tensions in Jaspers' work now been resolved? If not, give two examples of where they are still evident in modern philosophy.

Session 3 Conclusions: Jaspers, the *Methodenstreit*, and psychiatry today

Four tensions in Jaspers' notion of understanding

Our analysis of Jaspers' article 'Causal and "meaningful" connexions between life history and psychosis' has shown that there are four tensions running though his account of understanding. A first tension is broadly that between a Dilthean approach to understanding and a Rickert–Weber approach; a second is between different types of understanding; a third tension is around whether or not it is possible to reduce meanings to causes, to give a causal account of meanings; and a fourth tension is between Jaspers' 'values out' account of understanding and what in the terminology of Part I, we may now call the 'values in' account of Weber and Rickert.

First tension: Dilthey versus Rickert–Weber

The first tension, then in Jaspers' thinking, is between the different accounts of understanding given respectively by Dilthey and by Rickert and Weber. Thus, we saw in our answer to question 1 above, for example, that while using Dilthey's distinction between 'inner' and 'outer' sense to characterize the difference between understanding and explanation, Jaspers himself regarded this as 'wrong'.

His reason for concluding that Dilthey's distinction was mistaken derives from the Rickert–Weber rejection of the idea of two realms of reality (the 'mental' in which one finds meaningful connections, and the 'physical' in which one finds causal connections). In the Rickert–Weber approach there is only one realm of reality, any part of which can be subject to investigations that either attempt to understand it or causally explain it. For Rickert and Weber, the difference between understanding and explanation lies not in a difference of subject matter, but a difference in the approach taken to it, or the way it is 'perceived' (either regarding objects and events in their 'value relevance' or simply as instances of general concepts, indistinguishable from any other instance of the same concept).

Yet while drawing on this Rickert–Weber approach, Jaspers continues to place great emphasis on the Dilthean idea of 'empathy', an idea that both Rickert and Weber regarded as entirely misleading as to the nature of understanding. We can summarize the difference between the two approaches as follows:

- *The Dilthean approach*. In this approach understanding and explanation are distinguished in terms of the different realms of reality for which they are appropriate: psychic life we understand, nature we explain. What are primarily understandable are the 'meaningful connections' between mental states: we have an 'inner experience' of the meaningfulness of our own mental lives, and one seeks to understand another person empathically by re-living their mental states in our imagination. What is meaningful is essentially a private, subjective phenomenon that we have access to only within the inner sphere of our own mental lives.

- *The Rickert–Weber approach*. In the Rickert–Weber approach, understanding and explanation are distinguished in terms of the different perspectives taken to one and the same reality. In the natural sciences one disregards the value relevance of the objects and events studied; in human or 'cultural sciences' one seeks to evaluate the significance attaching to objects and events in a given situation in the light of the normative framework in force in that situation. The meaningfulness of objects and events is not a private, subjective matter, but something that is directly perceivable given an understanding of the values and norms that hold in a given situation.

Second tension: the varieties of 'understanding'

The second tension running through Jaspers' article derives from his failure to distinguish clearly between different types of understanding. At one extreme, we find Jaspers citing Nietzsche's highly conjectural thesis about the genesis of Christian morality as a paradigm example of a meaningful connection; at the other extreme, Jaspers thinks of understanding as a grasping of the immediate evidence of the meaningfulness of the words and actions we come across in everyday life. Thus one finds on the one hand a notion of understanding in which meaningful connections must be accepted as a simple given, and on the other a notion of understanding as interpretation, requiring a methodological hermeneutic circle to pin down the meaning of a particular action or event.

One way of avoiding this tension, suggested above, would be to distinguish between higher forms of understanding and more fundamental types. For example, trying to ascertain someone's motive for acting in a certain way would be a higher form of understanding—if one could not simply ask the person (or if one could not trust their reply!), then this type of understanding would remain a form of conjecture based on other observations. However, part of the very notion of a 'motive' is the idea that a certain belief or desire 'makes sense' of a certain action; that is, the connection between that belief or desire and the action in question is a 'meaningful' or 'understandable' connection. This would be a more fundamental type of understanding upon which the process of trying to ascertain someone's motives in a particular situation would be based.

Consider the commuter making his way north again. If seen in the distance striding purposefully along with many other suited 'gents' at 8.15 a.m. we might *hypothesize* that he is going to the station to go to work. That is one form of understanding we might successfully gain. It might be possible to catch up and ask him directly what he is doing. This will again give us an understanding that, under normal circumstances we would not class as a hypothesis. (Having studied philosophy one may overzealously argue that discounting the possibility that he is lying shows even this to be a hypothesis.) In order to get all the details exact, we might press him further as to why, if he wishes to go to work, he is heading north. His reply will be that he wishes to catch a train and he believes that the station is to the north. In principle we might want to make some further steps in his reasoning explicit: that, for example, he believes that the station, rather than a fish restaurant, is the best place to catch the train. But there will come a point where we do *not* ask: why, if you wish to catch a train and believe that you can best catch a train from a station are you going to the station? That rational connection we take for granted and not because we have questioned many commuters on their behaviour. Rather, it is the rational thing to do.

Third tension: can meaningful connections be reduced to causes?

A third tension we came across in Jaspers' thinking concerned the question of whether it is possible to give a causal account of a meaningful connection. While Jaspers emphasizes the need for psychopathology to combine both understanding and explanation, it was not clear whether this was for merely *practical* reasons (the then limited state of technology for investigating the workings of the brain) or because of an *in principle* irreducibility of meaningful to causal connections. Jaspers is torn in two directions here. On the one hand, he regards understanding and explanation as quite distinct, in that they approach a given phenomena from 'different sides'; on the other hand, he suggests it is only due to practical limitations that the two sides do not meet up, suggesting that what we label as a 'meaningful' connection is ultimately only a causal connection that we are not yet in a position to give a full account of. (Remember Jaspers' vivid analogy of two explorers approaching each other from opposite sides of a continent but never meeting because they were separated by impenetrable territory.)

A related tension concerned the question of how, in a particular case, we are to decide whether a phenomenon is more appropriately understood or causally explained. On the one hand we see Jaspers following the Rickert–Weber line that understanding and explanation are different types of perspective on one and the same reality, suggesting that any particular phenomenon can be both understood meaningfully and explained causally, depending on the perspective used. On the other hand, Jaspers argues that there are clear 'limits' to understanding, that is, there are cases where understanding is not possible and where a causal explanation must be used instead.

This idea of there being limits to understanding may be an echo of a more Dilthean approach: understanding is possible for one type of phenomena, explanation is possible for another. As a result, Jaspers tends to oversimplify the issue of when understanding or explanation is more appropriate: on the Rickert–Weber approach, there are no clear and distinct 'limits' to understanding. There are cases where a causal explanation is clearly appropriate (e.g. thunder) and cases where understanding is more appropriate (a patient's written expressions), but there are going to be many cases where the question of which perspective is appropriate will be inescapably a matter of open debate.

Fourth tension: values in or values out

We saw that one reason for the third tension in Jaspers' thinking is his neglect of the normative dimension to understanding that underpins the Rickert–Weber approach. That is, by regarding understanding as separable from any form of 'value judgement', Jaspers did not fully appreciate the normative dimension of what it means to regard an object or event as 'meaningful', a dimension that cannot in principle be captured in a causal analysis.

The conclusions for psychiatry

It is an indication of the importance of Jaspers' work on the conceptual foundations of psychopathology that many of the issues and tensions we have considered in the last two chapters reflect philosophical questions that are very much with us today. In the remainder of the book we will be looking in detail at questions such as the status of psychiatry as a science, the nature of causal explanation, the difference between a reason and a cause, the limitations of natural scientific perspectives on the mind, the reducibility or otherwise of mental phenomena to physical phenomena, and the importance in this respect of the relevance or otherwise of value judgements in the human sciences.

The role of value judgements was central to our exploration of concepts of disorder in Part I; and as noted above (at the end of the last session), we return to it again in Part IV in relation to psychiatric classification and diagnosis (Chapter 21). Among other themes in this part, then, our analysis of Jaspers' psychopathology—encompassing meanings as well as causes, understanding as well as explanation—has shown once more the need for psychiatry to take seriously the possible role of values in its psychopathological and diagnostic concepts. From the perspective of the traditional medical model, considered in detail in Part I, an acknowledgement of values is taken to be tantamount to a betrayal of medical science! Yet the work of both Rickert and Weber was driven (in part) by the idea that the human sciences, in necessarily making reference to the value-laden and normative dimensions of human life, are no less scientific for that. A 'human science', therefore, which is modelled exclusively on the aims and methods of a natural science, is at risk of being cut off from the very phenomena with which it is properly concerned: the meaningful experiences of real people.

Jaspers' insistence on the importance of meanings as well as causes in psychopathology thus re-engages psychiatry, as a uniquely human as well as natural science, with the experiences of real people. In this, as we have seen, although taking the method of empathy from Dilthey, Jaspers owes much to the philosophy of Weber. Yet in neglecting the basis of Weber's approach in Rickert's value-philosophy, Jaspers may have delayed the development of a more complete understanding of psychopathology in its meaningful as well as causal aspects.

Reflection on the session and self-test questions

Write down your own reflections on the materials in this session drawing out any points that are particularly significant for you. Then write brief notes about the following:

1. What are the four key tensions outlined in this session?

Reading guide

The *Methodenstreit*

Works on key figures in the *Methodenstreit* who influenced Jaspers include:

Dilthey

◆ See Hodges (1952) *The Philosophy of Wilhelm Dilthey*, and Makkreel's (1975) *Dilthey: philosopher of the human studies*.

Weber

◆ See Käsler's (1988) *Max Weber: an introduction to his life and work*, trans. by Philippa Hurd.

Rickert and Weber

◆ See Kuninski's (1979) 'The methodological status of the cultural sciences according to Heinrich Rickert and Max Weber' (trans. by T. Kadenacy), and Oakes' (1988) *Weber and Rickert: concept formation in the cultural sciences*.

Weber and Husserl

◆ See Muse's (1991) 'Edmund Husserl's impact on Max Weber', in *Max Weber: critical assessments*, vol. 2, edited by Peter Hamilton, pp. 254–263.

On the relationship between Jaspers and, respectively, Dilthey and Weber, see: Rickman's (1987) 'The philosophical basis of psychiatry: Jaspers and Dilthey', and Wiggins and Schwartz's (1994) 'The limits of psychiatric knowledge and the problem of classification', from *Philosophical Perspectives on Psychiatric Diagnostic Classification*, (ed. J.Z. Sadler, O.P. Wiggins, and M.A. Schwartz).

Neo-Kantianism

An excellent introduction (in English) to German philosophy of the period is Schnädelbach's (1984) *Philosophy in Germany 1831–1933* (trans. by Eric Matthews).

On neo-Kantianism generally, see Köhnke's (1991) *The Rise of Neo-Kantianism* (trans. by R.J. Hollingdale), and Malter's

(1981) 'Main currents in the German interpretation of the *Critique of Pure Reason* since the beginnings of Neo-Kantianism'.

The connection between Dilthey and Neo-Kantianism is explored in Makkreel's (1969) 'Wilhelm Dilthey and the neo-Kantians: the distinction of the *Geisteswissenschaften* and the *Kulturwissenschaften*'.

The modern *Methodenstreit*

Meares (2003) charts the shift from experiential to mechanistic models of human behaviour in the early years of the twentieth century. Yet concern about the relationship between causal explanations and meaningful understanding continue at a low level even within the British empirical tradition in psychiatry throughout the twentieth century (see, e.g., Hill, 1968; Bebbington, 1997). In philosophy, the debate about the difference between natural sciences and human sciences erupted again in the middle years of the twentieth century. The American philosopher of science Carl G. Hempel, to whose work we return in detail in Part III, argued in the 1940s that there is no difference between the formal structures of the explanations aimed at in the natural and human sciences, a view that was strongly opposed by another philosopher, William Dray. Key publications in the debate between them include:

◆ William Dray's (1957) *Laws and Explanation in History* and (1964) *Philosophy of History*.

◆ Carl Hempel's 'Explanation in science and in history' (1962), in *Explanation* (ed. by David-Hillel Ruben, 1993), and 'The function of general laws in history' (1942), in Hempel's (1965) *Aspects of Scientific Explanation and Other Essays in the Philosophy of Science*.

A good overview of the modern debate is von Wright's (1971) *Explanation and Understanding*.

Musalek (2003) shows the importance of content as well as form in empirical and clinical research in delusion. A balanced overview of the current position in psychiatry is given by Schwartz and Wiggins (2004). Heinimaa (2003) explores the limits of comprehensibility.

Recent 'classics' on the nature of the human sciences are: Alan Ryan's (1970) *The Philosophy of the Social Sciences*, Peter Winch's (1990) *The Idea of a Social Science and its Relation to Philosophy* (first published 1958), and Charles Taylor's (1985) *Philosophical Papers*: Vol. 2, *Philosophy and the Human Sciences*.

The modern *Methodenstreit* and psychopathology

We return in later chapters to recent works in philosophy, on causes and meanings in Part III and on reasons and causes in Part V. For the moment, note,

◆ the work by the philosopher-psychologist, Derek Bolton, and the psychiatrist, Jonathan Hill, on the possible reconciliation of meanings and causes in the information-carrying power of mental states (their-concept of 'intentional causation') and the explanatory potential of this approach for neuroscience-led developments in psychopathology. See Bolton and Hill (1997) Commentary on 'Reasons and causes', and also in *Philosophy, Psychiatry, & Psychology*, Bolton's (1997a) 'Encoding of meaning: deconstructing the meaning/causality distinction', with a commentary from an analytic perspective by Segal (1997), and a response by Bolton (1997b), and a commentary from a Continental perspective by Wiggins and Schwartz (1997), with a separate response by Bolton (1997c). Tim Thornton (1997) reviewed Bolton and Hill's work in *Philosophy, Psychiatry, & Psychology* in an extended article critiquing their concept of 'intentional causation', on 'Reasons and causes in philosophy and psychopathology', with a response by Bolton and Hill (1997). Bolton (2000) provided a further more detailed commentary on the issues.

◆ A special issue of *Philosophy, Psychiatry, & Psychology* edited by the Warwick philosopher, Christoph Hoerl (2001), on schizophrenia. This includes work from both Analytic (e.g. Cambell, 2001; Eilan, 2001) and Continental (e.g. Parnas and Sass, 2001) traditions, on the links between explanation, understanding and the disturbance of inter-subjectivity in schizophrenia. (See also Part V.)

◆ The importance of cultural factors in an increasingly globalized society, as explored by the American philosopher, Nancy Potter (2003a) in her *Moral Tourists and World Travelers*, with commentaries by Cassell (2003), Jaeger (2003), Spitz (2003), and with a response by Potter (2003b).

Jaspers' paper on 'Causal and "meaningful" connections' is revisited in the light of modern developments in neuroscience in Grant Gillet's (1990) 'Neuroscience and meaning in psychiatry'.

References

Bebbington, P.E. (1997). Psychiatry: science, meaning and purpose. *British Journal of Psychiatry*, 130: 222–228.

Blackburn, I.M. (1997). Commentary on 'The stoic conception of mental disorder'. *Philosophy, Psychiatry, & Psychology*, 4(4): 293–294.

Bolton, D. (1997a). Encoding of meaning: deconstructing the meaning/causality distinction. *Philosophy, Psychiatry, & Psychology*, 4(4): 255–268.

Bolton, D. (1997b). Response to the Commentary. *Philosophy, Psychiatry, & Psychology*, 4(4): 273–276.

Bolton, D. (1997c). Response to the Commentary. *Philosophy, Psychiatry, & Psychology*, 4(4): 283–284.

Bolton, D. (2000). Continuing commentary alternatives to disorder. *Philosophy, Psychiatry, & Psychology*, 7(2): 141–154.

Bolton, D. and Hill, J. (1997). Commentary on 'Reasons and causes'. *Philosophy, Psychiatry, & Psychology*, 4(4): 319–322.

Cambell, J. (2001). Rationality, meaning, and the analysis of delusion. *Philosophy, Psychiatry, & Psychology*, 8/2/3: 89–100.

Dilthey, W. (1976). *Selected Writings* (ed. and trans. H.P. Rickman). Cambridge: Cambridge University Press.

Dilthey, W. (1977). Ideas concerning a descriptive and analytic psychology. In *Descriptive Psychology and Historical Understanding* (trans. R.M. Zaner and K.L. Heiges). The Hague: Martinus Nijhoff, pp. 21–120.

Dray, W. (1957). *Laws and Explanation in History* Oxford: Oxford University Press.

Dray, W. (1964). *Philosophy of History*. Englewood Cliffs, N.J.: Prentice Hall.

Eilan, N. (2001). Commentary on 'Meaning, truth, and the self': A Commentary on Campbell, and Parnas and Sass. *Philosophy, Psychiatry, & Psychology*, 8/2/3: 121–132.

Gillet, G.R. (1990). Neuroscience and meaning in psychiatry, *Journal of Medicine and Philosophy*, 15: 21–39.

Gillett, C. and Loewer, B. (2001). *Physicalism and Its Discontents*. Cambridge: Cambridge University Press.

Heinimaa, M. (2003). Incomprehensibility. In *Nature and Narrative: an introduction to the new philosophy of psychiatry* (ed. K.W.M. Fulford, K.J. Morris, J.Z.S. Sadler, and G. Stanghellini). Oxford: Oxford University Press, Chapter 14.

Hempel, C.G. ([1962] 1993). Explanation in science and in history. In *Explanation* (ed. R. David-Hillel). Oxford: Oxford University Press.

Hempel, C.G. *Aspects of Scientific Explanation*. London: Free Press.

Hill, D. (1968). Depression: disease, reaction or posture? *Am. J. Psychiatry*, 125: 445–457.

Hodges, H.A. (1952). *The Philosophy of Wilhelm Dilthey*. London: Routledge and Kegan Paul.

Hoerl, C. (2001). Introduction: understanding, explaining, and intersubjectivity in schizophrenia. *Philosophy, Psychiatry, & Psychology*, 8/2/3: 83–88.

Jaspers, K. ([1913] 1974). Causal and 'meaningful' connections between life history and psychosis [Kausale und verständliche Zusammenhänge zwischen Schicksal und Psychose bei der Dementia praecox] (trans. J. Hoenig). In *Themes and Variations in European Psychiatry* (ed. S.R. Hirsch and M. Shepherd). Bristol: Wright.

Jaspers, K. (1997). *General Psychopathology* (trans. J. Hoenig and Marian W. Hamilton, 2 vols). Baltimore, MD: Johns Hopkins University Press.

Käsler, D. (1988). *Max Weber: an introduction to his life and work* (trans. by Philippa Hurd). Cambridge: Polity Press.

Köhnke, K.C. (1991). *The Rise of Neo-Kantianism* (trans. by R.J.Hollingdale). Cambridge: Cambridge University Press.

Kuninski, M. (1979). The methodological status of the cultural sciences according to Heinrich Rickert and Max Weber (trans. by T. Kadenacy). *Reports on Philosophy*, 3: 71–85.

Leavy, S.A. (1997). Commentary on 'The stoic conception of mental disorder'. *Philosophy, Psychiatry, & Psychology*, 4(4): 295–296.

Makkreel, R.A. (1969). Wilhelm Dilthey and the neo-Kantians: the distinction of the *Geisteswissenschaften* and the *Kulturwissenschaften*. *Journal of the History of Philosophy*, 7: 423–440.

Makkreel, R.A. (1975). *Dilthey: philosopher of the human studies*. Princeton: Princeton University Press.

Malter, R. (1981). Main currents in the German interpretation of the *Critique of Pure Reason* since the beginnings of neo-Kantianism. *Journal of the History of Ideas*, 42: 531–551.

Meares, R. (2003). Towards a psyche for psychiatry. In *Nature and Narrative: an introduction to the new philosophy of psychiatry* (ed. K.W.M. Fulford, K.J. Morris, J.Z.S. Sadler, and G. Stanghellini). Oxford: Oxford University Press, Chapter 2.

Mill, J.S. (1974). *Collected Works of John Stuart Mill*, Vol. VIII: *A System of Logic, Ratiocinative and Inductive* (ed. J.M. Robson). London: Routledge and Kegan Paul, Books IV–VI and Appendices.

Mordini, E. (1997). Commentary on 'The stoic conception of mental disorder'. *Philosophy, Psychiatry, & Psychology*, 4(4): 297–302.

Musalek, M. (2003). Meanings and causes of delusions. In *Nature and Narrative: an introduction to the new philosophy of psychiatry* (ed. K.W.M. Fulford, K.J. Morris, J.Z.S. Sadler, and G. Stanghellini). Oxford: Oxford University Press, Chapter 10.

Muse, K.R. (1991). Edmund Husserls impact on Max Weber. In *Max Weber: critical assessments*, Vol. 2 (ed. P. Hamilton). London: Routledge, pp. 254–263.

Nietzsche, F.W. (1996) *On the Genealogy of Morals*. Oxford: Oxford University Press.

Nordenfelt, L. (1997). Response to the Commentaries. *Philosophy, Psychiatry, & Psychology*, 4(4): 305–306.

Nordenfelt, L. (1997). The stoic conception of mental disorder: the case of Cicero. *Philosophy, Psychiatry, & Psychology*, 4(4): 285–292.

Oakes, G. (1988). *Weber and Rickert: concept formation in the cultural sciences*. Cambridge, MA: MIT Press.

Parnas, J. and Sass, L.A. (2001). Self, solipsism, and schizophrenic delusions. *Philosophy, Psychiatry, & Psychology*, 8/2/3: 101–120.

Potter, N.N. (2003a). Moral tourists and world travelers: some epistemological issues in understanding patients worlds. *Philosophy, Psychiatry, & Psychology*, 10(3): 209–224. Commentaries by Cassell (2003), Jaeger (2003), Spitz (2003), and with a response by Potter (2003b).

Quine, W.V.O. (1960). *Word and Object*. Cambridge: The MIT Press.

Rhodes, R. (1997). Commentary on 'The stoic conception of mental disorder'. *Philosophy, Psychiatry, & Psychology*, 4(4): 303–304.

Rickert, H. (1962). *Science and History: a critique of positivist epistemology* (trans. G. Reisman). New Jersey: D. Van Nostrand.

Rickert, H. ([1902] 1986). *The Limits of Concept Formation in the Natural Sciences: a logical introduction to the historical sciences* (trans. Guy Oakes). Cambridge: Cambridge University Press.

Rickman, H.P. (1987). The philosophical basis of psychiatry: Jaspers and Dilthey. In *Philosophy of the Social Sciences*, 17: 173–196.

Ryan, A. (1970). *The Philosophy of the Social Sciences*. London: MacMillan Press.

Schnädelbach, H. (1984). *Philosophy in Germany 1831–1933* (trans. by Eric Matthews). Cambridge: Cambridge University Press.

Schwartz, M.A. and Wiggins, O.P. (2004). Phenomenological and hermeneutic models: understanding and interpretation in psychiatry. In *The Philosophy of Psychiatry: a companion* (ed. J. Radden). New York: Oxford University Press, pp. 351–363.

Searle, J. (1969). *Speech Acts: an essay in the philosophy of language*. Cambridge: Cambridge University Press.

Segal, G.M.A. (1997). Commentary on 'Encoding of meaning'. *Philosophy, Psychiatry, & Psychology*, 4(4): 269–272.

Taylor, C. (1985). *Philosophical Papers*, Vol. 2, *Philosophy and the Human Sciences*. Cambridge: Cambridge University Press.

Thornton, T. (1997). Reasons and causes in philosophy and psychopathology. *Philosophy, Psychiatry, & Psychology*, 4(4): 307–318.

von Wright, G.H. (1971). *Explanation and Understanding*. London: Routledge and Kegan Paul.

Weber, M. ([1904] 1949). 'Objectivity' in social science and social policy. In *The Methodology of the Social Sciences* (ed. and trans. E.A. Shils and H.A. Finch). New York: The Free Press, pp. 50–112.

Weber, M. ([1917] 1949). The meaning of 'ethical neutrality' in sociology and economics. In *The Methodology of the Social Sciences* (ed. and trans. E.A. Shils and H.A. Finch). New York: The Free Press, pp. 1–49.

Weber, M. (1975). *Roscher and Knies: the logical problems of historical economics* (trans. G. Oakes). New York: The Free Press.

Weber, M. (1989). The concept of 'following a rule'. In *Max Weber: selections in translation* (ed. W.G. Runciman) (trans. E. Matthews). Cambridge: Cambridge University Press, pp. 99–110.

Wiggins, O.P. and Schwartz, M.A. (1994). The limits of psychiatric knowledge and the problem of classification. In *Philosophical Perspectives on Psychiatric Diagnostic Classification* (ed. J.Z. Sadler, O.P. Wiggins, and M.A. Schwartz). Johns Hopkins University Press, pp. 89–103.

Wiggins, O.P. and Schwartz, M.A. (1997). Commentary on 'Encoding of meaning'. *Philosophy, Psychiatry, & Psychology*, 4(4): 277–282.

Winch, P. ([1958] 1990). *The Idea of a Social Science and its Relation to Philosophy*. London: Routledge.

PART III

Philosophy of science and mental health

Part contents

Introduction to Part III

A key theme of this book is that a proper account of mental health practice, and indeed of health-care practice as a whole, requires what we called at the end of Part I, a full-field model. This is a model that focuses as much on the nature of the subjects involved in clinical interventions as on the objective facts that, in a traditional medical-scientific model of psychiatry, underpin and define professional expertise.

A full-field psychiatry

Some of the elements of this full-field model have been introduced in earlier parts of the book. Thus, in Part I, we introduced values alongside the facts of the traditional medical model, patients' experiences of illness alongside the traditional medical knowledge of disease, and an analysis of patients' experiences of illness in terms of action-failure (of a particular kind) alongside the traditional analysis of disease in terms of failure of function. In Part II, similarly, in our exploration of the philosophical origins of Jaspers' psychopathology in phenomenology and the *Methodenstreit*, we added meanings to the traditional causes, and understanding to the traditional causal explanations of disorder.

The importance of these elements in a full-field model, a model including subjects as well as objects, is evident enough: it is subjects who make and are sensitive to value judgements; it is subjects who experience and who understand, whose actions may fail, and for whom meanings are significant. Correspondingly, therefore, some of these elements of a full-field model will be examined further in later Parts of the book, notably values in Part IV (particularly in relation to diagnosis) and understanding in Part V (particularly in relation to its contribution to contemporary philosophy of mind).

A full-field science?

When it comes to science, however, as the focus of this part, it might be assumed that the subject, the experiencing subject, the subject who values and for whom individual meanings are significant, will drop out of the picture. In medicine, it might similarly be thought, it is not unreasonable that subjects should appear alongside and on an equal basis with the objects of scientific enquiry. After all, however 'scientific' medicine has become, it is always, at base, concerned with people. And one proper role of philosophy may be to help medicine, dominated as it is by objective science, to restore people, and the subjective perspectives of people as unique individuals, to their proper place at the focus of the clinical encounter. However, when it comes to science as such, disembodied from its applications in clinical medicine, then, it might be assumed, subjects will, as we said, drop out of the picture—it being after all in the nature of objective science, traditionally understood, that it places no particular requirements on, and is independent of, the subjects by whom it is developed and applied.

This assumption, however, of a subject-free objective science, is as we will see in this part, mistaken. To the contrary, a key theme of this part will be that subject- as well as object-related elements are central to the nature of science in general and are not limited to medical science in particular.

Epistemic values and the subject in sciences

One way to draw out the importance of the subject is to focus on the role of values in science. We touch on epistemic values, for example, the values (such as simplicity, elegance, etc.) that guide the development of scientific theory, at various points in this part. Epistemic values, like many other topics that we cover in this book, are contentious; and they are often discussed in the context of another contentious claim, namely that explanatory scientific theories are underdetermined by data. 'The underdetermination thesis', as it is often called, is the claim that any given body of data is in principle consistent with a large (possibly indefinitely large) number of explanatory theories (see Chapters 12 and 13). If, then, scientific theories are in this sense underdetermined by observational data, the choices we make between theories have to be constrained by something else—and epistemic values may play that part.

There is direct evidence that epistemic values are important in the development of scientific theory at least in psychiatry (see e.g. Sadler, 1996). Besides epistemic values, values of other kinds will be shown in this part to have a place in science: for example, in the 'context of interest' within which, as we will see in Chapter 14, scientific explanations are valid; and, in Chapter 16, where values, individual and social, will turn out to have a role to play in determining the research programmes that are taken up and the criteria by which progress in these programmes is judged to have been made. If, therefore, science itself turns on values of various kinds, it follows that the nature of the subject who has, and is sensitive to, the requisite values will play an important part.

From left- to right-field

A focus on the roles of values in science would thus have dovetailed neatly with the emphasis on values and subject-related, or, as we put it in Part I, 'left-field' concepts, elsewhere in the book. In this part, however, we will not be focusing on values as such. Rather, we will be switching attention from left- to right-field, as it were, and focusing on the importance of the experiencing subject even in 'hard' sciences such as engineering and physics. We show how the traditional model of science—making progress by inductive generalizations from perspective-free data—has had to be modified as philosophy, history, and other disciplines have given us a deeper understanding of the roles of subjects in how science really works in practice.

This deeper understanding, it is important to emphasize, is important in all areas of science, not just in psychiatry. However, some of its features—notably the central roles that it gives to the experiencing subject—provide a bridge between sciences of the mind, like psychiatry, and the (traditionally conceived) paradigms of natural science, like physics. Thus, for example, as we will see in

Chapter 14, it turns out that the 'hard' sciences, such as physics and engineering, rely, and rely *centrally*, on tacit (or implicit) as well as explicit knowledge. It should thus be no surprise—and certainly no criticism—to find that tacit knowledge is important in psychiatry too.

The storyline of Part III

The topics in the philosophy of science covered in this part broadly track the stages of the clinical process as outlined in Part I (Chapter 2). As we will see, at each of these stages, insights from the philosophy of science, in complicating the traditional model implicit in most psychiatric textbooks, provide a deeper understanding of the relationship between science and the experiencing subject in the clinical encounter.

Thus, *Chapter 11* outlines the traditional model of science in terms of four key stages: (1) data collection; (2) theory building, subdivided into 2A (defining patterns), and 2B (identifying causes); (3) theory testing; and (4) advancement of knowledge. Subsequent chapters then explore particular topics from the philosophy of science that deepen our understanding of each of these stages particularly as they are relevant to the clinical encounter: *Chapter 12* examines psychopathology and the theory dependence (the conceptual prestructuring) of observation (Stage 1); *Chapter 13* considers the relationship between reliability and validity in natural classifications (Stage 2A); *Chapter 14* looks at diagnosis as a form of explanatory scientific process in which tacit as well as explicit knowledge is crucial (Stage 2B); *Chapter 15* considers causal theories of disease, or aetiology, and the relationships between causes of and reasons for actions (Stage 2B again); and *Chapter 16* explores the concept of evidence-based medicine and the role of judgement in testing a knowledge claim in science (Stages 3 and 4). Finally, in a brief *Conclusions* we draw together the key themes of the part around the role of the experiencing subject and of individual judgement in the way that science really works.

Chapter outline of Part III

Given the number and complexity of the ideas introduced in this part, you may find it helpful to get an initial overview of the topics included in each chapter and of how these are related to the clinical encounter. The philosophical topics on which we focus in this part are drawn from among those for which there is already an established pay-off, at least in principle, for research and clinical practice. The topics chosen are far from exhaustive, however. We have little to say about probability, for example. Probability is an important topic, both in clinical work (in risk assessment, for example) and in research (being the basis of statistical 'tests' of significance). It is a topic, moreover, that is supported by a significant philosophical literature (see, for example, Hacking's (1990) *The Taming of Chance*). In this instance, however, the philosophical literature, other than

in relation to physics, has as yet had little impact on scientific research and practice, or indeed vice versa.

Chapter 11—Psychoanalysis: an introduction to the philosophy of science

We begin this part with a chapter that looks at the most cited psychiatrist of all time, Freud. First, we outline an intuitive and traditional model of scientific practice. Then, following the Austinian approach of 'philosophical fieldwork' outlined in Part I, we look in detail at a series of short extracts from Freud's work (the Project, and the case history of Dora). This approach shows that while Freud wrestled with the scientific status of his work he was hampered, at least in part, by attempting to fit his theories to the traditional model of science. That model, however, has subsequently been much modified by work in the philosophy of science. We highlight how some of the modifications in question are prefigured in Freud's own work. The final session of the chapter looks at alternatives to the scientific understanding of psychoanalysis, such as Ricoeur's hermeneutic reconstruction.

Chapter 12—Psychopathology and the theory dependence of data

The first stage of the psychiatric clinical process, and the basis of psychopathology, is observation. Observation plays a key role in underpinning the objectivity of science. On an intuitive view, which was formalized in the early part of the twentieth century by the Logical Empiricists, this role is ensured by a rigid distinction between theory and observation. The two-language model of Logical Empiricism, as it is called, is reflected in the development within psychiatry of structured and semi-structured interviews of known reliability (i.e. of known levels of agreement in observation) for the assessment of mental states.

Nevertheless, as we will see, more recent work in philosophy has undermined the Logical Empiricist's sharp distinction between observation and theory. Observation reports, it turns out, cannot be given in theory-free terms. The process or experience of observation, that is to say, is conceptually prestructured. Observation is always set within a framework of concepts and is thus, in this specific sense, necessarily theory-laden. The conceptual prestructuring of observation suggests that psychiatry, like any science, does not work (as the traditional model supposes) by relying on a neutral foundation of 'raw' data. What this in turn suggests, as we will see, is that while observations do indeed play a role in disciplining theory, the relationship between observation and theory is iterative rather than (as the traditional model supposes) linear.

Chapter 13—Natural classifications, realism, and psychiatric science

Perhaps the most pressing current issue in the philosophy of science as applied to psychiatry is the *validity* of psychiatric classification. This chapter examines the nature of validity primarily by way of an exploration of realism in the sciences, especially the physical sciences. The chapter looks at: (1) the influence of

Logical Empiricism on post-Second World War psychiatric classification through the work of the philosopher, Carl Hempel; (2) the connection between values and validity, arguing that despite the assumptions of the traditional model, the presence of values does not necessarily undermine the objectivity (hence validity) of psychiatric classification; (3) recent debates in the philosophy of physics about the reality of unobservables; and (4) the relevance of the debates about realism, particularly in physics, for the development of more scientifically valid classifications of mental disorder in psychiatry.

Chapter 14—Diagnosis, explanation, and tacit knowledge

A key stage in the clinical process is diagnosis. Diagnoses in medicine can be understood as being explanatory scientific theories that connect initial clinical observations and the results of laboratory test results to subsequent treatment and management. This chapter examines whether a fully explicit formal model of diagnosis, so understood, can be given or whether, by contrast, diagnosis always contains a tacit dimension. The first half of the chapter explores philosophical models of scientific explanation. The second half of the chapter develops the idea that there is a tacit dimension to diagnosis by looking to the role of tacit knowledge in the hard sciences. There is descriptive evidence that even engineering expertise depends on craft skills and other aspects of tacit rather than explicit knowledge. Consideration of Wittgenstein's later work suggests that there are also good theoretical grounds for believing that all forms of 'knowledge that' (explicit knowledge) depend on 'knowing how' (tacit knowledge).

Chapter 15—Causes, laws, and reasons in psychiatric aetiology

This chapter returns by way of the philosophy of science to a topic that we explored in Part II, namely the putative distinction between two kinds of knowledge important to psychiatry: understanding and explanation, or the space of reasons and the realm of scientific laws. If scientific laws are important in psychiatry, we saw in Part II, so too are reasons. But what exactly is the connection between them?

In the first half of the chapter we examine just what it means to say that, for example, a symptom is *caused* by a disease. We look back to the eighteenth century British empiricist philosopher, David Hume's, seminal puzzle about the origins of the very idea of causation and outline modern accounts that connect causation in one way or another, to natural laws. In the second half of the chapter, we examine philosophical work on the space of reasons: the special intelligibility that meaningful states and events have. Finally, in a concluding session, we examine two recent attempts in psychiatry to bring reasons and causes together: Bolton and Hill's thesis that reasons are encoded in brain states; and Brown and Harris' methodological innovations in their studies of the social origins of depression.

Chapter 16—Knowledge, research, and evidence-based medicine

The concluding chapter of this part looks at the underpinnings of evidence based medicine (EBM) in philosophical work on theory choice and the nature of progress in science. EBM can be understood as an attempt to formulate the best way to learn from experience and learning from experience involves inductive reasoning (see Chapter 5). Thus, in the first third of the chapter, we consider David Hume's original formulation of the challenge to induction and some of the ways in which recent authors have attempted to respond to his challenge. One of the general conclusions we draw from these responses to Hume is that the relationship between evidence and theory in scientific research is not as straightforward as the traditional model suggests. Evidence is itself just as much provisional as the theories it supports of falsifies. The most historically accurate accounts of scientific progress stress the contextual factors in *judgements* about what is supported and what is refuted by the evidence.

The middle third of the chapter examines models of knowledge drawn from philosophical epistemology. While attempting to sidestep Hume's problem of induction these models also suggest the communal, the social and interpersonal, nature of knowledge and its justification. Knowledge can 'rub off' on others. Equally, it depends on inherited assumptions and claims some of which simply have to be taken on trust before other claims can be put to empirical test.

The final third of the chapter examines the 'evidence hierarchy' of EBM. We suggest that it would be entirely within the spirit of EBM to regard the adoption of such a hierarchy as itself involving a scientific claim about the world and thus as being as much subject to test through fallible judgements as any other scientific claim. This brings us back once more to the importance of the subject and of individual judgement (scientific and clinical) in the way that evidence is both gathered and used.

In a brief concluding section we draw together the themes of Part III around the ineliminable roles of the subject and of individual judgement in science. These roles, identified and increasingly clarified by work in the philosophy of science and epistemology, are important in all sciences. They are writ large, though, in difficult sciences, sciences at the cutting edge, sciences, like psychiatry and theoretical physics, in which the problems with which we are concerned are as much conceptual as empirical in nature.

References

Hacking, I. (1990). *The Taming of Chance*. Cambridge: Cambride University Press.

Sadler, J. (1996). Epistemic value commitments in the debate over categorical versus dimensional personality diagnosis. *Philosophy, Psychiatry, & Psychology*, 3/3: 203–222.

CHAPTER 11

Psychoanalysis: an introduction to the philosophy of science

Chapter contents

The norms of mental illness are not 'anatomical and physiological' but 'psychosocial, ethical and legal'

Thomas Szasz, 'The myth of mental illness' (1960, p. 114)

The future of psychiatry, it seems, is biological

Editorial (Anon), 'The crisis in psychiatry',
The Lancet (1997, p. 349)

Science or non-sense? Along with other areas of human activity, medicine has reaped enormous rewards from science. Casting off myth and received authority, its history has been a history of progress—Vesalius, Harvey, Morgagni, Sydenham, Pasteur, Jenner, Currie, Fleming.... the great names ring down the centuries. Signs and symptoms are defined; diseases discovered; new treatments established; causal theories refined; and in this century in particular, all this has culminated in unprecedented improvements for many in life expectancy and freedom from disease.

Psychiatry and medicine: the standard view

Science or non-sense? Psychiatry, as the most medical of the mental health-care disciplines, has shared in this progress. It has been slower to get started, certainly—the brain after all is the most complex part of the body. But the last 50 years have seen it accelerating apparently along much the same path as bodily medicine. The symptoms of mental disorder have been defined; syndromes identified; new treatments established (both psychological and physical, including a range of powerful drugs); and, with recent developments in neuroscience and molecular genetics, the first glimmerings of credible biological theories of causation have appeared.

Yet the scientific status of psychiatry remains deeply controversial. Antipsychiatry, with Thomas Szasz, as in the first of the two quotes above (1960), considered it literally non-sense. This is too extreme a view, as we saw in Part I, but it is the coded message behind much of psychiatry's more 'popular' press, from lawyers, sociologists, patient groups, the media, and, even, its medical peers. Doctors themselves often treat psychiatry as the rump end of medical science—the *Lancet* editorial, in the second quote above (1997), went on to castigate psychiatry for pursuing the very biological paradigm on which the success of medicine itself has been built, arguing the need for a fusion of what the Editorial calls "narrow" neuroscientific and sociocultural approaches.

Psychiatry and medicine: changing the standard view

So is psychiatry science or non-sense? To answer this question, we will need to dig deep into the nature of science itself. This is what the philosophy of science is about. It shows that everything we normally take for granted about science—data, experiment, induction, etc.—is in fact rather more problematic than is generally recognized.

In the past this has not mattered practically. True, the insights of the philosophy of science apply to science as a whole. Indeed as we will see, important philosophical work, with clear implications for medicine, has been done in relation to such down-to-earth subjects as engineering. But the objects of scientific enquiry, in subjects such as these, have in the past generally been sufficiently simple to yield to a (methodologically) simple science. This is no longer the case. In a number of areas, from quantum physics through computing to neuroscience, we are finding ourselves in need of sharper and more sophisticated tools of enquiry. And the message of this and subsequent chapters in this part is that psychiatry is just such an area. It is not the rump end of medical science but at the cutting edge, and in need of cutting edge tools.

Psychoanalysis as a model

In later sessions of this introductory chapter we will explore this idea by looking at a long-running debate about the scientific status not of psychiatry but of psychoanalysis.

As an introduction to the subject, psychoanalysis offers a number of advantages. First, whereas (until recently) the scientific status of psychiatry has been attacked mainly by non-philosophers, there is a considerable philosophical literature on the nature of psychoanalysis. Second, this literature, although extending to other areas of philosophy as well, ranges over all the main issues traditionally covered by the philosophy of science. The scientific status of psychoanalysis, indeed, has been attacked at every point: its observations, it has been said, are not 'objective', its data are doubtful, its laws illusory, and its hypotheses are untestable scientifically. Third, each of these issues, although writ large in the debate over psychoanalysis, are also issues for the scientific status of psychiatry and mental health practice as a whole.

The debate about the status of psychoanalysis will thus serve as a highly relevant introduction to many of the issues in modern philosophy of science, while at the same time illustrating the need for a deeper understanding of the nature of science itself, of its strengths and indeed its limitations, for clinical work and research in psychiatry. Critical discussion of psychoanalysis also provides a motivation for different, explicitly non-scientific approaches, a sample of which we will outline briefly in the last session of this chapter.

The structure this chapter

Before tackling the issue of the scientific status of psychoanalysis directly, however, we will start this chapter with a session outlining the components of science, what it is to be 'scientific', and how psychiatry has identified with the scientific world view. Thus,

◆ *Session 1* examines our everyday 'pre-philosophical' assumptions about the nature of scientific disciplines. From this we derive a four-stage model of how science has traditionally been understood.

◆ *Session 2* looks at current assumptions about the scientific status of psychiatry, as exemplified in psychiatry textbooks and the American Psychiatric Association's classification of mental disorders, DSM (see Chapter 3), in the light of the traditional model set out in Session 1.

◆ *Sessions 3 and 4* examine Freud's case history of 'Dora' according to the four stages of the traditional model of science. The two sessions highlight difficulties that Freud had in reconciling his work with the traditional model. What emerges, though, is that (many of) Freud's difficulties in this respect actually reflect difficulties in the traditional model. Some of these difficulties are outlined in a preliminary way in this session. They form the basis for more detailed treatment in later chapters in this part.

♦ *Session 5* looks at alternatives to construing psychoanalysis as a science. These provide a third option for understanding the nature of psychiatry, i.e. as neither science nor non-sense, but, in one form or another, and at least in part, non-science. This option will not be examined further in this part (it corresponds broadly with Jaspers' twin-track psychopathology, in part II; and we return to a closely related topic, the relationship between causes and reasons, in Chapter 15).

Session 1 Science: What is it and what's the problem?

An Austinian approach to the nature of science

The problems raised by the status of psychiatry as a science are not (merely) philosophical problems but problems arising in everyday practice and research: they range from methodological aspects of research design, through concerns about the empirical status of psychological treatments (notably, though not only, of psychoanalysis), to disputes about the classification of mental disorders, and on to debates about the very validity of mental illness as a proper object of scientific study.

Getting started

This is ideal J.L. Austin country, therefore. The problems with which we will be concerned in this chapter, in explaining the scientific status of psychoanalysis, are problems arising in ordinary (i.e. non-philosophical) usage. Hence, as Austin recommended (Chapter 4), we can get started with these problems by examining ordinary usage. This 'philosophical fieldwork', to use Austin's phrase, will not be the end of the story, but it will be a good way to begin.

The problems raised by the scientific status of psychiatry, moreover, are problems arising, apparently, from the failure of concepts (i.e. in psychoanalysis), which (apparently) work well in other closely related contexts (i.e. as in general medicine). Like J.L. Austin's own work on excuses (Austin, 1956–7), therefore, which we looked at in detail in Part I, it could be that these (in Austin's terms) 'negative concepts' (the difficulties associated with a science of the mental) will prove to be 'wearing the trousers' (providing insights into the nature of science as a whole).

Knowing where we are going

It will be worth looking at this last point in a little more detail before getting started, in order to get a clearer sense of where we are going.

It is natural to think that where concepts are problematic this is because the concepts themselves are in some way muddled or confused. This, indeed, was the guiding assumption behind the whole debate about the concept of mental illness. The concept of mental illness is problematic in use while that of physical illness (by and large) is not. Hence, in the debate about mental illness, it has been almost universally assumed that physical illness is relatively transparent; and that the validity of mental illness turns, ultimately, on the extent to which it can be mapped on to physical illness. In other words, physical illness, because it is relatively unproblematic in use, has been taken to be a template against which the meaning of the relatively problematic (in use) mental illness has to be interpreted and its validity assessed.

Psychiatry second

Now, much the same set of assumptions lies behind the debate about the scientific status of psychiatry. The role, methods, application, outputs even, of science in psychiatry are all problematic. The role, methods, application and outputs of science, by contrast, are not problematic in, say, cardiology, gastroenterology, or indeed any other area of 'physical medicine'. Hence it is assumed that it is the scientific status of psychiatry that has to be justified; that psychiatry is an inferior or primitive science, lagging behind the sciences of cardiology, gastroenterology, and the like. Yet this is not the only possible interpretation of the facts. If psychiatry is more problematic scientifically, this could equally plausibly be because it is a more *difficult* science; cardiology, gastroenterology, and the like only *appearing* to be unproblematic because they are the scientifically simpler disciplines.

On the showing of the study of the concept of mental illness in Part I the latter interpretation seems more likely, i.e. that psychiatry is more problematic scientifically because it is the more complex science.

Psychiatry first

If this is right, this has the further consequences that examining the problems raised by science in psychiatry should lead to a better understanding of the role of science in medicine as a whole. For this was precisely Austin's point about negative concepts. Where concepts work unproblematically we are, as Austin said, blinded as to their meanings by a 'veil of ease and obviousness'. It is only where things go wrong that we can see through the veil. Austin, working on the philosophy of action, studied the (positive) concept of action through the (negative) concept of excuse (excuses all being examples of actions failing or going wrong). In the philosophy of science, similarly, psychiatry provides a whole series of instances where the concepts by which science is defined, and which work unproblematically in areas such as cardiology and gastroenterology, run into difficulty. Hence, where Austin studied action through excuses, this chapter will study science through psychiatry—though we will be learning lessons useful to psychiatry as we go along.

Describing the logical geography of science

The elements of science

On this upbeat note, then, we can get started. In J.L. Austin-style, the first thing is to get a sense of the logical geography. In this case, what this means is defining the conceptual elements of science, and these elements especially as they appear in the self-image of psychiatry as a science.

In the first half of this session we will be defining the logical geography through a series of exercises. Remember that it is important to do each of these for yourself before going on. This is partly because, as we have several times emphasized, learning philosophy is more like gaining a new skill than acquiring a body of knowledge; and we gain new skills primarily by practising them for ourselves rather than observing others.

In the case of science, though, these exercises are also designed to help us make explicit our own preconceptions about the subject. Science is so much part of our everyday culture, not only in health care but in all aspects of our lives, that we need to make explicit all the things we take for granted about it, before we can start to come to a better understanding of its nature.

EXERCISE 1 (20 minutes)

Write down some responses to the following questions:

1. What is science?

2. What characteristics must a discipline have to be a science?

Treat the exercise as a brainstorm, keeping your responses to words or brief phrases. This will help to bring out your own intuitive ideas about science. If you are a practitioner, your responses will reflect the conception of science and scientific practice that you have gained from your experience in mental health and more generally. If you are a philosopher, your responses will be influenced by your philosophical training, but try to focus on whatever experience you have of science as it is generally perceived (and especially in medicine—we will be coming to some examples of this in a moment).

A recent group of practitioners and philosophers produced the following list:

* 'experimentation and measurement'
* 'agreed method → cumulative knowledge'
* 'orderly progress, objectively valid, increasing refinement'
* '*not* mythology or metaphysics; testable means of understanding the natural world'
* 'discovery, certainty, truth'
* 'empirical'
* 'objective, value-free'
* 'accurate'
* 'analytic method'
* 'systematicity/structure'
* 'unity of science'
* 'testability'

Two key observations

If you compare this list with your own list, you will probably find a number of both similarities and differences.

EXERCISE 2 (10 minutes)

Compare your list with the one above, noting any similarities and differences. Then write down any general points that strike you about these lists. This is deliberately an 'open' question and hence one you may find difficult; but try it for yourself and write something down in reply before going on.

Most people come up with the following observations:

1. *The lists are incomplete*. Most people are usually able to produce quite quickly a long list of the elements of science. Notice, however, that such lists are rarely identical. The above list was produced by the collective efforts of about a dozen people, all of them 'into' philosophy, some of them philosophers, the rest with experience in a wide range of different disciplines relevant to mental health (including not only mental health practitioners of various kinds but also a lawyer).

   Even so, there are some obvious omissions. They may have come up with some elements of science that you missed: but you may well have thought of elements that they missed—data, observation, causation, natural laws, induction, reduction, variable, description, fact, classification, prediction, probability, quantification, refutation, and hypothesis, are a few examples!

   The first observation, then, is that although most people think they know what they mean by science, their understanding is incomplete. They think they do because they agree on a wide range of instances of the use of the term (physics, for example, is something that everyone agrees is a science). But when they try to define it, they come up with a long list of elements, which, although not dissimilar, are also far from identical.

   Thus far, therefore, matters stand very much as they did for the concept of bodily illness in Part I. There, too, people assumed (wrongly) that they knew what they meant by bodily illness because the use of the concept is generally unproblematic. The similarity between the two cases is deepened by the second observation.

2. *There is disagreement on elements*. Even granted a composite list, combining the elements of many different 'brainstorms', there will still be disagreement as to the elements by which science is defined. This is simply because for many of the elements there will be disagreement about whether or not they should be on the list at all. That is to say, exactly as in the case of bodily illness, there is disagreement as to which conceptual elements are *essential* to the meaning of the term, and which are not.

In the above list, for instance, there was disagreement among the group who generated it as to whether an 'agreed method' was really a mark of science. Those who said it was, talked of experimental method, controlled trials, and so on; those who said it was not, pointed to the frequency of disputes about 'appropriate' controls, to disagreements about what counted as an experiment, and to whether a plain observation, as in astronomy, was an 'experiment' at all. They further suggested that genuinely agreed methods were more characteristic of authoritarian disciplines such as magic and religion, rather than of science.

Taking these two observations together, then, this exercise reveals that, although science and the sciences are familiar enough, just exactly what a science *is*, what elements a subject must have to *be* a science, is far from self-evident. When pre-philosophically we reflect on this, we arrive at lists that are incomplete. And, besides such sins of omission, there are also sins of commission—other people include elements that we would exclude, and we include elements that they would exclude.

A traditional model of scientific practice

The practice of science

Discussions of scientific method, however, such as that noted above, usually lead to something over which there tends to be more consistency of approach, namely, how we should go about actually *doing* science. This is the subject of the next exercise.

EXERCISE 3   (30 minutes)

In this case, rather than a random brainstorm, try organizing your thoughts around the *practice* of science. Think of how you would (or have) tackled a scientific problem, and/or of the classics from the history of science. Don't be too specific, however. Think of examples in order to extract the general features of the scientific approach.

Do this exercise in two parts,

1. Write down the main stages of how a problem is tackled scientifically and of what you expect to get out of it; and then,

2. try to map on to these stages as many of the elements of science as you can (draw on your own list as well as the elements noted above).

Just what constitutes the practice of science, although less contentious than the defining elements of the subject, is of course not wholly unproblematic. None the less, in the first part of this exercise most people, thinking about concrete examples of how science proceeds, come up with a set of stages along the following lines:

◆ *Stage 1*: data collection

◆ *Stage 2*: theory building, by

● Substage (A) defining patterns, and/or

● Substage (B) identifying underlying causes.

◆ *Stage 3*: theory testing (involves further data, either at Substage A or Substage B),

◆ *Stage 4*: advancement of knowledge (negatively if the theory fails, positively if it succeeds).

In what follows we will take these four stages to exemplify a traditional model of scientific process. We will suggest that informative though it is, it is also oversimplified in important ways.

The periodic table and drug trials

A classic example of science that can be thought of as proceeding in this way is the development of our knowledge of chemistry. Probably the most important milestone in the emergence of modern scientific chemistry was the publication, in 1869, of the first Periodic Table of the Elements by the Russian chemist, Dimitri Mendeleev. This was a brilliant example of theory building by identifying a pattern, our Stage 2A. Mendeleev observed that the elements, ordered according to increasing atomic weights, showed repeating patterns (i.e. cycles or 'periods') of chemical reactivity: for example the most reactive elements in each column are at the top, and the most 'metallic' on the left. He was thus able to set them out in the now familiar Periodic Table with columns representing elements with similar chemical properties.

Mendeleev's Table was not merely descriptive, however. There were gaps in the pattern that allowed him to predict the existence and chemical properties of as yet undiscovered elements. The predicted elements constituted a magnificent example of Stage 3, theory testing; and their subsequent discovery fully vindicated Mendeleev's Table (Stage 4, advancement of knowledge). But Mendeleev was not working in isolation. He could not have

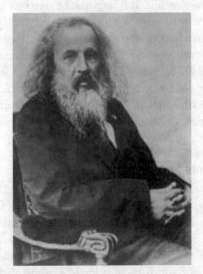

Fig. 11.1 Mendeleev

produced his table in the first place without the knowledge of chemistry accumulated by his predecessors in a more *ad hoc* way (i.e. Stage 1, data collection; though also involving descriptive and causal hypotheses that were to turn out to be mistaken, i.e. prior cycles of Stages 2, 3, and 4). His table, moreover, extraordinarily powerful as it was, contained anomalies that were only resolved when atomic theory, some 40 years later, made it possible to substitute a causal (or Stage 2B) theory for Mendeleev's descriptive (Stage 2A) account.

The key advance here was made by the young British physicist, Henry Moseley, working in Oxford just before the First World War (he was killed at Gallipoli). Moseley showed that the anomalies in Mendeleev's Table disappeared if the elements were ordered by atomic *numbers* rather than atomic *weights*. The atomic number of an element is the number of protons it contains (protons are one of the building blocks of the nucleus of each atom). This determines the number of electrons, which in turn determines its chemical properties. The atomic weight of an element, too, reflects the number of protons; but it also reflects the numbers of other building blocks, in particular, neutrons. The number of neutrons may vary to a small extent *within* elements, producing 'isotopes', i.e. chemically identical elements (because they have the same number and distribution of electrons) but with differing atomic weights (because they have different numbers of building blocks). It was the effects of the latter that explained the anomalies in Mendeleev's original Table, Moseley's work thus taking our knowledge of chemistry another major step forward, and indeed helping to lay the foundations for the subsequent reduction of descriptive chemistry to the highly mathematical quantum-mechanical model of atomic structure upon which modern chemistry as well as physics is built.

We have reviewed this historical story in some detail because it offers a paradigm of science that is more or less explicitly present in much of our thinking about what it is for a subject to be 'genuinely' scientific. It is important to see how similar is the practice of everyday science. The humble 'drug trial', for example, emerges from a background of data collection (Stage 1), through either a descriptive (Stage 2A, e.g. antidepressants), and/or a causal (Stage 2B, e.g. many classes of antibiotics) theory, as a test of the efficacy of a specific compound in a given clinical context (Stage 3). And this adds to our knowledge of therapeutics (Stage 4), either negatively (it doesn't work, or its side-effects are too many) or positively.

The elements and the practice of science

If we can agree broadly about the practice of science, however, the second part of Exercise 3, mapping the elements of science on to the practice of science, generates considerably more disagreement. Much of this reflects the diversity of views about the essential elements of science. But even for elements (such as data and objectivity), for which there is broad agreement that they are essential to science, there is often disagreement about the stage or stages of the traditional picture of the scientific process to which they are most relevant.

Even, therefore, where we can agree broadly about *how* science proceeds in practice, we remain deeply divided over precisely *what* is involved in this. The problem then, is 'not what we do, it's the way that we do it'!

One attempt to map the *elements* of science on to the *practice* of science is given in Table 11.1. See how far your 'mapping' corresponds with ours. Don't spend too long on this at this stage. We will return to it at the end of the chapter, after we have considered some of the arguments about the status of psychoanalysis as a science. As you will see, many of these arguments can be considered broadly within this framework. And in the next session, we are going to look at how the self-image of psychiatry as a science can be understood similarly, in terms of these elements as components of a practice organized along broadly these lines.

Table 11.1 A four-stage model of the practice of science

Stage 1: Data collection (observation)
  measurement, objectivity, accurate, observation, data

Stage 2a: Theory building—defining patterns
  empirical, analytic method, systematicity/structure, induction, description, fact, classification, prediction

Stage 2b: Theory building—identifying causes
  testable means of understanding natural world, discovery, explanation, testability, causation, natural laws, reduction, fact, prediction

Stage 3: Theory testing
  experiment and measurement; agreed method, quantification, refutation, objectively valid, value-free variable, probability; hypothesis

Stage 4: Advancement of knowledge
  cumulative knowledge, orderly progress, increasing refinement, not mythology or metaphysics, certainty, truth; unity of science

Reflection on the session and self-test questions

Write down your own reflections on the materials in this session drawing out any points that are particularly significant for you. Then write brief notes about the following:

1. If the difficulties about the scientific status of psychoanalysis (and hence of psychiatry) are *conceptual* difficulties, does this mean that psychoanalysis (and hence psychiatry) is a *defective* science, compared with, say, cardiology, or that it is a more *difficult* science?

2. When people write down their own ideas about what makes a discipline 'scientific', in what ways do they disagree? And what is the purpose of doing this if we are interested in the conceptual difficulties of psychiatric science.

3. What are the main stages of the scientific method, traditionally understood?

Session 2 Psychiatry as science

With the rise of modern biological psychiatry, many psychiatrists now take it for granted that their discipline has come of age as a science. Dynamic brain imaging methods, molecular genetics, advances in artificial intelligence, and increasingly sophisticated drugs, all seem to place psychiatry where physical medicine has been for some time, not merely among the sciences but at a stage (our Substage 2B) at which causal hypotheses about mental disorders, capable of direct testing, and generating progressive advancement of knowledge, are, at last, within our grasp.

The traditional model of science in a classic psychiatric textbook

Establishing our scientific credentials

This is not a false hope. But, as we will see, the model of science appropriate for psychiatry has to be considerably more sophisticated. It is important, though, to recognize just how recently the battle for scientific psychiatry was being fought, and the veritable labours of Hercules that were required to bring the discipline to its present level of development as a science. The extract below gives a vivid picture of the 'war-time spirit' of scientific psychiatry as recently as the 1960s.

EXERCISE 4   (30 minutes)

Read the extracts from the preface and introduction to:

> Slater, E. and Roth, M. (1969). *Mayer-Gross, Slater and Roth: Clinical Psychiatry* (3rd edn). London: Ballière Tindall and Cassell, pp. xiv–xv and 1–6

Link with Reading 11.1

When this edition was published, psychiatry was swinging from biological to psychological and sociological interests. Slater and Roth were primarily 'biological' psychiatrists and in these extracts they offer a no-nonsense defence of psychiatry-as-science and of (what they take to be equivalent) psychiatry-as-medicine.

As you read the extracts, make brief notes on:

1. Any words or phrases that mark out the authors' view of what it is to be 'scientific'; note how far these correspond with our cumulative list in Table 11.1 (above).

2. The kinds of knowledge they contrast with scientific knowledge.

3. Why they think it is important that psychiatry should be based only on scientific knowledge.

4. Why they think that a defence of scientific psychiatry should be necessary at all (in contrast to other areas of medicine).

Written with both clarity and passion, this is a detailed and sophisticated statement of the 'medical' model of psychiatry by authors whose scientific research has made enduring contributions to our knowledge of the brain basis of mental disorder.

Neither author, moreover, adopted this model unreflectively: Eliot Slater later developed a philosophy of the scientific basis of psychiatry (published in three parts as Slater, 1972, 1973, 1975). Martin Roth replied at length to criticisms of the concept of mental illness (for example, in Roth and Kroll, 1986); and, notwithstanding his perhaps somewhat negative comments about philosophy in this reading, he later became a staunch supporter of the new philosophy of psychiatry (he was the first Honorary President of the Philosophy Group in the Royal College of Psychiatrists). The remarks of Slater and Roth in these extracts thus help to make explicit what many in modern psychiatry take for granted about the scientific status of their subject. This comes through in the answers to each of the four questions in Exercise 4.

Question 1: psychiatry as a science

Starting with Question 1, Slater and Roth make no bones about the status of psychiatry not just as a science but as a *natural* science—the foundations of the subject, they say in the opening sentence of their introduction, 'have to be laid *on the ground of the natural sciences*' (p. 1, their emphasis).

This firm line is then reflected throughout the extracts in the language they use. Taking the two extracts as a whole, a large number of words and phrases in Table 11.1, are to be found somewhere in the text—for example, at the bottom of p. xiv, we find 'facts', 'hypotheses', 'explanatory', 'predictive power', and 'observations', all in a brief synopsis of the scientific method. To these are added, e.g. p. 3, 'causes' and 'effects' (para. 2); 'classification'

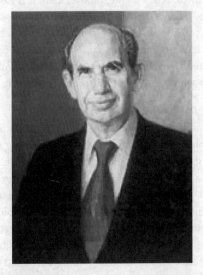

Fig. 11.2 Sir Martin Roth

(p. 4, para. 4); 'testable' and 'refutation' (p. 5, para. 2, with reference to Popper, see below), and 'quantitative relationship' (p. 5, para. 5); finally, on p. 6, we find a summary that broadly follows the four-stage model of the practice of science summarized above, in which 'facts' are gathered, 'precise' hypotheses derived, allowing 'critical' testing; only then will knowledge be advanced rather than 'every year a greater degree of confusion'.

Slater and Roth on the definition of science

On the other hand, when we compare different passages, it is considerably less clear precisely what the 'methods of science' (p. 1) consist in. On p. xiv, for example, science is described as not merely accumulating 'more facts' but as generating 'statements of increasing generality' and 'hypotheses . . . of an increasingly extensive explanatory and predictive power'; yet on p. 5, they endorse the view of the philosopher of science, Karl Popper, that 'the greater the explanatory power of a hypothesis, the less is its scientific usefulness' (they refer here to Popper's criticisms of psychoanalysis to which we will be returning in detail later in this chapter).

Slater and Roth would no doubt reply to this apparent contradiction, that a genuinely scientific explanation, even if all-embracing, is subject to 'critical testing', i.e. to being disproved (p. 6). But different words are used at different points to describe just what a *scientifically* critical test would be: 'new facts' (p. 2, para. 2), 'the impartial collection of careful clinical observations' (p. 2, para. 3), 'experiment' and 'observation' (p. 3, para. 4); 'objective test' and 'foundation of hard fact' (p. 6, para. 1); attributing a 'particular quality' to a sample (p. 6, para. 2); and the availability of 'control studies' (also p. 6, para. 2). Some passages, moreover, are contradictory: at one point the method of science involves 'recognizing similarities in phenomena which may, superficially, differ very greatly . . .', and from these deducing 'general laws' (p. 5, para. 3); but later we find that 'we deal, in fact, in terms of *differences*' (p. 5, para. 4, their emphasis).

Rather as in Exercises 1 and 2 above, then, it is easy enough to generate a long list of terms and phrases broadly associated with 'science', but considerably harder to pin down precisely what 'strict attention to scientific standards' (p. 2) means. This becomes even more obvious if we turn to the next question, concerning the subjects with which Slater and Roth contrast science.

Question 2: psychiatry as non-science

At a number of points in these extracts, Slater and Roth draw a clear contrast between science and what they take to be non-science. Thus, at the start of their introduction they note that their attempt to establish a scientific psychiatry must remain for the present largely promissory, as 'much of our clinical knowledge today belongs more to medical *art* than to science' (p. 1, para. 1, our emphasis). Similarly, further on they imply a sharp distinction between scientific disciplines and the humanities—philosophy and theology (p. 2, para. 2); economics, history, and literature (p. 4, para. 1).

The sciences basic to psychiatry

If psychiatry is a science, though, according to Slater and Roth, it is less clear on precisely which of the sciences they believe the subject should be based.

They start by urging an 'organic connexion between the natural sciences, biology, medicine and psychiatry' (p. 1, para. 1), but then (p. 1, para. 2) psychology (which many would take to be a science at least closely relevant to psychiatry) is identified with philosophy (which is elsewhere treated as one of the humanities). Psychology, indeed, is otherwise peculiarly absent from their account of a scientific psychiatry; and this notwithstanding, as they acknowledge, that (1) the data of psychiatry are psychological (p. 1, para. 4), and indeed, (2) that it is the role of 'psychological phenomena . . . as causes, signs and symptoms, or as curative agents' that mark out psychiatry from the rest of medicine (p. 6, first para. of the section of 'The field of psychiatry'). Cultural anthropology and sociology, on the other hand, which many would take to be closer than psychology to the humanities, are acknowledged to have a place, albeit somewhat grudgingly (p. 2, para. 5, *et. seq.*).

Individuals and scientific psychiatry

The difficulty of saying what is *not* science is clearest in Slater and Roth's treatment of individuals. On p. 3, para. 2, for example, where they endorse the virtues of biological medicine over sociology as the basis of psychiatric science, they argue that 'our knowledge of medicine gives us information about individuals; sociological knowledge gives us information only about groups, from which deductions about the individual are notoriously subject to error'. Yet on p. 4, para. 2, where they hold up physics as the paradigm of science, they say that 'An *excessive preoccupation with individuals* is heuristically sterile' (their emphasis). And they continue (para. 3) that in experimental biology, 'individual variation . . . will be classifiable, statistically, as "error" '.

We will return to the importance of the particular difficulty Slater and Roth have with individuals later in this session. It is a large topic, connecting indeed with the whole of the long-running debate about the relationship between the natural and the human sciences. For now, though, their difficulty with individuals underlines the point that it is easier to identify examples of sciences, and even of the elements of science, than to define precisely what it is to *be* scientific. Contrary to their conclusion, the requirements of 'a scientific approach' are far from 'simple' (p. 6, para. 2).

Question 3: Why should psychiatry be scientific?

Question 3 of this exercise was concerned with the importance of science in psychiatry. In a word, why bother?

Slater and Roth give a number of answers. The first is that a scientific foundation for psychiatry can help to protect the subject from the harmful effects of prejudice, whim, and fashion, so that 'lasting advances can be made' (p. 1, para. 1). Otherwise psychiatry will be 'swayed by every wind that blows' and there will be 'no standard of reference by which [new theories] may be criticised' (p. 3, para. 4).

Their second answer is that science gives psychiatry an appropriate focus. This is the 'boundary problem' that we examined in part I, the need to define where pathology ends and moral concepts begin (where 'mad' becomes 'bad'). Slater and Roth rightly point to the dangers of 'a grandiose and *unwarranted expansion of the scope of psychiatry*' once it is divorced from a medical scientific view (p. 4, para. 1, their emphasis).

To these perhaps unexceptionable answers, however, they add a third that is capable of being read as more self-seeking. On p. 2, in particular, Slater and Roth note the importance of the identification of psychiatry with medical science in giving the subject status. Before the First World War, they note, 'whoever took up psychiatry was considered a failure, a man unable to make his way in medicine or surgery'. Now, however, 'due to the cautious industry of responsible research workers and to the impartial collection of careful clinical observations . . . the psychiatrist is recognized as a physician of standing' though also (and somewhat contradicting their sterner comments on p. 4, just noted, about the restricted focus of scientific psychiatry) as . . . 'a counsellor in social problems of general interest'. Science, then, brings status and influence, as perceived by Slater and Roth, writing in 1969.

Question 4: Why the need for a defence?

This brings us to the final question in Exercise 4. Given the advantages science offers (as emphasized by Slater and Roth), and its evident successes in other branches of medicine, why should there be a need to defend the place of science in psychiatry? After all, no textbook of cardiology, say, or gastroenterology, would start with a defence and explication of the scientific method.

Slater and Roth give their reasons up front (p. 1). Their concern is to secure to psychiatry the benefits of scientific medicine. As on many other occasions in the hundred years of its existence, they say, 'psychiatry is in danger of losing its connexion with the body of medicine'. This is partly through impatience engendered by the urgent clinical contingencies of psychiatric practice. The primary concern of the practising psychiatrist 'is to treat and to help his patients': hence in place of the 'slow advance of science', there is a temptation to take 'shortcuts', to seize upon any 'new branch of scientific activity', or even 'a new philosophical movement', before it has been 'worked on by the methods of science' (p. 1, para. 3).

This impatience, of course, and the tendency to take shortcuts, is endemic to all areas of medicine. Psychiatry, however, is especially vulnerable because of its 'peculiar position . . . between medicine and neurology on the one side and philosophy and psychology on the other' (p. 1, para. 2). Little is said to spell out this position (it is clearly an aspect of the 'boundary problem'). But in the last paragraph of p. 1, it seems to amount to psychological 'data' being subjective and lacking precision; and to the particular extent to which 'mental terms' are 'open to varied interpretations' bringing with them the 'risks of vagueness and verbosity'.

Clearly, then, if this is the problem, there is potential here for philosophy; i.e. because the problems besetting scientific psychiatry, as identified by Slater and Roth, are no less than the 'problems of meaning' to which philosophical skills are apposite. Yet if philosophy, as we suggested in Part I, is (part of) the cure, Slater and Roth (here, at least) seem to suggest that it is (part of) the disease.

In the next part of this session, then, we will look at how far Slater and Roth's expectations have been fulfilled, and, more critically, at their attitude to philosophy.

As we noted earlier, Slater and Roth, although thoughtful and reflective about the philosophical issues raised by psychiatry, are in these extracts making a strong claim for psychiatry to develop as an exclusively scientific discipline, one based, moreover, like physical medicine, primarily on the biological sciences.

This is very much the line taken less explicitly by modern 'biological psychiatry'. It is important, therefore, to consider how far Slater and Roth, as experts in biological psychiatry, got it right.

Slater and Roth's expectations

In their preface, Slater and Roth themselves acknowledge that psychiatry seems to be developing as a science more slowly than other medical disciplines. Since the second edition of their textbook, they comment, hopes have faded for the biochemical basis of schizophrenia being clarified 'in the foreseeable future' (p. xiv). On the other hand, new psychotropic drugs are leading to useful hypotheses about the biochemistry of depression; powerful statistical techniques are being developed for analysing clinical data; and the 'basic clinical methods and clinical concepts' of psychiatry have been validated, to the confounding of the antipsychiatrists!

The model guiding the authors' identification of these trends is the standard scientific picture, to which they return in detail in their Introduction, of facts being organized into patterns from which underlying causes are discovered. Just as in physical medicine, then, while sociology and cultural anthropology may have a part to play (pp. 2–3), psychiatry should concentrate on its core agenda of clarifying symptoms and syndromes, and then using the methods of natural science to determine underlying disease processes. And developments in organic psychiatry (including what they describe as 'novel cerebral surgical techniques') are taken to support their view that this is the most fruitful line for psychiatry to follow.

Scientific psychiatry since Slater and Roth

The rise of biological psychiatry, especially with the development of modern brain imaging techniques and advances in genetic medicine, may seem to vindicate Slater and Roth's confidence in the future of a psychiatry based like general medicine on natural science. Since their 1969 edition, both descriptive psychopathology and the classification of mental disorders have become better established, and the brain sciences are now, if only recently, beginning to build on these advances by attempting to develop causal theories.

This picture, however, although one with which many psychiatrists would identify, has to be qualified in a number of respects:

- For all the advances in brain sciences since 1969, biochemically based *causal theories* remain promissory.

- Many, even within medicine, regard sociology and cultural anthropology as no less important than biology to the scientific basis of psychiatry. This has proved to be dramatically so in the development of 'community care', which Slater and Roth do not directly anticipate. Yet there is something about *mental* disorders generally that suggests a particular *need* for these disciplines, as the *Lancet* editorial (1997), quoted at the start of this chapter, so trenchantly suggested, arguing on *medical* grounds against an exclusively biological conception of psychiatry.

- Again, contrary to Slater and Roth's expectations, *organic psychiatry*, although still important, has not expanded in scope and influence. *Cerebral surgery* has proven of dubious value (thus far) for mental disorders: much of the supposed territory of organic psychiatry is now taken by liaison psychiatry, the particular focus of which is the *psychological* components of general medical disorders; and far from *psychopharmacology* expanding, many disorders treated in 1969 with drugs are now treated by psychological and cognitive-behavioural techniques (notably anxiety disorders and all but severe depression).

- Even *psychoanalysis*, a particular target of Slater and Roth's scientific agenda, has flourished—outside of medicine particularly, but it has become absorbed into many areas of medicine also. It is less partisan, less dogmatic, but many of the principles it embodied have now become incorporated into all areas of psychological treatment. This is an especially important development, since, as we will see later in this chapter, what is distinctive about psychoanalysis is, precisely, that it takes seriously the individual, their particular story, and, indeed, the meanings and purposes served by mental symptoms—that is, just those phenomena that Slater and Roth working within a traditional model, take to be directly antithetical to the scientific approach (e.g. p. xiv, para. 3).

- It is perhaps for this last reason above all, then, that as we saw in the first part of this book, *antipsychiatry*, far from being as Slater and Roth imply (p. xiv, para. 3) a spent force, is very much alive. Psychiatrists are still 'shrinks' to many; and for many, mental disorders are better dealt with by psychologists, mental health nurses, counsellors, therapists of various kinds, or, and this is perhaps the most important growth point of all, self-help and advocacy groups. Art, then, intuition and understanding, may be *more* important than the impersonal natural sciences to which Slater and Roth pin their colours.

A science appropriate to psychiatry

So, how goes the battle for medical-scientific psychiatry? It should be clear that science, *natural* science, is as important in psychiatry as in any other area of medicine. The *Lancet* editorial, organ of the medical hierarchy as it is, is at risk of throwing out the baby with the bath water when it appears to set itself against biological psychiatry.

But the last 30 years have shown us: (1) that the *particular* way science will develop in a difficult area such as psychiatry cannot be predicted with any confidence, even (perhaps especially) by those at the coal face of research (as Slater and Roth were at the time); (2) that science in a discipline such as psychiatry, a discipline centrally concerned with *people*, may be much less clearly demarcated, and certainly cannot afford to distance itself from, disciplines, which in an area such as physics would be taken to be *non*-science; and (3) that in its particular objects of study, again *persons*, it must accommodate (give some account of), rather than merely deny or exclude, the meanings and purposes by which individuals are individuated.

Back to philosophy of science

In each of these respects, then—unpredictable direction of advance; uncertain science/non-science boundary; and the importance of individuals—psychiatry is very different from areas of physical medicine such as, in our earlier example, cardiology and gastroenterology.

What are we to make of this? If we are committed, as many psychiatrists are committed (see the two short extracts at the start of this chapter), to the view that psychiatry will develop scientifically *just like* cardiology or gastroenterology, then we will take these trends as temporary aberrations—once the biochemical bases of schizophrenia, depression, and so on, have been clarified, we will expect to see disease theories of a conventional kind emerging, and the non-biological sciences (including psychology as well as sociology and cultural anthropology), not to mention the non-sciences (the 'arts' of the talking therapies), all fading away.

If, on the other hand, we are not committed to psychiatry developing in this way, following slavishly in the tracks of physical medicine, then these three trends could point to the emergence in psychiatry of a 'science', in the old sense of the word as a search for knowledge (Latin 'scientia' meaning 'knowledge' in the general sense), more appropriately tuned to its particular object of study, namely, persons. This does not mean, however, that psychiatry will collapse the other way, being absorbed not into biological medicine but into sociology and cultural anthropology, or even into psychology. For psychiatry, as we saw in Parts I and II, is 'on the cusp'; it is essentially *between* the medical and moral worlds.

There is no easy way in psychiatry, therefore, no collapse either to the human sciences or to the natural sciences. As to how things will develop in psychiatry, there is no guarantee that philosophy will contribute to the emergence of an appropriate science. But at the very least it should give us a deeper understanding of what it is to be scientific at all. What, then, are we to make of Slater and Roth's attitude to philosophy?

Slater and Roth on philosophy

To a superficial reading, Slater and Roth may seem to be taking the 'plain man's' line with philosophy, rejecting it as 'playing with words', as being of little practical relevance. The word 'philosophy' appears twice on p. 1, on both occasions with pejorative overtones: in para. 2, linked with psychology, and contrasted with 'medicine and neurology', and in para. 3, where new philosophical movements, meeting a popular response, are identified among the snares and distractions that divert the psychiatrist from the 'slow advance of science'. Philosophy appears again on p. 2 (para. 2), linked this time with theology.

Remember, though, that both Slater and Roth engaged, in different ways, in conceptual as well as empirical work (Slater, in his attempt to define the scientific basis of psychiatry, see above; Roth in his rejection of Szasz's arguments against the concept of mental illness, see also above); and in much of what they demand of psychiatry, their objectives are as much philosophical as scientific. Their call, in particular, for clearer definitions of the terms in which mental events are described (p. 1, para. 4), and their warnings of the dangers of 'vagueness and verbosity' (p. 2, para. 1), are no less than the objectives at least of analytic philosophy, as introduced in Part I. And as already noted, they rely explicitly on the work of the philosopher of science Karl Popper for support for their view of the nature of scientific method (p. 1, para. 2).

Their commitment, however, to a view of psychiatry following in the tracks of physical medicine, limits the use that they make of philosophy. Their general stance in this respect is clear at the start of their introduction where they observe that psychiatry is between medicine/neurology on the one hand, and philosophy/psychology on the other. For Slater and Roth this is a 'peculiar position', one from which psychiatry must be nudged into its correct place, firmly within traditional medicine. Yet psychiatry, as we have seen, has developed in recent years as strongly in the direction of psychology as of (biological) medicine. And the rapid growth of interest in philosophy and psychiatry around the world shows that philosophy, too, may become an increasingly important partner of psychiatry.

Slater and Roth need philosophy

And the need at least for philosophy of *science* in psychiatry is clear throughout this whole reading: it is clear in a general way in the variety of (and sometimes inconsistent) accounts that Slater and Roth give of what it is to be scientific (i.e. as noted above); but it is also clear in the plain errors in these accounts—no philosopher of science would have left out 'induction' in a résumé of the scientific method; and no philosopher, or indeed historian, of science, would identify with their picture of 'responsible researchers' engaged in the steady accumulation of raw facts, on the basis of which theories are developed entirely by formal processes of critical testing. As we will see, this is very far from what actually does, or indeed should, happen in science.

Much of the philosophical work in this area post-dated Slater and Roth's book. But not all of it did. Karl Popper, for example, to whom they refer, emphasized particularly the central importance in science of the wild, improbable, imaginative leap (see below). Similarly, contrary to their exclusion of meaning and purpose, Karl Jaspers, the founder of modern descriptive psychopathology,

but as we saw in Part II a philosopher as well as a psychiatrist, made much of the need for meaningful as well as causal accounts of mental disorders (e.g. Jaspers, 1974).

This is not meant as philosophical point-scoring off Slater and Roth. As we noted at the start of this session, by seeking to make explicit the preconceptions about science and the scientific method that most psychiatrists take for granted, they have taken us the first step towards a more sophisticated understanding of what is required of psychiatric science. By the same token, though, the difficulties in their own account show the contrary of their conclusion (p. 6, para. 1), that 'Its requirements are simple'. The requirements of a genuinely scientific psychiatry are exceedingly complex, empirically and conceptually.

Three responses to the complexity of science in psychiatry

Modern psychiatry and medical science

In recent years there has been a growing recognition that the application of science is not as simple in psychiatry as in other areas of medicine. Modern psychiatry has reacted to this in three main ways: (1) by denial—pretending the problem does not exist; (2) by proscription; and (3) by displacement. In the final part of this session we will look briefly at each of these.

Reaction 1: denial

One of the undoubted successes of the kind of painstaking approach to psychiatric science advocated by Slater and Roth is the greater reliability and consistency of modern systems of classification of mental disorders (to which we return in Chapter 13). However, in developing in this way, the authors of modern classifications have assumed that *all* the problems of psychiatric classification are, at root, empirical. This is illustrated in the next reading.

EXERCISE 6   (20 minutes)

Read the short extract from:

> American Psychiatric Association (1994). 'Introduction' in *Diagnostic and Statistical Manual* (4th edn). Washington, DC: APA, pp. xv and xvi

---

Link with Reading 11.2

What kind of programme do the authors of the DSM take its development to be? Make a note (as before) of all the words and phrases which mark out their commitment to the DSM being an exclusively scientific classification.

This is deliberately a short extract because we will look at classification in detail later on. But these two pages give a very clear (and fair) summary of how the whole project was conceived, namely as producing a practically focused tool (intended for 'clinical, research, and educational purposes', para. 1), which is 'supported by an extensive empirical foundation' (also para. 1).

There is much talk of 'formal evidence-based processes' (para. 3), of 'empirical evidence' (para. 5), and of 'data' (para. 6). Conceptual and methodological issues are recognized as being important; indeed, the whole system of work groups, conferences, and newsletters, was instituted to make the developmental process as open and explicit as possible. But the distinctive feature of the classification, the authors conclude, is that it is 'grounded in empirical evidence' (para. 7).

Fair enough, then, so far as it goes. There is nothing wrong with the empirical approach. But the model of science adopted here—of presuppositionless data, which if sufficiently comprehensively collated would lead to an observer-independent account of reality—is uncritically assumed. Even cross-cultural aspects of diagnosis are taken to be susceptible merely to a more comprehensive 'data set'. The authors of the DSM could be right in this. But they are wrong merely to assume it. And as we will see, their assumption is mistaken.

Reaction 2: proscription

The second way of dealing with the complexities of psychiatric science is proscription—that is, to acknowledge the complications but to proscribe them from the task in hand. This kind of response is illustrated by the next reading, the last in this session.

EXERCISE 7   (15 minutes)

Read the short extract from:

Gelder, M.G., Gath, G., and Mayou, R.A.M. (1983). Signs and symptoms of mental disorder. Chapter I In *The Oxford Textbook of Psychiatry* (1st edn). Oxford: Oxford University Press, p. 1

Link with Reading 11.3

◆ With this reading, note, (1) any similarities to Slater and Roth's characterization of psychiatry, and (2) any differences. What do you make of these?

As noted in Chapter 2, *The Oxford Textbook of Psychiatry* offers an authoritative review of current medical psychiatry. Like Slater and Roth, the emphasis is still very much on the importance of science—'data' (twice) and 'objectivity' come in the first three lines. Also, similarly to Slater and Roth, there is an emphasis on the importance of clear definition of terms. There is a difference of emphasis here, in that, over the intervening period, sufficient agreement has been reached on definitions of key symptoms, and also sufficient evidence of inter-rater reliability, to justify a whole first chapter.

There is an important difference in principle from Slater and Roth, however, in that, now, 15 years on, rather than downplaying the importance of 'intuitive understanding of each patient as an individual' (para. 1), this is emphasized as a key skill.

Why, then, do we call this 'proscription'? Because the sting in the tail is that intuitive understanding is portrayed as a skill that the psychiatrist acquires through a 'general understanding of human nature', rather than as a specialized 'clinical skill' distinct to psychiatry. Hence, only the latter ('the capacity to collect clinical data objectively . . .') can usefully be learned through a textbook. As with the DSM reading, this *could* be right. But it is stated without qualification as a matter of fact. And as we will see, at best it oversimplifies the distinction between the two kinds of skill, at worst it precludes from psychiatric training something that is essential to practice.

Reaction 3: displacement

That leaves displacement. Rather than denying or proscribing, this response to the complications of the scientific method in psychiatry is to push the problem to someone else! And in this case the fall-guy, as we will see in the next session, is psychoanalysis.

Reflection on the session and self-test questions

Write down your own reflections on the materials in this session drawing out any points that are particularly significant for you. Then write brief notes about the following:

1. Give four words or phrases, traditionally associated with what it is to be scientific, and claimed for psychiatry in its standard textbooks in the second half of the twentieth century.

2. With what is science often contrasted in these textbooks?

3. Why did the authors of these textbooks consider science (traditionally understood) to be so vital?

4. Have things developed as the authors of these textbooks expected?

5. What do subsequent developments suggest for the future?

6. Name two ways in which psychiatry has reacted negatively to the greater conceptual complexity of the discipline. (We noted three.)

Session 3 Scientific psychiatry and the case of psychoanalysis

The philosophy of science suggested by Freud's psychiatry

The main focus of this session will be on the status of psychoanalysis as a science. We will argue that there is much in common between the view of science adopted by the founder of psychoanalysis, Sigmund Freud, and the traditional model of science we have so far encountered. In his later writings, Freud did come to

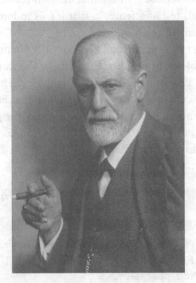

Fig. 11.3 Sigmund Freud

acknowledge the need for a more sophisticated view of science in psychiatry. But as we will see, his adherence particularly in the early years of the development of psychoanalysis, to the traditional model, left psychoanalysis vulnerable to charges that its observations are questionable as scientific data, its methodology suspect, and its theories untestable.

The aim of the discussion in this session, we should emphasize, is not to vindicate Freud's work against all criticisms. An assessment of the overall debate about the status of Freudian theory is clearly outside the scope of this book. The aim instead is to show that one source of a too swift criticism of Freud's scientific status is an oversimplified model of science and that replacing that model with a more sophisticated one shows continuity between many aspects of Freudian theory and more uncontentiously scientific theories. Attention to Freud, as we indicated above, will thus serve as a way of highlighting some of the modifications to the traditional model that need to be made, which will be outlined throughout this Part.

We will start with the third of the three responses mentioned above of modern psychiatry to the problem of applying scientific methods in mental health in general, namely displacement.

Reaction 3: displacement

At the end of the last session, we noted three ways in which psychiatrists have reacted to the recognition that 'the appliance of science' in psychiatry is not as straightforward as in areas of medicine such as cardiology and gastroenterology. We discussed two of these, denial and proscription. The third is displacement, i.e. as we said at the end of the last session, pushing the problem on to someone else.

Psychoanalysis is a clear target of Slater and Roth's introduction. Whenever they want to point out the *un*scientific, and contrast it with their model of a *scientific* psychiatry, psychoanalysis gets it 'in the neck'. On p. 1, psychiatrists are 'allured by the psychopathological theories of Freud . . .'; and on p. 5, joining with Popper, they criticize psychoanalysis for offering 'All-embracing explanations and concepts . . . of dubious value . . .'.

As noted in the last session, psychoanalysis, although changing to some extent in the forms (theoretical and institutional) in which it is presented, has certainly not withered away in the 30 years since Slater and Roth wrote these words. But it is perhaps no coincidence that at the present time, just as psychiatry is most keenly pressing its connections with biological medicine, it should at the same time be distancing itself from, if not the psychotherapies as a whole, at any rate the psychoanalytic theories of the father of the discipline, Sigmund Freud.

But why should psychoanalysis be such an easy target for those committed to a conventional model of science?

> ### EXERCISE 8 (30 minutes)
>
> Think about this question—why should psychoanalysis be such an easy target for those committed to a conventional model of science?—for yourself before going on. A full answer would cover most of the philosophy of science. But at this stage, make a brief checklist of any points you can think of under the four broad stages of the process of science we introduced in the last session: (1) observation; (2) theory building; (3) testing; and (4) progress.

Here are a few of the points that often come up. You may not agree with all of them, and you may well have thought of others. But the broad message is clear enough, that psychoanalysis looks very different from the sciences—like anatomy and physiology—on which general medicine depends.

Four failings of Freudianism?

Thus, in the terms of our preliminary and traditional four-stage model of the practice of science, some of the many charges laid at the door of Freudian psychoanalysis by supporters of the traditional view of science can be summarized as follows:

- *Stage 1* (*observation*): its data are peculiarly subjective (many of the most important observations in psychoanalysis are actually called 'interpretations').

- *Stage 2* (*theory building*): its descriptively defined categories of phenomena can vary radically from those of scientific psychiatry, and even between different schools of thought in psychoanalysis (e.g. the terms 'neurosis' and 'paranoia' were used by Freud with a much wider scope than medical psychiatry even in his day, and certainly much wider than is accepted today; differences in use still exist even within psychoanalysis—see the relevant entries in Laplanche and Pontalis (1973); and its causal theories are, largely, in terms of the very meanings and purposes conventional science eschews.

- *Stage 3* (*testing*): psychoanalysis has made little use of experiment, relying largely on clinical interpretation to vindicate its theories (and there may be difficulties of principle about what would count as proper controls—see, for example Eysenck and Wilson, 1973, pp. 32–33).

- *Stage 4* (*progress*): although its theories have changed in the 100 years or so of its existence, there has been little evidence of a growing corpus of widely accepted knowledge. It is true that there has been something of a truce in recent years between the different schools of psychoanalysis, but this has not been based on a growing theoretical consensus; on the contrary, the truce, as the writer and psychoanalyst Anthony Storr (1989, p. 123) put it, is an 'armed truce'.

Psychoanalysis, psychology, and neuroscience

On the face of it, then, psychoanalysis does not look right, it does not have the right 'tribal colours', for a medical science. Yet, as we will shortly see, psychoanalysis was conceived within scientific psychology and indeed precisely as the kind of psychology necessary to explain abnormal mental phenomena (such as hysteria). Moreover, Freud himself was trained as a neurophysiologist, and at least in his early work, he took himself to be defining psychological structures that would eventually be mapped on to brain mechanisms. Indeed, Freud's general aim continues to inspire similar attempts even today—see Melville Woody and James Phillips, 1995; we will return shortly to the issue of Freud's 'Project'.

The structure of the rest of this chapter

So is psychoanalysis a science, non-science, or, as many psychiatrists seeking scientific respectability by distancing themselves from their scientifically disreputable cousins would have it, plain nonsense?

In the remainder of this chapter, we will look at some of the many different answers that have been offered to this question, drawing particularly on relevant work from the philosophy of science. The rest of this session will cover Freud's views on the nature of a mental science, as set out explicitly in his 'Project', then as reflected in his actual working methods illustrated by one of his early case histories, the case of Dora. We will analyse this case under the four stages of the traditional model of science, taking Stage 1 (observation) and Stage 2 (theory development) in this session, and Stage 3 (theory testing) and Stage 4 (progress) in Session 4. This will cover some of the attacks on Freud's methods by philosophers of science and help highlight the modifications to the traditional model of the practice of science, the modifications we will be considering in detail in the remainder of Part III.

Finally, in Session 5, we will look at alternative 'readings' of psychoanalysis, notably as a hermeneutical (or interpretive) exercise, and through recent work in the philosophy of mind.

Freud's early hopes for a science of the mind

There is a huge literature about the scientific status of psychoanalysis in general and of Freud's theories in particular (Freud remains the most widely cited psychiatrist of all times!). Ironically, however, some of the literature on Freud fails the first (observational) test of science, in that it fails to look carefully at what Freud himself really said.

So, let's start with Freud, and his own early attempt to grapple with the problems of building a science of the mind, which he set out in his 'Project for a scientific psychology'. This turned out to be a highly controversial work, so much so that Freud himself, although intending it originally to be a 'credo' for psychoanalysis, tried to have it destroyed (written in 1895, when Freud was 39, it was not published until the 1950s). But see what you think. . . .

EXERCISE 9   (45 minutes)

Read the extract from:

Freud, S. (1966). Part I. General scheme. In *Project for a Scientific Psychology* (Standard Edition), Vol. 1. London: Hogarth Press, pp. 294–297

Link with Reading 11.4

As you read this extract, note down any words which indicate Freud's view of science. When you have finished, reflect for a moment on the similarities and differences between the view of science offered here, and the view taken by Slater and Roth in the previous session.

Note: in the legend on p. 294, the 'η' in Qη is the Greek letter Eta, or 'long e' (as in 'sleep'); the accent above the 'η' in the text is simply a pronunciation mark; φ = Phi, pronounced 'fie'; ψ = Psi, pronounced like the 'si' in 'sight'; ω = Omega. Also, note that the 'N' appearing in the last line of the introductory section (p. 295) is best understood as standing for 'nervous system' (see footnote 2, p. 296).

At first reading, and in the light of modern developments in psychiatry and neuroscience, it is far from clear why Freud should have felt compromised by his (relatively) youthful 'Project'. It offers, after all, what we should now regard as a sophisticated view of the requirements of a science of the mind. Like Slater and Roth and much of modern scientific psychiatry, Freud wanted to retain his commitment to science. That is, he wanted to conduct his research using the same scientific methodology as he had previously used as a neurolophysiologist. He wanted to make clinical observations, assemble facts, classify them, construct hypotheses, and arrive at general laws through testing his hypotheses against further data.

Freud as a conventional scientist

The first two sentences set the tone for the entire piece: 'The intention is to furnish a psychology that shall be a *natural* science: that is, to represent *psychical processes* as *quantitatively determinable* states of specific *material particles*, thus making those processes perspicuous and free from contradiction' (p. 295, emphasis added). Freud goes on: 'Two principle ideas are involved: [1] What distinguishes activity from rest is to be regarded as Q, subject to the *general laws* of motion. [2] The neurones are to be taken as material particles' (p. 295, emphasis added). Freud is here making an explicit commitment to the then recently advanced neurone theory of the brain, and, as can be seen from the stressed words, within a specific conception of science strikingly similar to that adopted by Slater and Roth.

Immediately following the first paragraph, we find further words giving us a traditional view of science: 'experiments' (p. 295, para. 2); 'observation' (p. 295, para. 3); 'generalize', 'structure', 'functions' (p. 296, para. 1); 'mechanisms' (p. 296, para. 2). He continues with similar terms in the pages that follow the above extract: 'discoveries' (p. 297, para. 2); 'system' (p. 298, para. 1); 'justification', 'hypothesis' (p. 298, para. 2); 'theory', 'explanation' (p. 299, para. 2); 'general' (p. 300, para. 1); 'assumptions' (p. 300, para. 2), 'correctly' (p. 300, para. 3), 'theory' (p. 300, para. 4); 'hypothesis', 'system', 'organization' (p. 302, para. 2); 'hypothesis', 'knowledge' (p. 302, para. 3).

If you compare this list of terms with the list appearing in Table 11.1 (above) you will find that there is a strong correlation. Freud's language is the language of conventional science. However, it is in some ways conceptually more transparent than that provided by Slater and Roth: Freud explicitly states that we should understand some of his claims as assumptions (p. 300, para. 2), and in the next paragraph he reminds us that there is a criterion of correctness against which his theorizing should be judged. The overall conclusion, though, must be that in the 'Project', Freud was taking a conventional view of science.

Freud's suppression of the 'Project'

As noted above, Freud rejected the 'Project' soon after completing it, and he never mentions it in his published work or in his surviving correspondence. It is thought he destroyed his own copy, but another copy survived in a letter Freud sent to Wilhem Fliess. The favourite theory for Freud's disenchantment with the 'Project', is that he came to realize that his then embryonic psychoanalytic method and theory could not hope to do justice to the theoretical model he had sketched out, and that as a result psychoanalysis would appear devalued. But it is also possible that he simply wanted to concentrate on more practicable projects. The neurosciences of the day, after all, were certainly not up to the demands he was placing on them.

Whatever may be the case, from shortly after writing the 'Project', Freud concentrated on developing his method and theory of 'psychical analysis' (first mentioned as such in his 1894 paper 'The neuro-psychoses of defence'; Standard Edition (SE), Vol. III, 1962, pp. 43–68). Freud's 'psychical analysis' became, by 1900, the theory and technique of psychoanalysis. But he frequently repeated his commitment to the principles and methodology of empirical science, and he never gave up the ideal that psychoanalysis should, in principle, be compatible with the scientific world view.

Freud's conception of psychoanalysis as a science

As we saw in the last exercise, Freud's 'Project' conforms to the traditional view of science. And this is very much the line that Freud takes, that of the traditional scientist, throughout much of his writings on psychoanalysis. For example, this is how he defined psychoanalysis in an article he wrote for an encyclopaedia in 1922:

> Psychoanalysis is the name (i) for the procedure for the investigation of mental processes which are almost inaccessible in any other way, (ii) of a method (based upon that investigation) for the treatment of neurotic disorders and (iii) of a collection of psychological information obtained along these lines, which is gradually being accumulated into a new scientific discipline.
>
> SE XVIII (Freud, 1955, p. 235)

Yet psychoanalysis, as we have already noted, was to turn out to be highly problematic from the perspective of precisely the traditional view of science Freud himself espoused. Just why Freud's fellow traditionalists were to turn against him, just why indeed psychoanalysis in general is so problematic from a traditional point of view, becomes clearer if we look, not at what Freud wrote *about* psychoanalysis, but at Freud himself *at work*. We cannot do this directly, of course, but Freud's case histories are vivid and detailed, and they include a good deal of his own reflections.

The case of Dora

In the next exercise we will read an extract from one of Freud's early case studies, the case of Dora. Dora was an 18-year old woman who was brought by her father to Freud for treatment. She presented with problems of obsessive thoughts about a friend of her father's, Herr K, whom she said she detested, and who, she said, had made an indecent proposal to her.

Freud treated Dora from 1896 to about 1900, that is, beginning immediately after he had written the 'Project', and during the period when he was conducting his own self-analysis. In the 'Dora' case study, a lengthy 'clinical picture' is given by Freud, which includes details of his approach, and then a discussion of her dreams. The dream analysis serves only to confirm the conclusions Freud has already arrived at on the basis of his therapeutic sessions with Dora, but we will describe them briefly by way of background to the reading that follows.

Dora's case study contains two dreams, which are heavily interpreted during her treatment. The first dream is of a house fire. Dora's father wakes her up to escape; her mother, however, wants to delay so that she can save her jewel case, but Dora's father refuses, saying that the survival of himself and his two children is more important than the jewel case. The dream ends when they reach safety outside the house.

This dream is interpreted by Freud as the expression of an unconscious love for Herr K accompanied by a wish to protect herself from his advances, and at the same time an accusation against her father for bringing her into contact with Herr K.

The second dream starts with Dora walking around a town she does not recognize; however, she reaches a house where she knows she lives, and in her room she discovers a note from her mother. This informs her that her father has died, with the explanation that, as Dora had left her parents' home without their knowledge, they had not wanted to bother her with news that her father was ill. But now he was dead, she could come home. She goes to the station and asks 'Where is the station?', receiving the reply 'Five minutes'. She sees a thick wood and enters it, where a man tells her 'Two and a half hours more', and offers to accompany her, which she refuses. She sees the station but cannot reach it, and feels anxious at not being able to progress. Then she finds herself at home, and in her flat the maidservant tells her that her mother and the others have already gone on to the cemetery.

Freud interprets this second dream as expressing an unconscious wish for revenge on her father, and also an unconscious wish to be deflowered by Herr K.

We are now ready to turn to Freud's account of the case of Dora. We will be reading a number of extracts from this case over the next few exercises.

EXERCISE 10   (75 minutes)

Read the extract from:

Freud, S. (1977). 'Dora' case study. In *Case Histories I*. The Pelican Freud Library, Vol. 8. London: Penguin, pp. 41, 45–49.

Link with Reading 11.5

As you read this and the other extracts from Freud (1977), write short notes on the following, using the stages of the scientific process identified in Table 11.1 above:

1. what does Freud say about his method of data collection, and how does it compare with the picture given in Stage 1, Table 11.1;

2. what is Freud's approach to theory-building, and can it be mapped on to Stages 2A and 2B;

3. how does Freud approach theory testing, and is his approach consistent with Stage 3?; finally,

4. what is Freud's view of the advancement of psychoanalytic knowledge, compared with that given in Stage 4?

For each of the four stages, note (1) Freud's use of language reflecting his commitment to a traditional view of science (as in his 'Project'), and (2) anything which, explicitly or implicitly, looks different or even incompatible with the traditional view.

Stage 1 of the traditional model of science: data collection

Freud is engaged in a careful search for what he takes to be objective data. Thus on p. 41 he talks of 'material from the histories of a large number of treatments'. On p. 42 he speaks of 'information'

and 'facts'. On p. 46 we find 'careful physical examination' (footnote 1); while on p. 47 we get 'facts which form the material of psychoanalysis' (para. 2), 'somatic data and symptoms' (para. 3), and 'empirical rule' (footnote 1). On p. 49 Freud begins a lengthy section entitled 'The clinical picture' in which he sets out the facts of the patient's history, utilizing information from the patient herself and her father.

So far so good. Freud is engaged in a process of data collection with which those committed to a traditional view of science (like Slater and Roth) would have no quarrel. However, there are two important differences between the process Freud is describing and the traditional view of data collection, (1) that it is theory dependent, and (2) that it is goal directed.

Look at this again for yourself before going on.

EXERCISE 11   (10 minutes)

Re-read the short section from p. 45 'I begin the treatment . . .' to p. 47, '. . . symptoms of the disorder'. Think again about any respects in which what Freud is doing here, in the way of Stage 1 observations, or data gathering, differs from the traditional conception of this as the first stage of the scientific process.

You may have identified other passages where these or other differences appear. But both the theory dependence and goal directedness of data gathering are clearly illustrated in this passage.

- *Theory dependence of data.* The first difference, then, from the traditional view of data collection, is that in Freud's account the data cannot be wholly prized free from the context of the theory (of psychoanalysis) in which they arise. For a 'fact' to be recognized or accepted, presupposes a theory within which it has its significance.

  Thus, Freud writes: 'I begin my treatment by asking the patient to give me the whole story of his life and illness' (p. 45). So far, then, this looks like traditional observation, or data gathering. Notice, however, what follows immediately after this: 'but even so the information I receive is *never enough to let me see my way about the case*' (p. 45, emphasis added). What else is needed, then, besides the plain story as told by the patient? In the next couple of pages, Freud tells us. Patients, he says, consciously conceal things they 'ought to tell' (p. 46), and they also unconsciously conceal information, which both possess 'great theoretical significance' (p. 46), and are 'theoretically requisite' (p. 47). In other words, the plain story told by the patient, the 'facts', cannot be accepted at face value. The story has to be understood, it has to be interpreted, in the light of the psychoanalytic theory of the unconscious.

- *Goal directedness of data.* Freud's second departure from the classical view of scientific data collection is a tacit, and at times explicit, acknowledgement that scientific method comes with its own aims—in this case, to afford an explanatory account that will inform and further advance treatment.

Thus he says: 'Whereas the practical aim of treatment is to remove all possible symptoms and replace them by conscious thoughts, we may regard it as a second and theoretical aim to repair all the damages to the patient's memory. These two aims are coincident. When one is reached, so is the other; the same path leads to them both' (p. 46). Freud seems to be saying here that it does not much matter which of two approaches is taken in treatment: the practical aim or the theoretical one. But the key point is that the aim of inquiry is to guide the inquirer to look for certain data, and to influence the interpretation placed upon the data obtained. In other words, what *counts* as a fact in psychoanalysis is determined, not by a disembodied process of objective observation, but by what satisfies the aim of successful treatment.

These two differences from the classical view of data—that Freud's data are theory dependent and goal directed—have been widely taken to undermine the scientific status of Freud's theory. They certainly make the data of psychoanalysis *look* very different from that of, say, chemistry. Indeed, they make psychoanalysis appear to be much closer to the subjective interpretations of art than the objective interpretations of science.

All data are theory laden and goal directed

But a central moral of modern philosophy of science is that, contrary to the traditional view, all data, even in disciplines such as chemistry, are theory laden and goal directed. This is the subject of Chapter 12. The hope that observations and theory could be clearly separated has proved a false hope. Science, contrary to the traditional model, is not like this. The idea that data are theory free and goal free has turned out to be an oversimplified picture of how science works.

These properties of data are not as evident in the physical sciences as in psychoanalysis, however. It may be that the *degree* of theory ladenness and goal directedness of psychoanalytic data (or some other *qualitative* difference) does indeed mark an essential difference between what Freud was doing and, say, Mendeleev's work in chemistry. It may be, moreover, that further work in the philosophy of science will restore something closer to the classical notion of theory-free and goal-free data. But the point is that, far from the theory ladenness and goal directedness of Freud's data being a knock-down argument against the scientific status of psychoanalysis, it anticipates (by some sixty-odd years), modern insights into the nature of science as a whole.

This raises two questions, (1) why should these features of scientific data, so belatedly recognized in the physical sciences, be relatively self-evident in psychoanalysis, and (2) why did Freud make so little of them?

Psychoanalysis as a difficult science

A non-specific, but important, answer to the first question, is that psychoanalysis, as a *mental* science, is more difficult than chemistry, as a *physical* science.

In what sense 'difficult'? A full answer to this would be book length. However, the core of the relevant sense of difficulty goes back to J.L. Austin's notion (from Part I) of the negative concept 'wearing the trousers'. That is to say, one way to understand the greater transparency of the properties of data in psychoanalysis, is that this is an area where the *concept* of a datum is problematic (because it is, say, stretched to its limit). You will recall that Austin argued that the best place to explore the meanings of our concepts is where they are problematic; it is in such contexts, Austin said, that we 'break through the veil of ease and obviousness' in which the meanings of our concepts are normally wrapped.

Psychoanalysis as a window on science

All this, remember, is not to say that psychoanalysis is or is not a science. It *does* show, however, that *whether* it is, is a trickier question than the traditional view of science would suggest. And it does show psychoanalysis, whether or not it is a science, in a very different light. It shows psychoanalysis, and more specifically Freud, not as struggling to adapt to the received paradigm of physical science, but as revealing, in the very difficulties he encountered, important features of the paradigm itself.

Rather like the (similarly problematic) concept of mental illness, then, in Part I, we have now repolarized our perception of psychoanalysis. Instead of being a reflection (at best) of a primitive or (at worst) of a degenerate science, the difficulties presented by psychoanalysis are seen to provide a window on the nature of science in general (whether or not, ultimately, one decides that psychoanalysis itself *is* a science).

Freud misses a trick

This brings us to the second question, then, why did Freud make so little of all this himself?

The short answer to this question is that, as we have seen, he was firmly committed to a traditional view of science. Like his critics, Freud believed—reasonably enough at the time—that the validity of his new science of the mind depended on its conforming to the paradigms of physics and chemistry. Hence, what we can *now* see as insights into the nature of science, remain half-submerged in his writings. They remain largely implicit rather than explicit, manifesting as tensions between the perceived need for 'objectivity' and the essentially subjective nature of the objects of inquiry (mental states and processes) with which he was concerned.

Freud, in these passages, then, gives an honest account of what he is about, he gives it to us 'warts and all'. The 'warts' leave him vulnerable to attack from those committed to a traditional view of science (not only Slater and Roth, but also, as we will see later, philosophers such as Sir Karl Popper). But in a more modern view of science, the 'warts' turn out, after all, to be a feature of science as a whole (and, many would argue, to be beauty spots rather than warts).

Moving on to Stages 2, 3, and 4

We have gone into this in some detail because the status of 'data' in psychoanalysis, as the key concept in Stage 1 of the traditional model of the scientific process, provides a particularly clear illustration of the way in which modern philosophy of science helps us think in a more balanced way about the status of psychoanalysis as a science. In the remainder of this session, and the next, we will be running through essentially the same line of argument in relation to the other three stages of the scientific process, theory building, theory testing, and the progress of science.

You may find it helpful to keep the general story line in mind as you work through this material. Thus, for each of the Stages 2, 3, and 4 of the traditional model of science, as for Stage 1, we will see

♦ *Freud the traditional scientist*, trying to impose a traditional model of science on what he is doing; but . . .

♦ *the materials of psychoanalysis* (people's experiences and behaviour) proving recalcitrant, refusing to accommodate fully to the traditional model, and, hence, differences from the traditional model of science breaking through. For Freud's purposes, of selling psychoanalysis as a traditional science, these differences are a potential embarrassment; but . . .

♦ *modern philosophy of science* has now shown the differences, contrary to the traditional view, to be implicit in the nature of science as a whole.

Later, in about 1916–17, Freud himself was to present these difficulties as an opportunity to extend the scope of science (see, e.g. his lecture 'Psychoanalysis and Psychiatry' in Freud, 1973, pp. 281–295).

Stage 2A of the traditional model of science: theory building—defining patterns

So let's move to Stage 2, theory building.

We divided Stage 2 into two substages, 2A (defining patterns), and 2B (identifying causes) (see Table 11.1 above). In practice, of course, these are not kept sharply distinct, but the idea (as illustrated in the last session by the story of the development of the chemical periodic table of elements), is that scientific theories develop, in the first instance by the identification of patterns of similarity and difference discernible in the 'raw' data, which, in the second instance, lead to the identification of underlying causes.

A clear example of Stage 2A (pattern recognition) comes early in Freud's account, when he identifies what he takes to be an anomaly in the emotional response of Dora to a proposal of marriage from Herr K. By the standards of the times, such a proposal should always stimulate a pleasurable response. So Dora would be expected to welcome Herr K's advances. In fact, she reacts with disgust, and this disgust then becomes disgust at the idea of Herr K having anything to do with her (prior to this she had been on friendly terms with him). Freud thus identifies a *pattern* of response here, which he regards as characteristic of neurosis, and which he terms 'reversal of affect' (p. 59).

Reversal of affect, defined in terms of a pattern of data (paradoxical emotion in response to a stimulus), thus renders intelligible the behaviour and mental experience of the patient, at least to the extent of identifying it with a class of similar cases.

Reversal of affect, moreover, is only one example of a broader, but still descriptive, category, namely that of any experience or behaviour that is inconsistently or incompletely described by the person concerned. This broader category emerges in Freud's account of Dora, as a criterion of neurotic pathology in general.

Distinguishing symptoms from normality

There are a number of explicit references to Freud's broader criterion for neurosis in the extract (see Exercise 10). On p. 46, footnote 1, for example, the criteria of normality are connected with the patient's ability to tell her story 'perfectly clearly and connectedly in spite of the remarkable events it . . . [deals] with'. Of course, even as Freud was employing this descriptive (i.e. Stage 2A) criterion—of gaps and inconsistencies as defining neurosis—he had in mind a (Stage 2B) theory about the *causes* of Dora's neurosis—which revolved around an experience that stimulated emotions in her that she found impossible to accept, and therefore had to be disguised in some way, even from herself. However, it is a descriptive (Stage 2A) criterion none the less. Freud is assimilating his observations about Dora to a general category within an overall descriptive classification of abnormal experiences and behaviour.

In this respect, therefore, Freud's method is no different in principle (albeit that it is different in the particular experiences and behaviours it marks out), from modern descriptive psychopathology, or indeed, general medicine. Thus, the seventeenth century English physician, Thomas Sydenham, identified symptoms and classified them into syndromes. The particular syndromes were to shift and change as medicine advanced; however, descriptively defined categories were an essential first step to identifying underlying causal processes. This 'first step', moreover, is, apparently, just the same as the first step in chemistry (identifying and classifying the elements by their properties).

On the face of it then, medicine in the eighteenth century, chemistry in the nineteenth century, and now Freud in the early twentieth century, are all involved in the same scientific process of identifying objectively existing patterns in objectively defined data. Or are they?

Classification and induction in science

The question of whether the patterns picked out in psychiatric classification are genuine, objective, or 'valid' (to adopt recent medical terminology) is a central theoretical concern for contemporary psychiatry and will be discussed at some length in Chapter 13. One recent attempt to ensure validity (as well as more directly 'reliability' or agreement) has been to concentrate on classifications that reduce to a minimum the theoretical assumptions made. The idea, as we saw in Chapter 3, is that classifications should pick out directly observational properties (symptoms and signs) rather than relying on theories of the underlying causes of disorder (aetiological theories).

But even if this is possible (arguments against will be deployed in Chapters 12 and 13) only some directly observable patterns can be projected reliably into the future. This is an aspect of the problem of induction discussed in Chapter 16. To anticipate a little, the point is that even assuming some general defence can be given of inductive reasoning—reasoning from particular cases to generalities—there remain concrete issues of which observed particular patterns can be more generally projected into the future. To exemplify this question the American philosopher Nelson Goodman (1983) set out what he called the New Riddle of Induction by inventing two new predicates: 'grue' and 'bleen', where 'grue' means green until, say, the year 2020 and blue afterwards, and 'bleen' means blue until then and green afterwards. Now the predicate 'grue' could be applied to all the healthy grass so far observed as far as past evidence is concerned as could 'green'. But the grass is either grue or green not both. (It either will or will not turn blue in 2020.) So what is it that supports our projecting its greenness into the future not its grueness? What is it that makes a predicate projectible? Giving an account of what patterns can be relied on to continue into the future is a genuine methodological problem even if Goodman's very clear example seems, for that reason, rather far fetched.

Induction and patterns of experience

Freud at work on Dora illustrates this key methodological problem. We return to this in a moment but will consider, first, the simpler case of a trial of a new drug treatment. In a drug trial, as in other areas of practical science, we take patterns to be 'objectively there' if they survive good experimental design, such as 'double blind control trials'. If we want to see whether a drug, A, produces an effect, B, we hide from both the experimental subjects and the experimenter the key information about whether the patients concerned are receiving the drug or a placebo (i.e. a preparation identical to A but lacking the active ingredient). If, then, the pattern 'A producing B' persists, we take it to be a pattern in the world rather than in the minds of those concerned.

Now, precisely the same principles have been applied in recent work on psychiatric diagnostic classification. We return to this in detail in Chapter 13. The central idea has been to clarify which syndromes (patterns of symptoms) are really there in the patient or are merely in the minds of the doctors concerned. But now notice this. Substituting psychopathological symptoms for drug A and response B, makes it much more difficult, perhaps even impossible, to avoid the whole pattern being accessible to those concerned (patients as well as doctors). In the case of the drug trial, someone quite separate makes up the placebo versus active drug packages. So this part of the pattern is readily isolated from the experience of both the patients and the experimenters. In the case of psychopathology, by contrast, the parts of any pattern (i.e. individual symptoms) cannot be separated in this way.

There are various ways that researchers have tried to get round this: using symptom checklists, interobserver ratings, and so on. But the basic point is that in psychopathology, separating out the parts of the pattern for separate recording is at the very least a great deal more difficult than in other areas of observational science. In Dora's case, Herr K's proposal could not have been a 'placebo'—whatever could that mean! Even if he was being

disingenuous, what Dora actually experienced *had* to be a genuine 'proposal of marriage' experience. So what she understood Herr K to be proposing, and her reaction to that proposal, as two key elements of the pattern in this case, were inevitably both within her experience.

In the case of pathological patterns of experience, moreover, there is yet a further complicating factor, the *interpretation* that is placed on the experience.

Induction and pathological experiences

This, too, is well illustrated by Freud at work on Dora. The next reading is a further extract from Freud's account of this case, a passage in which the interpretation that he places on the 'data' of Dora's experience and behaviour, is evident.

EXERCISE 12   (10 minutes)

Read the further short section from the case of Dora:

Freud, S. (1977). 'Dora' case study. In *Case Histories I*. The Pelican Freud Library, Vol. 8. London: Penguin, pp. 60–63

Link with Reading 11.6

◆ What interpretation(s) is Freud putting on the patterns of response he is describing here?

◆ He is not just describing these reactions, he is (implicitly) judging them in some way. In what way, do you think?

In this passage, Freud's observation of Dora's response is that it is not, merely, a rejection of Herr K's proposal; it is not merely a reaction of disgust. Crucial to his observation is that Dora's reaction is, somehow, *abnormal*. What we see, here, Freud says, is a 'reversal of affect', a reaction that is the reverse of what we should expect. This is why, along with other gaps and contradictions in Dora's story, her reaction to Herr K's proposal of marriage is taken by Freud as a symptom of neurosis.

In a word, then, the patterns Freud is concerned with are not just descriptive but normative. Just what norms are important in defining pathology, of course, takes us back to the whole question of the meanings of the concepts of illness, mental disorder, and so on, that we examined in Part I. However, it is clear in this case, at least, that what Freud 'sees' is normatively driven. In this, Freud, being very much a man of his times, takes it for granted that a 'normal' woman will and should be pleased and flattered by a proposal of marriage, even if it is one that she rejects. That would be a proper reaction. Dora's reaction, then, is abnormal.

Induction, values, and psychiatric diagnosis

Not only is psychiatric diagnosis norm-driven, but the norms involved are evaluative (good/bad) in nature. This follows directly from our work on concepts of disorder in Part I. As with concepts of disorder, so with diagnosis, this conclusion is not confined to psychiatry. As we will see, *all* diagnosis, in medicine as well as psychiatry, is in principle value-laden. The difference is simply that in psychiatric diagnosis the values are open and problematic. This is not a matter of poor science. On the contrary, it is a reflection of our diversity as human beings. Hence in the case of psychiatric disorders, there is far wider *legitimate* disagreement than in the case of the diagnosis of physical disorders.

Freud's work, represented by Dora's case, is no different from the DSM or ICD (our modern systems of classification) in being saturated with values. Though, with Freud, again as in DSM and ICD, the traditionally perceived importance of science being value free, has resulted in values not being recognized for what they are—they have been hidden or 'closet' values. This is, of course, all exactly as we should expect from the Austin/Wittgenstein notion of philosophical problems being 'illusions' of language outlined in Part I (see also Fulford, 1994; and Part IV of this book).

In this respect, then, if Freud is being unscientific in relying (tacitly) on norms, so is psychopathology in general, and indeed medicine as a whole. Physical medicine, if the ideas (from R.M. Hare and others) outlined in Part I are right, only *appears* to be value free because the values involved are, by and large, agreed and hence unproblematic. But does this leave psychopathology in practice (and all medical diagnosis in principle) outside the remit of science?

Epistemic values and the underdetermination of theory by data

The short answer to the question is 'no', or 'not obviously' at any rate, given the extent to which modern philosophy and sociology of science have shown science itself, even in areas such as physics and chemistry, to be norm-driven. The values concerned are diverse. They influence which research programmes are pursued, of course, but also such fundamental questions as the significance of 'data', and the very choice of theories. There are, as several philosophers of science have argued, further 'epistemic' values that are crucial to our choice of a particular theory. (See for example, Sadler, 1996, and the commentaries by John Livesley (1996) and Michael Luntley (1996).)

Epistemic values, moreover, are, in turn, an aspect of the broader ways in which theory choice is, in the American philosopher W.V. Quine's now famous phrase, 'underdetermined' by data. For any set of data (or observations), there will always be a number of alternative explanatory possibilities, and which theory we choose is therefore not determined *solely* by the data. Widely discussed epistemic values include economy, i.e. choosing the least elaborate theory, or using Occam's Razor, so-called after the fourteenth century Franciscan monk, William of Occam; and, even, elegance (especially in mathematical physics). And this underdetermination of theory by the data, in turn, reaching to an even more general level of consideration, is an aspect of the way in which the observer cannot (as the traditional model of science requires) be wholly separated out and divorced from the observed.

It follows, therefore, that if Freud's theories were underdetermined by his data, and if, even, his theories were partly determined by norms, this does not, in and of itself, put his theories beyond the scientific pale. In a traditional view of science, such characteristics would indeed put psychoanalysis beyond the pale. This is why Freud himself failed to make this explicit, though, as we have seen, he was clearer than many of his contemporaries that the notion of a *mental* medical science was more problematic than its physical counterpart. But modern work on the nature of science shows that here, at Stage 2A (pattern recognition) of the traditional picture of the scientific process, as at Stage 1 (observations of data), what Freud is doing in the case of Dora is not different in principle from what goes on in all areas of science, and that it is in fact very similar in practice to what goes on in other areas of psychopathology.

As before, this is not to prejudge the issue of whether psychoanalysis is a science. What it shows, though, is that on this ground at least, psychoanalysis is not obviously *non*-science. And indeed, as at Stage 1, from the perspective of modern philosophy of science, we see writ large in psychoanalysis something (the underdetermination of theory by data), which has only belatedly become recognized to be important in science as a whole.

This takes us to Stage 2B, *explanatory* theories.

Stage 2B of the traditional model of science: causal explanatory theories

Hidden causes of observed patterns

With Stage 2B of the process of science, you will recall, we start to develop theories about the underlying causes of the patterns we have identified (at Stage 2A) in the data (collected at Stage 1).

Here, Freud, and psychoanalysis in general, have been thought to be particularly vulnerable to charges of non-science. Many of the issues raised under Stage 2A apply also at Stage 2B: explanatory as well as descriptive theories are underdetermined by data; in explanatory as well as in descriptive theories epistemic values are important to theory choice; and in explanatory as well as descriptive theories, it is becoming increasingly clear that even (perhaps especially) in the paradigm science of theoretical physics, the classical separation of observer and observed can no longer be (unproblematically) maintained.

Freud's explanatory theories, moreover, at first sight look very similar in principle to those of chemistry and physics, in that all three explain surface phenomena in terms of underlying hidden factors. Thus, Freud observed gaps and contradictions as patterns in Dora's experience and behaviour. These required explanation. The explanations he offered were in terms of what have come to be called 'hidden variables'. The gaps and contradictions observed, Freud suggested, can be explained if we suppose that behind these, as 'surface' phenomena, there is a hidden (or not directly observable) mechanism, the *unconscious*. More specifically, a mechanism of *repression* may operate to block out traumatic memories from consciousness—hence the gaps, and hence the contradictions, in what can be consciously recalled.

Freud on hidden causes

What Freud is suggesting, then, looks very like (and he probably conceived of it as) an explanation in terms of hidden causes. He moves from pattern recognition (he talks of 'associations') to 'hidden variables' in the form of the operation of mechanisms that are ordinarily concealed from view. The symptoms of Dora's neurosis, which defy explanation in terms of our ordinary, common-sense understanding of mental functioning, can be explained by a set of causes operating in the unconscious.

Thus, Freud invokes the mechanism of repression, operating in the unconscious, to explain why Dora is unaware of the real nature of her feelings for Herr K. Freud believes that Dora is actually in love with Herr K; but, because to admit her love would be to transgress all the moral constraints she has internalized as part of her upbringing, her love for Herr K is repressed—contained within the unconscious (pp. 60–61; also pp. 88–89). This repression is incomplete, however, and from time to time evidence of it emerges in her dreams, thoughts, and behaviour. In particular, the mechanism of repression attempts to conceal the true nature of her feelings by disguising them as their opposite—i.e. disgust at the idea of relations with Herr K, rather than love for him.

Hidden causes and hidden reasons

In all this, Freud, the traditional scientist, is thus doing nothing odd or unusual. The apple (so the story goes) fell on Newton's head because of the (hidden) forces of gravity; the chemical elements fall into a well-defined periodic table because of the operation of (hidden) electron shells. Dora shows reversal of affect, and other gaps and contradictions in her conscious experience and behaviour, because of the operation of unconscious (hence, hidden) mechanisms such as repression.

Yet, closer examination suggests a crucial difference. In the physical sciences the hidden factors behind surface phenomena are, indeed, causes. In the case of human beings, on the other hand, the hidden factors are, characteristically, reasons. Human beings are subject, like anything else, to hidden causes. Human experience and behaviour may be driven by causes as obviously physical as, say, a brain tumour; and most people, nowadays, acknowledge the brain basis of *all* experiences and behaviour (see Part V). However, for human beings, unlike apples and chemical elements, the hidden factors to which in everyday life we attribute experience and behaviour, are not physical causes but reasons. Such attributions, indeed, broadly construed as encompassing wishes, desires, beliefs, meanings, and so on, have come to be called in recent times 'folk psychology'.

Freud on hidden reasons

Freud, in his account of Dora, uses the language of both kinds of hidden factor, of causes and of reasons. We have just seen several examples of his causal (mechanistic) language; but examples of his use of the language of reasons also run right through the case.

Later in the case history, for example, Freud claims that Dora's 'preoccupation with his (Herr K's) children was a cloak for something else'. In the language of causes, this would be an example of the operation of one of the mechanisms of repression, called displacement, whereby a painful or otherwise unacceptable experience is converted into something more acceptable. Freud was to develop his theory of unconscious mechanisms very much in these push–pull terms, Freudian psychodynamics indeed sometimes being compared with hydrodynamics. But in this instance, at least, the language that follows is of reasons. Dora is said to have become preoccupied with Herr K's children because she 'was *anxious to hide* from herself and from other people [that] she had for all these years been in love with Herr K' (p. 69, paras 1,2; emphasis added).

Other examples of Freud's reason-giving, or folk-psychological language, include ' "no" signifies the *desired* "yes" ' (p. 93, para. 2); 'a single symptom (may correspond) to several *meanings*' (p. 87, para. 2), and 'Dora had an unconscious *wish* to marry Herr K' (p. 149, para. 1).

Causes versus reasons?

Why should it matter that Freud uses the language of reasons? Why should this be taken to impugn the scientific status of psychoanalysis?

EXERCISE 13 (10 minutes)

Think about this briefly for yourself before going on. This exercise is not about general philosophical considerations. Try to think of a particular case or type of situation from clinical practice in which 'reasons-language' accounts and 'causes-language' accounts of human experience and behaviour have very different implications.

One important situation in which the two kinds of explanation have different implications is in attributions of responsibility. We started to look at this in Part I. The implication of saying that someone had reasons for something they did, is that they were responsible for it. But if someone's behaviour is said to be *caused* (e.g. by a brain tumour), the implication is that they are not responsible.

All this of course begs a range of deep metaphysical questions, about freedom, determinism, and so on. As a *practical* issue, however, the difference, where the death penalty is still in use, can mean literally the difference between life (with hospital treatment for someone whose behaviour was caused by their illness) and death (for a person found guilty of actions for which they are responsible).

Medicine versus morals

In terms of our conceptual map of psychiatry, therefore, introduced in Part I, Freud's use of reason-giving language could thus be seen as shifting psychoanalysis from the scientific world of medicine (as traditionally conceived) into the human world of moral agents.

It is this shift that lies behind one whole strand of criticism of the scientific status of psychoanalysis. An early exemplar of this strand of criticism was from no less a philosopher than Wittgenstein. In a series of lectures given in Cambridge in 1932–3, Wittgenstein (1982) commented on Freud's apparent 'muddle' over reasons and causes. Wittgenstein fails to acknowledge that Freud was working with an extraordinarily difficult problem concerning the conceptualization and explanation of mental processes, which even today continues to challenge philosophers working at the boundary between the philosophy of mind and the philosophy of science. Criticisms of this kind, however, have continued through those (such as the psychologist, Hans Eysenck) arguing that psychoanalysis is 'merely' story-telling or construction of plausible narratives, to the sophisticated reinterpretations of psychoanalysis by a number of French philosophers, as a hermeneutic or interpretive enterprise (e.g. Paul Ricoeur—we return to these later in the chapter, when we look at alternative accounts of psychoanalysis, as 'non-science').

Causes and reasons?

So, one way of taking Freud's use of reason-giving language is that it shows psychoanalysis, at Stage 2B of the scientific process, the stage of explanatory theories, to be a non-science. As with Stage 1 (observation) and Stage 2A (descriptive theories), though, there is a quite different way of taking Freud's use of reason-giving language, namely that it signals something important about science as a whole, something that modern philosophical work has shown is neglected or misunderstood in the classical model of science, but which breaks through in psychoanalysis (despite Freud's own commitment to the traditional model) because psychoanalysis, if it is a science, is a very *difficult* science.

Philosophically, Freud's use of reason-giving language, alongside and in the course of ostensibly developing a causal theory, anticipates a current debate, located somewhere between philosophy of science and philosophy of mind, about the relationship between reasons and causes. We return to this in detail later, in Chapter 15 in this part and in Chapters 23 and 24 in Part V.

Practically, Freud's use of reason-giving language anticipates an equally wide debate in psychology and the brain sciences about the appropriate 'level' of scientific explanations of human experience and behaviour. For some, 'folk psychology' will fade away as developments in neuroscience make talk of reasons metaphorical, rather as developments in physics have made talk of the sun 'coming up' metaphorical (the American philosophers Paul and Patricia Churchland are vigorous proponents of this view—see, e.g. Churchland, 1989).

For others, reacting against the positivism of early behavioural psychology, the language of reasons, cashed out now in the computational terms of cognitive psychology, is essential to any general science of the mind. This is no reinvention of Cartesian two-substance dualism (see Chapter 22). The idea, more straightforwardly, is that just as chemistry, although in principle reducible to physics none the less survives and indeed flourishes as a distinct level of explanation, so too for the mind. Whatever advances are made in our understanding of the brain, so this idea goes, the psychological will always remain necessary as a distinct level of explanation. The 'cognitive revolution', as it has come to be called, has been characterized as putting the mind back into psychology. In mental health, we could characterize it as putting mental states back into brains.

Reducing minds to brains, reasons to causes?

Reductionism is explained later in this Part (in relation to reasons and causes in Chapter 15) and again in Part V. But whatever the possibilities for mind–brain reduction, Freud's use of both kinds of language in the case of Dora, the language of causes and the language of reasons, is not in itself evidence that psychoanalysis is not a science. As at earlier stages of the traditional model of science, this is not to prejudge the issue of whether psychoanalysis is a science. The point is simply that both kinds of language, in the present state of our knowledge, are required for a science of the mind. Freud's use of both kinds of language reflects this and is not, therefore, a knock down argument against the status of psychoanalysis as a science.

As with the points considered at Stages 1 and 2A above, Freud himself is at best ambivalent about any watering down of the traditional model of science. Had he, though, been able to embrace this particular point more openly, not only would he have anticipated an important debate in the philosophy of science, he would have found himself in good scientific company. For the reasons/causes debate, in the guise of a contemporary debate about the status of human (as opposed to natural) sciences in general, was very much alive, at least among philosophers and psychologists, even in his day. Indeed, as we considered in detail in Part II, one of the founders of modern scientific psychopathology, the philosopher–psychiatrist Karl Jaspers, repeatedly emphasized the need for both causal and meaningful explanations in psychiatry (e.g. Jaspers, [1913] 1974).

Modern biological psychiatry, in the throws of its identity crisis as a medical discipline, has chosen to ignore Jaspers' 'meanings' and to run only with his 'causes'. Freud at work on Dora, and psychoanalysis in general, shows that this may well turn out to have been an aspect of the hemianopic (or half-field) view of medicine, in terms of which, we concluded in Part I, the 'medical' model has to be understood.

Psychoanalysis may or may not be a science, then. But Freud certainly made life difficult for psychoanalysis by his ambivalence about reasons and causes. This helped to make him an easy target for attack for those who (like Freud himself) are committed to the traditional model of science. But what mature reflection now suggests, is that the appearance of reasons-language alongside causes-language in Freud's account of Dora, is a signal of something important about the nature of the mental sciences as a whole.

Continued in our next

This leaves Stages 3 (theory testing) and 4 (progress of knowledge). These stages of the traditional picture have attracted more of the firepower of the critics of psychoanalysis, particularly among philosophers, than any others. It is to these that we turn in the next session.

Reflection on the session and self-test questions

Write down your own reflections on the materials in this session drawing out any points that are particularly significant for you. Then write brief notes about the following:

1. Name two (supposed) failings of psychoanalysis by the standards of the traditional model of science. (We listed four, one for each stage of the traditional model.)

2. What model of science did Freud have in mind in developing psychoanalysis?

3. What was Freud's case of Dora about?

4. Name the two ways in which Freud's initial observations of Dora depart from Stage 1 of the traditional model.

5. Name one way in which identifying patterns in the data of psychopathology (as in Freud's account of Dora) is more problematic than is supposed in Stage 2A of the traditional model of science. (We noted two.)

6. How is Stage 2B (explanatory theories) of the traditional model complicated in the human sciences as a whole?

Session 4 Theory testing and the progress of knowledge

In the last session we looked at Freud's methods as illustrated by one of his long case histories, the case of Dora. We saw that Freud's self-image was that of a traditional scientist. He believed, at least at this stage of his work, that psychoanalysis was a science of the mind in much the same sense as physics and chemistry are sciences of matter.

Freud's self-image of himself as a traditional scientist came through in his 'Project'. It was also evident in his actual working methods as he described these in his long report of the case of Dora. These methods, as we saw, mapped on to the first two stages of the scientific process, data gathering, and theory generation (descriptive and causal). At both these stages, though, the particular difficulties of working with the mind led to shifts away from the traditional model of science: the data turned out to be theory laden and goal directed; the patterns identified were normatively rather than just descriptively defined; and Freud's supposedly causal explanations were expressed in terms of reasons.

Completing the story

In this session we will complete the story of psychoanalysis as science by considering Stages 3 and 4 of the traditional picture of the process of science, theory testing, and progress. As with Stages 1 and 2, we will find shifts in Freud's working methods away from the traditional model. In respect of Stages 3 and 4,

indeed, these shifts will be larger and more obvious than for Stages 1 and 2—this is why philosophical attacks on Freud have concentrated on these aspects of his theory.

Even so, this does not show that his theory is *not* scientific. Rather, the changes anticipate recent insights from the philosophy (and history) of science into the nature of science as a whole. This, in turn, however, will not 'prove' that Freud's theory, or indeed psychoanalysis in general, *is* a science; still less will it prove that it offers a correct scientific theory of the mind. But it will, (1) show that the question of whether psychoanalysis is a science is a lot more difficult to answer than the traditional model of science would suggest, and (2) that Freud's difficulties understood now as arising from features of the nature of science as a whole, provide insights into the difficulties that, though less well recognized, are inherent in the nature of psychiatry as a science.

Stage 3 of the traditional model of science: theory testing

'Testing' psychoanalysis could mean one or more of a number of different things. It could mean simply investigating whether it works. This is important in health care. Major issues of resourcing, for example, turn on whether so-called therapies (of all kinds, not just of psychoanalysis) are clinically effective.

The question of clinical effectiveness is independent, though, of testing a particular theory. A therapy might work but for reasons independent of any particular theory of *why* it works—non-specific factors, such as the 'chemistry' between therapist and client, or listening and giving time, could be operative, for example. So what we are concerned with here is testing a specific theory.

Is psychoanalytic theory testable in this sense? Freud certainly thought it was (though with reservations—see the conclusions to this session). In the next reading we look at Freud testing his theory in the clinical context of his work with Dora.

EXERCISE 14	(10 minutes)

Read the five brief extracts from:

Freud, S. (1977). 'Dora' case study. In *Case Histories I*. The Pelican Freud Library, Vol. 8. London: Penguin, pp. 57, 69, 93, 94, 149–150

Link with Reading 11.7 [pp. 57 (1st extract), 69 (2nd), 93 (3rd), 94 (4th), 149–150 (5th)]

In each of these extracts, Freud is testing his theory in a particular way. Make brief notes on: (1) what 'test' you think Freud is using, and (2) whether you think this is sound scientifically. Finally, (3) can you associate Freud's method of testing his theory here with a particular school of philosophical thought about the nature of theory testing in science?

In the first extract (p. 57) Freud appears tentative and cautious about the theoretical significance of clinical information (e.g. '...seems to provide...', para. 3), while being emphatic about his existing theoretical claims: 'psychical trauma...which Breuer and I declared long ago to be the indispensable prerequisite for the production of a hysterical disorder' (para. 3). You will remember from Stage 2 (in the last session) that Freud's causal (or Stage 2B) theory was that such trauma became repressed, pushed into the unconscious; and from there, because repression is only partially effective, it produced the gaps and contradictions in the patient's account of themselves by which, at the descriptive (Stage 2A) level of theory, hysteria was defined (by Freud).

Interpretation as a test of theory

The picture here is thus of the careful scientist cautiously sifting clinical data. This is consistent with the model of scientific medicine advocated by Slater and Roth (1969) (in Session 2). And on p. 69, we find Freud actively testing his theory in the course of his treatment of Dora, by what has become known as 'the interpretation'. According to Freudian theory, because repressed material is never *fully* repressed, it may show itself by the way the patient reacts to being confronted with it. Freud's theory in Dora's case, is that the trauma that (now repressed) has produced Dora's hysteria, was the experience of finding herself, against all her 'better instincts', in love with Herr K.

Thus, Freud notes that Dora had been much preoccupied with Herr K's children and takes this to be a coded expression of her love for him. Her preoccupation with his children, he writes, was evidently a cloak for something else that Dora was anxious to hide from herself and from other people ... she had all these years been in love with Herr K. He puts this to her. And how does she react? He tells us, 'when I informed her of this conclusion she did not assent to it' (p. 69, paras 1,2). One might expect Freud to view this as a problem for his theory. But far from it. Writing later of the same moment in Dora's therapy, he says: 'My expectations were by no means disappointed when this explanation of mine was met by Dora with a most emphatic negative' (p. 93, para. 2). For, 'the "No" uttered by a patient after a repressed thought has been presented to his conscious perception for the first time, does no more than register the existence of a repression and its severity. If the work is continued, the first evidence soon begins to appear that in such a case "no" signifies the desired "yes" ' (p. 93, para. 2).

Consistently, then, on p. 94, referring again to his theory that Dora has repressed her love for Herr K, he indicates that towards the end of the analysis 'conclusive proof' of the correctness of his theory 'came to light'. That this 'coming to light' occurs towards the end of therapy implies that it is some time after his initial assertion that Dora was in love with Herr K. So he has not let Dora off the hook with her denial, and continues to look for evidence for his theory. And 'conclusive proof' comes when, on the last occasion he sees her, he remarks 'The fact is, I am beginning to suspect that you took the affair with Herr K much more seri-

ously than you have been willing to admit so far' (p. 149, para. 1). After checking a minor factual point with Dora, the rest of the exchange is all one-sided, with Freud giving a complex explanation of how Dora had an unconscious wish to marry Herr K, and that effectively she had 'engineered' the proposal from Herr K, and that she interpreted his behaviour as a serious proposal of marriage. Dora remains silent in response. She does not even bother to deny it. As this is the last time she turns up for therapy, Freud never sees her again. But Freud is still not dismayed. His interpretation of this outcome is that Dora and her father are out to sabotage what was up till then a successful treatment, 'just when my hopes of a successful termination of the treatment were at their highest' (p. 150, para. 2). In other words, breaking off the treatment at this crucial stage is conclusive proof of the operation of Dora's repressed love for Herr K.

Interpretation as confirmation

Extracted in this way from Freud's long and detailed case history, his proof may not seem to amount to much. It seems as though repression is a self-fulfilling hypothesis (this indeed is broadly what we will find Karl Popper arguing). However, Freud was not insensitive to evidence. At the time of Dora's case, he was working on his theory of sexual trauma, according to which the aetiology of hysteria always depended on a sexual trauma in early childhood. But Dora's case itself led him to modify the theory of hysteria he had developed with Breuer (Breuer and Freud, 1883–1895). Discussing this, he says, 'I have gone beyond the theory, but I have not abandoned it; that is to say, I do not consider the theory incorrect, but incomplete' (p. 57, n.2). In fact, Freud was prepared to abandon theories when the need arose— he was later to abandon the sexual trauma theory (the Freud/ Breuer model) altogether; and after that he also abandoned its successor, the so-called seduction theory, substituting for it the theory of unconscious wish-fulfilment (involving the process of unfulfilled desire, repression, unconscious fantasy, and wish-fulfilment), which became his mature theory of the production of psychoneurosis.

The approach to 'proving' his theories illustrated by the extracts, moreover, was in fact highly conventional by the standards of his day. Freud was a radical in that he attempted to provide a specific characterization of what the data should be for a science of the mind in terms of interpretations from the utterances and behaviour of the patient. But his view of how one should go about testing a theory is exactly the model adopted by the traditional model of science at the time. On this view, theories are tested by looking for confirming evidence, and the more instances of confirmation that are found, the stronger the claim of the theory to be correct. At the same time, the theory may be modified or developed to reflect the need to explain anomalous data. The overall picture is thus of a progressive accumulation of knowledge.

The idea that theories are confirmed (in Freud's terms 'proved') by evidence was the dominant view at this period. This approach was emphasized, for example, by the verificationism of the Logical Positivist movement in the philosophy of science in the 1920s, a form of scientific inductivism that in turn builds on the empiricist tradition in the philosophy of science.

Confirmation, inductivism, and empiricism

We return to this in Chapter 16, but, briefly, the idea is this. Scientific inductivism holds that deductive logic (the logic of the Aristotelian syllogism) cannot lead us to new knowledge, as the conclusions one draws are already implicitly contained in the premises (this is the 'uniformativeness' of deductive logic, in the sense discussed in Chapter 5). What is needed instead, therefore, is an inductive logic, which allows for the extrapolation from the premises of a conclusion that is conjectural. This means that science, instead of being characterized by the simple enumeration of observations and the identification of the deductions that are possible from the 'raw' data (this was the Aristotelian way of going about science), would be concerned with testing conjectures arrived at inductively. In other words, science would be as much about testing and experiment as about observation, enumeration, and deduction. This empiricist view of science was developed by a line of great British philosophers, including John Locke, David Hume, J.S. Mill, and Bertrand Russell. (An accessible introduction to the empiricist tradition in the philosophy of science is to be found in Losee, 1980.)

Freud, correspondingly, looked for evidence that would provide the data with which to explain the gaps and distortions he had detected in the story told by the patient. So he tested his theories by searching for confirming instances of their correctness. Dora's continued resistance to the idea that she was (or had been as a child) in love with Herr K was evidence in support of Freud's theory (it verified or confirmed his theory) that this traumatic emotion had been repressed. And the more she resisted the stronger the evidence for the theory became.

Popper's attack on confirmation in science

Criticism of the confirmation or verification approach to scientific evidence gathered pace in the 1950s and 1960s and forms the basis of a particularly influential criticism of Freud. The foremost proponent of the main alternative to verification, called 'falsification', was Sir Karl Popper (1902–94), one of the best-known philosophers of the twentieth century.

Sir Karl Popper was born in Vienna but moved to New Zealand in the late 1930s and then to Britain in the late 1940s. In 1949 he was appointed to the Chair in Logic and Scientific Method at the London School of Economics; and in 1976 he became the only philosopher to be made a Fellow of the Royal Society, in recognition of his contribution to scientific understanding (normally only scientists are admitted). In the 1920s Popper attended some meetings of the Vienna Circle (see chapter 12). But he was never a Logical Positivist, and he was uncomfortable with their verificationist views. He subsequently produced a philosophy of science based on a *falsificationist*

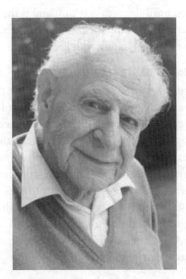

Fig. 11.4 Karl Popper

methodology (Popper, [1934] 1959). His most famous book is *Conjectures and Refutations* (1963).

As part of Popper's Falsificationist model, he demarcated science from non-science in terms of: (1) the validity of the theoretical constructs employed; (2) the predictive power of the theories involved; and, most importantly, (3) the susceptibility of the theories to being *falsified*. On this basis, he argued that psychoanalysis was at best a pseudo-science and at worst nonsense.

Falsification as demarcation

Popper argued that a genuine science always makes itself vulnerable to the risk of being falsified. The best examples of science are thus those disciplines that engage in a process of bold, imaginative conjectures, which are then exposed to attempts to refute them. Good theories survive these attempts, poor theories do not: they are falsified by the evidence produced in the testing process.

Science versus pseudo-science

Instances of confirmation, Popper argued, as distinct from refutation, are ineffective as tests of a theory. On the one hand it can seem that confirmation is available everywhere if you look hard enough. But on the other hand, confirmation of general scientific claims seems to be strictly impossible. Take the case of the claim that it is a natural law that all swans are white. Observing any finite number of white swans does not raise the probability that this law is true because it governs not only all the actual swans but all the swans that might have existed or may still exist and this is not a finite number.

By contrast, falsification seems to be a logically simpler matter: observing a single non-white swan shows that the proposed law-statement is false. A theory that is falsified is conclusively and permanently falsified, whereas a theory that is confirmed has simply survived until the next attempt, and if that fails, its supporters will carry on looking for confirmation elsewhere (this is exactly what we saw happening with Freud).

The emptiness of explanatory power

One of the critical points Popper makes is that the concept of 'explanatory power', a foundation-stone of the traditional view of science, is empty as a criterion of the scientific. Freud, for example, repeatedly emphasized how good psychoanalytic theory is at providing an explanation for almost every phenomenon. Popper, in contrast, says that such claims indicate not the scientific, but the pseudo-scientific: a theory that seems to explain everything explains nothing at all. This is because such a theory could be correct only in terms of the conceptual framework it provides—it is not grounded on any empirical base that would provide an independent source of 'test' data.

The rejection of psychoanalysis as a science

Popper suggests that psychoanalysis is not falsifiable and merely appears to be explanatory. This really does look like Freud's use of interpretation in Dora's case. Dora was 'damned if she did, damned if she didn't'. If she admitted her love for Herr K, Freud's hypothesis was confirmed; if she denied it, his hypothesis was confirmed.

Popper gives his own example of this 'Catch-22' when he asks us to consider how psychoanalysis would respond to an attempt at falsification. We can reconstruct Popper's account to bring out the point he is making with greater force. Imagine a case in which a man pushes a child into the water with the intention of drowning it. Psychoanalysis, claims Popper, would interpret this in terms of an unconscious motivation resulting from repression (he suggests the Oedipus Complex—see Dora's case study, pp. 90–91). The incident would be viewed as a confirming instance of psychoanalytic theory. But now suppose we learn that the original account was wrong—instead of trying to drown the child, the man was in fact attempting to rescue her. Does this falsify psychoanalysis? Of course not, says Popper, for psychoanalytic theory will simply shrug its shoulders and respond that, if the man was not after all trying to drown the child but instead trying to save it, then he had achieved a degree of sublimation of his unconscious motivations. So the incident is still a confirmation of the theory.

Because of this, psychoanalytic theories are not falsifiable. Ergo, psychoanalysis is not a science. Popper suggests it is more like astrology.

Falsifying falsification

The virtue of falsifiability looks to be a good aim for scientific theory and Popper's criticisms of Freud certainly seem justified given the latter's use of the 'interpretation', at least in the case of Dora.

But even Popper-inspired criticism of Freudian theory as unscientific does not amount to a 'knock-down' argument against the scientific status of psychoanalysis. For as we discuss further in Chapter 16, and as Popper himself and his followers came

increasingly to emphasize, falsification itself is not as clear-cut as suggested above. In a nutshell the problem is this: an observation and a scientific theory can indeed come into conflict. But this only falsifies the theory—shows it to be false—if the observation is true. And as will become increasingly clear throughout Part III, observations are themselves fallible claims made on the basis of a number of further theoretical assumptions. It may be that the observation claim itself is false because it presupposes a false theory, involves a false interpretation, or suffers some other kind of defect.

Popper's approach, then, has been very influential in science. But it is not without rivals. In turning now to Stage 4 of the traditional picture—scientific progress—we will outline one such rival account.

Stage 4 of the traditional model of science: scientific progress

The key development in modern understanding of the progress of science came with the publication in 1962 of a rival to Popper's theory in the form of the American historian of science, Thomas Kuhn's, *The Structure of Scientific Revolutions* (1962, 2nd edition, revised and enlarged, 1970).

Kuhn was frustrated by the lack of fit between philosophers' views of science and the historical record of how science actually progresses. The traditional account has it that theories are continuously developed and tested against a steadily accumulating body of data. This model is consistent with both verificationist and falsificationist accounts of theory testing. In practice, though, Kuhn argued, in most scientific research programmes matters are the other way around—instead of theory being

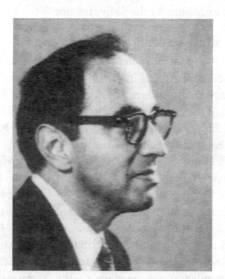

Fig. 11.5 Thomas Kuhn

driven by the data, what we take to be the relevant data are driven by the prevailing theory.

Normal and revolutionary science

Kuhn takes instances from the history of science to make his point. For example, he says, we might ask, 'how was oxygen discovered?'. The way philosophers, particularly inductivists, might answer this question is to draw attention to the support that laws about oxygen gained from the evidence available in the particular historical epoch. Kuhn points out, however, that the chemist who actually managed to prepare a reasonably pure sample of oxygen (Joseph Priestley) believed a wholly false theory about the nature of oxygen (Phlogiston Theory). At the same time, the scientist who developed the substantially correct theory of the nature and properties of oxygen (Lavoisier) was unable to produce a sample of the material. Data and the correct theory were thus largely disconnected.

This is an aspect of the theory ladenness of data that we encountered in Stage 1 of the traditional model (in Session 3). It leads, in Kuhn's historical account, to a picture of the progress of science not as a steady accumulation of ever-better theories, but rather as a kind of punctuated evolution. Kuhn argues that scientific disciplines go through long periods of relative stability in which the current theory (later to be called a 'paradigm'—see below) controls how data are used. In these periods of what he called 'normal science', parts of the prevailing paradigm may be changed in response to new data, but anything that challenges the paradigm itself is treated as an exception.

Every now and again, though, a problem emerges that threatens to destabilize the entire theoretical paradigm. Such a problem is called an *anomaly* by Kuhn. The existence of an anomaly presents an opportunity to construct radical theories that overturn the entire paradigm, ushering in a *revolution*.

Kuhn on normal science

Kuhn takes Popper's view of science to be representative only of 'normal' science. In *The Structure of Scientific Revolutions* (1970, pp. 92–110), Kuhn describes how in a period of normal science, scientists work within a 'disciplinary matrix' (or as it later came to be called, a 'paradigm'—see below, no. 4). Khun's disciplinary matrix has four elements:

1. A set of *symbolic generalizations* that function both to define terms and also as laws (for example, the term for electrical power, the Watt, is defined in terms of the voltage in a circuit multiplied by the current measured in amperes).

2. A set of *metaphysical beliefs* that constitute the model of reality adopted as received wisdom by members of the disciplinary matrix. The atomic model of the structure of the physical universe is an example. The strength of commitment to the model may vary within the group of members, so that it may be conceived of as a heuristic or an ontology, and within a given scientific community various models may coexist even in normal science. The models serve to characterize

what sorts of problem are legitimate for the science to address, what sort of explanations are considered legitimate, and the relative importance of different problems and explanations to the survival of a theory.

3. A set of *values*. These are what bind the diverse theoretical views of a scientific community together, and fundamentally apply to the nature of explanation and prediction, especially in terms of internal and external consistency. Values such as these will be of central importance to a community, others (to do with, say, whether science should be socially useful) will be less central. Even within a community, the expression of values may vary, so that notions such as plausibility, consistency, and simplicity may be applied differently.

4. A set of *exemplars* of scientific problem-solving, in terms of both method and outcome. Originally, Kuhn intended the term 'paradigm' to mean shared exemplars of this kind, but early commentators misread him to mean the disciplinary matrix as a whole, and this is the sense in which the term is now commonly employed (as Kuhn himself acknowledges in the postscript to the 2nd edition of his book).

A disciplinary matrix (or paradigm) thus serves to define the legitimate problems with which science is concerned, and the sort of solutions that are acceptable during a period of normal science (in Kuhn's terms).

Freud as a normal scientist

So how does Freud fare as a normal scientist in the case of Dora? Well, he is clearly operating with a set of *symbolic generalizations* (element 1 of the paradigm)—hysteria, repression, etc. Psychoanalysis, furthermore, offers a series of *metaphysical beliefs* by which its model of reality is defined (element 2): these beliefs include, of course, the unconscious. Then again, the community of psychoanalysts have a shared set of *values* (element 3): as noted earlier, these are often called epistemic values because they define what counts as a good theory—comprehensiveness was one of Freud's explicit values, but clinical effectiveness, as we saw in Session 3, is also important. Finally, the *exemplars* (element 4) of problem-solving methods and outcomes, include, respectively, the interpretation (one of Freud's key methods) and the removal of gaps and inconsistencies in the patient's account of themselves (a criterion of the best of all possible outcomes, a cure).

So Freud, at least at work on Dora, shows the key characteristics of Kuhnian normal science. This, although not absolving him from Popper's charge of producing self-verifying theories, puts a different slant on his reaction to exceptions. The picture Kuhn gives us is of normal science as a stable self-correcting dynamic system. The system allows us to tinker with the parts but not to challenge the whole. This is essentially what Freud is doing. Dora drops out of therapy, still refusing to accept that she was in love with Herr K—is Freud's theory wrong? No, according to Freud, on the contrary, this is clear evidence for resistance. Freud's approach is so meticulous and painstaking that it is easy to get the impression that he is seeking to test his theory of psychoanalysis as a whole (i.e. he is seeking to prove or disprove the whole thing). In fact his method of enquiry is almost entirely focused on the confirmation or disconfirmation of specific details or features of the theory, i.e. the theory as a whole is hardly ever called into doubt. Thus, difficulties of accommodating data into the theory are perceived as requiring extensions to the theory, rather than indicating its falsity. We saw this earlier with his changes to his theories of hysteria (some indeed prompted by the case of Dora). All these changes, however, represented only a series of modifications to the central claim of psychoanalytic theory: that unconscious mechanisms drive conscious experiences and behaviour and can be revealed and rendered intelligible by the psychoanalytic technique of interpretation.

(For an excellent discussion of how evidence apparently contradicting a supposed scientific law is handled in science in general, see Harré, 1993, especially pp. 56–78.)

After Kuhn

Kuhn, as a historian, has radically changed our perception of scientific progress and deeply influenced the development of the philosophy of science. His model has been subject to much criticism. He gives us, in particular, no useful account of just what makes an observation 'anomalous', and hence of precisely how a revolution in science is ushered in. But the basic picture he drew of science as a discontinuous rather than continuous process, and one in which large-scale theoretical structures are largely stable, is nowadays widely accepted.

Freud post-Kuhn

Granted this Kuhnian picture, then, Freud's working methods, and in particular the way he handles potentially disconfirming evidence, are less obviously unscientific than they would appear from the perspective of the traditional view of science. Indeed, as with the other stages of the process of science, Freud at work with Dora, although still struggling to preserve his image of psychoanalysis as a (traditional) science, is in effect displaying the stability of large-scale theoretical structures in science, a stability that has taken philosophers three-quarters of a century to identify and characterize.

Science and psychoanalysis

Taking this and the last session together, therefore, psychoanalysis, at least as illustrated by Freud's account of his work with Dora, has provided us with a window on the nature of science.

The findings at each of the four stages of the traditional view of the process of science are summarized in Table 11.2. This table makes a further important point, namely that, taking the findings at all four stages of the traditional picture together, gives us a *very different picture of the process of science itself*. The traditional model of science envisages data accumulating (at Stage 1) from which theories are developed (Stage 2) and tested (Stage 3), leading to a steadily progressive growth of knowledge (Stage 4). Modern work in the history and philosophy of science has effectively scrambled this neat picture: the data (Stage 1) and the models of testing (Stage 3) are in part driven by the theories (or paradigms) we hold (Stage 2); and as these paradigms are highly stable, requiring something really quite exceptional (an 'anomaly') to shift them, the pattern of scientific progress (Stage 4) is of long periods of normal (or paradigm-stable) science punctuated by occasional revolutions.

This 'modern' picture of science, it is important to add, remains subject to considerable debate. The demarcation problem, in particular, of what marks out science from non-science, remains unresolved. But as with many long-running issues in philosophy, the attempt to characterize science has shown our earlier views to be oversimple, thus leading us to a deeper or more realistic understanding of the subject.

Table 11.2 This table contrasts the traditional and modern views of science. At least in the early stages of his career, Freud perceived himself as a traditional scientist. Yet each of the shifts of understanding represented by the modern view of science are evident in his actual working methods, at least as illustrated by the case of Dora. For each of the Stages 1–4 in this table, Freud, although in effect identifying himself with the left-hand column (i.e. the traditional model of science) in fact displays all the features of the right-hand column (i.e. the model built up by modern work in the history and philosophy of science). Whether or not psychoanalysis is actually a science, it thus provides a window on the nature of science, offering insights that could be crucially important to any 'science of the mind', including psychiatry

Stages of scientific process	Traditional view of science	Modern view of science
1: Data collection (observation)	(i) Atheoretical (ii) and objective	(i) Theory dependent (ii) Contextual (iii) Driven by aims (goal directed)
2A: Theory building—defining patterns	Description—patterns of data (syndromes, in medicine)	Patterns defined also by values (e.g. epistemic values; also good/bad values in the case of pathology)
2B: Theory building—identifying causes	Causes/causal laws, explanation	Reasons/understanding also important
3: Theory testing	Experiment; verification	Experiment; falsification. Anomalies (rather than exceptions) are now needed to overturn normal science
4: Advancement of knowledge	Steady progress by accumulation of knowledge; Unified picture	Punctuated evolution; incommensurable paradigms

Science psychoanalysis and psychiatry

That this deeper or more realistic understanding could be crucially important to us in psychiatry is evident in the ease with which it has been derived from psychoanalysis. To return to the point made at the start of Session 3, the reason this picture is so readily discernible in psychoanalysis is because, to the extent that psychoanalysis aspires to being a science of the mind, it is, at the very least, a *difficult* science—much more difficult, indeed, than a science of, say, the chemical elements.

As we anticipated earlier in this session, then, this is a parallel to J.L. Austin's insight about the negative concept 'wearing the trousers'—it is where our concepts break down or are difficult to apply that we are most likely to gain insights into their full meanings.

We have thus, as we also anticipated, repolarized our assessment of the status of psychoanalysis. We started these two sessions, with psychoanalysis as the 'fall guy' to a psychiatry anxious to align itself with medical science and thus displacing its problems on to psychoanalysis. We should now see psychoanalysis no longer as a defective science but as a difficult subject. And the difficulties it so clearly displays are likely to be important in any discipline concerned with the mind. There are lessons here, therefore, for psychiatry itself.

All of which, as we have several times emphasized, is not to say that psychoanalysis *is* a science. It has indeed been subject to a number of quite different interpretations, many of which are closer to the arts than to science. It is to a sample of these that we turn in the final session of this chapter.

Reflection on the session and self-test questions

Write down your own reflections on the materials in this session drawing out any points that are particularly significant for you. Then write brief notes about the following:

1. What is the equivalent of 'testing' a theory in Freud's clinical work (as illustrated by his report of his work with Dora)?

2. What was the dominant account of scientific 'testing' of theories at the time of 'Dora'? Why did Popper reject this?

3. What was Popper's alternative account of scientific testing? Why did he consider that psychoanalysis failed to provide scientific tests of its theories?

4. Who was Kuhn? What was his key insight into scientific progress?

5. Does Kuhn's account of scientific progress increase or decrease the distance between psychoanalysis and a natural science such as physics? Either way, what does this tell us about the nature of science as a whole? And either way, what does it tell us about the scientific status of psychoanalytic theory?

Session 5 Psychoanalysis without science

In the last two sessions we have looked at Freud at work on the case of Dora. The conclusion we drew was that Freud viewed himself, at least at this stage in his work, as a traditional scientist. Yet many of the difficulties he encountered in trying to develop a science of the mind anticipated the modern view of science. These difficulties made him an easy target for critiques by conservatives in the philosophic and scientific communities, both in his own time and right up to the present day.

But such critiques leave a question hanging. If psychoanalysis is not a science, what is it? To repeat, it remains a matter of dispute whether or not it is a science. But if it proved not to be, what other options are there? Is the choice merely science or nonsense? We will see in this session that there are at least three other options for thinking of interpretative approaches to the mind. These might also serve as alternatives to the account of psychiatry as science that will be discussed in the remaining chapters of this part.

Three ways of being non-scientific

In this session we are going to look at three ways in which psychoanalysis has been presented as being non-scientific: (1) the *hermeneutic reconstruction*; (2) the view that psychoanalysis is a *failed science*; and (3) a recent theory by the English philosopher Sebastian Gardner based on modern philosophy of mind, which treats psychoanalysis as an extension of *ordinary or 'folk' psychology*. We will present these briefly and then consider each of them in more detail. Thus,

- *The hermeneutic reconstruction* is found in the work of certain French and German Continental philosophers, and also a number of psychoanalysts. Notable examples include the French philosopher Paul Ricoeur, the German philosopher, Jurgen Habermas, and the psychoanalyst, G.S. Klein. Below we will read an extract from the work of Paul Ricoeur (1970). The hermeneutic reconstruction treats psychoanalysis essentially as an interpretive exercise based on the imaginative symbolism found in language. It is notable for rejecting the view that psychoanalysis conforms to the traditional view of science. It claims rather that psychoanalysis rests in some way on a radical reconception of science, which owes more to a post-Kuhnian model.

- *Psychoanalysis as a failed science*—we will contrast the hermeneutic reconstruction of psychoanalysis with the view of the American philosopher of science, Adolf Grunbaum, who argues, (1) that the hermeneutic reconstruction of psychoanalysis is flawed, being logically and conceptually at odds with the views of Freud and eminent psychoanalysts, and (2) that psychoanalysis is in fact a *failed* science, in the terms in which Freud conceived science. Grunbaum, who is an arch-conservative in scientific terms (i.e. he rejects both the Popperian and Kuhnian models) comes to the conclusion that other than being a good example of a failed science, psychoanalysis is of no worth whatever.

◆ *Psychoanalysis as an extension of folk psychology*—finally, we will look at the work of the English philosopher of mind, Sebastian Gardner, whose reconstruction of psychoanalysis as an extension of folk psychology is set within Anglo-American analytic philosophy. Gardner (1993) argues that the merits of his reconstruction are independent of the status of psychoanalysis as a science, and thus is immune to Grunbaum's critical onslaught.

Ricoeur, Grunbaum, and Gardner

Before looking at the details of each theory, it will be helpful to set them in context by expanding a little on the line that each takes on psychoanalysis, and how they build on each other.

Paul Ricoeur offers an example of the hermeneutic reconstruction of psychoanalysis in his *Freud and Philosophy* (1970). He implicitly rejects the view that the merits of psychoanalysis as a hermeneutic method rest in any way on its status as a traditional science. Instead, he takes the view that Freud was working with a view of science that presages some of the radical post-Kuhnian models of science. These take science to be strongly relativistic in terms of content and truth—i.e. there is no one world view that represents how the world actually is. Although Freud himself denied that psychoanalysis constituted a *Weltanschauung* in its own right, there have been many who have interpreted it as implying a world view, especially a relativistic one—we all generate our own individual view of the world, and our own individual view may be fundamentally different from that of others. This is the sort of model adopted by some Continental philosophers of science, such as Jurgen Habermas, as well as by many sociologists of science.

Adolf Grunbaum rejects this view in his *The Foundations of Psychoanalysis* (1984). He has accused both Habermas and Ricoeur of offering a 'mythic exegesis of Freud's own perennial notion of scientificity' (Grunbaum, 1984, p. 93). He goes on to argue (1) that psychoanalysis as an interpretive method cannot be separated from psychoanalysis as a science, and (2) that, *contra* Popper, psychoanalysis is indeed a science, but a failed one. Taking (1) and (2) together, then, Grunbaum's view is that psychoanalysis has no credibility as either an interpretive method or a science.

Sebastian Gardner, building on the work of the philosophers James Hopkins and Richard Wollheim (see Reading Guide), has provided a detailed criticism of Grunbaum's position. Like Ricoeur, Gardner has produced a reconstruction of psychoanalysis that relies heavily on the notion that the symbolism of the unconscious has a kind of grammatical structure that allows it to be interpreted. Unlike Ricoeur, however, Gardner belongs to the Anglo-American analytic tradition in philosophy, which is perhaps why he claims that there is no need for a hermeneutic reconstruction along the lines proposed by Ricoeur.

In his book, Gardner (1993) argues (1) that psychoanalysis can be seen as an interpretive extension of ordinary ('folk') psychology, and (2) that this interpretive methodology stands independently of the issue of the scientific status of psychoanalysis. Much

of what is interesting about Gardner's view lies in the way he draws on issues in the philosophy of mind to construct his arguments. We will look at two short extracts from Gardner's book later on in this session, addressing (1) and (2) respectively.

In the concluding part of this session, we will reassess the relevance of the issue of the scientific status of psychoanalysis to modern philosophy of science. We will begin by looking at the work of Paul Ricoeur.

Psychoanalysis and the hermeneutic reconstruction

Ricoeur and the rehabilitation of psychoanalysis

Ricoeur's project was to make psychoanalysis philosophically respectable by showing how it successfully dealt with the problem of interpreting our response to the world and to ourselves. Ricoeur views psychoanalytic method as being primarily concerned with uncovering the hidden meanings behind the explicit story the patient is able to offer of his condition. Another way of putting this is to say that behaviour, experiences, and verbal expression, are inherently symbolic—they are interpretable as conveying meanings that lie underneath the surface—their full meaning is not transparent. This of course ties in closely at least with Freud's account of Dora—you will recall it was the gaps and contradictions in her account of herself with which he was primarily concerned.

Hermeneutics, as we saw in Chapter 4, is an important subdiscipline in Continental philosophy. It is concerned with the individual meaning generated in a specific instance of discourse, and also with the methodology by which the meaning can be

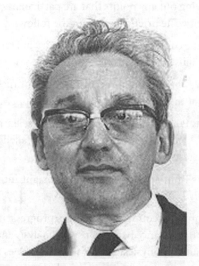

Fig. 11.6 Paul Ricoeur

extracted. Ricoeur thus draws on hermeneutics to develop his view that psychoanalysis is a kind of hermeneutics of the mind. In the next reading we will see Ricoeur (1970) arguing that there is an identifiable progression from the concerns and ideas of Freud's 'Project' to *The Interpretation of Dreams*, a progression that unmistakably bears the hallmark of hermeneutics.

EXERCISE 15 (30 minutes)

Read the extract from:

Ricoeur, P. (1970). Energetics and hermeneutics in *The Interpretation of Dreams*. In *Freud and Philosophy* (trans. D. Savage). London: Yale University Press, Book II, Chapter 2, pp. 87–93.

Link to reading 11.8

As you read this extract, write notes on the following:

1. What two changes does Ricoeur claim to have found between the 'Project' and *The Interpretation of Dreams*, and what are their consequences in terms of Freud's explanatory model?

2. What transformation in Freud's approach is revealed, according to Ricoeur, by these two changes?

3. What are the two tasks of interpretation, and what are their main characteristics?

In this extract, Ricoeur explains how Freud failed to arrive at the true significance of psychoanalysis (as a hermeneutic methodology) because he (Freud) remained, at the time of writing *The Interpretation of Dreams*, committed to the idea that psychoanalysis was a science. Ricoeur makes his point by first exploring his positive thesis: that *The Interpretation of Dreams* represents a shift by Freud away from a strict scientific reductionism to a more liberal theory of psychical processes.

Freud's move away from scientific reductionism

In question 1 of Exercise 15 we asked you to note the two changes in Freud's approach that Ricoeur identified as having occurred between the writing of the 'Project' and the writing of *The Interpretation of Dreams*. We can summarize these as follows:

◆ Whereas, in the 'Project', Freud had offered an energetic model of the psychical apparatus, in which the contents and processes of the mind were to be accounted for in terms of a cause–effect relationship between different 'anatomical' components, in *The Interpretation of Dreams* the psychical apparatus is *wholly* psychical—Freud no longer talks of 'cathected neurones' but in terms of 'cathected ideas' (Ricoeur, pp. 87–88).

◆ Whereas, in the 'Project', Freud's model of the content of the mind involves 'real' representations (i.e. direct representations of reality), driven in a deterministic way (hence the 'machine of

the Project'— Ricoeur, p. 88), in *The Interpretation of Dreams* Freud 'oscillates' between 'real' representations and '*figurative*' representations (Ricoeur, p. 88). By this Ricoeur means that Freud is presenting the mind as operating with a content that requires interpretation because it has more than one possible meaning.

The consequence of these two changes, Ricoeur implies, is that Freud can no longer be taken to be working with a scientific reductionist explanatory framework. Ricoeur argues that these two changes reveal a more 'radical transformation' in Freud's approach, to which we now turn.

The primacy of interpretation over explanation

Question 2 of Exercise 15 asks you to consider what this transformation consists of. It concerns, says Ricoeur, the relationship between explanation and interpretation (p. 88). In the 'Project', this relationship is left unclear—the interpretation of (observed) symptoms guides the explanatory model, but the precise relationship between interpretation and explanation remains unexplored. Indeed, the systematic explanation seems to be independent of the 'concrete work of the analyst' (i.e. what he actually does). But in *The Interpretation of Dreams* the explanation is explicitly 'subordinated' to the interpretation of the patient's utterances. In effect, the explanation in *The Interpretation of Dreams* is an explanation of the process of interpretation, during which the rules of interpretation are 'elaborated'. It is the work of interpretation (of the language in which the patient expresses his experiences) that is primary—without interpretation the 'dream-work' would not be revealed at all (p. 88). The primary issues, Ricoeur is implying, are (1) what the dream content *means*, and (2) what is signified by the symbolic processes operating in dreams.

There is thus an account to be had of the relationship between the exegesis of dreams and what is accomplished (psychically) in dreams. The issue is no longer about what processes are operating in the brain when psychic events such as dreams occur (which was Freud's concern in the 'Project'), but about what is involved in the claim that dreams have meaning.

Freud's positive and negative theses

The thesis that dreams (and other psychic events) have meaning is so central to the development of Freud's ideas that Ricoeur identifies it as advancing on two fronts, each with a positive and a negative claim. The first front is the opposition of the 'meaning' thesis to the view (popular at the time when Freud was writing *The Interpretation of Dreams*) that dreams are 'a waste product of mental life', and hence meaningless. Freud's negative claim here, says Ricoeur, is that this view is untenable: 'to understand dreams is to experience their intelligibility' (p. 88). The second front is the opposition of the 'meaning' thesis to the view (also popular at this time) that the appropriate explanation of dreams is in terms of some organic brain process. Again, Freud's negative claim here, according to Ricoeur, is that this view is untenable. The positive claim is that the content of dreams always affords more than one account, each with its own syntax and semantics, and that these accounts stand in relation to each other rather as two texts, which can be cross-translated (p. 89).

Ricoeur's point here is that, in *The Interpretation of Dreams* Freud is continuing a process, begun in *Studies on Hysteria*, of moving away from the notion that the symptom is a simple 'datum', towards the idea of the symptom as being variously interpretable, the true meaning being arrived at by adopting a method of interpretation appropriate to its content. In fact, in *The Interpretation of Dreams* Freud goes further than this, argues Ricoeur, by offering the view that (1) dreams reveal the 'mixed structure' (of meaning and sign) more clearly than is the case with symptoms (p. 89), and (2) dreams can tell us the meaning of symptoms, thus affording a 'general semiology', which integrates the normal and the pathological (p. 89).

What this results in, says Ricoeur, is an account of the relationship of 'meaning to meaning' (p. 90). But this means that interpretations will always be ambiguous, as more than one interpretation is always possible. We can get around this problem, says Ricoeur, by re-invoking concepts such as 'energy' and 'mechanism', but in a slightly different way than that in which Freud had used them in the 'Project'. The way we can now use them is in terms of dreaming being a mechanism through which certain work is carried out. This view affords a view of interpretation as having two tasks.

The two tasks of interpretation

The two tasks of interpretation are the focus of question 3 of Exercise 15. These two tasks can be summarized as follows:

- *Task 1*: 'discovering the thoughts, ideas or wishes that are 'fulfilled' in a disguised way' (p. 90). This is essentially about the *latent* content of dreams (i.e. their true meaning).

- *Task 2*: 'the "mechanisms" that constitute the dream-work and bring about the "transposition" or "distortion" ... of the dream-thoughts into *manifest* content' (p. 90, italics added). Later, Ricoeur says of the dream-work that it is characterized by 'disguise, distortion, and censorship' (p. 93).

In practice, though, this distinction is academic: what psychoanalysis shows is that the latent content of dreams is the same as the content of wakeful experience. What makes dreams so interesting, and so difficult to understand, is the way in which, in the dream-work, the mind is able to distance the manifest content (the level at which dreams are ordinarily experienced) from the latent content. Dreams are the expression of archaic motivational and mental structures, which are ordinarily repressed. Dream interpretation involves a regression to these earlier psychic mechanisms, and in this regression 'we are led from concepts of meaning to concepts of force by this relation to the abolished, the forbidden, the repressed ... Thus dreams, inasmuch as they are the expression of wishes, lie at the intersection of meaning and force' (p. 91).

Ricoeur thus presents the work of interpretation as achieving the reverse of the dream-work—undoing, in effect, the '*violence*

done to meaning' by the dream-work (p. 92, italics original). In order to understand this, says Ricoeur, we must combine the different discourses of the language of meaning and the language of force.

Combining the discourse of meaning with the discourse of force

Where the dream-work is concerned with rendering the true content of the dream thoughts hidden and inaccessible by disguising them in the manifest content of the dream, so interpretation is concerned with retracing the steps of the dream-work mechanism so as to arrive at the latent (true) content of the dream. This is explicitly about meaning—about the 'displacement of meaning to another region' (p. 91), and this is what is involved in Task 1. But it is impossible to achieve this without recognizing that Task 2 is inextricably implicated in Task 1. Freud, says Ricoeur, recognized this when he realized that in dreams there is a distortion of desires into images (p. 92). In order to understand how this distortion operates, we must 'combine two universes of discourse' (p. 92). For example, we talk of the *fulfilment* of a wish (the discourse of meaning), while at the same time acknowledging that its symbolic manifestation is a consequence of its *repression* (the discourse of force—p. 92). The distortion of meaning that occurs during the dream-work is, to use the same mixed discourse, a '*violence done to meaning*' (p. 92, italics original); likewise, the other two concepts that characterize the dream-work, disguise and censorship, are unintelligible without 'recourse to the same mixed language' (p. 93).

This mixed language, says Ricoeur later in the chapter, can be characterized in terms of the three aspects of regression Freud identifies: (1) temporal regression (the return to archaic mental and motivational structures, p. 91); (2) formal regression (syntax breaks down as logical relations are replaced by pictorial analogues; negation is replaced by the union of contraries in one object; a return to concrete pictorial expression; and the hallucinatory revival of perception—p. 95); and (3) topographical regression (the origin of mental experience and motivations is found in the unconscious rather than the preconscious or conscious—p. 105).

The hermeneutic model of theory change

It is worth considering the way in which Ricoeur's hermeneutic reading of Freud affords a model of theory change. Ricoeur notes later in his chapter that Freud's theory of dream interpretation is 'burdened', just as the 'Project' was, with a major theoretical belief arising from the commitment to a quasi-hallucinatory theory of dreams. This belief is in the reality of the childhood scene of seduction.

In the last session, when discussing Freud and theory change, we mentioned Freud's so-called seduction theory in the context of his shift from the trauma theory of psychoneurosis, through the seduction theory, to the theory of unconscious wish-fulfilment. The sexual trauma theory, which Freud developed in conjunction with Breuer (in the *Studies on Hysteria*, Breuer and Freud, 1883–1895 [1955]), was his main theoretical resource up till 1895, when, in response to the need to situate the trauma earlier and earlier in childhood, Freud changed to the seduction theory (to which he ascribed a major theoretical role between 1895 and 1897). However, for reasons that continue to be debated, Freud dropped the seduction theory in 1897 in favour of a theory that attributed the recovery of memories of childhood seduction to the effects of unconscious fantasy (in effect, the result of the repression of childhood sexual desires). This theory, of unconscious wish-fulfilment as an expression of repressed desires, particularly infantile sexual desires, which he developed progressively from 1897, became the foundation-stone of the mature theory of psychoanalysis.

Ricoeur discusses Freud's move from the seduction theory to the theory of unconscious wish fulfilment later in the chapter (immediately after the extract above on pp. 95–114). He claims that Freud's adoption of the seduction theory (as a replacement for the theory of sexual trauma, which was unable to explain why so many cases of psychoneuroses that Freud treated involved scenes of childhood sexual seduction) occurred because he 'gives the notion of symbol a ... restricted extension' (p. 97), and, furthermore, because he characterized dreams as 'the regression beyond memory images to the hallucinatory revival of perception' (p. 95). In fact, even at the time of writing the *Studies on Hysteria* Freud is already using a conception of a symbol being a 'mnemic substitute for a traumatic scene the memory of which has been suppressed' (p. 97, n.1). But he also sees that 'symbolisation is ... a distortion of the body through fantasies ... [and also] a revival of the primitive meaning of words' (p. 97, n.2).

However, in the first (1900) edition of *The Interpretation of Dreams*, Ricoeur argues, the concept of the nmemic symbol is narrowed so that it is restricted only to cultural stereotypes associated with the sexual symbolization of dreams, and that, moreover, the use of symbolism is totally subordinate to the dream-work, i.e. recourse to symbolization is a product of the dream-work. What happens in subsequent editions of *The Interpretation of Dreams* is that Freud progressively extends the scope of symbolism so that, ultimately, it is much wider than the original sense alluded to in the *Studies on Hysteria*. Ricoeur's account of these developments provides a hermeneutic model for theory change based on the progressive refinement of the conceptual basis of symbolism.

Refining the conceptual basis of symbolism

Ricoeur argues that Freud's belief in 'the reality of the childhood scene of seduction' (p. 95) is what underlies his confusion of 'fantasies with the nmemic traces of real perceptions, in which case topographical regression is a regression to perception and the proper dimension of the imaginary is lost' (p. 96).

As a result, Freud takes symbolism to be a product of the dream-work: 'the dream-work, when the imagination [*Phantasie*] is set free from the shackles of daytime, seeks to give a *symbolic*

representation [*symbolisch darzustellen*] of the nature of the organ from which the stimulus arises and the nature of the stimulus itself' (Freud, 1900, *The Interpretation of Dreams*, SE, Vol. IV, p. 225, parentheses and italics in original, quoted by Ricoeur, p. 99). The effect of taking this view of symbolism is that in 'this manner of "fantasying" the body reduces dreams to a useless activity' (p. 99). What then happens is that, in a series of re-editions (1909, 1911, 1914, 1919, 1921, 1922, 1930) Freud progressively expands the role of symbolism in the dream-work, but always in a subordinate setting (p. 99, para. 2, also n.21). What is happening here is that, in response to the need to account for the fundamental nature of symbolism in unconscious fantasy, Freud draws closer and closer to the view that symbolism is a special form of representation, requiring its own theory, quite separate from its use in the dream-work, so that the dream-work is now presented as making use of symbolism, which has already been accomplished elsewhere (p. 100; the relevant passages in *The Interpretation of Dreams* are to be found in SE Vol. V, pp. 347–349).

Unconscious phantasy and symbolism

According to Ricoeur, Freud by now has arrived at a view of symbolism as being the product of an innate capacity for unconscious fantasy, which finds expression in a general symbolic structure that permeates human culture: 'Wherever neuroses make use of such disguises they are following paths along which all humanity passed in the earliest periods of civilization—paths of whose continued existence today, under the thinnest of veils, evidence is to be found in linguistic usages, superstitions and customs' (*The Interpretation of Dreams*, SE Vol. V, p. 347). In fact, Ricoeur argues, it was almost inevitable that Freud should eventually arrive at this view, for a paragraph appears in the first edition, the ideas of which, although undeveloped at the time, form the nucleus of the later elaboration of a theory of symbolism: 'there is no necessity to assume that any peculiar symbolizing activity of the mind is present in the dream-work ... dreams make use of any symbolizations that are already present in unconscious thinking, because they fit in better with the requirements of dream-construction on account of their representability [*Darstellbarkeit*] and also because as a rule they escape censorship' (SE Vol. V, p. 347, quoted by Ricoeur, p. 100).

However, these theoretical developments allow Freud to restrict the conception of symbolism in dreams in another way. For, if symbolism supplies a set of cultural stereotypes, they have a precise place in a stereotyped code that is then utilized in dreams—their role in dreams is a 'pre-given fact of culture' (p. 101), affording a set of 'stenographic signs' (p. 102). Moreover, this allows Freud to argue that the interpretation of the meaning of symbols is merely an auxiliary function in the wider task of interpreting the dreamer's associations, says Ricoeur (p. 102). Ricoeur's project goes even further than this, in making the claim that the capacity for symbolism allows the creation of symbols as vehicles for new meanings.

Symbolism as the expression of infantile desires and the dawn of meaning

Ricoeur situates this claim in the context of what he argues is the orthodox Freudian view that symbols are nothing but the stereotypical expression of infantile ideas using archaic, culturally stable images. Ricoeur denies that symbolic meanings are merely 'vestiges' having 'nothing but a past' (p. 102).

In order to understand fully what Freud was doing in *The Interpretation of Dreams*, argues Ricoeur, it is necessary to view symbolism as affording 'new symbolic creations that serve as vehicles for new meanings'. Symbolism is thus also the 'dawn of meaning' (p. 102), which must be separated out from, and set against, the indestructible, timeless, infantile desires that are repressed in the unconscious but which seek expression in our fantasies, dreams and neuroses (pp. 103–114).

Ricoeur presents Freud's argument in chapter 7 of *The Interpretation of Dreams* as setting the entire psychoanalytic thesis in the context of our inability to escape from the overdetermination of indestructible, timeless, infantile desires—ultimately, however creative and ingenious is our capacity for inventing new meanings and symbols to express our situation, we are always condemned to remain aware that each of us is a '*Thing*', that is, at the mercy of our infantile desires.

Responses to Ricoeur

Ricoeur has been almost totally ignored by the scientific psychiatric world, and by much of the Anglo-American analytic philosophical world also. This is probably due to his addressing primarily a debate about the nature of hermeneutics rather than the debate about the status of psychoanalysis. This has not prevented the value of his work being recognized by many practitioners of, and writers on, psychoanalysis.

As an exception to the general rule, however, the hermeneutic reconstruction of psychoanalysis has attracted detailed criticism from the American analytic philosopher of science, Adolf Grunbaum.

Psychoanalysis as a failed science

Grunbaum's argument against the hermeneutic reading of Freud

Grunbaum's argument against the hermeneutic reconstruction of Freud is contained within his *magnum opus The Foundations of Psychoanalysis* (1984). This book aims to demonstrate that psychoanalysis (*contra* Popper) *is* a science, but that it is a *failed* science. Moreover, not only is psychoanalysis a failed science, but it can be viewed *only* as a failed science, i.e. there are no good reasons for viewing it as being anything other than a failed science. This rules out a hermeneutic reading of psychoanalysis, and a significant portion of the early part of the *Foundations* consists of a critical analysis of Ricoeur's argument in *Freud and Philosophy* (1970).

The title of one of the passages in Grunbaum's work discussed below ('Does the theory of repression furnish a "semantics of

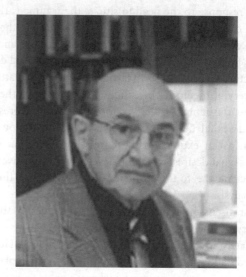

Fig. 11.7 Adolf Grunbaum

desire?" ') indicates that the point at issue is whether Ricoeur's analysis of Freud's concept of symbolism is true to Freud's actual use of the concept. This is itself central to two further issues— whether Freud's use of 'meaning' is consonant with Ricoeur's analysis, and whether Ricoeur's understanding of the mechanism of repression is true to Freud's theoretical model.

Meaning and causation

Grunbaum argues that the presence of what he calls 'thematic affinity' between the conjectured repressed thought and pathological behaviour provides no epistemological grounds for positing a causal link between the two—and yet this is precisely what the hermeneutic thesis requires (pp. 54–55). For if there is no such link, the hermeneutic thesis ceases to have any relevance to the psychoanalytic explanation of behaviour.

We will return to the issue of the relationship between meaning and causes later in this part.

Psychoanalysis and symbolism

Grunbaum begins the passage mentioned above, 'Does a theory of repression furnish a semantics of desire?', by noting that, on the orthodox reading of psychoanalytic theory, symptoms are taken to be the product of a defensive conflict between repressed ideas and the repressing ideas—that is, they are 'compromise formations', and are 'substitutive' (in a functional sense) rather than being semantically meaningful.

Grunbaum relies heavily in this passage on the explication of Freud offered by the English psychoanalyst Ernest Jones in 'The theory of symbolism' (1938). Freud himself did not view

Jones as a first-rank intellectual authority on psychoanalysis (see Grosskurth, 1991, pp. 189–190). However, this alone should not disqualify Grunbaum's reliance on Jones. In fact, Jones offers a distinction that seriously undermines Ricoeur's reconstruction of Freud. The distinction is between symbolism (as a means of disguising content) and sublimation (as a defence mechanism). Jones is categoric that with symbolism, when used in its ordinary psychoanalytic sense, there is no permanent symbolic structure at work (i.e. a general, indestructible cultural significance), and that it is only with sublimation (a less fundamental psychoanalytic notion) that appeal to an independent significance is made (Grunbaum, p. 61).

Grunbaum draws on Jones's distinction to make specific charges against Ricoeur as follows:

◆ *Ricoeur confuses epistemological issues with interpretational problems.* What matters, argues Grunbaum, is the basis upon which one can infer an origin from a trace of its existence (p. 63), in just the way that one infers retrodictively from a footprint in the sand that a human foot created it. Using the 'footprint in the sand' case as an analogy with psychoanalysis, Grunbaum argues that there are two substantive issues here: the interpretation of the footprint as a footprint (rather than, say, a chance impression made by the wind), and the epistemological inference from the footprint to the causal activity of the human foot.

A quite separate, and less substantive, issue concerns whether the footprint was made with the intention of communicating a specific meaning (for example, the footprint could have been traced out by someone as a 'sand-picture'). This issue is less substantive than the first two, because unless the first two are correctly dealt with, the issue of the specific meaning of the footprint cannot be addressed. What Ricoeur does, however, is to assume that the trace (symbolic meaning) qualifies as epistemically significant not on the basis of a *causal* link but a *semantic* one, which remains speculative (see below).

◆ *Ricoeur's notion of a 'semantics of desire' is a misreading of Freud.* Freud's use of 'meaning' as something's having a 'definite causal origin' (Grunbaum, p. 63) is antithetical to Ricoeur's model of symbolic meaning as being vested in the semantic status of a linguistic sign. Ricoeur is guilty, claims Grunbaum, of 'conceptual legerdemain' (p. 64) in assimilating the *cause* of the symbolic meaning of a symptom (in its role as having a substitutive function) with the *semantic* meaning of the linguistic constructions used to refer to it:

The footprint is *not*, as such, a vehicle of communication: it is not a linguistic sign or symbol; it does not semantically stand for, denote, designate, or refer to the past pedal incursion. When a language-user verbalises the inference of this event, then it is the *utterance* of this retrodiction—*not* the trace licensing it!—which has the semantic 'meaning' (p. 64, italics original)

Grunbaum even quotes Freud himself: 'A dream does not want to say anything to anyone. It is not a vehicle for communication' (Freud, SE Vol. 15, p. 231, quoted in Grunbaum, p. 64). This charge is closely connected with the following one.

◆ *Ricoeur conflates the manifestation of symptoms with linguistic designation of them.* The mechanism for this is Ricoeur's adoption of Husserl's view of wish-fulfilment as being a 'signifying intention' rather than the achievement of a desired outcome (Ricoeur, 1970, p. 30).

The problem here is that the susceptibility of a phenomenon to a descriptive semantics does not license the claim that the phenomenon is an expression of this linguistic semantics—yet this is precisely what Ricoeur claims. Ricoeur is assimilating the causal process of symptom formation and expression with the semantic formation and expression of symbolic meaning. The two cannot be legitimately assimilated, because to do so would also legitimate all sorts of other claims to finding 'indirect language' that would, in effect, undermine the whole process of science (for example, one might find oneself interpreting the headache of an undiagnosed subdural haematoma (a blood clot between the brain and the skull) as the expression of some unresolved unconscious conflict). Ricoeur conflates two aspects of the symptomatic expression of partial failure of repression, namely, the manifestation of such repressions, and the linguistic designation of them. The two are conceptually and logically quite distinct, and should not be conflated (Grunbaum, p. 65).

There is much more to Grunbaum's dismissal of Ricoeur's hermeneutic reconstruction—it occupies 26 pages, and is itself contained within a 94-page introduction that seeks to demolish the hermeneutic reconstructions of psychoanalysis offered by Habermas, Ricoeur, and G.S. Klein. A central claim of this critique is that the hermeneutic reconstruction of psychoanalysis is offered as a 'scientophobic' reading of Freud, which neglects his own commitment to the hypothetico-deductive inductivism which he took to characterize traditional science.

Grunbaum, however, is intent on offering a comprehensive demonstration of Freud's failure to comply with his own commitment to the canons of traditional science. As Grunbaum takes himself to have established that the hermeneutic reconstruction of psychoanalysis is neither logically nor conceptually valid, his conclusion is that psychoanalysis is nothing other than a failed science.

Grunbaum's attack on Freud

Grunbaum takes Freud's scientific credentials seriously. He also takes the theoretical claims of psychoanalysis seriously, as being scientific claims, just as he takes great pains to undermine the claims made by hermeneutic interpretations of psychoanalysis. This is to ensure that, if psychoanalytic theory fails as a scientific theory, it will not survive as *any* sort of theory (at least Popper was content to let psychoanalysis survive as a non-scientific theory!).

Grunbaum's *The Foundations of Psychoanalysis* has probably had more influence on the reputation of psychoanalysis as a science than any other published criticism. Its arguments are extremely complex, and the prose is dense and detailed. However, in 1988 Grunbaum published a précis of his argument, and it is to this that we turn in the next reading.

EXERCISE 16

Read the extract from:

Grunbaum, A. (1988). Precis of *The Foundations of Psychoanalysis*. In *Mind, Psychoanalysis and Science* (ed. P. Clark and C. Wright). Oxford: Basil Blackwell, pp. 10–13

Link with Reading 11.9

◆ Try to get a feeling for his approach from the start of Grunbaum's Precis of *The Foundations of Psychoanalysis*.

Grunbaum's rejection of Popper's critique

Grunbaum rejects Popper's claim that psychoanalysis is not testable empirically. Grunbaum and Popper disagree on two levels, however. First, they disagree in their interpretation of Freud's clinical methodology, and hence over the theoretical claims that followed from it. Second, they disagree over the correct methodology of theory testing in science. On both grounds, argues Grunbaum, Popper's view is flawed.

Popper interprets Freud's clinical methodology as giving rise to the theory of psychoanalysis (by a process of inductive logic), and argues that the confirmatory data necessary to support the theory were already defined by the theory, and therefore structured the expectations of the researcher to find just such data in the form of clinical observations ('interpretations'). This rendered psychoanalysis immune from falsification—it would always be the case that confirmatory data could be found, and potential falsifiers discounted on the basis of alternative interpretations. Given this, argues Grunbaum, it is a mere corollary 'that clinical data . . . cannot serve as a basis for genuine empirical tests' (p. 10). So why did Popper bother to target psychoanalysis? Grunbaum claims the real target was scientific inductivism, the method of inquiry first set out by the English philosopher and forerunner of the British empiricist tradition, Francis Bacon, in the early seventeenth century. Grunbaum is an arch-conservative who adheres to strict neo-Baconian principles of science.

Now, Popper's attack on inductivism fails, argues Grunbaum, because Popper is very selective about characterizing science: as Popper himself admits, the *evidence* that would falsify physics (generally cited as the most rigorous of sciences) is theory laden (because it must be specifiable using the terms of the theory), and, as such, any falsifications obtained are 'revokable' (p. 12—this means simply that if one revises the theory one can also downgrade the significance of any falsifying evidence). In this, physics is no different from psychoanalysis, and the fact that Freudians continue to discount falsifying evidence is a quite separate issue from the irrefutability of the theory they champion (p. 12).

In fact, Grunbaum goes on to argue, psychoanalytic methodology does afford a means of falsifying psychoanalytic theory empirically (i.e. extra-clinically), and on this basis, Popper is wrong about psychoanalysis being irrefutable, and, further, cannot use its supposed 'irrefutability' as a weapon against scientific inductivism—for scientific inductivists would agree with him on the invalidity of clinical validations of psychoanalysis, and on the need for extra-clinical testing.

Freud's Necessary Condition Thesis

Grunbaum's argument in support of the testability of psychoanalytic theory is drawn from the words of Freud himself. Freud had long been sensitive to charges that he used illicit suggestion on patients in order to get the results he desired. In 1917 he gave a lecture in which he addressed precisely these charges ('Analytic therapy', SE XVI, 1963; also in Pelican edition, Vol. 1, 1973). In this essay, Freud claims that it is not the conscious responses of the patient that may be cited as evidence (and which may be influenced by suggestion) but responses arising from the unconscious, and that arise only if the analyst's conjectures 'tally with what is real in him' (SE XVI, 1963 p. 452; Pelican Vol. 1, p. 505).

Grunbaum interprets this 'Tally Argument' to start from a 'bold premise' comprised of 'two causally necessary conditions' (p. 14):

1. that the psychoanalytic method is the *only* means of giving the patient a correct insight into (unconsciously generated) neurosis; and,

2. that this correct insight is causally necessary for the 'durable cure' of his neurosis: it should be noted that Freud himself (as one might expect) does not use the words 'durable cure', although he does employ phrases that might be interpreted as implying them, e.g. 'Through the overcoming of these resistances the patient's life is permanently changed, is raised to a high level of development and remains protected against fresh possibilities of falling ill' (Freud, 1963, SE XVI, p. 451; Pelican Vol. 1, p. 504).

The two parts of the premise of the Tally Argument constitute what Grunbaum calls the *Necessary Condition Thesis* (NCT) and it is upon the NCT that he bases his argument for the falsifiability of psychoanalytic theory. The NCT amounts to the claim that, if psychoanalytic techniques are correctly used, and if the analyst is able to present to the patient an interpretation that tallies with what is real in him, then the patient's symptoms will disappear, and, moreover, it is *only* psychoanalytic *theory* that can afford such an interpretation (i.e. psychoanalytic theory is the only theory that can account for the success of clinical psychoanalysis in gaining access to the unconscious in a therapeutically effective way).

The conclusions of the Tally argument

Grunbaum takes the Tally Argument to constitute the basis upon which Freud wanted psychoanalysis to qualify as a science. Further, Grunbaum argues that, if the NCT is granted, then certain conclusions can be drawn from the Tally Argument, provided it can be demonstrated that psychoanalysis does indeed achieve successful cures (p. 15).

If the patient has been cured, then, Grunbaum claims, it is reasonable to conclude that the interpretations offered to the patient at the end of treatment must have been correct (or at least nearly so); that the therapeutic success of psychoanalytic treatment can be cited as evidence for the correctness of both the clinical methodology and of the theory itself.

Further, therapeutic success indicates that the clinical data provided by 'successfully treated' neurotics are valid; and, as psychoanalysis is the only means of treating unconsciously generated neurosis, then its successes can be accepted as evidence of its correctness without the need for controlled trials or statistical comparisons.

Grunbaum's reconstruction of Freud's argument for the scientific status of psychoanalysis is impressive. The NCT effectively guarantees the validity of clinical evidence. Unfortunately, Grunbaum claims, Freud later rejected the NCT, calling the validity of clinical evidence into doubt, although he (Freud) never explicitly acknowledged this.

Freud's rejection of the Necessary Condition Thesis

Grunbaum argues (p. 16) that in 1926 Freud, in effect, rejected the NCT. This argument rests on two concessions made by Freud:

1. it was at least possible that unconsciously generated neurosis could spontaneously resolve; and,

2. that psychoanalysis, far from being indispensable to the cure of such neuroses, merely accelerated a spontaneous resolution (Freud, SE, Vol. XX, p. 154).

Grunbaum claims that later still, in 1937, Freud stated that a successful psychoanalysis does not guarantee that the same symptoms will not recur, and is not protection at all against the emergence of different symptoms—the effect of psychoanalysis is reduced to that of a palliative.

If this story is correct, Grunbaum suggests, it follows that (1) Freud cannot continue to claim that his clinical data are free from illicit suggestion; (2) the clinical data afforded by psychoanalytic theory are unreliable; and (3) the method of psychoanalysis is rendered dubious, so that successful treatment cannot be taken as evidence for the efficacy of the treatment—the resolution of symptoms could be spontaneous and have nothing to do with the treatment (p. 17).

Grunbaum's conclusion

Grunbaum draws the following conclusions from the argument he has offered. First, if the clinical data of psychoanalytic theory are unreliable, then some other means must be found of testing both theory and therapy. Extra-clinical methods could be used (statistical comparisons, control studies), but there will still remain the issue of how to distinguish clinically a genuine psychoanalytic success from a placebo effect.

Grunbaum concludes that any supporting evidence for the correctness of psychoanalytic theory or therapy derived from the clinical setting alone must be judged extremely weak; that proper testing of theory and therapy must be extra-clinical; and insofar as psychoanalysis is scientific, its standing at present must be judged precarious, on the basis of the lack of evidential support. But, despite all this, Grunbaum is emphatic that Freud, at least up till 1926, was a good scientific researcher, a conscientious seeker after truth, receptive to objections, and responsive to negative evidence.

Assessment of Grunbaum's arguments

Grunbaum's critique of psychoanalysis has been very influential—he is probably, at least in part, responsible for the decline in the clinical and institutional status of psychoanalysis in the USA over the last 20 years. He has, however, not had it all his own way. He has been criticized by contemporary philosophers of science for being narrow in his analysis, for misinterpreting Freud, and for imposing an ideology of science that is outdated. Grunbaum's is an ultra-orthodox view of science based on neo-Baconian canons, with which probably no contemporary science would comply! For example, physics, traditionally taken as the most rigorous of sciences, would have problems complying with Grunbaum's view of objectivity, which is too realist for contemporary particle physics.

Thus, Frank Cioffi, in a paper entitled 'Exegetical myth-making' in *Grunbaum's Indictment of Popper and Exoneration of Freud* (Cioffi, 1988, pp. 61–87), mounts a vigorous critique of Grunbaum. Cioffi's general criticism is that Grunbaum has simply not taken enough care to read through Freud's texts so as to arrive at a comprehensive knowledge of Freud's arguments and to interpret them correctly.

More specifically, Cioffi argues that Grunbaum's reconstruction of Freud's arguments in the form of the Tally Argument is quite simply wrong. Grunbaum does not recognize that Freud was not in a position to make any sort of claim of comparative therapeutic superiority (pp. 75–76), since Freud had no facilities to conduct comparative studies. Further, Grunbaum takes Freud's claim that he was responsive to negative evidence at face-value, when Freud in fact did not acknowledge the challenges mounted against him by his contemporaries such as Aschaffenburg, Kraepelin, and Janet.

In addition, Cioffi argues that Freud could not possibly have adopted the premises of the Tally Argument (which support the NCT) as to do so would have required him to explain how it was possible for him to make claims on the basis of the successful treatment of the 18 patients he cites prior to his rejection of the seduction theory, while the later Oedipal theory, which eventually supplanted the seduction theory, should be assessed on a quite different basis. For if they both achieved therapeutic success, then clearly therapeutic success cannot be used as a criterion of correctness of the theory employed; and, even worse, the claim that *only* psychoanalysis can provide a cure is plainly incoherent. Cioffi concludes that Freud could not possibly have supported the arguments Grunbaum assigns to him.

In fact, Freud never relied on therapeutic success as a criterion of the correctness of his theories, Cioffi argues. And if he did, one would expect his followers up to the time of his supposed abandonment of the NCT to also have cited therapeutic success as a validation of theory—but in fact this was not so, and Cioffi cites a list of Freud's influential followers who recorded their views on the subject, none of whom are investigated by Grunbaum.

The assumptions of modern psychoanalysis

Grunbaum could also be criticized for failing to acknowledge that psychoanalysis has changed a great deal since Freud. By contrast, an authoritative and balanced reassessment of Freud's work is given by the English psychiatrist and psychoanalyst, Anthony Storr, in his book *Freud* (1989). Thus, Storr notes that 'Modern psychoanalysts have recognized the difficulty of defining the exact nature of psychoanalysis' (p. 115). He then gives five basic assumptions that he says are 'perhaps as far as anyone can go today in trying to define what beliefs and theories are held in common by those calling themselves psychoanalysts' (p. 117). The five basic assumptions are:

- Psychoanalysis is a general psychology applicable to normal as well as abnormal cases.

- Psychoanalysis is primarily concerned with the individual's subjective experience, accountable in terms of a 'mental apparatus' that receives stimuli from the external world and the subject's own body; overt behaviour is of only secondary importance.

- Psychoanalysis is a theory of adaptation in terms of how the subject ('or ego') responds to the inner and outer world. Freud's 'Nirvana principle' (which stipulates that the aim of the psyche is to achieve the discharge of tension) has largely been replaced by a model based on the management of equilibria between conflicting stimuli or motivations.

- Psychoanalysts accept Freud's doctrine of determinism applying to mental activity, while also accepting that the aim of psychoanalysis is to increase the control individuals exercise over their lives.

- While psychoanalysts assume that 'some aspects of mental life are inaccessible to consciousness' (p. 116), some of these may surface 'in dreams, neurotic symptoms, slips of the tongue, and states of mind encountered in mental illness, most can only be brought into consciousness by the special techniques of recovery and interpretation that are an integral part of the psychoanalytic process' (pp. 116–117).

While Storr would not claim that this view is unproblematic, its claim to scientific status is strictly limited, being confined to the determinism of mental activities. There is no claim here that either the terms in which psychoanalytic interpretation is conducted, or the clinical methodology, or even the general theory of psychoanalysis, are scientific, at least in the terms of the traditional model as interpreted by Grunbaum.

The view that psychoanalysis should be judged on its merits in the context of present day standards of intellectual inquiry has been made philosophically respectable in Anglo-American analytic philosophy by the London-based philosophers Richard Wollheim and James Hopkins (see their collection, Philosophical

Essays on Freud, in the Reading Guide). Building on their work, the English philosopher Sebastian Gardner, of University College, University of London, has offered a critique of Grunbaum as well as an analytic-philosophy inspired reconstruction of psychoanalysis.

Psychoanalysis as an extension of folk psychology

Gardner's reconstruction of psychoanalysis

Gardner presents his project as aiming to integrate the debate about the status of psychoanalysis with the wider philosophical debate about the status of psychoanalysis as an epistemological enterprise as well as a theory of the mind. His starting point is an issue that has long troubled philosophers: what is the cause of irrationality? He argues that psychoanalysis offers the best prospect for an explanation of irrationality

Central to Gardner's reconstruction is an account of the symbolizing capacity of the mind. In the next reading (Exercise 17) we will look at an extract from Gardner's (1993) book in which he explains how this symbolizing capacity is exercised. In this passage Gardner is concerned to clarify what can be said actually to happen in this symbolizing activity. He distances himself in particular from the reading of symbolization taken by the French Continental philosopher, Jean-Paul Sartre. Sartre, like Ricoeur, takes *intentionality* as being a capacity of the unconscious. Gardner wants to stay closer to Freud's explicit view that the unconscious does not itself exercise intentionality (i.e. it is not trying to communicate). Instead, Gardner offers us a view of psychoanalysis as being an extension of ordinary (or 'folk') psychology, in that it provides an interpretive methodology that enables us to understand the symbolism we intuitively find in dreams, phantasy, and so on.

The passage begins with a discussion of how unconscious wish-fulfilment can be said to work—and this is where resort to a concept of symbolism is necessary, in the form of the operation of *censorship*.

EXERCISE 17   (30 minutes)

Read the extract from:

Gardner, S. (1993). *Irrationality and the Philosophy of Psychoanalysis*. Cambridge: Cambridge University Press, pp. 131–137

Link with Reading 11.10

As you read, write short notes on the following:

1. What characterizes Gardner's 'Symbolism I' and why does it lend itself to Sartre's charge of self-deception?

2. What are the four parts of Gardner's reconstruction of unconscious symbolism in 'Symbolism II'?

3. Why does Gardner reject the notion of an innate symbolizing function?

The structure of unconscious symbolism

In 'Symbolism I' Gardner starts with the assumption that the content of the unconscious is structured—hence the comment about the ability of (unconscious) wishes to recover representations from memory. In addition, in order to account for the symbolic content of dreams, we must import a notion of *censorship*, the idea that the true meaning of dreams is disguised. This, along with the assumption about the unconscious being structured, licenses the claim that unconscious processing involves 'syntactically characterisable' operations (p. 131).

Gardner then makes a distinction that is crucial: in order to make sense of the product of these operations as being 'bearers of meaning' (notice the similarity to Ricoeur's terminology here) we must make a distinction between *intra*-psychic symbolic relations (between different mental contents) and *extra*-psychic symbolic relations (between a mental content and an external object) (p. 132). What is interesting in the following passage is the way in which Gardner adopts what Dennett would call an 'intentional stance' in saying that 'desire assumes a disguise'. Gardner immediately softens this claim by saying that 'desires are 'plastic' and able to mutate by changing their object' (p. 132).

Gardner wishes to make clear why some writers, for example the French existentialist philosopher Jean-Paul Sartre, but also Ricoeur, have imputed an intentionality to the unconscious, which is not licensed by Freud's actual texts. For example, Sartre charges Freud with offering simply a clever (but wrong) account of self-deception. Gardner wants to show that this is incorrect, and offers a reconstruction of the symbolic mechanism in order to achieve this.

Gardner's reconstruction of symbolism

The issue here, according to Gardner, is how psychoanalysis can account for the unconscious being inaccessible to ordinary (i.e. non-psychoanalytic) thinking, yet not involve any functional partition of the mind (to accommodate the hidden censor) of the sort posited by Sartre. Also at issue here (although not explicitly acknowledged by Gardner) is the claim of psychoanalysis that it alone can render the unconscious transparent (which is precisely the claim made by Ricoeur).

Gardner's reconstruction of unconscious symbolism has four aspects.

1. *The symbolic mechanism exploits the prepositional/propositional border.* The substitution of an (unconscious) wish for a (conscious) desire occurs at the border between the unconscious and the conscious; however, this is also the border between prepropositional and propositional thought, where the substitution of the object of desire for the (symbolic) object of the wish occurs. No rational thought is required for either substitution (pp. 133–134).

2. *Desire involves the exercise of certain dispositions that are 'object-hungry'.* To have a desire is not necessarily to have an object appropriate to the satisfaction of that desire, although the disposition to satisfaction will mean that the desire will search for an object. However, this 'object-hunger' relies on no rational process, although it may be rendered rationally intelligible by psychoanalytic explanation. Desire is therefore 'plastic' in that it may change its object without rational motivation (pp. 134–135).

3. *The symbolic mechanism provides a path to the phenomenology of the object.* Rather than take a semantic path from symbol to object (like Ricoeur), Gardner opts for a phenomenological path: it is the 'shared phenomenology' between symbol and object that allows the symbolic mechanism to substitute the symbol for the object (p. 135).

4. *The apparent relation of meaning between symbols and objects is illusory.* Conceding nothing to Sartre (or Ricoeur), Gardner argues that the constant conjunction of symbol with object, and its role in the satisfaction of a desire (or wish) is insufficient justification for positing '*rules of meaning*' (p. 136, italics original), and, by implication, a semantics of desire (on the Ricoeurian model). All that can be posited is a symbolic gratification; however, this process is a causal one, and may fail if the symbol is inadequate. There is no disposition in dreams to communicate meaning. None the less, the shared phenomenology of symbol and object creates in the subject 'some sort of bond of comprehension', which may remain entirely implicit (p. 136).

The arguments offered by Gardner here are aimed specifically at undermining the claim (made both by existentialists such as Sartre and hermeneuticists such as Ricoeur) that there exists a systematic relationship between the system of symbolic meanings and the meanings to be found in ordinary language. He does this because he rejects the notion of there being an innate symbolizing function.

Gardner's rejection of the innate symbolizing function

Gardner goes on to argue, in a short section after the extract above, that psychoanalytic theory gives no credence to the view that there is some kind of innate symbolizing function necessary to support the claim (of the hermeneutic reconstructivists, and of Ricoeur in particular) that there is an innate capacity for unconscious fantasy, which finds expression in a general symbolic structure that permeates human culture, and gives rise to a motivational structure of indestructible desires. Still less is there a quasi-platonic system of entities (such as Jungian archetypes), which inform the unconscious and guide fantasy.

Interestingly, in arguing for this view, Gardner quotes exactly the same passage from Freud as Ricoeur used when arguing the opposite: 'there is no necessity to assume that any peculiar symbolizing activity of the mind is operating in the dream-work' (SE Vol. V, p. 347, quoted in Gardner, p. 137). This is possible because, where Ricoeur takes the only possible explanation for this state of affairs to rest on the presupposition of an innate symbolizing function, on the basis that there is a systematic, meaningful, relatedness between the symbolic and the non-symbolic, Gardner takes the view that it is not meaning that drives the relation between symbolic and non-symbolic, but causes. This licences a diametrically-opposite use of the quotation from Freud.

Gardner's argument about symbolism is part of a wider argument that centres on the issue of the explanatory relation between reasons and causes, which takes us right back to the debate about the relatedness of reasons and causes this time as applied to Freud. (We consider the much-contested relationship between reasons and causes later in this part (Chapter 15) and again in detail in Part V: the issues are related to those considered in Part II about the relation between meanings and causes.).

Reasons and causes are mutually inextricable

The case Gardner puts forward is that psychoanalytic explanation involves accounting for the causal efficacy of psychological properties. However, the only characterization of psychological properties we can give is 'profoundly dependent on semantic characterisations' (p. 138).

The point here is that our understanding of ordinary psychology commits us to accepting the causal efficacy of ordinary psycholog-ical semantics. For example, consider your psychological response to being verbally abused by a stranger. If you learn that the stranger is motivated by hatred for you, your response will be very different from your reaction if you are told that the man verbally abusing you is suffering from schizophrenia with delusions of persecution. Your response is different because you draw different conclusions about your abuser's motives and intentions in each case.

Gardner's proposal is that we need 'an alternative way of expressing the distinction between causal explanation in terms of reasons for action, and causal explanation involving only the notion of a weaker connection of content' (p. 138). Success in this enterprise would provide what Gardner aims for: an account of 'relations of meaning that are not rational, of the sort that psychoanalysis requires' (p. 139).

Such an account can proceed quite independently of the issue of whether psychoanalysis is a science, as it is conceptually licensed by the fact that ordinarily we can render our thought and behavi-our intelligible; and psychoanalysis, as an extension of ordinary ('folk') psychology, renders many of our apparently irrational instances of thought or behaviour intelligible. However, there is a need to address at least one of the charges made by Grunbaum, that Freud's interpretive methods, particularly free association, do not warrant an inference to unconscious causation.

Gardner's critique of Grunbaum

Grunbaum's specific charge against psychoanalysis is that the-matic affinity between conjectured repressed ideas and behaviour is insufficient to warrant the claim that there is a causal link between the two. Later in his book, Grunbaum uses this charge to support a demand for extra-clinical testing of psychoanalysis, on the grounds that only such testing is likely to reveal the extent of empirical support for the theory.

Psychoanalysis relies on the same presuppositions as ordinary psychology

Gardner's response is subtle but powerful. It may be summarized thus: there are presuppositions in the ordinary psychology which informs scientific psychology, which licence the general inference that, if there are 'affectively-charged connections of content' linking mental phenomena which are psychologically proximal, then there is a 'causal influence' between the two. The presuppositions by which the general inference is licensed are 'a priori considera-tions of mental order', without which 'the alternative is to view the mind as an atomised jumble of ideas, which would contradict its identification *as* a mind' (p. 143, italics original).

Gardner is saying, in effect, that the same preconditions for the positing of minds (in general) in ordinary psychology apply to psychoanalysis. And if the presuppositions of ordinary psychology (which in any case supply many of the assumptions of scientific psychology) are acceptable, then the presuppositions of psycho-analysis should be equally acceptable.

On this view, then, psychoanalysis is conceptually and logically continuous with ordinary psychology. If ordinary psychology is conceptually prior to scientific psychology, then so is psychoanalysis.

Psychoanalysis and extra-clinical testing

This is exactly why many theorists and practitioners of psycho-analysis view it as being immune to the results of extra-clinical testing. Such a view rests on the presupposition that extra-clinical testing will not provide evidence for the validity and veracity of psychoanalytic constructs or theory, because psychoanalytic theory is validated by its conceptual coherence.

Conclusions

The main focus of this session has been on psychoanalysis as a non-science, approached through the work respectively of Paul Ricoeur, Adolf Grunbaum, and Sebastian Gardner.

Gardner's work shows us that the debate about psychoanalysis in general should not be about what Freud said or did, but about the nature of psychoanalytic explanation and its ability to render intelligible the human mind. To do this we need to take into account the many developments in psychoanalytic theory and practice since Freud's death, including advances in the scientific and clinical testing of psychoanalytic theory and method.

In much of the rest of this part we will be concerned mainly with issues raised by scientific psychiatry and drawing on the philo-sophy of science. Non-scientific interpretations of Freud, however, provide a model for a different and potentially fruitful approach to the disciplines concerned with mental health: as interpretative ventures rather than aspiring to law-like aetiological theories.

The fact that such a different approach exists in no way dimin-ishes the importance of re-assessing the status of Freud as a scientific thinker. As we have seen in Sessions 3 and 4, Freud, at least at the time of Dora, was attempting to create a new science of the mind, and this science of the mind, if a science at all, turned out to be a very *difficult* science. It is the difficulties in a science of the mind that we will explore in more detail in subsequent chapters.

Reflection on the session and self-test questions

Write down your own reflections on the materials in this session drawing out any points that are particularly significant for you. Then write brief notes about the following:

1. Whose name is associated particularly with the hermeneutic reconstruction of psychoanalysis? How is this reconstruction related to debates about its scientific status?

2. What is emphasized in hermeneutic accounts of science generally.

3. Name a philosopher recently associated with a determined and sustained attack on psychoanalysis as a science. What line of argument is adopted?

4. What is 'folk psychology'? Which philosophers have recently explored the idea that psychoanalysis is properly understood as an extension of folk psychology?

Conclusions: a science fit for psychiatry

We started this chapter by asking whether psychiatry is science or non-sense. Our attempt to answer this question has taken a long route; from the 'logical geography' of science, our everyday conception of what it is to be scientific (in Session 1), to a more detailed look at how this conception is reflected in the self-image of psychiatry (illustrated, in Session 2, by the Introduction to Slater and Roth's classic textbook of psychiatry, *Clinical Psychiatry*, and the American DSM); and from there to an in-depth exploration of competing views about the scientific status of psychoanalysis (in Sessions 3–5).

From a two-valued to a three-valued question

In following this route we have highlighted the need for deeper understanding of the nature of science, and hence of what is involved in asking whether a given subject, such as psychiatry or psychoanalysis, is scientific. We have done this by anticipating some of the discussions that will be set out more fully in the rest of this part.

We have also seen, notably in the last session, that science is not the only way of 'making sense'; hermeneutics (with Ricoeur, for example), everyday 'folk psychology' (the basis of Gardner's approach from the philosophy of mind), and other disciplines, offer alternatives. Hence our original two-valued question has become a three-valued question: is psychiatry science, non-sense, or, in part at least, non-science?

This three-valued question, it must be said, flies in the face of the standard medical model. For Slater and Roth, you will recall, psychiatry was either a science or it was nothing. Yet, as a way of making sense, science itself, as we have found in the last three sessions, is considerably less transparent than has traditionally been supposed.

Freud's (scientific) difficulties with Dora

This came out clearly from our extended examination of Freud himself actually at work on one of his earlier cases, the case of Dora. At this stage in his career Freud was with Slater and Roth in believing that psychoanalysis was either a science or it was nothing. Hence we find Freud moulding his work with Dora to the four stages of the traditional conception of science, gathering data (Stage 1), building theories (Stage 2), testing his theories (Stage 3), and advancing knowledge (Stage 4).

Closer examination of each of these stages showed their application to Freud's work to be highly problematic. This, however, was not (as traditionalists about science have supposed) evidence that Freud, let alone psychoanalysis in general, is non-scientific. For the problems turned out to anticipate difficulties in the nature of science that modern philosophy of science has only lately, towards the end of the twentieth century, fully recognized. If Freud's 'data' are, often, 'theory dependent', so, modern philosophy of science has shown, are scientific data in general; if Freud's theories are driven by epistemic values, and if his 'causes' often look like 'reasons', so too do those in other areas of science; if his theory testing is less open to falsification than a traditional view of science (*a la* Popper) would require, this is now known to be a feature of all normal (*a la* Kuhn) science; and if psychoanalysis has shown no steady accumulation of knowledge, so, too, is the progress of all sciences now recognized to be one of punctuated, rather than of continuous, evolutionary change.

Psychoanalysis and a science fit for psychiatry

Some have taken all this to mean that science itself is, after all, non-sense. The point, though, is rather that, as a way of 'making sense', science is now recognized to be a far more problematic activity than the traditional conception (including our four-stage 'process of science') lead us to believe. The problems have been (relatively) inapparent so long as science was concerned with (relatively) simple sciences. As science now begins to tackle more complex areas, however, the difficulties, too, are becoming more apparent. This is true not just in traditionally 'soft' areas of science—such as psychoanalysis—but also at the cutting edge even of the hardest of hard sciences, theoretical physics (as we illustrate in the last session of the next chapter). Hence, if there are difficulties (as Freud found) in moulding psychoanalysis on to a traditional conception of science, so much the worse for the traditional conception of science.

Our choice of psychoanalysis for a case study introducing the range of topics covered by the philosophy of science, was driven partly by the richness of the philosophical literature in this area, but also by the fact that psychoanalysis has to some extent been treated as the 'fall guy' by psychiatry in its attempts to establish itself as a (traditionally conceived) medical-scientific discipline. Psychiatry, under attack from physical medicine for being 'unscientific', has sought to displace criticism on to psychoanalysis. This chapter has argued, consistently with our opening reference in Session 1 to J.L. Austin's aphorism of the negative concept 'wearing the trousers', that psychoanalysis, whether it be science, non-science or indeed plain non-sense, offers a window on the difficulties involved in developing a science in this, perhaps *the* most difficult of areas, a science not just of the mind but of disordered minds.

Reading guide

Introductions to philosophy of science and applied work on psychiatry

There are a growing number of introductions to the philosophy of science. Among more recent ones are: Bird (1998) *The Philosophy of Science*, Chalmers (1999) *What is This Thing Called Science?*, and Ladyman (2002) *Understanding Philosophy of Science*. The last is an informal guide, some of it written in dialogue.

Chapter 3 in William James Earle's (1992) *Introduction to Philosophy* provides a valuable synopsis.

Applied philosophical work on the scientific aspects of psychiatric diagnosis include: Sadler, J.Z., Wiggins, O.P., Schwartz, M.A. (ed.) (1994) *Philosophical Perspectives on Psychiatric Diagnostic Classification*. (See also Chapter 13.)

A useful collection of classic papers on the philosophy of science is Richard Boyd, Philip Gasper, and J.D. Trout (eds.) (1991) *The Philosophy of Science*.

Also of relevance is William Bechtel's (1988) *Philosophy of Science: an overview for cognitive science*.

Introductions to Freud and the philosophy of psychoanalysis

The bibliography on Freud and psychoanalysis is vast. If you have not read Freud before, a good place to begin is Anthony Storr's (1989) *Freud*. More partisan but with lots of detail is Richard Wollheim's (1973) *Freud*. A multi-faceted reference book containing articles on all aspects of Freud's thought, including a short summary by Grunbaum of his critique of the scientific status of psychoanalysis, is Edward Erwin's (2002) *The Freud Encyclopedia*.

The following are useful for in depth study: Charles Rycroft's (1972) *A Critical Dictionary of Psychoanalysis*, and Henri Ellenberger's (1970) *The Discovery of the Unconscious* (offers a comprehensive overview of the contribution of psychoanalysis to the development of dynamic psychiatry). Wollheim and Hopkins (1982) *Philosophical Essays on Freud*, and Hopkins (1988) 'Critical notes', offer extremely useful points

of entry into the philosophical issues generated by psychoanalysis. Paul Kline's (1972) *Fact and Fantasy in Freudian Theory* offers an accessible introduction to the issue of the scientificity of psychoanalysis.

Responses to particular interpretations of Freud

One of the best critical examinations of the opposition between the hermeneutic reconstruction of psychoanalysis and the views of Adolf Grunbaum is Carlo Strenger's (1991) *Between Hermeneutics and Science*.

An extremely useful book based on exemplary scholarly research is Laplanche and Pontalis' (1973) *The Language of Psychoanalysis*. Gianni Vattimo's (1997) *Beyond Interpretation* presents an excellent critique of the expansion of 'hermeneutics' to include diverse approaches within philosophy, especially the ideas of the German phenomenologist Martin Heidegger.

An excellent selection of critical papers on Grunbaum, with a response from Grunbaum himself, is given in Clark and Wright's (ed.) (1988) *Mind, Psychoanalysis and Science*.

Grunbaum published a follow-up to his *Foundations* (1984) book in 1993—*Validation in the Clinical Theory of Psychoanalysis*, still taking a strongly negative line on the scientific support for psychoanalysis.

Donald Levy's (1996) *Freud Among the Philosophers* explores both Wittgenstein's critique of psychoanalysis as well as Grunbaum's critique, and argues that both are ill-conceived.

A classic collection of papers on psychoanalysis, science, and philosophy is Sidney Hook's (1959) *Psychoanalysis, Scientific Method, and Philosophy*.

One of the early, but still highly useful, texts exploring the scientific testing of Freud's theories is Paul Kline's (1972) *Fact and Fantasy in Freudian Theory*. Kline's book was quickly followed by Eysenck and Wilson's (ed.) (1973) *The Experimental Study of Freudian Theories*, which came to the opposite conclusions: psychoanalytic theory was not supported by experimental evidence. This was followed a decade or so later by Eysenck's (1985) somewhat premature *Decline and Fall of the Freudian Empire*.

Seymour Fisher and Roger Greenberg's (1977), *The Scientific Credibility of Freud's Theories and Therapy*, provides a comprehensive survey of the scientific evidence for and against psychoanalysis. Bruno Bettleheim's (1982) *Freud and Man's Soul* remains a classic of humanistic interpretation.

Finally, a major post-Freudian thinker worthy of mention is the French psychoanalyst and philosopher Jacques Lacan's (1977a) *Ecrits* (trans. Alan Sheridan), and (1977b) *The Four Fundamental Concepts of Psychoanalysis* (ed. Jacques-Alain Miller, trans. Alan Sheridan). A useful introduction to Lacan and his work is provided in Malcom Bowie's (1991) *Lacan*.

For a detailed discussion extending his work as set out in the chapter, arguing that psychoanalysis is continuous with everyday 'folk psychology', see Gardner's (1995)

'Psychoanalysis, science, and consciousness', with commentaries by Hinshelwood (1995) and Snelling (1995).

For discussion of the status of Freud's early Project see Woody and Phillips' (1995) 'Freud's Project for a scientific psychology after 100 years: the unconscious mind in the era of cognitive neuroscience', with a commentary by Mohl (1995).

A particular version of an interpretational or hermeneutic approach to Freud is in Brockmeier's (1997a) 'Autobiography, narrative, and the Freudian concept of life history', with commentaries by Holmes (1997) and Robinson (1997), and a response by Brockmeier (1997b).

For an interpretation owing much to Nietzsche see Lehrer's (1999a) 'Perspectivism and psychodynamic psychotherapy', with commentaries by Pearson (1999), Hales and Welshon (1999), Lansky (1999), Lieberman (1999), and Mace (1999), and a response by Lehrer (1999b).

Baker (2003) provides a detailed critique of the widely canvassed view of Wittgenstein's philosophical method as a form of 'therapy'.

A useful recent review of Freud's contributions to western though is Bergo (2004). Edward Erwin's (1996) *A Final Accounting* assesses the successes and failures of Freudian theory judged by conceptual and epistemic standards.

References

American Psychiatric Association (1994). *Diagnostic and Statistical Manual of Mental Disorders* (4th edn). APA: Washington DC.

Anon (1997). Editorial: The crisis in psychiatry. *Lancet*, 347: 349.

Austin, J.L. (1956–7) A plea for excuses. Proceedings of the Aristotelian Society 57:1–30. Reprinted in White, A.R., ed. (1968) The Philosophy of Action. Oxford: Oxford University Press, pp. 19–42.

Baker, G. (2003). Wittgenstein's method and psychoanalysis. In *Nature and Narrative: an introduction to the new philosophy of psychiatry* (ed. K.W.M. Fulford, K.J. Morris, J.Z.S. Sadler, and G. Stanghellini). Oxford: Oxford University Press, Chapter 3.

Bechtel, W. (1988). *Philosophy of Science: an overview for cognitive science*. Hillsdale, NJ: Lawrence Erlbaum.

Bergo, B. (2004). Psychoanalytic models: Freud's debt to philosophy and his copernican revolution. In T*he Philosophy of Psychiatry: a companion* (ed. J. Radden). New York: Oxford University Press, pp. 338–350.

Bettelheim, B. (1982). *Freud and Man's Soul*. London, Penguin Books.

Bird, A. (1998) *The Philosophy of Science*. London: UCL.

Bowie, M. (1991). *Lacan*. London: Fontana.

Boyd, R., Gasper, P., and Trout, J.D. (ed.) (1991). *The Philosophy of Science*. Cambridge, MA: MIT Press.

Breuer, J. & Freud, S. (1955) The Standard Edition … *Studies on Hysteria*. (1883–1895) (transl. J. Strachey). London: The Hogarth Press.

Brockmeier, J. (1997a). Autobiography, narrative, and the Freudian concept of life history. (with commentaries by Holmes, 1997, pp. 201–204, and Robinson, 1997, pp. 205–208, and response Brockmeier, 1997, pp. 209–212). *Philosophy, Psychiatry, & Psychology*, 4(3): 175–200.

Brockmeier, J. (1997b). Response to the Commentaries. *Philosophy, Psychiatry, & Psychology*, 4(3): 209–212.

Chalmers, A. (1999). *What is this thing called science?* Buckingham, England: Open University Press.

Churchland, P.S. (1989). *Neurophilosophy*. Cambridge, MA: MIT Press.

Cioffi, F. (1988). Exegetical myth-making. In *Grunbaum's Indictment of Popper and Exoneration of Freud* (in the Clark and Wright volume, Mind, Psychoanalysis and Science). Oxford: Blackwell, pp. 61–87.

Clark, P. and Wright, C. (ed.) (1988). *Mind, Psychoanalysis and Science*. Oxford: Blackwell.

Earle, W.J. (1992). *Introduction to Philosophy*. New York: McGraw-Hill Inc.

Ellenberger, H.F. (1970). *The Discovery of the Unconscious*. New York: Basic Books. (London: Fontana, 1994.)

Erwin, E. (1996). A Final Accounting: Philosophical and Empirical issues in Freudian Psychology. Cambridge, Mass, USA: MIT Press.

Erwin, E. (ed) (2002). *The Freud Encyclopedia*. New York: Routledge.

Eysenck, H.J. (1985). *Decline and Fall of the Freudian Empire*. London: Penguin.

Eysenck, H.J. and Wilson, G.D. (ed.) (1973). *The Experimental Study of Freudian Theories*. London: Methuen.

Fisher, S. and Greenberg, R. (1977). *The Scientific Credibility of Freud's Theories and Therapy*. New York: Columbia University Press.

Freud, S. ([1894] 1962). *The Neuro-Psychoses of Defence* (Standard Edition), Vol. III. London: Hogarth Press.

Freud, S. (1955). *Standard Edition of the Complete Psychological Works Vol XVIII*. London: Hogarth Press.

Freud, S. (1963). *Analytic Therapy* (Standard Edition), Vol. XVI; also in 1973 Pelican edition, Vol. 1.

Freud, S. (1966). *Project for a Scientific Psychology* (Standard Edition), Vol. 1. London: Hogarth Press, pp. 283–397.

Freud, S. (1973). *Introductory Lectures on Psychoanalysis*. Pelican Freud Library, Vol. 1. London: Penguin.

Freud, S. (1977). 'Dora' case study. In *Case Histories I*. The Pelican Freud Library, Vol. 8. London: Penguin, pp. 41, 45–49.

Freud, S. (1900) *The Interpretation of Dreams* (Standard Edition), Vol. 4, p. 225 (cf Joyce Crick, Trans. 1999).

Fulford, K.W.M. (1994). Closet logics: hidden conceptual elements in the DSM and ICD classifications of mental disorder. In *Philosophical Perspectives on Psychiatric Diagnostic Classification* (ed. J.Z. Sadler, O.P. Wiggins, and M.A. Schwartz). Baltimore, MD: Johns Hopkins University Press, Chapter 9.

Gardner, S. (1993). *Irrationality and the Philosophy of Psychoanalysis*. Cambridge: Cambridge University Press.

Gardner, S. (1995). Psychoanalysis, science, and consciousness. (With commentaries by Hinshelwood, 1995, pp. 115–118, and Snelling, 1995, pp. 119–222) *Philosophy, Psychiatry, & Psychology*, 2(2): 93–114.

Gelder, M.G., Gath, G., and Mayou, R.A.M. (1983). Signs and symptoms of mental disorder. In *The Oxford Textbook of Psychiatry* (1st edn). Oxford: Oxford University Press, p. 1.

Goodman, N. (1983). *Fact, Fiction and Forecast*. Harvard: Harvard University Press.

Grosskurth, P. (1991). *The Secret Ring*. London: Jonathan Cape.

Grunbaum, A. (1984). *The Foundations of Psychoanalysis*. Berkeley, CA: University of California Press.

Grunbaum, A. (1988). Precis of *The Foundations of Psychoanalysis*. In *Mind, Psychoanalysis and Science* (ed. P. Clark and C. Wright). Oxford: Blackwell.

Grunbaum, A. (1993). *Validation in the Clinical Theory of Psychoanalysis*. Madison, CT: International Universities Press.

Hacking, I. (1990) *The Taming of Chance*. Cambridge: Cambridge University Press

Hales, S.D. and Welshon, R. (1999). Nietzsche, perspectivism, and mental health. (Commentary on Lehrer, 1999a) *Philosophy, Psychiatry, & Psychology*, 6(3): 173–178.

Harré, R. (1993). *Laws of Nature*. London: Duckworth.

Hinshelwood, R.D. (1995). Psychoanalysis, science, and commonsense. (Commentary on Gardner, 1995) *Philosophy, Psychiatry, & Psychology*, 2(2): 115–118.

Holmes, J. (1997). Commentary on 'Autobiography, narrative, and the Freudian concept of life history'. (Commentary on Brockmeier, 1997) *Philosophy, Psychiatry, & Psychology*, 4(3): 201–204.

Hook, S. (1959). *Psychoanalysis, Scientific Method, and Philosophy*. New York: New York University Press.

Hopkins, J. (1988) Epistemology and Depth Psychology: Critical Notes on The Foundations of Psychoanalysis, Part One, Section 2, p33, in P. Clark and C. Wright (eds) *Mind, Psychoanalysis and Science*. Oxford: Blackwell Publishers.

Jaspers, K. (1974 [1913]). Causal and 'meaningful' connections between life history and psychosis. In *Themes and Variations in European Psychiatry* (ed. S.R. Hirsch and M. Shepherd). Bristol: John Wright and Sons Ltd.

Jones, E. (1938). The theory of symbolism. In *Papers on Psychoanalysis*. London: Ballière Tindall.

Kline, P. (1972). *Fact and Fantasy in Freudian Theory*. London: Methuen.

Kuhn, T.S. (1962, 2nd edn/1970 revised and enlarged). *The Structure of Scientific Revolutions*. Chicago: Chicago University Press.

Lacan, J. (1977a). *Ecrits: A Selection* (trans. Alan Sheridan). London: Tavistock Publications.

Lacan, J. (1977b). *The Four Fundamental Concepts of Psychoanalysis* (ed. Jacques-Alain Miller, trans. Alan Sheridan). London: Hogarth Press.

Ladyman, J. (2002). *Understanding Philosophy of Science*. London: Routledge.

Lansky, M.R. (1999). Perspectives on perspectivism. (Commentary on Lehrer, 1999a) *Philosophy, Psychiatry, & Psychology*, 6(3): 179–180.

Laplanche, J. and Pontalis, J.-B. (1973). *The Language of Psychoanalysis*. London: The Hogarth Press.

Lehrer, R. (1999a). Perspectivism and psychodynamic psychotherapy. (With commentaries by Pearson, 1999, pp. 167–172; Hales and Welshon, 1999, pp. 173–178; Lansky, 1999, pp. 179–180; Lieberman, 1999, pp. 181–186; and Mace, 1999, pp. 187–190) *Philosophy, Psychiatry, & Psychology*, 6(3): 155–166.

Lehrer, R. (1999b). Response to the Commentaries. *Philosophy, Psychiatry, & Psychology*, 6(3): 191–198.

Levy, D. (1996). *Freud Among the Philosophers*. New Haven, CT: Yale University Press.

Lieberman, P.B. (1999). Perspectivism, realism, and psychotherapy. (Commentary on Lehrer, 1999a) *Philosophy, Psychiatry, & Psychology*, 6(3): 181–186.

Livesley, W.J. (1996) *Commentary on "Epistemic Value Commitments"*. Philosophy, Psychiatry, and Psychology, 3/3, 223–226

Losee, J. (1980). *A Historical Introduction to the Philosophy of Science*, (2nd edn). Oxford: Oxford University Press.

Luntley, M.O., (1996) *Commentary on "Epistemic Value Commitments"*. Philosophy, Psychiatry, and Psychology, 3/3, 227–230

Mace, C. (1999). On putting psychoanalysis into a Nietzschean perspective. (Commentary on Lehrer, 1999a) *Philosophy, Psychiatry, & Psychology*, 6(3): 187–190.

Melville Woody, J. and Phillips, J. (1995) Freud's project for a scientific psychology after 100 years: the unconscious mind in the era of cognitive science. *Philosophy, Psychiatry, & Psychology*, 2(2): 123–134.

Mohl, P. (1995). Freud's Project for a scientific psychology after 100 years. (Commentary on Woody and Phillips, 1995) *Philosophy, Psychiatry, & Psychology*, 2(2): 135–136.

Pearson, K.A. (1999). Perspectivism and relativism beyond the postmodern condition. (Commentary on Lehrer, 1999a) *Philosophy, Psychiatry, & Psychology*, 6(3): 167–172.

Popper, K. ([1934] expanded text, 1959). *The Logic of Scientific Discovery*. London: Hutcheson.

Popper, K. (1963). *Conjectures and Refutations*. London: Routledge.

Ricoeur, P. (1970). *Freud and Philosophy* (trans. D. Savage). London: Yale University Press.

Robinson, D.N. (1997). Commentary on 'Autobiography, narrative, and the Freudian concept of life history.' (Commentary on Brockmeier, 1997) *Philosophy, Psychiatry, & Psychology*, 4(3): 205–208.

Roth, M. and Kroll, J. (1986). *The Reality of Mental Illness*. Cambridge: Cambridge University Press.

Rycroft, C. (1972). *A Critical Dictionary of Psychoanalysis*. London: Penguin.

Sadler, J. (1996). Epistemic value commitments in the debate over categorical versus dimensional personality diagnosis. *Philosophy, Psychiatry, & Psychology*, 3(3): 203–222.

Sadler, J.Z., Wiggins, O.P., and Schwartz, M. A. (ed.) (1994). *Philosophical Perspectives on Psychiatric Diagnostic Classification*. Baltimore, MD: Johns Hopkins University Press.

Slater, E. (1972). The psychiatrists in search of a science; I Early thinkers at the Maudsley. *British Journal of Psychiatry*, 121: 591–598.

Slater, E. (1973). The psychiatrists in search of a science; II Developments in the logic and the sociology of science. *British Journal of Psychiatry*, 122: 625–636.

Slater, E. (1975). The psychiatrists in search of a science; III The depth psychologies. *British Journal of Psychiatry*, 126: 205–224.

Slater, E. and Roth, M. (1969). *Mayer-Gross, Slater and Roth: clinical psychiatry* (3rd edn). London: Ballière Tindall and Cassell.

Snelling, D. (1995). Psychoanalysis, science, and common-sense. (Commentary on Gardner, 1995) *Philosophy, Psychiatry, & Psychology*, 2(2): 119–122.

Storr, A. (1989). *Freud*. Oxford: Oxford University Press.

Strenger, C. (1991). *Between Hermeneutics and Science*. Madison, CT: International Universities Press.

Szasz, T.S. (1960). The myth of mental illness. *American Psychologist*, 15: 113–118.

Vattimo, G. (1997). *Beyond Interpretation*. Cambridge: Polity Press.

Wittgenstein, L. (1982). Conversations on Freud. In *Philosophical Essays on Freud* (eds R. Wollheim and J. Hopkins). Cambridge: Cambridge University Press.

Wollheim, R. (1973). *Freud*. London: Fontana.

Wollheim, R. (1981) *Sigmund Freud*. Modern Masters Series. New York: Viking Press (1971). Cambridge and New York: Cambridge University Press.

Wollheim, R. and Hopkins, J. (1982). *Philosophical Essays on Freud*. Cambridge: Cambridge University Press.

Woody, M.J. and Phillips J. (1995). Freud's Project for a scientific psychology after 100 years: the unconscious mind in the era of cognitive neuroscience. (Commentary by Mohl, 1995, pp. 135–136) *Philosophy, Psychiatry, & Psychology*, 2(2): 123–134.

CHAPTER 12

Psychopathology and the theory dependence of data

Chapter contents

Observation lies at the heart of psychiatry. The clinical process, as in the rest of medicine, starts with the careful articulation of symptoms of which patients complain, and signs: patients' appearance and behaviour, including speech. Theorizing about aetiology, both as part of the diagnostic and treatment/management process and as part of general clinical research, answers to data drawn from clinical observations.

Physics, philosophy, and psychopathology

This emphasis on the role of observation fits with the claim, discussed in Chapter 11, that psychiatry is scientific. A central component of the claim that a discipline is scientific is that it aspires to an objective account of the world. And, on the traditional model of science, neutral observation, at what we called Stage 1 of the scientific process, seems to be a precondition for objectivity.

Consistently, then, descriptive psychopathology, the signs and symptoms of mental disorder (outlined in Chapter 3), places particular emphasis on careful observation. Classification lies at the heart of psychiatry and psychiatric classification, coded in, for example, ICD-10 (WHO, 1992) and DSM-IV (APA, 1994), concentrates on the definition of syndromes in broadly observable terms (signs and symptoms). These classifications, furthermore, since DSM-III (APA, 1980), have directly emulated physics, the paradigm observational science, by seeking a basis in *operational* criteria.

Operational criteria were the brainchild of the American physicist and father of 'Operationalism' Percy W. Bridgman (1882–1961). Bridgman argued that there was a close connection between concepts and empirical tests for whether they applied.

> To find the length of an object, we have to perform certain physical operations. The concept of length is therefore fixed when the operations by which length is measured are fixed: that is, the concept of length involves as much as and nothing more than the set of operations by which length is determined. In general, we mean by any concept nothing more than a set of operations; the concept is synonymous with a corresponding set of operations.   Bridgman (1927 p5)

Bridgman's ideas were put forward by the philosopher Carl Hempel at a conference on psychiatric classification in 1959 that will be described more in Chapter 13. In the context of psychiatry, the emphasis on 'operations' was translated into observations or observable tests that, in principle, could be elicited by the 'operation' of asking certain questions in a particular way. One consequence of this has been to make clear the connections between syndromes and the observable signs and symptoms by which they are defined. So, for example, the DSM-IV (APA, 1994) criteria for schizophrenia begin:

A. Characteristic symptoms: Two (or more) of the following, each present for a significant portion of time during a 1-month period (or less if successfully treated):

- delusions

- hallucinations

- disorganized speech (e.g., frequent derailment or incoherence)

- grossly disorganized or catatonic behavior

- negative symptoms, i.e., affective flattening, alogia, or avolition

Note: Only one Criterion A symptom is required if delusions are bizarre or hallucinations consist of a voice keeping up a running commentary on the person's behavior or thoughts, or two or more voices conversing with each other.

The criteria specify the conditions that have to be satisfied for a diagnosis of schizophrenia to be made with the conditions spelled out in more basic terms, i.e. in terms of symptoms. The idea is that the symptoms can be identified prior to, and independently of, subsequent diagnosis by well-defined 'operations' of clinical interview and investigation. Rules then specify the connection between the diagnosis and symptoms and these connections (partially) characterize the nature of the concept of schizophrenia. That, broadly, is the debt to operationalism.

A key advantage of this approach to psychiatric diagnosis has been an increase in the *reliability* of psychiatric diagnosis. Writing in *A Research Agenda for DSM-V* (Kupfer *et al.*, 2002), Bruce Rounsaville *et al.* comment: 'When DSM-III was published in 1980, one of the most important advantages was a radical improvement in the reliability of psychiatric diagnosis by virtue of its provision of operational criteria for each diagnosis.' (*ibid* p. 13)

Reliability—which will be discussed more in Chapter 13—is a measure of consistency in diagnosis both between observers and over time. Concentrating on the connection between diagnoses and more basic observational symptoms should help provide a sound foundation for agreement in complex cases and thus for reliability.

There is a further feature of a broadly operationalist approach: the emphasis on atheoretical descriptions of signs and symptoms. Again since ICD-9 (WHO, 1978) and DSM-III (APA, 1980) there has been an emphasis on descriptions of symptoms that do not presuppose any particular aetiological theory. The hope has been that, consistently with the traditional model of science outlined in Chapter 11, a sound basis of descriptive psychopathology might provide a neutral framework for the subsequent development of psychiatric theory.

One of the lessons of this chapter, however, will be that notwithstanding improvements in reliability achieved through the move towards operational definitions, it is not possible completely to separate uncontentious observational elements of descriptive psychopathology from contentious theoretical models of aetiology. Diagnostic manuals such as DSM and ICD must, inevitably, include theoretical elements in their characterization of what is directly observable. That of course puts an extra burden on the authors of such classifications that the theories presupposed are *correct* but psychiatry is not alone in facing that burden.

There is another consequence of recognizing the blurring of observation and theory. It impacts on a worry about psychiatric observation that is summarized in the following passage:

> It is fashionable in some circles at the moment to decry the use of diagnostic labels, and to suggest that what doctors have to try to understand and treat are not diseases but problems, multi-faceted and unclassifiable. A knowledge of the biological, psychological and social processes involved in problem-formation is recognized as indispensable, but to give some thought to their taxonomy is said to lead inevitably to sterile pigeon-holing, inflexibility and inhumanity. Giving a name to a condition, according to this view, not only serves little useful purpose but in the case of mental illnesses it can be positively harmful, since the label is often also a term of opprobrium or one implying hopelessness.
>
> Wing *et al.* (1974, p. 1)

The worry can be summarized this way. If observation is connected to classification and diagnosis in the way exemplified by DSM, ICD, and the Present State Examination (PSE), then it involves a distortion because patients' experiences are forced into pre-existing categories rather than recognized for their individuality.

But while there are indeed cases where observations are reported in distorting ways, the implicit assumption that it would be possible to shed all preconceptions and simply 'drink in' a subject's experiences in all his or her individuality is impossible. As we will suggest, there are plausible arguments that all observation is always structured by prior concepts.

Plan of the chapter

◆ *Session 1* characterizes the theory dependence of observation through comments made about the nature of diagnosis in one of the first structured interview schedules, the PSE.

◆ *Session 2* charts the origins of the (supposed) separation of theory and observation in the two-language model of Logical Empiricism (this being a philosophical version of the traditional model of science—see Chapter 11).

◆ *Session 3* sets out arguments *against* the separation of observational statements and theoretical statements. In other words, these arguments demonstrate the theory dependence of observation by showing that the *language* of observation (the terms in which we report observations) cannot be clearly separated from the language of theory (whether psychiatric or drawn from physics).

◆ *Session 4* sets out arguments against the separation of theory and observation in the actual process and experience of observing. Like the arguments of Session 3, then, these are arguments supporting the theory dependence of observations, but in this case directed against the idea that observation is based on raw or brute data. Instead the session argues that observations are always conceptually structured..

◆ *Session 5* draws some conclusions about the theory dependence of observation in physics and psychiatry.

Session 1 The theory dependence of everyday observations and psychopathology

A practical exercise on the theory dependence of observation

The idea that impartial observation, as the basis of objectivity in science, is in important respects illusory, comes as something of a culture shock to most of us, at least in medicine, brought up as we are within a broadly traditional understanding of science. As we saw in Chapter 11, words like 'positivism' are associated with the idea, very much dominant in science as well as philosophy through much of the twentieth century, that it is of the essence of science that it should be based on 'clear' observations, on data that genuinely reflect features of the world 'out there', rather than the perspective of this or that particular observer. Hence we will begin with an exercise designed to bring out in a straightforwardly practical way some more mundane aspects of the theory dependence of observation.

EXERCISE 1

This exercise comes in two parts. It is the core of the session and thus it is particularly important to do it 'for real' before going on.

Part 1 (10 minutes)

Make comprehensive observations of a piece of furniture nearby: a chair perhaps. Make your observations as objective as possible. Write them down. Now mark those data which could be used for re-identifying this item at some time in the future.

Part 2 (30 minutes)

Think carefully about your answers to the exercises you have just completed. In what ways do they show that there are limits to how far we can be objective even about observations of everyday objects like chairs? Write down your own conclusions before going on.

In this exercise we are concerned with a relatively simple case of observation, compared with 'observing' mental states, for example. None the less, it brings out at least two ways in which observation is theory dependent, namely (1) that the data have always to be *selected*, and (2) there has always to be an assumed *level of precision*.

Two ways of observing chairs

That observations are theory laden in these two ways may seem, once one reflects for a moment, rather obvious. If we think about them in a little more detail, though, they bring out a rather less obvious and important general point about observation. Thus:

1. *Which data*? The first and most obvious sense, then, in which observation is theory dependent is that data have to be

selected. The instruction: 'make comprehensive observations' is impossible to satisfy. In this exercise, the most obvious observations include the size, shape, weight (or mass), colour, and location of the chair. But other possible observations include the orientation of the chair with respect to other pieces of furniture, nearby wildlife and distant stars. With a little ingenuity, more potential observations can always be added to any finite list.

This may seem merely an artificial and untroubling fact until one asks how, in practice, one avoids the need to try and record every possible observation. There is indeed a crucially important tension here, between, on the one hand, being overwhelmed with too many observations, and, on the other, restricting its range too narrowly. Patients with schizophrenia are often particularly good at making novel observations. They really do notice features of their environment that most of us would not. In the case of schizophrenia, this can lead to cognitive overload. But the same alertness to novel features of the environment is central to creativity, whether in science or the arts.

All in all, then, it is clear that observation, as the basis of science, in so far as it involves the correct selection of data, is not simply a matter of reflecting the world 'out there', a property (solely) of the thing observed, but is determined (in part and in some or more ways) by the particular context in which the observations are made. In certain contexts, one kind and quantity of data are appropriate, in other contexts, other kinds and quantities will be appropriate, and so on.

2. *Level of precision.* We will be considering 'context', as a feature of scientific method, at several points in this part. The second activity in this exercise makes explicit a key aspect of 'context', namely the purposes for which an observation is made. Here, we asked you to think about the data required to re-identify the chair in question. This particular purpose immediately gives, within the possible (infinite) range of observations, particular focus to which observation are appropriate. Orientation in space, for example, will not be helpful here. Whereas the kind of wood (or whatever material the chair is made) will be. This second activity, moreover, brings out second sense in which observation is theory dependent, namely that, for whatever data are selected, there must always be an assumed level of precision.

Thus, the observations that are relevant for re-identifying a chair may not include the more bizarre examples given. The first list may be adequate. But within this list, the right level of precision for your observations also depends on context. As you carried out the exercise, you might have noted, say, a particular style of chair leg as sufficient to re-identify the chair you were observing as against others in the room. But suppose you were concerned about someone swapping your chair for a similar one next door; then, perhaps, a particular scuff mark on the chair leg would become important.

Or, again, if you were an antiques expert, the precise way in which the leg was 'turned' could become crucial.

The normativity of observation

Both in the selection of data, therefore, and in an assumed level of precision, our observations, even for the relativity straightforward case of a chair, are not impartial. They are made from the point of view of a given observer in a given context and, importantly, for a given *purpose*.

This brings us to the general point illustrated by the two aspects of the theory dependence of observation, namely that observation, far from being neutral, turns out to be *normative*. To do something for a purpose is to acknowledge standards or criteria by which it can be said to be done well or badly, correctly or incorrectly, successfully or unsuccessfully. This is why, as in the above exercise, in speaking of observation, it is natural to use phrases such as the 'correct' selection of data and the 'right' level of precision. Such phrases, recalling Austin's concept of philosophical fieldwork (from Part I, Chapter 4), are linguistic-analytic signals that, notwithstanding the traditional model of science, observation, as the basis of scientific method, is theory dependent in the sense that what we observe necessarily reflects, not only the features of that which we observe, but a selection of those features that is driven by the purposes for which the observations in question are made.

The tip of the iceberg

To anticipate a little, it is important to note that there are still deeper ways in which observation is theory laden. As we will see later, philosophy of science has been concerned mainly, not with these *quantitative* aspects of the theory ladenness of observation, but with *qualitative* aspects. Both the selection of data and an assumed level of precision take for granted that there are determinate data 'out there': they assume that there are determinate objects (such as chairs and chair legs for example) out there; and that there are determinate properties (brown, square, etc.) in terms of which these objects can be described in different ways and to different levels of precision. But modern philosophy of science has shown that the very concepts used to frame observation reports (chair, leg, brown, square, etc.) themselves presuppose theory, and that the very experience of observing is determined (in part at least) by the theories one holds. We will come to the way in which concepts shape data in the next session.

The theory dependence of observation and the PSE

From chairs to descriptive psychopathology

First, though, we will compare observation of chairs with observation of psychopathology. We will be returning to psychopathology in the last session of this chapter. At this stage we just need to note that descriptive psychopathology, indeed observations of mental states in general, present still further complications beyond those presented by things such as chairs.

This exercise brings out some of the difficulties, over and above those involved in observing things such as chairs, in observing symptoms.

In the first place, it is clear that the sort of observations required for identifying symptoms varies dramatically. Some symptoms such as involuntary speech or action seem to be much more directly observable than others such as the hearing of voices. Behaviour is on the 'outside'; it is 'public' and available to inspection. 'Hearing voices' is inside someone's head; it is private and not (directly) available to inspection. This contrast is indeed conventionally expressed in medicine by the distinction between symptoms (which patients experience) and signs (which clinicians observe). But in the case of psychopathology, even 'publicly available' signs are problematic in ways that things such as chairs (which do not have mental states) are not. To take an obvious example, what appears to be involuntary speech, and hence pathological, may in fact be a piece of street theatre.

A traditional model of science

Much of psychiatry, particularly with the current vogue for 'biological psychiatry' assumes that observations of psychopathology are no more and no less problematic than observations of chairs, or, in a more nuanced way, that with a little effort observations of psychopathology can be made with more difficulty, perhaps, but in essentially the same way, as observations of chairs.

We will see in this part of this book that this is insecure science reflecting insecure philosophy! But the next reading represents a particularly clear and determined attempt to square the requirements of a traditional view of science with a sophisticated understanding of the difficulties involved in developing a science of mind.

The first author of this book, John Wing, was a psychiatrist and social scientist who based his work on a sophisticated understanding of the philosophical issues. His book, *The Reality of Mental Illness* (1978), represents a robust and detailed defence of medical psychiatry as a social as well as a biological science (the title is deliberately in opposition to Thomas Szasz's *The Myth of Mental Illness*).

Wing's basic commitment, which is made explicit in *The Reality of Mental Illness*, is to a medical model of mental disease in which psychiatry will eventually develop disease theories of the same broad kind as those in other medical specialities, such as cardiology. As in the rest of medicine, then, so here, a traditional model of science lies behind Wing's work. As we saw in Part I, psychiatry's image as a credible discipline is widely perceived as depending on this.

Observations as building blocks for theories

Much of Wing's work was thus concerned with establishing a sound observational basis for the development of psychiatry as a science traditionally understood. The PSE interview schedule, as it has come to be called, described in full in the book from which this reading is taken, was designed to do just that. Together with other similar schedules, it has been highly successful. As we will see, such schedules have been the basis of many of the most important developments in psychiatry over the last 20 years. As in other sciences, observations (here of psychopathology) have been the building blocks of scientific theories.

In the preface to the PSE, then, the broad message is that psychiatry needs to be put on a sounder scientific footing so that it can take its proper place among other medical sciences, and the basis of this is better observations. The commitment to foundational observations is evident in the references, for example, (1) to the 'good clinician' making a 'systematic exploration of the subject's mental state' in order to 'discover whether any of a finite number of abnormal mental phenomena are present'; (2) to the interviewer and patient coming to an 'exact description of the symptoms'; (3) to 'data', to 'coming closer to the truth' and,

SESSION 1 THE THEORY DEPENDENCE OF EVERYDAY OBSERVATIONS AND PSYCHOPATHOLOGY 293

shades of Chapter 11, in the sideswipe at psychoanalysis! It is also made explicit later in the book: for example, on p. 3, using the example of Kanner's original description of autism, we find 'No disease theory can be elaborated before the clinical syndrome has been recognised and labelled.'

Some normative considerations

In most psychiatric textbooks, as we saw in Chapter 11, the traditional model is taken for granted. Here, though, a more sophisticated approach is adopted. Despite the reference to 'the truth', the aim of the PSE is more modest. It is 'consistency' between observers achieved by formalizing (writing rules to capture) best diagnostic practice. This was an important aim at the time the PSE was being developed as a series of studies had shown that psychiatric observations were highly idiosyncratic. Different observers, or the same observer on different occasions, came up with quite different observations about the same case. Whatever the 'truth', therefore, we could have no confidence in such observations as building blocks for scientific theories.

The measure of success, therefore, the standard by which the authors of the PSE decided what the observations it produced were appropriate for their role in psychiatric science, is consistency, or, as it is usually called in medicine, *reliability*.

Can we rely on reliability?

Wing *et al.* (1974), then, although guided by a traditional notion of reflecting the truth that is 'out there' aimed only for a cautiously modest contribution to the observational route to this.

We will return to the nature of reliability in Chapter 13. But it is important to note how carefully the authors of the PSE, well aware as they are of the difficulties in a science of the mind, define the modest scope of their claims for it:

1. It is 'firmly in the European clinical school of psychiatry'— i.e., although the influence of this has 'spread widely' throughout the world, it has its origins in a specific social and cultural context and in studies of best practice in this tradition.

2. Similarly, although not everyone who used the PSE fully accepts it, they are willing to do so 'for the purposes of attaining compatibility with colleagues'—i.e. the particular purpose of these observations is specified.

3. Perhaps most important of all, it is not a passive process. This is, as noted earlier, an important prima facie difference between psychopathology and chairs. Chairs cannot engage in the observational process but the PSE (reflecting good practice in clinical interviews generally) directly involves the patient. To the extent that its aim is determining the presence of 'specific symptoms' (those identified as important in the European tradition) it inevitably involves a degree of 'cross examination'. But the aim of this is to engage the patient *with* the interviewer in the process of observation.

The PSE, along with other similar instruments, has sometimes been criticized as naively positivistic. Such criticisms fail to take account of the careful way in which the context and purpose of the observations the PSE generates are specified. Given, though, the traditional model of science that is evident in the Preface, and the thrust of Wing's more overtly conceptual work in *The Reality of Mental Illness*, the PSE is perhaps properly understood as sophisticated positivism: it represents a careful attempt to accommodate descriptive psychopathology to a model of medicine that, based as it is on a traditional model of science, aspires to a positivist paradigm. The middle part of this chapter (Sessions 3 and 4) will outline key arguments against positivism as a characterization of science in general. We return in Session 5 to the implications of these arguments for observation of psychopathology as the basis of a scientific approach to mental disorder and will help justify this antipositivist stance from a philosophical perspective.

Some problems deferred

Some of the underlying difficulties of determining other people's mental states on the basis of observation, including the problem of establishing whether other people have minds at all, will be investigated more thoroughly in Part V (see especially Chapter 27). We will find there that the public-private distinction, at least as conventionally drawn, is too sharp. But in the present chapter we are mainly concerned with the problems involved in all observation. For now, then, it is sufficient to note that mental health care shares with the physical sciences a central commitment to the importance of observation within a broadly positivist model of science according to which anything that threatens the impartiality of observation threatens the objectivity of its claims.

In next session, we will examine a particular version of the positivist model of science, Logical Empiricism, that dominated the first half of the twentieth century and that encapsulates an intuitive idea of how observation can be impartial. As already noted, Logical Empiricism is the most persuasive of many attempts to develop a conceptually sound version of the traditional picture of science. While there is no firm distinction 'Logical Empiricism' is the name given to a family of views derived from the Logical Positivism of the Vienna Circle but less firmly wedded to the latter's Verification Principle, which will be discussed below. Thus it can be thought of as starting with the Vienna Circle in the 1920s and continuing to be influential up to the 1950s and 60s. Its key aim was the articulation of the logic and structure of scientific theory and the separation of genuine empirical questions from others.

Having set out the elements of the model, then, in the next Session, and indicated its continuing influence in psychiatry, Logical Empiricism will be used as a stalking horse in the discussion of the theory dependence of observation that follows.

Reflection on the session and self-test questions

Write down your own reflections on the materials in this session drawing out any points that are particularly significant for you. Then write brief notes about the following:

1. What general issues does the exercise on observing a chair raise about the nature of observation and about the gathering of data? How does this complicate the traditional model of science?

2. What differences are raised by consideration of the PSE by comparison with the exercise on observing the chair?

3. How does the PSE fit with the traditional model of science outlined in Chapter 11?

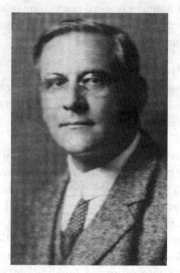

Fig. 12.1 Moritz Schlick

Session 2 An empiricist model of scientific theory

A good way to bring out the significance of the theory dependence of observation is to examine its impact on the Logical Empiricist model of science. As noted earlier, this model was prevalent in the first 60 years of the twentieth century and it incorporates a common sense view of the role that impartial observation plays in science. In particular, the Logical Empiricist model formalizes the traditional view of the importance of impartial observation. It presupposes that theory and observation can be separated. Setting out the consequences of the theory dependence of observation for this model shows the consequences for a worked out version of the traditional picture of science. This will show that both the process of observing and the recording of observations in observation statements presuppose some theory.

There is a second reason for sketching out the Logical Empiricist picture of science. This is that the understanding of science that has developed during the second half of this century is in part a response to *criticism* of Logical Empiricism. We can get a clearer understanding of recent work in the philosophy of science—and thus a better understanding of science—by contrasting it with Logical Empiricism. First, then, Logical Empiricism.

Logical Empiricism and the Vienna Circle

Logical Empiricism was developed by members of the Vienna Circle. The Vienna Circle was a group of philosophers and scientists who worked in the areas of philosophy, logic, mathematics, the natural and social sciences, and pioneered work in the philosophy of science in the analytic style. The circle published a manifesto, *The Scientific World View: The Vienna Circle*, in 1929.

The central figure in the Vienna Circle was Moritz Schlick, a professor of philosophy at the University of Vienna (later murdered by a student) but the group also included many of the most famous names in the philosophy of the first half of the twentieth century: Rudolf Carnap, Herbert Feigl, Philipp Frank, Kurt Gödel, Hans Hahn, Viktor Kraft, Karl Menger, Otto Neurath, Friedrich Waismann, and Edgar Zilsel. There were, in addition, various foreign 'guests', such as Hans Reichenbach, Carl G. Hempel (later to have a decisive influence on psychiatric classification, see Chapter 13), A.J. Ayer, Ernest Nagel, John von Neumann, Willard Van Orman Quine, and Alfred Tarski. There was also some peripheral contact with Ludwig Wittgenstein and Karl Popper.

What is Logical Empiricism?

The Logical Empiricist picture of science emphasizes the role of observations. In common with all forms of empiricism in philosophy, the key claim is that knowledge of the world is grounded in experience rather than in reasoning alone. Empiricism holds that while reasoning may have some part to play, all significant knowledge of the world is founded on experience.

Logical Empiricism adds to that basic emphasis on the role of observation a more precise account of how theoretical science is related to observations. Crucially, it assumes that the language with which observations are recorded is independent of the language of theory. The language of theory is then based upon the language of observation.

By making observational language independent of theoretical language (although not vice versa), Logical Empiricism attempts to explain how observation statements can be theory free and thus serve as an impartial basis for the development of scientific theory. This 'two-language model' will be discussed below.

Two different uses of observation

But before going on to the separation of observation and theory, it is worth first highlighting two different ways in which observations play a part according to two rather different models of science, both broadly within the Logical Empiricist tradition.

1. *Using observations to verify theories*: According to 'classical' Logical Empiricism, theory-neutral observation statements are invoked to provide positive support for theories. On this model, the aim of science is to provide justification for theories by marshalling positive evidence that they are true. Observations that accord with theories provide inductive support for them. We touched on induction in Chapter 5 and will return to it in detail later in this part (Chapter 16). A standard example of induction is the justification of the theory that all swans are white by citing the observation of several white swans. Given the open-ended and universal nature of theories such as this, no observation can establish once and for all their truth. But observations can be used, according to this model, to provide albeit non-conclusive inductive evidence of their truth. Given the crucial supporting role that observation plays, then, traditional Logical Empiricism emphasizes that observation itself must be impartial and theory neutral.

2. *Using observations to falsify or refute theories*: There is, however, another influential account of the role of observations in science, an account that can share with inductivism the two-language picture of classical Logical Empiricism, but that differs from it in one key respect. This alternative was developed by Karl Popper—an Austrian philosopher of science who was influenced by and influenced the Vienna Circle—in order to escape some of the philosophical problems that have plagued the idea of positive support. (These problems are generally called 'the problem of induction', although really there are several problems—see Chapter 16.) Popper's alternative is Falsificationism. According to this model, the purpose of science is not to provide positive evidence for the truth of theories by observation. Instead, observations serve to *refute* theories. A single observation cannot prove the truth of a universal claim (such as all swans are white). But it can (according to the original and most simple versions of Falsificationism) disprove a universal claim. Imagine, for example, an observation of black antipodean swans.

The virtues or otherwise of Falsificationism and its insistence that science aims to disprove rather than to prove theories is not what is at issue in this chapter. Both simpler and more sophisticated versions of Falsificationism will be discussed in the context of scientific progress and the role of evidence in research in Chapter 16. However, the advantages of Falsificationism of all kinds are clearest if it is assumed that the observations by which theories are taken to be falsified are themselves theory free.

In summary then, what is common to classical Logical Empiricism and at least simple, and thus the clearest, versions of Falsificationism, is that whether observations play a positive or negative role as the foundation of theory, the observations themselves are theory free.

The two languages model of Logical Empiricism

The two-language model of theory and observation

The key question, then, to return to the philosophical concerns of the Vienna Circle, is exactly how observations can play an impartial role in the assessment of theory. According to Logical Empiricism, part of the answer to this question is that there is a fundamental distinction between empirical and theoretical language.

It is this distinction that is at the heart of the two-language model of Logical Empiricism. According to this model, the terms that are used to report observations are distinct from, and more basic than, those used to make theoretical claims. The reason for this assumption is this. If the very meanings of the terms used to frame observational reports presuppose a theory, then it seems that those reports cannot be impartial tests of that or any other theory. If the very framework in which observations are reported presupposes that a theory is true, then it seems that those observation statements cannot be impartial tests of theory. (Whether this is true is a question to which we will return at the end of this chapter.)

Epistemology and semantics

Logical Empiricism thus attempts to ensure that theory does not infect observation by separating observation *language* from theoretical *language*. In other words, an *epistemological* thesis that one can know the truth of an observation statement independently of knowing the truth of any theory is underpinned by a *semantic* thesis about the meaning of observational and theoretical terms. Specifically, Logical Empiricism makes two semantic claims: (1) that observational concepts are defined in terms of experience only, and (2) that theoretical concepts are defined in terms of observational concepts.

Spelling this out a little, Logical Empiricism claims that the meanings of concepts used to report observations are thus, on this picture, given by definitional connections to experience. The language of observation reports is defined only by reference to what is directly observable and independently of theoretical explanations of what is observed. By contrast the language of theory is then defined by reference to observational concepts. Thus while theoretical language depends on observational language, observational language does not presuppose any theory.

Ideas: blurring the distinction between concept and experience

The connections between observational concepts and experience have at different times in philosophy been considered closer or more distant. In the seventeenth century it was widely assumed that the connection between concepts and experience was formed very directly at the level of individual concepts or words (i.e. rather than whole sentences, see below). The concept of redness, for example, was considered to be *extracted* from the experience of redness.

David Hume argued that our *ideas* all (or nearly all of them—for one exception see Chapter 16) derive from *impressions* that we receive in sensation or perception. But he also suggested that the only difference between impressions and ideas was one of 'vivacity' implying a very close connection between our thoughts or concepts and our experiences. Fellow British Empiricist John Locke (1632–1704) put forward a similar account. (See David Hume (1711–76) and his *Treatise of Human Nature* first published in 1739–40 (Hume, 1967) and *Enquiries Concerning Human Understanding and Concerning the Principles of Morals* of 1748 (Hume, 1975); and also see John Locke *Essay Concerning Human Understanding*, 1690 (Locke, 1989).)

In this century, such talk of 'ideas' has been abandoned and thus the direct link between individual terms or concepts and elements of experience cannot be maintained. Instead the connection between observational language and experience has been made at the level of *whole sentences*. The reason for this is simple and intuitive. The sentence is the smallest unit of language that can be 'compared with' the world because it is the smallest unit that can be used to *assert* anything. Thus the basic unit of meaning is the whole sentence whose meaning can be identified with the state of affairs that the sentence can be used to assert. Individual word meaning is really, on this account, an abstraction from sentence meaning and only in the context of a sentence does an individual word have meaning. In the philosophy of language, this thesis is generally referred to as Frege's Context Principle. We will return to some of the issues surrounding this in Part V.

The Verification Principle

In the philosophy of science, the most famous version of such 'whole-sentence' accounts is associated with Logical Empiricism and is called the Verification Principle. At its simplest the Verification Principle states that the meaning of a sentence is its method of verification.

The idea is that one can define the meaning of a sentence by using an account of how one would check that it was true. Thus, there might be a paradigmatic method of determining whether claims about, e.g., the lengths of everyday objects were true, a method of using a ruler according to a particular protocol, and thus giving the meaning of the sentence 'This chair is 100 cm tall'. This gives a very practical picture of the connection between the meaning of observational language and the process of making observations. It is clearly closely related to Bridgman's

Operationalism, which as we will see in Chapter 13 has had a profound influence on psychiatric classification.

Central to our interests in this chapter is that such an account suggests that observational language is theory free. The reason for this is that if the meaning of a sentence is given directly by a practical test, then it does not depend on theory. The meaning of the sentence is given by the test itself. This contrasts with a more recent view called the Duhem-Quine thesis (after Pierre Duhem and W.V.O. Quine), which claims instead that any such test always presupposes a body of surrounding theory. (See below.)

From observation to theory

Having defined observational language, Logical Empiricism can then define theoretical language using observational concepts. Theoretical language is thus defined through definitional connections or bridge laws 'upwards' from observational language. Theory presupposes observation but not vice versa. It is worth noting that this is an abstract idea expressed in logical terms. Few examples were ever actually set out.

It is also worth noting parenthetically two different approaches to theoretical statements both of which are consistent with this general approach to theoretical concepts. Theoretical statements may be regarded as simply convenient ways of organizing observational claims but not themselves true or false. On this account theoretical sentences do not strictly assert anything themselves but merely serve as heuristic devices for organizing and deriving observation claims. This view is a form of instrumentalism and was influential on some positivist philosophers of science. We will return to it in Chapter 13. Alternatively, theoretical statements can be regarded as capable of literal truth and falsity, although they could be analysed into a sufficiently complex list of observational claims.

Two languages and mental health

The details of the two-language model of observation are clearly very much *philosophical* details. But at the heart of the model is a codification of an *intuitive* separation of observation and theory. It is a formal model of a common-sense idea at the heart of the traditional model of science.

Correspondingly, therefore, as applied to mental health, and indeed medicine generally, the codification of the separation of observation and theory attempted by Logical Empiricism, provides what is at first glance an intuitively attractive account of the connection between symptoms and signs (descriptive psychopathology in mental health) and subsequent diagnosis. We noted the standard two-stage model of the diagnostic problem in Chapter 11. According to this model, Stage 1 is the identification of symptoms, signs (and perhaps the results of laboratory or other 'tests'), while Stage 2 is the matching of these observations to categories in our classification of disease. If Logical Empiricism is an accurate account of science, then, and if diagnostic assessment is indeed 'scientific', in the first stage of this process symptoms are described using an observational vocabulary which is independent of Stage 2, the subsequent assignment to a diagnostic category. Stage 2, according to Logical Empiricism, comprises a second and independent stage in which a theoretical interpretation is placed upon the symptoms.

As we will see in Chapter 13, this is the approach adopted by recent psychiatric classifications (such as the ICD and DSM). Recognizing that we lack satisfactory causal theories, these classifications are based largely on symptoms. But there is the hope and expectation that the categories so defined will eventually be linked 'upwards' to causal theories just as in areas of medicine such as cardiology they already have been.

Two senses of theory

But it is also worth noting a difference of emphasis between the philosophy of science more broadly and work on the nature of psychopathological or psychiatric classification. While the explicit aim of the psychiatric emphasis on observation has been to avoid premature *causal* theory, the aim of Logical Empiricism was to separate observation from *any* or all theory. These concerns are related and overlap but they are not identical and we will return to the distinction later in the chapter.

The PSE system discussed earlier is an attempt to codify and structure the gathering of data in clinical interviews. It comprises an ordered list of symptoms that are scored for severity and then taken as the foundation for subsequent diagnosis. As the authors comment, the system is supposed to form a 'clear-cut basis' (ibid: p. 10) for teaching, clinical work and research. The authors do not themselves make explicit claims that the symptoms are directly observational and presuppose no theory, but the suggestion of a 'clear-cut' basis for subsequent largely theoretical work strongly suggests such a distinction.

But is the two-language model right?

As we saw in Session 1, this view of the independence of observation and theory, although widespread in the sciences, is called into question by recent work on the theory dependence of observation. In fact, there are a number of different arguments against the independence of theory and observation, as we will see. One argument is to the effect that there is no distinction in kind between theoretical and observational language and thus that observation statements are themselves theory involving. They therefore fail to comprise a neutral basis for theory testing and there is no reason for supporters of rival theories to accept the same observation statements. It is with arguments of this kind that we will be concerned in Session 4. Another is that observation or perception more generally has to be understood to include conceptual elements and is thus not impartial with respect to our concepts.

The rest of this chapter will focus on several of these arguments. But it is worth recalling why the issue of the connection between the meaning of observational and theoretical terms is important.

Epistemology and semantics again

The real point at issue is whether and, if so, how observation provides a neutral and impartial test of theory thus underpinning the claims of scientific objectivity. In other words, it is whether observations can be used to test theories (or diagnoses) (whether by providing confirmation or refutation) independently of those theories (or diagnoses). In practical terms, this requires that if one wishes to test a theory by a relevant observation, knowing whether the observation statement is true must not require knowing whether the theory is true. This is an *epistemological* claim. The Logical Empiricists' *semantic* thesis that observation language is independent of theoretical language as a whole provides reassurance on this score and thus, if true, would partially explain the objectivity of science. But it is undermined by recent arguments. It is to these that we turn in the next session.

Reflection on the session and self-test questions

Write down your own reflections on the materials in this session drawing out any points that are particularly significant for you. Then write brief notes about the following:

1. What is the relation between Logical Empiricism and the traditional model of science outlined in Chapter 11?

2. What role does it ascribe to observation?

3. How does it attempt to use observation to underpin scientific objectivity?

4. What is the relation between the approach to theory and observation in Logical Empiricism and psychopathology? What role does 'theory' play in both?

Session 3 Arguments for the theory dependence of observation statements

Since the publication of ICD-9 (1978) and DSM-III (1980), psychiatric classification has concentrated on symptomatically defined syndromes in order to maximize the reliability of diagnoses and to provide a neutral starting point for aetiological theorizing. These have taken the form of observable tests. But there are powerful arguments to suggest that the distinction between theory and observation is not robust. As noted earlier, the arguments can be divided between those that concentrate on observation *statements* and those that concentrate on the process or experience of observation itself. The arguments, here as in most areas of the philosophy of science, focus on the physical sciences but they also apply to the biological sciences and indeed psychiatry.

Different statements of the theory dependence of observation

To anticipate a little, the traditional independence of observation and theory has been challenged in recent decades from a wide variety of philosophical angles. Typical claims made broadly in support of the theory dependence of observation include:

- there is no distinction of kind between observational and theoretical language;

- observation is theory laden;

- perception consists in the conceptual exploitation of sensations;

- the objects of perceptions are meanings;

- to know whether an observation statement is true requires knowing the truth of some theory.

These claims have in common the fact that they threaten the neat distinction between (impartial) observation and theory (to be tested against observation), which is presupposed by the traditional model of science. But they are strictly different claims that result from different arguments.

It is again worth remembering that the *semantic* questions, or questions of meaning, that will be discussed in this session gain their purpose from an *epistemological* thesis about the independence of observation from theory. Semantic claims, based on arguments about observation statements, aim to show that observation *reports* presuppose theory. (In Session 4 we will look more closely at the nature of observation itself and assess the possibility that it comprises the harvesting of raw or brute data. Again the session will only indirectly concern the epistemological thesis.)

Most of the claims about the theory dependence of observation in the list above are semantic: they turn on the *meaning* of observation statements or the *content* of perceptual experience. But the last claim, that 'to *know* whether an observation statement is true requires knowing the truth of some theory', is an epistemological claim. As we will see, although separable, there are also close connections between the semantic and the epistemological.

So why start, as in this session, with semantic arguments for the theory dependence of observation, rather than, as in Session 4, with the apparently deeper epistemological arguments?

Observation statements as public items and their unexplained connection to experience

One reason for starting with arguments concerning observation statements is that Logical Empiricism stressed the importance for an objective science of statements reporting observations as public items of language, as against observations themselves as private items of experience. Aside from a distrust of the private, however, a further motivation for starting with observational statements rather than observational experiences, was that Logical Empiricism lacked any clear account of how the two might be connected. What logical, rational, or evidential connection can there be between an experience and a statement? Statements can stand in rational or logical relations to other statements. They can be implied by other statements or contradict them. But how can they stand in any such relation to an experience or sensation?

This is an important issue to which we will return in Session 4. (Part of the answer has to do with distinguishing experiences from sensations.) However, the focus of this session is the question of whether observation language really can be distinguished from theoretical language as the naive account requires.

Duhem's argument: observations are made in theoretical terms

Physics as a paradigm case

One way to begin is to look to a paradigm of hard science: experimental physics. This is the focus of the key book by Pierre Duhem (1861–1916), a French philosopher of science and Pragmatist from the turn of the century, *The Aim and Structure of Physical Theory*.

EXERCISE 4   (5 minutes)

Look at the passage from:

Duhem, P. (1962). *The Aim and Structure of Physical Theory*. New York: Atheneum. (Extract pp. 145 and 147–8)

Link with Reading 12.2

On the assumption that it is descriptively accurate, what does the passage suggest about the relation between observation and theory? In particular,

- Does the relation depend on the facts particular to physics?

- Does the passage suggest any argument that observation statements *must* be couched in theoretical terms or just that they generally are?

- Does Duhem's description necessarily show that the Logical Empiricist semantic separation of observational and theoretical language must be false?

- What consequences does this have for theory testing and the specifically epistemological thesis that knowing the truth of an observation statement requires knowing the truth of some theory? Make some notes before going on.

Duhem powerfully suggests that observation statements are *typically* theory laden. However, he does not provide an argument that they *must* be. It is true that statements reporting what has occurred in an experiment typically or routinely employ theoretical concepts. Such claims require theoretical understanding both in order to know whether they are true and also what they mean. Duhem points out that what one can learn from the observation of an experiment depends on one's understanding of theory as well as complex practical procedures and that once one has mastered this repertoire, one's reporting of the experiment is in theoretical terms.

But the argument does not undermine the Logical Empiricist distinction between theoretical and observational language. Duhem's description of the habits of experimental scientists could be true even if that distinction could always be made. The fact that scientists typically report experiments using a theoretical vocabulary does not show that they *could not* report them using a pure observation language. A Logical Empiricist might argue that this is typically what happens if an experimental result is disputed. Scientists can 'retreat' from the theoretical interpretation of their experiments to a purely observational account of what was actually seen. In other words, although the results of experiments are typically reported using theoretical concepts, this does not show that they have to be or that such reports cannot be given in theory-free terms.

The Duhem–Quine thesis

The same goes for the underlying epistemological issue. The retreat mentioned above might correspond to retreat to basic independent observational knowledge. In other words this might be knowledge that requires no knowledge of other theory. In fact Duhem himself would have disputed this claim. He shared

with the later American Pragmatist W.V.O. Quine the view that theories can never be tested in isolation. Other 'auxiliary hypotheses', as Quine called them concerning, for example, the working of measuring equipment, are always in play. Consequently if an observation appears to contradict a theory under test it is always possible to hold that theory immune and reject instead one or other auxiliary hypothesis. This pragmatist thesis is known as the *Duhem–Quine Thesis*. Quine gives a clear statement of his view in his influential paper 'Two dogmas of empiricism'. Using the word 'reductionism' to refer to a verificationist theory of meaning, which connects statements to methods of verification (see above), he says:

> But the dogma of reductionism has, in a subtler and more tenuous form, continued to influence the thought of empiricists. The notion lingers that to each statement, or each synthetic statement, there is associated a unique range of possible sensory events such that the occurrence of any of them would add to the likelihood of truth of the statement, and that there is associated also another unique range of possible sensory events whose occurrence would detract from that likelihood. This notion is of course implicit in the verification theory of meaning.
>
> The dogma of reductionism survives in the supposition that each statement, taken in isolation from its fellows, can admit of confirmation or infirmation at all. My counter-suggestion... is that our statements about the external world face the tribunal of sense experience not individually but only as a corporate body...The unit of empirical significance is the whole of science.

While a verificationist approach to meaning (or 'reductionism') is consistent with a separation of theory and observation, Quine thinks that it cannot be put into practice because testing individual statements always takes place in a broader theoretical background, which might include, for example, theories about the working of instruments used to make the observations.

But plausible though Quine's view is, it relies on *first* dismissing Logical Empiricist claims that observation statements comprise a privileged basis for theory testing and thus we still need a clear argument against the semantic thesis.

By contrast with the claim that observations are *typically* reported using theoretical terms, there are arguments for a stronger claim that all observation statements must be stated in theoretical language. This stronger claim certainly contradicts the Logical Empiricist model described above. It is advanced by the contemporary American philosopher of mind and science, Paul Churchland (1942–).

Churchland's argument: translation of observation statements implicates theory

Churchland's philosophy of mind and science

Together with his wife Patricia, Paul Churchland is most noted for his work on the philosophical consequences of connectionist

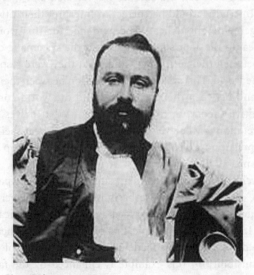

Fig. 12.2 Pierre Duhem

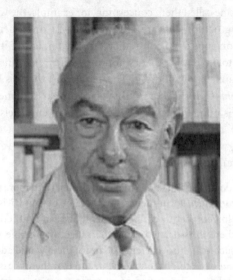

Fig. 12.3 W.V.O. Quine

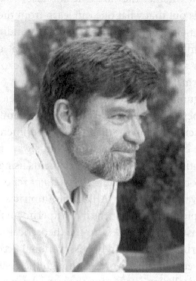

Fig. 12.4 Paul Churchland

models of brain architecture. One element of that work is his argument that folk psychology—the 'theory' with which we explain and predict others' behaviour—is a bad theory that should be replaced by a neurophysiologically informed scientific psychology. We will return to that in Part V. His argument in the following reading is related in one respect, however. It concerns the selection of theories which should inform our thinking about and observing the world.

EXERCISE 5   (30 minutes)

Read the short extract from:

Churchland, P. (1979). *Scientific Realism and the Plasticity of Mind*. Cambridge: Cambridge University Press (Extract pp. 8–10)

Link with Reading 12.3

◆ Summarize the arguments that Churchland offers concerning the connection between observational experiences and theory.

Paul Churchland offers two arguments to undermine the idea that the meaning of terms used to make direct observational claims depends on the observational experiences or sensations with which they are correlated.

His first argument turns on a thought experiment. Churchland claims that the sensations we have in colour experience could

be naturally produced in an alien species when its members directly experienced heat—perhaps through infra-red vision. If this were the case then the best interpretation or translation of their utterances would not be as incorrect judgements about colour—despite the similarity of their inner experiences of heat to our experiences of colour (or surface reflectance). Any such interpretation would be totally unreliable and fail to predict their utterances because there would be no systematic connection between the colours we detected and their utterances. Instead it would be correct to interpret their utterances as judgements about heat. The evidence for this would not be appeal to the alien's inner states but the systematic connections between their utterances and what they were responding to in the world. This systematic connection between their utterances and between their utterances and the world comprises a primitive theory, in this case of heat. What drives correct interpretation is whatever primitive theory of heat their utterances presuppose. The inner experiences thus drop out as irrelevant.

Churchland's second argument suggests that the experiences that we have and on whose basis we make direct perceptual judgements might be used to feed a different theoretical vocabulary. It could be, for example, that our 'sensations of heat' were used to drive judgements made using the vocabulary of caloric. The plausibility of this example is enhanced by the fact that although caloric is an outdated and false theory, the primitive theory of heat we generally use is also false in the light of physics but this does not stop us using it.

Churchland concludes that what matters to the meaning of observational claims is the (possibly primitive) theory presupposed by the use of concepts, not the sensations driving them.

Is descriptive psychopathology based on 'inner sensations'?

Churchland's examples concern direct perception of heat and colour and he argues that the experiences that we have when perceiving these might either indicate the presence of entirely different features of the world, or might be used to drive a different theoretical vocabulary albeit concerning the same features. In these examples it is clear what the sensations are that might be so used: sensations of heat and colour.

EXERCISE 6   (10 minutes)

♦ Are there similar sensations in the case of descriptive pathology?

♦ If there are not, what consequence does this have for applying Churchland's arguments to mental health?

Think about these questions before reading on.

It is much more natural to say that one has sensations of heat or sensations of colour than sensations of a patient presenting schizophrenia. Perhaps the nearest we come to such talk, is among phenomenologists: the German psychiatrist and phenomenologist, Alfred Kraus, for example, reminds us of the importance on occasion of the 'praecox feeling' in the diagnosis of schizophrenia (Kraus, 1994, 2003). How can the phenomenological-anthropological approach contribute to diagnosis and classification in psychiatry? But even in the case of 'feelings' like these, what is involved is not inner sensations so much as unanalysable (perhaps because tacit) judgements about what is externally the case: namely here that someone has schizophrenia.

The general point, then, is that direct perceptual judgement that a particular symptom is being manifested in a patient, does not correspond to a characteristic inner phenomenology on the part of the clinician, corresponding with simple sensations such as those of colour and heat. This point is not special to psychopathology, of course. The same might also be said, reverting to our example at the start of this chapter, in the case of the 'sensation of a chair'. By picking the cases that he does, therefore, Churchland makes it easier to imagine that qualitatively the same sensations might be enjoyed by aliens under different circumstances.

Many philosophers, however, including Quine, Dennett, Rorty, and Wittgenstein, would dispute the validity of reifying the inner feeling of judgements in this way. In the philosophy of the mind this disagreement focuses on the existence or not of raw feels or qualia, as they are called. This is not to say that Churchland supports qualia. In the philosophy of mind, Churchland himself is an opponent of qualia. But the arguments

he presents here are most easily understood as initially presupposing qualia in order then to dismiss their importance for observation statements.

A behaviourist reconstruction

Churchland's arguments, then, generalized from simple sensations (such as heat and colour) to the more complex observations involved in medicine and science, seem somewhat less persuasive.

Nevertheless, arguments similar to those that Churchland gives could be advanced by a more behaviouristic philosopher—such as Dennett, or someone influenced by Wittgenstein or Ryle, who denied that judgements involve an inner phenomenology over and above sensitivity to aspects of the world. Such philosophers deny that perception of redness involves both sensitivity to an outer colour in the world and also an inner raw feel or sensation of redness. They hold instead that the misleading talk of 'sensations of redness' is a misguided way of referring to the outer sensitivity. A reconstruction of the first argument would simply say that the correct interpretation in the first, alien, case can *only* be based on outer behaviour and consequently the meaning of observational terms will depend on the systematic underlying theory they hold. Similarly, in the case of Churchland's second argument, one could simply say that even direct perceptions are couched in a systematic framework and that this system comprises a form of theory.

Reconstructing Churchland's arguments from a more behaviouristic point of view helps to clarify what they establish. Inner experiences are irrelevant for the interpretation of reports of direct perceptions. Instead interpretation relies on the systematic connections on the one hand between different utterances and on the other between utterances and the features in the world. This picture of interpretation is akin to Davidson's idea of radical interpretation, which is discussed in Part V.

This undermines a central motivation for separating languages of theory and observation. That separation seems plausible on the assumption that observation language is defined using inner sensations. Churchland provides an argument against that assumption.

Nevertheless it remains possible, if less plausibly motivated, to suggest that the basic 'theory' of the world that underpins interpretation might itself be confined to directly observational features of the world. In other words a kind of 'a-theoretical theory'. To suggest that this is not a plausible possibility we will turn to one more argument against the independence of observational and theoretical statements, to end this section.

Hesse's argument: any division of theory and observation is itself theory relative

No distinction of principle: Mary Hesse

Establishing the theory dependence of observation statements, requires a principled argument that no distinction can be drawn between theoretical and observation languages. That is what Mary Hesse, the English philosopher and historian of science, attempts to offer in her book *Revolutions and Reconstructions in the Philosophy of Science* (1980).

Hesse presents a developmental story of how simple predicates (such as 'round' and 'green') are introduced and then become employed in a system of general laws such as 'balls are round' or 'in summer leaves are green'. As a result of the developmental process, she argues, this system of laws can introduce 'internal misfits and even contradictions', which in turn require revision in the definitions of predicates. Her claim is that no terms—'observational terms'—are immune to revision. She sums up her point thus:

> To summarise, the developmental story entails that no feature of the total landscape of functioning of a descriptive predicate is exempt from modification under pressure from its surroundings. That any empirical law may be abandoned in the face of counter-examples is trite, but it becomes less trite when the functioning of every predicate is found to depend essentially on some laws or other and when it is also correct that any correct situation of application—even that in terms of which the term was originally introduced—may become incorrect in order to preserve a system of laws and other applications. It is in this sense that I shall understand the 'theory dependence' or 'theory ladenness' of all descriptive predicates'.   Hesse (1980, p. 72)

In the next exercise we look at one of Hesse's examples from physics.

EXERCISE 7   (15 minutes)

Read the extract from:

Hesse, M. (1980). *Revolutions and Reconstructions in the Philosophy of Science*. Brighton: The Harvester Press (Extract pp. 77–78)

Link with Reading 12.4

♦ Extract from the historical detail the principled argument Hesse offers against a once and for all distinction between observational and theoretical arguments.

Hesse points out that the purpose of a distinction between theory and observation is to delimit an impartial test of theory. This is just to repeat the claim that the point of the Logical Empiricist two-language model, as a semantic model, is to provide reassurance on an epistemological issue about the impartiality of observation. But Hesse argues that what counts as an observation claim—what can be settled by observation—depends on which theory is presupposed. Her example in this reading is observations of time. For Newton, the simultaneity of two events was an objective and directly observable matter. For Einstein it was not directly observable because it also depended on considerations of relative inertial frames, the relative states of motion of observer and observed. For this reason simultaneity became perspective-relative. The concept of simultaneity was revised to become (more) theoretical.

A simpler case concerns observation of colours. Under normal circumstances judging the colours of objects does not seem to be a matter of theory. It is theory free. But it is also true that the colours of objects such as cars and buses can look different under different lights, although most of us would agree that the colours don't actually change: a red car is still red. Under abnormal conditions they can only be inferred given a suitable theory. Hence forming judgements about colours from direct perceptions requires that one knows that conditions are normal. But that conditions are normal is not itself a matter of simple observation.

Such a case exemplifies Hesse's claim. Relative to a background theory that conditions are normal we can say that colour perception is theory free. We do not need to *infer* the colour of observed objects. But this will not serve the purposes of Logical Empiricism of providing a theory-free language by which to test rival theories because the assumption that conditions are normal can be called into question and if it is that will change the status of colour judgement. If it is claimed that the atmosphere has been polluted and changed colour perception then judging the true colour of objects may become a theoretical inference.

The moral

The moral that Hesse invites us to draw is that there is no principled way of picking out an observation language because what *counts* as directly observable is itself a matter of theory. Any distinction between theory and observation is tentative and will not necessarily survive changes in theory. Consequently, it cannot

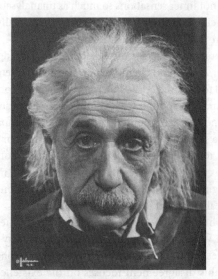

Fig. 12.5 Albert Einstein

be used to frame a theory neutral and impartial observation language. Any distinction presupposes theory and is thus not impartial.

Hesse's argument does not so much show that there cannot be a distinction between theoretical and observation languages as to present a powerful challenge to anyone attempting to define one. They must show that their observational terms are not observational merely in virtue of some assumed background theory. But it is difficult to see how this challenge could be met since the nature of the observational appears to depend on a range of theories. These include theories concerning human perceptual abilities or the working of scientific instruments when natural powers of observation are augmented by measuring instruments. But, as the example mentioned above suggests, what will count as observational will also depend on theories governing the particular subject matter of the science in question.

Hesse's argument and psychopathology

Hesse's argument applies to descriptive psychopathology in the following way. The aim of structured and semi-structured interviews such as the PSE was to establish a theory-neutral observational basis both to underpin diagnosis and to serve as a basis for research in broadly the way favoured by Logical Empiricism. But as Hesse argues, any such list of observable symptoms presupposes a background theory of what is and what is not observable. Thus it cannot act as an arbiter in cases where a difference of diagnosis or a different theoretical account of aetiology is the result of disagreement about what can and what cannot be directly observed. One physician's directly observable symptom or syndrome is another's mistaken theoretical construct.

What this suggests is that the idea of selecting directly observable psychopathological symptoms so as to provide a neutral basis for the construction and testing of theories cannot quite work. Not 'quite' because the judgement that certain phenomena are directly observable is itself a theoretical matter and thus the list arrived at need not survive a change of background theory. But that does not preclude devising, for example, classifications that are, to a first approximation, directly observable rather than a matter of inference according to best present theory. And thus the aim of devising classifications that are independent of premature causal theory is not ruled out. But even if that is successful it is not the same as suggesting that observation might be a matter of brute or raw data.

We return to the implications of the interweaving of the languages of observation and theory at the end of the chapter. First, though, we need to consider arguments showing that theory does not merely infect the sorts of observation statements codified in diagnostic manuals such as the PSE, but also the content of the experience or process of observation itself. It is to these that we turn in the next session.

Reflection on the session and self-test questions

Write down your own reflections on the materials in this session drawing out any points that are particularly significant for you. Then, looking back over the readings, write brief notes about the following:

1. What claim does the theory dependence of observation amount to?

2. What are the main claims advanced by each of Duhem, Churchland, and Hesse in the readings?

3. What conclusions should we draw for psychopathology?

Session 4 Arguments for the theory dependence of the content of the process or experience of observation

The previous session concerned arguments that aimed to show that the language used to frame reports of observations in science presupposes aspects of theory. To the extent that these arguments are successful they undermine the Logical Empiricist account of observation in which the languages of theory and observation are distinguished.

Logical Empiricism, as developed by the Vienna Circle, is important as a sophisticated attempt to provide a rigorous account of the first stage of the traditional model of science, as set out in Chapter 11, namely the making of observations that are themselves theory-neutral and hence can be used to test, or to differentiate between, rival theories. On the traditional model the initial description should be theory free if it is to serve as an impartial basis for theorizing. But the arguments discussed in the last session suggest that reports of observations (or observation statements), at least, cannot be, in the required sense, theory neutral.

But while, even if one accepts the force of those arguments, it is tempting still to think that there is something in the process or experience of observing that corresponds to gathering, or simply being struck by, brute data. Surely, the thought goes, when I open my eyes and take in my surroundings I am simply presented with a theory-free pattern of shades of light and colour, patterns in my two dimensional visual field. Theoretical interpretation comes later. In this session we will assess that assumption.

From selecting experience to experience itself

We have already had one indication that theory influences at least the selection of what we observe. You will recall that in the first exercise of this chapter, in which we 'observed' a chair, the particular features we picked out were determined partly by the chair 'out there', but also by our own prior 'theories', about what would be relevant for example, theories that are (pointing to one's head) 'in here'. What we decide to observe, then, depends to at least this extent on theory: relevant observations are chosen from the infinitude of possible features of our experience. We could not simply take note of everything and at every possible level of detail. This is uncontentious.

In this session, however, we consider arguments to the effect that theory also has a more intimate effect on observation: a phenomenological effect not just on what we select from our experience to attend to, but also on what we experience as such.

Empirical and conceptual sources

A final preliminary point is worth making. The arguments about the language of science described in the last session were derived from studies, historical and sociological as well as philosophical, of the 'hard' or natural sciences. The implication, therefore, was that if even in these disciplines, as paradigm sciences, no sharp distinction could be made between the language of observation and the language of theory, how much more so is this likely to be the case in the 'human' sciences.

The arguments to be described in this session, by contrast, although ostensibly concerned with the 'deeper' question of the natures of observation and theory themselves, have been influenced by the results of experiments carried out by psychologists on perception. In the previous session, then, philosophy had the role of challenging scientists to see that what they do, and hence how science works, is not quite (or at all) as they thought. In this session it is psychology, employing empirical research paradigms, which has helped to show that perceptions (the way in which we come to have experience) is not as any of us thought; and philosophy has then sought to explore why this is so. Both philosophers of mind and philosophers of science have based arguments on examples from basic psychological accounts of perception to more fundamental ideas about how experience in general has to be understood if we are to have rational contact with the world.

As between the last sessions and this session, then, there is a nice balance of empirical and conceptual, of understanding advancing through the interplay of experimental and analytic methods, of just the kind that is required, we suggested in Chapter 1, in mental health.

Card sorting: fallible but correctable perceptions

Before examining the main arguments, it will be worth getting clear what sort of connection between the perception, and prior theory is significant for the specifically philosophical concerns (albeit influenced by psychology) about the relationship between observation and theory. A passage from a book on the nature of science will help us to do this. The passage is taken from an accessible introduction to the philosophy of science written by Alan Chalmers who was based in the History and Philosophy of Science Unit of the Faculty of Science at the University of Sidney until his retirement in 1999.

EXERCISE 8   (5 minutes)

Read the passage from:

Chalmers, A.F. (1999) *What is this thing called science?* Buckingham: Open University Press (Extract p. 25)

Link with Reading 12.5

Think whether the phenomenon it describes has any analogue in descriptive psychopathology. Does it raise a significant threat to the objectivity of the description of symptoms?

Expectations and observations

This sort of experience is probably familiar to everyone in every day life as well as clinical experience. We are influenced in our direct perceptual judgements by our expectations. Accurate expectations about what we are likely to experience makes judgement quicker and more reliable. False expectations hinder it. This is a general phenomenon and is found as much in mental health care as anywhere else. The description above adds to this familiar phenomenon the potentially more interesting claim that the subject's experience—rather than just their dispositions to make judgements—itself changed. This claim will be more dramatic to those who think of inner experience on the model of sensations. Those of a more behaviouristic cast will want to assimilate experience and dispositions to judgements and thus will not think that anything extra has been added to the everyday phenomenon about expectations and reliability.

But even with these qualifications, the card identifying experiment does not present a fundamental threat to the objectivity of our direct perceptual judgements. It simply shows something that should be no surprise: that even direct perceptual judgements are fallible. This effect can be reduced through repeated checking, double blind testing and other modifications of experimental protocol. It is no part of the traditional account of scientific method that observation is infallible, just impartial with respect to theory. In the above example, repeated checking of observations effectively removes the taint of theory. But there are arguments to say that observation is necessarily impregnated with theory. This is what is claimed as a consequence of consideration of the duck–rabbit ambiguous figure, which is the subject of the next exercise.

The duck–rabbit figure undermines an intuitive but misguided model of perception

EXERCISE 9   (15 minutes)

Look at the illustrations below. What can you see? What does this suggest about the role of concepts in experience? Can we generalize to more everyday cases of observation. Are any observations independent of concepts? Think about the general lessons that can be learnt about observation from examples such as the duck–rabbit and the Necker cube.

The duck–rabbit

Wittgenstein (1953) introduces this figure in the second part of his *Philosophical Investigations* in this way:

I shall call the following figure, derived from Jastrow, the duck–rabbit. It can be seen as a rabbit's head or as a duck's.

And I must distinguish between the 'continuous seeing' of an aspect and the 'dawning' of an aspect.

The picture might have been shewn me, and I never have seen anything but a rabbit in it.   (p. 194)

Wittgenstein took the figure of the duck–rabbit from Joseph Jastrow (1863–1944) who was born in Warsaw but worked in the USA as an experimental psychologist. But figures of this sort were also a subject of 'Gestalt psychology' founded by the Czech psychologist Max Wertheimer (1880–1943).

Most people, when looking at the duck–rabbit, experience switches between perception of a duck and perception of a rabbit. The stimulus (the figure) has not changed, of course. But the very same features can be perceived either as a duck or a rabbit as though the picture itself had changed. Either aspect can dawn. If someone has not seen the ambiguity in the figure they might simply report that it is a rabbit (or perhaps a 'picture rabbit', a term Wittgenstein introduces). But if they do suddenly notice the duck aspect they might say 'Now it's a duck!'. Wittgenstein describes such an experience in a different case: 'I contemplate a face, and then suddenly notice its likeness to another. I *see* that it has not changed; and yet I see it differently. I call this experience 'noticing an aspect'. (ibid: p. 193)

What do cases of aspect dawning like this show?

Well, firstly, they establish the negative point that one common intuitive model of perception is false. According to this intuitive picture, to perceive something is to have an inner mental image of it. That mental image corresponds to raw brute data, impressed on a subject. But on this model, the best possible representation of seeing the duck–rabbit figure would thus simply reproduce it internally as a mental image. But that would not explain how we can perceive now the duck, now the rabbit aspect. The internal image could no more determine which aspect was perceived than the external picture can. (It is also worth thinking how reproducing the image inside the mind is supposed to 'solve' the problem of perception: how is the internal image itself perceived?)

Alongside that negative result, however, experience of the duck–rabbit figure also suggests the positive conclusion that our visual experience is, sometimes at least, affected by our conceptual resources. To see the protuberances in the figure as the rabbit's ears or as the duck's beak requires that one possesses the concepts of ears and beak. One needs to know what an ear or a beak is. This grasp of concepts, however, does not feature as a mere external feature of the experience of observing. It is not an interpretation of, or piece of ratiocination about, a neutral and prior image that is ambiguous between the duck and rabbit. Rather, the most basic experience is as of a *duck* or of a *rabbit* (or

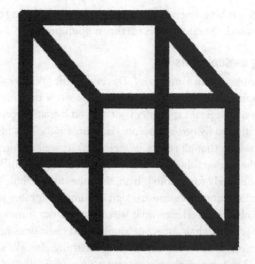

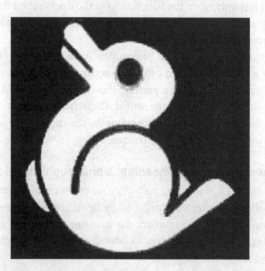

Fig. 12.6 A Duck-Rabbit and a Necker Cube

of a duck part or rabbit part if concentrating on a smaller area of the figure). That is the nature of the experience.

It may be tempting to think that there must be more basic components of perception from which our experiences are built up: typically, one might think that one perceives the lines that make up the figure and the rest is interpretation of these lines: a two component model. But in fact it takes some skill to learn to see the figure merely as lines. And our ability or lack of ability to reproduce it—to sketch it—suggests that our normal understanding of the figure is of a whole image: a duck or a rabbit from which we might then abstract the lines. (Compare copying letters in an alphabet one knows with, say, pictograms with which one is unfamiliar. This suggests that recognizing the letters as letters is more basic than recognizing them as lines.)

Furthermore, the experience of an aspect dawning, expressed in the utterance 'Now it's a rabbit!' suggests that there is no more basic way to describe that experience without referring to rabbits, their habitats, etc. The experience of seeing the rabbit aspect of the duck–rabbit is not one of interpretation of something directly seen. Instead, the rabbit aspect is thrust upon one.

Seeing as seeing-as

In a book called *Patterns of Discovery*, the Wittgensteinian philosopher of science Norwood Hanson drew the conclusion from psychological experiments of this kind that perception is always affected by one's concepts (Hanson 1958). This might be put by saying that all seeing is 'seeing-as'. As well as sometimes seeing the duck–rabbit *as* a duck, we also see ducks *as* ducks (and correspondingly for rabbits). If so, then the duck–rabbit switching phenomenon is an unusual sign of something more general: that we always experience what we observe under some conceptual aspect. The chair aspect of an observed chair does not need to dawn on us as we cannot see it *as* anything else. We see, not shapes that we secondarily interpret as a chair, but, directly, 'chair'. It is only when the stimulus, as in the duck–rabbit figure, is ambiguous, that we are aware of this 'seeing as', but it is a feature of perception as a whole.

The conclusion for the philosophy of science that Hanson draws is that observation cannot be separated or insulated from one's general conceptual repertoire including one's general theoretical understanding of the world. Consequently, what we see when we observe the world depends on the theories we already have. Seeing is conceptually structured.

Phenomenology and meaning: a philosophical aside

Hanson's conclusion—that perception is never a matter of receiving brute data but is instead conceptually structured—is correct. We will look at another argument for it at the end of this session. But it ignores some subtleties in Wittgenstein's discussion, which are also worth drawing out.

After introducing the duck–rabbit figure Wittgenstein goes on to say:

Here it is useful to introduce the idea of a picture-object. For instance, [bare sketch of a face] would be a picture-face.

In some respects, I stand towards it as I stand towards a human face. I can study its expression can react to it as to the expression of the human face. A child can talk to picture-men or picture-animals, can treat them as it treats dolls.

I may, then, have seen the duck–rabbit simply as a picture-rabbit from the first. That is to say, if asked, 'what's that?' or 'what do you see here?' I should have replied: 'a picture-rabbit'. If I had further been asked what that was, I should have explained by pointing to all sorts of pictures of rabbits, should perhaps have pointed to real rabbits, talked about their habits or given an imitation of them.

I should not have answered the question 'what do you see here?' by saying: 'now I am seeing it as a picture-rabbit'. I should simply have described my perception: just as if I had said 'I see a red circle over there'.   Wittgenstein (1953, pp. 194–195)

In these passages Wittgenstein hints at two important ideas that he elaborates later. One is that the relation between continuous aspect perception and aspect dawning is complicated. On the one hand, continuous aspect perception involves the spontaneous use of a description (for example, 'a picture-rabbit') rather than an interpretation of lines and shapes and thus shares some of the spontaneity of aspect dawning. But on the other, there seems to be nothing paradoxical about continuous aspect perception and in this it contrasts with aspect dawning when a description is wrung from one e.g. 'Now it's a rabbit!', when one simultaneously knows that nothing has changed. Wittgenstein suggests that the report in a case of aspect dawning is like an expression of pain, e.g. 'It hurts', which manifests the particular experience one is having.

Secondly, while aspect dawning suggests something about the 'logic' of perception and centrally that a two component model cannot work, Wittgenstein also suggests that it is a contingent feature of human vision. The fact that we can directly experience two aspects in the duck–rabbit is merely contingently true. He suggests that there could be subjects for whom this was impossible and who were 'aspect blind'. The hint of this idea in the passages above is the reference to standing to a picture as one does to a real human face, or children playing with pictures as with dolls. That suggests an immediacy of response in our normal phenomenology that might not be true of all possible subjects. To understand this it is useful to recall where this discussion takes place.

Wittgenstein's discussion of the duck–rabbit and aspect-perception takes place in the second part of his book *Philosophical Investigations* (1953). The first part contains an extended discussion of what it is to understand the meaning of a word. At the time, understanding the meaning of a word was widely regarded as involving some process of interpretation by 'reading off' from a set of rules. Wittgenstein, in the first part of *Philosophical Investigations*, shows that understanding a word cannot be explained as the successful interpretation of a rule because this leads to an infinite regress: one needs an interpretation of the interpretation.

In the succeeding discussion of perception Wittgenstein suggests that it would be possible to be 'aspect blind'. Someone who is aspect blind cannot experience a changing of aspects looking at, for example, the duck–rabbit. However, they would still able to understand such pictures as one does circuit diagrams. A further example he gives of the difference between those who are, and are not, aspect blind is between those who can experience meaning in a word and those who cannot. The kind of experience he means is that which can be lost by repeating the same word until it seems to loose its meaning. But even someone who can never hear the meaning directly in a word might still be able to use it perfectly correctly and thus know what it means.

Such understanding would be of an intellectual sort. It is tempting to say, in the visual case, that it would involve deriving what the picture is of from the lines by a set of rules rather than more immediately seeing the object in the picture. Someone who is aspect blind would then have to work out what the picture is rather as one has to work out what an information blueprint is about, i.e. by reference to a set of rules of interpretation But we know from the earlier part of *Philosophical Investigations* that Wittgenstein denies that understanding in general can be a matter of interpretation of a set of rules. So while the aspect blind would have to have a relationship to pictures akin to our relationship to blueprints, in neither case is that explained through having to interpret what is seen.

This suggests that the discussion of aspect dawning is not as simple as Hanson's account implies. Hanson is right to stress that perception—in both continuous aspect perception and aspect dawning cases—involves concepts and that the very possibility of aspect dawning suggests that a two-component model of vision is wrong. On that model, perception involves first taking in raw data and then interpreting it. But it cannot explain aspect dawning.

On the other hand, aspect dawning is a contingent feature of human perception. It would be possible, according to Wittgenstein, to be able to perceive but without having the phenomenological immediacy that we enjoy. For humans, at least, it is possible to relate to pictures, for example, as surrogates for fellow humans, to hear meaning directly in words and so on. Wittgenstein is keen to stress the importance of this engaged perspective on the world. It will be useful now to chart a disagreement between Hanson and Churchland, both of whom agree that observation is theory laden rather than a matter of brute data.

Hanson on seeing the sunrise

As we have seen, Hanson argues that all perception depends on one's general conceptual repertoire and consequently on the theories one holds about the world. As a result, he suggests that Tycho and Kepler saw something different at 'sunrise'. He suggests that the former saw the sun rise and the latter saw the earth turn because of their different theoretical commitments.

> Let us consider Johannes Kepler: imagine him on a hill watching the dawn. With him is Tycho Brahe. Kepler regarded the sun as fixed: it was the earth that moved. But Tycho followed Ptolemy and Aristotle in this much at least: the earth was fixed and all other celestial bodies moved around it. *Do Kepler and Tycho see the same thing in the east at dawn?* . . .
>
> [S]omething about their visual experiences at dawn is the same for both: a brilliant yellow-white disc centred between green and blue colour patches. Sketches of what they both see could be identical—congruent. In this sense Tycho and Kepler see the same thing at dawn. The sun appears to them in the same way. The same view, or scene, is presented to them both . . .
>
> [S]aying that Kepler and Tycho see the same thing at dawn just because their eyes are similarly affected is an elementary mistake. There is a difference between a physical state and a visual experience.
>
> Kepler and Tycho agree on [much] . . . Their visual fields are organized in much the same way. Neither sees the sun about to break out in a grin, or about to crack into ice cubes. (The

baby is not 'set' even against these eventualities.) Most people today see the same thing at dawn in an even stronger sense: we share much knowledge of the sun. Hence Tycho and Kepler see different things, and yet they see the same thing. That these things can be said depends on their knowledge, experience, and theories.

> Kepler and Tycho are to the sun as we are to [the duck–rabbit], when I see the [duck] and you see only the [rabbit]. The elements of their experiences are identical; but their conceptual organization is vastly different. Can their visual fields have a different organization? Then they can see different things in the east at dawn. Hanson (1958, p. 5–18)

The only way of resisting the conclusion that they saw something different would be to invoke the notion of a common brute datum as the two-component model postulates; however, that idea is rejected because of consideration of aspect dawning.

But is the claim that Tycho and Kepler see something different plausible? Do we all now see the earth turn rather than the sun rise?

Churchland on seeing the sunrise

Churchland (1979) takes issue with Hanson on this point. He claims that, as a matter of phenomenological fact, Tycho and Kepler, like the rest of us, see the same thing. None of us can help but see the sun rise. That 'theory' is too embedded to escape from merely by learning Kepler's alternative.

Churchland claims that we report observations using a theoretical language and that theory can affect perception, but he does not think that our experience is automatically transformed by any particular theory we hold. Thus although we may all report sunrise as the earth turning when attempting to speak accurately, Copernican theory does not inform our perceptions themselves. We have to re-educate ourselves to perceive in accordance with our theories. The connection between the act of perception and the theories we hold is not, according to Churchland, as close as Hanson claims it is. They agree that our perceptions are affected by our theories. They disagree on which theories our perceptions are affected by.

Churchland claims that one can teach oneself in certain conditions to 'see the earth spin' instead. This involves certain practical steps such as finding a suitable location in which the earth's horizon is unarresting and turning one's neck so that one's head points in a direction perpendicular to the ecliptic. It helps if there are planets visible so as to make the plane of the solar system clear. When successful it seems that the earth is spinning rather than the sun is rising. (Of course, unlike a fairground round, there are no physiological sensations of movement.)

What is the disagreement between Hanson and Churchland?

Both Hanson and Churchland agree that observation is theory laden but they disagree about how to apply that claim to the apparently simple case of the sunrise. What should we learn from this?

By looking in a little more detail at Wittgenstein's discussion of aspect perception we can adjudicate this debate. The disagreement does not threaten the basic idea that observation is not a matter of brute data but always, instead, conceptually structured. Concepts play a fundamental role in shaping of perceptual experience. But aspect perception also suggests that perception has a further (and contingent) immediacy, which is shown in the way perceptual experience of the duck–rabbit can 'flip' between the two aspects. (In addition, Wittgenstein suggests this is connected to our ability to experience meaning in the use of a word and lose it if the word is repeated.)

Churchland's account of the experiences one can have at sunrise look to a case of this latter phenomenological fact. Success in seeing the earth turn is like success in seeing the duck or rabbit aspect of the duck–rabbit. The criterion of achieving it might be saying 'Now it seems as though the earth is turning' like 'Now it is a duck'. If so, while it deepens our understanding of how perception, concepts, and experience are interconnected the disagreement between Churchland and Hanson is, strictly, orthogonal to the main issue, which is that, in Churchland's phrase, observation is a matter of the conceptual exploitation of the senses.

The coup de grace for Logical Empiricism?

This point marks a return to the Logical Empiricist emphasis on the importance of observation statements or reports. So it is worth recapping the argument of this session. Hanson argues that the experience of changes of aspect (of the duck–rabbit) shows that all seeing is seeing-as and thus directly concept-involving. That may be true—and we will look at another argument for it shortly—but it also neglects some of the subtlety of Wittgenstein's discussion. Wittgenstein's account of aspect blindness suggests that there is something immediate about human perception, which, in principle, need not be a feature of all perception. This in turn helps shed light on the disagreement between Churchland and Hanson who otherwise agree that experience involves concepts.

This leaves the following question. If conceptualized observation reports are what are relevant for theory testing and if these do not depend on the interpretation of neutral sense data (as Hanson, Wittgenstein, and Churchland all agree), how exactly are they connected to experience? This is the question to which the Logical Empiricists had no answer. And for that reason, there was something mysterious about the status of observation reports. Indeed, as we will note in Chapter 16, Imre Lakatos, drawing on this tradition, was forced to say that we adopt observation statements *by convention*. But surely, observation statements are derived, in some way, from experiences? We may choose to drive on the left or right by convention but surely there is more to observation statements than that?

One possible answer to this question is that sensations or experiences merely *cause* trained observers to make specific sorts of observation report. Sensations or experiences, that is to say, have a role as part of the causal process that leads to an observational report. This is the kind of account offered by behaviouristically minded philosophers like W.V.O. Quine (see his *Word and Object*, 1960). But it raises the question of what makes the report the *right* sort of report to make about the world. A merely causal story here makes reports of observations no more rational responses to the world than the noise made by an apple falling from a tree on to the ground. Reports of observations, if merely caused by sensations or experiences, thus seem unlikely to be any more *about* anything than the noise of the apple falling is *about* gravity. We will return to these matters in the philosophy of thought and language in Part V. But a final short description here will serve as a tempter to these philosophically deep waters.

More general considerations of the role of experience suggest that it is conceptually structured

McDowell is a contemporary philosopher who has written mainly on the philosophy of thought and language. *Mind and World* is a series of lectures in which he attempts to present a coherent overall metaphysical account of the connection between our experience of the world and the world—of mind and world (McDowell 1994). Broadly, he attempts to unite a Kantian framework with more recent analytic and continental philosophy. The first chapter focuses on the question of how our experiences can provide a rational test for our beliefs and thus serve to connect our beliefs with how the world is. McDowell's key thought, although somewhat understated, is that only if there *is* such a rational connection, can beliefs actually have the content or meaning that they *do*. Epistemology—in this case having reasons for beliefs—and the philosophy of thought and language go hand in hand.

McDowell thus reverses the normal order of philosophical batting. Most philosophers have sought arguments from the nature of perception to show how it is that we can have rational beliefs about the world. McDowell takes the fact that we do have rational beliefs about the world to show that it is in the essential nature of perception that it is conceptually structured.

But what is the Kantian framework?

The Kantian framework

One way to think about the relation of theory and observation in experience is to start with a slogan from Kant's first Critique: the *Critique of Pure Reason*. Kant says: 'Thoughts without content are empty, intuitions without concepts are blind' (Kant, 1929, p. 93, A51, B75).

This phrase expresses the interdependence of two aspects that together make experience possible: concepts and intuitions. Concepts are the responsibility of the faculty of spontaneity that looks after active judgement. Intuitions are the responsibility of the faculty of receptivity, which takes in how the world is. The slogan suggests that in empirical judgements, experiences of how the world is, the two aspects work in harmony. Thoughts require some intuitive content, and intuitions must be structured by concepts.

Some commentators such as Sellars and McDowell take it to express two further and potentially stronger claims. First, that thought in general is only possible because of the interplay of concepts and intuitions. In other words, experience is a condition of possibility of thought in general. Thus to say 'Thoughts without content are empty' is to say not that they are a special sort of empty thought but rather no thought at all. Secondly, that there is no such thing as pure receptivity. Experience is always a synthesis of conceptual and intuitive elements, but it would not be possible for us to have intuitions that were purely receptive—conceptual content is always involved.

Whether or not these stronger claims are accurate accounts of Kant—and we will return to McDowell's account shortly—the discussion of the thesis of the theory dependence of observation can be related to the slogan in this way. No observation is pure receptivity, a matter of merely passively taking in features of the world. Empirical judgements and the experiences they depend upon are always a synthesis of a worldly input in a conceptual form.

There is a further point worth making here that is also suggested by something else Kant says in a chapter on the 'The schematism of the pure concepts of understanding'. The point can be put in the following thoroughly un-Kantian way. Imagine that experiences are put together like this: the subconscious mind takes in some purely intuitive content, then selects an appropriate concept and synthesizes a conceptually structured experience such that a subject can, e.g., see that there is cat in front of her. The conceptualized content of the experience is given by what follows the 'that': *there is cat in front of me.*

But now consider how a suitable concept—'cat'—is to be picked. Not just any concept will do. The purely intuitive content cannot be squeezed into just any conceptual clothing. A cat does not look like an elephant, for example. So it looks as though a rule is needed that relates a class of intuitions to each general concept: cat, dog, elephant, etc. If so the particular intuition can now be compared with the rules and thus a concept selected. This, however, suggests a regress. The rule that connects the concept 'cat' to a class of intuitions will have to represent that class in some general way. And that looks to be a kind of concept. If so there will have to be another 'second order' rule to select which 'first order' rule should be used to select an appropriate concept. This initiates an infinite regress. One way out of this, although not Kant's way who, arguably devoted his third Critique in part to addressing this problem, is to block the regress at the start. Once

one has been initiated into a language, one's experiences are always conceptualized. Part of what it is to grasp a concept such as 'cat' is to have mastered an ability to have cat experiences. The pure intuition described in the thought experiment above is a myth. This is of a piece with the denial that observation can involve taking in raw data.

We will now turn to a sketch of McDowell's argument.

Foundationalism and Coherentism

McDowell provides a schematic argument that experience is always conceptually structured. He argues that observation *must* be always already conceptualized for there to be a *rational* connection between our beliefs about the world and the state of the world itself. Thus, he invites us to consider the alternative. Suppose that we conceive of observation as giving us *non-conceptualized* experience, then we have two possibilities:

1. Either experience merely *causes* us to have the beliefs we have and a causal connection is not a rational connection. This would be a form of Foundationalism in which the ultimate grounds for our beliefs would be brute unconceptualized sense data. McDowell calls this the Myth of the Given, arguing that without a rational connection to states of the world, our beliefs would not be *about* anything.

2. Or our beliefs are justified only by *other beliefs* in which case we do not have a grip on the world. McDowell calls this a form of Coherentism and dismisses it with the claim that it leaves our beliefs as no more than a 'frictionless spinning in the void' and thus, again, not *about* anything.

   The label 'Coherentism' picks up a distinction between two rival views of truth. Correspondence theorists suggest that truth is correspondence with a fact. A belief is true if it corresponds with the facts. But that leaves the problem of explaining what 'correspondence' and 'fact' mean in ways that do not simply presuppose, e.g. 'truth' and 'belief'. Coherentists claim that a belief is true if it coheres with other beliefs. But they then have to explain both what 'coherence' means and show that only true beliefs cohere.)

Concepts play a part in experiences as well as beliefs

Having thus rejected both Foundationalism and Coherentism, McDowell argues that the immediate output of observation must be always already conceptualized. The 'space of reasons' extends out to the most worldly part of our mind: our experience of the world. When we open our eyes, concepts that we have learnt actively to apply in judgements or beliefs are passively drawn into operation in experiences. McDowell argues that this enables us to be directly open to the world in experience. He goes on to claim that:

> [T]here is no ontological gap between the sort of thing one can mean, or generally the sort of thing one can think, and the sort of thing that can be the case. When one thinks truly, what one

thinks *is* what is the case. So since the world is everything that is the case . . . there is no gap between thought, as such, and the world. Of course thought can be distanced from the world by being false, but there is no distance from the world implicit in the very idea of thought. (p. 27)

Of course, this leaves the question of how one can distinguish what is true from what is false. That question might be asked in the philosophical context of a discussion of scepticism or in a practical context of choosing between diagnoses and would receive different kinds of answer. But McDowell aims to separate that question from the more basic question of how thought can make contact with the world. His answer is that providing one is not in error, the connection is very direct.

Observation and concepts for antipsychiatry

At the start of this chapter we mentioned a concern about psychiatric observation that runs as follows. If observation is connected to classification in the way exemplified by the PSE then it involves a distortion because patients' experiences are forced into pre-existing categories rather than recognized for their individuality.

With McDowell's argument in place, however, we can see that this objection trades on the false assumption that observation could ever be concept-free. As every observation is conceptually structured there is no possibility of completely unconstrained 'taking in' of patients' experiences.

Of course this is not to say that labelling is never distorting nor that the concepts in play at any time should not be critically reflected on and revised in the light of theory. However, it does help remove the false promise that observation could be carried out without preconceptions. It is precisely preconceptions that give observation its voice.

Unanswered questions

McDowell's picture leaves several questions to be thought through. Here are two:

1. Our experience is always already conceptualized because we are language users and thus already possessors of concepts that can be actively employed in judgements. These same concepts are then drawn passively into play when we open our eyes to the world. What then of the experience of non-language users?

2. What is the connection between McDowell's philosophical claim that experience cannot be broken down into non-conceptual elements and neurophysiological work on the underlying causal processes of vision?

We will return to these issues in Part V. In the final session of this chapter we will look briefly at some of the implications of these issues by comparing the complexity of observation in psychopathology with recent work revealing the complexity of observation in the hardest of the hard sciences: physics.

Reflection on the session and self-test questions

Write down your own reflections on the materials in this session drawing out any points that are particularly significant for you. Then write brief notes about the following:

1. How are concepts implicated in the experience or process of observation? What lessons can be learnt from experiments on the observation of bogus playing cards?

2. What lessons can be drawn from aspect figures such as the duck-rabbit?

3. What do they imply about the role of concepts?

4. What, if any, significance does our ability directly to experience the dawning of an aspect have for scientific observation?

5. How do general Kantian considerations count against the idea of raw data?

Session 5 The consequences for observation in psychiatry and in physics

Observation and theory, then, for any given science, are, if Hesse is right, interconnected in an essentially open-ended way: as theory develops so what counts as dry observation will change, in turn changing theory, and so on, without limit, or at any rate without a limit that can be either predicted or defined a priori, within the science itself.

It is important to emphasize that Hesse has in mind here, primarily, not the psychological and social sciences, but the hardest of hard sciences, physics. Her example cited above is taken from special relativity. A still deeper interweaving of observation and theory is evident in the development of quantum mechanics. The inherent limits on the observation of physical variables defined by the German physicist, Werner Heisenberg's (1901–76) complementary formalisms are well known: pairs of variables previously thought to be independent turn out to be complementary in the sense that, for a given experimental set-up, the more accurately you choose to observe one of a complementary pair of variables, the less accurately will you be able to observe the other: observe the *position* of a particle closely and its *momentum* (its state of motion) will be correspondingly uncertain.

Less well recognized than complementarity, but involving an even more radical break with a traditional understanding of observation, is what has become known as entanglement. As a feature of quantum mechanics, the puzzles generated by entanglement were first made fully explicit by a thought experiment

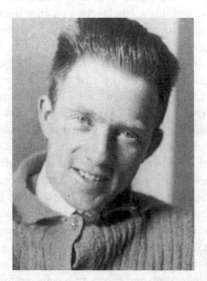

Fig. 12.7 Heisenberg

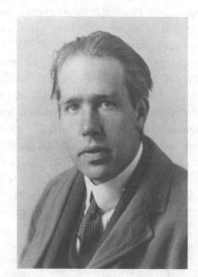

Fig. 12.8 Neils Bohr

called the Einstein–Podolsky–Rosen paradox, the 'EPR' paradox. It will be worth spending a few minutes on this. It takes us to the heart of the difficulties about observation in science, and indeed related difficulties about the nature of objectivity and the role of the subject, as these difficulties arise not speculatively in philosophy but in practice at the very cutting edge of physical theory.

As is well known, Einstein, early in his career, besides more or less single-handedly founding relativity, made crucial contributions to the development of quantum mechanics: his analysis of the spectrum of radiation given off by a hot but not glowing object, for example, the so-called 'black body radiation', was critical to establishing that energy is (under certain experimental set-ups, at least) 'quantised', i.e. broken up into discrete packets. Yet Einstein remained throughout his life deeply dissatisfied with quantum mechanics. Relativity, he believed, although novel, was consistent with a well-behaved traditional understanding of the world and of how science gives us access to it. Quantum mechanics, by contrast, Einstein insisted, is both probabilistic, and, more troubling still from a classical point of view, in some respects solipsistic—it winds the observer, and what the observer chooses to observe, in a most unclassical way into what is observed.

Einstein's concerns about the probabilistic nature of quantum mechanics were summed up in his famous aphorism 'God does not play dice'. Quantum mechanics works with probabilities: it gives, for example, the probability that a radioactive particle will decay over a given period giving off a particular pulse of radiation. Einstein argued that behind these probabilities there must be 'hidden variables', which, with future developments in

instrumentation, will translate the probabilities of quantum mechanics into the determinate observations and predictions of classical (including relativistic) physics. The situation with fundamental particles, Einstein argued, is in principle similar to, say, tossing a coin. Behind the apparently chance fall of a coin as heads or tails, lie hidden but none the less in principle observable variables—mass, energy, etc.—by which the actual path of an actual coin is rigidly determined.

Quantum mechanics denies Einstein's (common sense) determinism (putatively) underlying its probabilities. In quantum mechanics the probabilities—the fall of God's dice—go all the way back. There are no hidden variables. What you see (observe) is what you get.

Notwithstanding Einstein's opposition, the 'what you see is what you get' interpretation of quantum mechanics rapidly became the standard or 'Copenhagen' interpretation in the 1920s—'Copenhagen' because it was argued with particular effectiveness by the Danish physicist, Niels Bohr, who was based in Copenhagen. Bohr's arguments were based on complementarity. Tying down one of a complementary pair of variables more tightly will necessarily, according to quantum mechanics, loosen up the other. This, Bohr argued, showed that there cannot be a determinate set of discrete variables 'lying hidden behind' quantum mechanical observations.

Enter the EPR paradox! Einstein produced a whole series of counter-arguments to the Copenhagen interpretation, all of which Bohr was able successfully to counter, except one, the EPR paradox. The paradox arises from a 'thought experiment' devised by Einstein together with two graduate students, Podolsky and Rosen. We do not have space to go into the details here: published originally in *Physical Review Letters B*, an authoritative non-mathematical account has been given by the French theoretical physicist, Bernard d'Espagnat (1983). The essence of the EPR thought experiment is that it distinguishes, in principle, between, on the one hand Einstein's classical (hidden variables) interpretation of quantum mechanics, and, on the other, the Copenhagen or standard (no hidden variables) interpretation. The experimental set up in the EPR, that is to say, provides a test of the two interpretations, which does not depend on the demonstration (or failure to demonstrate) hidden variables as such. You set the experiment up: if you get one result there *are* hidden variables there waiting to be discovered; if you get a different result there are *no* hidden variables there waiting to be discovered.

The rub, though, has Einstein, Podolsky, and Rosen pointed out, is that the nul result, the standard Copenhagen no-hidden-variables result, was absurd. It required a direct and simultaneous influence of the observer (and of what the observer chooses to observe) not only in the immediate vicinity of the experimental set-up but also at (in principle) unlimited distances across the universe. Simultaneous action at a distance of this kind is bad enough from the point of view of a traditional model of science (it is literally impossible in relativity theory). That the experimental result, including such action at a distance, is a product not (just) of the physical system but of what the observer chooses to do, is tantamount to solipsism. Far from a clean separation of observer and observed, then, as in a traditional model of science, the results of the EPR thought experiment, if the experiment comes out consistently with the predictions of quantum mechanics, mean that the properties of a physical system (including parts of the system now at remote distances from the observer) are (in part) actually determined by the observations that the observer chooses to make. Absurd! Einstein concluded. Does the moon cease to exist, he said, in another famous quip, this time against the solipsism of quantum mechanics, when no one is looking at it?

Well, the absurd happened! To cut a long story short (given in full in d'Espagnat's book, above), in the 1960s a Northern Ireland physicist, John Bell, working at CERN (the Centre Européen pour la Recherche Nucléaire near Geneva), devised an ingenious mathematical treatment of the EPR paradox that made it possible in principle actually to carry out the EPR thought experiment; in the 1970s, with the development of lasers, the John Bell version of the original EPR thought experiment was carried out for real (by a number of researchers, but most decisively by Alain Aspect at the Institut d'Optique Théorique et Appliquée at Orsay in France); and the results, unequivocally, were *for* the 'absurd' (no-hidden-variables) Copenhagen interpretation of quantum mechanics and *against* Einstein's traditional and common-sense (hidden variables) interpretation.

What are the morals of this story for psychopathology as the observational basis of psychiatric science?

First, for theory. The EPR story shows the difficulties of observation and interpretation of experience in psychiatry, compared with bodily medicine, in a positive light. As we saw in Part I, these difficulties, in the twentieth century, were the basis of stigmatizing 'psychiatry second' attitudes. A traditional model of science, premised as it is on clear-cut objective observations as the basis of experimental tests of theory, inevitably led to pejorative comparisons between psychiatry and, say, cardiology as scientific disciplines. The EPR story shows, substantively, what Duhem, Quine, Churchland, Hesse, and others had suggested philosophically, that the traditional model, in this as in other respects, oversimplifies the nature of science. If, therefore, scientific progress at the cutting edge of the hardest of hard sciences, has complicated rather than resolved our understanding of the relationship between observer and observed, how much more will this be true with the added complications arising from the more explicit merging of observer and observed in the psychological sciences.

Just *how* observation and theory fit together, remains an open question. Even in quantum mechanics the Bell-Aspect results deepen rather than resolve this question. Any future physical theory must incorporate the Bell-Aspect results including their (by traditional standards) absurd implications. But just what such theories will look like remains to be seen. This indeed is an area in which the psychological sciences may, in the future, provide insights for the physical sciences rather than vice versa (Fulford, 1989, p 274). John Bell himself made the point strongly, in an interview with another theoretical physicist, Paul Davies, on the BBC's Radio 3 (Davies and Brown, 1986, p. 48):

Davies: So that these issues [about the nature of observation in physics] haven't been fully resolved, at least to your satisfaction?

Bell: Absolutely not. And the experiment of Aspect and the Einstein-Podolsky-Rosen correlations do not help to resolve this problem, but make it harder, because Einstein's view that behind the quantum world lies a familiar classical world was a possible (and now discredited) way of solving this measurement problem—a way of reducing the observer to an incidental role in the physical world.

Second, for practice. Important as the EPR/Bell/Aspect story is for showing the limitations of the traditional picture of observation in science, the story might seem to 'practical' men (recall Bertrand Russell's use of this term in Part I, p 114), too abstract and arcane to be of practical significance. The story was indeed, for a long time, neglected even by most physicists as being rather too close to mere philosophical 'playing with words'. Interesting, yes, was the standard line, even ingenious; but it could never be used for anything practical (like sending a signal). And certainly the original motivations behind the story were theoretical rather than, directly, practical. But as is the way with theoretically motivated research, there are signs, already, that the EPR/Bell/Aspect story could provide the window through which a whole new physics is opened up to us.

We return to the nature of progress in science, and to the way in which long periods of settled theory may suddenly and unexpectedly be disrupted, in Chapter 16. Einstein was responsible for one such disruption at the start of the twentieth century, with relativity; and (in part) for a second, in quantum mechanics. It may be that with the EPR/Bell/Aspect story, Einstein will end up as being (reluctantly) responsible for a third disruption, at the start of the twenty-first century! But the moral for psychopathology is that deep theory, explorations of the concepts underpinning research and practice in mental health, is not antithetical to practical outcomes. Such explanations are not driven by practical pay-offs. It may be that work of this kind is actually inhibited if connected too directly to practical pay-offs, at least of the kind defined by current science. But the lesson of history is that science progresses in practice through a combination of theory and observation, of conceptual and empirical studies, working together in a complex, and perhaps not fully codifiable, but none the less mutually interdependent way.

Third, no easy option. A third moral of the EPR/Bell/Aspect story for psychopathology, is that the theory dependence of observation is no easy option. Philosophers and perhaps even more sociologists of science, have sometimes appeared to conclude from their several demonstrations of the theory dependence of observation, that science is, in a word, bunk. This is unwarranted. Science is more complicated than in the traditional model. But it is not 'bunk' because it works: sociologists working in the 'strong' programme, notwithstanding their hostility to scientific truth, still went to brain surgeons for brain surgery. Nor, indeed, is even the distinction between observation and theory 'bunk'. Recall Putnam's point (from Part I, p 13), that such distinctions may not be dichotomies (capable of being driven all the way back). But they may still be useful tools for conceptual analysis. Useful, and, even, necessary: for of course the very demonstration of the theory dependence of observation implies the distinction (between observation and theory) some have taken it to deny.

So, work of this kind is not a way out of difficulty, but a way in. It sharpens up and highlights difficulties, producing results, theoretical and practical, not so much by 'solving' problems as by giving us deeper insights into some small part of the whole. There is a danger of obscurantism here, of course, of a retreat to what the Italian philosopher and historian of science, Paolo Rossi (2003), identifies as 'magical' thinking, insights reserved to the elite or chosen. As Rossi has so carefully charted, the scientific Renaissance of the fourteenth and fifteenth centuries consisted in a hard won climb up out of the thraldom of magical thinking towards '. . . logical rigour, experimental control . . . and the public character of results and methods . . .' (Rossi, 2003, p263). It was towards just such objectives for descriptive psychopathology that Wing and others, in developing instruments like the PSE, rightly aimed. It is towards the same objectives that a new philosophical psychopathology, building on twentieth century advances, must aim. The specifics will be different from quantum mechanics (the subject matters are different). But the principle is the same, that achieving a mature psychopathology will require, among other things, not the rejection of observation, but a deeper

understanding of its nature and role at the heart of science and hence of psychiatric science. It is to psychiatric science as reflected in current international classifications of mental disorder that we turn in Chapter 13.

Reflection on the session and self-test questions

Write down your own reflections on the materials in this session drawing out any points that are particularly significant for you. Then write brief notes about the following:

1. What general lessons for observation in psychopathology are suggested by recent work in physics (as in the EPR paradox)?

2. What role does this suggest for the PSE?

Reading guide

For further discussion of structured interviews see Farmer, McGuffin, and Williams (2002) *Measuring Psychopathology*.

Logical Empiricism and the Vienna Circle

A good account of the Logical Empiricist two-language model in a secondary text is Harold I. Brown's (1977) *Perception, Theory and Commitment*, especially chapters 1 and 3.

A useful collection on aspects of Logical Empiricism is Oswald Hanfling's (ed.) (1981) *Essential Readings in Logical Positivism*.

For an account of the Verification Principle in Logical Positivism see Waismann's 'Verification and definition' and Schlick's 'Meaning and verification' in Oswald Hanfling's (1981) *Essential Readings in Logical Positivism*.

The theory dependence of observation

Other accounts of the theory dependence of observation in the philosophy of science can be found in Bird's (1998) *The Philosophy of Science*, chapter 4, Chalmers' (1999) *What is This Thing Called Science?*, chapter 3, and Ladyman's (2002) *Understanding Philosophy of Science*, chapter 4.

A cognitive psychology approach is provided by William F. Brewer and Bruce L. Lambert (2001) 'The theory-ladenness of observation and the theory-ladenness of the rest of the scientific process', which responds to an influential paper by Fodor (1984, 'Observation reconsidered') in which he criticizes Churchland.

Perception and concepts

The view that all seeing is a form of seeing-as is defended from a phenomenological perspective in Mulhall's (1990) *On Being in the World*, which compares Wittgenstein and Heidegger. Wittgenstein's account is discussed in McGinn's (1997) *Wittgenstein and the Philosophical Investigations*.

McDowell's difficult book *Mind and World* is summarized by McDowell himself and discussed by a number of other philosophers in the *Journal of Philosophy and Phenomenological Research* (Vol. 58, 1998). Thornton's (2004) *John McDowell* is a secondary text covering his philosophical work as a whole.

The opposing view that at least some forms of perception turn on non-conceptual content can be found in Gunther's (2003) *Essays on Nonconceptual Content*.

References

APA (1980). *Diagnostic and Statistical Manual of Mental Disorders* (3rd edn, DSM-III). Washington, DC: American Psychiatric Association.

APA (1994). *Diagnostic and Statistical Manual of Mental Disorders* (4th edn, DSM-IV). Washington, DC: American Psychiatric Association.

Bird, A. (1998). *The Philosophy of Science*. London: Routledge.

Brewer, W.F. and Lambert, B. (2001). The theory-ladenness of observation and the theory-ladenness of the rest of the scientific process. *Philosophy of Science*, 68.

Bridgman, P.W. (1927). *The Logic of Modern Physics*. New York: Macmillan Press.

Brown, H.I. (1977). *Perception, Theory and Commitment*. Chicago, IL: University of Chicago.

Chalmers, A. (1999). *What is This Thing Called Science?* Buckingham: Open University Press.

Churchland, P. (1979). *Scientific Realism and the Plasticity of Mind*. Cambridge: Cambridge University Press.

D'Espagnat, B. (1983). *In Search of Reality*. New York: Springer-Verlag.

Davies, P.C.W. and Brown, J.R. (1986). *The Ghost in the Atom*. Cambridge: Cambridge University Press.

Duhem, P. (1962). *The Aim and Structure of Physical Theory*. New York: Atheneum.

Farmer, A., McGuffin P., and Williams, J. (2002). *Measuring Psychopathology*. Oxford: Oxford University Press.

Fodor, J.A. (1984). Observation reconsidered. *Philosophy of Science*, 51: 23–43.

Fulford, K.W.M. (1989). *Moral Theory and Medical Practice*. Cambridge: Cambridge University Press.

Gunther, Y.H. (2003). *Essays on Nonconceptual Content*. Cambridge MA: MIT Press.

Hanfling, O. (ed) (1981). *Essential Readings in Logical Positivism*. Oxford: Blackwell.

Hanson, N.R. (1958). *Patterns of discovery*. Cambridge: CUP.

Hesse, M. (1980). *Revolutions and Reconstructions in the Philosophy of Science*. Brighton: Harvester.

Hume, D. ([1739–40] 1967). *A Treatise of Human Nature*, Book I, Part 4 (ed. L.A. Selby-Bigge). Oxford: Oxford University Press.

Hume, D. ([1748] 1975). *Enquiries Concerning Human Understanding and Concerning the Principles of Morals*. Oxford: Oxford University Press, section VII.

Kant, I ([1781] 1829). Critique of Pure Reason (trans N. Kemp Smith) London: Macmillan.

Kraus, A. (1994). Phenomenological and criteriological diagnosis. In *Philosophical Perspectives on Psychiatric Diagnostic Classification* (ed. J.S. Sadler, O.P. Wiggins, and M.A. Schwartz). Baltimore, MD: Johns Hopkins University Press, pp. 148–162.

Kraus, A. (2003). How can the phenomenological-anthropological approach contribute to diagnosis and classification in psychiatry? In *Nature and Narrative: an introduction to the new philosophy of psychiatry* (ed. K.W.M. Fulford, K.J. Morris, J.Z. Sadler, and G. Stanghellini). Oxford: Oxford University Press, Chapter 13.

Kupfer, D.J., First, M.B. and Regier, D.E. (ed.) (2002). *A Research Agenda for DSM-V*. Washington, DC: American Psychiatric Association.

Ladyman, J. (2002). *Understanding Philosophy of Science*. London: Routledge.

Locke, J. ([1690] 1989). *Essay Concerning Human Understanding* (ed. P. Nidditch). Oxford: Clarendon Press.

McDowell, J. (1994). *Mind and World*. Cambridge, MA: Harvard University Press.

McGinn, M. (1997). *Wittgenstein and the Philosophical Investigations*. London: Routledge.

Mulhall, S. (1990). *On Being in the World*. London: Routledge.

Quine, W.V.O. (1960). *Word and Object*. Cambridge, MA: MIT Press.

Rossi, P. (2003). Magic, science, and equality of human wits. In *Nature and Narrative: an introduction to the new philosophy of psychiatry* (ed. K.W.M. Fulford, K.J. Morris, J.Z. Sadler, and G. Stanghellini). Oxford: Oxford University Press, Chapter 17.

Roth, M. and Kroll, J. (1986). *The Reality of Mental Illness*. Cambridge: Cambridge University Press.

Rounsaville, B.J., Alarcon, R.D., Andrews, G., Jackson, J.S., Kendell, R.E., and Kendler, K. (2002). Basic nomenclature issues for DSM-V. In *A Research Agenda for DSM-V* (ed. D.J. Kupfer, M.B. First,. and D.E. Regier). Washington, DC: American Psychiatric Association, Chapter 1.

Schlick, M. (1981). Meaning and verification. In *Essential Readings in Logical Positivism* (ed. O. Hanfling). Oxford: Blackwell.

Thornton, T. (2004). *John McDowell*. Chesham: Acumen.

Waismann, F. (1981). Verification and definition. In *Essential Readings in Logical Positivism* (ed. O. Hanfling). Oxford: Blackwell.

Wing, J.K. (1978). *Reasoning about Madness*. Oxford: Oxford University Press.

Wing, J.K., Cooper, J.E., and Sartorius, M. (1974). *Measurement and Classification of Psychiatric Symptoms*. Cambridge: Cambridge University Press.

Wittgenstein, L. (1953). *Philosophical Investigations*. Oxford: Basil Blackwell.

World Health Organization (1978). *Mental disorders: glossary and guide to their classification in accordance with the ninth revision of the International Classification of Diseases*. Geneva: WHO.

World Health Organization (1992). *ICD-10. International Classification of Diseases and Related Health Problems* (10th edn). Geneva: WHO.

CHAPTER 13

Natural classifications, realism, and psychiatric science

Chapter contents

A classification is a way of seeing the world at a point in time.
Norman Sartorius (1992, in the Preface
to ICD-10, p. vii)[1]

This chapter is about what science is about. It is about the real world 'out there' as distinct from our ideas about what is there. It is about what there *is* as distinct from our *beliefs* about what there is. It is about the objects—the entities and events—of which the real world is made up as distinct from the shapes that from this or that perspective we impose on the world. It is about what in philosophy has come to be debated by way of such contrasts as *objectivity* versus *subjectivity, realism* versus *idealism, essentialism* versus *nominalism.* (See Box 13.1 for brief initial definitions of realism and related terms.)

Natural classifications and what science is about

Classification, although of course not unique to science, is fundamental to the processes by which science seeks to find out what the world is really like. Classification lies at the heart of prediction and explanation. New phenomena are judged to be of the same kind as previously encountered phenomena and can thus be expected to behave in relevantly similar respects reflecting similar underlying causal mechanisms.

Scientific classifications come in many different forms. There can be groupings into rigid and mutually exclusive kinds, groupings on the basis of a number of possibly overlapping factors, groupings on the basis of mathematical quantities. But of any of these varieties of scientific classification we can ask: is it indeed a *natural* classification, a classification that, reflecting real, objective features of nature, provides insights into genuine causal mechanisms as a basis for explanation and prediction? Or is it, despite scientific appearances, an artificial classification that may be useful for us but that expresses *our* perspectives on the world as distinct from the nature of the world as it really is?

Natural classifications and what psychiatry is about

A natural classification, then, to adapt Sartorius' (1992) helpful aphorism (above), is the way in which a given science sees the world at a point in time. Small wonder, therefore, given the challenges of psychiatric science outlined in Chapter 11, that psychiatric classifications have been and remain deeply problematic. The two most widely used international psychiatric classifications of mental disorders are chapter V of the World Health Organization's (WHO) *International Classification of Disease* (current edition, ICD-10, WHO, 1992) and the American Psychiatric Association's *Diagnostic and Statistical Manual* (current edition, DSM-IVTR, American Psychiatric Association, 2000–TR stands for Text Revision; so this edition is DSM-IV, published in 1994, with mostly minor revisions). Corresponding,

[1] Chapter V, Mental and behavioural disorders, of the 10th Edition of the World Health Organization's *International Classification of Diseases* (ICD-10) is available in several different versions for different purposes. The version from which this quote is taken, *Clinical descriptions and diagnostic guidelines*, is the version used for general clinical and educational purposes. It is also the basis of all the other versions (WHO, 1992).

Box 13.1 Philosophical terminology: realism and related terms

The debate about the status of psychiatric classification is related to long-standing debates about realism throughout the history of philosophy. If you are new to these philosophical debates, the variety of terms and distinctions in this area can be somewhat bewildering. This is not helped by the fact that the terms and distinctions in question are sometimes used inconsistently. We give here a few illustrative examples (see also Reading Guide).

One early philosophical debate was concerned with properties:

◆ *Realists* argued that there really were universals—in the form of general abstract properties—out there in nature which were merely instantiated or realized in the properties of particular things (or 'particulars'). Thus the colour of a British post-box might be an instance of the universal (the general abstract property) redness. Plato was a realist about universals believing them to inhabit a realm separate from the natural world.

◆ *Nominalists* (such as William of Occam) argued that there were only particulars. The appearance of universals was a reflection of our linguistic practice of grouping together particular red things (British post-boxes, traffic lights at 'stop', etc.) but really there was nothing further—no general abstract property of redness—out there in nature.

Another early debate concerned the opposition to realism of *idealism.* Here,

◆ *Realists* (such as Locke, Hume, and other seventeenth century philosophers) denied idealism.

◆ *Idealists* argued that the world, or at least some central features of it, depended on our ideas of it rather than the other way round. Idealism is thus connected to the central role of ideas in seventeenth century British Empiricist theories of mind (see Part V). Thus a quick way of generating a form of idealism is to take the underlying realism implicit in Empiricist talk of people having ideas and impressions *of* the world and simply cancel the world out. Very roughly this was the eighteenth century philosopher, Bishop George Berkeley's strategy. It raises questions, among others, about who the subject of the ideas is. Kant (see Chapters 12 and 22) argued that how the world appeared to us, including its being spatially and temporally ordered, were products of the observing mind; however, he distinguished between the *empirical* self with which we normally identify ourselves and a *transcendental* self whose unknowable workings were responsible for this conceptual structuring (again, see Chapter 12).

Realism has more recently been opposed to other forms of antirealism such as antirealism about the past and the future,

about mathematics and about scientific theories. As we will see in Session 3, there are really a number of distinct debates here. One important distinction is between an *ontological* debate about realism and antirealism, and an *epistemological* debate. Ontology is about *what* is there. Epistemology is about what in principle we can *know* about what is there (i.e. in principle as distinct from any contingent limitations arising from, e.g. the limits of current instrumentation).

however, with the variety of alternatives to the psychiatric way of seeing the world of mental distress and disorder that we explored in Part I, there are competing classifications—psychological, psychoanalytic, and so forth. There are also those who, consistently with the view that mental disorders are really problems of living (also examined in Part I), reject outright psychiatry's medical-scientific way of seeing the world (Kutchins and Kirk, 1997).

Natural classifications and the validity of what psychiatry is about

Even, though, among those most committed to psychiatry's medical-scientific way of seeing the world, there are continuing debates about both the form and content of psychiatric classification. Many of these debates are authoritatively drawn together in *A Research Agenda for DSM-V* edited by three key figures in the DSM, the North American psychiatrists, David Kupfer, Michael First, and Darryl Regier (2002). We will be looking at the *Research Agenda for DSM-V* in detail in Session 1 of this chapter. But as Kupfer *et al.* point out in their Introduction, while psychiatry has seen dramatic improvements over the last three decades in the reliability of its classifications, and hence in their utility for purposes of communication, there has been little in the way of corresponding improvements in validity. Again, we return to these three key issues for classification—reliability, utility, and validity—in Session 1 (they are also defined briefly in Box 13.2). But the starting point of this chapter is that within psychiatry itself, as a medical-scientific discipline, there is deep concern about whether current psychiatric classifications are scientifically valid, and, hence, whether they are, in the sense of the term outlined above, *natural* classifications. Kupfer *et al.* put current concerns about validity at the very heart of their *Research Agenda for DSM-V*:

> 'Those of us' they say at the end of the first paragraph of their Introduction, 'who have worked for several decades to improve the reliability of our diagnostic criteria are now searching for new approaches to an understanding of etiological and pathophysiological mechanisms—an understanding that can improve the validity of our diagnoses and the consequent power of our preventive and treatment interventions'
>
> Kupfer *et al.* (2002, p. xv)

Strategy of the chapter

In this chapter we will be tackling the problems of validity presented by psychiatric classification, not directly, as they are set out in

Box 13.2 Psychiatric terminology: utility, reliability, and validity

Three terms are widely used in debates about the merits or otherwise of medical and psychiatric classifications. In descending order of difficulty of definition, they are utility, reliability, and validity:

- *Utility* is the extent to which a classification is 'good for purpose'. Easy to define, this concept is behind much of the debate about psychiatric classification, in part because of the diversity of purposes to which it is put, in part because of the diversity of values by which, as outlined in Part I, psychiatry itself is characterized.

- *Reliability* is the degree of agreement between users of a classification. Two main kinds of reliability are usually recognized. *Interobserver* or *inter-rater* reliability is the extent to which two or more observers agree about the classification of a given case on a given occasion. *Test–retest* reliability is the degree of agreement by a given observer in his or her classification of a given case over a period of time.

- *Validity* is a more complex notion. As noted in the text, broadly speaking the validity of a scientific classification is the extent to which it reflects the real world (or that aspect of the real world with which the science in question is concerned). Thus an alchemist's classification of chemical elements might have been very reliable, but it would have been a less valid classification in this sense than the chemical periodic table.

However, this 'absolute validity', as it might be called, is beyond the reach of many sciences, including psychiatry. Hence, 'lesser validities' are adopted, one or more of which might reasonably be taken to be a sign, albeit second hand, of absolute validity. In the psychiatric literature at least four kinds of lesser validity are distinguished (there are many others, e.g. concurrent validity, discriminantability, and, in the psychological literature a whole different approach through statistical tests.

- *Face validity*: the extent to which a classification appears to be of relevant features (which has consequences for the acceptability of a classification to its users; see e.g. Rust and Golombok, 1989, p. 78).

- *Construct validity*: roughly, the extent to which a classification relates to underlying theory. Thus, one commentator defines this form of validity as 'the extent to which the test may be said to measure a theoretical construct or trait' (Anastasi, 1968, p. 114). In medicine, reflecting the 'theory' that a patient's symptoms reflect an underlying pathophysiological causal mechanism, specific kinds of construct validity are often proposed. Thus in a classic paper, the American psychiatrists, Robins and Guze, emphasize the importance of family aggregation, reflecting presumed genetic factors (Robbins and Guze, 1970).

◆ *Predictive validity*: the extent to which the classification allows us to predict future properties: in medicine, these include prognosis (course and outcome) and response to treatment.

◆ *Content validity*: in respect of psychiatric diagnosis, Kendell (see Chapter 1) defines this as 'the demonstration that the defining characteristics of a given disorder are indeed enquired into and elicited before that diagnosis is made' (Kendell, 1975, p. 40).

The chemical periodic table, to return to our example above, has a high degree of validity in all these respects, it is prima facie relevant (face validity), it is strongly related to underlying theory (it has good construct validity, in the explanation of chemical properties based on electron 'shells'), it has high predictive validity (even to the extent of anticipating the existence of new elements), and it has good content validity (chemists really do enquire into the defining characteristics of an element before assigning it to a given class).

the *Research Agenda for DSM-V*, but indirectly, i.e. by exploring the potential relevance to these problems of a (far from exhaustive) selection of strands of work from the philosophy of science.

Brief plan of the chapter

The chapter is divided into four sessions dealing, respectively, with: (1) the influence of Logical Empiricism on current psychiatric classifications; (2) Bernard Williams' concept of an Absolute Conception and the significance of the traditional division between primary and secondary qualities for the place of values in a scientific classification; (3) recent philosophical work on realism in the philosophy of physics; and, finally, (4) the relevance of all these topics for the future development of scientific classifications of mental distress and disorder.

More detailed plan of the chapter

This is a relatively long chapter covering a good deal of new ground, both philosophical and psychiatric, so we will set out the overall line of argument briefly before starting on Session 1. Thus:

◆ *Session 1: Hempel and two New Agendas for Psychiatric classification*. We show, first, that the APA's current *Research Agenda for DSM-V* includes an embedded, albeit largely implicit, series of conceptual difficulties, that, together, make up the first of our new agendas, a **Conceptual** *Research Agenda for DSM-V*. The session then picks up on the themes of Chapter 12 by showing how developments in psychiatric classification over the last 50 years, culminating in and including the APA's *Research Agenda for DSM-V*, have been influenced by a core feature of Logical Empiricism, namely the separation of observational (or descriptive) statements from statements of theory. The standard story has been that Logical Empiricism influenced psychiatric classification directly through the work of one of its chief exponents, the American philosopher, Carl Hempel (we met Hempel in Chapter 12, of course). However, as we will see, there is a surprising twist to this story, a twist that will lead us to the second of our new Agendas for psychiatric classification, an agenda that we will call the *Conceptual Research Agenda for ICD-9*.

◆ *Session 2: Values, natural classifications, and the Absolute Conception*. Logical Empiricism, however, as we saw in Chapter 12, ultimately failed as a rigorous characterization of the traditional model of science. Hence in Session 2 we consider a more recent attempt to characterize the traditional model, Bernard Williams' 'Absolute Conception'. In the event, although superficially promising, this and other similar strands of work in the philosophy of science (for example on 'natural kinds', see Reading Guide), turn out not to be directly helpful in relation to the difficulties of psychiatric classification. These strands of work are indirectly helpful, on the other hand, in that they suggest the need for psychiatry to go beyond the traditional model, whether represented by Logical Empiricism or its more recent successors. In particular, arguments against the Absolute Conception, notably by the Pittsburgh-based philosopher John McDowell, suggest that, contrary to the traditional model, there is no obvious 'knock-down' argument why values may not have an entirely proper place in a natural classification.

◆ *Session 3: Scientific realism in physics*. We do not, however, pursue further the role of values in classification in this part of the book (we return to this topic in Part IV). Rather, in this part we move beyond the traditional model by exploring, in Session 3, a sample of ideas on the nature of science from the philosophy of physics— Van Fraassen's 'Constructive Empiricism', Boyd and McMullen's appeal to the 'inference to the best explanation', Cartwright's 'inference to the most probable cause', Hacking's work on realism and our ability to manipulate things, and Fine's 'Natural Ontological Attitude' (NOA). Despite their perhaps unlikely origins in the philosophy of physics, these strands of philosophical work turn out, in contrast to those considered in Session 2, to be directly illuminating in different ways for psychiatry.

◆ *Session 4: The third New Agenda – an agenda for an Extended Family of Classifictions*. In our concluding Session 4, therefore, we return to the current problems of validity facing psychiatric classification, and to the implications for these problems particularly of work in the philosophy of science modelled on the example of physics. By setting these implications from the philosophy of physics in context with our two new agendas developed in Session 1, we propose a third new Agenda, an *Agenda for an Extended Family of Psychiatric Classifications*, that, we argue, by analogy with the corresponding family of classifications in physics, will take us a step closer to satisfying current demands for improvements in the validity of psychiatric classifications by more closely reflecting what psychiatry, the *science* of psychiatry, is about.

Session 1 Hempel and two New Agendas for psychiatric classifications

In this session we will explore a number of key concepts in psychiatric classification by way of a mini 'history of ideas' of the ICD and DSM. But we will be looking forward not back. Our aim will be to identify the lessons from the history of ideas behind the ICD and DSM that will support future developments in scientific classifications of mental disorder.

Plan of the session

As this is a chapter-length session we will give a brief overview of the line of argument as it develops in each section.

With the first section, we start in the here and now with a reading (linked with Exercise 1) from the American Psychiatric Association's *A Research Agenda for DSM-V* (Kupfer *et al.*, 2002). The *Research Agenda for DSM-V*, as we noted in the introduction to this chapter, gives an authoritative picture of how, in the terms of Sartorius' (1992) aphorism at the start of this chapter, psychiatry sees the world of mental disorders at this point in time. Focusing in particular on Kupfer *et al*.'s Introduction, we draw out the philosophically-relevant aspects of their Agenda, thus developing the first of our new agendas, a *Conceptual Research Agenda for DSM-V*.

The second section, on *Hempel and the origins of ICD and DSM*, explores the history of ideas behind both DSM and ICD. In this section we jump back over 40 years, to 1959. This was the year of a joint WHO and American Psychopathological Association conference on classification to which the North American philosopher of science, Carl Hempel, made a crucial contribution, and from which, with the publication of ICD-8 in 1967 (WHO, 1967), a decisive shift in psychiatric classification was to be made from a theoretical (aetiology based) to a descriptive (symptom based) structure. A close reading of two passages from Hempel's paper (1961; see readings linked with Exercises 3 and 4) allows us to take a first look at a number of key concepts in scientific (including psychiatric) classifications: descriptive adequacy; Empirical Import; Systematic Import; objectivity; operationalism; and reliability.

These concepts, as set out by Hempel in his paper, have all turned out to be important in the subsequent development of ICD and DSM. But, and this is a big 'but', the direction in which ICD and DSM actually developed post-1959, proved, as we will see, to be very different from the direction anticipated by Hempel. There is a missing link in this story, therefore, which we identify in the next section (on *Hempel and the missing link to ICD and DSM*) with a reading from the transcript of the discussion that followed Hempel's paper.

Having identified the missing link, we are ready to derive a second new Agenda, which we develop in a section on a *Conceptual Research Agenda for ICD-9*. This Agenda is a counterpart of the agenda we developed in the first section for DSM-V. It is the philosophically-relevant Agenda for psychiatric classification as it stood at the time of the publication of the Glossary to ICD-8 in 1974 (WHO, 1974).

With our derived *Conceptual Research Agenda for ICD-9* in place, we then return to Hempel's paper, with a section on *Operationalism, reliability, validity, and a first look at what lies ahead*. As this rather long-winded title suggests, we look in detail, and at times critically, at Hempel's Logical Empiricist account of some of the concepts that have been particularly influential in the development of ICD and DSM through successive editions from ICD-8 to Kupfer *et al*.'s *Research Agenda for DSM-V* (2002). This suggests a number of preliminary ideas on the future development of psychiatric classification to which we will be returning in Session 4 of this chapter, after, as we indicate in a brief concluding section to this session, exploring in Sessions 2 and 3 of the chapter, various aspects of post-Logical Empiricist philosophy of science relevant to psychiatry.

The first new agenda – a conceptual research agenda for DSM-V

In this first section, then, we focus on the American Psychiatric Association's *A Research Agenda for DSM-V*. Published in 2002, it was edited as we noted in the introduction to this chapter, by three key players in the DSM, David Kupfer, Professor and Chair of Psychiatry at the University of Pittsburgh, Michael First, Associate Professor of Clinical Psychiatry at the Columbia University College of Physicians and Surgeons in New York, and Darryl Regier, Director of Research in the American Psychiatric Association. Our aim will not be to review the Agenda as it stands: as we will see, it is mainly an (authoritative) agenda for *empirical* research. Our aim, rather, will be to draw out, largely from Kupfer *et al*.'s editorial Introduction, the items on their agenda as they are relevant particularly to the possible contributions of *conceptual* research, alongside the contributions of empirical research, to the future development of psychiatric classifications. It is by drawing out these conceptually-relevant agenda items that we will develop the first our two new agendas for psychiatric classification, a *Conceptual Research Agenda for DSM-V*. This new agenda, although superficially very different from Kupfer *et al*.'s original *Research Agenda for DSM-V*, is, we will argue, already fully implicit within it.

We summarize our derived new agenda, *A Conceptual Research Agenda for DSM-V*, in Table 13.1. We will be referring to the agenda items in Table 13.1 *seriatim* as they emerge from our discussion of Kupfer *et al*.'s original. These agenda items (there are 12 in all) will help to guide you through the discussion. We suggest, however, that, consistently with the 'skills-development' approach of this book, you defer looking at the details of Table 13.1 until you have worked through the two exercises in this section and come to your own views on the conceptually relevant agenda items implicit in Kupfer *et al*.'s original agenda. Remember that, coming to these materials with your own particular background resources of knowledge, skills, and experience, you may well come up with different, and better, ideas than ours.

Kupfer *et al*.'s *Research Agenda for DSM-V*, then, has six main chapters based, in part, on a series of workshops convened jointly

Table 13.1 The First New Agenda – a Conceptual Research Agenda for DSM-V

		DSM-V (conceptual agenda)
(1)	Time-line	Back to DSM-III Forword to DSM-VI or even DSM-VII
(2)	Uses of psychiatric classification	Diagnosis by clinicians
(3)	Misuses of psychiatric classification	Reification of categories of mental disorder as diseases
(4)	Status of psychiatric science	Deficit model: current classification paradigm is 'limited' because it has proved to be 'almost wholly lacking in validity'
(5)	Concepts	Important: but not named for what they are. Conceptual issues are writ large but called, e.g. 'nomenclature' issues; and conceptual research methods are not mentioned.
(6)	Reliability	Run out of steam: only useful for improving agreement, hence communication between clinicians; as such, may even have worked against validity
(7)	Validity	THE BIG ISSUE: we need scientifically sound systems of classification; this means that they must become 'aetiologically based'
(8)	Structural solution	Aetiology-based: we need a 'fundamentally' new classification paradigm drawing on biological and clinical sciences
(9)	Process solutions	Empirical research: the route to vaildity is by way of empirical research to, (a) enrich the 'empirical database', and (b) facilitate the 'integration of findings' from different areas of biological and clinical research
(10)	Utility (of new classifications)	Better health-care services: a more valid (i.e. aetiology-based) classification will provide more powerful 'preventive and treatment interventions'
(11)	Overall tenor	Downbeat: as above, current paradigm is 'limited' and needs to be 'fundamentally' altered
(12)	Any other business	none

by the American Psychiatric Association and the National Institutes of Mental Health (NIMH—the principal source of Federal research funds for psychiatry in the USA). There were in all 40 North American authors of the six chapters of the *Research Agenda for DSM-V*, who, together with the three editors and two representatives of the NIMH, represented a wide range of expertise in North American psychiatry, psychology, and related clinical and research health-care disciplines. There were also four distinguished non-North American contributors, Bedirhan Üstün, the Coordinator of the ICD Revision Programme at the WHO, Robert Kendell from the UK (this is the Kendell of Part I), Margarita Alegria, Professor of Health Services Administration at the University of Puerto Rico, and Gavin Andrews, a Professor of Psychiatry at the University of New South Wales in Australia. Our first reading is from Kupfer *et al.*'s Introduction.

EXERCISE 1 (20 minutes)

Read the short passage from:

Kupfer, D.J., First, M.B., and Regier, D.E. (2002). Introduction. In *A Research Agenda for DSM-V* (ed. D.J. Kupfer, M.B. First, and D.E. Regier). Washington, DC: American Psychiatric Association, pp. xv–xvii

Link with Reading 13.1

As you read this passage, which comes on the first page of the Introduction, write down a checklist of as many agenda items for the DSM-V as you can identify from what the authors say. The passage includes the short section quoted, in the introduction to this chapter, in which the authors indicate the need for improved validity. So this is one item on their *Research Agenda for DSM-V*. But what do they mean by validity? And what other items on their agenda can you detect from this passage?

As noted above, it is important to write down your own ideas on this before reading on. This is important generally because of the skills-development aims of this textbook, as we have emphasized on many occasions. It is especially important here, in relation to psychiatric science, where, as we will see, we are very much at the cutting edge with no 'established corpus' of received ideas, and where, as Kupfer *et al.* themselves emphasize (see below), we are overdue for a fundamental shift of paradigms. So, your ideas are as likely to contribute to the required shift of paradigms as anyone else's!

In this passage, as noted in the introduction to this chapter, the big issue for the *Research Agenda for DSM-V* is identified by Kupfer *et al.* as the need for improved *validity*. We have included validity as Agenda Item 7 in Table 13.1. In this passage, a valid classification is spelled out by the authors to mean one that is an 'etiologically based, scientifically sound classificatory system.'

New agenda items

However, there are a number of further agenda items that we can glean from this passage. Thus,

1. *Reliability* (Agenda Item 6 in Table 13.1). Reliability, although something on which the authors emphasize they have worked 'for several decades', now seems to them to have run out of steam. To achieve validity, they say, we need 'new approaches'.

    So, what are the required approaches, according to Kupfer *et al.*,? They can be summarized under two further agenda items that we will call respectively, 'structural solutions' and 'process solutions'.

2. *Structural solutions* (Agenda Item 8 in Table 13.1). In seeking new approaches to psychiatric classification, Kupfer *et al.* suggest, we need to make *fundamental* changes in the basic structure of our classifications: we need, they say, to 'fundamentally alter the limited classification paradigm now in use'.

    Later on, Kupfer *et al.* add further details of the structural changes they envisage: their fundamental changes will involve basing the DSM-V (or later classifications) on categories that are defined by the findings from 'animal studies, genetics, neuroscience, epidemiology, clinical research, and cross-cultural services.' Correspondingly, therefore, among the six main chapters of the DSM-V Agenda, we find chapters on a 'Neuroscience research agenda to guide development of a pathophysiologically based' system of classification (Charney *et al.*, 2002, chapter 2), on 'Advances in developmental science' (Pine *et al.*, 2002, chapter 3); and, representing clinical as distinct from biological sciences, chapters on 'Personality disorders and relational disorders' (First *et al.*, 2002, chapter 4), 'Mental disorders and disability' (Lehman *et al.*, 2002, chapter 5) and 'Culture and psychiatric disorder' (Alarcón *et al.*, 2002, chapter 6).

3. *Process solutions* (Agenda Item 9 in Table 13.1). The processes by which these fundamental changes in the structure of our classifications will be brought about are, according to Kupfer *et al.*, those of empirical research designed, (a) to enrich the 'empirical database', and (b) to facilitate effective 'integration of findings' from the biological and clinical fields listed under 'structural solutions' above.

There is much work to be done here. But if successful, it will have, to come to a further Agenda Item for DSM-V, considerable *Utility* (Agenda Item 10 in Table 13.1). For the outcomes of empirical research of the kind proposed in the DSM-V Agenda will go to the heart of what health care is all about, improving, as Kupfer *et al.* put it, the 'power of our preventive and treatment interventions'.

Of course, none of this will happen overnight. Hence we have yet another Agenda Item for DSM-V, of *Time Line* (Agenda Item 1 in Table 13.1). Kupfer *et al.* are clear that we may not see improved scientific classifications, based on aetiological theories derived from empirical research in the biological and clinical sciences, until, perhaps, 'DSM-VI or even DSM-VII'.

The need for fundamental change?

The next reading (linked with Exercise 2) fills out Kupfer *et al.*'s Agenda for fundamental changes with two further passages from their Introduction. These passages come in a section that is titled the 'Need to explore the possibility of fundamental changes in the neo-Kraepelinian diagnostic paradigm'. This is a key section of Kupfer et al's *Agenda*. It is the second of two subsections of the section, titled 'Background', which immediately follows Kupfer *et al.*'s opening paragraphs (we included the first paragraph of the Background as the last paragraph of the reading in Exercise 1).

The first subsection of the Background explores the relationship between the DSM process and the 'research database'. Filling out our agenda items, respectively for Process Solutions and for Reliability above. This first subsection, (1) describes the field trials and other evidence-based processes that supported the development of DSM-III and DSM-IV, (2) observes that the focus in these classifications was on improved reliability, and (3) spells out what Kupfer *et al.* mean by improved reliability, namely agreement between clinicians: improved reliability, they say, ensures that '. . . multiple clinicians could come to the same diagnostic conclusions . . .'; and this in turn allows '. . . reproducible diagnosis in multiple clinical and cultural settings '(both p. xvi).

The second subsection of the Background, the subsection from which the next readings are taken, then develops Kupfer *et al.* 's theme of the need for fundamental changes to allow us to move on from reliability to validity. As we will see, this subsection fills out the *Research Agenda for DSM-V* still further by giving a particularly clear picture of how the authors perceive the current status of psychiatry's international classifications, their strengths and their limitations, at this point in time.

EXERCISE 2   (20 minutes)

Read the two passages from the Introduction to the *DSM-V Agenda* on why, in the authors' view, we need to explore the possibility of fundamental changes in the DSM and, by implication, the ICD:

Kupfer, D.J., First, M.B., and Regier, D.E. (2002). Introduction. In *A Research Agenda for DSM-V* (ed. D.J. Kupfer, M.B. First, and D.E. Regier). Washington, DC: American Psychiatric Association, pp. xviii–xix

Link with Reading 13.2

As you read these passages, go back to your checklist of items from the *DSM-V Agenda* in Exercise 1. Make notes on:

1. The way in which this passage expands on any particular items already on that Agenda. We expanded on the agenda

item for reliability in the lead up to this exercise (in Kupfer et al's *Agenda*, we noted, reliability is defined as meaning agreement between clinicians). Similarly, then, in this exercise, see what further expansions or clarifications you can find of other items in the *DSM-V Agenda*. Then,

2. Look for any new items that are added to the Agenda (if any). Finally,

3. Think about the general tenor of this passage: is it overall upbeat or downbeat?

A deficit model of psychiatric science

Taking our third question in Exercise 2 first, our question about the general tenor of this passage of Kupfer et al's *Agenda*, it is a remarkable passage in the extent of its self-criticism. The 'limited classification paradigm', as it was described in the first reading, now reappears in this reading as a classification that is more or less wholly lacking in any of the requirements of scientific validity ('not one laboratory marker has been found...', etc.). So dismissive is much of the passage in tone and temper that it would not be out of place among the writings of those who, in the antipsychiatry movement, have attacked the very status of the DSM as a medical classification. The downbeat tenor of the Introduction to Kupfer et al's *Agenda* is an important point of contact between philosophy and psychiatry to which we will return at the end of this chapter.

As to specific items on Kupfer et al's *Agenda*, to return to question 1 of Exercise 2, much of this passage is taken up with expanding on what we called above (under Exercise 1, Agenda Item 7), the 'big issue' of validity. The thrust of this passage, however, as just noted, is remarkably negative. The passage, then, to come to question 2 in the exercise, gives us a further agenda item, Agenda Item 4 in Table 13.1, namely how the status of psychiatric science is perceived. Kupfer *et al.*, in their introduction to their *Agenda*, present what might be called a 'deficit model' of psychiatric science: the problems of psychiatric classification, that is to say, are portrayed as a sign not of the *difficulty* of psychiatric science but of its *deficits*. The hope (of earlier classifiers in both ICD and DSM) was that reliability would lead on to validity. But this has not happened. The specific need, then, the particular deficit that needs, according to Kupfer *et al.*, to be remedied, is, as we saw earlier, for biological (e.g. genetic) categories of mental disorder comparable with, it is implied, the more valid (= scientifically sound, aetiology based) categories to be found in the (by implication non-defective) classifications of bodily medicine.

Kupfer *et al.* further imply that correcting the deficit in validity may actually be hindered by concerns about reliability. Thus in the first paragraph of this reading, they argue that the major advantage of a 'descriptive approach' is 'improved reliability', which in turn gives it its 'primary strength', which is its 'ability to improve communication among clinicians and researchers, *not* its validity' (emphasis added). In the second passage, similarly,

while Kupfer *et al.* acknowledge that there is value in improved 'diagnostic reliability', none the less, they point out, 'reification of DSM-IV entities... is more likely to obscure than to elucidate research findings.'

We will return later in this session to the relationship between reliability (of diagnostic criteria) and (scientific) validity. But it is important to note, in these and similar passages, how close Kupfer et al's *Agenda* comes to suggesting that improved reliability, far from being a step towards a more scientific classification of mental disorders, may have been achieved actually at the *expense* of progress towards (scientific) validity, thus contributing to the (perceived) deficits of psychiatric science.

Conceptual issues...

There is, however, an even more important agenda item in this passage, namely, *conceptual issues* (Agenda Item 5 in Table 13.1). The actual term 'conceptual' is not used by Kupfer *et al.* Indeed, although conceptual issues figure prominently in the *Research Agenda for DSM-V*, there is something of a reluctance throughout the *Research Agenda for DSM-V* to name them for what they are. None the less, as an agenda item, 'conceptual issues' are writ large in the two passages in this exercise. The very origins of our current problems (and hence the need for 'fundamental changes') is identified by Kupfer *et al.* at the start of the first passage in the reading, with what we might call the conceptual sins of the fathers: the 'neo-Kraepelinian approach' of focusing on syndromes rather than on aetiology. In the second passage, similarly, we find the concern that 'researchers' slavish adoption of DSM-IV definitions', and their 'reification of DSM-IV entities, to the point that they are considered to be equivalent to diseases', may have hindered research into aetiology. And in the final paragraph of the second passage, the proposed solution, directly echoing one of the roles of philosophy in healthcare outlined in our preface, is said to involve new 'ways of thinking' to achieve 'an as yet unknown paradigm shift' if we are to be more successful in uncovering the 'underlying aetiologies' of mental disorder.

...a plenty...

Given the importance of conceptual issues in driving Kupfer *et al.*'s call for fundamental changes in DSM, it is no surprise to find a substantive discussion of these issues later in the *Research Agenda for DSM-V*. The first chapter, by Bruce Rounsaville and colleagues (2002), although titled (consistently with the reluctance in the *Research Agenda for DSM-V* to name conceptual problems for what they are) issues of 'Basic nomenclature', actually includes discussions of such explicitly conceptual issues as the definitions of key concepts (including the concepts of mental disorder and illness) and the nature of validity. The discussion of validity in the chapter by Rounsaville *et al.*, furthermore, building on their discussion of definitions of key concepts, extends to such essentially conceptual topics as, (1) the need to develop a 'System for rating (the validity of) diagnostic categories', and (2) the 'Rationale for changing criteria'. There is also discussion in this chapter of: (1) conceptual aspects of the tension between dimensional and categorical approaches; (2) methods for reducing the discrepancies in categories and criteria between DSM and ICD; (3) cross-cultural aspects of DSM-V; and (4) the use of DSM-V in non-psychiatric settings. The latter is particularly interesting conceptually in that it signals the need to develop versions of the DSM that rely less heavily on 'clinical judgement' (p. 21).

...in all but name...

Conceptual issues are evident, too, in other more overtly empirical chapters of Kupfer et al's *Agenda*. Thus chapter 5, on 'Mental disorders and disabilities: time to re-evaluate the relationship?', starts with a discussion of what the authors themselves call the 'conceptual' separation of 'descriptive information regarding individuals' psychiatric presentation' into 'psychiatric symptoms' and 'functional impairment' (Lehman *et al.*, 2002, p. 201). Similarly, the final chapter of the *Research Agenda for DSM-V*, on cultural psychiatry, starts from 'the fundamental value of social context and meaning in the human experience', thus directly paralleling Jaspers' concern (explored fully in Part II) that psychopathology should encompass meanings as well as causal explanations (Alarcón *et al.*, 2002, p. 219); and this chapter concludes with the explicitly philosophical claim that the systemic approach of cultural psychiatry '... surpasses, despite some limitations, the mind-body dichotomy' (Alarcón *et al.*, 2002, p. 265).

The *de facto* importance of conceptual issues in the *Research Agenda for DSM-V*, makes it somewhat puzzling that the *term* 'conceptual' is so rarely used. There is no category for conceptual issues in the index (though the term does appear in some subcategories); the chapter on conceptual issues, as we noted above, is called 'Basic *nomenclature* issues for DSM-V' (Rounsaville *et al.*, 2002, p. 1, emphasis added); and the thrust of the editors' Introduction is very much to the effect that the *Research Agenda for DSM-V* is an agenda for *empirical* research: as you will see if you refer back to the first reading (linked with Exercise 1), even their one reference to an 'analytic' agenda is a reference, not to analytic research on concepts, but to a 'research and analytic agenda' for integrating the findings from basic science and clinical research into an enriched 'empirical database' (Kupfer *et al.*, 2002, p. xv).

...and in all but methodology

The thrust of Kupfer *et al.*'s Introduction, that this is not just a 'Research Agenda for DSM-V' but, specifically, an '*Empirical Research Agenda for DSM-V*', is carried through in the proposals for research outlined in their Chapter 1. This chapter, although covering, as noted above, a whole range of conceptual issues, makes proposals for research, that, even on the overtly conceptual problems raised by concepts of mental disorder, are limited to empirical field studies. Again, we return to the relevance of such studies at the end of this chapter. Combined with conceptual research methods, empirical field studies are a key part of what in Chapter 4, employing J.L. Austin's term, we called 'philosophical fieldwork'. But if the additional methodological and interpretive

resources of conceptual research are absent, such studies, however descriptively informative, are likely to compound rather than to illuminate the difficulties (and, as formulated in Part I, remember, they are very much *difficulties* and not deficiencies) of psychiatric science.

A new conceptual research agenda for DSM-V

In this first section of this session we have now built up an agenda for DSM-V, which although derived directly from materials in the original (Kupfer *et al.*'s Introduction together with supporting chapters), paints a very different overall picture. The original *Research Agenda for DSM-V*, although including conceptual issues, is largely taken up with empirical research. Even where, *de facto*, the *Research Agenda for DSM-V* is concerned with conceptual issues, it calls them, as we have seen, something else (issues of basic nomenclature) and it makes no mention whatsoever of conceptual research methods. Our new *Conceptual Research Agenda for DSM-V*, by contrast, emphasizes and draws out the significance of the conceptual issues identified in the original.

We summarize our new *Conceptual Research Agenda for DSM-V* in Table 13.1 (above). Later in this chapter we will be comparing this with a second new agenda, a *Conceptual Research Agenda for ICD-9*, using the same agenda items. We will come to our *Conceptual Research Agenda for ICD-9*, however, by way of an extended discussion of the history of ideas behind current classifications. This in turn will provide a foundation from which to assess the theoretical significance and practical consequences of the conceptual issues identified in this section as being implicit in Kupfer *et al.*'s *Research Agenda for DSM-V*.

Hempel and the origins of ICD and DSM

How, then, did we get to our current classifications of mental disease? What are their origins in the modern history of psychiatry? Kupfer *et al.*, in the Introduction to the *Research Agenda for DSM-V*, provide a clear account of the origins of their *Agenda* in successive revisions of DSM back to DSM-III (Kupfer *et al.*, 2002, pp. xvi–xviii). But of course DSM-III did not arise *sui generis*. In this section, therefore, we are going to push the story back a little further than DSM-III, specifically to the international conference on psychiatric classification in 1959 noted in the introduction to this session.

Back from DSM-III to 1959

Our purpose in going back to the 1959 conference is to look in some detail at the influence on the ICD/DSM story of the North American philosopher of science, Carl Hempel. Hempel, you will recall from Chapter 12, was one of the founders of the model of science developed by the Vienna Circle in the 1930s and 1940s, called Logical Empiricism. The central aim of Logical Empiricism, to establish a sharp separation between observational (or descriptive) statements and statements of theory, is directly reflected in the critical move in post-Second World War psychiatry, noted in the introduction to this session, from the theoretical (aetiology based) ICD-6 and ICD-7 to the descriptive (symptom based)

ICD-8. The link between Hempel and ICD-8 is generally taken to be the British psychiatrist, Erwin Stengel (see, e.g. Kendell, 1975, p. 93). As we will see, however, important as Stengel's influence on ICD-8 certainly was, there is a crucial missing link in this story. We will be uncovering this missing link in this section, and, in the process, taking an important step towards the derivation of our second new agenda, our *Conceptual Research Agenda for ICD-9*.

The background to Hempel's 1959 paper

First, then, Carl Hempel's role in post-Second World War psychiatric classification. As an internationally respected philosopher of science, Hempel was invited to present a paper at the conference on psychiatric classification organised by Joe Zubin (see Zubin, 1961) in 1959 in New York under the auspices of the American Psychopathological Association.

The aim of the 1959 conference was to contribute to a review process that would lead to the establishment of a classification of mental disorders, that, being acceptable on an international basis, would meet the WHO's requirements for comparative epidemiological studies and statistical reporting. Immediately on its foundation in 1945, the WHO had published a sixth revision of the *International List of Causes of Death* (which had previously been published by the French Government) renaming it as the *Manual of the International Statistical Classification of Diseases, Injuries and Causes of Death*, and including for the first time a classification of mental disorders (WHO, 1948). Most of the chapters in the new classification, those dealing with bodily disorders, were well received and readily adopted around the world. The mental disorders section, however, was one of the very few that proved to be problematic. Eleven years later it was found to have been adopted only in Finland, Peru, Thailand, and the United Kingdom. (We owe these historical details to chapter 7 of R.E. Kendell's authoritative book, *The Role of Diagnosis in Psychiatry*, 1975.)

The 1959 conference

Faced with these difficulties, the WHO commissioned the British psychiatrist, Erwin Stengel, to investigate and to make recommendations for a classification that would be more widely acceptable. It was in this connection that, at the 1959 conference, Hempel, as a philosopher of science, was invited to speak. Stengel was the first respondent to Hempel's paper and Hempel's insights into scientific classification, notably those dealing with the Logical Empiricist separation of observational (or descriptive) statements and statements of theory, appear, with full acknowledgements, in key sections of Stengel's subsequent report to the WHO (Stengel, 1959).

From 1959 to ICD-10 and DSM-IV

ICD-8 consequently appeared in 1967 (WHO, 1967), and, with the subsequent publication of a glossary (WHO, 1974), became the first predominantly symptom-based modern classification of mental disorders (the mental disorders section of ICD-7 was identical with ICD-6). The American Psychiatric Association adopted the ICD-8 nomenclature in its DSM-II (American Psychiatric

Association, 1968), abandoning, against much domestic opposition (Kendell, 1975), the predominantly psychodynamic-theoretical basis of DSM-I (American Psychiatric Association, 1952). ICD-9, which largely incorporated the ICD-8 glossary, followed in 1978 (WHO, 1978). The DSM-III (American Psychiatric Association, 1980) introduced explicit inclusion and exclusion criteria (the DSM-III Taskforce was led by Robert Spitzer). Finally, DSM-IV explicitly (American Psychiatric Association, 1994, p. xv), and ICD-10 implicitly (WHO, 1992), established evidence-based approaches to refining and modifying the categories in their respective classifications. (The DSM-IV Taskforce was led by Allen Frances, and the ICD-10 team at WHO was led by Norman Sartorius (who had previously worked on ICDs 7, 8 and 9) as Head of the Mental Health Section at the WHO.)

Hempel's 1959 paper

Hempel's paper, then, by so clearly flagging the Logical Empiricist separation of observation and theory at that crucial conference in 1959, had, on the face of it, a decisive influence on the subsequent development of both ICD and DSM. But what exactly did he say? In this section we will be looking at several extracts from Hempel's paper. It was published originally as part of an edited collection (see Hempel, 1961) but it has been reprinted a number of times, most recently in the edited collection by the American psychiatrist and philosopher, John Sadler and colleagues, in their *Philosophical Perspectives on Psychiatric Diagnostic Classification* (Sadler *et al.*, 1994). Sadler *et al.*'s book was published, with a foreword by Allen Frances, to coincide with the launch of DSM-IV and the collection includes a number of important contributions to the field. Our readings in this section are taken from Sadler *et al.*'s reprint of Hempel's paper (which is more or less identical with the original but with a number of helpful endnotes added by Hempel himself).

EXERCISE 3	(30 minutes)

Read the short extract from:

> Hempel, C.G. (1994). Fundamentals of taxonomy. In *Philosophical Perspectives on Psychiatric Diagnostic Classification* (ed. J.S. Sadler, O.P. Wiggins, and M.A. Schwartz). Baltimore, MD: Johns Hopkins University Press. (Extract pps 317–318.)

Link with Reading 13.3

This first extract comes early in Hempel's paper and gives an initial summary statement of two key requirements that he argues should be satisfied if a classification is to be genuinely scientific. The passage follows an opening section in which Hempel gives a brief but very clear review of the logic of classes relevant to classification and it is followed by two long sections in which Hempel discusses his two requirements in more detail.

The extract begins with the final paragraph of Hempel's introductory section. Here he distinguishes, very much along

Logical Empiricist lines, scientific *concepts* from the *language* in which those concepts are expressed (his 'vocabulary of science'). He then goes on to set out his two requirements.

As you read the extract, think about the following five questions:

1. What are the two requirements that Hempel places on scientific classifications?

2. How are these two requirements related to the Logical Empiricist model of science outlined in Chapter 12?

3. How are Hempel's two requirements related to the overall development of post-Second World War international psychiatric classification outlined above?

4. Is there anything that strikes you as odd about what Hempel has to say about psychiatric classification, given the storyline of this session, namely that we owe the essentially descriptive (symptom-based) form of current psychiatric classifications in part to his paper?

5. Similarly, given that the topic of this chapter is about what science is about, is there anything that strikes you as odd about the way Hempel describes the second of his two requirements?

Many of the key messages for psychiatric classification from Hempel's paper are captured by this brief extract. We will take our five questions in turn.

Five questions from Hempel's paper

1. *Hempel's two requirements.* The two requirements that Hempel places on a classification if it is to be scientific are that the terms (or vocabulary) in which it is expressed, and hence the concepts it reflects,

    (a) 'permit an adequate *description*' of the objects of the science in question, and

    (b) 'permit the establishment of general laws or theories by means of which particular events may be *explained* and *predicted* and thus *scientifically understood*;...' (Hempel, 1994, p. 317, emphasis in original).

    In his subsequent development of these two requirements, Hempel calls them respectively the 'Empirical Import' (or sometimes 'descriptive adequacy') and the 'Systematic Import' of a scientific classification. We will be exploring particularly the first of these two requirements, Empirical Import, in more detail later in this session.

2. *Logical Empiricism and Hempel's two requirements.* The origins of Hempel's two requirements in Logical Empiricism are clear: note, first, the emphasis on language—Hempel casts his two requirements in terms of the 'vocabulary' of science; and, second, the implied primary division into a language of

observation (here, 'description') and a language of underlying theory (here, 'general laws and theories').

3. *Hempel's two requirements and post-Second World War psychiatric classification.* Again, the link between Hempel's two requirements and developments in post-Second World War psychiatric classifications is, at least at first glance, clear. As described above, the key move in these developments was from, in Hempel's terms, the language of theory (aetiology) to a language of description (symptoms). In the second paragraph of the extract, furthermore, Hempel observes how (with 'some oversimplification') the development of a science can be understood as being marked by a progressive shift from descriptive to theoretical terms. It is a small further step, therefore, from this observation to a recognition of the need for a science to base its classifications on the stage that it is at in its development. Psychiatry, then, if lacking an agreed theoretical basis at this stage in its development, should base its classifications on symptoms (as in ICD-8 and subsequent classifications) rather than on theory (as in classifications prior to ICD-8).

4. *But what is odd about this?* What is odd about Hempel's paper, however, given Hempel's influence on developments in psychiatric classification, is that Hempel himself does not take this small further step. To the contrary, in this extract (para 3), he argues that with the development of psychodynamic theory, notably as the basis of the 'DSM' of the time (now called DSM-I), psychiatry is already following the route of general medicine from a descriptive to a theoretical stage in its development. Thus, citing an example (of conversion reaction) from the DSM of the day, Hempel notes that the diagnostic terms used are not observational but 'theoretically assumed psychodynamic factors'. And he goes on to compare the DSM in this respect favourably with physical theory (such terms as 'gravitational field', etc.).

Later in the article, it is true, Hempel speaks less favourably both of psychodynamic theory and of the DSM of the day. He says that the central concepts of contemporary psychodynamic theory 'lack clear and uniform criteria of application' (p. 318). But this criticism is merely by way of a preliminary to offering a remedy ('operationalism', as we will see in the next reading) rather than by way of rejecting psychodynamic theory in principle as a basis for psychiatric classification. Similarly, as to the contemporary DSM, the essence of Hempel's critique is not *that* it is a theoretical rather than descriptive classification, but rather that many of the terms it employs are value-laden, they have what Hempel calls 'valuational overtones' (p. 322). And he goes on to suggest that this, too, can be remedied.

We return to what Hempel has to say on values in psychiatric diagnosis in Session 2. For the moment, though, the point is that, far from suggesting that psychiatry should move to a more descriptive basis for its classification, the implication is that it is on the right track in following the rest of medicine from a descriptive to a more theoretical set of diagnostic concepts. Furthermore, Hempel sees nothing in principle against psychodynamic theory being the basis of psychiatric classification. Indeed he describes the gradual replacement of observational with explanatory theoretical terms in a genuinely scientific classification as being 'nicely illustrated' by the psychodynamically based DSM of the day (p. 326). And while he leaves it open as to whether the major theories used in the future in psychiatry will be 'biophysiological' or 'psychodynamic' (p. 327), he suggests that 'theories of either kind can satisfy the basic requirements for scientific theories' (p. 327), and he concludes with an express prediction that, whichever kind of theory is adopted, psychiatric classification will continue to shift from systems based on 'observable characteristics' to 'systems based on theoretical concepts' (p. 330).

All this is odd, then, given that, in the event, psychiatric classification moved sharply against Hempel's prediction, becoming more descriptive rather than more theoretical in orientation, and that, in the case specifically of the DSM, the move to a descriptive basis was achieved in the teeth of a domestic opposition intent on retaining psychodynamic theory.

5. *What is odd about Hempel's first summary statement of his two requirements?* What is odd about Hempel's first summary statement of his two requirements for a classification to be scientific, given that this chapter is about what science is about, is, in a word, that he makes no reference to realism: there is no requirement, explicitly at any rate, for a scientific classification to be about what is 'really there'. There is no explicit requirement even for a scientific classification to be 'objective'.

Interestingly, by contrast with his first summary statement, explicit references to the 'real' appear right at the start of Hempel's more detailed account of both requirements. The first sentence of his section on 'Empirical Import', as we will see in the next reading (linked with Exercise 4), is 'Science aims at knowledge that is *objective . . .*' (p. 318, emphasis in original). Similarly, at the start of his section on 'Systematic Import', he repeats the brief definition given in this first extract but with the crucial additional element that the 'general laws and theoretical principles' towards the generation of which a scientific classification should incline, should be such as 'reflect uniformities in the subject matter under study and which *thus* provide a basis for explanations, prediction, and generally scientific understanding' (p. 323, emphasis added).

We should not make too much of this, of course. Hempel's failure, in his first summary statement, to place any explicit requirement on a scientific classification to be about what science is about, is a natural enough slip even for perhaps the last great twentieth century philosophical champion of the traditional model of science. But Hempel's slip reminds us just how easily what science is about slips out of the picture when we are struggling with problems of classification. Again,

we will return to this point later. But if even Hempel, one of the founders of Logical Empiricism, can let what science is about slip below the threshold of visibility, how much more readily will this happen in a practical discipline, like psychiatry, that, whatever its scientific basis, is subject to a wide range of conflicting social and political pressures.

Hempel's first requirement for a scientific classification: Empirical Import

All the same, as the opening passages in Hempel's fuller treatment of his two requirements, cited above, make clear, Hempel *is* concerned with what science is about. So, how do his two requirements on a scientific classification, the requirements of Empirical Import and Systematic Import, help to ensure that a classification is indeed about what science is about, that it reflects, or aims to reflect, objective information about what is really there?

We will look first, and in most detail, at Hempel's first requirement, Empirical Import. As we will see, it is Hempel's discussion of Empirical Import that has most directly influenced the course of subsequent developments in psychiatric classification. Hempel's discussion of Systematic Import raises a whole series of key topics for our understanding of what science is about. However, we will look only briefly at these topics in this session, and mainly as they relate to validity, by way of preparation for more detailed discussions both in later sessions in this chapter (values, Session 2; and realism in physics, Session 3) and in later chapters in this part (explanation and scientific laws, Chapter 14; and causation, Chapter 15).

Descriptive adequacy and empirical import

First, then, Empirical Import. The next reading, which follows immediately on from the last reading (linked with Exercise 3), includes the concluding paragraph of Hempel's summary of his two requirements and the opening paragraphs of his longer treatment of his first requirement.

EXERCISE 4	(20 minutes)

Read the short passage from:

> Hempel, C.G. (1994). Fundamentals of taxonomy. In *Philosophical Perspectives on Psychiatric Diagnostic Classification* (ed. J.S. Sadler, O.P. Wiggins, and M.A. Schwartz). Baltimore, MD: Johns Hopkins University Press. (Extract, p 318).

Link with Reading 13.4

This is a very short passage from Hempel's paper but it has a great deal packed into it! As you read it think about:

1. The significance of the difference in the terminology Hempel uses of his first requirement in the paragraph before the subheading and in the subheading itself.

2. The sense that Hempel gives to that key word 'objective' as an aim of the kind of knowledge to which science aspires.

3. Hempel's criticisms of 'contemporary psychodynamic theories', in particular:

   (a) Are these criticisms justified in his own terms?

   (b) Why do you think Hempel introduces psychodynamic theory as an example at the start of a section on the Empirical rather than Systematic Import of a classification?

   (c) How is what Hempel says here about psychodynamic theory related to his comments in the last paragraph of the previous reading, the reading linked with Exercise 3. (Remember that these two passages about psychodynamic theory are separated in his paper by only a few lines.)

   (d) What are the implications of all this for the subsequent rejection of psychodynamic theory in the move from DSM-I to DSM-II.

Write down your own ideas on these points before going on.

Again, we will take the above three questions in turn.

1. *Hempel's terminology.* In the final paragraph of Hempel's summary introduction to his two requirements, he refers to the first as 'descriptive'; and 'descriptive adequacy', with appropriate variations, is the term he uses throughout his summary, including in the subheading to the summary (as in the reading above linked with Exercise 3). In the subheading to the next section, though, the term 'descriptive adequacy' has been replaced with 'Empirical Import'. There is a slide here, then, from the demand that a classification should be descriptively adequate to the idea that, in consequence, it has Empirical Import.

   The link between descriptive adequacy and Empirical Import in Logical Empiricism is, as we saw in Chapter 12, observation: it is observation statements that in Logical Empiricism are the basis for distinguishing between theories that are true as to 'what is there' and theories that are not; it is thus observation statements that have *empirical* content; and observation statements *describe* what is observed. This logical 'audit trail' will be important to us later when we came to the link between reliability (agreement in observational statements) and validity (being true to what is there). For the moment, though, it is important to note that the terms 'descriptive' and 'empirical' are so closely melded together in Hempel's thinking that they are used almost as synonyms.

2. *What Hempel means by 'objective'.* Hempel defines 'objective' in the first few lines of the section on Empirical Import consistently with Logical Empiricism. Thus 'objective' knowledge is the kind of knowledge that science aims to deliver, i.e. knowledge that is 'inter-subjectively certifiable, independently of individual opinion or preference, on the basis of data obtainable by suitable experiments or observations'.

   There are many qualifications and caveats between the lines of this definition that reflect refinements in the theory of

Logical Empiricism. Thus objective knowledge is not equivalent merely to intersubjective agreement: it is a matter, rather, of intersubjective *certification*; such certification, moreover, should not be on the basis of 'individual opinion', still less, anticipating Hempel's later concerns about values, 'preferences'; rather, certification should be on the basis of data that, if not actually to hand is 'obtainable' in principle (this is, roughly, the requirement of 'testability' in the traditional model of science, and, broadly, of 'verification' as discussed in Chapter 12); and, finally, though crucially, the data should be obtainable in principle on the basis of 'suitable experiments or observations', i.e. experiments or observations that are 'suitable' in the sense of being appropriate to the knowledge being 'certified' in the case in question (Hempel's word 'suitable' of course suggests one place at which, contrary to the tenets of Logical Empiricism, theory, in the form of conceptual prestructuring (see Chapter 12), 'infects' data). Hempel's next sentence then completes the connection between observation and description. For, he says, 'this' (i.e. intersubjective certification on the basis of observation) 'requires that the terms used in formulating scientific statements' (note the Logical Empiricist return to the importance of language) 'have clearly specified meanings and be understood in the same sense by all those who use them.'

At one level, all this makes perfect sense. If those involved in a process of intersubjective certification are using the same *terms* to describe their observations but with different *meanings*, whether through lack of clarity of meaning or for any other reason, then there will be no determinate way of knowing whether they agree or not. There are difficulties with this idea to which, with Hempel himself, we return later (see reading linked with Exercise 5 below). But the point for now is that Hempel does not specify that clear and agreed meanings are to be attached only to observational terms. He uses the generic 'scientific statements'. There is another slide here, then, for 'statement' could mean 'statement of observation' (i.e. *descriptive* statement) or 'statement of theory'. This slide is important to an understanding of the (apparent) criticism Hempel makes of 'contemporary' psychodynamics, by way of illustration, in the second half of the paragraph, and it is to this that we turn in the third part of this exercise.

3. *Hempel's example of psychodynamic theory.* Having defined what he means by 'objective' in the first half of the opening paragraph of this section, Hempel goes on to give an example. What is wrong with 'contemporary psychodynamic theories', he suggests, presumably with the example of conversion reaction (given a few lines above) in mind, is that their 'central concepts lack clear and uniform criteria of application'. As a consequence of this, therefore, 'there are no definite and unequivocal ways of putting the theories to a test by applying them to concrete cases'.

What is odd, then, and surely unjustified, about this example is not that it is critical of psychodynamically theory. It is rather that Hempel's criticism is directed, not against the observational basis of psychodynamically based diagnosis, but against its *theory*. Remember that this whole section is about the Empirical Import of a classification, i.e. its observational (or descriptive) basis, rather than its Systematic Import (Hempel's second requirement). Further, in the preceding section (in the reading linked to Exercise 3), Hempel appears to comment favourably on psychodynamic theory, by loose analogy with gravitational theory, as helping to move psychiatry along the course of true science from a descriptive to a systematic (or theoretical) basis for its classifications.

The appropriate response to Hempel's critique of contemporary psychodynamic *theories* in this section, therefore, is not, with DSM-II, to reject them; the appropriate response is rather to clean up their observational basis, in other words to provide the clear and uniform criteria of application that Hempel suggests they lack. This may be difficult to do: Hempel suggests later on that one attempt to provide such criteria (by Ellis, p. 321) fails. But, as we noted in the last exercise, Hempel expressly states at the end of his article that there are, in his view, no barriers of principle to adequate formulations of psychodynamic theory. And subsequent empirical studies, for example by the British psychiatrist and philosopher, Peter Hobson, have indeed shown that psychodynamic concepts are perfectly capable of being formulated in reliable terms (Hobson *et al.*, 1998).

Operationalism

In the next reading Hempel makes a key suggestion for how the Empirical Import of the terms in a scientific classification might be improved.

EXERCISE 5 (30 minutes)

Read the two passages from:

Hempel, C.G. (1994). Fundamentals of taxonomy. In *Philosophical Perspectives on Psychiatric Diagnostic Classification* (ed. J.S. Sadler, O.P. Wiggins, and M.A. Schwartz). Baltimore, MD: Johns Hopkins University Press

Link with Reading 13.5

This reading from Hempel's paper introduces a term—operationalism—from the philosophy of physics that has subsequently passed into the language of psychiatry. As you read these passages, think about precisely what operationalism means in physics, in particular its relationship to:

1. the Empirical Import of a classification understood, in Hempel's term in the first reading from his article, as descriptive adequacy; and

2. the relationship between the Empirical (descriptive) Import and Systematic (theoretical) Import of a classification and the relevance of this relationship to current concerns about the validity of psychiatric classifications as expressed in Kupfer *et al.*'s *Research Agenda* for *DSM-V*.

Operationalism, then, as Hempel describes in the first passage in this reading, was first fully set out by the physicist P.W. Bridgman in his book on *The Logic of Modern Physics* (1927). Essentially, operationalism seeks to make descriptive terms capable of unambiguous application by defining them by reference to the results of an operation: thus, in Hempel's example, the descriptive term 'harder than' means 'one material is harder than another if a sharply pointed sample of the former is capable of making a scratch on a sample of the latter'.

Operationalism and descriptive adequacy

In physics, then, this seems a sensible approach to providing clear criteria of the meaning of key terms, essentially because physics deals with things that, directly or indirectly, we can get hold of, and on which we can thus carry out operations. This indeed, as Hempel suggests in the second passage, is what makes the assertions of physics 'capable of objective test'. For, as he goes on to say, the ability to carry out operations is what gives the assertions of physics 'definite public criteria of application'. As a 'test' of the scientific, he further suggests, that is 'closely akin to the empiricist' (hence Logical Empiricist) 'insistence that meaningful scientific hypotheses and theories should be capable, in principle, of intersubjective test by observational data'.

This passage is important, not least, because it makes clear, again, the very tight link in Hempel's thinking between Empirical Import, or 'descriptive adequacy' as he also calls it, and Systematic (or theoretical) Import. Psychiatry has derived from Hempel's paper the need to establish a descriptively adequate set of criteria for its classifications. This, as Hempel suggests, is a pre-condition for objectivity, where objectivity means intersubjective agreement on whether a descriptive term applies in a given case. But the *point* of this is always integrally linked to providing a test of *theory*. It is this point, perhaps, that psychiatry, in focusing on descriptive adequacy has tended to lose sight of. It is this point, indeed, the point of advancing theory, that is behind current concerns, as in Kupfer *et al.*'s *Research Agenda for DSM-V*, about the *validity* of psychiatric classifications. Again, we return to validity and to its relationship with reliability below in the final part of this session.

Reliability

But before we get to linking up Empirical and Systematic Import, description and theory, we need to fill in a key step. For, as we saw earlier in this session, current concerns about the validity of psychiatric classification stand in contrast to claims, not, directly, of descriptive adequacy (Hempel's first term), still less of Empirical Import (his second term), but rather of reliability. In the next reading we look at the link in Hempel's paper between operational criteria, as one possible way of achieving Empirical Import in medical diagnosis, to a particular kind of difficulty that may arise in psychiatric diagnosis relevant to reliability.

Read the two short passages from:

Hempel, C.G. (1994). Fundamentals of taxonomy. In *Philosophical Perspectives on Psychiatric Diagnostic Classification* (ed. J.S. Sadler, O.P. Wiggins, and M.A. Schwartz). Baltimore, MD: Johns Hopkins University Press

Link with Reading 13.6

Here we want you to consider just one question.

♦ How strong or otherwise is the link Hempel makes between operationalism and reliability (agreement in the use of diagnostic terms—see Box 13.2).

This reading starts with a bald assertion that most medical diagnostic procedures are based on operational criteria. In the passage of his paper immediately preceding this reading, Hempel has given an example of a medical diagnosis based on carrying out a chemical test on a sample of a patient's urine. Fair enough, then. Such an 'operation' is capable (technical competence permitting) of unambiguous application (in most cases). Hempel then contrasts this example of a medical diagnosis with an example of a psychiatric diagnosis based on a characteristic subjective response, the 'praecox feeling', in the examiner. The 'praecox feeling', he says, does not satisfy the requirements of operationalism because its application 'is *not* independent of the examiner' (p. 312, emphasis in original; we return to Hempel on the praecox feeling later in this session).

Hempel on reliability

The link between operationalism of this kind and reliability in Hempel's paper is, however, surprisingly weak. 'Surprisingly' because, as we have seen, reliability has figured so prominently, and so prominently alongside claims to operationalism, in post-Second World War developments in psychiatric classification. Thus in the first passage in this reading, Hempel starts, as we have seen, by using the example of the 'praecox feeling' to mark the distinction between satisfactory operational diagnostic criteria in bodily medicine and unsatisfactory criteria in psychiatry. In the gap between the two passages in the reading, Hempel defines the link, that we looked at in the second paragraph of the reading linked with Exercise 5, between Bridgman's operationalism and empiricism. Then, in the second passage in this reading, Hempel starts by noting the interest in operationalism in psychology and sociology, reflected in the use of structured psychometric instruments; he follows this with a simple assertion, no more, at the start of the next paragraph that the 'concern' among 'psychologists and social scientists with the *reliability* of their terms reflects the importance attributed to objectivity of use' (p. 320, emphasis in original); and he then moves swiftly on in the rest of the paragraph to elaborate on the two main kinds of reliability (see Box 13.2) and how they are assessed.

This passage thus leaves entirely open precisely *why* or *how* reliability—agreement in the use of a term—is linked with either descriptive adequacy or Empirical Import as the focus of this section of Hempel's paper. We can only speculate on how Hempel might have unpacked this link. But it is important to be aware just how little Hempel himself makes of reliability, given the importance of reliability in current psychiatric classifications and its (not wholly satisfactory) relationship with validity—recall that Kupfer *et al.* (2002) imply, contra Hempel, that reliability has been achieved perhaps even at the expense of validity. This would be contrary to Hempel's expectations if Empirical Import (via descriptive adequacy) were indeed a step towards Systematic (or theoretical) Import and if reliability were sufficient for descriptive adequacy.

We return to the links between operationalism, reliability, and validity at the end of this session after we have explored how Hempel's ideas found their way (much modified) through into ICD-8 and, hence, set the agenda for psychiatric classification running towards its current status as summarized in Kupfer *et al.*'s *Research Agenda for DSM-V*.

Hempel and the missing link to ICD and DSM

We have now looked at a number of key points made by Hempel relevant to the subsequent development of psychiatric classification: (1) Hempel's two requirements for a scientific classification, Empirical Import (or descriptive adequacy) and Systematic (or theoretical) Import; (2) the connections Hempel makes between these and the objectivity of a science; (3) his comments on operationalism as a way of improving objectivity; and (4) the links he draws, such as they are, between objectivity, operationalism, and reliability.

At this point, reflect on what you have learnt about Hempel's paper thus far and the way in which, with ICD-8, psychiatric classification subsequently developed. In what respects has psychiatry adopted Hempel's message? In what respects has it not done so?

A rough 'audit' of Hempel's influence, on the basis of what we have read thus far, suggests that there is a broad consonance between his two requirements for a classification to be a scientific classification and how psychiatry's classifications actually developed with ICD-8. Hempel distinguished descriptive (or empirical) adequacy from theoretical (or systematic) import; and he noted that sciences tend to evolve from descriptive to theoretical stages. On the other hand, however, he also suggested that psychiatry, as a medical science was already showing positive signs of development towards a theoretical stage; and that, while the dominant theory at the time (at least in DSM), psychodynamic theory, needed to be operationalized, and while there were competing theories (notably biological theory), he none the less expected psychiatry to continue its established trend towards ever greater systematization. This of course was directly contrary to the direction psychiatry actually took. Similarly, although Hempel emphasized the potential of operationalism as a method for improving objectivity, and although this term did come into general use in psychiatric classification,

Hempel mentions reliability, which as Kupfer *et al.* (2002) note (above), and as we illustrate further in the Reading Guide, has occupied far more of the research agenda, only in passing.

A missing link

So there is a missing link. Hempel, and the influences generally of Logical Empiricism, are evident enough in ICD-8 and its successor classifications. But the particular effects of these influences, how they actually played out, suggest that some other factor must also have been involved. As already noted, Erwin Stengel is often credited with being the link between Hempel and ICD-8 (see for example Kendell, 1975, p. 93). Stengel was certainly influential on ICD-8. As noted earlier, he was the first respondent to Hempel's paper in the 1959 conference; and his remarks in that context were reproduced, in closely similar form, in his report to the WHO (Stengel, 1959). A closer reading of Stengel, though, in both places, suggests that he largely follows Hempel's line, i.e. suggesting that at the very least, psychiatric classifications will continue to be based on *both* symptoms (descriptive criteria) *and* aetiology (theoretical criteria). Again, then, there must be a missing link, some additional factor standing between what both Hempel and Stengel had to say about the future direction of development of psychiatric classification, and the direction that, in the event, it actually took.

The discussion following Hempel's paper

The next reading (linked with Exercise 8) is from a transcript of the discussion that was reproduced alongside the first publication of Hempel's paper in Zubin, 1961. We reference it here as Discussion, Various Contributors, 1961.

Stengel opens the discussion, covering essentially the material he was later to include in his report to the WHO, and a number of other contributors raise various points. About halfway through the discussion, in response to one of the points raised, Hempel picks up on what he had to say in his paper about the difference between a natural and an artificial classification, noting that the difference is not 'sharp and definitive, but a matter of degree; and secondly, that it is relative to the particular purpose which a classification is to serve' (Discussion, Various Contributors, 1961, p. 33). Hempel then goes on to develop his point, explaining that it is the *scientific* purposes of 'finding a system of laws or correlations by which explanations or predictions may be achieved', that was behind his requirement that if a classification is to aspire to be a natural classification, it must have, in addition to Empirical Import (or 'descriptive adequacy'), Systematic Import.

A decisive intervention

Hempel's comments in this passage of the discussion thus emphasize the extent to which, contrary to the direction that subsequent psychiatric classifications were to take, he focused on the importance of Systematic Import (rather than Empirical Import or descriptive adequacy) in a scientific classification. But it is at precisely this point that someone who has not yet spoken comes into the discussion. In a brief but decisive intervention, this person, (1) suggests a different way in which classifications

may be divided up; (2) connects this different way of dividing up classifications with the particular purposes served by an international psychiatric classification, and then, (3) delivers a punchline in the form of a specific proposal for developing ICD-8. In the next reading, we look at this decisive intervention in the discussion following Hempel's paper in full.

EXERCISE 8   (15 minutes)

Read the short extract from:

> Discussion, Various Contributors (1961). In *Field Studies in the Mental Disorders* (ed. J. Zubin). New York, Grune and Stratton. This extract comes on page 34.

Link with Reading 13.7

This reading is the whole of the decisive intervention by a person (at this stage unnamed) in the discussion following Hempel's paper. It is also the only intervention by this person. It occupies just half a page in a total of 28 pages, i.e. less than 3% of the 'column inches'. Yet it was indeed to prove decisive. As you read the passage, think about:

1. What the speaker takes from Hempel and what he does not

2. Precisely what the speaker's proposal for ICD-8 amounts to

Finally, who do you think the speaker is?

The speaker in this passage starts by connecting up what he (he is a 'he') has to say with Hempel's remarks by picking up on Hempel's point about the form of a classification, whether natural or artificial, being driven by the purposes it is intended to serve. Hempel, as we noted above, had talked about the purposes of scientific (or natural) classifications in general. The speaker in this passage, however, focuses rather on the particular purposes of particular sciences. Viewed in this way, he says, among scientific classifications 'we might properly distinguish between public classifications and private classifications'. It is the former, public classifications, that 'are most valuable for epidemiological work, since we need to make comparisons of findings in different countries, and unless there is uniformity of usage, that is impractical'. Private classifications, by contrast, although perfectly capable of uniformity of usage within a given group with a uniform background, are, none the less, only suitable for the usage of the group in question.

The speaker, therefore, in this passage, with his talk of 'epidemiological work' and of 'comparisons of findings in different countries', clearly has WHO's need for an international psychiatric classification in mind. But what does this mean for the basis of such a classification?

A decisive proposal for ICD-8

Here, again, the speaker draws on Hempel's insights into the nature of a scientific classification, but adapting them in a decisive way to meet the requirements of an international psychiatric classification. A scientific classification, he agrees with Hempel, should ideally be based on theory. For some private classifications, used by a group for whom a given theory seems 'workable', a theoretical basis may be appropriate. But no current psychiatric theory can meet the requirements Hempel has set out for adequate Systematic Import. Hence, the speaker suggests, coming to the punchline of his proposal for ICD-8, 'for the purpose of public classification we should eschew categories based on theoretical concepts and restrict ourselves to the operationalized, descriptive type of classification...'.

The missing link

Here, then, is an intervention capturing precisely the direction that psychiatric classification, from ICD-8 onwards, subsequently took...

...and the speaker turns out to be, as described in the transcript, one 'Dr Lewis'. This is none other than *the* Aubrey Lewis, then, Professor Sir Aubrey Lewis, the architect in the 1940s and 1950s of the Maudsley 'school' of rigorous scientific psychiatry, that we met in Part I: you will recall his analysis of concepts of disorder as 'part functions' (Part I, Chapter 2 Reading Guide) and his definitional attack on the concept of psychosis (Part I, Chapter 3, Philosophical Annotation on Insight).

Lewis adapts Hempel

Important, then, as Hempel's and in turn Stengel's influence was on ICD-8, it was from Lewis that the decisive move from theory-based to a descriptive- or symptom-based classification in ICD-8 came. Lewis, moreover, in suggesting this move, although drawing on Hempel's general insights into the nature and purposes of scientific classification, does so in an active rather than passive way. Lewis adapts Hempel's general insights into scientific classifications

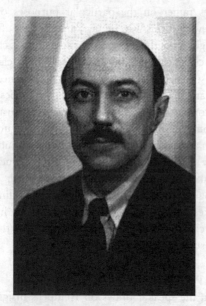

Fig. 13.1 Professor Sir Aubrey Lewis

to the particular needs of international psychiatry at the time for statistical reporting and for research based on the methods of epidemiological science.

Lewis later went on to make what the WHO, in the Preface to the ICD-9 (WHO, 1978, p. 5) described as a 'fundamental' contribution to the Glossary to ICD-8. We look at Lewis' own Preface to ICD-8 in detail below. Before coming to ICD-8, though, we need to fill in briefly how the story developed following Lewis' decisive intervention at the 1959 conference.

Not (yet) a 'done deal'

Lewis' proposed move to a predominantly descriptive basis for ICD appears to have gone down, with many of those at the 1959 conference, like a lead balloon. Lewis' intervention is picked up enthusiastically by some of the other delegates; but it is ignored or objected to by others (Hempel appears to ignore it); and although the Chair, Dr Reid, refers favourably to it in his summing up, as being 'in the interest of unambiguous communication and uniformity of use', he does so with qualifications; and he had rather more to say about the evolution of operational terms and about future scientific progress being based on the development of new instrumentation and corresponding advances in theory. It is an evolution of this (theoretical) kind, Dr Reid concludes, that is 'to be expected also in the domain of psychiatric research' (Discussion, Various Contributors, 1961, p. 49).

Similarly, in a separate summary of the discussion written by John Clausen (presumably at a later date), although there is reference to a possible move to a descriptive basis for psychiatric classification, Lewis is not credited with the suggestion, the objections to it are emphasized, and Clausen's summary, like the Chair's (Dr Reid's) summing up, ends with Hempel's comments on the need for progressive refinement of psychiatric classification in response to future developments in theory.

Dr Reid and John Clausen, it is important to emphasize, in making so little of Lewis' intervention, were both faithfully reflecting the discussion as a whole. Later in this part, in Chapter 16, we consider the factors that make or mar the chances of a scientific idea, however well founded, seeing the light of day. That Lewis was a tough and determined character who was in a position to see his suggestion through, was likely to have been a factor in this case. A second important factor was Lewis' ability to turn his general theoretical suggestion for a more exclusively symptom-based classification to good practical effect in the detailed development of the specific categories in the Glossary to ICD-8.

From Lewis with Sartorius through to ICD-10 and DSM-IV

This was indeed what Lewis did. What happened was that Lewis was invited to Geneva by the WHO and spent 4 days working intensively with Norman Sartorius to complete the Glossary to ICD-8 (Sartorius, 2004), building on an existing UK glossary (General Register Office, 1968) that had been produced by a small group (including Stengel) chaired by Lewis. DSM-II, as we noted earlier, subsequently adopted the ICD-8 nomenclature; ICD-9 incorporated the ICD-8 Glossary with a few minor changes; DSM-III took the idea of 'operational' criteria further with explicit inclusion and exclusion criteria for class membership; and ICD-10 and DSM-IV added an evidence-based approach to the process of developing and changing criteria and classes.

Hand in hand with these developments in psychiatric classification, as we noted in Chapter 12, have gone corresponding developments in structured and semi-structured instruments for assessing psychopathology. These instruments, to the extent that they seek to operationalize the observations on which clinical diagnosis depends in terms of carefully defined activities (or operations) for eliciting and recording symptoms, are, perhaps more so even than the criteria in modern psychiatric classifications, faithful to the principles of operationalism developed by Bridgman, referred to by Hempel, and embraced by Stengel and Lewis. Sartorius, as we saw in Chapter 12, was one of the three authors of the first semi-structured, internationally used and adapted mental state interview with known reliability, the PSE (Wing *et al.*, 1974). Sartorius was also to continue at WHO, eventually as the Director of the Mental Health Section, in which capacity he co-ordinated the production of both ICD-9 and ICD-10. But the decisive move, the (tactical) retreat from premature theory to a descriptive symptom-based structure for psychiatric classification, we owe, for good or ill, to Lewis.

For good or ill?

We say 'for good or ill', for of course, as we saw from Kupfer *et al.*'s *Research Agenda for DSM-V* at the start of this session, although psychiatry has indeed enjoyed the expected gains in reliability, and corresponding improvements in communication, at least among psychiatrists, and although there have been advances in epidemiological understanding, psychiatric classifications remain much embattled from without and contested from within. We will return to the current difficulties of psychiatric classification in a preliminary way in the final part of this session and again and in more detail in Session 4 of this chapter. We will now pause, though, for a moment to take stock of the agenda for psychiatric classification as it stood at the time of the publication of ICD-8. As we will see, the agenda at this time, the agenda that we will call our *Conceptual Research Agenda for ICD-9*, was considerably more upbeat than Kupfer *et al.*'s current *Research Agenda for DSM-V*.

The second new agenda – a conceptual research agenda for ICD-9

The next reading (linked with Exercise 9) is the Foreword to the Glossary to ICD-8 written by Sir Aubrey Lewis (as he had by then become). Published by the WHO in 1974, Lewis' Preface to the Glossary to ICD-8 was also included as a Foreword to ICD-9 '... in recognition of [the late] Sir Aubrey's fundamental contribution to that glossary [ie the ICD-8 Glossary], which constitutes the core of the glossary that is now an official part of the mental disorders chapter of the Ninth Revision [of ICD-9]' (WHO, 1978,

p. 5). It is the latter (the Foreword to ICD-9) that is reproduced in the reading below. As just noted, you will see that Lewis is considerably more upbeat about the research agenda for psychiatric classification at the time of the publication of the Glossary to ICD-8, than his successors, Kupfer *et al.*, some 30 years later, in their Introduction to the *Research Agenda for DSM-V*.

EXERCISE 9   (30 minutes)

Read Lewis' Foreword to the ICD-8 Glossary:

WHO (1974). *Glossary of Mental Disorders and Guide to their Classification, for use in Conjunction with the International Classification of Diseases*, 8th revision. Geneva: World Health Organization

---

Link with Reading 13.8

Lewis' Preface to ICD-8 is short but it packs, as you would expect from someone with Lewis' depth of knowledge and powerful discursive skills, a whole series of punches. As you read what Lewis says, think about the Agenda for psychiatric classification implicit in Lewis' Preface. Lewis of course does not use the term 'agenda'. None the less, his Preface amounts to a *Conceptual Research Agenda for ICD-9*.

In this part of the exercise you may want to use the agenda items listed in Table 13.1 (our Conceptual Research Agenda for DSM-V).

There are three stages to this exercise:

1. draw up your *own list of agenda items* as they are identifiable in Lewis' Preface. As before, it is important to complete your own list before referring to our suggestions below. Then,

2. *compare and contrast* Lewis' Agenda with that of Kupfer *et al.* (as summarized in Table 13.1). The main difference between them, as we have already indicated, is in their respective 'big issues', reliability (for Lewis at the time of ICD-8) and validity (for Kupfer *et al.* 30 years later in 'their' Research *Agenda for DSM-V*). But there are many other differences and also some important similarities between them. Finally,

3. consider the *wider influences* of the main difference between Lewis and Kupfer *et al.* in their 'big issues' (respectively of reliability and validity), i.e. how does the emphasis on reliability in Lewis' Agenda and the emphasis on validity in Kupfer *et al.*'s Agenda influence the ways they think about other items on their respective Agendas for psychiatric classification.

Lewis' Preface is a masterpiece of compression of thought. It is difficult to summarize what he says without writing a much longer piece! There are a whole series of points relevant to the research agenda for psychiatric classification at the time. We draw these points out here in the order in which they are given above in our *Conceptual Research Agenda for DSM-V*.

Thus, among the points Lewis manages to compress into this short piece are:

◆ *Agenda Item 1: Timeline*. Lewis, like Kupfer *et al.*, takes a long view: he notes that psychiatric classification stands in a long tradition, back to the second century BC.

◆ *Agenda Item 2: Uses of Psychiatric Classifications*. Lewis observes that classifications serve many purposes—note his observations on the 'multifarious needs' served by glossaries and classifications. But he focuses, like Kupfer *et al.*, on the uses of psychiatric classifications for diagnoses made by clinicians, in this case as the basis of international epidemiological research and statistical reporting.

◆ *Agenda Item 3: Misuses of Psychiatric Classifications*. Although a 'respectable' tradition, Lewis says, compiling glossaries, and by implication compiling classifications, also has a shadow side. The term 'glossary', Lewis continues, comes from the same root as to 'gloss over' or 'to gloze'. Hence we find pejorative associations with psychiatric classification, many of which, as listed by Lewis, remain all too familiar today: 'mere labelling', 'the neat complacency of classification', 'nosological stamp collecting', and a 'medical hortus siccus' (a dry garden).

Such name-calling is generally unwarranted, no doubt, but one particular reason for classifications falling into disrepute is, Lewis says, 'the excesses to which classification was pushed in the late 18th and early 19th centuries'. Beware, then, is Lewis' implication, similar excesses today as successive editions of both ICD and DSM trump each other in length and complexity. Kupfer *et al.* are concerned similarly with overextension, albeit a different kind of overextension, namely reification of the concepts in the DSM.

◆ *Agenda Item 4: Status of Psychiatric Science*. Lewis is clear that psychiatric classification is a more difficult case of medical classification. The 'modern psychiatric glossarist', he says, faces similar difficulties as the 'compiler of other medical classifications', only more so. Lewis' 'more so', however, is expressed, much as Kupfer *et al.*'s corresponding agenda item is expressed, in deficit terms: the difficulties of psychiatric classification are the same as for medical classifications, Lewis says, but 'aggravated by hazards arising from *paucity* of the objective data on which definition and diagnosis must depend': again, he [the modern psychiatric glossarist] has to *contrive* appropriate criteria…' (both second paragraph, emphases added).

◆ *Agenda Item 5: Concepts*. Lewis pinpoints one particular difficulty in producing a classification of mental disorders, namely in the concept of disorder itself. In this respect, then, in naming the conceptual difficulties for what they are, Lewis differs from Kupfer *et al.* There is no surprise in the fact that Lewis is alert to conceptual difficulties: you will recall his papers on diseases as 'part functions' and on the difficulties associated with the core concept of traditional psychopathology, psychosis, in Part I. What does come as a surprise, though, is that Lewis pinpoints the difficulty, not in any particular property of the concept of mental disorder (or of a mental disease, as he would have said),

but rather in the abstract status of concepts themselves. This is a surprise because, as Lewis himself makes clear, diseases in *general* (not just in psychiatry) are 'abstract concepts'.

This is how Lewis puts it: 'since diseases are in any case abstract concepts, it is no wonder that the disease constructs which psychiatrists work with have shimmering outline boundaries and overlap'. But put like this, it *is* a wonder, a *big* wonder, why the disease constructs with which *psychiatrists* work should have 'shimmering outline boundaries and overlap', while those of *bodily* medicine, which equally according to Lewis are 'abstract concepts', do not. (Remember that in this context Lewis is concerned with the *added* difficulty of psychiatric classification.) This brings us, therefore, in our Agenda, firmly to issues of reliability and of validity.

◆ *Agenda Item 6: Reliability*. As we have several times noted, where validity is the big issue for Kupfer *et al.*, in their *Research Agenda for DSM-V*, the big issue for Lewis is reliability. Interestingly, given the volume of research on reliability, Lewis does not confine himself to the need merely for reliability. Instead, he couches his remarks in terms of the wider need for psychiatry to improve the observational basis of its science. Thus, 'Observer variation', Lewis says in the second paragraph in the reading, 'is disconcertingly (note the deficit word) in evidence; [and] reliability is too low for scientific comfort' (yet another deficit phrase).

But if the observational difficulties that beset psychiatric science are defects (as just noted, Lewis, like Kupfer *et al.*, uses deficit words of psychiatric science), such defects, Lewis continues, are to an extent remediable, depending on whether they arise from '…inexact perception, personal bias, or divergency of the nosological systems or terms used'. So, Lewis says, in the next paragraph, 'The glossary put forward here, when faithfully applied, reduces the scope for error.' Why? Well, in providing for *con*vergence in the nosological terms used. But this is not a stand alone solution. It needs to be combined with constant attention to the need for 'accurate observation' rather than falling back on, in Lewis' words from his intervention in the 1959 conference (see reading linked with Exercise 9), '…the many hypothetical and unconfirmed schemas of 'psychodynamic mechanisms', and the concern with etiological inference…'. Thus it is, Lewis says, that 'since the disorders listed in this glossary are identified by criteria that are predominantly *descriptive*, its use should encourage an emphasis on careful *observation*' (emphases added).

◆ *Agenda Item 7: Validity*. Validity, although the big issue for Kupfer *et al.*, was important for Lewis, too. However, Lewis (although not using the word 'validity') takes it for granted that as a medical classification, a valid psychiatric classification will be concerned with diseases. The aim is to 'contrive appropriate criteria for differentiating one disease from another… a consistent scheme with which they [psychiatric diseases] will all fit'. Thus far, then, if we translate Lewis' 'diseases' into Kupfer *et al.*'s 'pathophysiological mechanisms', the two agendas are in agreement. A valid psychiatric classification, however, Lewis continues, reflecting his comments in the discussion following Hempel's paper, may take a wide variety of different forms. It may be descriptive or theoretical in structure: it 'may be based on clinical patterns (syndromes) or on clinical course; it may be psychodynamic, etiological (genetic), or pathological'. Lewis, then, is considerably more open in what he will allow as a valid scientific theory than Kupfer *et al.* (who focused on only the last two of Lewis' list).

♦ *Agenda Item 8: Structural Solutions.* As noted above (under Agenda Item 6, Reliability) Lewis, building directly on what he said in his intervention in the discussion following Hempel's paper during the 1959 conference, makes fully explicit that in the ICD-8 classification and its supporting Glossary, to repeat the key phrase quoted above, the 'disorders listed . . . are identified by criteria that are predominantly *descriptive* . . .' (again, emphasis added). Lewis, in contrast to Kupfer *et al.*, is thus confident of a 'reliability first, validity second' approach to building more scientific classifications of mental disorder.

♦ *Agenda Item 9: Process Solutions.* Lewis emphasizes the importance of collegiality (Lewis' 'spirit of cooperation'), of international collaboration (Lewis' 'international group of collaborators and advisors'), and of contributions from different perspectives (Lewis' 'advisors of such diversity of background and outlook'), all in his final paragraph.

Also important was the fact that all those involved had a shared aim. What drew everyone together, what secured collegiality, international collaboration, and diverse disciplinary perspectives, what allowed 'the emergence of an agreed version', albeit with some residual 'compromises and anomalies', was, in Lewis' closing phrase, the 'common recognition of an urgent need for better means of communication'.

♦ *Agenda Item 10: Utility (of new Classifications).* Lewis retains here his focus on the role of the new descriptively based classification as a tool primarily for improved international epidemiological research and statistical reporting by way of improved communication. As noted above, it is implicit that this will lead on as in other areas of medicine, to a variety of aetiological theories; but this is left unsaid; and of course, in his intervention in the 1959 conference, Lewis left open the possibility, with his distinction between public and private classifications, that other quite different classifications may serve the purposes of development of theory within different research programmes.

♦ *Agenda Item 11: Overall Tenor.* In his Preface, as we noted earlier, Lewis is a good deal more positive and optimistic than Kupfer *et al.* in their *Research Agenda for DSM-V.* Taking Agenda Items 9, 10, and 11 together, then, we can see that Kupfer *et al.* share with Lewis the goal of improved communication achieved through inter-disciplinary and international collaboration. The main difference between them, however, is that Kupfer *et al.*, while acknowledging (and indeed themselves contributing to) the improvements in the reliability of our classifications that have flowed from improvements in communication between clinicians, are, with the benefit of 30 years hindsight, considerably more downbeat than Lewis about the prospects for improvements in validity.

We summarize the above points in Table 13.2. This table also compares our *Conceptual Research Agenda for ICD-9,* as the second of our two new agendas, with the main points from our first new agenda, set out fully in Table 13.1, our *Conceptual Research Agenda for DSM-V* (as desired from Kupfer *et al.*'s *Research Agenda for DSM-V*).

What Table 13.2 brings out, to come to the third part of Exercise 9, is the importance of their respective 'big issues', reliability for Lewis in *ICD-9* and validity for Kupfer *et al.*, in *DSM-V*, in driving the similarities and differences between them on other agenda items. Thus, for Items 1–5 (the items coming before 'reliability') the two agendas, although separated by some 30 years, are in many respects remarkably similar: both (Item 1) adopt long timelines; both (Item 2) recognize the importance of communication between clinicians; both (Item 3) warn of misuses, respectively through overextension and by reification of categories; both (Item 4) assume a deficit model of psychiatric science; and both (Item 5) recognize the importance of conceptual issues (although Kupfer *et al.* do not name them as such).

From this point, however, their agendas diverge. For Lewis, improved reliability (Item 6) is a key step towards improved validity (Item 6), which, he assumes, will follow switching from a theoretical (aetiology-based) to a descriptive (symptom-based) classificatory structure (Item 8), settled by way of a collegial international process (Item 9), aimed at producing, in the first instance, 'public' classifications suitable for international epidemiological and statistical purposes (Item 10), but with a good prospect of ultimately leading to wider gains in validity (Item 11). Kupfer *et al.*, by contrast, starting from their perception that improved reliability (Item 6) has failed to deliver improved validity (Item 7), hope to cut directly to aetiology-based classifications (Item 8) by way of empirical research (Item 9) as the foundation for improved treatments (Item 10), all of which, in their estimation, the last 30 years of developments in psychiatric classification, and by implication psychiatric science, have singularly failed to deliver (Item 11).

Reliability and validity

Reliability and validity, then, are the fulcrum around which everything else on both agendas turns. This is why, in developing Table 13.1 as a summary of our *Conceptual Research Agenda for DSM-V*, we put these two items in the middle of the agenda, as a fulcrum or pivot, even though we dealt with them first. But how exactly are reliability and validity pivotal? As we saw earlier, translated and redirected by Lewis and Sartorius into the symptom-based classification of ICD-8, Hempel's ideas have been crucial to setting the course along which psychiatric classification has subsequently developed. But this course, in focusing on improved reliability (as an aspect of Hempel's Empirical Import) has been in the opposite direction to that anticipated by Hempel (towards ever-greater Systematic Import). In assessing, therefore, the relationship between the emphasis on reliability in Lewis' *Agenda for ICD-9* and the emphasis on validity in Kupfer *et al.*'s *Agenda for DSM-V*, it will be important to look carefully at what Hempel actually said about reliability and validity. We began to unpack Hempel's ideas on these two topics earlier in this session when (in

Table 13.2 The Second New Agenda – a Conceptual Research Agenda for ICD-9 – compared with the first new agenda

	ICD-9 (second new agenda)	DSM-V (first new agenda–table 13.1)
(1) Time-line	Back to 2nd century BC	Back: to DSM-III Forward: to DSM-VI/VII
(2) Uses of psychiatric classification	ICD primarily for diagnoses made by clincians as the basis of epidemiological research and statistical reporting	Diagnosis by clinicians
(3) Misuses of psychiatric classification	Overextension: i.e. where classifications are driven to excessive lengths	Reification of categories
(4) Status of psychiatric science	Deficit model: implicit in terms used to describe current diagnostic classification, e.g. 'paucity', 'contrive'	Deficit model
(5) Concepts	Concepts explicitly identified as problematic—but medical concepts in general, not concepts specifically of mental disorder (i.e. not differentiated from concepts of bodily disorder)	Important but not named as such
(6) Reliability	THE BIG ISSUE: poor, though remediable, reliability reflecting unsound observational base at the root of difficulties of psychiatric classification	Run out of steam
(7) Validity	Assumed to follow: wide variety of possible scientific theories assumed to follow improved reliability (provided observational basis remains secure) much as in bodily medicine	THE BIG ISSUE
(8) Structural solution	Improved reliability: achieved by switching from premature aetiology-based to descriptive symptom-based criteria	Aetiology-based
(9) Process solutions	Importance of collegiality, international collaboration, and incorporation of different perspectives, all within a shared aim	Empirical research
(10) Utility (of new calssifications)	'Public' (like ICD): for (international) epidemiological and statistical purposes. 'Private': for 'local' use in connection with development of theory.	Better health-care services
(11) Overall tenor	Up-beat: positive about the opportunities for improved reliability as the basis for international epidemiological studies, (and improved communication generally between researchers) which could contribute to improved validity.	Downbeat
(12) Any other business	none	none

Exercise 6) we looked at a key passage in his paper in which he introduced the idea of operationalism. In the next and final section of this session we look at a further passage from Hempel's paper, with a view to unpacking further, and to an extent critiquing, what Hempel has to say in the light of subsequent developments in psychiatric classification.

Operationalism, reliability, validity, and a first look at what lies ahead

First, then, we return to the key passage from Hempel's paper on operationalism.

EXERCISE 10 (20 minutes)

This reading follows on immediately from the passage we looked at in Exercise 6:

> Hempel, C.G. (1994). Fundamentals of taxonomy. In *Philosophical Perspectives on Psychiatric Diagnostic Classification* (ed. J.S. Sadler, O.P. Wiggins, and M.A. Schwartz). Baltimore, MD: Johns Hopkins University Press

---

Link with Reading 13.9

In the earlier passage, Hempel, you will recall, introduced the idea of operationalism, which, although derived from physics, offered one way of responding to the difficulties of psychiatric classification. Here, by contrast, Hempel focuses on some of the limitations of operationalism.

1. What are these limitations?

2. Do you agree with the consequences that Hempel draws from these limitations for the relationship between psychiatric classification and diagnosis?

3. What conclusions can we draw from Hempel's account of the limitations of operationalism for reliability and validity and, hence, the possible future direction of the development of psychiatric classifications?

Hempel's three limitations of operationalism

In this important passage Hempel notes three (although he says 'two,' see below) important limitations of the application of the principles of operationalism, as formulated by Bridgman, to psychiatry. The second of these limitations has been widely recognized in psychiatry (it is noted by Stengel, 1959, p. 612, for example), but, we will argue, also widely misunderstood. We will start with this second limitation, therefore, before turning to Hempel's other two limitations, which, we will argue, despite being less widely recognized in psychiatry, turn out to be even more important.

Limitation 1: mere observation

First, then, Hempel's second (and our first) limitation on operationalism: this is the limitation that, for psychiatry, the insistence on an operational specification of meaning '...has to be taken in a very liberal sense which does not require manipulation of the objects under consideration: the mere observation of an object, for example, must be allowed to count as an operation...'. Hempel then goes on a little later to spell out that this liberal sense of operationalism does not let us off the hook of defining criteria with '...reasonably precise meaning and (that) are used, by all investigators concerned, with high intersubjective uniformity...', that is, and here Hempel comes back in effect to reliability, '...a high degree of agreement among different observers...'. (Hempel, 1961, pp. 320–321).

It is Hempel's use of the phrase 'mere observation' in this passage that has descended, via Stengel (1959, p. 612) and others, into psychiatry as the justification for allowing the history taking and other clinical observations on which psychiatric assessments are based, to count as operations. Hempel, indeed, seems to warrant this directly, to the extent that, in the text cited in the paragraph immediately above, he appears to endorse such an interpretation of a 'liberal operationalism', provided that the criteria adopted in translating the 'direct observations' derived clinically into diagnostic categories, are reliable (provided, that is, they show '...a high degree of agreement between different observers').

Mere 'behaviourist' observations

However, if we look more carefully at the passage, it appears there is rather more in Hempel's mind than, 'merely', the interview processes on which psychiatric diagnostic assessments depend. Thus, in developing his point Hempel starts by asking us to consider the example of endomorphy. Endomorphy, he says, by way of illustrating what he means by a 'liberalized' operationalism, is defined by 'directly observable features'. Well, fair enough. But endomorphy is defined by certain *bodily* features. Hence, Hempel's example of what the 'mere observation' of a liberalized operationalism would amount to, is already a perhaps somewhat surprising step away from the application of operationalism to the features of *mental* states with which psychiatry is characteristically concerned. And two paragraphs later, Hempel's 'directly observable' becomes, for purposes of operational formulations of psychological terms '...*publicly* observable aspects of behaviour...' (emphasis added), which in turn is unpacked as '...publicly observable aspects of *behaviour* a subject shows in response to a specified publicly observable stimulus situation...' (emphasis added). Hempel's 'liberal' operationalism, then, is very far from being 'mere observation' if 'mere' means interviews of the kind on which psychiatry characteristically relies for its diagnostic formulations. By a 'liberal' operationalism, what Hempel

appears to have in mind is, rather, an essentially *behaviourist* interpretation of observation in the psychological (including by implication psychiatric) sciences.

Operationalism gets the credit but reliability does the work

To what extent, therefore, even the semi-structured interviews discussed in Chapter 12 (such as the PSE), let alone general clinical diagnostic assessment in psychiatry, can be considered to satisfy behaviourist principles, and hence Hempel's notion of a 'liberal' operationalism, is at the very least a matter for debate. 'Mere' observation may, indeed, be capable of satisfying operationalist principles in the psychological sciences. But strip away the language of operationalism, and it seems that much of the work of operationalism in improving the Empirical Import of psychiatric classificatory terms, as set out there by Hempel in his paper, falls back on the shoulders of reliability. The Empirical Import of psychiatric classificatory terms, that is to say, if we follow Hempel's unpacking of his point (as set out above), comes down, to repeat Hempel's concluding phrase cited above, '...a high degree of agreement between observers'.

Physics and psychiatry

Psychiatric classifiers, therefore, from Stengel onwards, may have been a little hasty in assuming that Hempel's phrase 'mere observation' warranted their oft repeated claim that modern psychiatric classifications reflect the principles of operationalism as developed by Bridgman for the case of physics. We will see later in this chapter, particularly in Sessions 3 and 4, that physics, and the philosophy of physics, have much to teach us in psychiatry, and for the best of reasons, namely that the two disciplines, physics and psychiatry, are alike in being peculiarly difficult sciences. But as we will also see particularly in Session 4, the differences between physics and psychiatry, notably that where physics is concerned with particles, psychiatry is concerned with people, mean that we have to exercise extreme care in applying any lessons learned from the one to the other.

In this instance, with Hempel's suggestion that operationalism may be helpful in psychiatry, we have seen that a careful reading of Hempel's own account of his suggestion, shows that it is, really, reliability that is doing the work. There is nothing extra that operationalism adds beyond the requirement (which of course is generic rather than a requirement specifically of operationalism) for the use of terms with '...reasonably precise meaning(s)...'. Recognizing that the work of Empirical Import is being done by reliability rather than by operationalism is important in principle for psychiatry today because of what we will argue below is the tendency, as in Kupfer *et al.*'s *Research Agenda for DSM-V*, to over-react to the (perceived) failure of reliability to deliver validity. First, though, we take a step back, to Hempel's first limitation on operationalism, as set out in this reading, what he calls (and what we renumber here as Limitation 2), the limitation of 'partial criteria of application'.

Limitation 2: partial criteria of application

Hempel's first limitation on operationalism, as set out in this reading, is that 'the operational criteria of application available for a term often amount to less than a full definition' (p. 320). This limitation on operationalism, as we noted above, is less widely recognized in psychiatry than Hempel's 'mere observation' limitation. There are two reasons why this might be so. First, it is a 'limitation', not of operationalism as it has to be 'liberalized' (Hempel's term) for purposes of application to the mental sciences, but of operationalism in *general*, including as it applies to the physical sciences. Hempel indeed gives the example of different thermometers being used across different ranges of temperature and being designed for different purposes. A thermometer, Hempel points out, provides an operational criterion of temperature. But no one thermometer can provide a complete operational definition of temperature. Indeed, while this or that thermometer may make an operational test possible in a given situation, 'there are reasons to doubt the possibility of providing *full* operational definitions for all theoretical terms in science…' (p. 320, emphasis in original).

Psychiatry, then, might reasonably have neglected this limitation on operationalism, it being a limitation that is inherent in operationalism itself rather than as applied specifically to psychiatric science. Moreover, the specific sense that Hempel gives to this limitation when he first introduces it, that the limitation arises from the 'partial criteria of application' of a concept, is, it would seem, readily and unproblematically transferable to psychiatry. Hempel's example of different thermometers, used across different ranges of temperature and designed for different purposes, is transferable more or less directly to psychiatry's wide variety of different semi-structured interview schedules (noted in Chapter 12) that, for a given area of psychopathology (such as depression), are used across different ranges of severity and are designed for different purposes (clinical, research, etc.).

As noted above, not much is lost to psychiatry through it being relatively unaware of the Limitation of Partial Criteria of Application. It might sometimes be helpful for those working with psychiatric diagnostic concepts to be more aware of this limitation of operationalism. This could help avoid, for example, the all-too-frequent assumption that a particular score on, say, the Beck Depression Inventory (which is a highly reliable instrument, Beck *et al.*, 1961), is sufficient to give an operationalized answer, across all kinds of depression and for all purposes, to the diagnostic question whether a given person is depressed.

Limitation 3: antecedently understood terms

Hempel, however, in the last paragraph of the reading, in developing his liberalized version of operationalism, comes to a further and quite different limitation of the operational definitions of terms, a limitation that, in contrast with the Limitation of Partial Criteria of Application, and more so even than the Limitation of Mere Observation, really is important for psychiatry. It is because this further limitation is so important for psychiatry, that we have characterized it here as a distinct third

limitation of operationalism, rather than, with Hempel, subsuming it to his Limitation of Partial Criteria of Application. The third limitation of operationalism, then, as set out by Hempel in this passage, is that 'It would be unreasonable to demand that *all* of the terms used in a given scientific discipline [can] be given an operational specification of meaning…' Why? Because '…then the process of specifying the meaning of the defining terms, and so forth, would lead to an infinite regress' (p. 321, emphasis in original). Why? Because, Hempel continues, 'In any definitional context (quite independently of the issue of operationalism), some terms must be antecedently understood…'.

Two key points for psychiatry

There are two key points for psychiatric classification to take from this important paragraph of Hempel's paper. The first key point is the point made above, that although merged by Hempel, the Limitation of Partial Criterion of Application, as illustrated by thermometers and semi-structured interviews, is very different in kind from the Limitation of Antecendently Understood Terms. The Limitation of Partial Criteria of Application is about the need for more than one equally well operationalized instrument (across different domains of a given variable and for different purposes). The Limitation of Antecedently Understood Terms, by contrast, is about a given definition—appropriate in and of itself for a given domain of application and for a given purpose—being, in and of itself, not fully operationalizable.

It is Hempel's *explanation* of this limitation that gives us the second key point for psychiatric classification that we should take from this paragraph. Recall how Hempel puts this: 'In *any* definitional context', he says, 'some terms must be antecedently understood' (p. 321, emphasis added this time). Put like this, then, Hempel's point in this passage on the limitations of operational definitions is thus nothing more nor less than precisely the point about, and hence carries all the importance for psychiatry of, the limitations of definitions in general that we explored in detail in Chapter 4 of Part I. Hempel indeed, in the parenthetical addition to his spelling out of his point, in the passage as quoted above, makes clear that this limitation is one that applies generally to all definitions and 'quite independently of the issue of operationalism' (p. 321).

Consequences for psychiatry

With Hempel's third (as we have numbered it) limitation on operationalism, then, the Limitation of Antecedently Understood Terms, go all the consequences for psychiatric science of the limitations of definition that we explored in Part I. It will be worth reminding ourselves of two of these consequences briefly as they apply to the definitions in scientific, including psychiatric scientific, classifications:

1. *'First define your terms'*. Once the limitations of definition are recognized, the 'first define your terms' assumption of traditional medical science becomes, with Austin and the 'philosophical fieldwork' of linguistic analysis, 'first look to the *uses*

of your terms'. Recall that in Austin's formulation, it is our ability to *use* high-level concepts (Hempel's *antecedently understood* terms) that allows the definitions of lower-level terms to be meaningful—in one of our examples from Part I, we can define the lower-level 'watch' only because we already understand, in the sense that we can already use, the higher-level 'time', even though the concept of time is deeply resistant to explicit definition. Correspondingly, therefore, in Hempel's terms, we can say that operational definitions of time in physics, in terms of accurate 'watches' such as atomic clocks, rely directly on an antecedent understanding (ability to use) the concept of time—for how, otherwise, with an extension of this point relevant to psychiatry's concerns with validity, would we know whether an operational definition of time was indeed of time or of something else; how, otherwise, to put the point in more familiar terms, would we know that, say, a watch (being a small instrument normally worn on the body and used for purposes of counting intervals of time) is indeed a kind of clock and not, say, a pedometer (being a small instrument normally worn on the body and used for purposes of counting intervals of space)! It is (generally) obvious in practice which is which. But it is only obvious because we understand the meanings of the relevant higher-level concepts, time and space, 'antecedently' as Hempel says here in Part III, and as evidenced by our ability to 'use' them as Austin said in Part I.

2. *Use and definition of terms in psychiatry.* In bodily medicine, the 'first define your terms' assumption of the traditional model works, by and large, fine, because, by and large, the relevant diagnostic terms for practical purposes are, in the formulation suggested by linguistic analytic philosophy, relatively low-level terms. In other words, the relevant diagnostic concepts in bodily medicine are, for example, the lower-level *heart* disease' not the higher-level '*disease*'. But of course in psychiatry, corresponding with its conceptually more difficult science, the higher-level concepts—illness, disease, dysfunction, disorder, etc.—are often precisely those that are relevant diagnostically. This is why there has been such vigorous debate about these concepts among those concerned practically, as users or as providers of services, within psychiatry, while in bodily medicine, by contrast, although there has been some debate at a theoretical level about the higher-level concepts, at a practical level debate has been considerably more limited. This is also why, to come to classification, the definitions in psychiatry's classifications so often appear muddled and incomplete compared with the definitions in the classifications of bodily medicine. The conceptual difficulties of psychiatric classification, indeed, as we saw in Part I, arise not only with concepts such as illness and disease, at the top of the medical hierarchy as it were, but with the concepts a level or two further down: thus 'delusion', as we saw, is more difficult to define than the lower-level 'delusion of guilt'; and, conversely, 'delusion', as a particular kind of psychotic symptom, is easier to define than 'psychosis'.

Conceptual difficulties: explicit and implicit

With these two considerations from Part I, therefore, taken together with Hempel's third limitation of operationalism (the Limitation of Antecedently Understood Terms), we are brought back squarely to the conceptual difficulties of psychiatric classification as recognized by Lewis (and summarized in Table 13.2, our *Conceptual Research Agenda for ICD-9*) and as they are implied by Kupfer *et al.* (and summarized in Table 13.1, our *Conceptual Research Agenda for DSM-V*). We are brought back squarely to these difficulties as *explicitly* conceptual difficulties about concepts of disorder (under Agenda Item 5). We are also brought back squarely to them as *implicitly* conceptual difficulties about reliability (under Agenda Item 6) and about validity (under Agenda Item 7). We will not, here, attempt a full explication of the conceptual difficulties raised under the latter two agenda items, either separately or taken together (the latter being the conceptual difficulties raised by the links between reliability and validity). Exploring these difficulties, even using the resources only of Logical Empiricism, would take us into all the deep difficulties about realism, essentialism, and so forth, with which this chapter as a whole, and the background philosophical traditions on which it draws, are concerned. We will return to some of these later. For the moment, though, we will note just two implications, the first for reliability (Agenda Item 6) and the second for validity (Agenda Item 7), by way of a promissory note for a further exploration of the potential relevance of the philosophy of science for psychiatric classification in Session 4.

Reliability

Reliability, as we have several times noted, although the big issue for psychiatric classification with Lewis in 1974, becomes, by the time of Kupfer *et al.*'s *Research Agenda for DSM-V* in 2002, at best a side-show, at worst a possible barrier to the big issue for DSM-V, validity. The implication, then, is that with future psychiatric classifications, reliability might have to be sacrificed for purposes of improving validity. A careful reading of Hempel's paper, and of the way in which his ideas were translated by Lewis and Sartorius into psychiatric classification in the ICD-8 and ICD-9, suggests that any inclination to trade reliability for validity, risks throwing out the baby with the bath water.

We return to the risk of throwing out the baby of reliability in Session 4, when we develop our third new agenda for psychiatric classification, drawing, particularly, on work in the philosophy of physics. For now, though, the key point about reliability to take from a more careful reading of Hempel's paper is that *reliability is a small but still necessary step to validity*. Thus, neither Hempel nor Lewis and Sartorius intended that reliability should become the focus of research on psychiatric classification at the expense of validity. On the contrary, Hempel explicitly, and Lewis and Sartorius implicitly, turned to reliability only as a *step*, and a *small* step at that, towards improved validity. Hempel, in particular, as we have seen, sketches, no more, only a tangential link between reliability and even Empirical Import, let alone Systematic (theoretical)

Import. Reliability, however, *is* none the less important. It may be only a *step*, it may be only a *small* step, but it is a *necessary* step. We will indicate below, in Session 2, some of the many ways in which reliability and validity (at least as reflected in objectivity) are linked. But the importance of reliability as a small but necessary step to validity is signalled here by the fact that notwithstanding Hempel's limited references to reliability, in his own presentation of operationalism, it is reliability (and not operationalism) that, as we saw earlier, ends up doing the (empirical) work.

Hempel's example of the 'praecox feeling' makes the point. And it is a point, as it turns out, against himself! Earlier in his paper, as we saw in the reading linked with Exercise 6, he had criticized the praecox feeling as the basis for a satisfactory diagnostic criterion, because, he said, it is a matter of *feeling* not of observation. And of course compared with the criteria for endomorphy (Hempel's example), the praecox feeling is, to any obvious reading, more subjective. But if the real work of operationalism is being done by reliability, what matters is not whether a criterion is based on observations that are more or less subjective, but on whether the criterion in question is based on observations that are reliable. The praecox feeling may or may not be reliable (i.e. capable of being identified with a high degree of agreement between observers). But it is reliability that is the key issue in Hempel's own terms.

Validity

Recognizing that reliability is what is doing the work of 'operationalism' in psychiatry is important for psychiatric classification because, if we get too hung up on 'operational' criteria, rather than relying on reliability, we risk cutting ourselves off from whole rafts of observational data that may have crucial significance for the development of theory. This is why, as we said, talk of trading reliability for validity risks throwing out the baby with the bath water.

There is indeed more than one baby here. First, there is the 'baby' of phenomenology and related disciplines. As just noted, the subjective praecox feeling may or may not be reliably identifiable. But all of phenomenology, on which as we saw in Part II descriptive psychopathology is based, is about the structure of subjectivity. Phenomenology, furthermore, as we noted in Part I, has recently been making a strong comeback into mainstream psychiatry in part as a direct response to the needs of the new neurosciences; and the new 'mental sciences', as we might call them, all the many new methods now available for the rigorous study of subjectivity, are already producing results, which, combined with the results of the new neurosciences, have considerable potential significance for the advancement of psychiatric scientific theory (Fulford *et al.*, 2003).

Second, and closer perhaps to the immediate concerns of current psychiatric classifications, there is the 'baby' of the concepts of traditional psychopathology, some of which, without regard to their reliability, and hence potential for the development of theory, have already been expelled from our classifications for want of clear explicit definition. The concept of psychosis, as we saw in

Part I, is the prime case in point. Psychosis is indeed difficult to define. This is why, as Lewis himself originally advocated (Lewis, 1934), the concept was (ostensibly) dropped between ICD-9 and ICD-10. Yet, at least as expressed in such paradigm psychotic symptoms as delusion, psychotic loss of insight is identifiable with a high degree of reliability (Wing et al., 1974) (see Chapter 3). The concept of psychosis, then, has, as we could now say in Hempel's terms, considerable Empirical Import and hence may also have considerable (albeit still only potential) Systematic Import.

Third, and finally, there is the 'baby' of psychoanalysis. As we noted above, Hempel, although critiquing the (as he saw them) subjective terms in which the psychodynamic categories of the DSM of his day were defined, implied that psychiatry's response to this should be to 'operationalize' the terms in question, not to reject psychodynamic theory as such. So far as Hempel's influence on psychiatric classification is concerned, therefore, it seems that psychodynamic theory has been eliminated from ICD and DSM on the basis of a misunderstanding. There may be other reasons for not basing an international psychiatric classification on psychodynamic concepts. But Hempel's (supposed) critique of their Empirical Import is not one of them. Hempel's criticisms of psychodynamic theory, as we saw earlier in this session, were criticisms, not of its status as a theory, but of what he perceived to be the poorly defined terms in which, at the time, it was formulated. Yet these terms, to cite again the work of Peter Hobson (1998) and others, whatever their Systematic Import, have no less Empirical Import (to the extent that they are no less capable of reliable use) than many of the symptom categories in the PSE.

Again, our point here is not to endorse or otherwise this or that theoretical approach, this or that theoretical concept, but rather to be clear that we increase, rather than decrease, our chances of achieving validity by taking, with Hempel, Lewis, Sartorius, Spitzer, Frances, and others concerned with the development of our current classifications, the first step of reliability.

Conclusions: from logical empiricist to post-logical empiricist philosophy of science

In this session we have explored (in reverse order) the agenda for psychiatric classification as it stood with Lewis at the launch of the Glossary to ICD-8 (our *Conceptual Research Agenda for ICD-9*, see Table 13.2) and the agenda for psychiatric classification as it stands today, as represented by Kupfer *et al.*'s Research Agenda for DSM-V (our *Conceptual Research Agenda for DSM-V*, see Table 13.1). We have also examined the origins of both agendas in Logical Empiricism as represented by Hempel's key paper to the 1959 conference on psychiatric classification, as translated and developed through the work of Lewis, Sartorius, Spitzer, Frances, and others.

In the final session of the chapter, we will bring together our two new agendas, our conceptual agendas respectively for ICD-9 and for DSM-V, with a third agenda, an agenda for what we will call an Extended Family of Psychiatric Classifications. This third agenda seeks to build on the strengths of both earlier agendas (for ICD-9 and DSM-V) by drawing on the resources not just of Logical Empiricism, but also of post-Logical Empiricist philosophy of science. For Logical Empiricism, as we saw in Chapter 12, although a determined and rigorous attempt to identify the essential features of scientific method, ultimately failed to provide a full and final characterization of what science is about. Recent decades have thus witnessed a vigorous development of post-Logical Empiricist philosophy of science, on which, in addition to the (still pertinent) resources of Logical Empiricism, we can draw in developing our understanding of what psychiatric science, and hence psychiatric classification, is about.

It is with post-Logical Empiricist philosophy of science, therefore, that we will be occupied in the next two sessions. Post-Logical Empiricist Philosophy of Science covers a wide range of different approaches. Some approaches are realist in tone, others antirealist. Some seek to secure a broadly traditional model of what science is about, others attack one or other aspects of this model. As we should expect from the considerations of Part I, what will become clear is that there is no simple equation or code that can fully capture what science is about. But as we should also expect from Part I, taken together, these different approaches will add up to a rich potential resource for investigating the complex 'concept + data' driven problems that are at the heart of what psychiatric science is about.

Reflection on the session and self-test questions

Write down your own reflections on the materials in this session drawing out any points that are particularly significant for you. Then write brief notes about the following:

1. What is the 'big issue' on the agenda for those developing the next edition of the DSM (the DSM-V)?

2. What broad kind of issue is evident in the DSM-V Agenda but not named as such?

3. What feature of Logical Empiricism has been carried over into modern international psychiatric classifications?

4. Which American philosopher was particularly influential in this respect? Which British psychiatrist? And which official of the WHO?

5. Which classification was the first to show a direct influence of Logical Empiricism and in what way?

6. What have subsequent classifications added from the account of what it is to be scientific outlined by the philosopher referred to in question 4?

7. What was the 'big issue' on the agenda of psychiatric classification in the run up to ICD-9?

8. What are the three limitations of operationalism identified by the philosopher referred to question 4? Which of these are generic and which are limitations specifically of operationalism in psychiatric science?

9. Name at least two ways in which the development of modern international psychiatric classifications has proceeded differently from expectations since ICD-9? (We noted four.)

Session 2 Values, natural classifications, and the Absolute Conception

In this session we return to one of the recurring themes of this book, namely the role of values in psychiatry. We explored the role of values in relation to concepts of disorder in detail in Part I, and, though less extensively, in relation to Jaspers' psychopathology in Part II. Here the presence of values goes to the heart of the focus of this chapter on what science is about. The familiar intuition, which as we noted in Chapter 11 is a core though usually tacit feature of the traditional model of science, is that, like oil and water, the objectivity of science is immiscible with the subjectivity of values. It follows, therefore, according to this traditional model, that if psychiatry is value-laden it cannot be objective; and that, correspondingly, if its classifications are value-laden they cannot be natural classifications.

Are values and science like oil and water?

It is the oil-and-water intuition about values and science that, as we will see, is behind the line that Thomas Szasz (1972) takes in one of his arguments against the reality of mental illness. It is the oil-and-water intuition, too, that motivates the arguments of those, like R.E. Kendell and Christopher Boorse, who, as we saw in Part I, have sought to exclude values from at least the scientific 'core' of psychiatric theory. But is the familiar oil-and-water intuition about science and values well founded philosophically? Is it really true that the presence of values in a discipline puts it beyond the remit of science?

In this session we will be looking in detail at an attempt by the British philosopher, Bernard Williams, to show that values and science are indeed immiscible. At the heart of the objectivity of science, Williams argued, is an 'Absolute Conception' of the world. Scientific progress consists in approximating ever more closely to the Absolute Conception by progressively shedding the conceptions of the world that we form from (i.e. relative to) this or that particular point of view. Williams based his argument on the progressive replacement in science of secondary qualities (like colours) with primary qualities (like the wave length of light). Secondary qualities, he argued, being perspectival, have no place in the Absolute Conception, and neither therefore (others have argued) have values.

Williams, you will recall from Part I, was one of those 'depressive' philosophers who have been unduly pessimistic about the practical effectiveness of philosophy. His argument for the Absolute Conception can thus be considered to be part of his overall programme of marking the contrast between what he took to be the effectiveness of science compared with the impotence of philosophy. As we will see later in this session, however, there are philosophical counter-arguments to William's Absolute Conception, and, indeed, free-standing arguments to the effect that values and science are not immiscible at all.

Plan of the session

The plan of the session is this. We look first at what Hempel says about values and science in his 1959 conference paper (from Session 1): he is surprisingly mild on values, given his background in Logical Empiricism. We pair Hempel's arguments with some interesting observations on the objectivity or otherwise of humour by the British philosopher, Crispin Wright. We then contrast Hempel's argument with the familiar intuition (the oil-and-water intuition) as deployed by Szasz. This leads into a detailed examination of Williams' Absolute Conception and of some of the arguments, particularly by John McDowell, against it. The bottom line of the session is that there is no 'knock down' argument to support the intuition that values and science are immiscible. In the conclusions to this session, we look briefly at the implications of this bottom line for the role of values in psychiatric classification. We consider the role of values in psychiatric classification in detail in Part IV.

Hempel, Crispin Wright, and Szasz on values and science

Given the extent of debate about the role of values in concepts of disorder, and the centrality of this issue particularly in the psychiatry/antipsychiatry aspects of the debate, Hempel has surprisingly little to say about values in his paper to the 1959 conference on psychiatric classification. True, much of the debate about concepts took off in the 1960s. However, the issues were there, and not unimportant philosophically, all along: in the long-running is-ought debate in ethics, for example (see Part I); in the *Methodenstreit* and, consequently, in Jaspers' work (see Part II); and as a particular (critical) focus of the positivist movement in the philosophy of science in the 1920s and 1930s, of which Logical Empiricism was a development.

Hempel, then, writing as a philosopher of science, and for a conference on the difficulties of psychiatric classification, might have been expected to have had a good deal to say about the role of values. In fact, what he says comes largely in just one short paragraph fairly late in the paper.

> ### EXERCISE 11 (20 minutes)
>
> Read the paragraph from Hempel's paper in which he discusses the role of values in psychiatric classifications:
>
> Hempel, C.G. (1994). Fundamentals of taxonomy. In *Philosophical Perspectives on Psychiatric Diagnostic Classification* (ed. J.S. Sadler, O.P. Wiggins, and M.A. Schwartz). Baltimore, MD: Johns Hopkins University Press
>
> Link with Reading 13.10
>
> 1. How are Hempel's comments here connected with his general arguments about the objectivity of a classification and the ways in which this may be undermined (think about the two requirements he placed on a scientific classification, as outlined in Session 1).
>
> 2. What is the significance of the relatively low priority Hempel gives to the role of values?

In Session 1 we noted that Hempel placed two requirements on a scientific classification. The terms employed in a scientific classification, Hempel said, (1) should have Empirical Import, that is they should have clear, public criteria of application, and (2) they should have Systematic Import, they should lend themselves to the formulation of general laws that reflect underlying uniformities in nature. Both of these requirements in Hempel's account can be understood as reflecting different aspects of the more general requirement that scientific classifications should be *objective*.

Hempel's two requirements for objectivity

Hempel's account of scientific classifications thus suggests two routes by which classifications may fail to be objective. The first route is that they may fail to provide clear-cut standards for classificatory judgements: lack of reliability, as we have seen, is connected with this route in Hempel's account. The second route is that they may fail to track underlying natural uniformities. This is a failure of validity, then, a failure to reflect valid insights into the way the world really is.

Two threats to objectivity

You will recall that in his paper Hempel draws only a weak link between his first requirement for a classification to be scientific (hence objective) and reliability. There *is* a link, as we saw in the last part of Session 1; and the link, as we will see in this session, is at least in part by way of *values*. But to see this, and hence to understand what Hempel is saying in this passage about the 'valuational' aspects of psychiatric classification, we need to fill out a little Hempel's own account of the link between objectivity and the reliability of classifications.

Values and loss of objectivity: route 1 (via reliability)

As we saw in Session 1, Hempel touches on the issue of reliability in his section on Empirical Import, called earlier in his paper 'descriptive adequacy'. Unless, he says in one of the passages examined in Session 1 (reading linked with Exercise 6), there are clear rules for applying descriptions, for fitting the phenomena under investigation into descriptive categories, then the classification in question will not be *reliable*. Hempel discusses the two main meanings of reliability—test–retest and inter-rater reliability—noted in Box 13.2 above. If a classification is *not* reliable, then a single investigator might make different judgements about the same case on different occasions given the same information (test–retest *un*reliability); or two investigators may disagree in the application of a classificatory term in the face of the same, and indeed all relevant, information (inter-rater *un*reliability).

Disagreements of these kinds will have practical consequences for psychiatric treatment and research. They will undermine any possibility of consistency in treatment both over time and between clinicians, and, thus, across different geographical areas. As such, though, all this says nothing directly about objectivity.

A link between lack of reliability and lack of validity

But there is another feature of this kind of disagreement, which Hempel himself does not stress but which *does* have important consequences for the objectivity of a classification. The key point, to put it first in the negative, is that, *absent objectivity, none of the divergent judgements in the use of (an unreliable) classification need be mistaken*. This is because, if the standards that govern the correct use of a classification are themselves flexible or open-ended, then the fact that judgements differ with respect to classifying a given phenomenon by reference to those standards need not imply that the standards have been broken. Flexible standards can bend without being broken. But of course, to come now to the positive side of the point, it is precisely such flexibility in the use of a classification that undermines any claim it might have to objectivity. For without the idea that when two judgements differ as to how a given phenomenon should be classified then at least one of the judgements must be mistaken, the difference between a true (valid) and false (invalid) claim about what is 'really there' in the world is fatally undermined.

In other words, a breakdown of reliability not only causes difficulties because of the practical consequences—on the surface, as it were—of that breakdown of agreement, it also suggests a deeper underlying malaise. Flexible standards for judgements imply that those judgements do not track underlying objective features of the world. This is not to say that in *every* case where there can be disagreement without mistake then nothing objective is being judged. Disagreements about *how much* evidence is needed to support a diagnosis might be subject to vagueness at the boundary. Judgements about colours are vague across boundaries in an analogous way without undermining their objectivity (although there may be other reasons to doubt their objectivity, as we will see below). But if disagreement does *not* imply error, and not just because of vagueness of this boundary sort, then this undermines the claims to objectivity (and hence validity) of the judgements in question.

Is humour objective?

The link between reliability and objectivity can be illustrated by an example. It is at least arguable that the classification of things (events, stories, jokes) into those that are funny and those that are not, is not reliable and thus not objective in the sense just outlined. People's senses of humour vary widely. Thus, if two people who share all the relevant facts about how a joke is supposed to work, and who grasp the allusions being made, still disagree about whether it is funny, *neither need have made a mistake*. They may, and indeed ordinarily would be said to, simply differ in their sense of humour. Unlike the items marshalled into scientific classifications, few think that there are objective comic facts. So there seems to be a connection between, on the one hand, the idea that in some cases disagreement (unreliability) in judgements need not imply that a mistake has been made, and, on the other hand, the thought that the subject matter of such judgements is not objective.

Cognitive command and objectivity

The example of comedy comes from the British philosopher and logician, Crispin Wright's, *Truth and Objectivity* (1992). Wright suggests that one mark of the objectivity of at least certain kinds of judgement is that they possess 'cognitive command'. An interesting feature of Wright's book is that he suggests several different tests for different sorts of objectivity and provides no reason to think that these different tests will apply to the same sorts of judgements. In other words, he thinks that there might be kinds of judgement that possess one sort of objectivity (provided by cognitive command, for example) while other kinds of judgement possess different forms of objectivity altogether. In the following passage, he is concerned only with the 'test' of 'cognitive command'. He sets up the link between the possibility of genuine agreement in judgement and 'cognitive command' initially by way of the reciprocal link between mere differences of opinion and 'cognitive shortcomings'. This is how Wright puts it:

> It is a priori [i.e. roughly, true by definition—see Chapter 5] that differences of opinion formulated within the discourse [in question], unless excusable as a result of vagueness in a disputed statement, or in the standards of acceptability, or variation in personal evidence thresholds, so to speak, will involve something which may properly be regarded as a cognitive shortcoming. (p. 144)

Values and reliability

If this principle is a priori then the type of judgement in question possesses one kind of objectivity. To recapitulate, this principle is designed as a test for the objectivity of the subject matter of a class of judgements. Think of the reciprocal connection first. If agreement between judgements of a certain class is *commanded* by their subject matter, i.e. the relevant objective facts, if they are in this sense genuinely matters of *cognising*, then disagreements will have to imply that someone has made a *mistake*. Wright suggests that the converse also holds. If there is a genuine notion of mistake at play, then that notion implies a kind of objectivity. Conversely, if there is not (and not just because of boundary-vagueness), then this kind of objectivity (hence validity) is lacking.

'Cognitive' in psychiatry and in philosophy

To understand this passage we need to pause for a moment on that key word 'cognitive'. In psychiatry, as we saw in Chapter 3, 'cognitive' is used, as in the Mental State Examination, of the 'cognitive functions' of orientation, attention, memory, and general IQ, as distinct from such functions as affect, volition, perception, and belief. Wright, by contrast, uses 'cognitive' in this passage, as it is generally used in philosophy, to mean, roughly, that which is known, where knowledge in turn means 'justified true belief', of which the paradigm cases are always beliefs about the world. This is what lies behind his initial apparently rather question-begging conditional, 'If it is a priori . . .'. Most philosophers, Wright is able to assume, will take it for granted that if a judgement is a matter of genuine 'cognising', i.e. of *knowing* something about (= having justified true beliefs about) the world, then it is indeed true by definition that the truth or falsehood of that judgement is, in Wright's sense, *commanded*.

With this point of clarification in place, the force of Wright's example of humour is now clear. The judgement that a joke is or is not funny is not 'commanded' by any objective feature of its subject matter, i.e. of the joke in question. There is no 'cognitive shortcoming', then, involved in a difference of opinion; no one need have made a mistake about whether the joke in question is or is not funny. By contrast, judging the time the joke took to tell, for example, really is 'commanded' by an objective feature of the world (ordinarily understood), namely the actual passage of time that telling the joke really took. Here, correspondingly, it is possible to be mistaken about an objective feature of the world, to 'get it wrong'. And to be mistaken, or to get it wrong, is a matter, in Wright's term, of 'cognitive shortcoming'.

Granted, then, the above point of clarification about the meaning of 'cognitive', and Wright's example of humour, his claim that 'cognitive command' is an a priori test of one kind of objectivity, seems fair enough. It is a different matter just how the test could be applied in practice other than in a question begging way. Wright is not concerned with this. But in capturing clearly one important intuition about objectivity (that it is possible to be right or wrong about objective features of the world), Wright helps to unpack the idea behind Hempel's comments on values in his 1959 paper.

Back to Hempel on values

We are now ready to come back to what Hempel says in the reading linked with Exercise 11 about values and the reliability of psychiatric classification, and to fill in the link to objectivity.

Hempel, then, in the above passage, suggests that one source of unreliability in psychiatric classifications is what he calls their 'valuational aspect'. As examples he picks out such notions as: 'inadequacy of response, inadaptability, ineptness and poor judgement', which were all used to characterize the signs of Inadequate Personality in DSM-I. These seem not to be straightforwardly matters of fact but to involve value judgements by clinicians. And Crispin Wright's notion of 'cognitive command' fills in the implied link to objectivity. For if Hempel is right, the values involved in psychiatric diagnosis might lead to lack of reliability (i.e. because clinician's values may differ). By analogy with humour, then, such diagnostic judgements may lack 'cognitive command', which, if Wright on humour and Hempel on values are right, suggests that such judgements do not reflect objective features of the world, and hence that, in this sense, they lack validity.

As already noted, there is a further question about how a judgement would be 'tested' for cognitive command in practice. But leaving this aside, it is still important to ask, at least of values, whether Hempel *is* right? Is it necessarily the case that values lead to unreliability? The considerations of Part I, drawing particularly on Hare's work, suggest that while values *may* lead to discrepant diagnostic judgements, often they will not do so. Specifically, values will not lead to unreliability where they are *shared*. This of course leads back to the bottom line of the implications of Hare's work for the debate about mental illness. For it suggests, consistently with the 'full field', fact + value, model to which we came in Part I, that classifications of bodily disorders are, despite appearances, not value-free. They appear to be value-free only because and to the extent that they embody values that, in contrast to the values in classifications of mental disorders, are widely shared.

We return to the practical significance of the role that values may play in psychiatric classifications at some length in Part IV. But it is worth noting Hempel's attitude to them in this paper. He argues that the formulation of more reliable classifications that are not valuational is 'very desirable' but not an 'easy task'. It is thus not something to be insisted on from the start but rather something towards which we should aim as an eventual goal. This is a natural corollary of the traditional model. Our conclusion in Part IV, by contrast, will be that as values are there and essential, rather than seeking to eliminate them, we should make them explicit with a view to working with them in a more rigorous and effective way.

Values and loss of objectivity: route 2 (via validity)

Exactly what working with values in a more 'rigorous and effective way' means in this context will be a key topic for Part IV. But Hempel's two requirements allow a second link between values and loss of objectivity, via validity. This as we have seen is the basis of the familiar oil-and-water intuition about values and science. It is on the oil-and-water intuition that Szasz draws in the next reading in developing one of his arguments against the reality of mental illness.

Read the extract below from:

Szasz, T.S. (1972). The myth of mental illness. *The Myth of Mental Illness*. Paladin (Extract pp. 14–17.)

Link with Reading 13.11

We examined Szasz' arguments in detail in Part I. In this reading, think particularly about three questions:

1. What sort of argument does Szasz advance against the reality of mental illness in this passage as against or in addition to his arguments in Part I?

2. How, in particular, does Szasz employ the idea that values undermine objectivity to advance his argument?

3. What role does causality play in his argument?

4. Are his arguments sound?

Szasz's core argument

At the heart of this passage is Szasz' core argument against the reality of mental illness that we explored in detail in Part I, namely his claim that mental illnesses are defined by reference to value norms ('psycho-social, ethical and legal'), whereas (real) bodily diseases are defined by factual norms ('anatomical and physiological').

This core argument, as we saw in Part I, is highly effective in that it relies precisely on the 'medical' model that is common ground between Szasz and his opponents, such as R.E. Kendell. Both sides in the debate about mental illness, as we saw in Part I, have generally taken it as a given that bodily diseases (whether thought of as entities or processes) are, like atoms, weather systems, and stars, objective elements in the real world 'out there' and independently of anything we might think of them. Given, then, the overtly value-laden nature of mental illness compared with bodily illness, the burden of proof falls very squarely on those who, in Szasz' phrase in this piece, believe that 'mental illness is just as "real" and "objective" as bodily illness'.

Realism and Szasz's core argument

Here, though, Szasz tops and tails his core argument from Part I using the language of scientific realism. Thus, the passage opens by pointing out that in the modern world people struggle not so much with *biological* (implies objective) as with social (implies, at least as in Szasz' core argument, evaluative) challenges; he continues with a critique of the idea that mental illness could be a *cause* of a deformity in the personality (we look at the substance of Szasz' argument from causation in a moment); similarly, it is, he urges, absurd to use *medical* (again implies objective) means for a problem that is 'psycho-social and ethical'; this, he says, reflects the 'currently prevalent claim that

'mental illness is just as '*real*' and '*objective*' as bodily illness'; which claim, if true, would, Szasz argues, mean that we could 'catch', 'have or harbor it' [a mental illness], that one could 'transmit it to others' and 'get rid of it'.

Now, there is much that, as in Part I, could be said both for and against Szasz' position in this passage. He overstates his case, no doubt, in places: an attitude, for example, such as racism, although defined in part by values, can be, as Szasz says a disease can be, 'caught', 'had or harbored', 'transmitted to others' and 'got rid of'. So these are certainly not attributes that are confined to and hence provide a marker of 'real and objective' entities. In support of Szasz' position, on the other hand, writing as he is in the late 1960s and early 1970s, it is worth pointing out that he is truly prescient in his remarks about the overuse of medical treatments such as medications. Szasz' final comment, furthermore, about mental illnesses being 'communications' has a powerful resonance with the claims of both Lewis in ICD-8 and of Kupfer *et al.* (2002) in *A Research Agenda for DSM-V*, that the great success of modern more reliable psychiatric classifications is to improve communication (see Session 1 above)! But the key point to take from this passage is that, just as Szasz relies in his core argument against the reality of mental illness on the distinction between evaluative and descriptive (or scientific) norms, so, here, in reinforcing his core argument, he relies on a largely direct appeal to the widespread traditional intuition that values are immiscible with what science is about, i.e. to repeat Szasz' phrase, ' "real" and "objective" ' features of the world.

The force of Szasz' direct appeal to realism

Szasz' appeal to the traditional oil-and-water intuition about science and values is thus, with one partial exception (see below), direct: he does not (here) attempt actually to argue from one or other component of philosophical realism (objectivity, etc.) to the non-reality of mental illness. He just relies directly on the oil-and-water intuition that values (and hence the value-laden mental illness) equal non-science (and hence that the value-laden mental illness cannot be a species of the (as he takes it to be) scientific concept of disease.

Szasz' direct appeal to the oil-and-water intuition, moreover, is effective in much the way that his core argument is effective, i.e. by relying on the assumptions of his opponents. His core argument, as just noted, takes off from the traditional medical model. The burden of proof thus falls on those who (taking the traditional medical-scientific model for granted) believe that mental illness, despite being value-laden, is, really, as value-free as bodily illness (in the traditional model) is taken to be. Similarly here, then, the appeal to the traditional oil-and-water intuition puts the burden of proof on those who (taking the traditional oil-and-water intuition for granted) believe that mental illness, despite being value-laden, is, really, as much a matter for medical-scientific intervention as bodily illness. The message, in both cases, is put up or shut up!

Szasz' argument from causality

There is of course a third way, here as in Part I, between Szasz and his opponents, which is to resist tradition, the traditional medical-scientific model in Part I, the traditional oil-and-water intuition here. Before turning to this third way, however, it will be worth looking at the one actual argument from scientific realism that Szasz advances in this passage. Although presented only briefly by Szasz, it is an important argument because it is concerned with an element of realism, causality, that figures large in medical science. We will be examining causality in detail in Chapter 15. In this passage, Szasz deploys the argument that causality often appears in the views of those who defend the reality of mental illness both as cause and as effect. Mental illnesses are defined by reference to disturbances of behaviour (they are used to identify features of, or more specifically deformities of, personality). But mental illnesses are also, Szasz points out, invoked *causally* to explain those same disturbances of behaviour. Since, then, Szasz concludes, nothing can cause itself, the concept of a mental illness is incoherent.

Again, this is a powerful argument. In this case, however, the strength of the argument depends on the premise that mental illnesses really are merely short hands for behaviour. An alternative position would be to claim instead that, although mental illnesses are identified via behaviours, they are not identical *with* those behaviours but are instead their underlying causes. As we will see in Part V, the contemporary American philosopher Donald Davidson defends a conception of mental states of just this sort. As he points out, we often describe events by their effects. The act of firing a gun may also be described as an act of murdering a president. The same can apply to describing mental states. However, this does not require a behaviourist identification of mental states and behaviour.

Szasz' argument in this passage, whether or not he needs to place any weight on it, does provide one clear way of understanding, a *causal* way of understanding, what the denial of the reality of mental illness amounts to. Realism about mental illness of this causal kind involves the claim that mental states play an underlying causal role in the production of behaviour. This conception of what the reality of mental illness would amount to is thus related via causality to Hempel's discussion of the Systematic Import of a natural classification. Szasz in this passage can be interpreted as adding to his core argument that mental illness is (because value-laden) a myth, the claim that a classification of mental disorders cannot be a natural classification because it does not describe any kind of underlying mental causal mechanisms, and hence that, in Hempel's terms, it lacks (at least this causal kind of) Systematic Import.

A third way?

Returning, then, to Szasz' core argument, and to the reinforcement of his core argument with the appeal to realism, what is our third way here? In Part I, our third way was to resist the assumptions of the traditional medical-scientific model by drawing on the work of Hare and others in the Oxford 'school' of linguistic analytic philosophy. Szasz (1972) took the more value-laden connotations of mental illness to show that mental illness is a myth; his opponents, such as Kendell, took these same value-connotations to be merely provisional on the development of a more advanced psychiatric science. Our third way was to show that if the medical concepts—illness, disease, dysfunction, etc.—are indeed value terms, then, simply in sharing the logical properties of value terms in general (as described by Hare, Warnock, Urmson, Foot, and others), the uses of these concepts in psychiatry would necessarily be more value-laden than in bodily medicine, not because psychiatry is less scientific than bodily medicine, nor because it is concerned merely with 'problems of living', but because human values are more diverse in the areas with which psychiatry is concerned (emotion, belief, sexuality, etc.) than in the corresponding areas with which, in acute hospital-based medicine at least, bodily medicine is concerned (severe bodily pain, imminent threat of death, etc.).

Opening up a space

Here, in responding to Szasz' reinforcement of his core argument with the language of realism, our third way is to resist the assumptions of the traditional oil-and-water immiscibility of science and values by drawing on more recent work in the philosophy of science and epistemology. We will not be able to do more than take a few preliminary steps along this particular third way. The topic, after all, realism, is considerably wider and more multifacetted than the relatively well-defined topic, the is-ought debate, on which we drew in Part I. Even more so than in Part I, therefore, our objectives in opening up a third way are modest. Our objectives here as in Part I, are not to 'prove' that the third way is right. The is-ought debate, after all, continues; and debates about realism, although now often badged as epistemology rather than philosophy of science, having continued for over 2000 years, show no sign of running out of steam.

Our objective, therefore, here as in Part I, is the more modest objective of opening up a space between traditional polarities, a space for new intellectual enquiries, a space for new practical initiatives. The space opened up in Part I, by drawing on the resources of Oxford linguistic-analytic philosophy in the middle decades of the twentieth century, is already becoming occupied by new models of service delivery and of clinical skills training, models to which we will come in Part IV. The space to be opened up here, although considerably more complex and less well explored, has a corresponding potential for occupation by new (or at any rate newly expanded) ways of understanding psychiatric science, new ways of understanding psychiatric science that, we will suggest in Session 4 of this chapter, are overdue for at least partial incorporation into psychiatry's classifications of mental disorder.

From Szasz to Williams and McDowell

So, what are the arguments from the philosophy of science (and epistemology) that will open up a third way between Szaszian antirealism and psychiatry's realism about mental disorder?

In the next part of this session we will examine one particularly carefully framed philosophical argument that some have taken to provide grounds for believing that science and values are like oil and water, Bernard Williams' argument for an 'Absolute Conception' of the world. We say 'some have taken' because, as we will see, Williams' argument is aimed primarily at excluding from science the secondary as distinct from primary qualities (a primary quality is, e.g. the wavelength of light, a secondary quality is, e.g. the colour we see). However, the Australian philosopher (also at Oxford) J.L. Mackie (1977, p. 15), for example, is among recent philosophers who have taken Williams' argument about secondary qualities to provide an argument for the exclusion of values from science.

By way of context, it is important to be aware that other philosophers have taken very different lines on the relationship between values and science: the English philosopher, Jonathan Dancy, for example, has argued that there are grounds, independent of and in some respects in opposition to any arguments by extension from secondary qualities, for believing that there are 'moral facts' (Dancy, 1993). Here, though, we will confine ourselves to, (1) Williams' argument for an Absolute Conception as a potential 'knock down' philosophical argument to show that values and science are immiscible, and (2) a counter-argument from the Pittsburgh-based philosopher, John McDowell, a counter-argument that, in being applicable equally to secondary qualities and to values, will serve our modest objective of opening up a third way in the form of a space between Szasz and psychiatry, a space for potential occupation by an enriched model of psychiatric science.

Bernard Williams and the Absolute Conception versus John McDowell

Williams' argument for an Absolute Conception comes in his book on Descartes. He outlines what he means by the 'Absolute Conception' in the next reading (linked with Exercise 13). Williams, as we will see, presupposes a knowledge of the long-standing philosophical distinction between primary and secondary qualities. Familiar in classical philosophy, this distinction was reintroduced into modern philosophy in the seventeenth century by the British Empiricist philosopher, John Locke (1632–1704), as the distinction between things such as shape, weight, mass, or velocity, which seem to belong to things independently of observers, and other things such as taste, smell and colour, which depend on our particular psychological features and other properties. The distinction was made more popular in the seventeenth century by the rise of an atomistic natural philosophy promoted, among others, by the chemist Robert Boyle (1627–91).

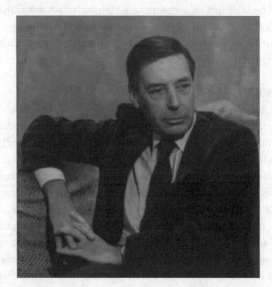

Fig. 13.2 Bernard Williams

EXERCISE 13   (30 minutes)

Read the two extracts from:

Williams, B. (1978). *Descartes: the project of pure inquiry*. London: Penguin (Extracts pp. 64–65 and 244–246.)

Link with reading 13.12

Think carefully about Williams' argument for an Absolute Conception and what that conception is of.

◆ What are the implications of Williams' account of secondary qualities for the role of values in psychiatry?

Again, it is important to work through the reading critically before going on to what *we* have to say in answer to this question.

The objectivity of knowledge

Williams develops his account of the Absolute Conception in this reading in order to explain more fully what he takes to be an everyday understanding of what knowledge (as justified true belief) consist in. This involves the idea that justified (as district from accidentally) true beliefs answer to a world which is independent of our beliefs. 'Knowledge is of what is there *anyway*'. It is this basic assumption about the independence of the subject matter of justified true beliefs or knowledge that seems to be threatened by the thought that mental illnesses are partially constituted by societal and other values. In such a case it seems that the object of one's knowledge is precisely *not* objective or independent, is not there 'anyway'. The Absolute Conception is supposed by Williams to constitute a filling out of what it is that our beliefs answer to when we say that they answer to the world. It is part of an explanation of what the objectivity of justified true beliefs, or knowledge, amounts to.

The argument for the Absolute Conception

Williams' way of substantiating the Absolute Conception develops from the following thought experiment. Two people, A and B as Williams calls them, both have different but equally true beliefs about the world. Perhaps their different beliefs stem from the fact that they are looking at the same thing but from different perspectives. If so, then it must be possible to give a larger account of the set up, an account that includes how A and B's beliefs, as different representations of the same thing, are related both to each other and to the thing of which their respective beliefs are representations. But this larger account is itself a *representation* of the world that includes A and B and explains how their beliefs are related to each other and to the world. Hence, in giving the larger account, we form a conception of a *representation* of the part of the world in question (construed broadly to include both A and B and A and B's representations), which is distinct from our conception of that *part of the world* itself. Thus the larger story maintains the contrast between, on the one hand, a representation *as a* representation of the world, and, on the other, the world of which the representation is (merely) a representation.

But now it can be seen that postulating two people, A and B, with different beliefs is unnecessary for the thought experiment. The new representation can itself be the subject of a broader account of how it itself relates to, but is distinct from, the world it represents and to other true representations of the world that could be given. Clearly this process can be iterated until, finally, it includes the relation between one representation (the Absolute Conception) and all other possible representations. The conclusion that Williams draws, is that only if one can form this *Absolute Conception* of the world, which includes how all possible true representations are related to it, can one have a proper conception of any individual item of knowledge since that must include the contrast between representation and the world. Reflection on the latter escalates into the former.

The dilemma facing the Absolute Conception

Williams' conclusion can be clarified by examining a dilemma that the Absolute Conception raises. This concerns how the content of the 'Absolute Conception' can itself be filled out. Without some additional substantiation, there is a risk that the phrase remains empty, meaning vacuously merely 'what true representations represent'. But if so, then according to Williams, it will be impossible to understand the contrast between a representation and the independent reality from which it stands distinct. On the other hand, any specific account of reality that we may be tempted to offer runs the risk of being merely another of our *representations*

reflecting our local perspective and thus not a characterization of an independent reality after all.

Williams' own suggestion for evading both horns of this dilemma is to invoke the progress of science. This allows the non-local characterization of the Absolute Conception as that which is progressively revealed by science. This will include the findings of physics, chemistry, and biology—or whatever sciences succeed them—concerning the fabric of the world in a narrow sense, but we can also add in neurology, psychology, and psychiatry (cf. p. 245). These latter sciences will play a role in explaining both how it is possible to acquire the knowledge of the world we have obtained and also how it was possible to form the preceding *false* beliefs which have littered the history of science, as these also, in a broader sense, are a part of the world or world history. We will return to an assessment of this suggestion shortly. What is important for now are the consequences it suggests both for secondary qualities and for values.

Primary and secondary qualities

One way of interpreting the history of science is to conclude that some of the features that humans have previously taken to form part of the world—in the narrower sense—turn out to have been instead local features of our perspective on the world. Thus while it was once assumed that the world really was coloured, we now 'realize' that colour is an artefact of the way in which humans and some other animals perceive the world. We can thus now entertain the thought that a combination of, perhaps, physics, neurophysiology, and psychology will, in the future, describe not just how light and bodies interact but also how we see in colour, how we once projected this experience on to the world, and how we later realized that this was wrong and came to develop the account of the world and ourselves that we are now contemplating.

On Williams' picture, the difference between primary and secondary qualities is this. Primary qualities are those that will be required by a future physics to describe the behaviour of the fundamental fabric of the world. Secondary qualities are those that are features merely of our local perspective on the world, of how the world appears to us with our particular sense organs. The progress of science is in part characterized by an increasing ability to describe the world in a way that prescinds away from our specific sensory experiences and describes it instead as though from no particular perspective. (Secondary qualities will still feature in scientific accounts but only as items to be explained in the history of science. They will be part of the broader world history that includes our history but not part of a narrower natural history of the world as it really is.) Thus any account couched instead in secondary quality terms is not fully objective because secondary qualities are not proper parts of the world.

Values and the objectivity of diagnosis

The philosophical model presented here of what is involved in the very idea of knowledge provides one connection between the presence of values in psychiatric classification and its supposed failures of objectivity and realism. The idea, for example as developed by Mackie (1977) is that, by analogy with secondary qualities, values reflect features of our perception of the world and thus cannot properly be regarded as part of the world (in the narrow sense) that is independent of us. As science aspires towards an account of the world that prescinds away from local features of our perspective and uncovers what would also be discovered by *any* scientific inquiry, whatever the details of the individuals or species carrying it out, any classification that relies on mere values, like any classification that relies on mere secondary qualities, cannot be properly objective.

EXERCISE 14 (15 minutes)

Before going on, think about the account that Williams (1978) provides. Is the Absolute Conception itself a coherent idea? Does it really provide a principled reason for denying the objectivity of secondary qualities?

Critically reflect on how Williams suggests that we can form a conception of the world in this way. Think in particular about the way he deploys the distinction between primary and secondary qualities. What is the significance of the fact that, as we flagged in the run up to Exercise 13 above, Williams' takes knowledge of this distinction for granted.

One criticism of Williams' account of the Absolute Conception is, precisely, that he merely presupposes his key distinction between primary and secondary qualities rather than providing an independent argument for it. What the Absolute Conception does is rather to give a further *interpretation* of that distinction on the assumption that it exists. Thus one way of attacking the conclusion that secondary qualities cannot form part of an objective account of the world would be simply to deny that there is any such distinction as that which is expressed by the traditional distinction between primary and secondary qualities. For our purposes, of understanding the role of values in psychiatric classifications, corresponding analogical moves include:

1. to deny that psychiatric classifications are (at least) essentially value-laden: this as we have seen is the nub of what those defending an essentially value-free model, like Kendell and Boorse, seek to do; or

2. to claim that despite being value-laden, those values were somehow independent of us and objective features of the world: although not deployed directly in the psychiatry/antipsychiatry debate, there is a large literature in ethical theory claiming, in one way or another, that there can be what amount to moral 'facts' (see, e.g. Dancy, 1993; McDowell, 1998).

But there is a different approach altogether to denying the Williams-inspired conclusion, an approach that we owe to John McDowell. It is to this that we turn next.

John McDowell's account

John McDowell is the contemporary South African born, Oxford educated, and now Pittsburgh-based philosopher of mind,

language, and metaphysics, that we introduced in Chapter 12. McDowell, as we noted, has written mainly short papers on a number of different but inter-related themes. What might be called his metaphysical world view is set out in a book of lectures, *Mind and World* (1994), the first chapter of which we examined in Chapter 12.

McDowell's arguments against Williams' Absolute Conception come in his paper 'Aesthetic value, objectivity, and the fabric of the world'. This paper, from which the next reading is taken (linked with Exercise 15 below), was written in part as a response to J.L. Mackie's book *Ethics: inventing right and wrong* (1977), and comes also in a different collection of his essays, called *Mind, Value, and Reality* (1998). The general thread of McDowell's arguments in this book concern whether values can be found in the world or have, as Mackie supposes, to be projected on to it. In this context, McDowell gives, as we will see, two arguments against Williams' Absolute Conception. Before coming to the specifics of these arguments, we will briefly fill out the background to them as set out in McDowell's paper.

Secondary qualities as *sensory* qualities

McDowell's starting assumption is that there is indeed a fundamental distinction between primary and secondary qualities. To this extent he agrees with Williams. McDowell argues that secondary qualities, unlike primary qualities, have to be characterized by appeal to our experiences.

Note that a different approach might have been to deny that supposed secondary qualities such as colour really do differ in kind from primary qualities. P.M.S. Hacker, an Oxford philosopher who has written extensively on Wittgenstein, argues in his book *Appearance and Reality* (1987) that there is no such distinction. Colours such as red are defined by appeal to red *samples* and not by appeal to our inner *experiences* on looking at red objects. They are thus similar to supposed primary qualities such as length, which are also defined by appeal to public samples.

But McDowell agrees with Williams that there is an important difference. To be red, for example, is to be experienced as red. He defines secondary qualities in general in this way:

A secondary quality is a property the ascription of which to an object is not adequately understood except as true, if it is true, in virtue of the object's disposition to present a certain sort of perceptual appearance: specifically, an appearance characterisable by using a word for the property itself to say how the object perceptually appears   McDowell (1998, p. 133)

McDowell, following the Oxford philosopher of thought Gareth Evans, calls secondary qualities so understood 'sensory' qualities (Evans, 1980). It is this connection to a subject's experience that will play an important part in his criticism of the Absolute Conception (see below).

One further terminological point is important, however. McDowell also calls secondary or sensory qualities 'subjective'. He defines a subjective property thus: 'A subjective property, in the relevant sense, is one such that no adequate conception of what it is for a thing to possess it is available except in terms of how the thing would, in suitable circumstances, affect a subject—a sentient being'. (McDowell, 1998, p. 113).

So secondary qualities are sensory and subjective. But while this may be an intuitive assimilation, McDowell's use of the term 'subjective' does not mean that a quality so described cannot be 'out there' as part of the fabric of the world. McDowell's diagnostic distinction between objective and subjective does *not* simply amount to what is found in the world and what is projected onto it. His idea is that a quality may be both subjective in the sense described above—i.e. conceptually connected to our experiences—but also the sort of thing that makes up reality.

In part his challenge is simply to point out this conceptual possibility. In other words, in a classic philosophical move, he points out that while we may assume that if a quality depends conceptually on our experiences it cannot really be out there, be a valid quality, actually this assumption may not be well founded and needs an argument. Secondarily he undermines one argument for this, which depends on the Absolute Conception and to which we will now turn.

Recall the dilemma that the Absolute Conception faces. On the one hand, to serve as a genuine contrast to representation in characterizing the objectivity of representation, the Absolute Conception must mean more than merely: 'whatever our representations represent'. But on the other hand the Absolute Conception cannot be substantiated by merely invoking one of our local representations. That will collapse the necessary contrast between our local representations and what our local representations are of.

Williams invokes science to escape this dilemma. We have a conception of the conception science will eventually give us in terms of non-local absolute concepts. (It is a kind of meta-conception.) Part of the moral of this is that secondary qualities drop out from the account of features of the world (in the narrow sense) and appear merely as aspects of our local perspective on the world to be explained (as they are part of the world history in the broader sense). Secondary qualities cannot form part of the fabric of the world and thus are not properly objective or real. Our primary interest here is that the same argument could be applied to psychiatric classifications if these depend on human evaluations.

We will now turn to McDowell's main argument against this. McDowell advances two lines of criticism against Williams's Absolute Conception. We will look at his account of the first (in the next reading) and summarize the second below.

- What is McDowell's argument against the possibility of fitting secondary or subjective qualities into the Absolute Conception?
- Think how this argument might be extended to cover values as well as secondary qualities.

McDowell's first argument against Williams

The reading covers McDowell's first main argument against Williams' Absolute Conception. On Williams' picture we aspire towards moving from our local perspective to what the American philosopher, Thomas Nagel, has called, in a book of the same name, the 'view from nowhere' (Nagel, 1986). But while the Absolute Conception is supposed to *contrast* with our local perspective, it also has to *include* it as even our local representations need explanation. But how can secondary, or as in the Evans/McDowell reformulation *sensory*, qualities be explained except by *adopting* the relevant perspective? Knowing what it is that is to be explained, requires adopting the perspective from which ex hypothesis they make sense. Thus there is a tension in the very idea of the 'view from nowhere' implicit in the Absolute Conception.

McDowell's argument turns on the assumption that secondary qualities are properly understood as sensory qualities and are thus subjective in the sense defined above. If so, then it seems that the only way of characterizing secondary qualities will be by adopting a subjective, i.e. *local*, perspective. It would be a separate matter to describe, e.g. the physics of light that might underpin colour. But to understand the secondary quality of colour itself, to understand the subjective sensory quality of colour, McDowell suggests, requires that we understand what it is like to *have* colour experiences. And that is part of a local perspective, which, in direct contrast with the central requirement of Williams' Absolute Conception, is precisely *not* available to all possible subjects.

In the case of values, there is nothing akin to the physics of light. And thus it appears that there will be even less that an Absolute Conception can describe given that it is not allowed to describe our responses to the world. Surely, then, runs the implication of McDowell's argument against Williams' Absolute Conception (as developed in respect of values by Mackie), there is no prospect of understanding values without understanding how things matter to us as subjects.

McDowell's second argument against Williams

McDowell's second argument against Williams' Absolute Conception, a little later in his paper, disputes the idea that invoking the progress of science can be of any help with the dilemma of which Williams is aware in developing his Absolute Conception. The dilemma, you will recall, ran thus: on the one hand, to serve as a genuine contrast to representation in characterizing the objectivity of representation, the Absolute

Conception must mean more than merely 'whatever our representations represent'; however, on the other hand, the Absolute Conception cannot be substantiated by merely invoking one of our *local* representations. Williams invokes the progress of science to escape from the horns of this dilemma: the progress of science, Williams points out, consists of a progressive substitution of local perspectives (secondary qualities) in favour of ever-more non-local perspectives (primary qualities); however, our ability to have a conception of progress of this kind, Williams argues, depends on our already having a conception of an absolutely non-local perspective (Nagel's view from nowhere, Williams' Absolute Conception) with which all local perspectives are contrasted.

The problem that McDowell points out with using the progress of science in this way, is that it depends on giving an account of science—so as to form a conception of the Absolute Conception—which falls prey to essentially the same sort of dilemma that arises in trying to characterize the world (of which our representations are representations) directly. In other words, invoking the progress of science, while it may get us off the horns of Williams' original dilemma, leaves us just as firmly stuck on the horns of a new dilemma that is no less fatal to the claims of the Absolute Conception to preclude secondary qualities from science. The two dilemmas indeed, Williams' original dilemma and the new dilemma pointed out by McDowell, have essentially the same form. The Williams' original dilemma, the dilemma that Williams invoked the progress of science to resolve, was the dilemma that, on the one hand, if we describe the world in a concrete way, if we simply say that the world which our representations are of is thus and so, then we merely use other of our *local* representations and thus fail to describe the *Absolute* Conception; however, if, on the other hand, we say that the world is just whatever our representations are of, we fall into vacuity. Agreed, says McDowell. But invoking the progress of science, far from getting us off the horns of this dilemma, impales us even more firmly on the horns of a new dilemma, a dilemma in essentially the same form, which arises when we attempt a characterization of science itself that is sufficient for Williams' purposes. McDowell's new dilemma is that, on the one hand, if we describe science in a concrete way, spelling out specific methods for example, we are simply using features of our *local* perspective on science and thus fail to describe anything that could be part of Williams' Absolute Conception; but on the other hand, if we say 'science is whatever gives us (non-local) access to the world', we again fall into vacuity.

Conclusions to the session: no knock-down argument

The line of argument of this session has had a restricted purpose: to show that, to date, no one has come up with a knock-down argument to support the assumption of the traditional model that values and science are, like oil and water, immiscible.

Williams' and McDowell's arguments

Williams' Absolute Conception is a sophisticated attempt to provide such an argument. Williams, as we have seen, focuses on the traditional distinction between primary and secondary qualities; and his conclusion, that secondary qualities have no place in science, has been taken by others (such as Mackie) to show, equally, that values have no place in science. McDowell's counter-arguments to Williams, building on Evans' interpretation of secondary qualities as sensory (hence essentially subjective) qualities, suggest that the key step in Williams' argument, of invoking the progress of science to get us off the horns of a dilemma on which we are impaled by the Absolute Conception, leaves us impaled on a new dilemma with essentially the same pair of horns. Williams' Absolute Conception, then, sophisticated as it is, fails to provide a knock-down argument against subjectivity, as a hallmark of secondary qualities, and hence values, having a place in science.

Other arguments

There are other lines of argument that are relevant here: as noted above, we have said nothing about 'natural kinds', for example, as a possible route to *excluding* values from what science is about; nor, conversely, have we considered 'moral facts', as explored by Dancy and others, as a possible route to *including* values in what science is about. Again, we have said nothing, here, about values and science (evaluation and description) having, perhaps, complementary roles. This is the line of argument that we will be developing in Part IV. The claim, made particularly in Chapters 20 and 21 of Part IV, that values have a role in diagnosis, although consistent with the bottom line of this chapter, that no one has yet come up with a knock-down argument against values having a proper place is science, is not dependent on that bottom line. The arguments of Part IV depend, rather, on the Hare–Putnam-based account of the medical concepts developed in Part I, as concepts that combine distinguishable (though not necessarily separable) elements of evaluative and of descriptive meaning, with the evaluative elements of meaning becoming practically (as well as theoretically) important where, as in psychiatric diagnosis, the operative values are diverse rather than shared.

Fact and value in Part IV

That model, then, the fact + value, the full field model of Part I, being the model that will be applied to psychiatric diagnosis in Part IV, leaves it entirely open whether the classifications underpinning psychiatric diagnosis should fully include, fully exclude, or partially include and partially exclude, values. Current practice includes examples of both versions of the latter: the ICD, for example, partially excludes values by separating off issues of good and bad functioning in a classification, the ICF (or International Classification of Functioning, WHO, 2001), which, although described as being part of the same family of classifications as the ICD, is published separately; the DSM, by contrast, more fully includes values by including criteria of good and bad functioning within the body of the classification itself (e.g. its Criterion B for schizophrenia, see Part IV).

Facts in physics

Again, we return to the significance of such overtly evaluative criteria appearing at the heart of psychiatry's most self-consciously scientific classification (the significance is entirely positive) in Part IV. For now, though, for purposes of focusing in this part on what science is about, we will turn from post-Logical Empiricist attempts to exclude subjectivity and values from science, as a way of trying to hang on to a traditional model, to post-Logical Empiricist philosophy that has been engaged with taking a fresh look at science itself, in the form of the paradigm natural science, physics. It is with post-Logical Empiricist philosophy of physics, then, that we will be concerned in the next session, before returning, in Session 4, to developing our third new agenda, our agenda for an *Extended Family of Psychiatric Classifications*.

Reflection on the session and self-test questions

Write down your own reflections on the materials in this session drawing out any points that are particularly significant for you. Then write brief notes about the following:

1. What did Hempel say about values in science?

2. How does this compare with what Szasz says about psychiatry?

3. Why did Crispin Wright argue that humour is not objective?

4. What is Bernard Williams 'Absolute Conception'?

5. How did Williams' employ the distinction between primary and secondary qualities?

6. What implications did J.L. Mackie (and others working in ethics) draw from Williams' account of the Absolute Conception for the place of values in science?

7. Give one of John McDowell's arguments against Bernard William's Absolute Conception (we noted a preliminary and two main arguments).

8. What is the implication of John McDowell's work for the place of values in science?

Session 3 Scientific realism in physics

This session will examine the debate about realism in the philosophy of science that has largely focussed on physics. It will consider the arguments for and against taking a realist attitude (of one kind or another) to the entities—such as atoms and electromagnetic fields—that are the basis of theory in the physical sciences.

Why physics?

The session will function at one level as 'time out' from the problems of classification in psychiatric science. It will put much needed air and space around those problems by exploring the extent of the comparable problems in physics. One consequence of this will be to provide a basis for shifting attitudes from the deficit model of psychiatric science, evident as we saw in the agendas for both Lewis for ICD-9 and Kupfer *et al.*, for DSM-V, to a *strengths* model. A further consequence will be to derive a number of specific lessons for the future development of classifications in psychiatry and the wider mental health movement. We will not be drawing these consequences in this session, however (we return to them in Session 4). In this session, we will be exploring the problems of realism in physics in their own right as a way of deepening our understanding of what science itself, in general and in physics as the hardest of hard sciences, is about.

Plan of the session

The session starts with the background to current debates in Logical Empiricism and a philosophical successor to Logical Empiricism, Constructive Empiricism. Something of the complexity of modern debates is reflected in the fact that Constructive Empiricism, in the work particularly of the Dutch-born philosopher (who works at Princeton University) Bas (B.C.) Van Fraassen, combines, as we will see, semantic and metaphysical forms of realism with a version of epistemological antirealism. Constructive Empiricism then leads into a discussion of three different realist responses to the epistemological antirealism of Constructive Empiricism: realism about explanations (Boyd and McMullen); realism about causal explanation (Cartwright); and realism about what can be manipulated (Hacking).

The session concludes with the work of the American philosopher of physics, Arthur Fine, on what he calls the Natural Ontological Attitude or NOA. Fine, as we will see, rejects both realist and antirealist positions in the traditional debate about what science is about. He argues that the traditional debate is premissed on an impossible-to-achieve perspective from *outside science*, that philosophers should instead confine their attention to what *particular* scientific disciplines are about, and that they should work by engaging directly in the *practices* of particular scientific disciplines. (Fine himself has contributed to the detailed interpretation of modern physical theory.)

Logical Empiricism and Constructive Empiricism

Logical Empiricism, positivism, and instrumentalism

First then, Logical Empiricism and one of its philosophical successors, Van Fraassen's Constructive Empiricism.

In the early part of this century, as we saw in Chapter 12, many philosophers of science advocated an instrumentalist and positivistic attitude towards science. They argued that theoretical claims about the world did not function as literally descriptive claims. In part, this emphasis was the result of the precise way in which observation was credited with a central role in science as described in Chapter 12. As we saw, the Logical Empiricists attempted to defend the central role of impartial observation by distinguishing between an independent language of observational concepts and a dependent language of theoretical concepts. Given this distinction, it was plausible (although by no means mandatory) to construe statements framed with observational concepts as making genuine empirical claims while construing theoretical statements as merely playing a heuristic role in organizing the former. When so construed, theoretical statements are not themselves fact stating or capable of truth and falsity. They play a part that is not one of assertion but rather as an instrument for organizing genuinely fact stating claims.

Such a view reflects a positivistic attitude to the connection between meaningfulness and verification. As theoretical statements cannot themselves be directly verified and receive whatever confirmation or refutation indirectly via observational statements, they were regarded by many as possessing a different kind of meaning from verifiable observational statements.

While positivist and instrumentalist attitudes are still found among philosophically influenced practising scientists, they are nowadays rare among philosophers of science. One reason for this is the attack on the distinction between theory and observation, explained in chapter 12, that undermines the possibility of marking a firm semantic distinction between the meaning of observation statements and that of theoretical statements. If theoretical and observational statements are made in the same language—if complete separation is not possible between theoretical and observational concepts—then theoretical statements cannot be sharply marked out as playing a different kind of role from observation statements. The difference between theory and observation is a matter of degree.

Scientific realism—the current orthodoxy

In place of a positivistic and instrumentalist view of scientific theory, the current orthodoxy is a form of realism about science called scientific realism. As we will see, 'realism' describes more than one philosophical position. The varieties of realism and antirealism, and their different combinations in the views of different authors can be somewhat bewildering—hence we have summarized the key positions that we will discuss in this session in Table 13.3. We will approach the issues via one particular attack on realism that shares some of the features of a positivistic view but which also shares some of the underlying metaphysical assumptions of scientific realism.

Constructive Empiricism—a current form of scientific antirealism

The following short extract is taken from Bas Van Fraassen's influential book published in 1980, *The Scientific Image*. Van Fraassen is a contemporary philosopher of science who has also written on the nature of probability and on the philosophy of quantum physics. In this reading, however, he focuses more generally on what the aim of science should be.

Table 13.3 Realism and antirealism in the philosophy of physics

Philosopher	Position	Strapline
Van Fraassen	(1) Ontological realist (2) Semantic realist (3) Epistemological antirealist	There really are things (like electrons) we can't see and in the same sense that there really are things (like chains) we can see
Boyd/McMullen	Ontological, semantic and epistemological realists	inference to the best explanation
Cartwright	Realist about causes (hence also causally effective 'unobservable' entities)	Inference to most probable cause
Hacking	Realist about what can be manipulated	What can be manipulated is real
Fine	Realism and antirealism equally flawed because they attempt to stand outside particular sciences—hence what is valid is a matter for local determination within the theory and practices of a particular science	Natural Ontological Attitude (NOA)

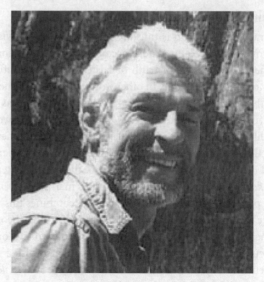

Fig. 13.3 Van Fraassen

Van Fraassen's relation to realism

Van Fraassen's position is a form of antirealism. But it is important to be clear just what it is that he denies. As he says on p. 187, one element of a *realist* attitude to science is that science aims to give us a 'literally true story of what the world is like'. But this claim itself involves two aspects according to whether one focuses on the claim to (scientific) truth about the world or the language in which that claim is expressed:

> This [ie the two aspects of the realist claim] divides the antirealists into two sorts. The first sort holds that science is or aims to be true, properly (but not literally) construed. The second holds that the language of science should be literally construed, but its theories need not be true to be good. The antirealism I shall advocate belongs to the second sort. (p. 187)

Semantic and metaphysical forms of realism

Van Fraassen's position is thus *not* the same as a positivistic or instrumentalist account. Those accounts deny that theoretical statements are capable of truth or falsity but serve a different, purely organizational, role. In other words they can be 'true' in so far as they organize successfully, but this is not the same as literal truth (i.e. giving us a literally true picture of what the world is really like). By contrast, Van Fraassen accepts the realist view that theoretical scientific statements are either true or false when construed literally. Just as they appear to do, theoretical statements really *do* make claims about the world. This marks out a *semantic* realist position. Furthermore, Van Fraassen combines this with a further metaphysical view about the nature of truth. Theoretical statements are true (or false) in virtue of how the world *is* or what the facts *are*. Truth is a matter of correspondence with a mind-independent objective world. This is a form of 'ontological' realism, therefore, realism about what there is 'out there'.

Constructive Empiricism is *epistemological* antirealism

But Van Fraassen combines his semantic and ontological realist views with a form of *epistemological* antirealism. Although

theoretical statements are construed as (really) either true or false in virtue of the world, we can never arrive at sufficient evidence to discover or to know which statements are true and which are false. Thus, we should refrain from committing ourselves to the truth of theoretical statements. To do so is to take an unnecessary risk. Instead science should aim merely to arrive at theories that are *empirically adequate*. Acceptance of a theory should similarly involve merely belief that it is empirically adequate. A theory is empirically adequate if and only if 'what it says about the observable things and events in this world, is true—exactly if it *saves the phenomena* (emphasis added). And 'saving the phenomena' means accounting comprehensively for our observations. We should aim at nothing beyond this.

In his writings, Van Fraassen gives considerable theoretical underpinning to the two key terms in this account of what science is about, 'empirical adequacy' and 'saving the phenomena'. The latter phrase, by the way, is not original to Van Fraassen (although Van Fraassen gives it a particular meaning within his theory): it appears in the title of a book published originally in 1908 by the great French philosopher, physicist and mathematician, Pierre Duhem (whom we met in Chapter 12, see Duhem, 1985), and dates back via Ptolemy to Plato. At all events, you can get something of the force of his position from the traditional contrast between *phenomena*, as that which appears to us (through sight, hearing, etc.), and *numena*, as that which is really there and the source or origin of phenomena. In terms of this contrast, Van Fraassen's Constructive Empiricism says, in effect, that science is about the phenomena not the numena. You will see the parallels here with positivism and instrumentalism. But what Van Fraassen adds to these positions is an original and particularly clear analysis of how one can be at the same time an *ontological realist* (about what is there) and *semantic realist* (using 'real' with the same meaning of observable objects like chairs as of unobservable objects like electrons) and yet an *epistemological antirealist* (denying that there is anything one can know about what is really there beyond what appears to be there, i.e. the phenomena).

Empirical adequacy is enough?

So characterized, then, Constructive Empiricism is prescriptive. It says that one should not accept the truth of theoretical statements in science to the extent that this involves accepting anything over and above the empirical adequacy of the theory within which the statements in question are made. But this prescription is not arbitrary and results from epistemological arguments about what can and cannot be known. In *The Scientific Image* chapter 1, Van Fraassen's argument for Constructive Empiricism takes the form of a series of attacks on epistemological realism. In effect he argues that as believing in the (ontological) truth of theories involves more than believing merely in their empirical adequacy, there should be an argument for this extra step and that no such argument is successful.

An argument for Constructive Empiricism

On a first encounter, however, this may seem an unusual way of apportioning the burden of proof. As Constructive Empiricism is counter-intuitive, a positive argument, rather than or in addition to Van Fraassen's negative arguments against realism, might be needed to motivate it. One such argument might run as follows:

1. At any given time, the only evidence for a theory is the set of relevant observations already made.

2. For any finite body of observations, there is always more than one theory that is consistent with it. These different theories differ in what they say about unobservables. (They might also differ in what they say about future observables, but we will ignore this point for the moment.)

3. As the only evidence for theories concerns the observable realm, there is no way of deciding which theory correctly describes the unobservable realm.

4. Thus we should not take the risk of choosing between these different theories and accept instead what they all have in common: their descriptions of the observable realm. We should, in other words, adopt Constructive Empiricism.

5. However, as all the consequences that can matter for us are observable we also loose nothing by this.

The underdetermination of theory by data

As we will see, this argument is not watertight because it rests on premises that can reasonably be doubted. However, the basic assumption that drives it—and which will not be questioned in what follows—is the thesis of what has become widely known from the work of the twentieth century American Pragmatist W.V.O. Quine (1975) as the Underdetermination of Theory by Data.

There are stronger and weaker versions of this thesis. At its strongest it claims that even given all the *possible* evidence that we could amass, there would remain more than one theory consistent with it. Some care has to be taken in how one construes 'all possible evidence'. If it means simply 'all the facts' then it is hard to see how this would not determine which theory were true. Instead it has to be construed—even in this strong version of the thesis—as meaning 'all the evidence that it is possible for we *humans*, having extended our senses through instruments, to amass'. But there is a weaker thesis that will serve our present purposes. It is the claim that for any *finite* body of evidence, there is always more than one theory consistent with it.

Even this weak reading of the Underdetermination Thesis appears to justify Van Fraassen's claim, then. Thus, theories that are consistent with the data will have to differ one from another in what they say either about future observable matters or about unobservable matters. A version of Constructive Empiricism that restricted our beliefs to past observable states of affairs would be one that followed Hume's sceptical attack on induction. This would be a radical position that denied that we could know anything about the future. Van Fraassen's position is more reasonable.

Granting that induction is sometimes possible, he concentrates instead on those aspects of theories that concern unobservable matters and says that we should withhold judgement on these. The reason for this restriction is the claim that the only rational method of judging between theories is evidence, and that, by definition, there cannot be evidence that concerns the unobservable realm. That would require that the realm were not unobservable.

Coupled with the claim that we cannot have knowledge of the unobservable realm, Van Fraassen also suggests that we lose nothing by abstaining from judgement about it. All that can interest us are the observable consequences of theories, because these are the only aspects that have practical consequences. Thus we should not take the risk of commitment to particular accounts of unobservables but neither is this of any practical loss.

We will shortly he going on to outline three critical responses to Van Fraassen below. But it is important—as ever in philosophy—to think through in advance and for yourself whether Van Fraassen's is a good argument, and if not, why not.

EXERCISE 17   (15 minutes)

How convincing are the arguments for Constructive Empiricism? Is it a satisfactory account of science? What realist counter-arguments to Constructive Empiricism are possible? Make a note of any such counter-arguments, and think what further arguments Van Fraassen might offer in reply, before reading on.

Here are two common counter-arguments to Van Fraassen's Constructive Empiricism. The first depends on the discussion in Chapter 12 on the Theory Dependence of Observation. The second concerns the way in which theories can be combined. Constructive Empiricism has answers to both these criticisms but they are worth looking at briefly before coming directly to modern accounts of scientific realism. As elsewhere in philosophy, the criticisms help to clarify the account (here, a form of antirealism) to which other accounts are a response—in this case the three forms of realism to be considered below.

Constructive Empiricism and the theory dependence of observation

The brief presentation above of Constructive Empiricism presupposed a sharp distinction between the observable and the unobservable. But, as the arguments in Chapter 12 show, no such distinction can be drawn. In so far as there is a distinction it is both one of degree, not of kind, and one which itself presupposes a background of theory. Changing the theoretical background changes what is deemed directly observable and what is a matter of inference. So, can an argument for Constructive Empiricism be advanced even without such a sharp distinction?

Van Fraassen's approach is to distinguish two senses of observable. In some cases we cannot observe an entity with the naked eye because it is too far away. While it is not directly observed, it is observ-*able* in that, if one travelled closer to it, one would be able to observe it. In other cases, however, there is no possibility of direct observation. Thus sub-atomic particles, for example, are not observable. Van Fraassen then suggests that one should advocate Constructive Empiricism about the latter only.

As we will see later, this response is vulnerable to the objection that we can literally see through microscopes. (This is the point made by Ian Hacking below.) But another response is available. Rather than maintaining a distinction between theory and observation, one could, instead, accept that there is a scale ranging from the purely observable (relative to some background theory) to the purely theoretical. A Constructive Empiricist prescription can now be reformulated as follows. Adopt a degree of belief in a theoretical statement in proportion to its degree of observationality.

Degrees of belief

Talk of 'degrees of belief' may seem obscure and artificial. But it is simply a codification of an everyday phenomenon. If I take an umbrella out on a Spring day it does not mean that I am certain that it will rain. I may not even think that it is as likely as a fifty per cent certainty. Providing the 'cost' of taking the umbrella—its inconvenience and such like—is sufficiently low, then it will be worth taking even if I think that the chances are very remote. But if I am certain that it will not rain, and there is even the smallest inconvenience attached to taking the umbrella, then it would be irrational to take it.

Another way of making my degree of belief explicit is by examining the bets I would be prepared to make. If I think that the chances of it raining are fifty per cent then I should be indifferent between a gamble in which I am rewarded if it rains and one in which I am rewarded if it does not. Degrees of belief can be formally codified using preparedness to accept bets. But for now all that matters is an informal understanding of the idea. This can then be pressed into the service of Constructive Empiricism.

Constructive Empiricism about novel predictions from combined theories

The second preliminary argument against Constructive Empiricism turns on the effect of combining theories. Put simply the challenge is this. If one takes a Constructive Empiricist attitude to a theory then one should believe only its observable consequences. Thus if one adopts this attitude to two theories one should believe the combination of their observable consequences. But the observable consequences of the combination of two theories is not necessarily the same as the combination of the observable consequences of the two theories considered in isolation. The reason is this. The unobservable (or theoretical) component of one theory may 'interact' with either the theoretical or observable component of the other to generate fresh observable consequences, i.e. consequences that flow from neither theory working in isolation from the other. Given this fact, it seems that Constructive Empiricism is an inadequate philosophy of science because it cannot account for the fresh predictions that result from combining theories.

This issue will receive further discussion later. But for now the following response is sufficient. The combination of theories does nothing to change the basic position. The observational consequences of their combination still underdetermines the microscopic (unobservable) realm. Thus there is still no reason to believe in anything more than the empirical adequacy of the theories in question whether we consider them working together in combination or separately in isolation.

Three current scientific realist defences against the antirealism of Constructive Empiricism

The next three short extracts provide arguments against Van Fraassen's Constructive Empiricism. The first by the American philosopher of science, Richard Boyd, represents the orthodoxy of scientific realism. The following two are both qualifications to such straightforward realism. This first paper, however, attempts to defend head on a form of inference that Van Fraassen rejects.

EXERCISE 18	(20 minutes)

Read the extract from:

Boyd, R. (1999). On the current status of scientific realism. pages 195–222. In *The Philosophy of Science* (ed. R. Boyd, P. Gasker, and J.D. Trout). Cambridge, MA: MIT Press (Extract pp. 207, paras 3–5)

Link with Reading 13.15

♦ How does Boyd's account of scientific realism counter the arguments for Constructive Empiricism?

♦ What extra ingredient does he introduce?

Boyd introduces an extra ingredient to considerations of the relation between theory and observational data. The Underdetermination Thesis played a key role in the brief sketch of an argument for Constructive Empiricism above. The Underdetermination Thesis is based on the claim that there is more than one theory that is *consistent* with any finite body of evidence. But that claim is remarkably weak. It simply means that there is more than one theory that is not incompatible with the data, that there is more than one theory whose falsity is not implied by the data. Thus the claim that there is more than one such theory may come as no surprise.

The relation of theory and evidence: consistency versus inductive support

Normally in science, in contrast with the Underdetermination Thesis, we think that there is a stronger relation between data and theory than mere consistency. We think of data as *supporting* theory. Data provide positive evidence or warrant for our beliefs. That is what is involved in taking events in the past as a *reason* for holding beliefs about what will happen in the future. Inductive inference involves not just eliminating theories that are inconsistent with past events but also using past events as a guide to choosing between the consistent theories that remain. The fact that Van Fraassen accepts that this is possible is shown by his acceptance of theories that make predictions about future observable matters. But this leaves the problem, according to Van Fraassen, that in the case of unobservables, so long as they remain genuinely *un*observable, we cannot begin to establish inductive generalizations linking them with observables because we are never in a position to check them.

Inference to the best explanation

But as Boyd points out, there is another kind of relation between theory and data, a relation provided by *explanation*. If a theory enjoys explanatory success, then, according to Boyd, it is likely to be true, or likely to be largely or approximately true. This suggests that there is a way of supporting detailed claims about unobservable realms. One looks for the best explanation of observable phenomena whether or not it employs unobservable or microscopic features. This is the nub or strap-line of modern Scientific Realism, that we should be realist about whatever it is (observable or unobservable) that supports an inference to the best explanation.

McMullin on lunar mountains

Another realist philosopher, Ernan McMullin (1987, pp. 51–73), gives the example of Galileo's explanation of the changing shadows on the moon that invokes lunar mountains. Because lunar mountains are the best explanation of the shadows, there is good reason, given the existence of the shadows, to believe in the existence of the mountains. This example would be classed by Van Fraassen as concerning observables because lunar mountains could eventually be observed with the naked eye. But the same kind of explanation-based strategy could also be applied in microscopic cases (such as subatomic particles) that are not directly observable even in principle.

In the case of Galileo and lunar mountains, the qualification 'best' in inference to the best explanation, may seem superfluous. Knowing what we know now, what other explanation of their shadows could there be? But given the status of the astronomical telescope as a scientific instrument at the time, even in this case an alternative might have been to explain the observed phenomenon away as a mere artefact of the instrument. Mere 'noise' is often an appropriate rival explanation in the case of putative observations made with complex modern instruments (whether space telescopes, vats of cleaning fluid for the detection of neutrinos or electron microscopes). Furthermore, while the shadows of mountains was a perfectly reasonable explanation, many others were available: the greening (or silvering) by algal growth (rather as Earth's appearance changes with the seasons); a change in chemical and reflective properties of the lunar surface in response to heat and light; etc. Again, knowing what we know now, these alternative theories would have dropped away. But it has always

been a difficulty for Scientific Realism, that it relies on past performance and is able to say little or nothing about current difficulties or the direction that future developments of theory should take. Past performance, as the financial adverts remind us, is no guarantee of future performance!

Summary so far

Scientific Realism is typically regarded as the combination of semantic, ontological, and epistemological views. We have already seen that Van Fraassen holds realist views about both the semantics and the ontology of science. Scientific statements, literally construed, are either true or false. And they are true or false in virtue of the state of a mind-independent world. What we can *know* about the world, however, is always limited: one reason for this limitation being that for any given set of observations, more than one theory is possible. Hence Van Fraassen is an antirealist about what we can know about the world, he is an epistemological antirealist. Realists, such as Boyd and McMullin, seek to counter Van Fraassen's epistemological antirealism by arguing that we can indeed claim to know the truth, or approximate truth, of the full range of scientific statements. As we have seen, the key tool for this claim is explanatory success or more specifically inference to the best explanation.

The issue of whether explanatory success can ground claims about the truth of scientific claims across the board is also contested—in a different way from Van Fraassen—by the contemporary American philosopher of science and of physics, Nancy Cartwright.

Cartwright's attack on the validity of scientific laws

> **EXERCISE 19** (30 minutes)
>
> Read the extract from:
>
> Cartwright, N. (1999). The reality of causes in a world of instrumental laws. pp. 379–386. In *The Philosophy of Science* (ed. R. Boyd, P. Gasker, and J.D. Trout). Cambridge, MA: MIT Press (Extract pp. 379–380)
>
> Link with Reading 13.16
>
> ◆ How does Cartwright's position differ on the one hand from Scientific Realism, on the other from the epistemological antirealism of Van Fraassen?

Two arguments against inference to the best explanation

Cartwright suggests a middle path between full Scientific Realism as advocated by Boyd, McMullin, and others and the epistemological antirealism of Van Fraassen. Roughly speaking, she is a realist about those unobservable entities that are invoked to give the best causal explanation of observable effects. She rejects

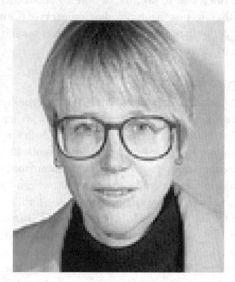

Fig. 13.4 Nancy Cartwright

inference to the best (theoretical) explanation but accepts inference to the most probable cause. There are two general arguments that underpin this distinction.

1. *Cartwright's general claim about theoretical explanation.* Theoretical explanation is, she suggests following Van Fraassen, a matter of providing a unifying account of diverse phenomena. In the physical sciences this is provided by mathematical theories from which statements about observable phenomena can be derived. But such theoretical explanations do not presuppose the truth of the explanatory theory. That a description of an observable phenomenon can be derived from a theory coupled with the fact that the description is true, does not imply that the theory is also true. The truth of a description of a phenomenon derived from a given theory, is no more a guarantee of the truth of that theory, than is the fact that one philosophical paper precedes another true philosophical paper a guarantee that the former is also true. Truth is an optional extra. (This is a contentious claim about explanation as we will see in the Chapter 14. Others argue that for an explanation to count as an explanation it has to be true.)

2. *Cartwright argues that there are, in theoretical physics at least, very often more than one, strictly incompatible, theoretical accounts that could, in principle, be applied to the same phenomena.* Scientists take a pragmatic attitude to choosing which theoretical treatment to use depending on which is most appropriate to any particular case. Appropriateness in this case depends on ease of mathematical application as well as

accuracy. But if the theories used in explanation had to be true, then no such pragmatic attitude would be consistent. Scientists would have to determine which was the *right* theory or withhold explanation.

Theoretical versus causal explanation

Cartwright differs from Van Fraassen, however, in distinguishing theoretical explanations from causal explanations. Causal explanation, she argues, does provide reason for believing in the existence of the entities that are invoked in the explanation (hence this is sometimes called entity realism). The key difference between the two kinds of explanation is that (higher-level) explanatory theories do not bring about the (lower-level) descriptions that can be derived from them, but causes do bring about their effects. Thus if a causal explanation were to fail to pick out real entities, it would fail as an explanation. By contrast, if a high-level theoretical explanation turns out to be false it might none the less organize the lower-level descriptions of the world in an efficient and clear manner.

Cartwright's favoured examples concern the 'gap' between the Schrödinger equation in quantum physics and its application in particular problems. She suggests that, as a matter of fact, there are a number of different and conflicting assumptions and approximations that allow physicists to connect the high-level equations of theoretical physics with the practical applications of the theory in, for example, work on electronics. But they cannot all be true, because they conflict. Cartwright suggests that high-level theories or laws do not make lower-level theories true in the way that claims about causal entities can make true claims about observable phenomena.

Of course from some perspectives, belief in neither may seem very attractive. But this helps reiterate an implicit point that all these argument forms are, from a logical point of view, invalid: i.e. true premises can lead to false conclusions. As we saw in Chapter 5, the conclusions of a valid argument in logic are true because those conclusions are derived by nothing more than 'unpacking' the premises of the argument. In the case of a scientific argument, by contrast, the conclusions (about this or that underlying cause) are derived by inference (substantive but therefore fallible inference) from descriptions of an observed effect (serving as premises).

An objection to the distinction

We will return to the analysis of scientific explanation in Chapter 14. But it is worth noting here a natural general objection to Cartwright's claim that theoretical explanation does not require the truth of the explanatory theory. Surely if a theory is false, it cannot provide an explanation of anything. Here is an analogy. A false belief cannot form the basis of knowledge. There is no such thing as false knowledge, just apparent knowledge which, in fact, is not knowledge at all. Likewise, an 'explanation' based on a false theory is not an explanation at all but rather merely an *apparent* explanation that is not one at all.

Aside from simply rejecting the claim that truth is an essential part of any explanation, Cartwright has two responses to this objection:

1. One has already been mentioned. It is to note that in fact this is not how high-level theoretical explanations are regarded by scientists. They take a pragmatic attitude to the multiple and mutually inconsistent theoretical treatments that are available.

Now one might respond to this by saying that while this may be what happens *in fact*, it *ought not* to. Perhaps it reflects the present incomplete stage of scientific knowledge. Cartwright's second response provides a clue to why she thinks that this is not the reason for such a pragmatic approach to high-level theories.

2. Cartwright claims that it is *no coincidence that high-level laws are all false.*

Explanation versus truth as the goal of science

The argument for this startling claim (put forward especially in chapters 2 and 3 of Cartwright's *How the Laws of Physics Lie*, 1983) is that explanation and truth are incompatible goals. To be explanatory a theory must abstract from the descriptions of individual cases, an underlying pattern. An example is Newton's law of gravitational attraction that states that the force exerted on any particle in the universe by any other is proportional to the product of their masses divided by the square of their distance apart. But such a theory neglects other forces that also act on particles, such as electromagnetic forces. To be accurate one would have to say 'all other things being equal', or *ceteris paribus*, the force is proportional to.... But as other things are rarely equal, such a law, although true, would not be explanatory. In general the higher the level the theory or law, the more explanatory but the less true will it be.

Vector addition as a counter-argument?

Again there is a natural counter-argument. One might say that the law of gravitational attraction gives the force due to gravity and that the resultant force acting on a particle depends on the vector sum of this force and all other forces. Aside from some specific arguments against the reality of the component forces involved in that calculation Cartwright's general argument is that there is no general analogue of vector addition for laws with *ceteris paribus* clauses. Snell's law, which governs refraction, applies only to isotropic media and so should be read as relying on a *ceteris paribus* clause. But if other things are not equal, if the media are not isotropic there is no mechanical way of producing an appropriate refinement. In general there is no neutral way of combining the effects of different *ceteris paribus* laws, which all apply to some specific circumstance.

Cartwright's view of nature

This view is a reflection of a more fundamental view of nature which is best expressed in Cartwright's (1983) own words:

> I imagine that natural objects are much like people in societies. Their behaviour is constrained by some specific laws and by a handful of general principles, but it is not determined in detail even statistically. What happens on most occasions is dictated by no law at all. This is not a metaphysical picture that I urge. My claim is that this picture is as plausible as the alternative. God may have written just a few laws and grown tired.
>
> Cartwright (1983, p. 49)

Or again:

> The laws that describe this world are a patchwork, not a pyramid. They do not take after the simple, elegant and abstract structure of a system of axioms and theorems. Rather they look like—and steadfastly stick to looking like—science as we know it: apportioned into disciplines, apparently arbitrarily grown up; governing different sets of properties at different levels of abstraction; pockets of great precision; large parcels of qualitative maxims resisting precise formulation; erratic overlaps; here and there, once in a while, corners that line up, but mostly ragged edges; and always the cover of law just loosely attached to the jumbled world of material things. For all we know, most of what happens in nature occurs by hap (sic), subject to no law at all. What happens is more like an outcome of negotiation between domains than the logical consequence of a system of order.
>
> Cartwright (2000, p. 1)

Is realism about entities really distinct from realism about theories?

It is worth noting that this view is an expression of a form of antirealism that is not merely epistemological but also (despite Cartwright's protestation and her commitment to realism specifically about entities) ontological. It is not merely a prescription about which elements of science one should believe but also a claim about how the world is. Although she is a realist about entities, she believes that they really exist and that we can know about them (and is thus both an ontological and epistemological realist about entities), yet she also thinks that the world really might lack a kind of underlying order or structure. We will return to ontological antirealism shortly. First, however, it is worth considering a further objection that might be raised against Cartwright's position, namely that the distinction presupposed by a combination of entity realism and theory antirealism is unstable. Surely, runs the objection, to be a realist about entities requires believing in the theories that are used to identify the entities. Electrons, for example, are just those things of which our relevant atomic theories are true.

There is some truth in this objection. The distinction between theory and entity realism cannot be as sharp as Cartwright suggests. On the other hand, our theories about electrons have changed almost beyond recognition during the course of the twentieth century but we still take them to have been concerned throughout with the very same things. The original theories are now understood not to have been true, but not to have been so completely false that they were not describing anything real. It is just that we believe we now have a better idea what elections are 'really' like. The case of electrons thus differs from that of theories about phlogiston, for example, which are now taken to have been so false that they did not even refer to anything. (Although Putnam reports the suggestion that even those theories can be saved from complete vacuity providing they are construed as describing valence electrons, see Putnam, 1996, p. 15).

Hacking's view of nature

There is, however, another motive for distinguishing between explanatory theories and causal-explanatory theoretical entities, and that concerns our practical engagement with the world. This is the view expressed by the Vancouver born, Toronto-based philosopher of science, Ian Hacking.

The following passage complements the previous one in that both Hacking and Cartwright share a suspicion of theory and a contrasting commitment to (causally efficacious) entities. But Hacking develops further the role of experimental manipulation of entities. (This is based on Hacking's original book, *Representing and Intervening*, 1983.)

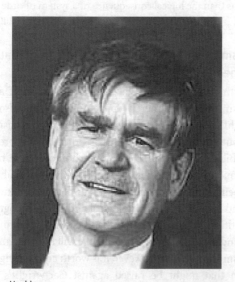

Fig. 13.5 Ian Hacking

EXERCISE 20   (30 minutes)

Read the extract from:

Hacking, I. (1999). Experimentation and scientific realism. pp. 247–260. In *The Philosophy of Science* (ed. R. Boyd, P. Gasker, and J.D. Trout). Cambridge, MA: MIT Press (Extract p. 248).

Link with Reading 13.17

◆ To what extent is the kind of practical manipulation Hacking describes applicable to psychiatry?

Realism and practical manipulation

Hacking agrees with Cartwright that successful explanation does not provide much justification or warrant for the truth of a scientific theory. But he argues that successful theoretical explanation is not the only way to confirm the existence of specific unobservable particles. One can also develop techniques to measure and manipulate them. It is this practical hands-on component that helps support a form of realism about entities very like that of Cartwright. These practical techniques are based on a general understanding of the causal properties of unobservables. Thus 'the "direct" proof of electrons and the like is our ability to manipulate them using well-understood low-level causal properties.'

Hacking's example in the paper from which this extract is taken is the development of the PEGGY II electron gun. It is because this successful machine relies on spraying electrons, that no one could plausibly deny the existence of electrons. This is true despite the fact that the theories used to describe the machine may well not be correct. The ability to manipulate and the ability successfully and correctly to explain do not go hand in hand.

Links to later chapters

Hacking's claims about entity realism are connected to two subjects which will be discussed later but which are worth flagging now.

1. One is the degree of tacit knowledge in scientific work that often goes unnoticed. This is particularly apparent in the case of debugging PEGGY II where there is no checklist to determine in advance what factors are relevant—and what are not—to proper working. This will be discussed in Chapter 14.

2. The other is the way machines can serve as black-boxed embodiments of scientific claims about the world. Once one has built a machine that either measures some 'unobservable' or manipulates it to measure something else, then doubts about its status seem flimsy. Bruno Latour, the French sociologist, describes this rhetorical use of machines in *Science in Action: how to follow scientists and engineers through society* (1987). We will describe briefly other aspects of this sociological approach to science in Chapter 16.

But while entity-realism seems plausible in the context of physical and engineering science it is less directly applicable in psychiatry. This is an issue that has been hanging over us since considering Cartwright: to what extent can a distinction between realism about theories and realism about entities be drawn for a science of the mind? Hacking adds to that question the further dimension that, in some sciences, the entities postulated in theories can eventually be the subject of practical manipulation. But is there any analogue of this in psychiatry that could be used to address the issue of the validity of psychiatric classification?

The natural ontological attitude: assessing scientific validity from the inside?

The discussion of scientific realism so far has focused on the epistemological claim that we can come to know about hidden or unobservable aspects of the world via science. But it is worth remembering that this claim is made against a background of ontological realism. It is to ontological realism and antirealism that we will now turn by considering the American philosopher, Arthur Fine's, Natural Ontological Attitude or NOA.

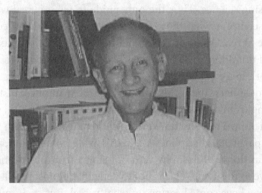

Fig. 13.6 Arthur Fine

EXERCISE 21 (30 minutes)

Read the extract from:

Fine, A. (1999). The natural ontological attitude pp 261–277. In *The Philosophy of Science* (ed. R. Boyd, P. Gasker, and J.D. Trout). Cambridge, MA: MIT Press (Extract pp. 271–272.)

Link with Reading 13.18

♦ What is the Natural Ontological Attitude?

The circularity of inference to the best explanation

Fine begins by arguing against the effectiveness of realism as an account of the success of science. The epistemological antirealist is characterized by Fine as resisting the claim that a successful explanation is likely to be true. This fits Van Fraassen. Realists claim, by contrast, that realism is the only account of science that does not make its success a miracle. But the argument used to support epistemological realism is thus of the following form: *scientific realism explains the success of science and thus it is likely*

to be true. In other words it trades on just the inference from explanatory success to truth that epistemological antirealists deny. Fine's key claim is thus that deploying realism to explain the success of science simply reiterates the form of reasoning that is in question.

Notice that the issue about realism is precisely the issue as to whether we should believe in the reality of those individuals, properties, relations, processes, and so forth, used in well-supported explanatory hypotheses. In the case at hand—psychiatric classification—it is whether we should take the categories set out to answer to genuine structural features of our mental lives and mental health and ill-health.

Now what is the hypothesis of realism, as it arises as an explanation of scientific practice? It is just the hypothesis that our accepted scientific theories are approximately true, where 'being approximately true' is taken to denote an extra-theoretical relation between theories and the world. Thus, to address doubts over the reality of relations posited by explanatory hypotheses, the realist proceeds to introduce a further explanatory hypothesis (realism), itself positing such a relation (approximate truth). Surely, Fine argues, anyone serious about the issue of realism, and with an open mind about it, would be behaving inconsistently if he were to accept the realist move as satisfactory.

The natural ontological attitude

But, although Fine argues against traditional epistemological realism, he does not support a form of epistemological antirealism either. Instead he argues that the debate between realism and antirealism is itself the result of a mistaken metaphysical urge. What both realists and antirealists should—and he claims typically do—accept is a 'homely line'. This 'homely line' Fine calls the Natural Ontological Attitude (or NOA). NOA is what scientists working in a particular science find it natural to take for granted about what is real. This core position comprises an acceptance of well-grounded scientific claims as having the same status as everyday knowledge claims. Philosophers, Fine argues, of whatever realist or antirealist persuasion, take over and assume this NOA. But realists and antirealists go on to qualify this common core with further and different metaphysical claims. The difference between realists and antirealists, then, Fine argues, is that they go on to add to the common core further and unsupportable ontological additions.

Does Fine's argument apply to Van Fraassen and Cartwright?

Before going on to summarize those ontological additions, it is worth emphasizing that Fine's homely line would not be acceptable to Van Fraassen. He, by contrast, distinguishes between claims that would be regarded as of equal status by Fine because his distinction between claims made about observables and unobservables is revisionary of ordinary scientific practice. Things are less clear with regard to Cartwright and Hacking. There is some reason to believe that Cartwright's distrust of high-level explanatory scientific theories is itself an accurate reflection of scientific practice. This is certainly one of the arguments she presents for it. Scientists are, she suggests, pragmatically open to the use of any of a range of different and incompatible theories, selecting between them on the basis of usefulness. On the other hand, a sharp distinction between realism about theories and entities would be revisionary in that a well-established theory might well be accepted as having the same status as the claim that electrons exist.

Philosophical glosses

Fine then suggests that realists and antirealists add to the basic core position a further philosophical gloss. Antirealists might add an idealist theory of existence that is tied to human experience. Or they may construe the truth of a belief as coherence with our other beliefs or as being a useful belief, as some Pragmatists claim. Each of these modifications reinterprets the common core. Recall, however, that Van Fraassen suggested that there were two forms of antirealism. The first sort holds that science is or aims to be true, properly (but not literally) construed. The second holds that the language of science should be literally construed, but its theories need not be true to be good. On Fine's account, antirealism is of the former kind. Van Fraassen claimed that his Constructive Empiricism was of the latter. We will return to this distinction shortly.

What realism adds to the Natural Ontological Attitude

Fine's characterization of what a realist adds to the common core is simpler: 'what the realist adds on is a desk-thumping, foot-stamping shout of "Really!"'. The reason for this is that:

> The realist, as it were, tries to stand outside the arena watching the ongoing game [of science] and then tries to judge (from this external point of view) what the point is. It is, he says, about some area external to the game. The realist, I think, is fooling himself. For he cannot (really!) stand outside the arena, nor can he survey some area off the playing field and mark it out as what the game is about.
>
> (p. 131)

And antirealism?

In another paper, Fine (1984) offers a parallel criticism of anti-realists in the philosophy of science. Again he assumes that antirealists do not enter the nitty gritty of scientific disputes. They assume the same core beliefs about scientific entities as realists—the Natural Ontological Attitude again—but, like realists, offer a particular interpretation of their status. Where the realist adds a 'table thumping "Really"', the antirealist offers a particular account of what the truth of claims about entities or theories consists in. Rather than taking it to be a matter of correspondence with the facts—as realists typically do—they define it merely as an acceptable belief.

> [S]cientific anti-realists…, recently, have tried to promote some kind of consensus-cum-pragmatic picture. I will try to give this picture a canonical representation so that we can identify the features that these particular anti-realisms have in common. So

represented, it portrays the truth of a statement P as amounting to the fact that a certain class of subjects would accept P under a certain set of circumstances. If we let the subjects be 'perfectly rational' agents and the circumstances be 'ideal' ones for the purposes of the knowledge trade…, then we get the picture of truth as ideal rational acceptance…

> For the antirealism expressed in the idea of truth-as-acceptance is just as metaphysical and idle as the realism expressed by a correspondence theory.
>
> (pp. 360–361)

Natural Ontological Attitude without Philosophical additions

Realism and antirealism, then, attempt to add something to a common homely line, their shared NOA. Ergo, Fine suggests, the best philosophical response is to adopt the homely line, the NOA, as such, without adding anything further to it. One should adopt merely a NOA that is faithful to the beliefs and commitments of practising science. Thus the only guide to what is real within a given science is what those working within that science come to believe is real. What is real is defined solely by the praxis and related unfolding view of what is real which is internal to scientific work in a given area.

Philosophers, then, this line of argument implies, instead of working from an assumed perspective outside of science, should get stuck in. They should work in close partnership with scientists in particular disciplines—and this as we noted above, is what Fine has done. Philosophy cannot bring a fruitful external perspective to this issue. This is not to deny that philosophical reflection may have some bearing on what is real. But such reflection should be a proper part of scientific method and not an attempt at an Archimedean perspective from outside science.

But what is Fine's Natural Ontological Attitude really directed against?

Fine's account is attractive because of its simultaneous distancing from both realism and antirealism and because of its emphasis on a naturalistic solution. The degree of realism one should adopt to a subject matter should depend on the local scientific case for it. But it is also clear that Fine is characterizing a different kind of debate from the one with which we have been most concerned earlier in this session. The NOA is distinguished from realism and the latter is characterized as trying to say something further, something illicit. But in the discussion of Constructive Empiricism above, belief in specific claims about unobservables—which comprises a rejection of that form of ontological antirealism and which would often be part of a NOA—was called realism. Fine's description of realism appears to be not merely an opposition to a specific epistemological antirealist attack on some class of beliefs—unobservables, high-level theories—but a further claim in its own right. It is an attempt to step outside our practices and provide them with further philosophical foundations. While Fine is successful in casting doubt on the coherence of any such move, it is not clear that anyone should want to make it.

This point can be spelt out like this. Boyd and McMullin argued (as described above) that the best explanation of the success of science was that its theories (about unobservables) were approximately true and that this suggested that those theories were indeed approximately true. If this argument is construed as a piece of scientific reasoning—perhaps a standard piece of arguing from effects to inferred causes to block Van Fraassen's worry—it surely lies within the NOA and does not amount to a further tendentious form of realism.

If, on the other hand, it is adopted as an attempt to provide additional reassurance that the claims that science makes as true really are true, then it does amount to a further gratuitous form of realism and Fine's argument against it is well directed. What would be the point of this further claim? Against what position could it be directed? The most obvious answer is that it could be used against an ontological antirealist: someone who denied that we could begin to describe a world independent of us, that apparently world-involving claims are really claims about sense-data or ideas.

Thus Fine might be seen as running together issues that are best characterized as part of an epistemological debate and issues from an ontological debate. But his solution to both is a form of philosophical quietism. To determine those elements of a science in which one should believe, one should turn to the science itself. One should reject philosophical prescriptions about which beliefs are sound and which are not. A dispute about which scientific beliefs are sound is a matter for local resolution within the science concerned. One should refrain from attempts to provide extra-scientific foundations for resolving such disputes by saying, for example, that science as a whole must be right because it is successful. That amounts merely to a table-thumping cry of 'really!' and adds nothing to the debate.

Conclusions of the session

What conclusions can we now reach at the end of this session? We have seen that there has been considerable debate about the kind of inference that is justified within science in general, or at any rate particularly within physics, broadly speaking from observable to unobservable matters. Van Fraassen argues that such inference is never justified. McMullin argues that it is justified whenever it is grounded in an explanation of observable phenomena. Cartwright argues that it is justified but only if the explanations in question cite the causes of observable phenomena and not just higher-level theories from which the explanandum can be derived. Hacking adds to Cartwright's causal explanation, the importance of our ability directly to manipulate the (unobservable) causes in question.

Fine takes a different line which starts by diagnosing what he takes to be the problem with this kind of reflection in general. Fine suggests that if arguments about realism and antirealism are construed as attempts to validate—or undermine—scientific reasoning from a perspective outside science, then, although they highlight some of the difficulties of scientific reasoning, they cannot succeed in legislating for good scientific practice. This is because it is impossible to take the sort of external perspective on science that these arguments seem to require. We should thus be content with, Fine concludes, and work within, the NOA (Natural Ontological Attitude) found in and proper to a given science.

If on the other hand, reflections of the kind outlined in this session are seen as continuous with and part of a scientific perspective, then they are useful in a modest way: as reminders of the sorts of consideration that can be brought to bear in the sort of informal reasoning that even the hard sciences such as physics have to employ. This is broadly how, in the next and final session of this chapter, we will be using the ideas outlined in this session in relation to psychiatric classification. It is worth pointing out, however, that the specific suggestions of both Van Fraassen and Cartwright about what inferences one should draw, seem too simplistic. Sometimes belief in unobservables is justified in the circumstances and sometimes not. Sometimes there is good evidence for high-level theories and sometimes not. In fact, as we will see in Chapter 16, high-level theories often play a role as methodological guides and are held immune from refutation by the evidence. They serve as guides to the development over time of research programmes rather than as simple descriptions of the world.

Reflection on the session and self-test questions

Write down your own reflections on the materials in this session drawing out any points that are particularly significant for you. Then write brief notes about the following:

1. What are the three key elements of Van Fraassen's 'constructive empiricism'?

2. What is 'empirical adequacy' as defined by Van Fraassen?

3. Among other 'post-Logical Empiricist' philosophers of science, what key ideas about what science reveals are associated with each of the following:
   (a) Boyd and McMullen
   (b) Cartwright
   (c) Hacking.

4. Is Arthur Fine a realist or antirealist about science? What is the Natural Ontological Attitude?

5. On which science has recent philosophical work on validity (realism) been particularly focused? How are the implications of this work relevant to issues of validity in psychiatric classification?

6. What key idea relevant to issues of validity in psychiatric classifications do we owe to Fine?

Session 4 The third New Agenda – an Agenda modelled on the Philosophy of Physics

As psychiatry entered its post-Second World War phase in the development of its classifications, with the publication of ICD-6 from the WHO, it shared with the rest of medicine, and indeed with most other scientific disciplines, the traditional model of science outlined in Chapter 11. Theoretical physics aside, it was at this period still common ground among scientific disciplines, that what we get from empirical research is, if not *the* right way of seeing what the world is really like, then at any rate an ever closer *approximation* to the right way of seeing what the world is really like.

From one to many pictures

The philosophical project of Logical Empiricism, in the middle decades of the twentieth century, as we described in Chapter 12, aimed to put the traditional model of science on a rigorous basis by way of an in principle separation of the language of observation from the language of theory. The failure of Logical Empiricism, and subsequent work over the last 50 years in the philosophy of science, a sample of which we have examined in the last two sessions of this chapter, has shown that what we get from science, and hence what is captured in a scientific classification, is, in the terms of Sartorius' aphorism at the start of this chapter, not one but many ways of seeing the world. Somewhat like a photograph, then, the ways of seeing the world that we get from a science depend, among other things, on what kind of camera we use and on where we choose to point the camera. The picture also depends, as we will see in Chapters 14 and 15, on the judgements we make, implicit and explicit, when it comes to interpreting the resulting image.

From one to a family of classifications

One conclusion, then, from post-Logical Empiricist philosophy of science is that, in psychiatry as in physics, we need, at least in the present state of the development of the field, more than one picture, more than one classification. This conclusion is indeed anticipated to some extent by the WHO in its growing Family of International Classifications (the FIC, see http://www.who.int/classifications/en). In addition to the original International Classification of Diseases (the ICD, of which the Mental Disorders section is one chapter), the WHO's 'extended family' of classifications now includes an International Classification of Functioning (ICF) and a Classification of Psychosocial Stressors (CPS, at http://www3.who.int/icf/icftemplate.cfm). The American Psychiatric Association, similarly, includes within the one DSM family 'album', additional diagnostic criteria and nosological 'axes' covering much the same extended family members as the WHO's FIC (DSM includes criteria for social and occupational functioning, for example, to which we return in Part IV; and a separate axis for psychosocial stressors). Established clinical practice in psychiatry, too, reflects the need for more than one way of seeing the world in its diagnostic formulations. As we saw in Chapters 2 and 3, a diagnostic assessment in psychiatry is often summarized as a

'formulation' in which descriptively defined disorders (phobia, obsessional disorder, etc.) are separated out from possible aetiological factors (psychological and social as well as biological).

Is it rocket science?

So, someone may say, the bottom line is that we need more than one way of seeing the world—that's hardly rocket science! But a second conclusion from post-Logical Empiricist philosophy of science is that, well, actually, in psychiatry as in physics, classification, to the extent that it reflects the ways that we see the world at a point in time, really *is* rocket science.

Post-Logical Empiricist philosophy of science has replaced the relatively simple picture of the traditional model with something more like a kaleidoscope. We have touched on some of the complexities involved in understanding what science (notably physical science) is about, as revealed by post-Logical Empiricist philosophy of science, in Session 3. We will be looking at these and at other aspects of this complexity in more detail in later chapters in this Part. But this second conclusion—that psychiatry, like physics, is a very *difficult* science—is fundamental in its own right. Run the story of psychiatric classification only from the publication of DSM-III, and the disaggregation of psychiatry's classifications into a family of different ways of seeing the world has all the implications of failure carried by Kupfer *et al.*'s (2002) *Research Agenda for DSM-V*. Take the story back a few years further to the critical move, with the Lewis/Sartorius ICD-8, from an aetiological to a descriptive basis for a classification designed primarily for the purposes of international epidemiological and statistical studies, and the subsequent evolution of psychiatric science towards a family of classifications reflecting different ways of seeing the world appropriate for other and different purposes, becomes a success. Take the story back further still, with Lewis to the second century BC, and the emergence for the first time of a genuine *family* of classifications, in place of the two millennia of disparate and often competing ways of understanding mental distress and disorder that we reviewed in Chapter 7, becomes a truly *remarkable* success.

Risks and challenges

There are risks and challenges here, of course. Families, especially extended families, all too readily become dysfunctional. We return below to a number of pointers from the philosophy of science to the requirements for developing and sustaining a fully functional family of ways of understanding mental distress and disorder. One particular challenge, furthermore, to which as we saw Kupfer *et al.*'s (2002) *Research Agenda for DSM-V* clearly points, is that measured against the standards of the 'nuclear families' of bodily medicine, the well-defined unitary classifications of cardiology, gastroenterology, and so forth, measured against these traditional nuclear families of bodily medicine, the extended family of psychiatric classifications may appear dangerously 'free thinking', a nosological equivalent of the threat to traditional family life posed by the 'post-modern' anything goes.

This is a serious threat to which, again, we return below (under Agenda Item 9, on 'process issues') and at the end of the chapter.

How we respond to this challenge, we will argue, how we respond to the challenge of living within a diverse family of classifications, will critically determine whether psychiatry's extended family of ways of understanding mental distress and disorder is a functional or dysfunctional *scientific* family. But as to the *need* for an extended rather than traditional nuclear family in psychiatry, this is a reflection, no more and no less, of the fact that the psychiatric sciences, like the physical sciences, are, inherently and irreducibly, difficult sciences, delivering, at least at this stage in their development, different and not always fully commensurable ways of seeing the world.

Physical science and psychiatric science

We should be careful not to push the parallels between physics and psychiatry too far. The parallels are there, and, we will suggest below, important. But there are also antiparallels: in physics rigorous conceptual thinking is readily formalized in available mathematics; in physics the domains of application of different pictures of the world are in general easily distinguished (relativity for the large scale, quantum mechanics for the small scale—although the interface between these pictures remains highly problematic); and, crucially, in physics the 'objects of study' are particles, whereas, in psychiatry, the 'objects of study' are people—not, as the use of the term 'objects of study' might imply, theoretical entities or abstract scientific concepts, but *real* people. This last difference between psychiatry and physics is one that we have already seen, in Part II, adds a whole extra dimension of difficulty to psychiatric science, the dimension of personal meanings, of significance, of empathy and of understanding. We pick up on this extra dimension of difficulty later in this part, in Chapter 15 on Reasons and Causes, and again in Part V.

The third agenda – an agenda for an extended family of classifications

In the remainder of this fourth session we will be drawing together some of the indications particularly from post-Logical Empiricist philosophy of science for the further development of an extended family of ways of understanding mental distress and disorder, an extended family that seeks to build on the families already emerging from the ICD and DSM processes.

The indications from the philosophy of science for the future evolution of psychiatric classifications are conjectural, of course, and wide open to refutation in the event. Physics, the paradigm science from which these conjectural indications are largely taken, is, as we noted immediately above, in key respects different from psychiatry. One of the lessons, furthermore, from the 1959 conference on classification described in Session 1, is that the best informed conjectures from the philosophy of science are open to refutation in the event. Hempel's confident conclusion that psychiatry would proceed along its established course towards ever-more theoretical classifications, was refuted, in the event, by psychiatry going in precisely the opposite direction. The purpose of conjecture, though, as the British philosopher of science, Sir Karl Popper, pointed out (Popper, 1963—we met Popper in Chapter 11 and return to him in Chapter 16), is not to be 'proved right'. It is rather to establish hypotheses that can then be 'refuted'

(or otherwise) in the event. The purpose of conjecture, which Popper argued in science could and should often be *wild* conjecture, is precisely to lay oneself open to refutation in the event. As we will see in Chapter 16, the Hungarian philosopher of science, Imre Lakatosh, took this idea further, suggesting that it was at the heart of the distinctive way in which progress is made in science.

And it may be your ideas (your wild conjectures, even) rather than ours, that, as we have repeatedly emphasized in this book, turn out to be the ones that emerge and flourish! Before, therefore, pursuing further our ideas for an Extended Family of Psychiatric Classifications, the next exercise asks you to take some time going back carefully over the materials in this chapter by way of developing your own ideas on how psychiatric classifications should develop from here.

EXERCISE 22   (30 minutes)

In this exercise we want you to take a broad overview of the materials covered in this chapter (including, where relevant, their underpinnings from other sections of the book) and to consider their implications for the future of psychiatric diagnostic classification.

Consider in particular two questions:

1. what contributions might the philosophy of science have to make to future developments in psychiatric classification, and

2. how best might these contributions be made?

In answering these two questions, use the agenda items adopted above for our Conceptual Agendas respectively for ICD-9 (Figure 13.2) and DSM-V (Figure 13.1). What are the similarities, and what are the differences, between these two Agendas and a new philosophy-of-science driven *Agenda for an Extended Family of Classifications*?

By way of example, we have already covered ideas relevant to three of the first four items on the Agenda in the above run-up to this exercise. The *Agenda for an Extended Family of Classifications* will take, under Agenda Item 1, its time line, with Aubrey Lewis, from at least the classical period, albeit concentrating, with DSM-V, on the modern history of ideas. Under Agenda Item 2, the Uses of Classification, the *Agenda for an Extended Family of Classifications* will adopt, again with Aubrey Lewis, a 'horses for courses' approach, recognizing the need for different classifications for different purposes. Unlike, however, both the ICD and DSM Agendas, the *Agenda for an Extended Family of Classifications*, under Agenda Item 4 (we return to 3 below) will admit any charge of deficit scientific status only to the extent that theoretical physics, too, in adopting a family of ways of seeing the world at this point in time, is vulnerable to a charge of deficit scientific status. (We return to this key issue in more detail below.)

So, at this point on the Agenda, it is over to you.

As before, write down our own ideas using the agenda items adopted above for both ICD-9 and DSM-V, before reading on. This is a 'Star Trek' exercise in which we 'boldly go', as the famous split infinitive has it, where no one has been before. So, be bold; you may well have better ideas than us!

Here are our ideas for a future Extended Family of Classifications of Mental Disorder, as guided by ideas from the philosophy of science. As in the exercise, we have ordered our ideas broadly according to the agenda items developed for the corresponding Conceptual Research Agendas for ICD-9 and DSM-V. Table 13.4, below, gives a comparative table of the three agendas summarizing the main continuities and differences between them. As you read through the following materials critical review our suggestions under each agenda item and compare them with your own.

Agenda Item 3. The Misuses of Classification

We start, then, picking up from the agenda items covered in the run up to Exercise 22, with Agenda Item 3, the Misuses of Classification. Here, post-Logical Empiricist philosophy of science puts a rather different interpretation on the concerns of both the ICD-9 and DSM-V Agendas. In the ICD-9 Agenda, Lewis was concerned with classifications becoming overextended. In the *DSM-V* Agenda, Kupfer *et al.*, as Editors (in their Introduction), and indeed Rounsaville *et al.* in chapter 1, were concerned with inappropriate reification of psychiatry's diagnostic concepts. Both sets of

Table 13.4 The Third New Agenda – an Agenda for an Extended Family of Classifications – compared with first and second new agendas

Agenda Items	ICD-9 (agenda 2 above)	DSM-V (agenda 1 above)	Extended Family of Classifications (agenda 3)
(1) Time-line	Back: to 2nd century BC	Back: to DSM-III Forward: to DSM-VI/VII	Back: at least to ICD-8 Forward: to ICD-12/DSM-VI
(2) Uses of psychiatric classification	Epidemiological and statistical	Diagnosis by clinicians	Multiple: different uses of different (coexisting) classifications in different contexts and for different purposes
(3) Misuses of psychiatric classification	Overextension	Reification of categories	Multiple: What counts as a 'misuse' of a scientific classification is context and purpose specific
(4) Status of psychiatric science	Deficit model	Deficit model	Strengths model: Deficit model is *rejected outright* in favour of a strengths model as the basis of progress
(5) Concepts	Concepts recognised as problematic	Important; but not recognised	Strengths model opens up resources for conceptual research hand in hand with empirical research
(6) Reliability	THE BIG ISSUE	Run out of steam	Reliability a small, but still *necessary*, first step to validity
(7) Validity	Assumed to follow reliability	THE BIG ISSUE	Multiple validities appropriate for an *Extended* Family of Classifications but all based on scientific criteria
(8) Structural solution	Descriptive symptom-based criteria	Aetiology based	Different classificatory structures needed for different purposes and ranges of application
(9) Process solutions	Collegiality, international collaboration, different perspectives and a shared aim	Empirical research	THE BIG ISSUE: *two* rules of (observational) science: (1) challenge received authority, and (2) listen instead to what the world (whether of 'particles' as in physics or of 'people' as in psychiatry) has to say.
(10) Utility (of new classifications)	'Public' classifications (like ICD): for (international) epidemiological and statistical purposes. 'Private' classifications: for 'local' use for particular research programmes and other specific purposes.	Better health-care services	Improved face validity: 1) results in improved communication between professionals and patients and between different professional groups, and 2) a step to improved construct validity
(11) Overall tenor	Upbeat	Downbeat	Upbeat, based on: (1) observational science, (2) challenge to received authority, (3) enough time
(12) Any other business	none	none	*New resources*: from the neurosciences, the mental sciences, national policy initiatives, and international networks *Next steps*: depend on (1) continued research initiatives, and (2) a successful 'Renaissance science' challenge to received authority

concerns, in the context of the ICD-9 and DSM-V Agendas, represent conflicts with the traditional model: Lewis' implied contrast is between the overextended classifications of medieval taxonomy and the neat compression of information in such classifications as the chemical periodic table; the DSM-V's explicit contrast is between psychiatry's descriptive categories and the aetiological information packed into the disease concepts of bodily medicine in disciplines such as cardiology.

Post-Logical Empiricist philosophy of science, while endorsing these concerns as potential misuses of classification, suggests that the difference between use and *misuse*, between appropriate and *in*appropriate uses of classification, is context and purpose dependent. We return to this idea below, under issues of validity. It arises partly from the difficulty of 'fixing' the sense in which a scientific classification is properly about what science is about (i.e. the 'real' world); partly from the work of Arthur Fine and others suggesting that what is 'real', and hence which classifications are valid, is a matter for local determination within particular scientific disciplines; and partly from issues of utility, i.e. the many different ways in which values comes into science, including, the 'context of interest' of explanations (see Chapter 14), the epistemic values that Quine and others have argued are necessary (though of course not sufficient) determinants of theory choice, and the pragmatic considerations that arise in applying the results of scientific research in this or that particular practical context.

All of which, to repeat an oft-made but oft-needed point, is not to say that 'anything goes'. Post-Logical Empiricist philosophy of science gives no warrant to that version of postmodernism that would have us believe that any classification, any way of seeing the world, is as 'good' as any other. Certainly, a classification can become overextended: some have argued that with their increasing size and complexity, both ICD and DSM are perilously close to becoming overextended, at least for clinical purposes. Certainly, too, classificatory concepts can be inappropriately reified: the considerations of Part I of this book amount to a critique of the inappropriate reification of concepts of disorder, equally by opponents and supporters of the concept of mental illness, where 'inappropriate' reification means taking disorders to be real in the way that stars and stones are real independently of human values. But the key point here is that what counts as a *misuse* of a classification, what makes a classification *over*extended, what is *inappropriate* reification of classificatory concepts, is not something to be judged against a generic standard of what a scientific classification should be like. What counts as a misuse of classificatory concepts has to be judged rather on the particulars of a given science according to the state of development of that science and the purposes for which the classification in question is to be used.

Agenda Item 4. Status of Psychiatric Science

An easy one, this, to a first approximation at least—as noted in Exercise 22 (above), what is good enough for the complex science of theoretical physics (i.e. a family of ways of seeing the world), is good enough for the complex science of psychiatry.

Given, however, the importance of correcting the deficit model of psychiatric science, as a key aspect of the twentieth century stigmatization of psychiatry as an 'also ran' to bodily medicine (see Part I), it will be worth spelling out just how radically an *Agenda for an Extended Family of Classifications of Mental Disorder*, drawing particularly on the philosophy of physics, differs from both Lewis' *Agenda for ICD-9* and Kupfer *et al.*'s *Agenda for DSM-V*, in its view of how the status of psychiatric science should be understood. The ICD-9 and the DSM-V Agendas, as we have seen, are alike in embodying deficit models of psychiatric science, and hence of psychiatric classifications. The *Agenda for an Extended Family of Classifications*, by contrast, drawing on the resources of a philosophy of science focusing on physics, not only rejects any form of deficit model but also actively embraces a *strengths* model.

The move from deficit to strengths model in the *Extended Family of Classifications of Mental Disorder* is anticipated by earlier discussions in this book: the 'full-field' picture of the conceptual structure of psychiatry to which we came in Part I, offers, we argued by extension from Austin's observations on the heuristic significance of conceptual difficulties in general, a window on conceptual elements of medicine (patients' experiences, agency, and values) that, although important in all areas of health care, remain partially hidden and hence (relatively) neglected in areas of bodily medicine where these elements are (relatively) unproblematic. Similarly, then, here, the added difficulties of psychiatric classification may indeed turn out to provide a window on aspects of medical classification, medical ways of seeing the world, that, although important, have tended to remain relatively hidden because they are relatively unproblematic and hence have been relatively neglected (to date) in other (less conceptually difficult) areas of medicine.

Three steps to a strengths model

So how, exactly, do we get from deficits to strengths? The move from a deficit to a strengths model of psychiatric classification, as developed here particularly by way of the resources of the philosophy of physics, involves three steps. The *first step* is the recognition of the structural similarities between psychiatry and physics: (1) their shared conceptual as well as empirical difficulties (in neither discipline are the meanings of their key terms of art—time, space, particle, mental, illness, etc.—capable of full explication beyond operational definitions for particular purposes); (2) their shared difficulties about the separation between observer and observed (remember the EPR (Einstein–Podolsky–Rosen) paradox in Chapter 12); and (3) their shared need for more than one classification, more than one way of seeing the world.

That psychiatry shares with theoretical physics these structural similarities, however, is capable of different interpretations. This brings us to the *second step* in the move from deficit to strengths model, a step that depends crucially on post-Logical Empiricist philosophy of science. In a traditional understanding of science, the structural similarities between psychiatry and theoretical physics point, perhaps surprisingly, to a deficit model of the physical sciences rather than to a strengths model of psychiatric science. This is surprising because the physical sciences are the traditional paradigm of hard sciences and theoretical physics is at the cutting edge of the physical sciences. However, the difficulties of definition of the key terms of art in theoretical physics, its problems of separating observer from observed, and its need for more than one (mutually incommensurable) way of seeing the world, are all, by the standards of the traditional model of science, signs of deficit as much for theoretical physics as for psychiatry. (Recall in this respect, from Chapter 12, that Einstein conceived the EPR paradox precisely to show that quantum mechanics is, literally, absurd by the tenets of traditional scientific realism. See also d'Espagnat, 1976.)

Post-Logical Empiricist philosophy of science, by contrast, stands this story on its head. Focusing on what, in particular, theoretical physics is *really* like, as distinct from what it *should* look like according to the traditional model, post-Logical Empiricist philosophy of science shows that these structural features, although particularly transparent in psychiatry and physics, are indeed features of *all* sciences. As Austin would have anticipated, we notice these structural features of all sciences where they cause difficulty. But the fact that they cause difficulty in, of all sciences, theoretical physics, suggests that difficulties with these structural features are not a feature of a deficient science but, to the contrary, of a science at the cutting edge. By extension, therefore, the appearance of the same structural difficulties in psychiatry suggests that psychiatric science, too, is a science at the cutting edge.

There are, as we noted above in the run-up to Exercise 22 at the start of this session, important differences as well as similarities between theoretical physics and psychiatry. These differences bring us to the *third step* in the move from a deficit to a strengths model of psychiatric science. For the third step is to see that, by the lights of post-Logical Empiricist philosophy of science, the differences between theoretical physics and psychiatry, as much as the similarities, are a sign of the strengths of psychiatric science not of deficit.

The strengths—rather than deficit—implications of the differences between theoretical physics and psychiatry are well illustrated by the relatively value-laden nature of psychiatric science. Thus, as we saw in Session 2 of this chapter, post-Logical Empiricist philosophy of science has shown that the traditional opposition between science and values (their supposed immiscibility as we called it), is not sustainable: attempts to hang on to a traditional value-free model of science have (so far) failed; and, conversely, the importance of values has been directly demonstrated in a number of key stages of the scientific process (including observation, theory choice, and applications of the outputs from science to practice).

A key difference, however, among the differences that we noted above between physics and psychiatry, is that psychiatry is concerned not with particles but with *people*. This, indeed, we said, is a *key* difference between what psychiatry is about compared with what physics is about. Combine, therefore, the post-Logical Empiricist demonstration of the presence of values in all areas of

science, with the demonstration in Part I of this book that psychiatry is value-laden because (following Hare) it is concerned with aspects of human experience and behaviour (emotion, sexuality, belief, etc.), in which human values are characteristically diverse, and the value-laden nature of psychiatric classifications emerges, not as a sign of a deficient science, but as a sign of a science that is properly reflective of a key aspect of the nature of what, as a science, psychiatry, in contrast with physics, is really about, i.e. people.

From deficit to strengths to progress

We have spent some time on this particular Item on the Agenda for psychiatric classification because the deficit model of psychiatric science is so deeply embedded in the lay as well as scientific (including psychiatric scientific) mind. The move from deficit to strengths model, correspondingly, is liable to be dismissed as wishful thinking equally by psychiatry's opponents and by its supporters. Merely adopting a strengths model is no guarantee of progress, of course. But the move from deficit to strengths model is the basis of a series of further moves, summarized in the rest of our Agenda for an *Extended Family of Classifications*, that together open up the space within which, we argued at the start of this session, progress will become possible.

Agenda Item 5. Concepts

The importance of moving from a deficit to a strengths model of psychiatric science in opening up the space needed to make progress possible is well illustrated by the different ways in which concepts of disorder are treated, on the one hand in the ICD-9 and DSM-V Agendas, and, on the other, in the Agenda for an *Extended Family of Classifications*.

The ICD-9 and DSM-V Agendas both recognize the importance of conceptual difficulties in relation to psychiatric classification. For both, though, working within a deficit model, these difficulties are inevitably taken to reflect deficiencies in psychiatric science. To this point, then, the deficit model does no more than take us back to the considerations of Part I. However, the importance of moving to a strengths model becomes clear when we come, in chapter 1 of Kupfer *et al.*'s *Research Agenda for DSM-V*, to the proposals advanced there for tackling these difficulties. For despite implicitly acknowledging the conceptual nature of these difficulties, the proposals in the *DSM-V Agenda* for tackling them are limited, as within a traditional model of science they are necessarily limited, to proposals for empirical (rather than conceptual) research.

Conceptual alongside empirical methodologies

We return to the specifics of the DSM-V proposals for empirical research on concepts below (under Agenda Item 9, Process). However, the point for now is that in limiting itself to the deficit model of psychiatry embedded in the traditional model of science, Kupfer *et al.*'s *Research Agenda for DSM-V* thereby cuts itself off from the now considerable resources available for conceptual research in general and research on values in particular. Just how productive working with these additional resources will prove to be, only time will tell. However, as we saw in Part I, Austin's concept of philosophical fieldwork, which is entirely consistent with *starting* with empirical studies of broadly the kind proposed by Rounsaville *et al.*, in Chapter 1 of the *Research Agenda for DSM-V*, has already yielded tangible results (Colombo *et al.*'s, 2003, work on models of disorder, and other examples in the Reading Guide to Chapter 4); and, as we will see in Part IV, similar work on values is already finding its way into policy and practice in mental health in a number of countries around the world.

Agenda Item 6. Reliability

Reliability, as we saw in Session 1, was the big issue for the ICD-9 Agenda. Correspondingly, much of psychiatric science in the last three decades of the twentieth century (covering the periods of both ICD-9 and -10, and DSM-III and -IV) has been concerned with improving the reliability of our diagnostic methods in relation both to assessments of psychopathology, as we saw in Chapter 12, and, as we noted in Session 1 of this chapter, in relation to the categories in our diagnostic classifications (references to a sample of classic reliability studies are given in the Reading Guide).

The danger now, though, so long as psychiatry continues to operate within the limited space provided by a deficit model of its science, is, as we noted in the final part of Session 1 of this chapter, the danger of throwing out the baby with the bathwater, the danger of losing what we had gained. The danger is that our hard won improvements in reliability will be thrown out with what is perceived within a deficit model of psychiatric science as the failure of validity. This 'failure' has been the basis of growing criticisms from, among others, but importantly, some of those most directly concerned in the new neurosciences (e.g. Hyman and Fenton, 2003). But the danger of losing what we had gained is also signalled in Kupfer *et al.*'s *Research Agenda for DSM-V* itself, by the frustration that shows through in the language used to describe this supposed failure—you will recall the shift in Kupfer *et al.*'s terminology between the two readings early in Session 1, from a 'limited' classification paradigm (linked with Exercise 1) to a long catalogue of total 'failures' of validity (linked with Exercise 2).

Reliability is only a step...

The danger here, of losing the gains that with so much hard labour we have made, is mitigated by going back to the very modest claims for reliability made by Hempel and Lewis at the time of the 1959 conference. Hempel, you will recall, made only a more or less passing reference to reliability as something that, as a concern particularly of the social and psychological sciences, coincided with the importance of the concepts on which scientific classifications are based having, as one of his two key requirements, Empirical Import. Lewis, similarly, when he introduced into the discussion following Hempel's paper, his distinction between public and private classifications, emphasized that international agreement (i.e. reliability) in the use of a classification was important only for the limited purposes (which of course were the WHO's purposes in developing ICD) of international epidemiological work and statistical reporting.

...but a necessary step

Reliability, then, as an aspect of the observational basis of a science, and even within Logical Empiricism as a version of the traditional model that placed so much emphasis on the observational basis of science, is only a step towards what science is really about, the development of theory. It is important in this respect not to lose sight of the excitement and sense of promise that went with the appearance of new and more reliable classifications, outside as well as within psychiatry: the *New York Post* (28 July 1963) heralded Robert Spitzer's work as Chair of the DSM-III Taskforce, under a headline 'Approach Holds Promise for Standardized Diagnostic Aid', describing DSM-III as 'a tool which may become the psychiatrist's thermometer and microscope and x-ray machine rolled into one'.[2]

The disappointment that things have not moved so fast and so far as anticipated, is, as we have seen, at the heart of current disenchantment, at least as expressed in Kupfer *et al.*'s *Research Agenda for DSM-V*, with our present day classifications. Hempel, no doubt, would have shared the frustration of today's psychiatric scientists, among others, both those without and those within the DSM process, that the anticipated progress from reliability to validity, has been, at best, faltering. But, and this is the big 'but' that we explored in the last part of Session 1, reliability, even as measured by a more careful reading of Hempel, *is* a step. Just exactly what that step consists in and how it may lead to validity is a matter for further debate. It may be that reliability, as Kendell argued in his 1975 book on classification, is a limiting step, i.e. that validity can never be greater than reliability (Kendell, 1975). It may be that reliability, as we concluded in the last part of Session 1 of this chapter, is a necessary step to the ultimate shared goal of validity. Either way, though, miss the first step of reliability, and we risk finding ourselves back where we started, in a nosological Tower of Babel.

Agenda Item 7. Validity

If the big issue for Lewis' *Agenda for ICD-9* was reliability, the big issue for Kupfer *et al.*'s *Research Agenda for DSM-V*, as we saw in Session 1, is validity. Given, as noted under Agenda Item 6 (Reliability), the disappointing (from the traditional point of view) rate of conversion of reliability into validity, the emphasis on issues of validity in the *Research Agenda for DSM-V* is no surprise. What is a surprise, though, at first sight, is the line on validity taken in chapter 1 of the *Research Agenda for DSM-V*, by Rounsaville and colleagues (2002) on conceptual issues (the chapter, you will recall, titled 'Basic nomenclature issues for DSM-V'). The surprise is that so much of the discussion of validity, although explicitly focused on the 'uses of validity in psychiatric nosology' (p. 7), is taken up, not, as one might expect from the traditional model, with explanatory theories, with prediction, with underlying regularities, and with hidden entities and causal laws. The discussion, when it comes to the crunch, the crunch of the 'Rationale for Changing Criteria' in the move from DSM-IV

---

[2] With thanks to Giovanni Stanghellini for spotting this.

to DSM-V (pp. 10–11), is largely taken up with social and political issues.

Social and political validators?

'Traditionally', this section starts, 'when changes in criteria in a diagnostic system are contemplated, the positive features of such changes (e.g. improvements in reliability or validity, greater ease of use, or superior discriminatory ability) are emphasized'. Well, if that is 'traditional', surely, with suitable extensions of the 'e.g.' (expanding, e.g., validity to face, predictive and construct validity), these are not merely 'positive' features but features of what science, and hence the categories in a scientific classification, are all about. Yet Rounsaville *et al.*, instead of enlarging on the requirements for scientific validity, list some the 'disadvantages' of changing categories, disadvantages that, at first glance, appear to have little or nothing to do with what science is about: (1) confusing busy clinicians; (2) having to change report forms; (3) prejudicing the cumulative capacity of research (because meta-analyses require stable categories over time); (4) having to trade being thought 'old fashioned' against the need for longitudinal studies; (5) the need to develop new structured interviews; (6) the spawning of 'cottage industries' to assess the validity of new categories when research budgets are so limited; and (no surprise this one given the deficit model) (7) 'the possibility that frequent changes of diagnostic category can potentially discredit the revision process and increase the chances of the DSM becoming a subject of ridicule' (all from pp. 10–11). Small wonder, then, that Rounsaville *et al.* conclude, in the final paragraph of this section, that no 'compelling guidelines' for changing criteria can be given. They note, instead, a number of points to be taken into consideration, points that are important but again more of a political and social than (traditional) scientific nature (e.g. bias among committee members and the pressures of career advancement).

There are warning signs here, then, under this agenda item for validity as under the last for reliability, of the scientific baby being thrown out with the bath water. Faced with the failure (as the deficit model of psychiatric science sees it) of the ICD and DSM processes to date, Rounsaville *et al.* in this chapter of the *Research Agenda for DSM-V*, appear to be at risk of giving up on what science is about (what the world is really like) and of retreating to what science is decidedly not about (what we, individually and collectively, would like the world to be really like). Rounsaville *et al.*, it is important to emphasize, in their opening reference to the 'traditional validators' noted above, call these 'positive features'; and the points they make in the concluding paragraph of this section of their chapter, are all points of warning against prejudicing good scientific process by social and political factors. The baby is to this extent still in the bath. However, their discussion of the traditional validators occupies considerably fewer column inches than those devoted to the social and political factors guiding (in their view) category change. Moreover, their bottom line observation on the traditional validators, in an earlier section of their chapter, was that, since the traditional validators often

point in different directions (predictive validity, for example, pointing in a different direction from family aggregation), assessing the validity of this or that category necessarily depends on a prior choice between validators, a choice which, they say, 'Unfortunately . . . is fundamentally a value judgement' (Rounsaville *et al.*, 2002, p. 8).

Validity is of course a large topic that has generated a considerable and often ingenious literature within psychiatry as well as in related disciplines such as psychology and sociology (see, for example Robbins and Guze, 1970; and Schaffner 1986 and 1993 in the Reading Guide). Our aim in this chapter, however, has not been to review this rich literature, but rather to indicate the potential resources from the philosophy of science for further strengthening the psychiatric literature on validity. Hempel, for example, drawing on the resources of Logical Empiricism and related positivist literatures in the philosophy of science, has much to offer that remains highly relevant: his check-list of key criteria for Systematic Import, for example, his Systematicity Check List as it might now be called, still bears detailed study (Hempel, 1961, pp. 327–328). And the further resources of more recent post-Logical Empiricist philosophy of science open up yet further interpretive resources for current debates.

Differentiating claims

Post-Logical Empiricist philosophy of science, for example, suggests a number of interpretations of the recent claim by Kendell and Jablensky (2003), reflecting similar claims in both the ICD-9 and DSM-V Agendas, that clinicians should think of diagnostic categories as 'simply concepts, justified only by whether they provide a useful framework for organizing and explaining the complexity of clinical experience in order to derive inferences about outcome and to guide decisions about treatment' (Kendell and Jablensky, 2003, p. 5). Kendell and Jablensky may, for example, be advocating something like Van Fraassen's Constructive Empiricism: a form of agnosticism about whether psychiatric classification is really valid. On the other hand, the success of a classification (if it is successful) in guiding treatment, in successfully intervening in subjects' health, might provide arguments for supposing the classification to be valid, arguments that would follow the work of Cartwright and Hacking in emphasizing, respectively, causal-predictive power and practical manipulation of unobservable entities (in this case disease entities). Or, again, Kendell and Jablensky may be claiming something stronger: that classificatory categories could not possibly be anything more than 'mere concepts', constructs that are neither true nor false to the 'real' world but merely help to organize data. That would be a form of instrumentalism. If so, then Fine's work suggests that the claim risks foundering on an attempt to step outside the NOA (Natural Ontological Attitude) proper to psychiatric science.

To those responsible for developing the next editions of psychiatry's classifications, rich as the additional interpretive resources of post-Logical Empiricist philosophy of science may be in principle, in practice these resources may seem merely to add further and unwarranted complications to an already daunting task. Certainly the issues *are* complicated. The burden of this chapter is after all that just below the surface, as it were, of the problems of validity in psychiatric classifications, lie the deep philosophical issues of realism, idealism, essentialism, and so forth, issues that in two and half millennia the brightest and best have been able to explore only in small part, and issues that in the hardest of hard sciences, theoretical physics, are today very much where the scientific action is. We pick up on further closely related and equally problematic issues, particularly as they relate to scientific theory (Hempel's Systematic Import), in later chapters of this part: the nature of explanation in Chapter 14, of causal explanation in Chapter 15, and of progress in science in Chapter 16.

No compromises

Still, if the issues *are* complicated, it would surely not be consistent with the demand for rigour in science that, for 'practical' purposes, the issues should be artificially simplified. We would not consider compromising the evidence-base of our science. Neither should we compromise its conceptual base. All of which is not to say that everything should somehow go on hold while a two-and-a-half-millennium debate about realism is suddenly and conveniently resolved! To the contrary, as in all areas of science, we should get on with doing what is do-able. And there are indeed 'quick wins' to be had in the move from a deficit to a strengths model of psychiatric science drawing on the resources of post-Logical Empiricist philosophy of science. Some of these quick wins, it is true, will perhaps not be so very quick in that they will require a shift of paradigm in the processes by which psychiatric science, and its corresponding classifications, are developed. We return to 'process' issues below, under our Agenda Item 9 for the *Extended Family of Classifications*, towards which, we have argued, developments in both ICD and DSM are already pointing.

But some quick wins to be had

Other quick wins, however, in moving from a deficit to a strengths model of psychiatric science, could be more or less immediate. Break, for example, the Procrustean bed of a single way of seeing the world assumed by the traditional model, and Rounsaville *et al.*'s observation that different validators may point in different directions ceases to be, as in a deficit model of psychiatric science, a source of confusion and conflict, and becomes, in a strengths model, a resource (i.e. of different ways of seeing the world across different domains of application and for different purposes). Break, similarly, the assumption of the traditional model that values and science are immiscibility, and the fact that, as Rounsaville *et al.* point out, the choice of validators involves value judgements, ceases to be, as in a deficit model of psychiatric science, a matter for regret (recall Rounsaville *et al.*'s word, 'unfortunately'), and becomes in a strengths model an insightful observation of the extent to which, in psychiatry as in physics, we may need, at least in the present state of development of our respective sciences, different ways of seeing the world for different purposes. Break,

finally, the assumption of the traditional medical-scientific model that the (rightly celebrated) successes of the explanatory 'disease entities' (categorical and continuous) of the sciences underpinning bodily medicine warrants the adoption of essentially similar explanatory entities in the very different (and very much more difficult) sciences underpinning psychological medicine, break this myth and Rounsaville *et al.*'s conclusion noted above that 'no compelling guidelines' can be given for changing the categories in a psychiatric classification, ceases to be, as in a deficit model it inevitably is, an acknowledgement of (at least temporary) failure, and becomes in a strengths model a direct parallel of Arthur Fine's conclusion from symmetric issues in the physical sciences, that validity is irreducibly an issue for local debate and local assessment and balancing of the evidence.

Agenda Item 8. Structural Solutions

With Lewis, in our *Conceptual Research Agenda for ICD-9*, the structural 'solution', as we have seen, was to move from a theoretical (aetiology-based) to a predominantly descriptive (symptom-based) classification. In Kupfer *et al.*'s *Research Agenda for DSM-V*, there are suggestions that it may be time to move back the other way, to reintroduce theory: e.g. Kupfer *et al.*'s talk of the need for 'fundamental changes' (2002, p. xviii), for 'an as yet unknown paradigm shift' (2002, p. xix). There is of course, as Hempel emphasized in his 1959 paper (published in 1961), everything to gain in moving on when the time is right from a descriptive to a more theoretical stage in the development of a science. The concern, though, with this move as it is discussed in Kupfer *et al.*'s *Research Agenda for DSM-V*, is that it is motivated, not, as Hempel would have required, by explanatory success, but, consistently with the deficit model of psychiatric science, by (perceived) explanatory failure. We have noted a wide variety of the deficit terms used in Kupfer *et al.*'s *Research Agenda for DSM-V*. The danger, then, in making a move back to theory, if the move is motivated by a deficit model of psychiatric science, is that we will end up back where we started in the 1950s, in, as we put it above, a nosological Tower of Babel.

When the time is right...

It is no part of the role of philosophy to determine when the time is right for a structural change in a science. Fine's work, as we have seen, on the NOA and realism in physics, makes this point particularly clearly. Hempel, too, in his 1959 paper, held back from providing other than generic criteria for judging when the time is right for moving from Empirical Import to Systematic Import. As to specific theories, furthermore, as to whether psychiatry should develop on the basis of biological, psychodynamic or some other theory or combination of theories altogether, Hempel, as we noted above, made a point of staying strictly neutral.

There is, though, without anticipating future substantive developments in psychiatric theory, at least one clear structural implication of post-Logical Empiricist philosophy of science for psychiatric classification, a structural implication that as we will see, underpins the crucial 'process' issues to which we will turn in a moment. The structural implication in question has to do with the nature of the Extended Family of Classifications to which, we suggested above, developments in both ICD and DSM are already pointing.

...as judged by those directly concerned

Thus, in the traditional model, with its core assumption of one (true) way of seeing what the world is really like, any family of classifications must have a 'head of family'. There must be, as it were, a top classification, closer to what the world is really like than other classifications, and a classification to which, therefore, other classifications are subordinate. We need to be clear here: it is essential to the scientific process (as we will see in Chapter 16) that there should be lively competition between different ways of seeing the world. But the competition has to be run by the rules of science. And what we learn from post-Logical Empiricist philosophy of science, guided remember by the example of physics, is: (1) that the rules of science allow for heterogeneous classificatory structures, different ways of seeing the world, to coexist (across different domains of application and for different purposes); (2) that where competition does arise, there is no pre-assigned vantage point from outside the science in question by which the 'winner' at a given point in time is to be judged; and (3) that 'winning' is a matter for local judgement between—and this takes us directly to the key point for process—the stakeholders directly concerned.

Agenda Item 9. Process Solutions

With the structural issues in place, there is a simple, though fundamental, and to some of those concerned fundamentally ill-conceived, point to make about process. The fundamental point about process is this: if the development of an Extended Family of Psychiatric Classifications, guided by post-Logical Empiricist philosophy of science focusing on the model of physics, must involve, as we put it immediately above, 'the stakeholders directly concerned', then the stakeholders directly concerned includes those who are *most* directly concerned, namely those who *use* services as well as those who (in whatever role) provide them. Patients, therefore, their families and communities, as well as researchers, practitioners, managers, policy makers, and the executive, should be involved in the development of an *Extended Family of Classifications* if this is to be firmly based on rigorous scientific principles.

Subject to the rules of science

If there is one 'big issue' on the Agenda for an *Extended Family of Classifications*, this is it. As just noted, however, the point about process, fundamental as it is, will be considered by many, including many of those most deeply involved in bringing psychiatric classification to its present stage of development, to be ill-conceived: Robert Spitzer, for example, who, as Chair of the DSM-III Task Force, introduced clear inclusion and exclusion criteria for the first time, considered the involvement of patients and family members in the DSM-V process 'political correctness

gone mad' (Spitzer, 2005, in reply to Fulford *et al.*, 2005). Perhaps Spitzer is right. But it is important to be clear that as a point about process, this is no 'post-modern' appeal to a policy of anything and everything goes, but an argument in *scientific validity*. This is because any claim to membership of the *Extended Family of Classifications*, to the extent that it lays claim to being a *scientific* classification, must conform to the rules of science. Post-Logical Empiricist philosophy of science, guided by the model of physics, has shown the rules of science to be more complicated and less capable of formal codification than had previously been realized. Observation, in particular, as we saw in Chapter 12, has turned out to be conceptually structured; the extent, similarly, to which key terms both of observation and theory can be 'operationalized', as Hempel, no less, reminded us in his 1959 lecture, has turned out to be subject to in principle limits; and, as we will consider further in Chapter 16, there is a good deal more to progress in science than observational tests of theory alone. But there *are* rules, none the less. And none of the complications to these rules identified in post-Logical Empiricist philosophy of science, justifies a return to the obscurantism of what the Italian philosopher and historian of science, Paolo Rossi, has called the 'magical thinking' from which Renaissance physics had to work so hard to escape (Rossi, 2003). Post-Logical Empiricist philosophy of science has indeed shown that there is more to the difference between science and magic than had previously been appreciated. But that there is more to science than had previously been appreciated is, as Rossi argued, a reason for building on, not for reversing, the achievements of Renaissance physics.

It is from the achievements of Renaissance physics, then, that the argument for involving all stakeholders on an equal basis in the future development of psychiatric science, at least to the extent that this is an argument in scientific validity, derives. It will be worth setting out the argument in a little more detail as it is from this shift in process, a shift from the authority of this or that group of experts to the shared authority of *all* stakeholders, that the added value of an *Extended Family of Classifications*, guided by the insights of post-Logical Empiricist philosophy of science, is most directly derived. The argument, as we will see, can be thought of as embodying two key rules of scientific process as exemplified by the achievements of Renaissance physics.

Rule 1: challenging received authority

The argument, then, starts from the achievements of Renaissance physics and the fact that these were two-sided, or bivalent, achievements. One side of the achievements of Renaissance physics, the side that is best remembered today, was to establish the precedence of observation in the development of theories about what the world is really like. It is to this side of the achievements of Renaissance science that we remain true when we hang on firmly, despite all the difficulties, to the principles of observational science (including the need for reliable observations). But the other side to the achievements of Renaissance science, the side that is less well remembered today, was the overthrow of received authority. It is this second side of the achievements of Renaissance science that, transposed from the *particles* with which Renaissance physics was concerned to the *real people* with whom present day psychiatric science is concerned, generates the argument in validity for the involvement of all stakeholders on an equal basis in psychiatric science. The 'authorities' in the two cases are different, of course. For Renaissance science, the received authority was the authority of the established religion. In present-day psychiatry, the received authority is the authority of the established scientific disciplines, biological, psychological, and social. But there is a received authority in both cases. In both cases, similarly, received authority is justified, not by scientific validity, but by the need for 'good order': the good moral ordering of society by established religion in the Renaissance; the good medical ordering of policy and clinical decision making in current health-care practice. And in both cases the implications for *observational* science are the same, namely that science, observational science, succeeds in giving us a valid picture of the world by setting aside received authority and attending directly to what the world—whether a world made up of particles or of people—has to tell us.

Rule 2: listening to what the world (of particles or of people) has to say

Again, it is important to be clear here—this argument, to the extent that it is an argument in scientific validity, is no postmodern *laizzez-faire* appeal to a policy of anything and everything goes. There is no warrant here for everyone doing their own brain surgery or their own brain imaging! Expertise in the natural sciences, expertise on what the world—of particles, or livers and lungs, or indeed brains—has to tell us, expertise gained by listening carefully to what the world has to say, and expertise that includes the skilled use of instruments and the skilled interpretation of what those instruments reveal, expertise in all these areas is indeed genuine expertise (though as we will see in Chapter 16, there is rather more influence of received authority even in the sciences of particles than is generally acknowledged!). In these sciences, then, the natural sciences, a valid picture of the world is one that, in Crispin Wright's (1992) evocative phrase (from Session 2), is 'commanded by' the way the world really is. But transpose Crispin Wright's concept of cognitive command from particles, as the proper concern of physics, to people, as the proper concern of psychiatric science, and the corresponding scientifically valid way of seeing the world is one that is 'commanded' by the way *people* really are; and the expertise required to see the way people really are, is, or at the very least must centrally include, people themselves, *real* people, as patients, families, and communities, with direct experience of mental distress and disorder; people, then, as *experts*, not by professional or scientific training, indispensable as such experts are, but, to borrow a phrase from one of the UK government's current policy initiatives outlined later, 'experts by experience' (see Resources, below).

Agenda Item 10. Utility (of New Classification)

There are of course many other arguments, besides the above argument in scientific validity, for involving all stakeholders on an equal basis in the development of psychiatric science. There are arguments in equity, for example (Sadler and Fulford, 2004). Perhaps the most direct argument, though, is the observation that, to date, in failing to involve all stakeholders, in failing to listen carefully enough to the people with whom psychiatric science is most directly concerned, psychiatry has so regularly got things, from the perspective of its patients, so disastrously wrong.

We discussed the gap between patient and professional in psychiatry in Part I as a gap of models: the radical antipsychiatry movement, of which there is no corresponding counterpart in, say, cardiology, was motivated by a particularly radical gap in models. We consider the gap between patients and professionals in psychiatry again in Part IV in terms of a gap of values. The counterpart of these gaps here, in psychiatric science, is a communication gap arising from a gap in face validity—a gap between (many) patients and professionals in, to return to Sartorius' metaphor, their respective ways of seeing the world.

Improved face validity

It is not difficult to see how a communication gap between patients and professionals might be opened up in a psychiatric science that is guided by the 'one right way of seeing the world' assumption of the traditional model. Lewis, you will recall, in arguing at the 1959 conference for a symptom-based classification, stressed the need for improved communication for purposes of epidemiological research and statistical reporting. And it is gains in communication that, right through to the *Agenda for DSM-V*, have been perceived as the principal return from the enhanced reliability of modern psychiatric classifications. However, the communication in question has been, from Lewis right through to DSM-V, between professionals, and indeed mainly between doctors, not between doctors and other professional groups, still less between professionals and patients.

And improved construct validity

The need, then, corresponding directly with the need identified in Part I in terms of models, is not to abandon this or that way of seeing the world of mental disorder. The need, rather, is for a range of different ways of seeing the world through which different professional groups, representing expertise in different scientific ways of seeing the world of mental distress and disorder, are able to match their expertise appropriately to the equally diverse ways of seeing the world of mental distress and disorder represented by individual patients. Improved communication is of course of considerable value in its own right clinically. Scientifically though, improvements in face validity arising from improvements in communication between all stakeholders, could turn out to be a crucial further step (a crucial further step on from reliability) to the ultimate goal of improved construct (or theoretical) validity.

Agenda Item 11. Overall Tenor

It will be clear by now that, if Lewis in the *ICD-9 Agenda* is generally upbeat, and if Kupfer *et al.* in the *DSM-V Agenda* are somewhat downbeat, the *Agenda for an Extended Family of Classifications* will be definitely upbeat, though, as we will see, it is upbeat with strings.

Four upbeat lessons

The upbeat lessons drawn above from post-Logical Empiricist philosophy of science, guided primarily by the example of the physical sciences, are that: (1) psychiatric science is a difficult not defective science; (2) as such it demands the best of conceptual as well of empirical methods; and (3) psychiatry's models of validity, its ways of seeing the world, will be enriched by the full engagement of all stakeholders in the further development of psychiatric science. These three lessons give us reason enough to be upbeat. And we can add to them the further lesson from Part I, that the difficulties faced by psychiatric science today, arising as they do from psychiatry's irreducible engagement with people (rather than with the parts of people, their hearts, lungs, brains, etc.), will be the difficulties faced by the rest of medical science tomorrow.

Based on: (1) observational methods

The upbeat tenor of the Agenda for an *Extended Family of Classifications*, however, as noted above, comes with strings. One string is the point to which we have returned several times in this session, the need to remain true to the principles of observational science, albeit that these principles stand to be developed and deepened if they are to be applied in a valid as well as reliable way in a difficult science like psychiatric science.

(2) Challenge to received authority

A second string is the counterpart of the first, namely that hand-in-hand with the principles of observational science, as established in Renaissance physics, goes the overthrow of received authority. It is fundamental to the successful development of a fully functional *Extended Family of Classifications* that there should be no dominant way of seeing the world to which all other ways of seeing the world must be subsumed. In recent history, it has been the 'medical' model, a model based on the models of cardiology and other sciences of bodily medicine, that has been dominant in psychiatry. Before that, at least in the USA, it was psychoanalysis. The modern rise in authority of a variety of other models (noted in Part I), a variety entirely to be welcomed to the extent that it provides a balanced heterogeneity of models corresponding with the diversity of models represented by individual patients and carers, carries the risk of collapse into one or another new hegemony. This risk, if history is any guide, is all too real. The antipsychiatry movement was motivated by the myth of mental illness. However, as the German historian and psychiatrist, Paul Hoff, has eloquently put it, throughout its history psychiatry has shown itself to be all too capable of replacing one myth with another (Hoff, 2005).

(3) Enough time

A third string is the need for a long view. It is natural, faced with the reality of mental distress and disorder, to look for immediate returns on research. There are, as we noted above, quick wins to be had from opening up the additional intellectual space of a strengths model of psychiatric science created for us by post-Logical Empiricist philosophy of science. But the substantive development of theory in this most difficult of sciences is bound to take time. The research leading to improved reliability took decades, not years. We should not expect improvements in validity in an any less generous time scale. The new neurosciences, certainly, just in *being* new, promise un-looked for advances. Combined with the new mental sciences outlined in Part I, and reviewed briefly below (under 'Resources'), the currently hoped-for advances in the neurosciences may well result in improvements in validity, in better ways of seeing the world of mental distress and disorder; better as judged by those most directly concerned, patients, their families, and communities. These are exciting times, then, times that indeed hold out tantalising glimpses of Kupfer *et al.*'s 'as yet unknown paradigm shift' (p. xix). It may be that the shift will happen overnight. These things after all are by definition unpredictable. But we should not be surprised, or disappointed, if the looked-for paradigm shift takes a little longer.

Agenda Item 12. Any Other Business

Under 'Any Other Business' in the Agenda for an *Extended Family of Classifications*, are 'resources' and 'next steps'.

Resources

Much of our third agenda, our Agenda for an *Extended Family of Classifications*, like its predecessors in ICD and DSM, has been taken up with the tough challenges of psychiatric classification. And the challenges are tough indeed reflecting as they do the combined empirical and conceptual challenges of psychiatric science. But the 1990s, as we indicate in Chapter 29 of this book, and as Fulford et al., 2003, describe in detail, witnessed an explosion of new resources for meeting these challenges. We summarize these resources here under four broad categories: (1) the new neurosciences; (2) the new mental sciences; (3) new national policy initiatives; and (4) new international networks.

1. *New neurosciences.* The resources of the new neurosciences— behavioural genetics, psychopharmacology, and brain imaging— are one of the keys to the development of more effective mental health services in the twenty-first century. Yet science, as we saw particularly in Part I, despite its many dramatic successes in medicine, has had an increasingly bad press recently. One clear task for the new philosophy of psychiatry, therefore, developing as it has hand-in-hand with the new neurosciences, is to help provide a framework for a synergistic rather than mutually destructive relationship between researchers, practitioners, and (as the ultimate stakeholders in mental health) patients, carers, and others who use mental health and related

social care services. Without such a synergistic relationship, the danger is that the resources of the new neurosciences are as likely to compound as to relieve the problems of mental distress and disorder.

2. *New mental sciences*. A key resource from the new philosophy of psychiatry for the development of a synergistic relationship between the neurosciences and its stakeholders, is the wide range of methods now available for the rigorous study of subjectivity, of the meanings and personal significance of individual experience. Many of these methods, as we noted in Part I, besides being potential research partners to the new neurosciences, are already paying dividends clinically: discursive, hermeneutic, and phenomenological methods are all cases in point (for details see Reading Guides, particularly to Chapters 3, 4, 9 and 10; also the work on values in Part IV). The hope must be, therefore, that the new mental sciences, as they might be called, will continue to grow alongside and in partnership with the new neurosciences, as a resource for mental health care.

Specifically in relation to classification, the proposals by Juan Mezzich, the Peruvian Professor of Psychiatry at the Mount Sinai Hospitals, New York, for an 'idiographic classification' (Mezzich, 2002; also Mezzich *et al.*, 1996, and Mezzich *et al.*, 2003) complement the existing WHO Family of Classifications, establishing the basis for a more comprehensive approach to psychiatric assessment. Mezzich has wide experience of international classification, having been a member of the workgroups developing DSM-III, DSM-IV and ICD-10, chair for many years of the WPA classification section, and currently chair of the WPA-WHO workgroup on International Classification and Diagnostic systems. As WPA president from September 2005, it is therfore particularly significant that his proposals already include not only key elements both of the subjective aspects of mental disorder that are the focus of the new mental sciences, but also of the expanded policy and practice initiatives currently emerging in a number of countries around the world.

3. *New national policies*. Policy and practice initiatives, although not important in a traditional model of psychiatric science, are a crucial resource for the development of an *Extended Family of Classifications*, guided by a post-Logical Empiricist philosophy of physics, but concerned with people rather than particles.

It is important to be aware just how fast and far things have already moved. Thus, mental health policy in a number of countries has recently been expanded to embrace new initiatives in such areas as health promotion, psychosocial interventions, and recovery practice. In the UK, national policy is explicitly user-centred and multidisciplinary (Department of Health, 1999) and the work of the UK government's mental health policy implementation body, the National Institute for Mental Health in England (NIMHE), includes: (a) work

streams in such areas as recovery, social inclusion, black and minority ethnic services, spirituality, values-based practice (to which we return in detail in Part IV), and (b) crucially for classification (Agenda Item 9, above), 'experts by experience', a programme aimed at developing leading roles for patients and informal carers in the development and implementation of services and in many areas of research.

4. *New international networks*. Complementing these national developments has been the emergence and strengthening of new international networks. The importance of international collaboration in the development of psychiatric classifications has already been noted: Aubrey Lewis, you will recall from Reading 13.8, made a point of commenting on the fundamental importance of the strongly 'collegial' international effort that led to ICD-8. Improvements in international travel, and the development of the World Wide Web, provide new opportunities for building on the success of such initiatives. The philosophy of psychiatry, notably, has developed through the work of a number of national and subject-based groups around the world. The recently launched *International Network for Philosophy and Psychiatry* (the INPP) will provide crucial communication and co-ordination support for these groups.

Among established international organizations, the World Psychiatric Association (WPA), with its energetic regional groups and subject-based sections, provides a strong international basis for the development of an *Extended Family of Classifications*, incorporating, but also adding to, the 'families', respectively, of the ICD and DSM classifications. The WPA has already established, under the chairmanship of Juan Mezzich, a Conceptual Workgroup for Classification to spearhead work on classification. Supported as the Workgroup is by the WPA's sections respectively for Classification, for Psychopathology, and for Philosophy and the Humanities, and including as it does in its membership neuroscientists, philosophers and 'experts by experience' from many countries around the world, the WPA's Conceptual Workgroup is an exemplary example of the resources already available for building on the successes of psychiatric classification in the twentieth century to produce an *Extended Family of Classifications* as the basis for a twenty-first century science-based but also user-centred psychiatry.

Next steps

As we 'go to press', a number of small but potentially significant next steps towards the development of an *Extended Family of Classifications* have already been taken. In addition to the work just noted of international organizations, such as the WPA, there have been already three conferences specifically on new approaches to psychiatric classification.

1. *The Dallas Conference*. As early as 1997, John Sadler, Professor of Psychiatry and Director of Medical Education at UT Southwestern Medical Centre, convened an international

conference in Dallas on philosophical aspects of psychiatric diagnosis. Besides philosophers, patients, psychiatrists, and neuroscientists, the conference included key culture carriers from the successes of twentieth century psychiatric classification, notably the Chair of the DSM-III Task Force, Robert Spitzer. (The proceedings of this conference are published in Sadler, 2002).

2. *The NIMHE conferences.* In the UK, the NIMHE (see point 3, above), although a policy implementation rather than research-funding body, has sponsored two international research meetings, one in London in 2003, the other in Windsor in 2004. Although concerned primarily with the role of values in psychiatric diagnosis (to which we turn in Part IV), the rationale for NIMHE's support for these meetings was the need for an expanded basis for psychiatric classification consistent with the expanded policy objectives for mental health adopted in the UK (noted under point 3 of 'Resources' above).

   The network of researchers, policy makers, and stakeholders established through these two meetings, and with their direct links into policy and practice in the UK, will thus be well placed to contribute to the work of the Conceptual Workgroup for Classification established by Juan Mezzich in the WPA.

   As with the Dallas conference, the two NIMHE meetings included, in addition to researchers from both empirical and phenomenological traditions, representatives of all stakeholders in mental health (users of services, clinicians, and researchers) as well as leading figures in the development of twentieth century approaches to psychiatric diagnosis and classification (Norman Sartorius and Julian Leff, for example), and, in this instance, key figures from the WPA, including Juan Lopez-Ibor, Ahmed Okasha and, specifically concerned with the new classifications, Juan Mezzich and the Secretary of the WPA's Classification Section, Claudio Banzato.

3. *The WPA Conceptual Workgroup on Classification.* As noted above under 'Resources' (point 4), the establishment by the WPA of a Conceptual Workgroup for Classification, supported by the WPA's strong structure of regional and subject-based groups, could prove to be a key step towards the development and implementation of an *Extended Family of Classifications* for international use in mental health. A series of meetings of the network has already been planned in different countries around the world within a framework for collaborative action between the WPA, the WHO (on ICD) and the DSM-V Taskforce.

So, where will these 'next steps' lead? This will depend, among other key factors, on the scientific research programmes that develop within psychiatry over coming decades. A scientific classification, after all, must reflect as well as help to shape, the science to which it relates. Where these next steps will lead will also depend on the outcome of the interplay of social and political forces represented by the disparate models of mental health that we explored in Part I. The traditional model of science would have it that these two kinds of factor—the research programmes of science and social and political factors—are unconnected. As we will see in Chapter 16, however, the connections between them are, to the contrary, crucial. It is to the connections between scientific and social and political factors, therefore, in the future developments of psychiatric classification, and to these connections as identified in this chapter in a post-Logical Empiricist model of science guided by the example of physics, that we now turn in a brief concluding session.

Reflection on the session and self-test questions

In this session we developed an Agenda for an *Extended Family of Classifications* drawing on the philosophy of science as represented particularly by the history and philosophy of physics. Write down your own reflections on the materials in this session drawing out any points that are particularly significant for you. Then write brief notes about the following:

1. What 'big issue' did our Agenda for an *Extended Family of Classifications* identity as important in the agenda for ICD-9? Why was this important also for the 'big issue' on the agenda for DSM-V?

2. What class of issue did we name in our new agenda that is both explicit and *named as such* in the agenda for ICD-9, but explicit and *not* named as such in the agenda for DSM-V?

3. What is the 'big issue' on our Agenda for an *Extended Family of Classifications*?

4. In our Extended Family of Classifications: (a) What is the assumed status of psychiatric science relative to the sciences in other areas of medicine? (b) What new category of methods of investigation become available in addition to empirical methods? and (c) What is the role of patients and other users of services?

5. What role will patients and other users of services have in our new agenda as an agenda specifically for a future *scientific* classification of mental disorder?

Conclusions: being about what science is about

'A classification', as Norman Sartorius (1992) reminded us epigrammatically in the quote from the Preface to ICD-10 at the start of this chapter, is 'a way of seeing the world at a point in time'. As we come to the end of the chapter it will be clear that the operative word in Sartorius' epigram is the indefinite article 'a'— '*a* classification is *a* way of seeing the world at *a* point in time'.

The assumption of the traditional model of science, an assumption derived from such paradigms as the Chemical Periodic Table, has been that, as science is about what the world is really like, a scientific classification should be, not *a* way, but *the* way of seeing the world, our currently best shot at seeing what the world is really like at *this* point in time.

From 'the' to 'a'

The shift from 'the' to 'a', from the definite to the indefinite, from one to many scientific ways of seeing the world at a point in time, starts, so far as the philosophy of science is concerned, with the failure of Logical Empiricism, and related broadly positivist programmes, to provide a formal codification of what science is about, an abstract test, external to the practice of this or that discipline, by which a uniquely scientific way of seeing the world might be distinguished from other ways of seeing the world that, although perhaps authoritative and important in other ways, are not consistent with the uniquely scientific way of seeing the world.

Logical Empiricism, as we saw in Chapter 12, focused on the role of observation in science. Genuinely scientific ways of seeing the world, in the paradigm of Renaissance physics, start from observation, from looking and really *seeing* what the world is like, and, thereby, differentiating between true (valid) and false (invalid) theories about what the world is like. Logical Empiricism, then, failed to the extent that it failed to find an unambiguous way of distinguishing observation statements from statements of theory. But this 'failure', the storyline of Chapter 12 suggests, was, in fact, a brilliant success. For it opened the way to a deeper understanding of the relationship between observation and theory in science, a recognition that, (1) observation itself is theory laden in the specific sense of being conceptually prestructured; hence that, (2) while observation—looking and really seeing—remains, as in the paradigm of Renaissance physics, the basis of differentiating between scientifically valid and invalid ways of seeing the world, none the less, (3) as observation itself is conceptually prestructured, it follows that the relationship between observation and theory is not linear but iterative, and, in consequence, (4) that there may be at any one time, and as there is at the present time in physics, more than one scientifically valid way of seeing what the world is really like.

From Logical Empiricist to post-Logical Empiricist science

In Chapter 12 we found evidence of the brilliant success of the failure of Logical Empiricism in the development, in the second half of the twentieth century, of reliable observational methods for psychiatric science. The PSE, we noted, and other 'semi-structured' schedules for identifying and recording mental states, provide vivid illustrations of the conceptual prestructuring of observation: recall Wing *et al.*'s (1974) account of the development of the PSE as an operational formalization of good clinical practice among clinicians working in a broadly European psychiatric tradition. In this chapter we have found further evidence of the brilliant success of the failure of Logical Empiricism in the development, also over the second half of the twentieth century, of psychiatry's two major international scientific classifications of mental disorder, the ICD and DSM, successive editions of which have built on Lewis' translation, in the 1959 conference, of Hempel's Logical Empiricist account of scientific classifications into the need for what he called 'public' and 'private' classifications for different scientific purposes. Lewis' translation of Hempel, we can now see, and the subsequent evolution of both ICD and DSM towards their respective families of classifications, and the further evolution from these families to the *Agenda for a Extended Family of Classifications* outlined in Session 4 of this chapter, are all direct parallels of the corresponding translation in post-Logical Empiricist philosophy of science, guided by the paradigm specifically of physics (as in Session 3 of this chapter), from the single valid scientific way of seeing the world assumed by the traditional model of science, into many valid scientific ways of seeing the world.

Cutting against the grain

The shift from 'the' to 'a' valid scientific way of seeing the world, and hence from one to an *Extended Family of Psychiatric Classifications*, will cut against the grain with those who have other and different agendas. It will cut against the grain, for example, with those whose personal, professional, financial, or political interests lie in promoting this or that particular way of understanding mental distress and disorder. It will cut against the grain, similarly, with those whose personal, professional, financial, or political interests lie in overthrowing this or that particular way of understanding mental distress and disorder. Corresponding with the 'full field' model to which we came in Part I, an *Extended Family of Classifications* will build on, not replace, established ways (including the established medical way) of understanding the world of mental distress and disorder.

The move from 'the' to 'a', however, the move from one to an *Extended Family of Psychiatric Classifications*, will cut most deeply against the grain with those who are convinced, honestly convinced, that, in broad outline at least, they already know what is *the* right way to understand the world of mental distress and disorder. The shift from 'the' to 'a', the honestly convinced may acknowledge, has been guided by the paradigm of Renaissance science as currently embodied in theoretical physics. The shift from 'the' to 'a', the honestly convinced may further acknowledge, is but one aspect of the discovery of radical uncertainty that is perhaps the unique intellectual heritage of the twentieth century—recall the EPR paradox in physics from Chapter 12, and, from Chapter 6, the still deeper uncertainties in mathematical logic identified by the Gödel undecidability theorems. The shift from 'the' to 'a', the honestly convinced may additionally acknowledge, provides no warrant for the relativization of scientific knowledge so often (and illegitimately) promoted under a banner of 'postmodernism'. The point, after all, the honestly convinced may continue, of recognizing (with Chapter 12) the conceptual prestructuring of observation, is, as Hesse (1980) argued, not to abandon the basic scientific discipline of observational testing of candidate explanatory theories, but to recognize that such 'testing' is effective only to the extent that it is carried out within a given range of candidate explanatory theories, candidate ways of seeing what the world is really like. The point, similarly, the honestly convinced may finally concede, of recognizing (with this chapter) the undetermination of theory by data, is, to extend Hesse's point, not that *any* theory may be determined by the data, but that the data serve, on the one hand to exclude from among a given range of candidate explanatory theories those that are false (invalid), i.e. because they conflict with and hence are not determined by the data at all, while, on the other hand, and at the same time, leaving wide open the range of possible future explanatory theories that may be *true*.

Back to Renaissance science

All these points, then, about the shift from 'the' to 'a' way of seeing the world scientifically, the shift from one to an *Extended Family of Psychiatric Classifications*, those who are honestly convinced they already know in broad outline what the world is really like, may acknowledge. And yet, the honestly convinced may go on to say, for *practical* purpose, for the purposes of good order in a practical discipline such as psychiatry, there is a need, if not for one way of seeing the world, at least for a *dominant* way. In physics, particularly theoretical physics, those who are honestly convinced may point out, theoreticians have the luxury of being able to 'play' with different ways of seeing the world. This 'play' may, indeed, in the long run prove to be highly productive scientifically, i.e., in giving us new and powerful ways of seeing the world. But where physics is for particles, psychiatry, as this chapter after all has repeatedly emphasized, is for people. And the practical contingencies of a discipline that is concerned not with particles but with people require, the honestly convinced may suggest, not play, however productive in the long run, but a clear line of authority to ensure good order in the development and delivery of services as the basis of effective day-to-day clinical care. Granted, therefore, the honestly convinced will conclude, that we (we the honestly convinced) already have, if not *the* scientific way of seeing the world, at any rate our current best shot at *the* scientific way of seeing the world, then the requirement for good order in clinical care leads directly to the need for a clear line of authority derived from our (the honestly convinced's) way of seeing the world...

...which is precisely the point at which, as we saw in Session 4 of this chapter, with the successful *overthrow* of a received authority justified by the honestly convinced in the name of good order, modern observational science, in the form of Renaissance physics, first came in. Building, therefore, an *Extended Family of Psychiatric Classifications,* a family of equal members, and a family in which membership is secured not by way of received authority but by way of the disciplines of rigorous observation-based ways of seeing the world, will be nothing if not all about what science is about.

Reading guide

The absolute conception

- The absolute conception is introduced by Williams in both *Descartes: The Project of Pure Inquiry* (1978), and *Ethics and the Limits of Philosophy* (1985).

- It is discussed by the philosopher Hilary Putnam (1995) in *Renewing Philosophy*, and by McDowell (1998) in *Mind, Value, and Reality*.

Realism in the philosophy of science

- A good introduction is Bird (1998) *The Philosophy of Science* (chapter 4).

- The definitive collection on scientific realism is Leplin (ed.) (1984) *Scientific Realism*, but it is also discussed in Papineau (1987) *Reality and Representation* and Laudan (1977) *Progress and its Problems*.

- Realism based on the argument from explanation is the main subject of Lipton (1991) *Inference to the Best Explanation*.

- Cartwright's work is further developed in *The Dappled World* (2000).

A valuable collection of articles on causal explanations in healthcare in the Swedish philosophers, Ingmar Lindahl and Lenart Nordenfelt's (1984) edited collection in the *Philosophy and Medicine* book series.

Natural kinds

One debate that has not been touched on in this section concerns whether disease is a natural kind. Some of the concerns of that debate should now be clear. The concept of disease groups together diverse conditions, but does this reflect fundamental and underlying similarities or is it instead that these have in common something that reflects our local interests in what affects us. See for example.

- Reznek (1987) *The Nature of Disease* (chapters 1–4);

- Reznek (1995) Dis-ease about kinds: reply to D'Amico (*Journal of Medicine and Philosophy*); and

- D'Amico (1995) Is disease a natural kind (*Journal of Medicine and Philosophy*).

You should now be in a position to assess the underlying argument here.

Psychiatric classification and diagnosis

Introductions to current systems of psychiatric classification and to diagnosis are included in all the major textbooks of psychiatry (noted in the Reading Guide to Chapter 2). As detailed in the chapter, the current version of the WHO's classification of mental disorders, is chapter 8 of the 10th edition of the *International Classification of Disease* (WHO, 1992). The WHO website (http://www.who.int/en) gives details of its family of classifications, including the ICF, the *International Classification of Functioning, Disability and Health* (2001). The American Psychiatric Association's current classification is a revised version of its DSM, the fourth (revised, 2000) edition of the *Diagnostic and Statistical Manual* (DSM-IV-TR—'TR' for text revision). The DSM is complemented by a valuable range of additional publications to support research and teaching—see the DSM-IV-TR Library section in the American Psychiatric Association website. As noted in the chapter, both ICD and DSM classifications are currently undergoing revision with a view to publication of new editions around 2010. Cultural issues are reviewed by Kleinman (1996) and by Mezzich *et al.* (1996), and the case for personalized 'idiographic' classifications in Mezzich (2002) and Mezzich *et al.* (2003).

Psychiatric classification remains contentious and the issues discussed in this chapter have generated a huge literature. A recent authoritative analysis, including a novel approach to the nature of validity is the American philosopher and psychiatrist, Kenneth Schaffner's (1993) *Discovery and Explanation in Biology and Medicine*. See also his (1986) edited collection *Logic of Discovery and Diagnosis in Medicine*. As noted in the chapter, Kendell and Jablensky (2003) examine validity and utility from a psychiatric perspective. Cooper (2003) provides a critical review of the Research Agenda for DSM-V.

Sadler *et al.*'s (1994) *Philosophical Perspectives on Psychiatric Diagnostic Classification* is an edited collection including chapters on many of the key conceptual issues. Sadler's (2002) more recent edited collection, *Descriptions and Prescriptions*, provides a further valuable resource with a focus particularly on the role of values (see Part IV, especially Chapters 20 and 21). Regular reviews and updates are published in *Current Opinion in Psychiatry*, both in the *History and Philosophy* section, and in specific clinical topic areas. Jennifer Radden (1994) reviewed key philosophical issues in *Philosophy, Psychiatry, & Psychology*. The opening chapters of John Sadler's (2004a) *Values and Psychiatric Diagnosis*, give a comprehensive and very readable update, including a detailed discussion of the issue of validity. Kutchins and Kirk (1997) present the case against psychiatric diagnosis. Sadler's (2004b) 'Diagnosis/ antidiagnosis' provides a succinct overview of current debates.

A classic but still invaluable source for both historical and conceptual issues in classification is R.E. Kendell's (1975) *The Role of Diagnosis in Psychiatry*. This book was written at a time when the debate between psychiatry and antipsychiatry was at its most polarized (1975 was also the year of Kendell's reply to Szasz that we looked at in detail in Part I). It includes discussions of the 'pros and cons' of diagnosis (chapter 1), of the relationship between diagnosis and concepts of disease (chapters 2 and 5), of issues of reliability and validity (chapter 3) and of practical utility (chapter 4), and of quantitative methods (chapter 8), including a forward-looking discussion of the role of computers (chapter 11), of the choice between categories and dimensions (chapter 9), and of the problems generally of defining diagnostic criteria (chapter 10). Specifically on the history of current classifications, Kendell's two chapters on 'International differences in diagnostic criteria' (chapter 6) and on 'The international classification' (chapter 7), provide a wealth of detail. John Cooper (1999) describes the development of the WHO programme of classifications. For further details of the WHO programme of classification, see Sartorius, 1976, 1991 and 1995, and Kramer *et al.*, 1979.

Kendell's book (especially chapter 3) also draws together in an easily accessible form details of the many early studies of psychiatric diagnosis that have been important in shaping current classifications, including:

1. *Wake-up calls* of the need for a more rigorous approach, for example: (a) Temerlin's (1968) experiment, in which an audio-tape of an actor talking normally was consistently interpreted as 'psychotic' by an audience of psychiatrists and psychologists primed to expect pathology, and (b) Rosenhan's (1973) experiment, in which a number of social scientists, having had themselves admitted as patients to psychiatric hospitals, found that everything they did (including keeping notes of their experiences) was interpreted by staff as symptoms of illness.

2. *Studies of reliability*: for example (a) the *Philadelphia Study* (Beck *et al.*, 1962), an early American study of reliability that established a rigorous methodology for quantifying various sources of diagnostic disagreement (differences of interview technique, different weightings of responses, loose diagnostic criteria, etc.), and (b) the *Chichester Study* (Kreitman *et al.*, 1961), a similar study in the UK. Early versions of the PSE (see chapter 12) were also important in establishing the reliability of individual symptoms (e.g. Wing *et al.*, 1967).

3. *International collaborative research*, for example: (a) the *US-UK Diagnostic Project* (Cooper *et al.*, 1972), a collaborative study of differences in rates of diagnosis between Britain and America. These had been recognized previously (see Kramer, 1969; Kramer et al., 1979) but this collaborative research design allowed the differences in rates of diagnosis of psychiatric disorders to be fully mapped out for the first time using structured interview methods; (b) the *International Pilot Study of Schizophrenia* (or IPSS, WHO, 1973), which extended the US–UK project internationally (see also Part IV).

References

Alarcón, R.D., Bell, C.C., Kirmayer, L.J., Lin, K-M., Üstün, B., and Wisner, K.L. (2002). Beyond the funhouse mirrors: research agenda on culture and psychiatric diagnosis. In *A Research Agenda for DSM-V* (ed. D.J. Kupfer, M.B. First, and D.E. Regier). Washington, DC: American Psychiatric Association, pp. 219–282.

American Psychiatric Association (1952). *Diagnostic and Statistical Manual of Mental Disorders* (1st edn, DSM-I). Washington, DC: American Psychiatric Association.

American Psychiatric Association (1968). *Diagnostic and Statistical Manual of Mental Disorders* (2nd edn, DSM-II). Washington, DC: American Psychiatric Association.

American Psychiatric Association (1980). *Diagnostic and Statistical Manual of Mental Disorders* (3rd edn, DSM-III). Washington, DC: American Psychiatric Association.

American Psychiatric Association (1994). *Diagnostic and Statistical Manual of Mental Disorders* (4th edn). Washington, DC: American Psychiatric Association.

American Psychiatric Association (2000). *Diagnostic and Statistical Manual of Mental Disorders*, Fourth Edition, Text Revision. Washington, DC: American Psychiatric Association.

Anastasi, A. (1968). Psychological Testing, 3rd ed. New York: The Macmillan Company.

Beck, A.T., Ward, C., Mendelson, M., Mock, J., and Erbaugh, J. (1961). An inventory for measuring depression. *Archives of General Psychiatry*, 4: 561–571.

Bird, A. (1998). *The Philosophy of Science*. London: UCL.

Boyd, R. (1999). On the current status of scientific realism. In *The Philosophy of Science* (ed. R. Boyd, P. Gaspar, and J.D. Trout). Cambridge, MA: MIT Press, pp. 195–222.

Bridgman, P.W. (1927). *The Logic of Modern Physics*. New York: Macmillan Press.

Cartwright, N. (1983). *How the Laws of Physics Lie*. Oxford: Oxford University Press.

Cartwright, N. (1999). The reality of causes in a world of instrumental laws. In *The Philosophy of Science* (ed. R. Boyd, P. Gasker, and J.D. Trout). Cambridge, MA: MIT Press, pp. 379–386.

Cartwright, N. (2000). *The Dappled World*. Cambridge: Cambridge University Press.

Charney, D.S., Barlow, D.H., Botteron, K., Cohen, J.D., Goldman, D., Gur, R.E., Lin, K-M, López, J.F., Meador-Woodruff, J.H., Moldin, S.O., Nestler, E.J., Watson, S.J., and Zalcman, S.J. (2002). Neuroscience Research Agenda to Guide Development of a Pathophysiologically Based Classification System. In *A Research Agenda for DSM-V* (ed. D.J. Kupfer, M.B. First, and D.E. Regier). Washington, DC: American Psychiatric Association, pp. 31–84.

Colombo, A., Bendelow, G., Fulford, K.W.M., and Williams, S. (2003). Evaluating the influence of implicit models of mental disorder on processes of shared decision making within community-based multi-disciplinary teams. *Social Science & Medicine*, 56: 1557–1570.

Cooper, J.E., Kendell, R.E., Gurland, B.J., Sharpe, L., Copeland, J.R.M. and Simon, R. (1972). *Psychiatric diagnosis in New York and London*. Maudsley Monograph Series No. 20. London: Oxford University Press.

Cooper, J. (1999). Chapter 2 in *Promoting Mental Health Internationally*, edited by Girolamo et al. London: The Royal College of Psychiatrists, Gaskell Press.

Cooper, J. (2003) Editorial: Prospects for Chapter V of ICD-11 and DSM-V. *British Journal of Psychiatry*, vol 183: 379–381.

D'Amico (1995). Is disease a natural kind. *Journal of Medicine and Philosophy*, 20: 551–569.

Dancy, J. (1993). *Moral Reasons*. Oxford: Blackwell Publishers.

Department of Health (1999). *National Service Framework for Mental Health—Modern Standards and Service Models*. London: Department of Health.

d'Espagnat, B. (1976). *Conceptual Foundations of Quantum Mechanics*, (2nd edn). W.A. Benjamin Inc.

Discussion, Various Contributors (1961). In *Field Studies in the Mental Disorders* (ed. J. Zubin). New York, Grune and Stratton, pp. 23–50.

Duhem, P. (1985). *To Save the Phenomena: an essay on the idea of physical theory from Plato to Galileo*. Chicago: University of Chicago Press.

Evans, G. (1980). Things without the mind. In *Philosophical subjects: essays presented to P.F. Strawson* (ed. Z. van Straaten). Oxford: Clarendon Press.

Fine, A. (1984). 'And not anti-realism either'. *Nous* 19, 51–65. (reproduced in *Scientific Knowledge: basic issues in the philosophy of science* ed J.A. Kournay (1998). Belmont, California: Wadsworth Publishing Company, pp. 359–368.)

Fine, A. (1999). The natural ontological attitude. In *The Philosophy of Science* (ed. R. Boyd, P. Gasker, and J.D. Trout). Cambridge, MA: MIT Press, pp. 261–277.

First, M.B., Bell, C.C., Cuthbert, B., Krystal, J.H., Malison, R., and Offord, D.R. (2002). Personality disorders and relational disorders: a research agenda for addressing crucial gaps in DSM. In *A Research Agenda for DSM-V* (ed. D.J. Kupfer, M.B. First, and D.E. Regier). Washington, DC: American Psychiatric Association, pp. 123–200.

Fulford, K. W. M., Morris, K. J., Sadler, J. Z., and Stanghellini, G. (2003). Past improbable, future possible: the renaissance in philosophy and psychiatry. In *Nature and Narrative: an introduction to the new philosophy of psychiatry* (ed. K.W.M. Fulford, K.J. Morris, J.Z. Sadler, and G. Stanghellini). Oxford: Oxford University Press, pp. 1–41.

Fulford, K.W.M., Broome, M., Stanghellini, G., and Thornton, T. (2005). Looking With Both Eyes Open: Fact *and* Value in Psychiatric Diagnosis? *World Psychiatry*, 4: 2,78–86.

General Register Office (1968). *A Glossary of Mental Disorders. Studies on Medical and Population Subjects.* No. 22, London: HMSO.

Hacker, P.M.S. (1987). *Appearance and Reality*. Oxford: Blackwell.

Hacking, I. (1983). *Representing and Intervening*. Cambridge: Cambridge University Press.

Hacking, I. (1999). Experimentation and scientific realism. In *The Philosophy of Science* (ed. R. Boyd, P. Gaspar, and J.D. Trout). Cambridge, MA: MIT Press, pp. 247–260.

Hempel, C.G. (1961). Introduction to problems of taxonomy. In *Field Studies in the Mental Disorders*. New York: Grune and Stratton, pp. 3–22. (Reproduced in Sadler, J.Z., Wiggins, O.P., and Schwartz, M.A. (1994). *Philosophical Perspectives on Psychiatric Diagnostic Classification*. Baltimore, MD: The Johns Hopkins University Press, pp. 315–331.)

Hempel, C.G. (1994). Fundamentals of taxonomy. In *Philosophical Perspectives on Psychiatric Diagnostic Classification* (ed. J.S. Sadler, O.P. Wiggins, and M.A. Schwartz). Baltimore, MD: Johns Hopkins University Press.

Hesse, M. (1980). *Revolutions and Reconstructions in the Philosophy of Science*. Harvester.

Hobson, R.P., Patrick, M.P.H., and Valentine, J.D. (1998). Objectivity in psychoanalytic judgements. *British Journal of Psychiatry*, 173: 172–177.

Hoff, P. (2005). Die psychopathologische Perspektive. In: Bormuth M, Wiesing U (eds) *Ethische Aspekte der Forschung in Psychiatrie und Psychotherapie*. Deutscher Aerzte-Verlag, Cologne. Pp:71-79

Hyman, S.E. and Fenton, W.D. (2003). What are the right targets for psychopharmacology? *Science*, 299: 350–351.

Kendell, R.E. (1975). *The Role of Diagnosis in Psychiatry*. Oxford: Blackwell Scientific Publications.

Kendell, R.E. and Jablensky, A. (2003). Distinguishing between the validity and utility of psychiatric diagnoses. *American Journal of Psychiatry*, 160: 4–12.

Kleinman, A. (1996). How is culture important for DSM-IV? In *Culture and Psychiatric Diagnosis: a DSM-IV perspective* (ed. J.E. Mezzich, A. Kleinman, H. Fabrega, and D.L. Parron). Washington: American Psychiatric Press Inc., Chapter 2.

Kramer, M. (1969). Cross-National Study of Diagnosis of the Mental Disorders: origin of the problem. *American Journal of Psychiatry*, 125 (suppl.), 1–11.

Kramer, M. Sartorius, N. Jablensky, A., Gulbinat, W. (1979). The ICD-9 Classification of Mental Disorders: A Review of its Development and Contents. *Acta Psychiatrica Scandinavica*, 59: 241–262.

Kreitman, N., Sainsbury, P., Morrissey, J., Towers, J., and Scrivener, J. (1961). The reliability of psychiatric assessment: an analysis. *Journal of Mental Science*, 107: 887–908.

Kupfer, D.J., First, M.B., and Regier, D.E. (2002). *A Research Agenda for DSM-V* (ed. D.J. Kupfer, M.B. First, and D.E. Regier). Washington, DC: American Psychiatric Association.

Kutchins, H. and Kirk, S.A. (1997). *Making Us Crazy: DSM—the psychiatric bible and the creation of mental disorder*. London: Constable.

Latour, B. (1987). *Science in Action: how to follow scientists and engineers through society*. Cambridge, MA: Harvard University Press.

Laudan, L. (1977). *Progress and its Problems*. Berkeley, CA: University of California.

Lehman. A.F., Alexopoulos, G.S., Goldman, H., Jeste, D., and Üstün, B. (2002). Mental disorders and disability: time to reevaluate the relationship? In *A Research Agenda for DSM-V* (ed. D.J. Kupfer, M.B. First, and D.E. Regier). Washington, DC: American Psychiatric Association, pp. 201–218.

Leplin, J. (ed.) (1984). *Scientific Realism*. Berkeley, CA: University of California.

Lewis, A.J. (1934). On the psychopathology of insight. *British Journal of Medicine and Psychology*, 14: 332–348.

Lindahl, B.I.B. and Nordenfelt, L. (ed.) (1984). *Health, Disease, and Causal Explanations in Medicine*, Vol. 16. In *Philosophy and Medicine Book Series* (series ed. H.T. Engelhardt and S.F. Spicker). Dordrecht-Holland: D. Reidel Publishing Company.

Lipton, P. (1991). *Inference to the Best Explanation*. London: Routledge.

Mackie, J.L. (1977). *Ethics: inventing right and wrong*. New York: Viking.

McDowell, J. (1994). *Mind and World*. Cambridge, MA: Harvard.

McDowell, J. (1998). Aesthetic value, objectivity, and the fabric of the world. pp. 122–130, in. *Mind, Value, and Reality*. Cambridge, MA: Harvard University Press.

McMullin, E. (1987). Explanatory success and the truth of theory. In *Scientific Inquiry in Philosophical Perspective* (ed. N. Rescher). New York: University Press of America, pp. 51–73.

Mezzich, J.E. (2002). Comprehensive diagnosis: a conceptual basis for future diagnostic systems. *Psychopathology*, 35(2–3): 162–165.

Mezzich, J.E., Kleinman, A, Fabrega, H., and Parron, D.L. (ed.) (1996). *Culture and Psychiatric Diagnosis: a DSM-IV perspective*. Washington, DC: American Psychiatric Press Inc.

Mezzich, J.E., Berganza, C.E., Von Cranach, M., Jorge, M.R., Kastrup, M.C., Murthy, R.S., Okasha, A., Pull, C., Sartorius, N., Skodol, A., and Zaudig, M. (2003). IGDA. 8: Idiographic (personalised) diagnostic formulation. In *Essentials of the World Psychiatric Association's International Guidelines for Diagnostic Assessment (IGD)*. *The British Journal of Psychiatry*, 182(Suppl. 45): 55–57.

Nagel, T. (1986). *The View from Nowhere*. Oxford: Oxford University Press.

Papineau, D. (1987). *Reality and Representation* Oxford: Basil Blackwell.

Pine, D.S., Alegria, M., Cook, E.H. Jr, Costello, E.J., Dahl, R.E., Koretz, D., Merikangas, K.R., Reiss, A.L., and Vitiello, B. (2002). Advances in developmental science and DSM-V. In *A Research Agenda for DSM-V* (ed. D.J. Kupfer, M.B. First, and D.E. Regier). Washington, DC: American Psychiatric Association, pp. 85–122.

Popper, K. (1963). *Conjectures and Refutations*. London: Routledge.

Putnam, H. (1995). *Renewing Philosophy*. Harvard, MA: Harvard University Press.

Putnam, H. (1996). In *Words and Life* (ed. J. Conant), (3rd edn). Harvard University Press.

Quine, W.V.O. (1975). "On Empirically Equivalent Systems of the World". *Erkenntnis*, 9, pp. 313–328.

Radden, J. (1994). Recent criticism of psychiatric nosology: a review. *Philosophy, Psychiatry, & Psychology*, 1(3): 193–200.

Reznek, L. (1987). *The Nature of Disease*. London: Routledge.

Reznek, L. (1995). Dis-ease about kinds: reply to D'Amico. *Journal of Medicine and Philosophy*, 20: 571–584.

Robbins, E., and Guze, S.B. (1970). Establishment of diagnostic validity in psychiatric illness: its application to schizophrenia. *American Journal of Psychiatry*, 126: 983–987.

Rosenhan, D.L. (1973). On being sane in insane places. *Science*, 179: 250–258.

Rossi, P. (2003). Magic, science, and equality of human wits. In *Nature and Narrative: an introduction to the new philosophy of psychiatry* (ed. K.W.M. Fulford, K.J. Morris, J.Z. Sadler, and G. Stanghellini). Oxford: Oxford University Press, Chapter 17.

Rounsaville, B.J., Alarcón, R.D., Andrews, G., Jackson, J.S., Kendell, R.E., and Kendler, K. (2002). Basic nomenclature issues for DSM-V. In *A Research Agenda for DSM-V* (ed. D.J. Kupfer, M.B. First, and D.E. Regier). Washington, DC: American Psychiatric Association, pp. 1–30.

Rust, J. and Golombok, S. (1989). *Modern psychometrics*. London: Routledge.

Sadler, J.Z. (ed.) (2002). *Descriptions and Prescriptions: values, mental disorders, and the DSMs*. Baltimore, MD: Johns Hopkins University Press.

Sadler, J.Z. (2004a). *Values and Psychiatric Diagnosis*. Oxford: Oxford University Press.

Sadler, J.Z. (2004b). Diagnosis/antidiagnosis. In *The Philosophy of Psychiatry: a companion* (ed. J. Radden). New York: Oxford University Press, pp. 163–179.

Sadler, J.Z. and Fulford, K.W.M. (2004). Should patients and families contribute to the DSM-V process? *Psychiatric Services*, 55(2): 133–138.

Sadler, J.Z., Wiggins, O.P., and Schwartz, M.A. (ed.) (1994). *Philosophical Perspectives on Psychiatric Diagnostic Classification*. Baltimore, MD: Johns Hopkins University Press.

Sartorius, N. (1976). Modifications and New Approaches to Taxonomy in Long-Term Care: Advantages and Limitations of the ICD. *Medical Care*, 14: 109–115, Supplement 5.

Sartorius, N. (1991). The classification of mental disorders in the Tenth Revision of the International Classification of Diseases. *European Psychiatry*, 6: 315–322.

Sartorius, N. (1992) in the Preface to World Health Organization (1992). *The ICD-10 Classification of Mental and Behavioural Disorders: Clinical Descriptions and Diagnostic Guidelines*. Geneva: World Health Organization.

Sartorius, N. (1995). *Understanding the ICD-10 Classification of Mental Disorders. A Pocket Reference*. Science Press Limited, London. (Also published in Polish, Russian and Ukrainian).

Sartorius, N. (2004). Personal Communication (at the World Psychiatric Association conference in Florence, November 10–13, on *Treatments in Psychiatry: an Update*).

Schaffner, K.F. (ed.) (1986). *Logic of Discovery and Diagnosis in Medicine*. Pittsburgh Series in Philosophy & History of Science. Berkley, CA: University of California Press.

Schaffner, K.F. (1993). *Discovery and Explanation in Biology and Medicine*. Science & Its Conceptual Foundations. Chicago: University of Chicago Press.

Spitzer, R.L. (2005). Recipe for disaster: professional and patient equally sharing responsibility for developing psychiatric diagnosis. *World Psychiatry*, 4:2, p89.

Stengel, E. (1959). Classification of mental disorders. *Bulletin of the World Health Organization*, 21: 601–663.

Szasz, T.S. (1972). The myth of mental illness. *The Myth of Mental Illness*. St Albans, England: Paladin.

Temerlin, M.K. (1968). Suggestion effects in psychiatric diagnosis. Journal of Nervous and Mental Disease, 147: 349–353.

Van Fraassen, B.C. (1980). *The Scientific Image*. Oxford: Oxford University Press.

Van Fraassen, B.C. (1999). To save the phenomena. In *The Philosophy of Science* (ed. R. Boyd, P. Gasker, and J.D. Trout). Cambridge, MA: MIT Press, pp. 187–194.

Williams, B. (1978). *Descartes: the project of pure inquiry*. London: Penguin.

Williams, B. (1985). *Ethics and the Limits of Philosophy*. Cambridge, MA: Harvard University Press.

Wing, J.K., Birley, J.L.T., Cooper, J.E., Graham, P., and Isaacs, A.D. (1967). Reliability of a procedure for measuring and classifying 'Present Psychiatric State'. *British Journal of Psychiatry*, 113: 499–515.

Wing, J.K., Cooper, J.E., and Sartorius, N. (1974). *Measurement and Classification of Psychiatric Symptoms*. Cambridge: Cambridge University Press.

WHO (1948). *Manual of the International Statistical Classification of Diseases, Injuries, and Causes of Death* (ICD-6). Bulletin of the World Health Organization, Suppl. 1, Geneva: World Health Organization.

WHO (1967). *Manual of the International Statistical Classification of Diseases, Injuries, and Causes of Death* (ICD-8). Geneva: World Health Organization.

WHO (1973). *International Pilot Study of Schizophrenia*. Geneva: World Health Organization.

WHO (1974). *Glossary of Mental Disorders and Guide to their Classification, for use in Conjunction with the International Classification of Diseases*, 8th revision. Geneva: World Health Organization.

WHO (1978). *Mental Disorders: glossary and guide to their classification in accordance with the ninth revision of the International classification of diseases*. Geneva: World Health Organization.

WHO (1992). *The ICD-10 Classification of Mental and Behavioural Disorders: clinical descriptions and diagnostic guidelines*. Geneva: World Health Organization.

World Health Organization (2001). *International Classification of Functioning, Disability and Health*. Geneva: World Health Organization.

Wright, C. (1992). *Truth and Objectivity*. Cambridge, MA: Harvard University Press.

Zubin, J. (ed) (1961). *Field Studies in the Mental Disorders*. New York: Grune and Stratton.

CHAPTER 14

Diagnosis, explanation, and tacit knowledge

Chapter contents

The central role of diagnosis

In this chapter we move from symptoms of mental disorder and their classification to the diagnostic process: how we come to explain or claim knowledge of someone's condition. Diagnostic explanation in medicine, as we saw in Chapter 3, is partly in terms of syndromes (identifying a patient's symptoms with a recognized pattern that carries implications for treatment and prognosis) and partly in terms of aetiology (causal information).

In general medicine, diagnostic explanations are more in terms of aetiology; in psychiatry and nosology, they are more in terms of symptoms and syndromes (they are 'descriptive', in the sense of that term used in ICD and DSM, see Chapter 13). Either way, though, diagnostic explanations are perceived as a species of scientific explanation. This prompts the question, therefore, just what a sound scientific explanation consists in. This question, as we will see, has been the subject of close scrutiny in the philosophy of science, and, although no definitive answers have been given, a number of key points have been established which are relevant to our understanding of the nature of scientific explanation in general and hence of diagnostic explanation in particular.

Diagnostic difficulties

As with many other aspects of medicine, psychiatric diagnosis has proven peculiarly problematic. One reason for this, highlighted above (Chapter 13), is that the aetiological theories, available in general medicine, have been much harder to establish for the brain. Hence psychiatry, from ICD-9 and DSM-III onwards, has focused, consistently with a traditional model of the process of science, on what can be directly observed, i.e. symptoms and signs. An important benefit of this, as we saw in Chapters 12 and 13, has been clearer specification of the rules (criteria) for establishing a given diagnosis. This in turn has led to improvements in reliability, which, it is (reasonably) assumed, reflects a closer approach to objectivity in psychiatric diagnosis, and, as a further aim, to the future establishment of causal accounts comparable with those available in other (non-neurological) medical disciplines. But this prompts the following general question that will be examined in the first half of this chapter. Can scientific explanations in general, and hence diagnostic explanations in particular, be analysed to provide an objective measure, a standard of correctness that any diagnosis has to pass? Is there a logical recipe that governs the form of every diagnosis? Can diagnosis, as a species of scientific exploration, be fully codified?

The focus of the first half of the chapter

To consider this question the chapter will begin by examining formal models of explanation from the philosophy of science. The reason for this is that both diagnosis and explanation share a common element. Both are ways of bringing bodies of general knowledge to bear on particular cases or facts. Work in the philosophy of science has produced a number of formal models of explanation that may thus shed light on diagnosis, as a species of explanation.

The main conclusion from the first half of the chapter, in Sessions 1 and 2, will in fact be a negative conclusion, namely that the project of full explicit codification of what counts as a sound scientific explanation, is not fully completable. This is an important conclusion particularly for psychiatric diagnosis, because it shows that, for all the benefits explicit codification has brought, something more, something additional to the critera spelled out in our official classification, will be needed for sound diagnostic explanation. This is not because psychiatric diagnostic explanation is unscientific but because of a feature (i.e. resistance to full explicit codification) that it shares with scientific explanation in general.

This leaves a gap, however, between the explicitly codified rules of diagnostic classification and their applications in diagnostic practice.

This suggests a second general question to be addressed in this chapter: Can diagnostic expertise in general be codified? Or does it, by contrast, rely on an element of tacit or implicit knowledge that resists such codification?

These two questions—about the possibility of a formal model of diagnosis drawing on work on explanation, and about the role of tacit knowledge—are distinct. But we will look at both in this chapter because, if developing a formal model of diagnosis is not finally successful, it suggests, at the very least, the possibility of a role for tacit knowledge that might also be independently supported by philosophical argument. That is what we will find. Philosophical models of explanation suggest a role for both laws and for causality in a proper understanding of diagnosis. But they also suggest the importance of tacit knowledge embodied in experience and practical skills.

The plan of the chapter

The plan of the chapter, then, is this:

1. The first session will examine Hempel's logical model of explanation: the Deductive-Nomological (DN) model.

2. The second session will concern two less formal models of scientific explanation that stress the role of causation and also context.

3. The third session will examine arguments for the claim that there is an element of uncodifiable tacit knowledge present in engineering and physical sciences.

4. Finally in the last session we will turn to the issue of whether a science of the mind presents particular problems for the formal regimentation and representation of knowledge and how it is applied to particular cases. This last session will provide a link between the phenomenological account of diagnosis explored in Part II and the scientific approaches discussed here. It will also lead directly into the discussion of reasons and causes in the next chapter, Chapter 15.

Session 1 The Deductive-Nomological model of explanation

Diagnostic explanation: descriptive and causal

To get started it is necessary first to have some clear idea of what is involved in diagnosis. That is the purpose of the first exercise.

EXERCISE 1   (15 minutes)

Think about the nature of medical diagnosis. What does diagnosis add to a description of signs and symptoms? What makes a diagnosis correct? What is the purpose of diagnosis? Look at the DSM-IV criteria below and think whether the general conclusions apply in this case.

DSM-IV diagnostic criteria for Attention-Deficit/ Hyperactivity Disorder

A. Either (1) or (2):

1. six (or more) of the following symptoms of **inattention** have persisted for at least 6 months to a degree that is maladaptive and inconsistent with developmental level:

   a. often fails to give close attention to details or makes careless mistakes in schoolwork, work, or other activities

   b. often has difficulty sustaining attention in tasks or play activities

   c. often does not seem to listen when spoken to directly

   d. often does not follow through on instructions and fails to finish schoolwork, chores, or duties in the workplace (not due to oppositional behavior or failure to understand instructions)

   e. often has difficulty organizing tasks and activities

   f. often avoids, dislikes, or is reluctant to engage in tasks that require sustained mental effort (such as schoolwork or homework)

   g. often loses things necessary for tasks or activities (e.g., toys, school assignments, pencils, books, or tools)

   h. is often easily distracted by extraneous stimuli

   i. is often forgetful in daily activities

2. six (or more) of the following symptoms of **hyperactivity-impulsivity** have persisted for at least 6 months to a degree that is maladaptive and inconsistent with developmental level:

   Hyperactivity

   a. often fidgets with hands or feet or squirms in seat

   b. often leaves seat in classroom or in other situations in which remaining seated is expected

   c. often runs about or climbs excessively in situations in which it is inappropriate (in adolescents or

adults, may be limited to subjective feelings of restlessness)

   d. often has difficulty playing or engaging in leisure activities quietly

   e. is often 'on the go' or often acts as if 'driven by a motor'

   f. often talks excessively

   Impulsivity

   g. often blurts out answers before questions have been completed

   h. often has difficulty awaiting turn

   i. often interrupts or intrudes on others (e.g., butts into conversations or games)

B. Some hyperactive-impulsive or inattentive symptoms that caused impairment were present before age 7 years.

C. Some impairment from the symptoms is present in two or more settings (e.g., at school [or work] and at home).

D. There must be clear evidence of clinically significant impairment in social, academic, or occupational functioning.

E. The symptoms do not occur exclusively during the course of a Pervasive Developmental Disorder, Schizophrenia, or other Psychotic Disorder and are not better accounted for by another mental disorder (e.g., Mood Disorder, Anxiety Disorder, Dissociative Disorder, or a Personality Disorder).

Diagnosis, explanation, and causal information

Medical diagnosis is usually based on the signs and symptoms presented by a patient to a clinician. But the aim of diagnosis is usually more than just the articulation and description of those signs and symptoms. It usually involves a further inference. This, however, is disguised in the recent concentration in DSM and ICD on operational criteria for diagnosis.

Consider two contrasting cases. One informal indication of diabetes used especially among itinerant workers in the middle of the twentieth century was the presence of white spots on footwear.

This works as an indication because of the following connections. Diabetes raises the level of sugar dissolved in urine. Whether or not suffering from diabetes, men sometimes splash their footwear when urinating. In the case of diabetics, however, when such splashed urine dries it leaves a precipitate of sugar: a white spot on the footwear. And, because they are, at some remove, *effects* of it, these spots are an *indicator* of diabetes.

In this case there is a clear gap between the signs and what they are signs of. Diabetes does not *comprise* having white spots on the footwear. It takes an inference, a judgement, to move from them to the underlying illness condition.

Things seem less clear in the criteria for attention-deficit/ hyperactivity disorder (ADHD) set out above. In this case there is more of a temptation to say that ADHD is not so much indicated by the behavioural criteria as simply being, or being constituted by, that pattern of behaviour. If so, it may seem that no further inference is required once the signs are articulated. But, in fact, whether or not that is a fair characterization there would still be a judgement in place even so in moving from the specific signs and symptoms of a particular patient to the general diagnosis of ADHD. The application of the general concept to the specific presentation is still a work of judgement.

Thus on the assumption that there is a further inference involved in diagnosis, what sort of inference is it? What constrains it? We will consider two suggestions. The first is that a diagnosis provides an *explanation* of symptoms. The other is that diagnosis aims to provide *causal information* about the symptoms.

By taking diagnosis to be a form of explanation we can shed light on it by looking at some of the more influential philosophical work on explanation. While both of the influential models of explanation considered below have difficulties they suggest the importance for explanation of both laws and of causality. (The problems turn on how *exactly* these play a role.) At the same time one of the morals that looking at these models will raise is that an explanation is offered in a particular context and given particular interests. This does not itself strictly imply that explanation, and thus diagnosis, necessarily contains a tacit element but it is suggestive.

Hempel's formal models of explanation

The classic model of explanation, which has dominated the philosophy of science during most of the twentieth century, is Hempel's DN model. You will recall Hempel's influence on psychiatric classification in Chapter 13. The effect of his work on scientific taxonomy by the psychiatrists working on ICD and DSM was to shift away from a premature aetiological focus to a descriptive or symptom-based approach.

Hempel's model of explanation dovetails with the Logical Empiricist model of science because it provides a *logical* recipe for satisfactory explanation. The recipe specifies the logical structure in which the sentences that comprise an explanation have to stand. By providing a required formal structure, the model aims to provide necessary and sufficient conditions for scientific explanation. It aims to establish what a satisfactory explanation is in a general and objective manner, independently of the particular subject matter being explained. Hempel described his model in many different papers, making various adjustments.

EXERCISE 2   (20 minutes)

Read the short extract from:

Hempel, C.G. (1999). Laws and their role in scientific explanation. In *The Philosophy of Science* (ed. R. Boyd, P. Gasker, and J.D. Trout). Cambridge, MA: MIT Press, pp. 299–315 (extract pp. 301–302)

Link with Reading 14.1

◆ What are the key conditions that, according to Hempel, any explanation has to meet.

Two sorts of explanation

Hempel characterizes two forms of explanation: DN explanation and Inductive Statistical (IS) explanation. To begin with we will focus on the former because the central ideas behind it are clearer.

Explanation as a logical argument

In very general terms, the key idea behind the DN model is that explanation is a *sound argument that establishes the truth of its conclusion*. The sentence that describes the event to be explained (the explanandum sentence) forms the conclusion of an argument whose premises (the explanans sentences) are sentences that state general laws and initial conditions. By equating explanation and logical argument, Hempel aims to use logical machinery to stipulate the form of any satisfactory explanation. In other words, Hempel's model is an abstract or formal model that aims to account for all forms of scientific explanation independently of their subject matter. Thus, on the one hand, the model promises to deliver an objective model of adequate explanation. On the other, it presupposes that explanation can always be so codified. This general assumption needs to be substantiated.

Hempel's two conditions

In *Philosophy of Natural Science* (Hempel, 1965), Hempel puts forward two quite general conditions for satisfactory scientific explanation:

1. explanatory relevance;
2. testability.

The first is explicated through the notion of giving grounds for belief. The explanatory information provided should afford good grounds for believing that the phenomenon to be explained did, or does, occur. It is a *necessary condition* for explanation that the information that is offered is relevant to what occurred.

The second condition requires that information offered as explanation should be substantial and make a real claim about the world. Hempel exemplifies this through a contrast with the vacuous explanation of gravitational attraction as a natural tendency in the universe. Such a claim lacks content and makes no concrete claim about the world. Crucially, as far as logical empiricism is concerned, it is incapable of being tested. (This emphasis on testing reveals the verificationist aspirations of Logical Empiricism.) The statements constituting a scientific explanation must be capable of empirical test.

Hempel's four conditions

These two conditions are further explicated and augmented elsewhere in Hempel's *Aspects of Scientific Explanation* (Hempel, 1966). There he lists four conditions:

1. the explanation must be a valid deductive argument;
2. the explanans must contain essentially at least one general law;
3. the explanans must have empirical content;
4. the sentences constituting the explanans must be true.

The first three are called *logical conditions of adequacy*. The last is called the *empirical condition of adequacy*. The former concern the *structure* to which explanations must adhere. One can imagine establishing that these are met without knowing anything of the nature of the world in which we live. The latter, however, connects explanation to this world. To establish that it is met requires knowing what the world is like, which facts obtain.

Explanation is a 'success' concept...

This way of explaining the difference between the two sorts of conditions does, however, risk one distortion. Hempel stresses that explanations must be true as opposed to being highly confirmed by evidence. In other words explanation is a 'success concept'. This idea can be explained by another example of a success concept: knowledge.

...like knowledge

The traditional analysis of *knowledge* has three components:

1. justified

2. true

3. belief.

If a candidate as a piece of knowledge lacks any of these components or if any one of these conditions is not met, then it fails to count as knowledge. This means that if a belief is not true, even if it is justified by available evidence, it is not knowledge. Similarly, if is true but not justified (a lucky guess perhaps), it is not knowledge. Thus our claims to knowledge are fallible in a strong sense. If they are false they are not merely 'false-knowledge' but not knowledge at all. The same goes for explanation on Hempel's model. The requirement that the explanans is true implies that putative or supposed explanations in which this condition is not met, such as explanation of diseases by reference to humours, are not just false explanations, but not explanations at all.

An example explanation

Hempel's first two conditions on explanation stipulate the kind of logical argument that explanation is supposed to consist in. A simple example might comprise:

1. the general law that objects acted upon by a net force accelerate in the direction of that force at a rate inversely proportional to their mass;

2. the initial claim that some such object was subjected to a net force of such and such;

3. and the conclusion that it accelerated in such and such a manner.

Given the initial condition and the general law then the conclusion follows by the logical argument form called *Modus Ponens* (see Chapter 5). In this logical structure, if the premises are true, then the conclusion *must* also be true. Thus the premises make it rational to believe the conclusion. The argument gives grounds to believe that the conclusion is true.

These characteristics concern DN explanation proper. Such explanation requires deduction from exceptionless laws. If the DN model were supposed to serve as a model of all scientific explanation then it would be seriously flawed for the following reason. There are many fields of science that do not provide exceptionless laws and instead employ merely statistical or probabilistic laws. The laws of most if not all of the special sciences such as geology, economics, psychology are either formally statistical or couched with 'ceteris paribus' clauses. (The latter include examples such as: in general, a wandering river erodes its banks.) But the unavoidability of statistical laws is not merely a reflection of imperfect nature of these sciences. As we are all by now very familiar, the physics of the very small (quantum physics) suggests that probabilistic laws are an inevitable consequence of the nature of the world rather than merely the result of our ignorance. As a result of this, Hempel proposed his second model alongside that of the DN account: the IS model.

The Inductive Statistical model

The IS model is similar to the DN model in that it is based on the intuition that an explanation is an argument that would support the truth of the explanandum. But the argument in this case is merely a statistical or probabilistic argument for the likelihood of the conclusion. IS explanations are not strictly valid arguments because the truth of the premises does not guarantee that the conclusion—or explanandum—must be true. While at first sight this might seem a minor difference it has at least one paradoxical consequence of which Hempel was aware. The same event can be given contradictory 'explanations' depending on how it is described.

One example runs as follows (taken from Brown, 1977, p. 58):

Consider a case in which Jones contracts a streptococcal infection and is treated with penicillin. One explanation of what happens next can be formed in the following way. The general, statistical law is: the probability of recovering from a streptococcal infection when treated with penicillin is close to one. This can be conjoined with the particular fact that Jones has a streptococcal infection and was treated with penicillin. The result is an IS explanation of the fact that Jones recovers from the streptococcal infection.

But if Jones is over 80 years old a different and contradictory explanation can be framed. In this case the general law is that the probability of a man over 80 years old not recovering from a streptococcal infection is close to one. The particular condition is that Jones is over 80 years old and has a streptococcal infection. What is explained is that Jones does not recover from streptococcal infection.

Thus whatever the outcome in this case, an appropriate IS explanation can be given. By contrast with DN arguments, two different explanations can be formed with true premises but leading to contradictory results. Thus the apparent similarity between the two forms of argument disguise fundamental differences.

For our purposes in this chapter, however, the differences between the IS and DN models are less significant than their similarities.

Think back to the criteria for ADHD set out at the start of this session. How would a diagnosis for ADHD be formalized using Hempel's model of explanation. What would be the explanans and explanandum? How would laws of nature figure? How might the difference between DN and IS be relevant?

Explanation and the codification of diagnosis

We are now in a position to see how the DN and IS model might shed light on diagnosis. Observed symptoms take the place of the explanandum. They are what have to be explained. General laws are provided by psychiatric theory and any particular conditions are provided, for example, by aspects of patient history. A successful diagnosis is thus one which makes clear how the observed symptoms derive from these general laws together with particular facts about the patient's life. A diagnosis sheds light on symptoms by showing how they are part of a more general picture and the way it does this can be codified or formalized by using Hempel's model.

In the case of ADHD, for example, the explanandum might take the form of signs and symptoms from a clinical encounter or a case vignette. They are what will be explained by the diagnosis. The explanans is the combination of the general laws and particular conditions. In this case, the general laws are those that describe the general behavioural features of sufferers of ADHD and the fact that the service user has ADHD. Thus the conjunction of the particular claim that a particular person has ADHD and with the general claim that anyone with ADHD will present with such and such signs and symptoms implies that the person in question will present with such and such symptoms.

With this model in mind we can see how the general laws present may be statistical rather than deductive. Looking back to the behavioural criteria we can see that they are disjunctions. Thus just because someone has ADHD does not imply that they have the sign: 'often fidgets with hands or feet or squirms in seat'. That is one of nine criteria, six of which have to be present to satisfy merely one disjunct of the overall criterion A. So at best, the diagnosis raises the probability of that sign.

Providing this analogy between explanation and diagnosis holds good—and it seems to—and providing that Hempel's formal models of explanation are sound, then it seems that a formal model can be specified for medical diagnosis. The hope, remember, is that if a formal model can be provided then diagnosis will be shown to be capable of objectivity. It will no more (and no less!) depend on subjective features of psychiatrists—on what chunks of information they choose to give and what general laws they choose to quote—than science in general depends on subjective features of scientists.

This is, of course, not to say that diagnoses might not go astray as a result of personal biases any more than that attempts at explanation might prove to be false and result from scientific error or bias. But they will fail by failing to meet up to the public and objective standards established by the formal logical model of what a diagnosis ought to be.

Objections to Hempel's model

Hempel's models have been very influential in the philosophy of science; however, they have also been subject to much criticism. Van Fraassen—a contemporary analytic philosopher of science whose work on realism was discussed in Chapter 13—summarizes a number of these, which are discussed below, in *The Scientific Image* (1980, pp. 97–112).

Van Fraassen raises a number of objections to the simple DN and IS models of explanation. Most of these objections are long standing and well known to both proponents and critics. We will focus on four examples. Their purpose here is not simply to point out that these particular models of explanation are flawed. Perhaps the models can be modified so as to escape these particular criticisms. (Hempel himself has continued to fine tune them for many years.) Rather the objections will serve to deepen our understanding of explanation in general and thus of diagnosis in mental health care.

Four counter-examples

The objections are:

1. The flagpole example: Is there a symmetric explanation for both the height of a flagpole and the length of its shadow?

2. The barometer example: Is explanation symmetric in the way that providing reasons for belief seems to be?

3. Birth control pills: Can the fact that contraceptive pills prevent pregnancy explain why a man who takes them does not himself become pregnant?

4. Syphilis and paresis. What is the explanatory relation between having untreated syphilis and developing paresis?

We will explain them in turn. In the first three examples the conditions for DN explanation can be met for cases that, pre-philosophically, we would deny were bona fide explanations. The fourth presents a slightly different case.

The flagpole

In the flagpole example, there are general laws governing trigonometry that can be applied to the straight path of light, straight flagpoles impeding it and the straight shadows that result. There are also particular facts. These comprise the angle that light from the sun makes with the ground, the height of the flagpole and the length of the shadow. Pre-philosophically there is one particular fact that can legitimately be explained among these by the other two. We can explain the length of the shadow with respect to the angle of the sun and the height of the flagpole. This explanation can be formalized in accord with the DN model. Given the general laws, and two of the particular facts (the angle of the sun and height of the flagpole) the third (the length of the shadow) can be derived.

But according to the DN model this is not the only way to assemble the laws and facts into an explanation. The model implies that either the angle of the sun, or the height of the flagpole can be explained by invoking the other fact in conjunction with the length of the shadow and the laws of trigonometry. Both of these 'explanations' accord with the DN model's prescriptions concerning the logical form of explanation. Neither, however, accord with our pre-philosophical intuitions about explanation. Intuitively there is an asymmetry about what can be explained here. The length of the shadow is explainable using the other facts and laws. But an explanation of why the flagpole is the height that it is or why the sun's light strikes the earth at its particular angle to the plain of the ground will have no use for information about the length of flagpole's shadow.

This asymmetry might also be expressed in this way. There is an asymmetry between explanation and the provision of grounds for belief. Knowledge of the length of the shadow and the height of the flagpole provides *reason to believe* that the angle of the sun is such and such and likewise for the two other particular facts. Any of the pairs of particular facts can, given the laws of trigonometry, provide reasons to believe the remaining fact. But only one fact can be *explained* by the other two. Thus, contra Hempel's original idea, explanation and having reason to believe are not symmetric.

The barometer

This last point is encapsulated in the barometer example. A barometer embodies a way of predicting the weather on the basis of current atmospheric pressure. It provides reasons to believe that the pressure is such and such and thus that the weather will be so and so. But that the barometer gives a certain reading does not explain why the pressure is such and such and why the weather will be so and so. Instead, pre-philosophically we should say that current pressure explains both the barometer's reading and the future weather, the former by simple physical laws, the latter by complex meteorological laws. But despite this, the DN model allows that any of these particular facts could be explained given the others and the laws.

Male birth control

Jones takes his wife's contraceptive pills. No one who takes contraceptives falls pregnant (let us assume). So Jones does not become pregnant.

The birth control example presents the following problem. It meets the logical conditions on explanation provided by the DN model. But, intuitively, it fails as an explanation. As men do not themselves become pregnant in any case, the fact that Jones takes his wife's birth control pills is irrelevant to his not becoming pregnant. In the earlier statement of conditions concerning explanation, Hempel attempted to preclude cases like this by stipulating that the explanans should be *relevant* to the explanandum. But the way this is 'unpacked' in the more explicit statement of four conditions is not successful. There, relevance is replaced by the prescription that the explanandum should follow logically from the explanans. That condition is met in the birth control example.

As our intuitions diverge strongly from the DN model in these three cases it is important to determine why this is so.

Causation

The most pressing objection to the possibility of explaining the height of the flagpole by citing its shadow is that this gets things the wrong way round. The shadow depends on the flagpole and not vice versa. This dependence is *causal*. The height of the flagpole is part of the condition that *causes* the shadow to be the length that it is. The shadow by contrast does not causally affect the flagpole's height or the sun's angle. Similarly, the barometer reading is caused by atmospheric pressure but does *not* cause it.

The general moral that these cases suggest is that one cannot explain causes in terms of their effects, although one can explain effects by citing their causes. The asymmetry of the relationship between cause and effect explains the asymmetry highlighted in these examples between explanans and explanandum.

Reasons for belief and causation

It is worth noting that the provision of reasons to believe does not depend in this asymmetric manner on causal relations. Causes can give reasons to believe in effects *and vice versa*. Barometer readings are caused by atmospheric pressure and thus serve as instruments that respond to and detect it. In fact this is the general principle behind detecting instruments. They are designed in such a way that their readings are the causal effects of the phenomena they detect. But knowledge of causes can also provide reasons to believe that their effects will obtain. Thus knowledge of the height of the flagpole (*inter alia*) provides reason to believe that the shadow will be of a certain length. Likewise, knowledge of underlying pathologies can give reason to believe that their causal symptoms will come about but equally, knowledge of symptoms, can give reason to believe in specific underlying pathologies.

Modifying Deductive-Nomological explanation?

One response to these counter instances is to augment the basic DN model by the claim that the explanans cause the explanandum. In the next session we will examine the general plausibility of this suggestion. But note that Hempel's aim was to provide a topic-neutral account of explanation through the provision of a purely formal and logical recipe for constructing good explanations. Adding in causation as an extra ingredient threatens that neutral account. It will impose a causal element into *all* forms of explanation. But is that a plausible claim? Think especially about those cases in psychiatric explanation that turn on the meaningfulness of certain sorts of action or reaction. There is a long-standing view in both the philosophy of science and of mind that reason explanations involve a different sort of intelligibility to subsumption under law. (We will return to this issue in Chapter 15, which will contrast subsumption of events under causal laws with rationalizing them by placing them in the 'space of reasons'.) Consider also that many diagnoses in neurology as well as psychiatry assimilate a case to a symptomatically defined category rather than specifying an underlying causally defined aetiology.

Before going on to consider the role of causation in explanation further below, remember that there is a different sort of reaction available to counter-instances to the philosophical model of explanation so far discussed. This is to give up the hope that there is a unified account of explanation that all proper explanations are instances of. It is too soon to adopt such a position yet, but it is worth keeping in mind that the assumption that every concept has an analysis is a *philosophical* assumption and rather a dubious one at that.

Syphilis and paresis

The fourth criticism listed above concerns syphilis and paresis. This example was introduced to philosophers in 1959 by the philosopher Michael Scriven. Scriven took the facts to be these: paresis or neurosyphilis occurs in patients that have progressed through the primary and secondary stages of a syphilis infection without antibiotic treatment. About one patient in four develops paresis. This is the only route to paresis. (Changes in empirical findings concerning paresis do not affect the basic point raised.)

EXERCISE 5   (15 minutes)

Consider the following questions:

♦ Can we explain why someone has paresis by saying they have untreated syphilis?

♦ Does this fit the DN or IS model from Hempel?

♦ Does the putative explanatory power depend on context?

♦ How does this case differ from the example of ADHD as regards Hempel's models?

The idea that we can explain the development of paresis by citing untreated syphilis turns on the thought that had the subject not contracted syphilis, or had it been treated, then they would not have developed paresis. Untreated syphilis is a causal step towards paresis and by preventing it, one can prevent paresis. So to that extent it looks as though it can sometimes be at least part of an explanation. Clearly this at least accords with the causal component of explanation that has been isolated above. At least

part of the reason for saying that untreated syphilis explains paresis is that there is a causal connection between them.

But on the other hand, the fact that a patient suffers untreated syphilis does not provide reason to believe that he or she will develop paresis because the chances of developing it are small. Most subjects with untreated syphilis do not develop the condition. So again the example highlights a difference between explanation and have reasons for belief in the effect. In this case, it does not even seem that the explanans makes the explanandum likely.

We will return to the question of context later. But the question highlights the fact that there may be differences in the explanatory power of the explanans given the context. Think of the differences between asking the question of why Jones has paresis if Jones visits his general practitioner versus asking it if Jones is on a hospital ward for those with previously untreated syphilis.

There are a number of differences between this case and that of ADHD discussed above. In this case, the putative explanation of paresis is *causal*. It is an aetiological account albeit probabilistic (in 1959 at least). By contrast the ADHD case looks to fit the DN or IS model even though it seems to turn on *pattern recognition* at the level of syndromes rather than underlying causal mechanism.

We will develop some of these points by looking to a more explicitly causal model of explanation in the next session.

Reflection on the session and self-test questions

Write down your own reflections on the materials in this session drawing out any points that are particularly significant for you. Then write brief notes about the following:

1. What is it that diagnosis adds to a description of a patient's signs and symptoms? Why might diagnosis involve a form of inference? If so, what form of inference?

2. What is the nub of Hempel's model of explanation? What kind of thing is an explanation?

3. What role do laws play? How does explanation relate to prediction?

4. What should we learn from the counter examples to Hempel's formal models?

Session 2 A causal model of explanation

David Lewis, an influential American metaphysician, develops the causal strain in explanation that the counter examples to the DN model bring to light. Philosophical theories of the nature of causation will be the subject of Chapter 15. Here we will concentrate on the role of causation in explanation.

The key idea on which Lewis' account is based is that events or facts are explained by providing information about their causes. This accords with the intuition above that explanation and causation are interconnected. Rather than adding a further causal condition to the DN or IS models, Lewis simply says that explanation comprises provision of causal information however that is provided. This change of approach marks a further fundamental difference.

More or less explanation

Lewis' example of crash investigation supports his claim that the notion of *complete* explanation is of no practical significance. As explanation is, according to Lewis, the provision of causal information and as there is no practical limit to the causal information that could be provided short of a history dating back to the Big Bang, explanation is always partial. All explanations provide less than the full causal story and what they do provide is selected on the basis of one's explanatory *interests*. Thus in different contexts, different explanations might be given for the same car crash.

Take the example of a car crash whose causal history includes both of the following facts (and an almost infinite number of other factors). The driver had consumed sufficient alcohol to slow his or her reactions and the car was equipped with ordinary brakes that, in the event, locked on. All other things being equal, if either the driver had not consumed alcohol or the car had possessed an antilocking braking system, the crash would not have occurred. Depending on one's interests in biology or engineering one might thus say that the explanation of the crash was alcohol consumption or having poor brakes. Providing that both these features played a causal role, neither is straight-forwardly a better candidate for *the* explanation. Both are partial explanations but citing one or the other may be more relevant given one's interests.

The importance of Lewis's 'explanatory interests' in causal explanations may seem to run counter to the 'objectivity' of science. But so far as medicine at least is concerned, the Swedish philosopher, Ingmar Lindahl, has produced direct empirical evidence for precisely this interest-led feature of causal explanations in his empirical study of attributions of causes of death in hospital records (Lindahl and Johansson, 1994). In the context at least of

medicine, then, Lewis' theoretical work on scientific explanation in general, combined with Lindahl and Johansson's empirical study, provides a clear illustration of the goal-directedness of science noted in Chapter 11. This in turn connects with one of the key themes of this book, spelled out particularly in Part I (on Concepts) and Part IV (on Values), of the pervasiveness and importance of evaluation, alongside description, at least in the medical sciences.

Causal information and diagnostic validity

Thus the attraction of something like Lewis's approach can also be seen in contemporary thinking about diagnostic categories in psychiatry. Robert Kendell and Assen Jablensky put the following suggestion in 'Distinguishing between the validity and utility of psychiatric diagnosis' (2003):

> [A] few diagnostic categories in psychiatry are almost universally accepted as valid. Most of these categories designate causes of mental retardation or dementia, such as Down's syndrome, fragile X syndrome, phenylketonuria, Huntington's disease, and Jacob-Creutzfeldt disease. (p. 8)

They go on to suggest that a test for validity is:

> [i]f the category's defining characteristics are more fundamental—that is, if the category is defined by a physiological, anatomical, histological, chromosomal, or molecular abnormality—clear, qualitative differences must exist between these defining characteristics and those of other conditions with a similar syndrome. (p. 8)

The suggestion is that a diagnosis is paradigmatically valid if distinguishing causal information is available to support it.

Kendell and Jablensky (2003) do not address the context dependence of explanation present in Lewis's account. But we can begin to see how such context dependence will be less visible in cases where there is background agreement on the kinds of causal information under scrutiny in the medical profession. That might, for example, focus attention on factors that can be changed, physiological factors (rather than broader causal factors) and so on. In other words, it is possible to borrow Lewis's focus on causation and downplay his context dependence.

Some putative counter-instances

This context dependence of explanation is an important point to which we will return shortly. Whatever its prima facie attractions, however, as a model of diagnostic explanation, Lewis's general claim that explanation comprises the provision of causal information must be reconciled with some apparent counter examples. Lewis himself considers some of the following cases, which will be outlined below.

1. Teleological explanation: Is teleological explanation possible?

2. Fermat's least time principle and the gas laws: Do all explanations drawn from contemporary physics fit Lewis's account?

3. Biological teleological explanation: Is putative teleological explanation possible?

4. Intentional explanation: Does the explanation of action in terms of desires for the future fit the model?

5. Mathematical explanation: Can explanation in non-causal disciplines be accommodated?

Teleology

As the key claim is that explanation turns on causality, there can be no genuinely teleological explanation. A teleological explanation is one that explains by citing a telos or goal. But to explain an event by citing its goal is not to cite its causes as one of the marks of causality is its temporal ordering. Effects cannot precede their causes.

The Greek fourfold notion of causality

Teleological explanation dates back to the Greeks. In Greek philosophy there are four notions of causality: efficient, final, formal, and material. The concept of causation as it occurs in contemporary analytic philosophy is most closely associated with the Greek efficient cause. The other aspects have now been separated from causality. Roughly speaking, the final cause corresponds to the general telos or purpose of something. The formal cause is the form or idea lying behind it. The material cause corresponds to the underlying substance. Thus if we consider the 'causes' of a ceremonial cup then the efficient cause might be the hammering of the silversmith; the final cause might be the purpose of celebrating the gods through drink; the formal cause might be the design idea the smith had in mind; and the material cause might be the silver involved. Clearly, this rich fourfold notion of causality is only dimly related to our much slimmer notion of causation. But in so far as there is a relation it is that our idea of causation corresponds to the Greek idea of efficient cause and that we lack a genuinely teleological notion of causation.

Teleological explanation is still a live issue in psychiatry because of attempts to use it define psychiatric disorder; see, e.g. Megone, 2000.

Teleological explanation in physics?

In apparent contradiction of the claim that there can be no such thing as teleological explanation there are examples of explanation in physics, biology, and psychology, which seem to be future directed. If Lewis's account is correct then despite appearances, none of these cases can really be teleological. This is what he attempts to establish. In each case, the basic strategy is the same.

The problem with both Fermat's least time principle and the gas laws, is that events are explained (the passage of light, the behaviour of gases) by invoking future states of affairs. Light travels through those points that lie on a path that comprises the quickest way through a refracting medium. Gases tend towards the ratios of temperature, pressure and volume given by the law PV/T = constant. Both therefore appear to be teleological.

Teleology is only apparent in physics

Lewis's response is to deny that such explanations rely only on the laws explicitly cited. Instead, he suggests, their explanatory force stems from the causal account that, he argues, must be assumed implicitly to underlie these regularities. The laws themselves describe in a convenient form the result of purely causal processes. The explanation may *appear* teleological, therefore, but it is not.

Thus Fermat's least time principle is a heuristic for calculating the path of light that is itself made true—assuming that it really is true—by underlying non-teleological causal processes. Likewise the gas laws express relationships between volume, pressure and temperature which are themselves the macroscopic result of underlying microscopic causal interactions between gas molecules. The genuinely causal regularities that govern the behaviour of individual gas molecules give rise to, and can be used to explain, the regularities that govern gases when considered at the macroscopic level. In both these cases, the explanatory power of apparently teleological physical laws or principles derives from the genuinely causal regularities that make them true. It is because there are laws linking the causal processes with the higher level teleological principles that we can use those higher principles as explanations at all. Their teleological explanatory power is thus, according to Lewis, derivative of causal explanations.

Teleological explanation in biology?

While apparently teleological explanation is rare in the physical sciences, it is much more common in the biological sciences. Here, however, Lewis's strategy is more familiar. Perhaps the most striking feature of natural selection as an explanation of biological diversity is precisely that it attempts to show how apparently purposive adaptation is really the result of normal efficient causal processes. In the light of this theory, purposive explanations of adaptation are not completely excluded. But they receive reinterpretation. The explanation of biological features through their functions or teleology is really a shorthand for a longer and properly causal account of the selective advantages produced by random genetic variation.

The debate about the nature of teleological biological explanations has recently re-surfaced in psychiatry over the nature of dysfunctions in the characterization of mental illness. One side of the debate, represented, for example, by Wakefield (2000), claims that a proper understanding of biological function and dysfunction allows psychiatry to be purged of any evaluative notion. The other side, represented, for example, by Fulford (2000), argues that a proper understanding of biological function maintains its evaluative status.

Intentional explanation

The case is less clear-cut in the case of intentional psychological explanation: the explanation of action through the intentions of the agent involved.

The nature of this kind of explanation will be the subject of further discussion in the Part V. Here, however, the important point is that explanation of action is typically provided through consideration of what the purpose of the action is. One might explain the adding of seasoning to a casserole by saying that the cook wanted to improve its flavour and believed that adding seasoning would bring that about. This seems to be a typical form of explanation of actions. The act of adding seasoning *during* the cooking is explained by its intended effect *later on* when the food is to be eaten. That this is a standard feature of action explanation is uncontentious. But it presents a prima facie difficulty for Lewis's model of explanation because it appears to be a case of genuinely teleological explanation.

Reasons as causes

Lewis's response is to defend his model of explanation by subscribing to a particular view of the philosophy of mind. This view is in no sense outlandish or outré. It is in fact an element of the current orthodoxy in the philosophy of mind. Nevertheless it is an important feature of Lewis's model of explanation that it does have this action at a distance in the philosophy of mind. Future directed mental states—such as the desire to improve the taste of the casserole—are really, on this view, *encoded* in present tense physical states of the body. These occurrent states cause the actions that they explain through physical and genuinely non-teleological causal connections. Thus even the intentional explanation of action turns out to be, on this philosophical interpretation, a species of causal explanations and thus to fit Lewis's model.

Rationalizing explanations

The example does, however, suggest a further limitation of Lewis' model. Intentional explanation is a combination of two elements. On the one hand it can be used to explain actions or events and the best model we have of the explanation of events is causal explanation. On the other hand it relies on the provision of *reasons* for actions. This suggests that intentional explanation is a species of rational explanation. The mental states of agents *support*, *justify*, or *undermine* one another. Mental states are in this sense normative.

Mathematical explanation

It is this normative element in intentional explanations that does not fit easily with Lewis's account. Lewis provides no insight into the *rational* power of reasons. Similarly, he provides no insight into the *normative* explanations of why such and such a conclusion follows from premises or why a particular figure is the correct result of a mathematical calculation (e.g. the result is two, *because* one plus one equals two). Logical and mathematical explanations are not causal explanations, as required by Lewis, but they are explanations none the less.

This is a limitation in Lewis's account rather than evidence that it is wrong. While causal information may be relevant to the explanation of why events in the causal order happen, it is not relevant to normative explanations. To explain the explanatory power of normative explanations, a different account

is needed. The limitation might be characterized like this. Causal explanation is needed to account for why events occur but not (except in some cases) what about them makes them the events they are. Thus they can be used to explain why a batsman in a game of cricket was dismissed Leg Before Wicket (because the bowler bowled a fast ball and the batsman did not keep his eyes on the ball) but not what about event permitted it to be classified LBW (because the ball bounced where it did before hitting the leg). Again, we return to this point later in this part, in Chapter 15 on Causes, Laws and Reasons, and in Part V.

Hempel and Lewis: a rapprochement?

But there is a more pressing problem for our purposes here. The aim of this chapter is to examine the relevance of models of explanation in the philosophy of science for the purpose of formalizing diagnosis. But Lewis's account appears to be too woolly to help in this matter. The claim that explanation comprises providing causal information does not itself suggest how this should be brought about. Perhaps it is true that diagnosis also relies on pinpointing the *causes* of the symptoms recorded by descriptive psychopathology. If so then the model provides some insight into diagnostic practice. Certainly, as Hempel (1999) pointed out, there is a sense in that the descriptive categories on which ICD and DSM are largely based, are promissory on future discoveries of underlying causes, much as the descriptive categories of Victorian medicine, such as dropsy (accumulation of fluid in the lower legs), have now been replaced by a range of different aetiological categories (heart failure, liver disease, and so forth). But Lewis' formal model of explanation does not show precisely how diagnostic explanation relies on causation (actual or promissory) and thus how diagnosis might be an objective, rule governed practice. It does not point to a substantial methodology for diagnosis.

In fact, having stressed the differences in emphasis between his account and the DN model, Lewis suggests that there could be a rapprochement between his and Hempel's accounts. There is no reason why causal information could not be provided by DN explanations. Providing that these deliver *elements* of the causal history of the explanandum and are not thought of as comprising *the* explanation, they can provide (partial) explanations.

Lewis's model and the codification of diagnosis

But, for the purpose of codifying diagnosis, there is a profound objection to Lewis's model that relates back to a feature highlighted earlier. As Lewis denies that there can be such a thing as *the* explanation of an event, what passes for 'the' explanation in the context of everyday life depends on the context of interests that guide research. A formal model of explanation, including diagnostic explanation, thus depends (*inter alia*) on a formal account of context. But as Van Fraassen (1999) argues in the reading linked with Exercise 7, there seems to be no prospect of the context of explanation itself being formalized.

Van Fraassen's emphasis on the context of explanation

EXERCISE 7   (30 minutes)

Read the extract from:

Van Fraassen, B. (1999). The pragmatics of explanation. In *The Philosophy of Science* (ed. R. Boyd, P. Gasker, and J.D. Trout). Cambridge, MA: MIT Press, pp. 317–327 (extract pp. 324–325)

Link with Reading 14.3

♦ Think of the consequences of this reading for the prospect of codifying explanation and thus diagnosis.

Explanation is a three-place relation

The moral that Van Fraassen (1999) draws is that explanation is not a simple relation between a fact and a body of theory and antecedent conditions as Hempel (1999) suggests. Likewise, if Lewis's claim that explanation turns on the provision of causal information, this does not imply that the relation of explanans and explanandum can be codified. Instead, Van Fraassen suggests, explanation is a three-place relation between theory, fact, and context. This is because explanation is, on this account, an answer to an implicit why question. As such, explanations need to be evaluated with respect to their implicit questions. But there is no single context for all questions of the form: why P? What exactly is being asked for is fixed by the particular context of interests.

Syphilis and paresis again

Consider again the syphilis and paresis example. Having untreated syphilis can be an explanation of developing paresis because it is necessary (although not sufficient) for developing the latter that one has the former. If a patient had not had syphilis she would not have developed paresis. But as an *explanation* this is only successful against a background assumption that it is unusual to have untreated syphilis. On a hospital ward in which everyone has syphilis, the explanation of why only Jones has developed paresis cannot simply be that she (like everyone else) has syphilis. In that context, the question involves an implicit contrast with the other patients. Why has she, in contrast to the others, contracted that disease? It may be that there simply is no explanation of that fact. Outside the context provided by the hospital ward, however, syphilis does provide an explanation because contracting it explains why Jones in contrast to her co-workers develops paresis.

Of course one issue that this example raises is an issue of principle that concerns the presence or not of other causal factors. It seems intuitive to think that if the chances of developing paresis given untreated syphilis are small, then there must be other factors in play when sufferers do develop it (factors that are missing for those who do not). And this in turn raises an interesting question of how to interpret statistical claims. If the chances of a particular group developing a particular condition are 80%, are the chances 80% for individuals within that group (i.e. there is a genuine element of indeterminacy) or are they determined as either 100% or 0% for each individual and the 80% figure overall is a measure of our ignorance of the particular details? Whatever the answer to that question of principle for each such claim, however, we do use statements of probability to explain events. But as the discussion of Hempel's IS model of explanation suggested above, such explanations suffer the complication that different probabilities apply depending on how an individual is picked out. (In the example above Jones has a nearly 100% chance of recovering from a streptococcal infection if described as a member of the general population but nearly 100% chance of not recovering if described as over 80 years old.)

Thus in the absence of completely deterministic explanations—which seem unlikely in medicine—the context will play an important part in explanation. In fact, according to models of contrastive explanation, context is important even in deterministic explanation.

Contrastive explanation

The Cambridge Professor of Philosophy of Science Peter Lipton presents a related account by focusing explicitly on contrastive explanations. In these, one aims to explain why one thing happened rather than another. Thus explanation involves both the fact that actually obtained and a foil that did not. As Lipton convincingly argues in his *Inference to the Best Explanation* (1991), contrastive explanation cannot be reduced to a more basic form. (But unlike Van Fraassen, Lipton assumes, although he does not flesh this out, that there can also be non-contrastive explanation in accord with Lewis's account. He does not counter Van Fraassen's claim that such explanation is also always implicitly contrastive.)

The strength of Lipton's account is that once a suitable foil is selected, he shows the sort of causal information that is required for a contrastive explanation. It is information about the cause of the fact and the absence of a corresponding cause in the history that leads to the foil. Such explanation works by pinpointing what it is that makes the difference between the one thing happening and the other not happening. But as Lipton admits, he provides no recipe for how to choose one contrast rather than another. He simply demonstrates that some choices will not furnish a suitable explanation because they are too different. The fact and foil must share much of their causal history because otherwise 'we do not know where to begin to answer the question'. But this will still leave an infinite number of possible foils. Lipton's point is that choosing one contrast rather than another is context dependent in a way that (thus far) resists explicit codification. So the explanation 'works' in the relevant context but between 'consenting adults', who are consenting because they share the same (largely tacit) context.

The end of diagnosis?

The suggestion that context plays an ineliminable role in the evaluation of explanation suggests that explanation cannot be formalized in a logical recipe. This suggests that diagnosis is also unformalizable. The connection runs as follows. Van Fraassen (1999) suggests that it makes no sense to talk of *the* explanation of an event because what would be a relevant explanation will depend on local matters of substance rather than general abstract features of explanation. Similarly, what makes a diagnosis the right diagnosis is not just that it explains the symptoms but that it is the right and relevant explanation in the clinical circumstances. These will include the possibility of supplying a suitable prognosis and the possibility of treatment. Van Fraassen's work suggests that while this context guides diagnosis, it cannot be codified. Does this imply that diagnosis is a tacit skill? And if so does this mark out mental health and health practice in general as less than rational or less than scientific?

Remember, however, that the arguments discussed here have all been developed with the sciences of physics and engineering in mind. To the extent, therefore, that the process of diagnosis is scientific, it shares with physics and engineering the limitations that recent philosophy of science has identified. It is a different model of science rather than non-science that we are converging on.

There is a further important theme that you may have noticed in this session. The stress on the role of context for explanation suggests that values impact on science here. But we began the part saying that we would not focus on values in science (although epistemic values were briefly mentioned in Chapter 11), but instead on the role of judgement in science even when explicit value judgements were not to the fore. Values seem, however, to return when we look at explanation. Does this imply that science contains values because it contains explanations? Van Fraassen himself does not think this is so. Because explanations rely on a particular context of interest, which is not itself a scientific matter, he says that 'science *contains no explanations*' (Van Fraassen, 1999, p. 325). In other words, one response to the question just asked attempts to keep science value free by suggesting that

explanation itself is not part of science itself. The natural opposing view is to preserve the connection of science and explanation and follow where the practical context of interests guides us. It is to this we will turn in the next session.

Session 3 Clinical skills and tacit knowledge

Two aspects to diagnosis

We have seen that the most influential models of explanation provided by work in the philosophy of science do not provide a regimented codification, which could apply to diagnosis. They do not provide a model of just what a complete diagnosis would consist in. That is not to say they offer no insights. Hempel's model suggests that explanation is connected to laws of nature. It is by appealing to laws that an explanation has the content it does. Lewis suggests that explanation is connected to the provision of causal information. Thus far, these insights are consistent with a traditional medical-scientific understanding of clinical diagnosis. The discussion suggests that successful diagnosis should be underpinned by laws of nature (biological, chemical, and indeed physical), and that it should explain a patient's symptoms by describing (or implying) what causes them.

Less familiar, though, in a medical context, is the idea that scientific explanations depend, according to Van Fraasen, on a context of interest. If this is right, scientific explanations in general, and hence diagnostic explanations in particular, cannot be formalized. That is to say, as there is no way of giving a formal specification of the relevant context (context being essentially particular), and as context is (if Van Fraassen is right) essential to scientific explanation, there can be no fully explicit and complete set of rules for identifying a 'good' scientific (including diagnostic) explanation. What is a good explanation in one context of interest may not be in another.

The implication for the project of codification of psychiatric diagnosis (as in ICD and DSM) is clear. Important as the project of codification has been in improving the reliability of psychiatric classification, diagnostic practice can never be fully captured by explicit 'rules', however carefully spelled out (operationalized).

Again, this is not to undermine the status of psychiatry as a science. The context dependence of scientific explanation is a feature of scientific explanation as a whole. It may be more important to recognize that explanation is context dependent in psychiatric science than in other areas (i.e. because the practical impact of context may, as a feature of the greater difficulty presented by sciences of the mind, be greater). That, as they say, is another story. But the point for now is, simply, that scientific explanation in general is not explanation of a kind that can be fully codifiable; hence we should not expect diagnostic explanation, if scientific, to be fully codifiable.

This conclusion thus leaves us with a question. What else, besides following a set of rules, is involved in diagnosis? What do

---

Reflection on the session and self-test questions

Write down your own reflections on the materials in this session drawing out any points that are particularly significant for you. Then write brief notes about the following:

1. What is the heart of Lewis's suggestion about what explanations have in common? How does his account relate to Hempel's?

2. What are the consequences of Lewis's model for a formal codification of explanation.

3. What does Van Fraassen add to this picture?

we have to fill the gap between theory (i.e. the codified rules of a psychiatric classification) and practice (i.e. the diagnostic explanations given by practitioners in individual cases)?

In the last two sessions of this chapter we will turn to one possible candidate for filling the gap between theory and practice, namely tacit knowledge built up through clinical experience and embodied in clinical practice skills. That tacit knowledge may be important in the gap between theory and practice in medical (including psychiatric) diagnosis is, as we will see, suggested by arguments from both the philosophy and sociology of science to the effect that tacit knowledge is important in the gap between theory and practice in *all* sciences.

There is of course no strict connection between the context dependence of scientific explanation and the tacit knowledge of practical skills. Tacit knowledge, though, as we will see, like the context dependence of explanation, has been shown to be a feature of the paradigm 'hard' sciences such as physics and engineering. If, then, tacit knowledge is important in physics and engineering, it is entirely consistent with the scientific status of medicine (including psychiatry) that tacit knowledge should turn out to be important in these disciplines as well. Though as we will see in the concluding session of this chapter, when it comes to diagnostic explanations specifically of *mental* symptoms, i.e. as in psychiatry, there is an added element of difficulty, foreshadowed in Chapter 11 by the tension between scientific and hermeneutic (meaning-driven) accounts of psychoanalysis, an element of difficulty arising from the fact that such symptoms may demand what Karl Jaspers (in Part II) identified as (meaningful) understanding as well as (causal) explanation.

An empirical investigation of the role of tacit knowledge in applied physics

One of the clearest demonstrations of the role of tacit knowledge in the hard sciences is to be found in the work of the contemporary British sociologist, Harry Collins. The sociology of science will be the subject of Chapter 16. As we will see, the very idea that there can be a distinctive sociological investigation of science raises important questions, both about its underlying assumptions and its relation to the philosophy of science. Investigating those issues, in a later chapter, will help shed light on the scientific enterprise generally. But one preliminary issue concerning the nature of the sociological of science is worth advertising in advance of that later discussion.

Two views of the role of sociological investigation

There have, historically, been two views of the role of sociological analysis of science. On one view, sociology complements philosophical analysis. Philosophy of the science articulates the rational structure that scientific progress ought to take. This is then mapped on to historical or sociological analysis of what has

actually happened. Where there are divergences it is up to historical or sociological analysis to explain why the scientists concerned did not follow the path of rationality as dictated by philosophy. The assumption behind this approach, which was historically supported by the sociologist Carl Mannheim, is that rationality is its own explanation. Once one has pointed out that an action was rational in the light of the demands of scientific method, no further explanation is needed of why it took place. All that needs sociological explanation is failure of rationality.

On the other view, there is no trans-historical standard of rationality by which to judge the progress of science and it is the task of sociological analysis to determine just what, in any given context, was judged to be rational and why. This second view is clearly a more radical view and gives greater weight to sociological findings. Collins subscribes to this more radical view. But in what follows, while we will see some of the evidence that might be used to support the radical view, it is not necessary to assume that it is correct.

Background to the extract

The short extract linked with Exercise 8 below gives a feel of Collins' work in his book *Changing Order* (1985). The book as a whole is concerned with a key aspect of scientific process: replicating findings. Replication plays a role in science in general like reliability in medicine. Collins takes it to be the mark of scientific respectability that a finding can be replicated. His argument concerns the abilities of scientists involved in successful replication and the role of tacit or implicit knowledge.

In chapter 3 of his *Changing Order* Collins discusses the case of replicating a new kind of laser. While it might have been assumed that publishing the technical details of such lasers in an engineering journal would provide trained scientists with the ability to construct one, this proved not to be the case. In fact new lasers were built only by those who had direct practical experience of a working laser in another laboratory. Was this because insufficient details had been given? The extract below suggests some general reasons for the uncodifiability of the whole of the expertise involved.

EXERCISE 8 (20 minutes)

Read the extract from:

Collins, H. (1985). *Changing Order*. London: Sage (extracts: pp. 66–67, 69–71)

Link with Reading 14.4

- What is the connection between replication and objectivity?
- What reasons does Collins suggest for there being a tacit dimension to knowledge?

Think about whether and how these might apply to clinical expertise.

Replication and objectivity

Collins suggests that replication is a central test of the objectivity of scientific claims, especially claims based on experimental results. For an experimental result to be objectively established it must be possible for others to replicate it. (This matches the connection between validity and reliability discussed in Chapter 13.)

Scientific knowledge is both general and impartial. Its results should be reproducible because it concerns the *general* working of the world in accordance with universal principles and principles should be indifferent to the particular experimental scientists concerned. (Science does not subscribe to the personality cults of witchcraft, see, e.g. Rossi, 2003.) If an experimental result cannot be reproduced, this suggests that it is not a reliable indicator of how the world really works but a mistaken interpretation, a result of some error somewhere in the original experiment.

According to Collins, scientific practitioners generally misrepresent what is involved in replication. They assume that experimental protocol can be satisfactorily and fully recorded in the written research papers published in journals and that these contain sufficient information to enable others to replicate results. But this is not in fact so.

Knowledge cannot be linguistically represented

Collins's key claim is that the knowledge necessary for replication both is not and cannot be completely linguistically codified. Some necessary knowledge is practical and tacit. It is not conveyed in the formal representation of experiments found in both research journals and science textbooks. Rather, it can only be communicated through practical demonstrations and personal contact.

It is worth examining the reasons suggested in the extract for the presence of a tacit dimension. Perhaps the most powerful point is the suggestion that noting some and ignoring other differences between different lasers is crucial. Seeing some physical differences as playing an important role and seeing others as completely inessential presents a real problem for codifying scientific expertise. Listing all the things to be ignored, for example, would be an infinite task.

Collins's summary of his own empirical findings

Collins goes on to draw more radical conclusions than those we have highlighted. He summarizes his findings in the following six points:

1. Transfer of skill-like knowledge is capricious.

2. Skill-like knowledge travels best (or only) through accomplished practitioners.

3. Experimental ability has the character of a skill that can be acquired and developed with practice. Like a skill it cannot be fully explicated or absolutely established.

4. Experimental ability is invisible in its passage and in those who possess it.

5. Proper working of the apparatus, of parts of the apparatus *and of the experimenter*, are defined by the ability to take part in producing the proper experimental outcome. Other indicators cannot be found.

6. Scientists and others tend to believe in the responsiveness of nature to manipulations directed by sets of algorithm-like instructions. This gives the impression that carrying out experiments is literally a formality. This belief, suspended at times of difficulty, recrystalizes upon the successful completion of an experiment.

These claims go further than we have a justification for. Claims 4 and 5, for example, suggest that because an ability cannot be fully written down it is both impossible to establish ('absolutely') and is invisible in its transfer. But in general we do not think that it is impossible to assess practical skills using practical examination and there seems to be nothing particularly mysterious in transmitting such skills through practical instruction. This is part of a standard medical training.

But whether or not all his conclusions are justified, his claim about the central role of a tacit dimension is important. What makes Collins's analysis particularly striking is that it is advanced as a result of the investigation not of an interpretative or social science but of the 'hard' science of engineering. He is not merely saying that there is some tacit knowledge in some of the softer sciences but that tacit knowledge is a necessary feature of replication in the whole of science.

The status of Collins's remarks

Such a general claim deserves to be taken with some scepticism. Collins's work is based on empirical research and thus, by the same scientific standards that he articulates, stands in need of replication. What is more, a general claim of the sociology of science is that social factors—including interests and values—have a profound influence on scientific investigation. Thus one might expect a professionally optimistic sociologist to 'discover' that his subject matter—hard science—contains aspects that can only be investigated using sociology. Here, however, our purpose is not to establish the general scientific credibility of Collins's claim. Instead it is to raise Collins's claim as an interpretative tool for examining mental health care and to investigate whether there are conceptual or philosophical reasons to support it.

Replication and diagnosis

The connection between Collins's discussion of replication and our concern with explanation and diagnosis is this. Replication requires that the same experimental results are reproduced by other experimenters in other contexts. The most direct method of attempting this is to reproduce the same experiment using the same equipment and the same methods. It is for this reason that details of experimental methods are given in technical papers in scientific journals. But, according to Collins, such papers can never fully explicate what the relevant 'sameness' comprises.

The number of factors that could in principle be specified in describing the original experimental set-up is unlimited and thus could not all be set down. Instead such descriptions presuppose an unrepresented set of assumptions that have to be communicated as practical know-how.

The same general issues are repeated in the case of explanation and diagnosis. Diagnosis requires identifying particular medical conditions as the *same* as others of the same diagnostic classification. The general lesson that Collins's account of replication suggests is that no account of sameness in the case of diagnosis can be given that does not rely upon uncodifiable presuppositions. Sameness in the case of diagnosis cannot be codified. In other words, Collins arrives at a similar claim to that arrived at above through the discussion of formal models of explanation. The result of that discussion was that explanation could not be codified in a formal model because it is essentially contextual and depends on a background of assumptions about what is relevant and of interest. Collins's claims add to that the thought that formal models of diagnosis could not be successful because diagnosis presupposes an uncodifiable background of practical skills and assumptions about what is relevant.

Theory and practice

Because the example discussed is that of building a laser, Collins's claims about the role of tacit knowledge might seem to apply only to the *practical* elements of science. Those are areas where the presence of a tacit dimension is least surprising. Diagnosis also has such a practical element. It is the practical application of medical knowledge in specific cases for practical purposes. But, according to some philosophers and historians of science, tacit knowledge also plays a part in guiding the theoretical side of sciences. One such author is the historian and philosopher of science whose work we touched on in Chapter 11, Thomas Kuhn. His book *The Structure of Scientific Revolutions* (1962) has been very influential in the debate about the development of scientific theory and the possibility of growth or progress.

The central role of tacit knowledge in Kuhn's account of science

Normal and revolutionary science

To understand Kuhn's claims here it will be necessary first to review very briefly his general account of science as outlined in Chapter 11. Kuhn argues, on the basis of historical analysis, that scientific activity falls into two kinds. In the main, scientists are engaged in 'normal science'. This comprises the articulation and application of stable dominant theories and meta-theoretical assumptions to new areas. Kuhn calls this background the dominant paradigm (although he also and confusingly uses that word for many other things including, for example, worked examples). During such periods, no serious attempt is made to refute or even defend the theoretical background, which is instead simply presupposed. However, these stable periods of normal science are punctuated by brief periods of revolutionary theory change. Sparked both by the accumulation of anomalous results and by the development of rival theories or even rival meta-theoretical assumptions, the dominant orthodoxy is cast aside and a new theory or set of theories put in its place. Only during these revolutionary periods is the truth of what will become the new scientific background called into question.

Given this general account of science, Kuhn suggests in the reading linked with Exercise 9, that normal science is guided by entrenched tacit knowledge.

EXERCISE 9	(30 minutes)

Read the extract from:

Kuhn, T.S. (1962). *The Structure of Scientific Revolutions*, Chicago: University of Chicago Press (extract pp. 46–47)

Link with Reading 14.5

♦ What is the connection between normal science, puzzle solving and tacit knowledge?

Puzzle solving

In this extract, Kuhn (1962, pp. 46–47) suggests that the main activity carried out in normal science is puzzle solving. What is characteristic of puzzle solving is that the nature of the solutions sought is already partly determined by the dominant theoretical background. Even more importantly, puzzles are selected because they are soluble by the lights of the background theory or paradigm. Solving them is thus not a matter of great surprise but rather serves as a test of the theoretical or experimental prowess of the scientist in question. It also serves to extend and make more explicit the paradigm. (Problems that mattered to previous paradigms may be rejected as the product of bad science or bad metaphysics or they may simply be ignored until a subsequent revolutionary change makes them into important puzzles again.)

Kuhn goes on to suggest that puzzle solving highlights the role of tacit knowledge in theoretical science. One of the central skills that is acquired by puzzle solving is learning to recognize how to apply the background theories to new cases, what assumptions or approximations count as reasonable, what would constitute a satisfactory solution, and so forth. In other words, explicit knowledge of a regimented theory is insufficient to be counted as a competent scientist. One must also have the 'know-how' required to *apply* high level theories to particular cases. A key element of this is to recognize that apparently different puzzles can in fact be treated in the same or analogous ways.

Four areas of tacit knowledge

That is only one of the ways in which scientific research work is guided by tacit knowledge. Kuhn (1962) also suggests that scientific work is guided by a set of underlying assumptions or commitments in four ways:

1. At a practical level, research is guided by commitments to particular kinds of instrument, experiment, or tests.

2. Laws and theories...

3. ...and higher level meta-theoretical or metaphysical assumptions determine what is taken to be the subject of science, what sort of thing there is—atoms in a plenum or fields of force—and thus the sort of account to be developed.

4. ...Finally, the values that are constitutive of being a scientist: weight placed on rationality, coherence, quantification, observation, and measurement.

Kuhn's argument for the tacit status of these commitments

It might seem that these commitments are imposed upon scientists working within a particular tradition in the form of *explicit* rules or codes. But Kuhn (1962) argues that they are, in fact, implicit and tacit. He provides two main arguments for this claim. The first is empirical. Historical inquiry has simply failed to discover evidence of sufficient numbers of *explicit* rules to explain the coherence of scientific traditions. Therefore the rules must be *implicit*. (Note, by the way, that Kuhn himself reserves the word 'rule' for explicit rules.)

Secondly, Kuhn suggests how it might be that the rules are implicit. Scientific training, from its beginnings in school-work to PhD level and beyond, is by example and application. Terms are introduced together with the theoretical context in which they have their life. Theories are introduced alongside applications in the solution of problems or puzzles. Most of a scientific education comprises learning how to apply theories to problems. If these 'finger exercises' are successful, a trainee scientist learns to see similarities between cases that permit the application of familiar puzzle-solving techniques. However, this does not require that he or she has abstracted an explicit rule about what it is that makes cases similar *except* that the same sort of solution can be applied.

This point can be put in a way that Kuhn does not. The reason why some knowledge must be tacit is that explicit knowledge of rules or principles would be insufficient. One can know a theory without knowing how to apply it to solve a problem. Similarly, one might know a general principle without being able to apply it in particular cases. But the latter ability is just what is required in normal science.

A conceptual argument for the essential contribution of tacit knowledge

Are there philosophical arguments for a tacit dimension?

While Kuhn's (1962) account broadens the issue of the role that tacit knowledge plays in science it is still, like that of Collins (1985), an empirical account albeit derived from historical rather than sociological sources. What we need now is to see whether

there are philosophical reasons to think that science must be like that and that Kuhn and Collins are more than contingently correct.

Sameness in Wittgenstein's later philosophy

The key idea in both Collins' (1985) and Kuhn's (1962) work is that both practical and theoretical expertise relies on a perception of the relevant similarity of different situations. Collins highlights this by looking at the similarity and difference between working and non-working lasers and the components from which they are built. Kuhn discusses the sameness of different physical situations for the solving of scientific puzzles. Diagnosis clearly also involves seeing sameness in the form of illness between different patient presentations. Is there reason to believe that this must always involve a tacit dimension? Or could an explanation of similarity be given without any hostages to fortune?

The Cambridge-based Austrian philosopher Ludwig Wittgenstein (1889–1951) in his *Philosophical Investigations* (1953), provides just such an argument. The key argument is contained in one hundred or so central paragraphs that discuss following a rule. The general moral of this discussion is beyond the scope of this chapter, but some of its negative results are clear. (In the introduction to Collins' book from which the extract above is taken, he explicitly appeals to just these sections of Wittgenstein's work to serve as a philosophical framework for his own empirical research.)

Wittgenstein (1953) sets up the discussion by considering what it is that guides a speaker to apply a word consistently over time in accord with its meaning. One could imagine that the word was a descriptive term for a form of observable psychopathology. If so to apply it correctly would require a sensitivity to the signs and symptoms presented. But it will also require that one understands what the word means so as to know to which signs and symptoms it applies. Wittgenstein then questions how we can understand this latter element.

Understanding appears to combine two elements: what is grasped in a flash and what is applied over time.

But we *understand* the meaning of a word when we hear or say it; we grasp it in a flash, and what we grasp in this way is surely something different from the 'use' which is extended in time!

(§138)

[I]sn't the meaning of the word also determined by this use? And can these ways of determining meaning conflict? Can what we grasp *in a flash* accord with a use, fit or fail to fit it? And how can what is present to us in an instant, what comes before our mind in an instant, fit a *use*?

(§139)

The problem is thus to explain the connection between what occurs in a flash and the use one makes of a word over time. The problem now is that if one models the understanding one has as a kind of inner definition or instruction that will only guide correct behaviour if one can explain how one understands that inner definition or instruction. It appears that that requires that one knows how to interpret the inner sign and that generates a regress.

Consider, for example, how we might explain understanding the meaning of a simple signpost such as a pointing arrow. If one understands the sign—if one has grasped its meaning—then one understands, centrally, which way it points. It points towards, rather than away from, the arrowhead. So, schematically, one might attempt to represent that meaning in the mind of someone who has understood the signpost with a pointing arrow, pointing in the same direction as the signpost. But, of course, that representation will only represent pointing in the direction of the arrowhead if one already understands how to interpret it. And the problem is that specifying the correct interpretation of the inner representation—through another representation—would generate a vicious regress.

Summary of the problem

Using a word in accord with its meaning requires that one uses it in the same, or in a relevantly similar, way on each occasion. But how is one's use of a word guided by what it means? What does understanding a meaning consist in? Wittgenstein (1953) argues that it cannot consist in having any symbol in mind. Any symbol could be interpreted in a multitude of different ways. So if having a symbol in mind is to play a role in understanding it will have also to be augmented by a particular interpretation. This, however, simply pushes the question back one stage. What is it to have an interpretation in mind? Is this to possess a further symbol that redescribes or interprets the first symbol? If so then this new symbol could be interpreted in any way and will need to be augmented by a further interpretation.

Understanding a series

This point can be brought out by considering what understanding the correct continuation of the rule of successively adding two could comprise. It cannot involve the conscious entertaining of the whole of that series as it is unlimited. But any *representation* of it could be misinterpreted. In everyday life the instruction: 'write 2, 4, 6, 8, 10, 12, and so on' is unambiguous. But it could be misinterpreted to mean what we would mean by 'add 2 starting at 2 up to 1000 and 4 afterwards'. One might add the rule: 'ensure that the units are always follow the following series: 2, 4, 6, 8, 0 ...' But even this rule might be misinterpreted because it is open ended. Of course we might protest that if one were to continue 18, 20, 23, 26 then the units are not the same as those prescribed. But the problem is to explain what this assertion of *sameness* amounts to. (Consider the case of adding 10. Here one might say that the units should always follow the series 0, 0, 0, 0 ... Now it

may seem to us bizarre that anyone might 'follow' this rule by writing a number that ends in anything other than a nought. But the question is: what about this symbol *compels* our interpretation and precludes the deviant rule follower. Each nought, after all, is different—is a different nought in a different place—from the one before even if to us they are relevantly similar.)

The negative moral

The purely negative moral that Wittgenstein (1953) draws is that no amount of adding further disambiguating clauses will escape the fact that each new clause has to be *understood in the right way* if it is to be successful and could not be misinterpreted. Clause A requires disambiguative Clause B; but Clause B requires disambiguative Clause C; and so on ad infinitum. But there is no infinite regress in practice. In practice we do know what it means to continue a series, apply a rule or use or word. Thus it seems that attempting to specify what it means to continue a series, apply a rule or use a word in the same way by using words (or other explicit symbols), always leaves something out, that 'something' in which our given knowledge must (in part) consist.

Wittgenstein (1953) summarizes this in the following way:

> It can be seen that there is a misunderstanding here from the mere fact that in the course of our argument we give one interpretation after another; as if each one contented us at least for a moment, until we thought of yet another standing behind it. What this shows is that there is a way of grasping a rule which is *not* an *interpretation*, but which is exhibited in what we call 'obeying the rule' and 'going against it' in actual cases.   (§201)

A positive corollary

Wittgenstein's positive characterization of understanding links it directly to a practical ability. Understanding the meaning of a word is identified with being able to use it correctly. This practical orientation is emphasized in Wittgenstein's otherwise surprising suggestion that understanding is not a *mental* process or state at all. What this suggests is that there is a tacit dimension that underlies even linguistic representation. Even if the project of codifying all aspects of scientific method were to be successful it would still presuppose that degree of tacit knowledge.

Meaning and tacit knowledge

The claim that the meaning of a word is tacit may appear to be contradicted the following everyday fact: for normal speakers and learners of a language, knowledge of meaning *is* something that can be put into words, i.e. made explicit. One can explain what words mean in both the same and different languages. Wittgenstein, however, is by no means arguing that meaning is private and ineffable. (That is a picture of meaning he explicitly attacks.) So in that sense it is not tacit. But it is tacit in that such explanation presupposes our normal and shared responses to explanations of meaning. What these shared responses amount to are agreement in how to use words that cannot be expressed *in* words in a non-question begging way. Knowledge of meaning is tacit in that it goes beyond mere interchange of symbols.

Wittgenstein's discussion of rules has important implications for the role of tacit knowledge in scientific claims for the following reason. Whenever an activity is rule governed it will rest on a basis of tacit knowledge or know-how. This will apply at all levels of practicality or theoreticity: from correctly applying a mathematical formalism or deducing a result, to the rule governed classification and recognition of signs and symptoms in medical diagnosis. All will depend upon implicit knowledge of how to go on. Any attempt to express this knowledge will itself depend on implicit knowledge left unexpressed.

Reflection on the session and self-test questions

Write down your own reflections on the materials in this session drawing out any points that are particularly significant for you. Then write brief notes about the following:

1. What support do Collins and Kuhn provide for thinking that there is a role of tacit knowledge in scientific practice?

2. What specific arguments does Collins provide from his investigation of replication in engineering?

3. What is the basis of Kuhn's arguments for the importance of tacit knowledge?

4. Do Collins and Kuhn provide principled reasons for thinking that this is an essential feature of scientific knowledge?

Session 4 Tacit knowledge, diagnosis, and a possible link to phenomenology?

In this chapter, we have seen that there are reasons for believing that scientific explanations, and hence diagnostic explanation, may not be fully codifiable. We have also seen that there are good reasons to think that all scientific work—both the more theoretical and the more applied—presupposes tacit expertise and knowledge. This suggests that psychiatric diagnosis must likewise depend on an element of tacit knowledge that could never be fully captured in a formal or linguistic codification. But that conclusion as derived in this chapter applies to diagnosis in all areas of medicine. In this last session, therefore, we consider the particular nature of diagnosis in psychiatry. We ask whether the fact that psychiatry is concerned with the mental implies that psychiatric diagnosis has a further and special tacit dimension?

The following exercise links with a reading by the German psychiatrist and phenomenologist, Alfred Kraus, who takes up this suggestion in a specific way. Kraus (1994) argues that there is a *phenomenological* element in psychiatric diagnosis. What that means will become apparent shortly. But note that this is just one way in which psychiatric diagnosis might involve tacit elements. Kraus argues that it is because of the nature of psychiatry that it involves skills that can only be described using phenomenology and that a consequence of that is that they cannot be explicitly codified, as attempted in recent versions of ICD and DSM.

EXERCISE 11   (20 minutes)

Read the extracts from:

Kraus, A. (1994). Phenomenological and criteriological diagnosis. In *Philosophical Perspectives on Psychiatric Diagnostic Classification* (ed. J.S. Sadler, O.P. Wiggins, and M.A. Schwartz). Baltimore, MD: Johns Hopkins University Press, pp. 148–162. (extracts: pp. 152, 154)

Link with Reading 14.6

♦ What arguments does Kraus advance against the explicit regimentation of symptoms that underlies diagnosis using DSM or ICD?

♦ Do these turn on the particular subject matter of psychiatry?

Top-down or bottom-up?

Kraus (1994) argues that diagnostic systems such DSM and ICD miss out an important element of psychiatric diagnosis. This is the result of their fundamental structure. Because the model presupposed by these manuals is one in which diagnoses are built up from a number of individual and conceptually independent symptoms they cannot capture top-down and holistic elements of diagnosis.

One criticism that Kraus makes of what he calls this criteriological approach to diagnosis, is that rather than providing a reliable foundation, the connection between individual symptoms and conditions lacks specificity. There remains widespread disagreement about the correlation between individual symptoms and underlying syndromes. By contrast, according to Kraus, a top-down holistic model is more specific because it allows a correlation between schizophrenia and *particular kinds* of catatonia or delusional structure. Correlations are not between schizophrenia and delusions in general but delusions with a specific schizophrenic colouring. But this connection can only be established with a top-down rather than criteriological model of diagnosis.

Conjoining symptoms: more than the sum of the parts

A further inadequacy of the bottom-up model is that symptoms can only be added together through conjunction. But no mere conjunction of individual symptoms—a 'Chinese restaurant menu' approach—can capture the full sense of psychological wholeness that the individual parts add up to. For that, one again needs, according to Kraus (1994), a holistic approach. This is not to say, however, that particular elements cannot be identified in a holistic diagnosis. It is just that the individual elements have a different logic. One way of marking this distinction (not Kraus's) is to contrast parts that are independent pieces and parts that are essential aspects. The pieces of a jigsaw add up to a whole, but each piece can exist independently of the others. By contrast a musical note has both a tone and a pitch, but neither aspect can exist independently of the other. Thus according to a holistic approach, psychological symptoms are interdependent aspects of a psychological unity.

Kraus combines with these two comments on the limits of a criteriological model of diagnosis a further philosophical explanation of the difference in approach. This is why he contrasts the criteriological with a *phenomenological* rather than merely a holistic model. This concentrates not on psychiatric diseases but on the mode of being of whole persons, the 'whole of the being in the world of schizophrenics or manics'. Thus the phenomenologically based diagnosis of schizophrenia turns on an overall assessment of the patient—a 'praecox feeling'—as having a very different form of 'being-in-the-world' (see also Reading guide).

Heidegger on 'Being-in-the-world'

The term 'being-in-the-world' is taken from Heidegger's account of the nature of human beings in his early work *Being and Time* ([1927] 1962), which he describes as a piece of phenomenology. (Heidegger was introduced in Chapter 10.)

Heidegger argues there that it is an essential feature of humans that they inhabit a world that they did not choose but that has practical significance and thus meaning for them. It is through the use of 'handy tools' in temporally extended practical projects that humans make sense of themselves, their lives, and their eventual deaths. Being-in-the-world symbolizes this embeddedness in mundane activity and contrasts markedly with Descartes's view that human beings are essentially disembodied thinkers. Heidegger suggests that Descartes's account of bodies as mere objects in a three-dimensional space, rather than as things with significance and purpose, has influenced our thinking about everything we encounter and ourselves. We think of each other and even ourselves as objects whether or not we also adopt Descartes's claim that we are thinking objects. The criteriological approach to mental illness might well be thought to a phenomenologist as exemplifying this Cartesian objectivist attitude.

Phenomenology is only one kind of holism

But while a phenomenological account provides one possible explanation of the difference between a criteriological and a holistic account of diagnosis, phenomenology is not the only way to mark that contrast. All one needs for that purpose is to recognize that the symptoms one picks out may be mutually dependent aspects of a psychological whole rather than independent symptoms produced by underlying causes. No bottom-up procedure will capture a diagnosis made on the basis of an irreducibly holistic judgement in which individual 'symptoms'

are, as we put it above, interdependent aspects or moments of a psychological whole.

Kraus's (1994) phenomenological approach is worth comparing in this respect with the debate between 'theory theory' and 'simulation theory' as different approaches to understanding other minds, described in Chapter 27. While theory theory supposes that the ability to 'read' another mind turns on an implicit theory that licences inferences from observable signs (behaviour) to underlying mental states, simulation theory denies this. Instead simulation theory suggests that one has access to others' minds by putting oneself imaginatively in other people's positions. As we will see, there are reasons to think that such an ability cannot be codified whether or not one subscribes to a phenomenological approach to psychiatry.

If phenomenology is not the only form of holism, however, it is one that, as we saw in Part II, has been particularly influential in the history of ideas specifically about *psycho*pathology, about, as in the title of Andrew Sims' classic text (see Chapter 3), symptoms 'in the mind'. And as we also saw in Part II, it was Karl Jaspers above all, as a phenomenologist and founder of modern descriptive psychopathology, who argued that with mental symptoms, at least, it was essential that medical explanations were concerned as much with meanings as with causes. With meanings, then, or reasons, we have at least one kind of extra element of difficulty involved in providing explanations, diagnostic or otherwise, of *mental* symptoms. In Chapter 15, correspondingly, we will examine the role that meanings or reasons play in psychiatry and contrast their structure with that of causal explanation.

Reflection on the session and self-test questions

Write down your own reflections on the materials in this session drawing out any points that are particularly significant for you. Then write brief notes about the following:

1. What does the reading in this session drawn from the phenomenological tradition add to the discussion of tacit knowledge so far?

Reading guide

◆ A good overview of explanation is provided in book length form in Salmon, W. (1989) *Four Decades of Scientific Explanation*.

◆ A useful collection of original essays on the philosophy of explanation is Ruben's (ed.) (1993) *Explanation* and Cornwell's (ed.) (2004) *Explanations*.

◆ The pragmatic aspect of explanation is discussed in Lipton's (1991) *Inference to the Best Explanation*.

Tacit knowledge

◆ The locus classicus for tacit knowledge is Polanyi ([1958] 1974) *Personal Knowledge: towards a post-critical philosophy*.

◆ And tacit knowledge is discussed by Ryle (1949) *The Concept of Mind* (especially pp. 25–61), Dretske (1991) *Explaining Behavior: reasons in a world of causes*, and Reber (1995). *Implicit Learning and Tacit Knowledge: an essay on the cognitive unconscious*.

◆ And in a practical context, by Luntley (2002).

Interdisciplinary work on psychiatric diagnosis

◆ A broader perspective is provided by Sadler (2004) 'Diagnosis/antidiagnosis' and Phillips (2004) 'Understanding/explanation', both in Radden (ed.) (2004) *The Philosophy of Psychiatry*, and Spitzer (1994) 'The basis of psychiatric diagnosis' in Sadler *et al.*'s (ed.) (1994) *Philosophical Perspectives on Psychiatric Diagnostic Classification*.

References

Brown, H. (1977). *Perception Theory and Commitment.* Chicago, IL: University of Chicago Press.

Collins, H. (1985). *Changing Order.* London: Sage.

Cornwell, J. (ed.) (2004). *Explanations.* Oxford: Oxford University Press.

Dretske, F. (1991). *Explaining Behavior: reasons in a world of causes.* Cambridge, MA: MIT Press.

Fulford, K.W.M. (2000). Teleology without tears: naturalism, neo-naturalism and evaluationism in the analysis of function statements in biology (and a bet on the twenty-first century). *Philosophy, Psychiatry, & Psychology,* 7: 77–94.

Heidegger, M. ([1927] 1962). *Being and Time* (transl. J. Macquarrie and E. Robinson). Oxford: Blackwell.

Hempel, C.G. (1965). *Aspect of scientific explanation.* London: Free Press.

Hempel, C.G. (1966). *Philosophy of natural science.* London: Prentice-Hall.

Hempel, C.G. (1999). Laws and their role in scientific explanation. In *Philosophy of Science* (ed. R. Boyd, P. Gasker, and J.D. Trout). Cambidge, MA: MIT Press, pp. 299–315.

Kendell, R.E. and Jablensky, A. (2003). Distinguishing between the validity and utility of psychiatric diagnosis. *American Journal of Psychiatry.*

Kraus, A. (1994). Phenomenological and criteriological diagnosis. In *Philosophical Perspectives on Psychiatric Diagnostic Classification* (eds J.S. Sadler, O.P. Wiggins, and M.A. Schwartz). Baltimore, MD: Johns Hopkins University Press, pp. 148–162.

Kuhn, T. (1962). *The Structure of Scientific Revolutions,* Vol. II, No. 2. Chicago, IL: University of Chicago Press.

Lewis, D. (1986). Causal explanation. In *Philosophical Papers,* Vol. II. Oxford: Oxford University Press pp. 214–240. (Reprinted in Ruben, D.-H. (ed.) (1993). *Explanation.* Oxford: Oxford University Press, pp. 182–206.)

Lindahl, B.I.B. and Johansson, L.A. (1994). Multiple cause-of-death data as a tool for detecting artificial trends in the underlying cause statistics: a methodological study. *Scandinavian Journal of Social Medicine,* 22(2): 145–158.

Lipton, P. (1991). *Inference to the Best Explanation.* New York: Routledge.

Luntley, M. (2002). Knowing how to manage: expertise and embedded knowledge. *Reason in Practice,* 2(3): 3–14.

Megone, C. (2000). Mental illness, human function, and values. *Philosophy, Psychiatry, & Psychology,* 7/1 pp. 45–65.

Phillips, J. (2004). Understanding/explanation. In *The Philosophy of Psychiatry* (ed. J. Radden). Oxford: Oxford University Press.

Polanyi, M. ([1958] 1974). *Personal Knowledge: towards a post-critical philosophy.* Chicago, IL: University of Chicago Press.

Reber, A. (1995). *Implicit Learning and Tacit Knowledge: an essay on the cognitive unconscious.* New York: Oxford University Press.

Rossi, P. (2003). Magic, science, and equality of human wits. In *Nature and Narrative: an introduction to the new philosophy of psychiatry* (ed. K.W.M. Fulford, K.J. Morris, J.Z.S. Sadler, and G. Stanghellini). Oxford: Oxford University Press, Chapter 17.

Ruben, D. (ed.) (1993). *Explanation.* Oxford Readings in Philosophy. Oxford: Oxford University Press.

Ryle, G. (1949). *The Concept of Mind.* Chicago, IL: University of Chicago Press.

Sadler, J.Z. (2004). Diagnosis/antidiagnosis. In *The Philosophy of Psychiatry* (ed. J. Radden). Oxford: Oxford University Press.

Salmon, W. (1989). *Four Decades of Scientific Explanation.* Minneapolis: University of Minnesota Press.

Scriven, M. (1959). Truisms as the grounds for historical explanation. In *Theories of History* (ed. P. Gardiner). New York, pp. 443–468.

Spitzer, M. (1994). The basis of psychiatric diagnosis. In *Philosophical Perspectives on Psychiatric Diagnostic Classification* (ed. J.Z. Sadler, O.P. Wiggins, and M.A. Schwartz). London: Johns Hopkins University Press.

Van Fraassen, B. (1980). *The Scientific Image*. Oxford: Oxford University Press.

Van Fraassen, B. (1999). The pragmatics of explanation. In *The Philosophy of Science* (ed. R. Boyd, P. Gasker, and J.D. Trout). Cambridge, MA: MIT Press, pp. 317–327.

Wakefield, J.C. (2000). Aristotle as sociobiologist: the 'function of a human being' argument, black box essentialism, and the concept of mental disorder. *Philosophy, Psychiatry, & Psychology*, 7: 17–44.

Wittgenstein, L. (1953). *Philosophical Investigations*. Oxford: Blackwell.

CHAPTER 15

Causes, laws, and reasons in psychiatric aetiology

Chapter contents

Introduction

The previous three chapters have examined some of the lessons we can learn from the philosophy of science for a deeper understanding of:

1. clinical observation (as of signs and symptoms);

2. classification of symptoms; and

3. diagnosis based on those symptoms.

In each case we have been concerned with issues that, although particularly prominent in psychiatry, are generic to medicine as a whole. In this chapter, by contrast, we will be concerned with a complication to diagnostic assessment that, traditionally at least, has been identified particularly with psychiatry, namely the role that reasons as well as causes may play in how we understand the aetiology of mental disorders.

Why this is a complication

Why is this, as we put it a moment ago, a 'complication'? Essentially because the two ways of attributing aetiology, in terms of reasons and/or in terms of causes, leave psychiatry at one and the same time drawing on two different, and not necessarily compatible, ways of making symptoms intelligible.

Thus, on the one hand, like the 'hard' physical and biological sciences, psychiatry aims to discover the natural laws that govern the structure and interactions of psychiatric phenomena. These include the laws that govern the *causal* relations that may obtain. But on the other hand, psychiatry also aims to fit many of those phenomena into a different pattern of intelligibility, a pattern that is defined by their significance, social functions, and personal meanings. This second pattern, then, is interpretative or hermeneutic. Crucially it is also normative in a sense that will be further explained below.

We can distinguish these two different forms of intelligibility as the *realm of law* and the *space of reasons* (following, as we will see below, the work of the philosophers Wilfrid Sellars and, more recently, John McDowell). The complication, indeed the series of complications, which allegiance to these two forms of intelligibility at least threatens to raise can be simply put. The principles that govern these two different ways of making sense of the world—the world of law-like causal relations and the world of meaningful relations—are, prima facie, different. So how can they be reconciled as part of a unified discipline? Or is it instead that the causal and perhaps more biological elements of psychiatry are distinct from or discontinuous with its more hermeneutic or interpretative elements? If they are distinct, can psychiatry's concern with both reasons and also with causes be reconciled? Or, alternatively, do we have to choose between them? Do we have to choose either to view symptoms *only* as *effects* that carry meanings at most metaphorically. Or should they be viewed as literally having *meaning* in themselves, being perhaps meaningful responses to events in a patient's or client's life but either *not* part of the *causal* order or at least not subject to *laws of nature*?

Reasons and causes in science

We met these complications, in various guises, at several points earlier in this book, notably in Part II, in the tensions, as between meanings and causes, evident in Jaspers's foundational work on psychopathology. Those tensions, as the British philosopher and psychologist, Derek Bolton, has recently pointed out, are still unresolved in psychiatry (Bolton, 1997a). We should not, though, be too surprised by this. For as we saw in Part II, the tensions in Jaspers' work were a direct reflection of a long-running debate in the nineteenth century (the *Methodenstreit*) about method in the human (or social) sciences. And debate about the relationship between reasons and causes in general, as we will see in this chapter, and again in Part V on the philosophy of mind, continues to this day.

As with other topics examined in this part, therefore, although problems about the interrelation between reasons and causes are particularly evident in psychiatry, we should approach these problems as a sign, not that psychiatry is, somehow, unscientific, but rather that it is, in this as in other respects, a peculiarly *difficult* science.

Reasons and causes in the philosophy of mind

One response to the problems about the interrelation between reasons and causes is to argue that it is more apparent than real. This, as we will see in Part V, is one line on these problems that has recently been developed particularly among those working in the philosophy of mind. One idea is that mental states, properly understood, are just the sorts of things that can be, at one and the same time, causes and also reasons. Mental states, that is to say, are states with both physical properties, which can be subsumed under natural causal laws, and also rational and intentional 'properties', which can be fitted into the space of reasons. This, then, is an ontological approach, focusing on the nature of mental states, on the kind of thing that a mind is. Such ontological solutions, in attempting to grant mental states two sets of prima facie incompatible attributes, face severe difficulties that will be discussed in Part V.

Reasons and cause in the philosophy of science

If responses to the problem of reasons and causes from the philosophy of mind have been largely ontological, responses from the philosophy of science have, by contrast, been largely methodological. Approaches from the philosophy of science, that is to say, have been concerned, not with difficulties about what is, but with the issues that arise for those *disciplines* that investigate laws of nature (including causal laws) and those that investigate patterns of meaningful behaviour.

Overview of the storyline of Chapter 15

The storyline of the chapter (set out in more detail below) runs broadly from causes to reasons and back again.

The starting point: Hume

Thus we start (in Session 1) with what is widely regarded as the mainspring of modern philosophical work on the nature of causation, the eighteenth century British empiricist philosopher, David Hume's, sceptical claim that, in effect, there is no such thing as a causal connection. Hume, as we will see, argued that the idea we have of causation is actually nothing more than a gloss (an epiphenomenal gloss) that we put on our experiences of things occurring together: an approach based on regularity.

Humeans and non-Humeans

Hume's regularity or constant conjunction theory, as it has come to be called, has been developed in various ways by subsequent generations of Humean philosophers. The challenges that 'constant conjunction' theories face is to explain how genuinely *causal* conjunctions differ from more accidental generalizations. Hence there have also been many Humean philosophers, differentiated by their different approaches to analysing the essential feature(s) of a genuinely causal generalization. In *Session 1*, we explore a range of ingenious approaches to analysing causation that draw in different ways on the idea that causal connections are, in one respect or another, nomological, i.e. that they are a species of law. In *Session 2*, we examine two rather different approaches to analysing causation, one in terms of counter-factuals, the other in terms of probability.

From causes to reasons...and back again

None of these approaches, as we will see, is wholly successful, although each is in different ways illuminating for medicine and psychiatry. They show, in particular, that attributions of causation, contrary to the traditional model of science, are both context-dependent and normative (the causes we attribute are in part driven by the interests we have). In these respects, then, causes and reasons, notwithstanding their prima facie differences, begin to appear rather similar! *Session 3* thus turns from causes to reasons, looking at recent influential accounts, both of the differences between them, and, at how, prima facie differences or not, they might none the less be reconciled at least in psychiatry.

More detailed structure of Chapter 15

In more detail, the chapter is divided into three main sessions. Sessions 1 and 2 are concerned with different ways of analysing causation, respectively, in terms of regularity, or more precisely, natural laws (Session 1) and of either counter-factual conditionals, or of probability (Session 2). Session 3 is concerned with reasons and with whether and in what way reasons are related to causes.

Session 1

This is concerned with the origin of much of the philosophy of laws and causes in David Hume's famous (and as we will see still not adequately refuted) sceptical account of causation. At least according to one interpretation, Hume argued that a so-called causal connection is nothing more than a psychological gloss that we put on what he called 'constant conjunction'. Causation, according to Hume, is, and is nothing more than, things regularly occurring together.

Hume's sceptical attack will help put in place recent philosophical work on the relation between causes and laws. While not all philosophers agree that causation should be *analysed* in terms of laws (i.e. *mean* linked by laws), most think that where there is a causal relation between individual or particular events, there must also be a general regularity, or law, linking events of those types. Thus the hope is that light can be shed on the nature of individual causation by looking at the higher level of regularities that comprise natural laws. There remain, however, difficulties with the distinction between those observed regularities that correspond to genuine laws of nature and those that are mere accidental generalizations.

Session 2

This considers two further approaches to understanding causation. One attempts to define causation in terms of what are called counter-factual conditionals and the other in terms of probability. Counter-factual conditionals are conditionals (if...then statements) that run counter to the facts. Consider the claim: *If* John F. Kennedy had not been assassinated *then* Lyndon B. Johnson would not have become president. This expresses a claim about what would have happened if something else, which did not in fact happen, had happened. One thought is that these can be used to explain causation (Kennedy's assassination was the *cause* of the swearing in of Johnson).

The second, probability based, approach is to define causation as the raising of the chances of effects. This approach is familiar in health-care research in the form of statistical 'tests' of the significance of experimental or survey findings. The assumption guiding such tests, an assumption directly reflecting Hume's 'constant conjunction' account of causality, is that the less likely it is that a result could have been obtained by chance, the more likely it is that the result reflects an underlying causal process.

Neither of these approaches, through counter-factual conditionals or through probability, has yet been fully successful in explaining causality (acting as a rival to a regularity approach). But as the session concludes, even if they were, there would still be reasons for thinking that there is a general connection of the kind explored in Session 1, i.e. a connection between causes and regularities or, more precisely, laws.

Session 3

This examines the 'space of reasons'. By contrast with the idea of subsuming causal events under a structure of natural laws, the human sciences (such as history) have traditionally been thought to embody a different organizational principle. Rather than understanding phenomena by fitting them into a structure of causal laws, the human sciences attempt to understand the meanings of phenomena. Thus the structure they embody is not one of causal laws but a rational structure of reasons.

The session outlines recent work in philosophy picking out the key features of the space of reasons and arguing that these show it to be different in kind from the realm of law, including the realm of causal laws. However, the session concludes by examining two approaches that seek to respond, in different ways, to reasons and causes at least as they arise in psychiatry. Bolton and Hill argue that reasons are encoded in brain states and thus a principled reconciliation is possible. In other words, they try to show that there is not a gulf between the space of reasons and the realm of law. The former is, properly speaking, part of or a special case of the latter.

Brown and Harris, by contrast, present a model of the social and psychological origins of depression that combines reasons with causes in a way that takes for granted their joint operation. In other words they suggest that, although there is a distinction, both can operate together in an informative way in psychiatry.

Session 1 An introduction to philosophical accounts of causation

Causation in physical disease and mental illness

Causality plays a central role throughout medicine. Physical diseases cause symptoms, disability, and death. Diseases are themselves caused by biological infections, poor diet, underlying social conditions, or inherited susceptibility. Treatment is often thought of as a causal intervention in the patient's health whether through chemical, surgical, or other means. Sometimes the causal pathways or mechanisms involved in these processes are well known and sometimes they are not. But even when they are not, it is a working assumption for many that some such causal mechanism must exist and that it is one role of medical research to find it.

There is, however, much debate about whether, and if so how far, any such causal medical model can be usefully applied to *mental* illness. One of the issues in the debate about whether one should talk of mental *disease* or mental *illness* is the applicability of causal models of aetiology (see Part I). Are mental illnesses the result of underlying causes or should they instead be identified with deviation from social norms and suchlike? Can they be subsumed under either deterministic or even probabilistic laws or are they instead to be understood as a partially rational response to psychological trauma subject only to interpretation? A satisfactory resolution of that debate requires, as one of its ingredients, a proper understanding of causation itself.

Is causation important for science?

Although this will be one of the subjects of this chapter, it is worth flagging in advance the fact that opposing claims have been made about the connection between causation and natural laws in the natural sciences. Intuitively, causation seems to have a central role in the conceptual tool bag of science. This claim was, however, criticized by the philosopher Bertrand Russell early in the twentieth century. He argued that causality was useful only in

the early stages of science after which it is replaced by a concern with laws of nature that make no reference to cause and effect. Providing science can structure phenomena under law-like relations, and chart the relations between physical quantities or properties, there is no need to talk about the individual causal relations between events.

As we have already seen in Chapter 13, this view of the priority of laws over causes has in turn been criticized by Nancy Cartwright. She argues that one should not take a realist attitude to the high-level laws of physics, for example, but should take a realist attitude only to those entities that *cause* observable effects. It is also clear that in the technological *application* of science at least, causality has a central role. If one wants to make something happen, to bring about a desired effect, then one needs to know what will bring it about, or cause it. As medicine is in this respect a practical or applied discipline, causality looks, prima facie, to be an important part of its conceptual structure.

Other philosophical accounts of causation, however, as we will see in this session, have stressed a *connection* between it and laws of nature rather than a priority one way or another. This in turn suggests a key connection between the kind of nomological systematicity found in scientific disciplines and the use in these disciplines of causal concepts. Natural sciences attempt to articulate the structure of natural laws that gives shape to and unifies the diverse phenomena they study. These in turn underwrite the causal interconnectedness of natural phenomena.

Structure of the session

So this session starts by looking at the kind of assumptions naturally made about the concept of causation taking as its example a reading from a medical journal article (Rizzi, 1994). It then looks at Hume's sceptical account of our idea of causation and, in particular, causal necessity or, as we might informally put it, causal glue. Hume argues that when one looks for the source of our idea of a causal glue connecting events together, one cannot find it. And thus he gives three definitions of causation that do not rely on such a notion and that he took to be equivalent, two of which stress the connection between causation and regularity or generalization.

We then look at a recent Humean account that attempts to relate causation to the logical notions of necessity and sufficiency (neither of which quite coincide with Hume's target conception of a causal glue type of necessity). While this serves as a useful model for refining our concept of causation we find that it is, again, dependent on a notion of regularity. But as the final part of the session outlines, whereas some regularities or generalizations correspond to genuine laws of nature that might indeed underpin causal relations, others are merely accidentally true. Thus if a regularity version of Hume's account of causation is to work we need an independent account of the difference between natural laws and mere accidents. We examine two such accounts.

Causal reasoning in medicine

Causation in diagnosis

The first reading in this chapter (linked with Exercise 1 below), which is taken from a recent edition of a medical journal, illustrates the role of causal reasoning in physical medicine. It picks up the theme of the previous chapter (Chapter 14), about the nature of diagnosis, but adds an explicitly causal dimension. What is important about this extract for our purposes is not its main argument but what it takes for granted about the nature of causation.

EXERCISE 1   (20 minutes)

Read the short extract from:

Rizzi, D.A. (1994). Causal reasoning and the diagnostic process. *Theoretical Medicine*, 15: 315–333 (extract: pp. 315–317)

Link with Reading 15.1

◆ Identify some of the background claims and distinctions that are made concerning the nature of causality.

◆ List some of the connotations of 'causality' suggested at the start of this paper.

Rizzi (1994) shares a general assumption that was discussed in Chapter 14. Like most forms of *explanation* in the physical sciences, medical *diagnostic* explanation involves a causal element. With symptomatically defined diseases, as we saw in Chapter 14, the causal element is implicit. However, the assumption behind diagnostic explanations of a patient's condition is that a causal agent is present that is waiting to be identified to which suitable treatment can be fitted. A fuller explanation of why that agent was present and what other factors contributed to the disease will take the form of a fuller causal explanation. Thus Rizzi's account of different forms of diagnosis deployed for different purposes resembles Lewis's account of having more or less explanation (see Chapter 14).

Rizzi also suggests, again consistently with the themes of Chapter 14, that the kind of causal explanation offered of the same disease will vary depending on the interests of the clinicians concerned: whether general practitioners or medical researchers. Similarly, he argues that the simple model in which for any disease there is a corresponding causal agent is mistaken. These wider themes in the paper can, however, be put to one side for the moment.

Connotations of causation

Rizzi's (1994) paper—both in the short extract above and later in the paper—takes for granted certain claims about the nature of causation that will be discussed during this chapter. Some of these are that:

1. There is an important distinction but also a relation between singular cases of causation and general causal relations (p. 316).

General causation and singular causation are co-dependent (p. 321).

2. Individual causal factors may not be the cause but are still in some sense non-redundant elements of effective causal complexes (p. 317).

3. Causes explain their effects (p. 321).

4. Causes and effects possess a form of 'necessity' (p. 323).

5. Causation relates events (p. 324).

6. It is reasonable to claim that there are no absolute causal facts (p. 331).

Rizzi goes on to argue that the correct causal model for the medical sciences has to be broadened from that which is generally found in the natural sciences. But to understand and assess that claim requires an understanding of the philosophical background.

The history of the modern philosophy of causation: David Hume

The Humean origins of the problem

The modern history of causation began with the eighteenth century British empiricist philosopher, David Hume's discussions in his *Treatise of Human Nature* [1739–40] and his *Enquiries Concerning Human Understanding and Concerning the Principles of Morals* [1748]. These two works contain substantially the same philosophical material. The *Treatise* was not well received by Hume's contemporaries. In his own phrase it fell 'dead-born from the press'. Hume took this to be the result of its presentation rather than the ideas it contained. Thus the *Enquiries* is a later revision that differs more in style than content, although for our purposes it presents a clearer account of causation than the equivalent sections in the *Treatise*.

To understand Hume's account of causation it is necessary first to have some understanding of what would nowadays be described as his philosophy of mind (mentioned already in Chapter 12).

Ideas

Hume populates the mind with two sorts of entity: ideas and impressions. There is some difficulty in ascribing a precise view to Hume's notion of *ideas*. In modern terms *ideas*, or thoughts, are construed to be either the bearers of mental content or the content itself. Ideas are thus either the vehicles of thought or the thought itself. This distinction between the bearer of content and the content itself will be important in the Part V. For now, think of the distinction between a written sentence and the meaning it bears. It is unclear whether Hume thinks of ideas on the model of the sentence or its meaning.

Impressions

Impressions, by contrast with ideas, are directly experiential. It is through our impressions that we have access to the world. Except for the fact that Hume uses this word for both ideas and impressions, it would now be usual to call impressions 'perceptions'. Hume also calls them feelings and sentiments. Unconvincingly, he suggests that the main difference between impressions and ideas is one of *vivacity*. The key claim, however, is that ideas are derived from impressions. With a couple of exceptions, all complex ideas can be derived, via simple ideas, from impressions (the exceptions are causality, as we will see, and unexperienced shades of colours lying between previously experienced shades).

There are some fundamental difficulties with views, like Hume's, which populate the mind with free standing and independent mental states. Once mental states or ideas are conceived as existing independently of how the world is, this opens up both a sceptical question about how we can know that our ideas represent the world *correctly* but also, more fundamentally, how they come to have any representative powers *at all*. We will return to these issues in Part V. For now, what is relevant is the *use* to which Hume puts the distinction between ideas and impressions, both conceived as free-standing mental entities.

Hume's philosophical methodology

Hume suggests that because ideas are fainter than impressions, they can be confused, leading to errors in reasoning. Impressions having more vivacity, by contrast, cannot. This leads to a central methodological principle: for any problematic idea 'enquire from what impression that supposed idea derived' (p. 22). It is this that guides the subsequent discussion of causation.

The account of causation

Having grasped the picture of mind that underlies Hume's methodology and his suggestion for investigating difficult (philosophical) ideas, we can now turn to Hume's account of causation.

EXERCISE 2	(30 minutes)

Read the extract from

Hume, D. ([1748]1975). *Enquiries Concerning Human Understanding and Concerning the Principles of Morals.* Oxford: Oxford University Press, section VII, pp. 63–64

Insert reading 15.2 here

♦ How good is Hume's style of argument concerning causation?

♦ What conclusions does Hume draw about causation?

What is the source of the impression of a necessary connection?

Hume's account takes as its premiss the claim that a key component of the concept of causation is that of the *necessary* connection between cause and effect. Hume suggests, however, that this idea is puzzling and problematic. What does it amount to to say that one event necessitates another? How can we find this out? Following the methodological principle set out above, Hume suggests that in order to clarify our understanding of this 'idea'

of necessity, we should look to the corresponding 'impression' from which it is derived. This leads him to consider the different possible sources of our idea of necessity in impressions derived from both outer sense (experience of the outside world) and inner sense (experience of mental phenomena).

Hume does not conduct an exhaustive empirical survey. Instead he considers the sort of experience that may possibly be available. However, this inquiry does not turn out to be of any help. To begin with, our experience of the outer world does not provide the right sort of impression:

> When we look about us towards external objects and consider the operation of causes, we are never able in a single instance, to discover any power or necessary connection; any quality which binds the effect to the cause, and renders the one an infallible consequence of the other. We only find, that one does actually, in fact, follow the other.   (p. 63)

As Hume remarks, events in the world appear to be independent of one another. We do not observe in them—at least when considered individually—any further power from which we could derive subsequent effects. 'Solidity, extension, motion; these qualities are complete in themselves, and never point out any other event which may result from them.' (p. 63)

Nor, according to Hume, is any experience provided by our inner sense of help. Hume rejects the idea that a necessary connection or causal power is experienced when we move our limbs or in the action of the will using six different arguments. But the key idea is that no inner experience of the action of the will can provide an impression of a necessary connection. Mental events, like the physical events experienced in outer sense, appear to be independent of one another and of actions. They are conjoined but not connected. It is quite consistent with any mental event that any other event succeed it.

This result appears to put Hume's general claim that ideas are derived from impressions under threat. If there is no impression from which the idea of a necessary connection is derived, how could one even undertake the search that Hume describes. Hume's own response does not immediately seem to address this point. Instead he suggests that our idea of causality derives not from any single case but from the general connection between events of one sort and events of another sort. If a general relation is observed then:

> we make no longer any scruple of foretelling one upon the appearance of the other... We then call the one object, *Cause*; and the other, *Effect*... It appears, then, that this idea of a necessary connection among events arises from a number of similar instances which occur of the constant conjunction of these events.   (p. 75)

In effect Hume's method works in a negative way. When we go from the (less vital) idea of causal necessity to the (more vital) impressions from which the idea is derived, it becomes clear that all there is, is constant conjunction. Whatever our initial assumption, there is no further sense of causal necessity.

Is there an impression of necessity?

There are two immediately striking features about the suggestions that Hume makes here. One is the naturalistic and descriptive tone of the solution. As a matter of fact we are habituated to moving from the 'cause' event to the 'effect' event by repeated experience. Hume's account of causation is built on a foundation of habits of thought. Secondly, he emphasizes the importance of a *general* relation between types or kinds of events for the definition of *individual* or *single* causal relations between pairs of individual or token events. Singular causal relations depend on general relations. Many recent philosophers have embraced a 'regularity' theory of causality. But, as we will see, it is not clear that this is an accurate view of Hume's account.

One difficulty, which was raised above, can now be put like this. If the idea of a necessary connection between one event and another results from the habitual expectation of events of the second kind on presentation of events of the first sort does this not undermine Hume's claim that every simple idea derives from a corresponding impression? However, Hume preserves the connection between ideas and impressions even in this case, while slackening any connection between impressions and something worldly that corresponds to them. He says: 'This connection, therefore, which we *feel* in the mind, this customary transition of the imagination from one object to its usual attendant, is the sentiment or impression from which we form the idea of power or necessary connection. Nothing farther is in the case.' (p. 75)

It is important to note that, given his sceptical search, 'the feeling of connection' cannot literally be an impression of some connection that is present either in the outer world or in the mind. It is not an impression that is of or responsive to a worldly fact. It is just a feeling—perhaps of inevitability—that is produced in the mind after experience of repeated conjunctions of events. But given this connection between the idea of a necessary connection and this 'impression' it is not clear that Hume himself proposes a true regularity theory analysis of causation. Such an analysis provides a definition of the meaning of causation in terms of regularity (see below). But it seems plausible that Hume's appeal to regularity is as a precondition for the concept but not part of its meaning. Without regularity there would be no feeling from which the idea of a necessary connection is drawn. But that latter idea is not of regularity. And thus Hume's account is not strictly a regularity analysis of causation. Nevertheless, most Humean accounts of causation take some form of regularity claim for granted.

Hume's three accounts of causation

In fact Hume provides three characterizations of causation in the *Enquiries*:

1. an object, followed by another, and where all the objects similar to the first are followed by objects similar to the second. (p. 76)

2. Or in other words where, if the first object had not been, the second never had existed. (p. 76)

3. an object followed by another, and whose appearance always conveys the thought to that other. (p. 77)

None of these definitions is equivalent. The first is the basis of a regularity theory of causation. The third unpacks Hume's claim that the concept of causation depends on habits of thinking rather than direct experience or the product of reasoning. The first and the third cast light on Hume's account from both objective and subjective perspectives. The second is different, however. Like the first it is a claim about the metaphysical status of causality. But it approaches this from a different perspective. We will explore the relation between this idea and a pure regularity thesis below.

The analysis of causal claims

Two senses of necessity

One of the issues that has so far not been touched upon is what is meant by the claim that a cause and effect stand in a necessary connection. In fact this is a central problem in the philosophical explanation of causation that will be discussed throughout this session (and will not be finally resolved). But it is important first to distinguish between two different distinctions with which it might be confused: necessary versus contingent, and necessary versus sufficient:

1. *Necessity as 'not possibly not'*. A truth is a necessary truth if it could not have been otherwise, if it is not possible that it is not true. This sense contrasts with contingency. This is not the sense of necessity that underpins the necessary connection of cause and effect. As Hume points out, it is *logically possible* that any state of affairs might result from any other. Causal relations are contingent. Smoking might not have been a cause of cancer, for example. If smoking does cause cancer, that is not a necessary truth, by contrast with, for example, the truths mathematics explores, or statements that are true by definition (known as 'analytic truths'). An example of the latter would be 'All bachelors are unmarried men'. (See also Chapter 5.)

2. *Necessity as 'without which not'*. If one event is necessary for another event in this sense, then for the second to occur the first must occur. Without the first event, the second event would not occur. On the other hand if the first is necessary for the second, the second is sufficient for the first. If we know that the first event is a necessary precondition of the second, and if we know that the second occurs, then we can conclude that the first must also have occurred. Necessity and sufficiency are related and complementary notions. As we will see, the 'without which not' sense of necessity, although apparently similar to causal necessity, is not identical with it.

To reiterate, something might be necessary for something else in the second sense while this dependence might not be a necessary fact in the first sense. In order to leave a building it may be necessary to go past the security guard—there may be no other way out; however, this fact is contingent on there being no escape through a window. Had the architect been less thorough, such an escape might have been possible.

Causation, necessity, and sufficiency

So much then for the two senses of necessity. What has this to do with causation? Even on the assumption, following Hume, that necessity is an ingredient of the concept of causation, what precisely is the connection? Given that causal relations are contingent and thus not necessary in the first sense, then the two most obvious options are that causes are *necessary* conditions for their effects in the *second* sense or that causes are *sufficient* conditions for their effects. Combining these options gives a third position: a cause is a necessary and sufficient condition for its effects.

But there are problems with any of these approaches when set out so baldly and the next reading (linked with Exercise 3), by J.L. Mackie, will help to show this. One problem is that a cause cannot be a necessary condition (in the second sense) for an effect if there is any other way in which the effect could come about. A similar problem is that a cause cannot be a sufficient condition if its effectiveness depends on its being combined with other factors, or the absence of other factors. J.L. Mackie's influential article puts forward a more sophisticated and guarded view of causes that clarifies and avoids these difficulties.

Mackie, a fellow at Oxford from 1967 to his death in 1981, wrote mainly on the British Empiricists, the nature of causation, and on ethics. In this article he explores a broadly Humean model of causation.

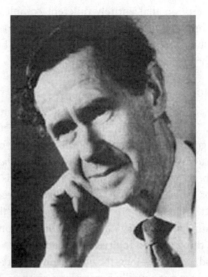

Fig. 15.1 J.L. Mackie

EXERCISE 3 (30 minutes)

Read the short extract from:

Mackie, J.L. (1993). Causes and conditions. In *Causation* (ed. E. Sosa and M. Tooley). Oxford: Oxford University Press, pp. 33–50 (extract pp. 33–35)

Link with Reading 15.3

◆ What does Mackie mean by an INUS condition?

◆ Could this account capture the use of causation that is made by medical science?

Short circuits cause house fires?

The key idea behind Mackie's INUS condition analysis of causation (defined below) is captured by the following problem. Suppose that experts agree that a house fire was caused by an electrical short circuit. They do not think that the short circuit was either necessary or sufficient for the fire; but necessity and sufficiency do have something to do with it. So what is the 'force' of the claim that it caused the fire? The INUS condition is supposed to reconcile these different elements.

The short circuit was not necessary for the fire because the fire could have come about in a different way: through a short circuit somewhere else or through arson for example. And it was not sufficient because in the absence of oxygen and flammable material or in the presence of an efficient sprinkler system, it would not have come about.

It is worth pausing here to ask whether it would have been the same fire had it had a different origin. This is related to asking what the identity conditions of fires are; do they include their causes? One might say that it is necessary (both 'without which not' and 'not possibly not') for the coming into being of a human that they have some or other biological father. Now consider a particular child. Was it necessary for its coming about that it had the specific father that it did? By analogy with Mackie's comment that a short circuit elsewhere could have caused the same fire, one might say no: it might have had a different biological father. But in fact, most people have the intuition that having your own particular biological parents is a necessary condition for being you. This intuition can be partially unpacked by saying that one would not have the same genetic material unless one did and that genetic material is an essential (although not sufficient) feature of being the person you are. And thus, by analogy, it may be that a short circuit elsewhere would have caused a *different* fire. But we will put this issue aside here and return to the notion of identity in Chapter 23 in Part V.

Electrical faults INUS house fires!

Instead, Mackie suggests that the short circuit was a necessary ingredient of a particular complex condition that was itself sufficient for the fire. Thus, given that there were no other short circuits, the complex condition that brought about the fire had to include just this short circuit. That short circuit had to be combined with the presence of flammable material and the absence of sprinklers to bring about the fire, but, so combined, the whole complex was sufficient. It was, however, not a necessary condition for the fire on the assumption that entirely different complex conditions could have brought about the fire. Hence the short circuit is an *Insufficient* but *Necessary* part of an *Unnecessary* but *Sufficient* condition for the fire: an *INUS* condition.

The need for a causal field

Mackie goes on to refine the account by adding in reference to a *causal field*. The key difficulty this is designed to remove is this. Unless one goes so far as to build the effect into the complex that is supposed to cause it, no causal complex can be *sufficient* to bring anything about. One way of thinking about this is to consider the (perhaps vanishingly small) temporal gap between the cause and its effect. As long as there is any such gap, then the cause can never be sufficient or *enough by itself* to bring about the effect. If the right thing were to intervene in that instant—such as the hand of God, perhaps—then the effect could be pre-empted. So even if this does not actually happen in a given case, the causal complex normally cited would not, properly speaking, be a sufficient condition.

Mackie suggests that when we say that A caused P, we tacitly imply that this is relative to a further background set of conditions—or 'causal field'—in which intervention by the hand of God, or whatever, is precluded. Thus A might be sufficient in relation to that background. This tacitly presupposed background is important in searching for general causal relations. So, for example, if one is attempting to discover the cause of influenza, one might be interested only in the case of human beings and not rats, or one might be interested in why, given the presence of the virus, some humans caught influenza and others did not: 'In all such cases, the cause is required to differentiate, within a wider field in which the effect sometimes occurs and sometimes does not, the sub-region in which it occurs: this wider region is the causal field.' (p. 39)

Adding in the idea of a causal field rules out a complete *analysis* of causation in independent terms. What it suggests is that Mackie is instead demonstrating the connection between our use of concepts of causation, necessity and sufficiency. It is a matter of charting connections rather than reducing the concept of causation to something supposedly simpler. If the only purpose of philosophy were the reduction of higher level to lower level concepts then this would be a failure. But in fact most philosophical accounts aim more modestly to show the interconnections between concepts. In that context, talk of causal fields remains a refinement to Mackie's general picture.

There is, however, a more fundamental objection to Mackie's position that also motivates the subject matter of a paper by Nancy Cartwright's paper (1983, see Exercise 6) that will be discussed in the next session. The emphasis on even post facto sufficiency has the consequence that indeterministic causation cannot be accommodated within the model. If a state of affairs merely makes another more probable but still less than a probability of 1

then it is not sufficient for it and cannot be a cause of it if Mackie is correct. But typically we *do* think that causes can merely make their effects more probable. According to contemporary accounts of physics, nuclear decay is a matter of probability less than 1. Thus in principle even if the bomb worked as it was designed to in every humanly controllable way dropping the atom bomb on Hiroshima did not raise the chances of an explosion to 1. It remained some small amount less than that. But if so it was not sufficient for the effect. Nevertheless we still generally think that it caused the explosion.

Mackie's use of counter-factuals as telescoped arguments

To return to the main lines of Mackie's account (i.e. putting aside causal fields and the question of whether causes are sufficient for their effects), he suggests that singular causal relations are related to necessity and to sufficiency through two sorts of conditional statements. Thus he suggests that the example 'a short circuit here was a necessary condition of a fire in this house' is closely related to the *counter-factual* conditional 'If a short circuit had not occurred here this house would not have caught fire'. (Recall from Chapter 14: a counter factual conditional is a conditional statement—if . . . then . . .—whose antecedent runs counter to the facts.)

And 'A short circuit here was a sufficient condition of a fire in this house' is closely related to the *factual* conditional "Since a short-circuit occurred here, this house caught fire" '. Thus Mackie forges a link between the idea of one event causing another and specific sorts of conditionals holding between them. We will focus on counter-factuals of the sort: had the cause not occurred then neither would the effect. This is a counter-factual conditional because the antecedent runs counter to the facts as, in actual fact, the antecedent did occur.

As we saw above, Hume (1975) used just such a claim to characterize causality in addition to making other comments that look closer to a regularity theory (without apparently realizing that there was any great difference between them). Thus it looks as though Mackie wishes to explain the problematic notion of causation through the idea of counter-factual connections. But this impression is misleading. Mackie goes on to suggest that such conditional claims are in turn 'telescoped' arguments that employ (although often only by implicit implication) universal generalizations or laws. (As we will see not all universal true generalizations are laws but we will set this issue aside for the next few paragraphs.)

In other words, although Mackie's account seems at first sight to be a counter-factual account it really relies on the idea of universal true generalizations or laws of nature. The counter-factuals that are true are true in virtue of underlying natural laws. To return to the context of philosophical analysis, the problematic notion of causation is unpacked in terms of counter-factuals, but these are in turn explained through the more fundamental notion of laws of nature. These are what fix counter-factual possibility. The very idea of one event causing another depends on there being a law of nature connecting events of the former and latter kind. Necessity at the individual level is analysed by appeal to *nomic* or law-governed necessity.

Counter-factuals or laws of nature?

So one way of thinking about the different possibilities of philosophical analysis here is this. Having spotted the connection between causal relations and specific counter-factual claims one can either:

1. invoke a primitive notion of counter-factual possibility to explain causation directly, or

2. explain counter-factual possibility in terms of a more basic notion of laws of nature.

In fact, in either case, some further philosophical work has to be done. Even in the first case, something more has to be said about which counter-factuals hold true and in virtue of what. In the second, the notion of a law of nature has to be further unpacked, and, as we will see, distinguished from mere accidentally true generalizations.

We will turn (again) to the work of the American philosopher David Lewis a little later to consider an example of the first strategy. But for now we will focus on the second strategy and consider how Hume's problem arises again at the level of laws.

INUS conditions and laws

As we have seen, although INUS conditions look at first sight to define causation by invoking a more primitive notion of counter-factuals, Mackie presents a different account of those to that of Lewis. In the paper discussed above, Mackie suggests that counter-factuals are telescoped arguments based on universal true generalizations or laws. In other words, at its base, Mackie's account is a regularity theory.

But this raises a further question—set to one side above—because a regularity theory depends on an account of what makes the right sort of regularity at the level of laws. What distinguishes a universal true generalization that reflects a genuine law of nature from a universal true generalization whose truth is a matter of accident or coincidence? The one answer that the Humean (relying only on the impression of constant conjunction) cannot invoke is that only in the former case does the generalization reflect the fact that some properties (of forces, perhaps) necessitate others (such as accelerations). Humeans have undermined the idea of causal necessity and replaced it with the weaker notion of conjunction or regularity.

The analysis of laws of nature

Laws and accidents

David Papineau, Professor of Philosophy at Kings College London, has provided a useful summary of the debate in his paper 'Laws and accidents' that is discussed below (Papineau, 1986).

EXERCISE 4 (10 minutes)

Read the short extract from:

Papineau, D. (1986). Laws and accidents. In *Fact, Science and Morality* (ed. G. MacDonald and C. Wright). Oxford: Basil Blackwell, pp. 189–218 (extract pp. 190–191)

Link with Reading 15.4

◆ What is the problem that Papineau's sets out to solve?

◆ Why is this a problem for Humeans?

What's the problem?

Papineau focuses on issues that arise at the level of generality rather than individual causal relations. The key question is what distinguishes those generalizations—those universal true generalizations—which are or reflect laws of nature, and those that are merely accidentally true, true by coincidence. But this is closely related to the nature of causality because the necessary connection for which Hume looked between cause and effect might be expected to connect the properties linked in laws of nature. There is a Humean approach to laws that mirrors the Humean approach to causes.

Another way of putting this point is this. Even though Hume suggests that we ascend from particular instances of cause and effect to the general coincidence of types of events, this does not provide any fresh materials *in the world*, with which to analyse the connection between causes and effects. So accounting for natural *laws*, which describe the relation between properties—such that a change in one property will change the other—faces a similar Humean challenge: What *connects* properties in laws given that we can never observe any causal glue? And if the Humean response is that—properly speaking—nothing does, what is the difference between law-like correlations and accidental or coincidental correlations? These are the questions Papineau addresses.

What distinguishes a law of nature from an accidentally true generalization?

What distinguishes a law of nature from an accidentally true generalization? One might say that when there is merely an accidental correlation the antecedent does not *make* the consequent happen. It just happens by coincidence. Papineau gives the following example. Every time he has gone to the football ground at Highbury no goals have been scored. He will thus never go again. Thus there is a universally true generalization: every time Papineau goes to Highbury the score is nil nil.

But the score at Highbury is not nil nil *because* Papineau is in the crowd. It is merely accidentally true. Hume's analysis of causation, however, does not seem to be able to distinguish this case from a genuine causal regularity. Hume's appeal to the level of generality rather than instances to account for causation does not introduce any fresh ingredients at the new level to bind events of one sort with events of another. They are merely constantly conjoined (and for Hume also contiguous and temporally related). Or so Papineau suggests. So a different response is needed to distinguish laws from accidents.

Laws support counter-factuals

A different response is to point out (echoing this element of both Mackie's and Lewis's (see below) views on causation) that laws support counter-factuals while accidents do not. Laws tell us something about other possible worlds while accidents do not. (This is the same sort of claim that is made about causal relations.) But as Papineau points out, this suggestion leads to a dilemma. If counter-factuals are read at face value then a Humean (who thinks that laws are in some sense *just* constant conjunctions) has to explain why they should hold across other possible worlds. But if counter-factuals are just a figure of speech, then while it may be analytic that laws are classed as 'sustaining counter-factuals', the Humean has to explain why they, but not accidents, are introduced or talked about in this way. In general, Humeans face the task of explaining 'why some constant conjunctions are better than others' (p. 191).

Neither of these points tell *against* saying that laws sustain counter-factuals. In fact, this is a good diagnostic test for whether one thinks of a generalization as a law or as an accident. But it is only a *first* philosophical move. Papineau goes on to discuss two different Humean strategies for explaining what this distinction really amounts to before examining recent non-Humean examples. He summarizes this move succinctly in the *Oxford Companion to Philosophy*:

> At first sight it might seem easy to develop the Humean strategy. Cannot we simply require that laws be truly general, and not restricted to such things as what happened to a particular person in a particular city at particular times? However, this does not get to the heart of the matter. For even if we formulate our example in general terms, not mentioning me or Paris, but specifying a certain kind of person and city, it may still be that the only instances of these kinds in the universe are still, by accident, constantly conjoined with rain. Conversely, there seem to be examples of laws which are restricted in space and time, such as Kepler's law that the planets move in ellipses, which is specific to our solar system.
>
> A better suggestion is that accidents, unlike laws, are no good for predicting the future. This is not because accidental patterns cannot stretch into the future, but rather because, when they do, we cannot know that they are true. J.L. Mackie has argued that laws differ from accidents in that they are inductively supported by their instances, whereas accidents can only be known to be true after all their instances have been exhaustively checked.
>
> However, even if Mackie's criterion is necessary for lawhood, it is not clear whether it is sufficient: couldn't some inductively anticipatable patterns still be accidents? Perhaps a better Humean solution is that proposed by F.P. Ramsey, and later revived by David Lewis: laws are those true generalizations that can be fitted into an ideal systematization of knowledge—or, as Ramsey put

it, laws are a 'consequence of those propositions which we should take as axioms if we knew everything and organized it as simply as possible in a deductive system'. Accidents are then those true generalizations which cannot be explained within such an ideal theory.

Two Humean strategies

To unpack that passage, one idea about how to distinguish laws from accidents thus turns on the relation between different generalizations. According to Richard Braithwaite (1900–90), a Cambridge professor of philosophy, a generalization is a law if it fits within an established deductive scientific system. But this makes lawhood depend on what we take (at a particular time) the laws to be and not the other way around. So a better approach is one taken by the philosopher Frank Ramsey (1903–30, a contemporary of Wittgenstein at Cambridge, who died young) and later by David Lewis. A law is a generalization that fits into a deductive system that optimizes the conflicting requirements of simplicity and universality.

Simplicity and universality are in tension because a simple system would only contain only those generalizations that fitted a single deductive system: perhaps the laws of theoretical physics. But that would miss out on laws from other sciences, such as geology, which resist such assimilation into that deductive system. So the idea is that the optimal balance of these conflicting virtues would yield all but only the laws and exclude all merely accidentally true generalizations. The main problem with this idea is that it is by no means clear that we can make determinate sense of what optimizing simplicity and universality would be. It is not supposed to be merely good general advice ('treat as laws only those generalisations that fit into an optimised science . . . !') but actually to specify what is and what is not a law.

The alternative Humean account, put forward by Mackie, connects the problem of laws and accidents to the problem of induction. The key claim here is that laws, but not accidents, are *inductively supported* by (even a subset) of their instances. As we saw briefly in Chapter 13 in the discussion of scientific realists it is arguable that there is more to the notion of evidence for a theory than the mere *consistency* of the evidence and the theory. Theories are not just consistent (or not) with empirical findings. Those findings *support* some of the theories with which they are consistent better than others.

This idea of inductive support can be further illustrated by mentioning briefly Nelson Goodman's New Riddle of Induction (Goodman, 1983). Goodman invents two new predicates: 'grue' and 'bleen' where 'grue' means green until, say, the year 2020 and blue afterwards and 'bleen' means blue until then and green afterwards. Now the predicate 'grue' could be applied to all the healthy grass so far observed as far as past evidence is concerned as could 'green'. But the grass is either grue or green not both. (It either will or will not turn blue in 2020.) So what is it that supports our projecting its greenness into the future not its grueness? What is it that makes a predicate projectible? (Note that the quick response that grue and bleen are time dependent while green and blue are not is not decisive. A supporter of grue and bleen will point out that 'green' means grue before 2020 and bleen afterwards and thus is time dependent itself.)

Mackie suggests that whatever the answer to that question is, it can be used also to distinguish laws from accidents. Laws are couched in projectable predicates and are thus supported by their instances while accidents are not.

The epistemology of causation

Having sketched two Humean accounts of the difference between laws and accidents, Papineau goes on to consider a non-Humean account. Roughly, this is an account that, contrary to Hume, postulates that there really is a kind of causal glue, a necessitating link between properties and this is what is reported in statements of laws.

Papineau himself argues that even if that were to make sense (contrary to Hume, again) there would be no warrant to believe in such necessary connections because we could not be in a position to gain knowledge of them. His reason for this claim is that the best interpretation of what a non-Humean adds to the Humean account is that of carrying information about other possible worlds.

Now talk of possible worlds—to which we will return below and in more detail in Chapter 23—is a convenient way to illustrate the distinction between contingent and necessary truths (necessary in this case meaning not possibly not rather than without which not). A contingent truth is one that just happens to be true. The US flag is red, white and blue, but it might not have been. It is true in only some possible worlds. We can say that there are possible worlds where it is a different colour. But the fact that two plus two is four is true in every possible world because it is a necessary truth. It is not possible that it is not true.

But while some philosophers think that such talk of possible worlds is just a convenient way of speaking, others think that they really exist. All these other possible worlds are 'out there' in some sense. Papineau argues that supporters of non-Humean approaches to necessitating relations have to believe in possible worlds in this literal sense if they are to explain what causal necessitation means. But since there can be no (causal) contact between different possible worlds, we can never know the (putative) non-Humean facts about laws or causation that (non-Humeans argue) exceed those given in the Humean account.

Literal versus metaphysical construals of possible worlds

Papineau's argument that non-Humeans have to take talk of possible worlds literally (as existence claims about other non-actual worlds) is this. Non-Humeans do have to account for the meaning of their claim that there is a necessitating relation between properties linked in laws. As Humeans such as Mackie also talk of possible worlds non-Humeans have to distinguish themselves in

some way. Papineau suggests they must take possible worlds to be real. (But if so then as we cannot be in causal contact with other possible worlds we should not *believe* in necessitating conditions.)

The moral?

There is something strange about this argument, however. Note the ad hominum point that Lewis famously believes possible worlds are real and yet supports Humeanism. As Papineau reports earlier in his paper, a Ramsey–Lewis model of laws explains why laws hold across possible worlds without implying the existence of any non-Humean ingredient connecting properties. In any case, a possible world reading of the necessitating relation seems wrong because it is supposed to be a relation in *this* world. It seems that non-Humeans cannot appeal to possible worlds to explain this and hence what sense can they give to it. In other words, it is arguable that non-Humeanism is worse off than Papineau suggests.

On the other hand, neither of the two Humean distinctions between laws and accidents is completely satisfactory. The Ramsey–Lewis model depends on optimizing the opposing virtues of simplicity and universality. But what sense can we apply to this advice? How could we decide what the right balance between, for example, extending the system to include more laws at the risk of increasing the total number of free-standing independent deductive systems? Although its opposing virtues have an intuitive appeal, it is not at all clear how they should be applied to real cases.

The Mackie (1993) account, however, writes a cheque on the solution to the New Riddle of Induction. Effectively it reduces two philosophical problems to one. But it does not actually supply an answer to that one problem. The solution to the problem of the distinction between laws and accidents thus remains wide open.

Reflection on the session and self-test questions

Write down your own reflections on the materials in this session drawing out any points that are particularly significant for you. Then, looking back especially at the reading from Hume, write brief notes about the following:

1. What role does causation have in medicine?

2. What is the philosophical puzzle about causation? Does Hume solve it?

3. How does Mackie's analysis of causation as an INUS condition relate to Hume's brief definitions?

4. What general problem about laws does a regularity theory of causation raise?

Session 2 A probabilistic view of causation?

Two strategies for explaining causation again

In this session we look at two more recent attempts to explain the nature of causation. We then return to the connection between causes and laws and thus the structure of 'the realm of law'.

We saw above that there were two obvious strategies inspired by the connection between causation and counter-factual conditionals:

1. invoke a primitive notion of counter-factual possibility to explain causation directly, or

2. explain counter-factual possibility in terms of a more basic notion of laws of nature.

Mackie takes the second line, but this raises questions about how we can characterize those generalizations that are laws from those that are mere accidental true generalizations. David Lewis takes the other view to which we will now turn.

Lewis's work on explanation has already been discussed in Chapter 14. That discussion focused on the idea that an empirical explanation should cite some of the causal history of the event or fact to be explained. In his paper 'Causation', Lewis ([1973] 1993) complements that claim with a sketch of how the concept of causation should itself be analysed. Having looked at some of the advantages and disadvantages of Lewis's strategy, we will return to the prospects of something like Mackie's (1993) account with its underlying regularity or law-based analysis.

Lewis bases his approach on the following thought:

> Hume defined causation twice over. He wrote 'we may define a cause to be an object, followed by another, and where all the objects similar to the first are followed by objects similar to the second. Or in other words where, if the first object had not been, the second never had existed.' Descendants of Hume's first definition still dominate the philosophy of causation: a causal succession is supposed to be a succession that instantiates a regularity... It remains to be seen whether any regularity analysis can succeed... I have no proof that regularity analyses are beyond repair, nor any space to review the repairs that have been tried. Suffice it to say that the prospects look dark. I think it is time to give up and try something else.
>
> A promising alternative is not far to seek. Hume's 'other words'—that if the cause had not been, the effect never had existed—are no mere restatement of his first definition. They propose something altogether different: a counter-factual analysis of causation.   Lewis (1993 p. 193)

Causation and counter-factuals

The key idea behind the strategy is this. Lewis accepts the characterization of causation given by Hume in counter-factual terms. But rather than attempting to explain the counter-factual in terms of regularity (in line with Hume's other characterizations as well as most post-Humean philosophy on the subject), Lewis

bites on the bullet and attempts to explain counter-factuals in other terms. This he does through the idea of different possible worlds.

But to get a feel for the difficulty here, it will be useful to pause and think about what a counter-factual is about and what makes it true or false.

EXERCISE 5   (10 minutes)

Think for a moment about counter-factual conditional claims.

First, what is a conditional claim? Write down a statement with the characteristic if... then... form. Now think up a conditional whose antecedent (first bit!) runs counter to the facts, i.e. is not true. Write it down. Now think about how the statement works. What is it about? What facts does it answer to? How would you decide whether the counter-factual conditional you have written down was true or false?

When you have read about Lewis's account of counter-factuals below ask yourself whether it is an objective or valid account in the sense discussed thoroughly in Chapter 13. Does it answer to something independent of human judgement?

What is the problem with counter-factuals?

What is the problem with counter-factuals? Why do they need an analysis? Take again the example mentioned at the start of this chapter:

> *If* John F. Kennedy had not been assassinated *then* Lyndon B. Johnson would not have become president.

This expresses a claim about what would have happened if something else, which did not in fact happen, had happened. It may be true or false. (Perhaps there is reason to think that he would have become president in the longer term in any case.) But if it is true, what is it true in virtue of? What makes it true?

Consider the simpler claim:

> John F. Kennedy was assassinated

This is true. We might happily say that the sentence 'John F. Kennedy was assassinated' is true because it is a fact that John F. Kennedy was assassinated. There is a good question about how explanatory this is of the notion of truth because it is unclear that we have any clearer idea of *facts* than *truth*. (Perhaps the best we can say is that facts are what true sentences state. But that requires that we already understand the concept of truth and so this approach to facts could not also be used to explain truth.) But it does seem more plausible to say that it is true because of how the world is than to say that the first claim is true because of how the world is. The reason for that is that in this world Kennedy was assassinated. So with what can the *counter-factual* conditional be compared? Hence the need for an analysis of what makes a counter-factual true.

Lewis agrees with Mackie (and everyone else) that there is a close connection between causal relations and counter-factuals, but he offers a novel account of the latter. This is spelt out as follows:

> If p were true then q would be true' is itself true iff (if and only if) there is a possible world where both are true which is more similar to this world than any where p is true and q is not. Or: a counter-factual is non-vacuously true iff it takes less of a departure from actuality to make the consequent true along with the antecedent than it does to make the antecedent true without the consequent. (p. 197)

One way of thinking of this general strategy is as follows. (Don't worry if this does not help!) Lewis accepts Hume's claim that we cannot make sense of a this-worldly necessary connection between cause and effect (a kind of causal glue). So instead he attempts to deploy a notion of necessity in terms of relations to other possible worlds. In so doing he moves towards the sense of necessity that means not-possibly-not. (But he does not attempt to define causal relations as holding across *all* possible worlds. Counter-factuals are defined in terms of relations to certain close possible worlds.)

One cost of a possible world analysis of counter-factuals

There are, however, serious 'costs' attached to this solution. One is spelling out the idea of relative similarity of possible worlds. Van Fraassen (1980) points out that Lewis's analysis requires a prior understanding of *relative similarity to actual world history*. Thus it requires assessment of what is more similar. But, Van Fraassen suggests, this is an essentially context dependent issue.

> If the plant had not been sprayed
> (and all else had been the same)
> then it would not have died...

> It is true in a given situation exactly if the 'all else' that is kept 'fixed' is such as to rule out death of the plant for other reasons. But who keeps what fixed? The speaker, in his mind. There is therefore a contextual variable—determining the content of that tacit *ceteris paribus* clause—which is crucial to the truth-value of the conditional statement. Let us suppose that I say to myself, *sotto voce*, that a certain fuse leads into a barrel of gunpowder, and then say out loud, 'If Tom lit that fuse there would be an explosion.' Suppose that before I came in, you had observed to yourself that Tom is very cautious, and would not light any fuse before disconnecting it, and said out loud, 'If Tom lit that fuse there would be no explosion.' Have we contradicted each other? Is there an objective right or wrong about keeping one thing rather than another firmly in mind when uttering the antecedent 'If Tom lit that fuse...'? It seems rather that the proposition expressed by the sentence depends on a context, in which 'everything else being equal' takes on a definite content. (p.116)

In Van Fraassen's example, is it the case that if Tom had lit the fuse then the bomb would have exploded, or is it the case that if Tom had lit the fuse he would have already disconnected it from the bomb? If we know that Tom is cautious then the latter may seem the most important factor in assessing relative similarity.

But what hope is there of settling questions of relative similarity objectively?

A second cost of a possible world analysis of counter-factuals

Of course, examples like this trade on intuitions. But as Lewis (1993) intends to analyse the very idea of one thing depending causally on another—which one would ordinarily think of as an objective matter—on ranking of relative similarity, some account of how this is to be calibrated is required. But it is not forthcoming. There is another price to pay for a possible world analysis of counter-factuals: a belief in possible worlds. This point can be put by asking what is the foundation of our understanding here? Do we understand counter-factual claims because we have an antecedent understanding of possible worlds and their relative similarity relations? Or do we instead only understand the *facon de parler* of possible worlds because we already have an understanding of counter-factual claims? Lewis wants to claim the former, but to make a distinction he has to claim that he takes talk of possible worlds literally. They really exist, it is just that they are not actual. Actuality is itself an indexical term. (*We* say of *this* world that it is actual. Our counter-parts on other worlds may use the same words to say a different but parallel thing.) But how convincing is the claim that we can 'unpack' the supposedly more problematic conception of causation in terms of the supposedly less problematic idea of other equally real but non-actual possible worlds?

In a sense similar to one that will be explored in Chapter 16, Lewis's counter-factual and possible world account of causal relations and hence of causation is more a 'research programme' than a single instance of philosophical analysis. Thus objections of Van Fraassen's type serve more to show the work that would have to be carried out rather than to refute Lewis claim in one blow. Nevertheless, the prospects look equally bleak for the prospects of formalizing the primitive notion of relative similarity of possible worlds as Lewis claims they do for a regularity analysis of causation.

Causation and probability

We touched on an important criticism of Mackie (1993) earlier. This is that Mackie's model is a limited form of sufficient condition while we now acknowledge the role of causal relations that are not sufficient, in a logical sense, for their effects.

Recall that on the INUS account, a cause involves a condition that is unnecessary but, given an assumed causal field, is sufficient for its effects. It is sufficient in the circumstances. But many sciences invoke notions of causation that are weaker than this. They construe causation as a relation that can occur even if the cause only makes the effect *probable*. The next approach to analysing causation discussed in this chapter considers just such a proposal and argues against it to the effect that causation cannot be definitionally reduced to a probabilistic or statistical notion.

EXERCISE 6   (20 minutes)

Read the short extract from:

Cartwright, N. (1983). Causal laws and effective strategies. In *How the Laws of Physics Lie*. Oxford: Oxford University Press, pp. 21–42 (extract: pp. 23–25)

Link with Reading 15.5

♦ What are Cartwright's arguments against a probabilistic account of causation?

♦ If correct, why would they imply that causal laws could not be derived from 'laws of association'?

If a cause need only raise the chances of its effects (by some amount yet to be specified) might it be possible to *define* causes this way: as conditions that raise the chances of other events or facts. Of course *this* possibility is not a consequence of indeterminacy: causation may resist any such definition. But it is an attractive suggestion for a philosophical account of causation.

This is one of the projects that Nancy Cartwright considers and rejects. She claims that it is impossible to extract causal relations from statistical correlations without building in some prior assumptions about what causes what. A consequence of this (if it is true) is that causation cannot be defined from statistical 'laws of association'. Cartwright's conclusion, to which we will return shortly, is that causation resists definition and is *sui generis*.

One of the reasons for Cartwright's claim is illustrated by the example of a letter from an insurance policy: 'It simply wouldn't be true to say, "Nancy L D Cartwright . . . you own a TIAA life insurance policy you'll live longer." But it is a fact, none the less, that persons insured by TIAA do enjoy longer lifetimes, on the average, than persons insured by commercial insurance companies that serve the general public.' (p. 22)

Cartwright claims that one needs the notion of causation to ground that of an 'effective strategy' in order to distinguish between the fact that there is an association between having a life insurance policy and living longer and the further fact that taking out a policy is an effective strategy for living longer.

The argument against reduction

Cartwright's (1983) key argument against the reduction of causation to a probabilistic relation is this. Suppose that two factors are connected as indeterministic cause and effect. It may seem therefore that a cause ought to increase the probability and thus observed frequency of its effect. But this may not happen in fact if there are other causal factors at work. 'Background correlations between the purported cause and other causal factors may conceal the increase in probability which would otherwise appear.' (p. 23)

In her example, if smoking is correlated with a sufficiently strong preventative factor, the expected increase in the probability of heart disease among smokers will not show up. But how is

this to be ruled out without specification that other *causal* factors are absent? Cartwright suggests that the best that can be done by way of a probabilistic analysis of causation is: ' "C causes E" if and only if C increases the probability of E in every situation which is otherwise causally homogenous with respect to E.' (p. 25)

However, this cannot serve to *define* causation because it presupposes the idea of causal homogeneity. There is clearly a connection between probability and causation. We use statistical tests of probability of non-random association as 'probes' for causal relations: e.g. the association between smoking and lung cancer identified by Sir Richard Doll as an epidemiologist led to subsequent research on the underlying causal mechanisms. Cartwright is not undermining that connection. But she does claim that we cannot define causation in terms of probability. It is worth recalling from Chapter 13 that Cartwright argues that there is a close connection between explanation and the citing of causal factors. Having renounced the aim to reduce the concept of causation to whatever raises the chances of its effects, Cartwright still stresses the claim that a causal explanatory factor must increase the chances of is effects (relative to a background that holds constant all other *causal* factors).

Laws of association and effective strategies

In the second part of her paper, Cartwright (1983) goes on to argue that a parallel difficulty faces any attempt to define effective strategies for achieving ends simply in terms of probabilities. Causal laws are needed in characterizing effectiveness because they pick out the right properties on which to base one's conditional probabilities. Otherwise, a strategy can appear to be an effective strategy—to reduce heart disease—because of a statistical connection that is in fact the result of a different but correlated causal factor.

Cartwright's conclusion is that there is a connection between causation, strategies for attaining one's ends, and raising probabilities. But she argues that this does not allow the definition of either of the first two in terms of the third. The objectivity of causal laws is what the effectiveness of means-end strategies depends on and also what their accurate statistical measurement depends on. But this leaves causality undefined: a primitive concept in our description of the world.

Epistemology again

The fact that causation could not be defined in terms of probabilistic relations would not imply that statistical findings could play no role in the *epistemological* matter of finding out about what causal relations hold in the world. But it would imply that this inference—like many in science—involved an element of holism or bootstrapping. The interpretation of statistical correlations is only a reliable guide either to causal relations or to effective strategies if one already knows what is the right way to partition the facts or conditions that are statistically correlated. 'Only partitions by causally relevant variables count in evaluating causal laws' (Cartwright, 1983, p. 38). On the other hand, statistical correlations are still a valuable source of evidence for causal relations, but only if one already knows some other causal information.

It is worth stressing again, that the philosophy of causation has by no means reached a settled stage. There are competing research programmes, one of which aims to characterize causality in probabilistic terms. But if Cartwright is right then not only does the reduction of causation to probabilistic relations fail, but so does any reduction. Causation is a primitive notion that defies analysis in other terms. It is connected to the raising of probability but not in such a way that allows its elimination (i.e. by translating causality into probability). As we will see shortly, this does not sever the connection between causes and laws.

Hume's challenge again

Think again about what the arguments have so far shown. Hume's argument attempted to show that there was something wrong with the way we think of causation as part of the world. The notion of necessary connection could not be traced back to any experiences of the world or of the interaction of the mind and body. Given this negative result he then at least seemed to offer positive definitions of causation that replaced any such worldly component with an alternative picture of both how the concept of causation originates and what it amounts to, i.e. a relation of 'constant conjunction' of events. The problem with these characterizations, however, is that they seem to give us less than we want from the notion of causation and, by extension, from laws of nature.

There is, however, a different response available to Hume's critical inquiry into the impressions that supposedly ground the concept of causation. One need not accept that the failure of Hume's reduction of the concept to anything more primitive undermines its reality or our pre-philosophical understanding of its nature. One might instead accept that the reduction of causation is impossible while taking this simply to reaffirm its *primitive* status in our ontology. We understand the world to contain both causal relations and laws of nature over and above the coincidences and statistical relations we observe. These are connected to the notion of making something happen, bringing it about, sustaining counter-factual claims about what would have happened and so on. But none of these related notions allows a conceptually unproblematic independent definition of causation.

The connection between causes and laws remains

A further connection between causes and laws

Even if such a non-reductionist realism about causality is the right moral to draw from the debate, however, it does not undermine the close if not definitional connection between causes and laws. The American philosopher of mind and language Donald Davidson (1917–2003) whose work will be discussed throughout

Part V argues for just such a connection in 'Laws and cause' in *Dialectica* 49 (1995, pp. 263–279).

Singular causal relations and epistemology

Davidson (1995) argues that the thesis that there is a connection between causes and general laws need not turn on a denial of the phenomenological claims that we can directly perceive that one event has caused another without evidence from similar cases. In other words he turns his back on arguments inspired by Hume's examination of the source of an impression of necessity. This is an important point. Davidson does not subscribe to an *epistemological* argument that turns on this claim and concludes instead that causation must mean something else. Epistemology is not important in Davidson's argument so he can afford to say that we can directly perceive singular causation.

This point is worth taking a little slowly. Davidson reports the philosopher John McDowell as saying that, without a particular picture of the relation of language to the world with which language deals, there is no reason to deny—as Hume denies— that singular causal relations are 'given in experience'. Now the details of that philosophical picture—it is called 'scheme-content dualism'—do not matter here. But McDowell draws the conclusion that it is only with some such philosophical theory in place that one will want to deny that one can observe singular causal relations. If this is so, then Hume's sceptical inquiry into the grounding of our concept of cause presupposes doubtful philosophy and its outcome might just as well be the denial of that philosophy as the denial that we can experience individual causes.

Davidson's response is to concede that point but maintain that it does not undermine Hume's basic claim that where there are causes there must also be laws and that this is consistent with an epistemology in which direct detection of singular causes is possible. He goes on to discuss informal experiments by the philosopher C.J. Ducasse in which audiences do report epistemologically one-off causal relations.

Changes and laws

Davidson (1995) suggests these experiments lead to a definition of causation that is something like this. 'If c is the only change in situation S which precedes the only subsequent change e in S, then c is the cause of e.' (p. 271). At first sight this looks very different from Hume's characterization of causation in terms of regularity. But Davidson argues that the difference is more apparent than real once one also realizes that the recognition of something as a change requires some background assumptions about what counts as no change:

> It is not surprising, then, that singular causal statements imply the existence of covering laws: events are changes that explain and require such explanations. This is not an empirical fact: nature doesn't care what we call a change, so we decide what counts as change on the basis of what we want to explain, and what we think available as an explanation. In deciding what counts as a change we also decide what generalizations to count as law-like. (p. 273)

This is a Wittgensteinian point. The key idea is that there is no 'theory neutral' perspective from which to judge that two events or actions are relevantly similar or that there has been no relevant change in nature that calls for explanation. The notion of sameness and difference is always relative to a rule. Judging that objects are the same in respect of colour turns on the rules of colour ascription. For example, one would not complain to a car manufacturer that there was something wrong with its paint if it seemed to change colour under sodium light. Judging that two objects are moving in the same way turns on the rules of kinematics. Thus if a body continues to move in a straight line at uniform speed, we no longer think that anything needs explanation. It is changes that need explanation. But our post-Newtonian view differs from that of the Greeks who did think that an explanation was needed for why, e.g., arrows continued to move. Davidson suggests that these points also imply that to understand the kinds of changes that stand in causal relations presupposes a background that gives sense to these through an idea of contrast.

Causation and explanation

The conclusion Davidson (1995) draws is that whatever our awareness of individual or singular causal relations in the world, there is still a fundamental relation between causal relations and laws. In drawing this conclusion Davidson provides support to a claim that has been implicit in the last two sessions. There is a close connection between the concept of *causation* and causal *explanation*. Davidson highlights this connection through the idea that causes have to be picked out as changes against an unchanging background. It is the changes that stand in need of particular explanation and thus have to be charted as effects of antecedent causes. Our concept of cause is thus informed by what we take to need explanation and what can be used as part of that explanation.

Conclusions? Four responses to Hume

We can now take stock. The material of this session and the last has concerned the recent philosophical discussion of causation and, to a lesser extent, its relations to laws of nature. Hume's discussion has been crucial in the history of the subject but the correct response to the problems Hume highlighted remains unclear.

1. One approach seeks to offer a regularity theory of causation following one of Hume's own characterizations. Such analysis faces a related problem at a higher level of generality: what distinguishes laws from mere accidental correlations, given that one cannot say without some further explanation that the antecedent conditions in laws make subsequent effects happen. However, even if the problem of separating laws and accidents could be solved—both conceptually and epistemologically—there remains a further problem according to Cartwright (1983). One cannot milk the concept of causation from laws of association.

2. Another strategy is to take Hume's suggestion that causes are connected to counter-factual conditionals. Now this connection is also exploited in broadly Humean regularity theories.

Such theories attempt to explain counter-factual conditionals as truncated arguments using general laws. But Lewis (1973), as we saw above, attempts to characterize them independently of general laws and thus dodge the problems just summarized. He faces different and grave difficulties, however, in spelling out just how the relative similarity of different possible worlds is to be 'measured' if his solution is to provide any genuine insight.

3. A third option is to define causation in probabilistic terms. We have not examined this in any detail because it faces Cartwright's (1983) objection: How is the relation between causality and probability to be spelt out in terms which do not involve partitioning according to causal factors? (In addition it is worth noting that if probability is taken to be underwritten by probabilistic laws, the problem of laws and accidents will recur in this third case.)

4. A fourth possibility is to accept the current failures of analysis of causation as indicative of something deeper. Perhaps causation cannot be given a reductionist analysis and is simply a primitive concept in our ontology. This does not mean that it cannot be given any further characterization. It is connected to counter-factual reasoning, to the idea of making things happen and, as we have just seen, to explanations of a certain sort.

The connection of causes and laws in psychiatric diagnosis

Causation has played a part in the two previous chapters: in the very idea of a fruitful classification that can help reveal aetiology, and in the nature of diagnosis. This chapter has examined the concept of causality in more detail. Whatever final analysis might be arrived at, there does seem to be an important connection between causes and laws. At the very least, laws play a central role in the epistemology of causation and thus the development of psychiatric aetiology will turn on the development of body of

Reflection on the session and self-test questions

Write down your own reflections on the materials in this session drawing out any points that are particularly significant for you. Then write brief notes about the following:

1. What was Hume's second definition of causation and how does it suggest an alternative to a Regularity Theory of causation?

2. How successful is Lewis' account of a counter-factual?

3. How else might causation be defined?

4. What connections might remain between causation and general natural laws?

psychiatric laws. We also saw that one of the virtues of a classif-icatory system emphasized by Hempel and discussed in Chapter 13 was that it should fit existing laws and suggest new laws (in effect, construct validity). Thus the discovery of laws seems to be an essential feature of a conception of psychiatry as a successful science. But is that all there is to psychiatric understanding?

Session 3 The realm of law and the space of reasons

So far this chapter has been concerned with the nature of causes and their connection with laws of nature. Causation is an import-ant ingredient in medical and psychiatric aetiology. Finding the causes of psychiatric symptoms is an important aim of medical research and promises to be a step towards a psychiatric classif-ication based on deeper underlying similarities and differences rather than merely what can be observed on the surface, as the extract from Hempel suggested in Chapter 13.

Causes and explanation

Furthermore, whatever its precise nature, there are plausible arguments to suppose that some relation exists between causation and lawhood. Thus one strand of psychiatric research promises to aim at the subsumption of psychiatric phenomena under laws. This is (or should be) part of the aim of a scientific psychiatry. We have also seen from Chapter 14 that on one prominent model, there is also a relation between such subsumption under laws and scientific explanation. Whether or not the formal Deductive-Nomological model is really adequate to accommodate all scientific explanations (and to preclude non-explanations), what seems right about it is that subsumption under laws is at least one way of explaining things. It is one way of revealing an underlying pattern in otherwise diverse phenomena.

This session, however, picking up on the themes of Part II of the book, will focus on a different pattern, which, following Wilfrid Sellars and John McDowell, we can call fitting events into the normative 'space of reasons'. The key question is whether the pattern provided by the 'space of reasons' is fundamentally different from and discontinuous with the 'realm of law'. We will explore this question by charting four different views of the rela-tion between the space of reasons and realm of law.

Plan of the session

The first two views discussed embody a shared response to this question. The first, expressed in McDowell's *Mind and World* (1994), emphasizes the difference between causes and reasons as different modes of intelligibility while in no way denigrating the realm of law.

The second emphasizes the consequences of the distinction between reasons and causes or laws for the social sciences. Peter Winch's influential *The Idea of a Social Science and its Relation to Philosophy* (1958) argues that meaningful behaviour resists incorporation in a causal law-like social science and requires a different model.

An opposing view argues that the two kinds of approach can be reconciled. The contemporary UK psychologist and philosopher, Derek Bolton, argues that reasons and causes can be assimilated in information-rich causal sciences on the assumption that the brain encodes meanings. If so then what McDowell (1994) calls the space of reasons is really just a part of the realm of law.

The fourth view that will be discussed is from Brown and Harris's (1978) now classic empirical study of the *Social Origins of Depression*. It provides a less ambitious assimilation. Brown and Harris argue that meaningful events can cause depression, although they make no attempt to unite the structure that imparts meaning to the events with the structure of causal laws that connects those events to subsequent depression.

McDowell's (1994) account of the distinction between the space of reasons and the realm of law

The background to *Mind and World*

The first view, then, is drawn from John McDowell's collection of lectures *Mind and World* (1994). The first lecture of this collec-tion was discussed in Chapter 12 on the theory dependence of data. It introduced the idea that perception involves the inelimin-able interplay of two ingredients that are not separable. Drawing on Kantian philosophy, McDowell characterizes these as the 'faculty of receptivity' and the 'faculty of spontaneity'. Talk of receptivity is meant to capture the idea that perceptual experi-ence is passive in that we open our eyes to how things are in the world. But McDowell follows Kant in claiming that even here, our *conceptual* abilities are also—albeit passively—drawn into play. Experience is always already conceptualized. These conceptual abilities are the very ones used in active judgements—the domain of the faculty of spontaneity.

The reason for this last claim—that concepts are passively drawn into play in experience—is that only so is it plausible that perception can have *rational* consequences for the beliefs that we form about the world. The only model we have of rational rela-tions between mental states is that which holds between concep-tualized beliefs. Thus if these are to be in rational contact with how the world is, then they will have to be grounded ultimately in conceptualized experience, in which the state of the world is taken in through experience.

In the short extract below (linked with Exercise 7) McDowell (1994) further characterizes the conceptual order, its character-istic form of intelligibility and its relation to that form of intel-ligibility that rose to prominence in the seventeenth century in the West: the realm of law. The idea is that in what is often called the 'Scientific Revolution' of the seventeenth century, the rapid development and rise of influence of the natural sciences, also promoted a particular way of understanding or rather explain-ing the natural world: charting laws of nature. This kind of understanding is different from that involved in the interpretation of texts that was central to the discussion of the Methodenstreit and Jaspers in Part II of this book. Furthermore, the rise of natural science defeated the previous view of even the natural world as a kind of text with built in meaning. But while McDowell applauds the technological achievement of natural science he argues that we should not take it for granted that that is the only way of discovering what is real. That, however, leaves the problem of relating understanding and explanation.

EXERCISE 7   (60 minutes)

Read the extract from:

McDowell, J. (1994). *Mind and World*. Cambridge, MA: Harvard University Press, (extract pp. 70–72)

Link with Reading 15.6

- Try to extract the broader distinction between the space of reasons and realm of law.

- What is McDowell's attitude towards the naturalness or otherwise of the former?

McDowell's concern is with the connection between nature and what is natural on the one hand, and with meaning and what is meaningful, on the other. As he points out, it was a hard-won achievement to separate the kind of intelligibility found in the natural sciences from those deployed in the interpretation of texts. We no longer believe, as the mediaevals did, that nature is a book of quasi-moral or mystical lessons for us. Instead the kind of intelligibility that characterizes the natural sciences is distinguished as answering to different organizational principles which are, in part, the subject matter of the philosophy of science.

A central tension

McDowell argues that the structure that governs our use of concepts is distinct from, is *sui generis* by comparison with, the realm of law. This presents a tension, however, because we also tend to think that nature can be completely described in scientific terms. We think that the realm of law exhausts nature. The tension arises from the fact that our use of (meaningful) concepts cannot be fitted into that structure (i.e. the structure of the realm of law) and thus can seem to be unnatural (outwith nature).

As we saw in Chapter 12 on observation, McDowell argues that perception involves concepts. Perceptual experiences are always conceptually structured. Thus on the one hand, perceptions seem to lie outside nature because concepts cannot be fitted into the realm of law. But on the other hand, perceptions seem to be part of the ordinary course of nature, a natural feature of human life. And thus there is a tension.

To repeat, the problem is that if concepts are an essential part of perception or sensibility, and if concepts cannot be explained from the perspective of the realm of law implicit in the natural sciences, then perception cannot be fully explained using the natural sciences. This may suggest that perception of the world is not itself a *natural* phenomenon. McDowell is centrally concerned with perceptual experiences but the same general point applies to all concept use in, for example, reasoning. Because the space of reasons appears, at first sight at least, to be different from the realm of law, if we assume that nature can be fully described using the latter, then reasoning seems to be unnatural.

McDowell goes on to suggest that there are three different responses to this tension that are typically made in philosophy.

First response to the tension: bald naturalism

Bald naturalism, according to McDowell, is the attempt to show how the conceptual structure of the space of reasons—'relations of justification and the like'—can be framed in the terms appropriate to the realm of law. In other words, it attempts to provide a translation of meaning-laden terms into a purely law-like idiom. Although McDowell does not say this, a baldly naturalistic view would be one which like the work of the US philosopher Jerry Fodor in the philosophy of thought and language, attempted to 'naturalise' intentional concepts by showing precisely how meaning is the result of 'natural' causal or law-like relations (see Part V, Chapter 24). (In fact things are more complicated than this. Fodor does not so much attempt to explain the structure of rational or reason relations in terms of causal processes as the more modest aim of showing, in purely causal law-like terms, how it is possible for our thought processes to track rational relations. This is not quite the same thing as explicating that rational structure in causal terms.)

Surprisingly, McDowell does not offer much in the way of explicit argument against bald naturalism in *Mind and World*. His aim in these lectures is instead to explore the challenges to a philosophical perspective that already accepts that the space of reasons is genuinely distinct from that of laws. But there is an argument that he gives elsewhere that the two structures cannot be mapped onto one another. This is that such a mapping would require that the rational structure of reasons could be codified: it could be organized into a prescriptive, deductive structure of general principles that is independent of context. But while certain areas of rationality have been given a codification—Frege's predicate logic being the best example—this is not plausible in general. Rationality must include, as well as deductive relations, both inductive support and perceptual evidence. In neither case is there much prospect for a context-neutral characterization of reasons for belief.

Second response to the tension: anomalous monism

The remaining two responses considered by McDowell disagree with bald naturalism in that they take the different structures of the space of reasons and the realm of law as genuinely distinct. The first, however, which McDowell ascribes to Davidson, takes it that although the two conceptual structures are genuinely distinct, they can both hold of the same subject matter at the level of particulars. This is the purpose of Davidson's answer to the mind–body problem: anomalous monism, which will be described more fully in Chapter 23. The very same states are both mental— governed by rational principles—and also physical—occupants of the realm of law.

McDowell's objection to this picture turns on the naturalness that the picture ascribes to experience. If being a natural phenomenon turns on being explicable within the realm of law and if the faculty responsible for conceptual abilities—the faculty of spontaneity—'functions in the space of reasons' then 'spontaneity cannot permeate the operations of sensibility as such' (p. 75), and 'So if we go equating something's place in nature with its location in the realm of law, we are debarred from holding that an experience has its conceptual content precisely as whatever natural phenomenon it is.' (p. 76).

It is quite difficult to interpret these passages so as to determine what the precise objection to Davidson's reconciliation of reasons and causes (or laws) is. But as we will see in Part V, it turns on the following concern. If mental states are identified with free-standing internal states of the body, then their intentional or meaningful properties, their 'aboutness', becomes mysterious.

McDowell argues that there is a common strand from Descartes, through Locke, to modern functionalist accounts of mind and other forms of representationalism. In each case, mental states, including experiential states, are construed as 'self-standing configurations in an inner realm' (McDowell, 1986, p. 151). The motivation for this, he suggests, is that it allows for a science of man that can appeal to 'states of the organisms whose intrinsic nature can be described independently of the environment' (p. 152):

> Now this intellectual impulse is gratified also in a modern way of purportedly bringing the mind within the scope of theory, in which the interiority of the inner realm is literally spatial: the autonomous explanatory states are in ultimate fact states of the nervous system, although, in order to protect the claim that the explanations they figure in are psychological, they are envisaged as conceptualized by theories of mind in something like functionalist terms. This conception of mind shares what I have suggested we should regard as the fundamental motivation of the classically Cartesian conception; and I think this is much more significant than the difference between them.
>
> McDowell (1986, p. 153)

But, he argues, so construed the mind goes 'blank or blind' because it is impossible to see how such free standing internal states can be about anything. They can be caused by and cause changes in the outside world, but that is not to say that they stand in rational meaningful relations as well as causal relations to states of the world.

Third response to the tension: resonating to reason is in our nature

The third position is the one that McDowell wishes to advocate. It accepts that there is a genuine contrast between the structure that governs reasons and that operative in the realm of law and does not help itself to the quick ontological fix of postulating a neutral subject matter. Instead, McDowell argues that we have to broaden our conception of what is natural so as to include the fact that we as natural animals can 'resonate' to the demands of reason. This is part of our 'second nature': 'To see exercises of spontaneity as natural, we do not need to integrate spontaneity related concepts into the structure of the realm of law; we need to stress their role in capturing patterns in a way of living.' (1994, p. 78).

McDowell goes on to deploy an analogy with moral judgements to try to underpin this picture.

A parallel with moral judgement

McDowell suggests that the best way to think about moral judgements—a way he attributes to Aristotle—is to regard as the purpose of a moral upbringing the opening up of recipients, through the development of practical wisdom, to the moral demands of situations that are 'there anyway'.

> The ethical is a domain of rational requirements, which are there in any case, whether or not we are responsive to them. We are alerted to these demands by acquiring appropriate conceptual capacities. When a decent upbringing initiates us into the relevant way of thinking, our eyes are opened to the very existence of this tract of the space of reasons.   (1994, p. 82)

McDowell goes on to criticize one of the motivations for rejecting the underlying moral realism that he advocates. This is the thought that reality can be conceived as though from a position external to our language, concepts, and practices. So conceived, we would be able to think (and philosophize) about the relationship between the conceptual structure of our language and the world. What is more, we might try to ground such theorizing by thinking of nature from the perspective of scientific thinking (the realm of law, or perhaps Williams's Absolute Conception as discussed in Chapter 13). If so we might try to characterize the nature that is there independently of us as comprising only what is revealed by the natural sciences, and thus not the sort of nature that can make rational or moral demands on us. From this perspective, ascribing the source of moral demands to the world (and thus in that sense objective) rather than to us (and thus fully subjective) seems to be simply mistaken.

But McDowell rejects the idea that it makes sense to think about the world from any such extra-conceptual perspective. The problem is that once such a perspective is entertained in which the world is construed as lying outside the edges of the thinkable, it becomes impossible to see how our thought can be rationally constrained by states of affairs in the world. What is more, the fact that thought is rationally constrained by the world is necessary even for the kind of thinking that finds its expression in the realm of law. Subsuming events under laws is a distinct form of intelligibility to placing them in rational relations; however, it nevertheless presupposes that the relation between thinking and the world is rational, is the sort of thinking characterized by the space of reasons and not the realm of law.

This is why McDowell sometimes says in *Mind and World* that there are no limits to the conceptual sphere. This follows from the claim that experience is the direct presence of the world to us and the claim that only if experience is always already conceptualized can it make rational demands on our thinking.

McDowell: the space of reasons is part of the natural order

We are now in a position to take stock of McDowell's (1994) claims about the space of reasons. McDowell (1998) argues that the space of reasons comprises a way of thinking about aspects of the world, which is fundamentally distinct from the causal way of thinking that has (justifiably) risen to prominence in the West since the Scientific Revolution of the seventeenth century.

> Disenchanting that part of the natural world described by the realm of causal law was an intellectual achievement. But we should not limit what is natural to that which can be fitted into the framework of causation. Thus our own responsiveness to reasons (including moral reasons) is a natural part of our being even though it cannot be described in terms ultimately reducible to causal or other natural laws.
>
> But it is one thing to recognize that the impersonal stance of scientific investigation is a methodological necessity for the achievement of a valuable mode of understanding reality; it is quite another thing to take the dawning grasp of this, in the modern era, for a metaphysical insight into the notion of objectivity as such, so that objective correctness in any mode of thought must be anchored in this kind of access to the real ... [It] is not the educated common sense it represents itself as being; it is shallow metaphysics.   McDowell (1998 p. 182)

Two kinds of intelligibility: two methods of investigation

If McDowell is correct then there are two distinct forms of intelligibility that govern different kinds of natural phenomena. This suggests that disciplines investigating these different kinds of phenomena will have to have different kinds of structures and different kinds of concepts. In other words, the conceptual distinctions between the space of reasons and realm of law will have a methodological correlate.

Broadly speaking, the social sciences—those disciplines concerned with charting meaningful relations between events—will be methodologically distinct from natural sciences—those disciplines concerned with subsuming events under general laws. This corollary of McDowell's argument provides a connection with the *Methodenstreit*, the long-running nineteenth century debate about method in the social (or, more broadly, human) sciences, which, as we saw in Part II, was one of the main influences on Jaspers's foundational work in descriptive psychopathology. That the natural and human sciences have different methodologies, as a corollary of McDowell's arguments, is also precisely the conclusion for which the British philosopher Peter Winch argued in 1958 in his influential

book: *The Idea of a Social Science and its Relation to Philosophy*. Because Winch offers a further characterization of the prima facie difference between the natural and human sciences, his work is useful to us here in thinking about a proper understanding of psychiatry as a science combining, to a unique degree, the space of reasons with the realm of law.

Winch's account of the difference between the natural and social sciences

Peter Winch

Winch (1927–98) was one of the first generation of Wittgensteinians who attempted to deploy arguments from the later Wittgenstein's work—mainly *Philosophical Investigations* (1953)—in more applied areas of philosophy. In *The Idea of a Social Science*, Winch (1958) argues that the social sciences—broadly construed—cannot and should not be modelled on the natural sciences because they employ a different form of understanding. In the preface to the 1988 reprinted edition, Winch suggests that he does not mean by this the distinction between explanation and understanding as developed by the nineteenth century German philosopher Max Weber and incorporated into Jaspers's psychopathology (see Part II). Rather he has a deeper point. Only if there is an antecedent or background level of understanding can the sort of deficiency of understanding that an explanation might fill, be intelligible.

This presupposed background understanding is 'expressed in the concepts that constitute the subject matter we are concerned with. These concepts ... also express certain aspects of the life characteristic of those who apply them.' One of the key aims of Winch's book is to chart just what this background understanding is like.

Reasons and rules: the normativity of the space of reasons

A further preliminary point is important. Winch argues that a central element of understanding meaningful behaviour is an understanding of the nature of rules. For this he draws on Wittgenstein's lengthy discussion of rules, rule following and understanding in the *Philosophical Investigations*. He makes three claims:

1. Rules are central to social science because actions are constituted *as* the actions that they are by the rules that are operating. Thus, to give one of his examples, putting a cross on a piece of paper is an act of voting given the right context of rules. Sound patterns, similarly, are constituted as meaningful assertions (words, etc.) given the rules of spoken language.

2. Explaining an action by citing a rule presupposes a grasp of the rule not just by the social scientist but also (to a first approximation) by the agent whose behaviour is being explained.

3. Rule following is grounded in implicit practical knowledge of what actions count as going on in the same way. Rule following cannot rest entirely on explicit linguistically codified knowledge because that explicit knowledge would require further implicit knowledge of how the written prescription is to be interpreted.

Rules also have a further (generally) implicit but important feature. They are *normative*: they prescribe correct and incorrect moves. In the example mentioned above they prescribe the difference between a successful vote and a spoiled ballet paper. Only certain actions count as casting a vote. So if understanding an event involves relating it to a rule, this form of understanding involves a notion of correctness. It involves understanding what makes it correct or appropriate as a piece of voting behaviour. This is not the same as saying that most votes are cast at a particular time of day or night or by a particular socio-economic proportion of the electorate. That may be discovered by empirical study. But the normative rules that characterize an event as an act of voting are not provided by any such statistical generalizations.

With these claims in place, Winch goes on to argue that social science is fundamentally dissimilar to natural science.

Winch's key argument

Winch's key argument is that because explanation of meaningful action in terms of rules presupposes a grasp of the rules and concepts in question by the people whose actions are being explained or understood, social science deploys fundamentally different kinds of generalizations to natural sciences. They are not universal true generalizations under which events can be subsumed. They are instead open-textured patterns of behaviour, which by virtue of the normative rules acquired by shared use in the social context of development grant actions with meaningful intelligibility.

Winch's cat

One of the examples that Winch gives is characterizing the behaviour of a cat as writhing. As he says, the very same movements might be plotted out in great detail in a physical vocabulary. But the two statements could not be substituted one for another. They belong to different conceptual frameworks.

Now one might think that what is missing from the purely physical description of the movement of the cat is the fact that the cat is a conscious animal. And that may be true. Perhaps the concept of writhing is reserved for conscious beings. But the key point here is more modest: writhing is connected as a matter of its meaning with pain and ascriptions of pain can be used to *explain* or *rationalize* certain forms of (subsequent) behaviour. By contrast the purely physical description does not sustain these rational connections.

Winch's conclusion

Winch concludes that it is thus a mistake to think that the social sciences can or indeed should ever aspire to being causal sciences on the explicit assumption here that causes are to be explained nomologically, i.e. as or in terms of natural laws. He goes on to suggest that the kind of intelligibility they deploy is more akin to philosophical understanding.

Now it is worth thinking about this conclusion. A central argument Winch deploys is that, in social science, it is the understanding possessed by the objects of study (human subjects, people) of their own behaviour that plays a key role and that this is not reflected in say the physics of billiard ball motion. The social scientist has to understand social behaviour by understanding it, at least in part, through the understanding that the agents he or she studies have. But why does that point preclude understanding in terms of laws? Why, for example, could not social science explanations fit Hempel's Deductive-Nomological model of explanation and invoke laws?

The answer, as far as Winch and McDowell are concerned is this. The kind of understanding that makes sense of actions is not *codifiable* as a set of laws. It contrasts with the factors that govern billiard ball motion because those factors are codifiable in a Newtonian physics of forces. Now one of the conclusions of Chapter 14 was that explanation in the physical sciences is not fully codifiable and thus it might seem that there are no differences between understanding and explanation, the space of reasons and the realm of law. But a difference remains. However one selects factors from the causal history of an event to explain it relative to one's context of interests, it is natural to think of that history as governed by the tapestry of relevant natural laws. The interaction of all the physical and other natural scientific properties can be codified in natural laws. By contrast, according to McDowell and Winch, there is no equivalent codification of the factors that constitute the space of reasons. This space is not so well regulated.

Furthermore, the social science form of understanding involves an implicit *normative* notion. It turns on matters not correctness and incorrectness. It is not just that most acts of voting take place in a particular way: rather it is a matter of our shared and largely implicit rules of meaning that only specific marks in specific contexts are to count as voting. To vote is to mark a ballot paper *correctly*.

McDowell Winch and psychiatry

It is worth thinking what the consequences would be for psychiatry if McDowell's and Winch's argument were correct. Psychiatry, as we explored in detail in Part II, involves elements that belong to both sides of Winch's distinction. It aims to discover the causal laws governing the operation of the brain and its responses to both surgical and drug intervention. But it also seeks to *make sense* of people's experiences: to characterize their experiences as meaningful responses to psychological trauma, for example. The first sort of intelligibility corresponds to what McDowell would call the realm of law and the second to the space of reasons. Thus if these two highly influential philosophers are right, it would seem that psychiatry is an essentially divided discipline: a mixture rather than a compound of the two elements.

An opposing view: Bolton's claim that meaning is encoded in neural processes

McDowell's and Winch's conclusion has, however, been resisted. Its key assumption is that there is a characteristic difference between rule-governed reasons and law-like causes. Thus the most direct way to attempt to resist it is to argue that there is no simple distinction between reasons and causes: that reason explanation can be a species of causal explanation. This is just the methodology that underlies work in the philosophy of mind (more specifically the philosophy of thought or content) by authors such as Fodor and Millikan. In our field, a recent example is the book by the philosopher/psychologist and psychiatrist team of Derek Bolton and Jonathan Hill called *Mind Meaning and Mental Disorder* (1996). (A good expression of the overall view is Bolton, 1997.)

Rethinking the dichotomy

Bolton's work, to which we have referred several times, is a sustained attempt to undercut the distinction between the space of reasons and the realm of law. The key idea is that the distinction cannot be reconciled by attempting to explain either side in terms of the other: favouring either side of the distinction and attempting to reconstruct the other in its terms. (Ironically, given their substantial disagreement about reasons and causes, this is a metaphilosophical point about dichotomies also shared by McDowell.) Rather, then, than reducing one to the other, Bolton and Hill (1996) argue, we should recognize that neural states have the specific property of encoding meanings. Neural states are thus at one and the same time in both the realm of law and the space of reasons. Or, to put the same point the other way round, with neural states the dichotomy between the realm of law and the space of reasons breaks down.

Bolton's attempt to reconcile reasons and laws

Bolton's conclusion is that a genuine resolution to the tension implicit in psychiatry requires a rethinking of the philosophical battle lines that he characterizes in the following strong terms:

> The split between science and meaning [which twentieth century psychiatry inherited from the *Methodenstreit* through Jaspers] was bound to lead to assault by the one side against the other for excluding it: sympathy with meaning led to outrage against scientific psychiatry, and adherence to science led to contempt for speculations about meaning. This mutual hatred—if that is not too strong a word—was a sign that the split had become intolerable.   (p. 256)

Bolton argues that 'post-modern' accounts of meaning are too restrictive in their dismissiveness of the neurological underpinnings of meaning. And on the other hand, recent views that mature cognitive science would dismiss meanings in favour of causes are similarly restrictive. The latter argue that because causal relations turn on the local physical properties of neural states there is no need to invoke any encoded meanings in those

neural states when accounting for their causal powers. The 'syntax will do for the purpose of causal explanation, and putative encoded meaning drops out as irrelevant.' (p. 258)

Bolton's objection to the argument that syntax if sufficient is that explanation can be broader or narrower depending on what it is that is to be explained.

> If you want to explain, for example, how a rat finds its way to the goal box, the answer will involve positing some state of the rat which encodes information about the route to the box. If you want to explain how it moves its leg, then positing a non-intentional process will do: the muscle contracts because of some physico-chemical processes.   (p. 259)

Thus given the thesis that neural states can encode meanings and the need for broader explanations, there is positive reason to preserve a meaningful element in causal explanations in cognitive science.

How do brain states encode meaning?

What, however, is much less clear, as one of us has argued elsewhere is how it is that the thesis that neural states encode meanings is supposed to be explanatory (Thornton, 1997). The problem is this. The notion of encoding makes perfect sense in some contexts: intentionally translating a sentence in one language into another semantic structure, for example. However, Bolton makes no attempt to cash the notions of encoding out in the context of neural states. In what sense, precisely, do neural states carry meaning? Bolton seems content with arguing that they must do so in order to underpin meaningful but causal explanation of behaviour. But this is just to assume that the reconciliation he requires can in fact be effected. It is not to say *how* it is to be effected.

One way to see this point is to consider what the force is of Bolton's suggestion that the scope of what is to be explained imposes constraints on the nature of the explanation. Consider, not a rat, but the explanation of the route taken by an adult human across a large city such as London. This may involve ascribing to her many different and interacting beliefs about various features of the city. This explanation will contrast with a physiological explanation of the movement of one of her legs. But it is not obvious that both explanations will be causal. The first involves content-laden mental states, but it is a matter of philosophical dispute, (1) about whether that explanation is causal, and (2) about how, if it is, its causal elements and its meaningful elements combine. It may be that the explanation is both causal and rational. But if so, then the properties that underpin the causal and the rational are distinct or come apart (as appears to be the case in Davidson's account, which will be discussed in Part V).

Bolton suggests that the explanation of the rat's behaviour will be both causal and information-involving. However, it may be that these two features also come apart—as seems intuitively more plausible in the human case—rather than being different aspects of the same explanation. As with other long-running debates in philosophy, then, Bolton and Hill's challenging concept of encoded meanings has driven our ideas forward (their book includes detailed treatments of various kinds of psychopathology, for example) without, finally, resolving the deep issues with which the debate is concurred.

Reasons and causes in psychiatric research: George Brown's Approach

Does there need to be a philosophically sophisticated reconciliation?

While much work would have to be done to show that the kind of normative, idealized patterns of the space of reasons could be reduced to the nomological structure of the realm of law, that has not stopped work being done in psychiatry deploying both elements. The following extract is from an empirically based study of depression among women. While the details of the findings are interesting in their own right, it is the implicit connection between meanings or reasons and causal laws that is of interest to us in this chapter.

EXERCISE 8   (30 minutes)

Read the extract from chapter 15 of:

  Brown, G.W. and Harris, T. (1978). *Social Origins of Depression*. London: Tavistock Publications, (extract pp. 233–238)

Link with Reading 15.7

◆ How are reasons and causes assimilated in this paper?

Davidson's and Bolton's different reconciliations

As described above, philosophers such as Derek Bolton attempt to undercut the distinction of kind between the two realms of intelligibility that McDowell (following Sellars) labels the 'space of reasons' and the 'realm of law'. Now McDowell suggests that Davidson's Anomalous Monism (to which we will return in detail in Part V) is an attempt to reconcile reasons and causes by showing that, although the two modes of intelligibility are genuinely distinct, they share a common subject matter. (In fact, reasons are a *subset* of nomic events.) But Bolton's project (shared by philosophers such as Jerry Fodor, Ruth Millikan, and others) is more ambitious: to show how the two modes of intelligibility are in fact continuous. Information-rich causal sciences comprise a bridge between the space of reasons and the realm of law (not that Bolton puts it in these terms). We also saw that there were grounds to be sceptical about whether Bolton has been successful in reconciling reasons and causes in this way.

In their work on depression, Brown and Harris (1978) subscribe implicitly to a different and much more modest reconciliation. Their work thus serves as another attempt to answer the question with which this chapter began: can psychiatry form a unified discipline or is it essentially a disjunction of two different research and diagnostic methods?

The above extract sketches out the results of an inquiry into the aetiology of depression and proposes a causal model (of sorts) as a result. The causal model is given as a kind of flow chart on p. 238. Vulnerability factors lead to ongoing low self-esteem and these together with a precipitating or provoking agent produce depression via a sense of hopelessness or by way of unworked-through grief.

Brown and Harris's reconciliation

As already noted, Brown and Harris' is an influential theory of the aetiology of depression. What is important for this chapter, however, is that the elements of the causal model are themselves charged with meaning. Thus the authors talk, for example, of the importance not of external events but of the way women '*respond* to external events and difficulties' (p. 237, emphasis added), of the '*need* for *meaning*' and, more transparently of all, of the 'loss of important sources of *value*' (p. 244, emphasis added). These are the component parts of their causal model but they depend for their characterization on a different kind of context to a context of causal laws. The required context is that in which events make sense or have meaning: the rational space of reasons. Interestingly, also, it is the patient's own assessment of the meaning or significance of an event which is important (p. 234). It is possible that a major blow will not have a later depressive effect if one thinks that one has, at the time, stood up well to adversity.

Thus Brown and Harris (1978) attempt to mobilize elements that have to be recognized by their role in the space of reasons in a causal model, which itself is part of the realm of law. This results in a hybrid conception of psychiatry in that two sorts of assessment stand in an uneasy relation. Crucially, the presence of meaningful elements threatens the kind of universal laws to which a causal science aspires. If Winch and McDowell are correct and the space of reasons that governs meanings cannot be codified into a set of natural laws then some of the basic elements of Brown and Harris's causal model—meanings—will resist incorporation into universal laws: their characterization will turn on the particular context. Think of when rejection by one's lover might lead to helplessness and sense of worthlessness and when it might lead instead to heroic resignation. What laws will govern this if it turns on the context of meaning and significance that the agent places it in?

Brown and Harris' model illustrates a general issue. We have seen that there is a tradition in the philosophy of science for thinking that where there are causes there are also underlying laws. (We have also seen some conflicting views.) Now laws of nature are generally thought of as something like true universal claims. (Again there are interesting opposing views, but such a view is a benchmark of lawhood.) So the challenge of a hybrid view of the *causes* of depression is to reconcile a convincing account of the sociological detail (in which meanings play an important role) with this aspiration to the universal law-based status for such a discipline. The problem is something like this: the more meanings play a role in the way we understand the origins of a condition, the less immediately obvious is it that a law-based account will be possible of the causes of that condition.

Brown and Harris, it is important to add, are well aware of the difficulties here. Brown has indeed contributed to the wider literature on the difficulties of investigating meanings in the social sciences. And although writing in places in this literature of causal factors, Brown and Harris call their book, not The Social *Causes* of Depression' but 'The Social *Origins* of Depression'. Then again, that their choice of terminology is no coincidence is evident from their description of how they devised their interview protocol: rather than exploring meanings as such, they sought to identify factors that would have a similar meaning for most people most of the time. In other words, Brown and Harris attempted to stabilize meanings, to convert the particularity of individual personal meanings into general causal factors by confining themselves to meanings that, as it were, are (more or less) universal.

As a methodological approach to reconciling reasons (or meanings) with causes, then, this is ingenious and well-grounded theoretically; and Brown and Harris' model, as we have emphasized, has been heuristically powerful (though as with all scientific theories, debate continues about the precise role that some of the factors they identified, notably 'life events', play in depression). As an approach, moreover, it is consistent with those accounts of causation that emphasize (contrary to the traditional model), the context dependence and normativity of causal attributions. Their approach indeed suggests an account of the relationship between reasons and causes in which reasons approximate to causes in inverse proportion to the extent of their context dependence and normativity. In other words, reasons approximate to, or at any rate approximate in *appearance* to, causes where context *inde*-pendent and, crucially, where the interests they express are much the *same* for anyone.

Read, therefore, for interests, 'values, and the limitations of Brown and Harris' approach, ingenious as it is, will be evident from the considerations of Part I. For a key conclusion of Part I was that mental health differs, overall, from bodily health, in the relative *diversity* of the values by which concepts of mental disorder are (partly) defined.

Once, therefore, we move away from the artificially constrained circumstances of a research project and into the more open fabric of day-to-day clinical practice, for Brown and Harris's model to provide aetiological insights it must be combined with direct understanding of the individual meanings given to events by those concerned. Brown and Harris's results certainly guide us over the kind of factors with which we should be concerned in seeking to understand the origins (aetiology) of someone's depression. But, in the terminology of Part II, the understanding this gives is, indeed, *understanding* of personal meanings rather *explanation* in terms of general causal laws.

Reflection on the session and self-test questions

Write down your own reflections on the materials in this session drawing out any points that are particularly significant for you. Then write brief notes about the following:

1. What is the difference between the 'space of reasons' and 'realm of law'? Can they both describe aspects of the real world? What is the connection between these and what is really real and how does this relate to psychiatry?

2. What distinction between the natural and social sciences does Winch outline?

3. How does Bolton attempt to reconcile reasons and laws?

4. How do Brown and Harris attempt a reconciliation?

Reading guide

Note from philosophy of medicine's literature the edited collection, Lindahl and Nordenfelt (ed.) (1984) 'Health, disease, and causal explanations in medicine.' Vol. 16 in Engelhardt and Spicker *Philosophy and Medicine Book Series*.

Hume's philosophy of causation

♦ Hume's philosophy is described in a number of introductions, including Pears' (1990) *Hume's System*, and Stroud's (1977) *Hume*.

♦ Hume's account of causation is discussed in detail in Strawson's (1989) *The Secret Connexion: causation, realism and David Hume*.

More recent philosophy of causation

♦ The state of the philosophical debate about causation is reflected in a set of essays in Sosa and Tooley's (ed.) (1993) *Causation*.

♦ Recent criticism of Lewis's counterfactual account of causation include: Menzies (1996) 'Probabilistic causation and the pre-emption problem'; Menzies (1999) 'Intrinsic versus extrinsic conceptions of causation', in Sankey's (ed.) *Causation and Laws of Nature* (pp. 313–329); and Schaffer (2000) 'Trumping preemption'.

♦ A good example of a probabilistic theory of causation is Mellor's (1991) *Matters of Metaphysics*.

♦ For a valuable edited collection relevant to health care, see Lindahl and Nordenfelt (1984).

The social sciences

- An introduction to the philosophy of the social sciences is Papineau (1987) *For Science in the Social Sciences*.

- McDowell's distinction between the space of reasons and realm of law is criticized in Rorty (1998) *Truth and Progress* (chapter 7).

- Bolton's work is developed in book length form in Bolton and Hill (2004) *Mind Meaning and Mental Disorder*. He develops his ideas further in *Philosophy, Psychiatry, & Psychology* in Bolton's (1997a) 'Encoding of meaning: deconstructing the meaning/causality distinction', with commentaries by Segal (1997) with a response by Bolton (1997b), and by Wiggins and Schwartz (1997) with a further response by Bolton (1997c).

- The hermeneutic aspect of psychiatry is stressed in Schwartz and Wiggins (2004) 'Phenomenological and hermeneutic models: understanding and interpretation in psychiatry', in Radden (ed.) *The Philosophy of Psychiatry*.

References

Bolton, D. (1997a). Encoding of meaning: deconstructing the meaning/causality distinction. (With commentaries by Segal, 1997, with a response by Bolton, 1997b, and by Wiggins and Schwartz, 1997, with a further response by Bolton, 1997c). *Philosophy, Psychiatry, & Psychology*, 4(4): 255–268.

Bolton, D. (1997b). Response to the Commentary by Segal (1997). *Philosophy, Psychiatry, & Psychology*, 4(4): 273–276.

Bolton, D. (1997c). Response to the Commentary by Wiggins and Schwartz (1997). *Philosophy, Psychiatry, & Psychology*, 4(4): 283–284.

Bolton, D. and Hill, J. (1996; 2nd edn 2004). *Mind, Meaning and Mental Disorder: the nature of causal explanation in psychology and psychiatry*. Oxford: Oxford University Press.

Brown, G.W. and Harris, T. (1978). *Social Origins of Depression*. London: Tavistock.

Cartwright, N. (1983). *How the Laws of Physics Lie*. Oxford: Oxford University Press.

Davidson, D. (1995). Laws and cause. *Dialectica*, 49: 263–279.

Goodman, N. (1983). *Fact Fiction and Forecast*. Harvard, MA: Harvard University Press.

Honderich, T. (ed) (1995) *The Oxford Companion to Philosophy*. Oxford: Oxford University Press.

Hume, D. ([1748] 1975). *Enquiries Concerning Human Understanding and Concerning the Principles of Morals*. Oxford: Oxford University Press.

Hume, D. ([1739–40] 1967). *Treatise of Human Nature*. Oxford: Oxford University Press.

Lewis, D. (1973). Causation. *Journal of Philosophy*, 70: 556–567 (Reprinted in *Causation* (ed. E. Sosa and M. Tooley). Oxford: Oxford University Press, 1993, pp. 193–204.)

Lindahl, B.I.B. and Nordenfelt, L. (ed.) (1984). *Health, Disease, and Causal Explanations in Medicine*, Vol. 16. In Philosophy and Medicine Book Series (series ed. H.T. Engelhardt and S.F. Spicker). Dordrecht, The Netherlands/Boston, MA: D. Reidel Publishing Company.

Mackie, J.L. (1993). Causes and conditions. In *Causation* (ed. E. Sosa and M. Tooley). Oxford: Oxford University Press, pp. 33–50.

McDowell, J. (1986). Singular thought and the extent of inner space. In *Subject Thought and Context* (ed. J. McDowell and P. Pettit). Oxford: Oxford University Press, pp. 137–168.

McDowell, J. (1994). *Mind and World*. Cambridge, MA: Harvard University Press.

McDowell, J. (1998). *Mind, Value, and Reality*. Cambridge, MA: Harvard University Press.

Mellor, D.H. (1991). *Matters of Metaphysics*. Cambridge: Cambridge University Press.

Menzies (1996). Probabilistic causation and the pre-emption problem. *Mind*, 105: 85–117.

Menzies (1999). Intrinsic versus extrinsic conceptions of causation. In *Causation and Laws of Nature* (ed. H. Sankey). Kluwer Academic Publishers, pp. 313–329.

Papineau, D. (1986). Laws and accidents. In *Fact, Science and Morality* (ed. G. MacDonald and C. Wright). Oxford: Basil Blackwell, pp. 189–218.

Papineau, D. (1995). Laws. In *Oxford Companion to Philosophy* (ed T. Honderich) Oxford: Oxford University Press.

Papineau, D. (1987). *For Science in the Social Sciences*. Basingstobe Palgrave.

Pears, D. (1990). *Hume's System*. Oxford: Oxford University Press.

Rizzi, D.A. (1994). Causal reasoning and the diagnostic process. *Theoretical Medicine*, 15: 315–333.

Rorty, R. (1998). *Truth and Progress*. Cambridge: Cambridge University Press.

Schaffer, J. (2000). Trumping preemption, *Journal of Philosophy*, 9: 165–181.

Schwartz, M.A. and Wiggins, O.P. (2004). Phenomenological and hermeneutic models: understanding and interpretation in psychiatry. In *The Philosophy of Psychiatry: a companion* (ed. J. Radden). Oxford: Oxford University Press.

Segal, G.M.A. (1997). Encoding of meaning. (Commentary on Bolton, 1997a) *Philosophy, Psychiatry, & Psychology*, 4(4): 269–272.

Sosa, E. and Tooley, M. (ed.) (1993). *Causation*. Oxford: Oxford University Press.

Strawson, G. (1989). *The Secret Connexion: causation, realism and David Hume*. Oxford: Oxford University Press.

Stroud, B. (1977). *Hume*. London: Routledge and Kegan Paul.

Thornton, T. (1997). Reasons causes in philosophy and psychopathology. *Philosophy, Psychiatry, & Psychology*, 4: 307–317.

Van Fraassen, B. (1980). *The Scientific Image*. Oxford: Oxford University Press.

Wiggins, O.P. and Schwartz, M.A. (1997). Encoding of meaning. (Commentary on Bolton, 1997b) *Philosophy, Psychiatry, & Psychology*, 4(4): 277–282.

Winch, P. (1958). *The Idea of a Social Science and its Relation to Philosophy*. London: Routledge.

CHAPTER 16

Knowledge, research, and evidence-based medicine

Chapter contents

Introduction

Like other areas of medicine, treatment and management within psychiatry has increasingly been influenced by the growth of evidence-based medicine or evidence-based practice. A recent review article in the *British Journal of Psychiatry* starts with this observation.

> Clinical effectiveness, evidence-based medicine (EBM) and related terms were the politically correct medical slogans of the 1990s. For many they are 'buzz-words' conveying a modern progressive approach and in some circles it is unwise to express scepticism. Evidence-based medicine is being embraced by all specialities and there has been a strong signal that psychiatry is joining the movement by the introduction in 1998 of a psychiatric journal dedicated to evidence-based practice.
>
> Williams and Garner (2002. p. 8)

The authors go on to express some guarded scepticism about the scope of the application of EBM to psychiatric care. They argue that 'too great an emphasis on evidence-based medicine over-simplifies the complex and interpersonal nature of clinical care' (ibid., p. 8). What is striking is the degree of caution expressed in making this modest criticism. Why is EBM so influential and what limitations might it possess?

At heart, EBM concerns how best to learn from experience. So this chapter will start by looking back to a very influential if abstract way of raising that general question: the eighteenth century Scottish philosopher David Hume's notorious 'problem of induction'. It will then examine two different kinds of response to the challenge raised there. This will help shed light on the nature of knowledge itself and the social character both of the production and transmission of knowledge. In turn this will suggest that while evidence plays a bottom-up role in supporting scientific theories, there is also a 'top-down' influence on evidence by theory. This interplay of factors calls for judgement by scientific practitioners.

One response to the problem of induction is contained within the philosophy of science. It involves methodological routes to scientific conclusions. (One cannot say routes to scientific *knowledge*, however, because Popper's influential falsificationist account denies that positive reasons for belief can be given in the face of Hume's problem.) Examining some of the conflicting responses made within the philosophy of science will highlight the role of the broader scientific context to the evidence that can be offered for scientific medical claims.

The second kind of response is contained within a different branch of philosophy: epistemology. This branch concerns discussion of the nature (logos) of knowledge (episteme). Responses within epistemology to the problem of induction have tended to argue against the problem. That is, they have attempted to show that there is no real problem once the nature of knowledge if properly understood. By examining some responses made within this branch of philosophy we aim to show how knowledge can be a product of social processes and can be socially transmitted.

The connection between practical debates surrounding EBM and the more abstract problem of induction is that EBM concerns the issue of how best to learn from past experience and to apply past findings to future practice. The strategies generally favoured by EBM are based on the use of evidence derived from randomized clinical trials (RCTs). Now it may seem obvious that randomized trials comprise the best method of arriving at clinical findings, and indeed there are good arguments for this method. However, as the chapter will argue, RCTs should not be thought of as ways of simply harvesting available data in accordance with a priori reasoning about proper scientific method. Instead they have their place within a broader context of scientific theory that influences both the methods used for gathering data and the interpretation of that data. Indeed, as Chapter 12 argued, it is misleading to talk of data in this way as though there were a way of gathering facts *before* interpreting them. A proper understanding of the role of evidence in scientific psychiatry suggests the need to balance both bottom-up and top-down interdependence of evidence and theory.

Hume's problem of induction

The first session will explore how Hume's sceptical argument appears to undermine knowledge based on induction. Inductive reasoning—reasoning from particular facts to generalizations—plays a prima facie important role in science (although there are philosophers, as we will see, who deny this). Deductive reasoning—reasoning from general principles to other general principles or to particular facts—is important as well (as in the Hypothetico-Deductive method deployed in diagnosis), but it is induction that appears to be closely tied to the very idea of an *empirical* science. Even on the assumption that induction plays a role in empirical science, it cannot be the whole story, because scientific reasoning also involves the postulation of new and sometimes unobservable entities. But it does play a role in grounding or warranting (as it is sometimes called in philosophy) scientific laws.

Hume's problem of induction is a direct sceptical attack on the justification of this sort of reasoning. He argues in effect that induction can only be justified by induction itself and that that is question-begging.

Induction and the philosophy of science

Session two will then examine one strand of thinking in the philosophy of science, particularly associated with the late Sir Karl Popper, which starts with an assumption that inductive inferences cannot support knowledge claims and thus that science should be construed as a systematic structure of conjecture and *refutation*. The positive idea of evidence supporting theories is replaced by an emphasis on the use of evidence to reject false theories. This turns on the simple idea that while no finite amount of confirming instances can entail the truth of a universal generalization, a single counter-instance can entail that it is false. In fact, however, this simple thought cannot yield the precise methodology that it might, at first, suggest. For reasons that build on the discussion of the theory dependence of observation of Chapter 12, even refutation is more difficult than it might seem.

Responding to these difficulties, another famous figure in modern philosophy of science, Imre Lakatos, developed falsificationism into a sophisticated model of a historically extended process of developing theories within competing research programmes. But as Lakatos admits, this does not yield a *prescriptive* methodology.

Partly as a response, historians and sociologists of science, including most famously Thomas Kuhn argued in the 1970s that there were no applicable trans-historical patterns of scientific rationality and that understanding of scientific practice should instead concern itself with the local perspective on what was deemed rational by the practitioners of science themselves. Most interestingly, perhaps, they have the courage of their conviction and also say that this is the perspective which should be applied to the sociology of science.

But, whatever their efficacy in resolving the problem of induction, what these discussions do help to show is that there is more to theory testing than simply gathering data and forming inductions on the basis of it. Evidence is interpreted in the light of background theories that are supported by, but also support, evidential claims.

Induction and epistemology

While, within the philosophy of science, the response to the problem of induction has focused on methodological strategies, philosophical epistemology has concentrated instead on rethinking the assumptions about knowledge that make induction appear problematic. One such assumption is that knowledge is self-intimating: that when one knows something, one knows that one knows it. Another is that knowledge requires that the knowing subject can supply a justification for their knowledge claims. Session 3 will examine the success that more recent work in epistemology has had in resolving the problem of induction.

Although the focus will be responses to the problem of induction Session 3 will highlight the dependence of individual inquirers or scientists on other people in acquiring knowledge. Knowledge, in the phrase of the philosopher the late Gareth Evans rubs off on other people 'like an infectious disease'.

In fact, what should become clearer during the course of this chapter is that there is something to be said for both approaches: epistemological approaches show how Hume's scepticism can be defused by adopting a more realistic picture of knowledge while the philosophy and sociology of science show the kind of practical arguments that count in actually selecting theories.

Evidence-based medicine

Session 4 will examine the consequences of these discussions for the role of evidence in medicine. Starting with an examination of some of the assumptions underlying clinical trials, the final session will look at recent emphasis on EBM and the nature of

the evidence in question and the strengths and weaknesses of this approach in light of advances in our understanding of the nature of science provoked by Hume's original problem. It will also summarize how issues raised throughout this part have an impact on a better understanding of EBM. Underlying the simple idea that medical practice should be based on the best available evidence is the real complexity, and the element of uncodifiable scientific judgement, in the generation of such evidence.

Plan of the chapter

* *Session 1* puts discussion of EBM into the context of the philosophical origins of the problem of induction in Hume's work.

* *Session 2* charts responses to Hume's problem drawn from the philosophy and sociology of science. Such responses suggest a number of rival models of scientific research and rationality, which emphasize the top-down influence of theory on evidence as well as more expected bottom-up dependence of theory on evidence.

* *Session 3* sets out some responses to the problem of induction drawn from philosophical epistemology. These help suggest a connection between a more realistic contemporary understanding of the nature of knowledge and its social transmission.

* *Session 4* looks to Mill's methods as a way of examining the origins of research evidence in controlled trials and thus the ineliminable role of good judgement in assessing evidence.

But before starting that detailed analysis we will turn to a positive expression of the virtues of EBM for psychiatry.

Session 1 Evidence-based medicine, Hume, and the problem of induction

EXERCISE 1	(30 minutes)

Read the whole of the short paper

Geddes, J.R. and Harrison, P.J. (1997). Closing the gap between research and practice. *British Journal of Psychiatry*, 171: 220–225

Link with Reading 16.1

* What is the purpose and rationale for EBM in mental health care?

The aim of evidence-based medicine

Geddes and Harrison (1997) present a very clear account of the motivation for adopting EBM. There is, they argue, a 'knowledge gap' between the accurate information generally employed by clinicians and the decisions that they make partly on the basis of it. In other words, clinical decisions are underdetermined by the readily available (pre-EBM) evidence. This is not to say that the decisions are therefore made arbitrarily. The gap is instead filled by other factors: 'the conceptual aetiological school to which we subscribe' and 'the combination of experience and habits which we accumulate' (p. 220). However, these factors vary from clinician to clinician, which thus undermines the inter-rater reliability of diagnosis and treatment. Nor are they empirically tested guides. Hence, instead, the need for EBM to guide diagnosis and treatment.

Evidence-based medicine and randomized clinical trials

'EBM is the "conscientious, explicit and judicious use of the current best evidence in making decisions about the care of individual patients" ' (p. 220) The kind of evidence in question is that provided through clinical trials. But there are issues about how to assess or rank conflicting evidence. The paper asserts that RCTs, or better still systematic reviews of RCTs, are the most reliable study design for the evaluation of treatments' (p. 221). But because such trials are not always available, Geddes and Harrison (1997), following widely accepted principles of EBM (see, e.g. Sackett *et al.*, 2000), suggest that there is a hierarchy of kinds of evidence that can also be pressed into service. It is as follows:

1a. Evidence from a meta-analysis of RCTs

1b. Evidence from at least one RCT

2a. Evidence from at least one controlled study without randomization

2b. Evidence from at least one other quasi-experimental study

3. Evidence from non-experimental descriptive studies, such as comparative studies, correlation studies and case–control studies

4. Evidence from expert committee reports, or opinions and/or clinical experience of respected authorities.

Complexities in the use of evidence-based medicine

It is worth noting that despite the presentation of this hierarchy of forms of evidence, the whole tenor of the paper is that EBM is not a mechanical procedure that removes the need for intellectual effort on the part of the clinician. To the contrary, he or she must be able to search out sources of evidence, assess their quality or reliability, assess their relevance to the clinical case at hand, and interpret what conclusions should be drawn from the evidence. But despite this emphasis, there still remains a danger that the concentration within EBM on RCTs disguises some of the complexities of scientific method discussed so far. An awareness of these helps to immunize against the assumption that things are as clear-cut as less nuanced accounts of EBM may sometimes seem to suggest.

The origins of the problem of induction: David Hume

We will start with Hume's (1975) sceptical attack on the foundations of induction, although Hume himself does not use that term. It is contained in a section that precedes his discussion of causation, which was the subject of Chapter 15, but it is related. As we will see, Hume suggests that knowledge can be divided into either demonstrative relations of ideas or matters of fact. The latter are established on the basis of causal relations that are in turn founded on experience (by contrast with deductive demonstration). He is then concerned to establish their credentials for establishing matters of fact (causal relations) through experience.

EXERCISE 2 (15 minutes)

Read the extract from

Hume, D. ([1748]1975). *Enquiries Concerning Human Understanding and Concerning the Principles of Morals*. Oxford: Oxford University Press, section iv (extract pp. 37–38)

Link with reading 16.2

◆ What is the kernel of Hume's sceptical argument?

Hume's fork

Hume starts the section from which this extract is taken with the bold claim that all the objects of human reason can be divided between relations of ideas and matters of fact. This distinction, generally known as 'Hume's Fork' sets up the contrast that will be important between the status of knowledge claims that can be arrived at through deductive demonstration and those for which a merely inductive warrant can be provided.

It is worth noting briefly two features that characterize the distinction.

1. Truths that comprise relations of ideas do not depend on, or presuppose, any existence claims. Thus the claim that the square of the hypotenuse is equal to the sum of the squares of the other two sides is a truth that is independent of whether there are any right-angled triangles in the universe.

2. The negation of truths that comprise relations of ideas produces claims that could not have been true and cannot be 'distinctly conceived by the mind'. By contrast, the negation of matters of fact could have been true and thus can be so conceived. This amounts to saying that relations of ideas express necessary rather than just contingent truths (see also Chapter 5).

Three kinds of truth

A distinction of this sort has been influential throughout empiricist philosophy. Consider the three binary distinctions:

1. epistemological: a priori versus a posteriori

2. metaphysical: necessary versus contingent

3. semantic: analytic versus synthetic.

One appealing assumption has been that these different ways of sorting truths all sort them into the same sets. Thus all truths that can be known a priori (that is, without experience) are necessarily true and their truth is fixed by the concepts used to frame them (they are analytically true in virtue of their meaning). Equally, all truths that require experience to be known, and are thus a posteriori, are also contingent and synthetic (i.e. their truth requires both a contribution from their meaning and from the world).

There are also prima facie plausible arguments for the alignment of these distinctions. For example, if a truth is a priori then one does not need to know which possible world one inhabits in order to know its truth. (Experience teaches us which of the many possible worlds we actually live in.) This suggests in turn that it must be a necessary truth (one that holds in *all* possible worlds). Furthermore it seems plausible that it must be analytic, because its truth clearly does not require a worldly contribution and thus must be fixed entirely by its meaning.

Despite these arguments, the neat alignment of truths has also come under attack. The Prussian philosopher Immanuel Kant (1724–1804) argued that there were synthetic truths which could be known a priori including mathematics. In this century, the American philosopher W.V.O. Quine (1908–2000) attacked the assumption that the distinctions are well founded clear-cut distinctions of kind and the logician Saul Kripke (1940–) argued that some a posteriori truths are, nevertheless, necessary (such as that water is H_2O). We will return to the consequences of Kripke's arguments in Part V. For now all that matters is noting that drawing the distinction allows Hume to focus the issue of the foundations of matters of fact. (If the distinctions do not align or are not even firm this will not solve the general problem Hume raises for justifying empirical knowledge. It merely changes the form it takes because there ceases to be a clear contrast between fallible a posteriori reasoning and the supposedly certain a priori and deductive reasoning.)

Knowledge by induction versus knowledge through the testimony of the senses

Having drawn the distinction between relations of ideas and matters of fact, Hume (1975) then focuses his attention on the status of knowledge of matters of fact. In fact, the focus is narrower still: on knowledge of what lies 'beyond the present testimony of our senses, or the record of our memory' (p. 26). Thus he does not here investigate the status of direct observational knowledge of particular matters of fact—knowledge made available by my opening our eyes to the world—or even our memory of such particular facts. On the one hand, this sets up an implicit contrast between observation and induction. The latter appears less reliable than the former. And indeed, as we will see later, induction in general will never have a stronger justification than observation in general because inductive inferences take observations as their premises. On further reflection, however, the concepts used to frame observation reports are typically laden with theory (see Chapter 12). They can in individual cases thus be overturned on the basis of enough inductive counter-evidence.

Hume (1975) suggests that such reasoning is founded on the relation of cause and effect. It is this relation that underpins reasoning beyond our direct observations and binds unobserved facts to observed facts. 'Were there nothing to bind them together, the inference would be entirely precarious.' (p. 27). However, Hume goes on to question what grounds our knowledge of cause–effect relations. He argues that this cannot be a piece of a priori reasoning and is instead based on our experience. Hume argues both that cause–effect relations concern separate events and thus no amount of inspection of the cause-event can yield knowledge of what effect it will lead to and also that the negation of cause–effect relations does not produce any logical contradiction or a state of affairs that cannot be distinctly conceived. Having cleared the ground in this way, Hume goes on to discuss how experience rather than a priori demonstration can ground our knowledge of cause–effect relations.

Hume's problem of induction

Section iv, part II contains the sceptical discussion of induction. Hume begins by asking, on the assumption (for which he has just argued) that the foundation of our knowledge of matters of fact (aside from the case of direct perception) is knowledge of cause–effect relations, what underpins that relation? His answer is experience. This seems like a good answer and in everyday contexts would mark the end point of inquiry. But Hume, like a good philosopher, then asks a further question: 'what is the foundation of all conclusions from experience?' (p. 32). He suggests that he will argue that our knowledge of matters of fact is not founded on *reasoning* from past experience.

Taking as his example the connection between the sensible or observational properties of bread and its 'secret power' to provide nourishment, Hume argues that experience can play only a direct role in establishing that there has been such a connection in particular cases in the past, but questions how experience can underpin the extension of a more general connection 'to future times, and to other objects'.

> These two propositions are far from being the same, I have found that such an object has always been attended with such an effect, and I foresee, that other objects, which are, in appearance similar, will be attended with similar effects. I shall allow, if you please, that the one proposition may justly be inferred from the other: I know, in fact, that it always is inferred. But if you insist that the inference is made by a chain of reasoning, I desire you to produce that reasoning.   (p. 34)

Hume goes on to argue that inductive inferences cannot be demonstrative because their negations make good sense. The course of nature could (logically possibly) change. Thus a deductive defence of induction appears to be unconvincing because too strong. But on the other hand inductive defences of induction also appear hopeless because they are circular. Hume suggests that empirical reasoning:

> proceed[s] upon the supposition that the future will be conformable to the past. To endeavour, therefore, the proof of this

last supposition by probable arguments, or arguments regarding existence [ie inductive arguments about matters of fact], must be evidently going in a circle, and taking that for granted, which is the very point in question.   (pp. 35–36).

The problem in a nutshell

So stepping back from the details of Hume's argument we can set out the problem as follows. Suppose that the premiss is that all bread previously tested has been nourishing and the conclusion is that all future bread will be nourishing. Hume's challenge is to explain what form of inference justifies the conclusion.

The natural suggestion is that experience grounds the *rule* of inference as well as the *premiss* (in this case that all bread previous tested has been nourishing). It does this because of the more general piece of direct experiential knowledge that correlations between (in this case) sensible qualities and secret powers have held over time. This general experiential finding is then used to ground the inference from past to future in the specific bread case. But as Hume points out: using experience to ground the rule itself presupposes that very rule as an inference. Why should the fact that such correlations have held in the past support the claim that they will hold in the future unless an inductive inference is justified here as well?

Hume (1975) says:

When a man says, I have found, in all past instances, such sensible qualities conjoined with such secret powers: And when he says, Similar sensible qualities will always be conjoined with similar secret powers, he is not guilty of a tautology, nor are these propositions in any respect the same. You say that the one proposition is an inference from the other. But you must confess that the inference is not intuitive; neither is it demonstrative: Of what nature is it then? To say it is experimental, is begging the question. For all inferences from experience suppose, as their foundation, that the future will resemble the past . . . It is impossible, therefore, that any arguments from experience can prove this resemblance of the past to the future; since all these arguments are founded on the supposition of that resemblance.   (pp. 36–37).

Inductive justification of induction

This passage suggests the following alternatives. For experience to yield a principle that will underpin reasoning from observed to unobserved cases we need an argument of the following sort.

- Premiss 1: Correlations have held in the past (observed cases)
- Conclusion: Correlations will hold in the future (unobserved cases)

Now by itself this argument is neither demonstrative nor deductive (it is not a valid argument). If experience of the stability of past correlations is to warrant the claim that they will continue to be stable, it does this in virtue of an *inductive* inference. But that was the very rule that this argument was supposed to justify rather than presuppose.

Deductive justification of induction

On the other hand, Hume suggests that such arguments presuppose that the future will resemble the past. Now putting aside the details of how it resembles it, if this were true, inductive arguments would be successful. But how is this fact supposed to help justify those arguments? The obvious answer is that if this is introduced as a second premiss, the argument becomes a valid demonstrative argument.

- Premiss 1: Correlations have held in the past (observed cases)
- Premiss 2: The future resembles the past (unobserved resemble observed cases)
- Conclusion: Correlations will hold in the future (unobserved cases)

But if it is to underwrite a true conclusion, this valid argument requires the truth of the second premiss, which is, as Hume points out, not a necessary truth or a truth that can be arrived at demonstratively. It requires a further inductive argument to justify it. So in either case, there appears to be no non-circular argument for inductive reasoning from experience.

> **EXERCISE 3**   (15 minutes)
>
> Take some time to think through the issues raised by Hume's argument. What are we to make of broadly Humean sceptical arguments directed at inductive reasoning? Hume appears to show that a substantial fraction of our knowledge claims about empirical matters are unjustified. But does this matter? Is it merely a game, a piece of word play?

Knowledge and justification

Hume's (1975) argument suggests the following worry. If we make a knowledge claim about unobserved events on the basis of observed events we open ourselves up to the challenge of providing grounds. Now there are first and second moves available to us. We can justify our claim about the *unobserved* by citing our experience of the *observed*. Hume can then challenge us to say how exactly experience of what has been *observed* has a bearing on what has so far *not been observed*. We can then say (as our second justificatory move) that we have more general experience (i.e. we have *observed* the following) that *observed* matters have always (in the past) been a good guide to initially *unobserved* but subsequently observed matters.

Prior to reading Hume this looks to discharge the burden of providing grounds for our original claim. However, Hume shows that this second justificatory claim only works if we can take it for granted that past experience is a good guide to future experience, or that what is observed is a good guide to what is unobserved, and that is just what he is challenging us to justify. At this point we have apparently no further arguments to make and the chain of justifications comes unstitched backwards from here. If we cannot justify induction in general, we cannot justify it in the particular case at hand. Thus we cannot say what the relevance of our past experience is to our claim about the unobserved and thus we cannot justify that supposed knowledge claim. Thus we must admit that we do not know it despite our pre-philosophical inclinations.

The 'justified true belief' analysis of knowledge

This way of setting out the virulence of Humean scepticism reveals a hidden assumption that will be questioned later in the chapter: in order to know something it appears that we must either *know* that we know it or at least be *able* to know that we know it. Why is this at all plausible as an assumption? The answer is that at first sight it seems to be implicit in our concept of knowledge.

We distinguish between knowledge and mere true belief. If someone knows something it is not enough that they have true beliefs, something else needs to be added. (Note that truth and belief both appear to be *necessary* features of knowledge. One cannot know something that one does not believe. And one cannot know something falsely, although one can *think* one knows it: a case of merely *believing* falsely.)

Suppose, to use a well known example, I claim to know that the name of the President of the United States starts with a 'C' and that this is in fact true (as it was when the President was called 'Clinton'). Now suppose my reason for believing this is that I think his name is 'Churchill'. Although I have a true belief (the President's name does, at the time considered, start with a 'C'), it is not *knowledge* because it is held for the wrong reason. In this case the supporting belief is false and that is what undermines the first knowledge claim.

But knowledge claims can also be undone by faulty reasons even when the reasons involve true beliefs. Suppose I correctly believe that the President's name is Clinton but I believe this because, on the night of his election, a superstitious supporter of an opposing candidate who did not want to prejudice the final result declared to me that Clinton had already won. As a result, I believe that the name of the President of the United States starts with a 'C' and this is in fact true. And I believe it because I believe that his name is 'Clinton'. That is the justification, and it is a true belief. But it does not justify the first belief because I have *arrived at it* for the wrong reason: I would have believed it even if Clinton had not eventually won the election. So it is not itself justified.

Knowing that one knows

This sort of reasoning suggests that if knowledge is a belief that is true, and in addition justified, then that justification must be a belief (which is had or is available to be had by the subject of the first belief), which must itself both be true and be justified. This leads to the initially attractive assumption that if knowledge is justified true belief—a view that dates back to Plato—then the justification must also be known (it must be a justified true belief). In that case, however, its justification will also have to be known. This leads to a regress. And it is this regress that feeds Humean scepticism because of his argument that one cannot provide an independent justification for induction. If one cannot do that—at the metalevel—then one cannot justify the claim that experience justifies ground level claims about future sunrises and the nourishing value of bread because knowledge at that level requires in addition that one knows that one knows. (The importance of this assumption for Hume will become clearer in the third session where it will be questioned.)

The point of philosophical scepticism

So the problem can be put like this. Some fairly low level and intuitive reasoning about knowledge leads us to believe that it requires justification and that justifications themselves have to pass muster. But an equally simple argument from Hume seems to show that inductive knowledge cannot pass this test. Thus it should not be counted as knowledge. Because the arguments concerned are so simple minded but concern something as central to us as the concept of knowledge, it is not convincing simply to dismiss this as a mere word game. If the arguments are wrong, it should be possible to show where they go wrong. If not, however, the only other conclusion is that paradoxically our reasoning itself leads to an unpalatable result. (Hume's own response here was precisely to play down the role of reason in general: to conclude that sceptical reasoning showed the limitations of reasoning.)

Now one response to any case of philosophical scepticism is to refuse to take its conclusion seriously in the sense of taking it to be true. Typically, a key feature of philosophical scepticism is that such conclusions are so radical that they cannot be accepted in practice in daily life—we could not put one step in front of the other if the past were not, or could not be assumed to be, for practical purposes, a guide to the future. But the point of philosophical scepticism is rather to force us to think more critically about such everyday assumptions of daily life. Philosophical scepticism is in this respect a kind of conceptual probe or microscope that helps us to open up and gain a more critical understanding of these everyday assumptions.

In Part I, we saw how the sceptical attacks of Szasz and others on the concept of mental illness led to a deeper understanding of that concept with important consequences for research and practice in mental health. Hume's 'problem of induction', similarly, has led to a deeper understanding of what is involved in relying on knowledge derived from experience (as in EBM). It is precisely, therefore, *because* the consequences of Hume's sceptical attack on induction are so radical that we should take his arguments seriously.

One way of taking Hume's arguments seriously is to question whether, if his conclusion is so radical, there must be something wrong with the premises that lead to it. That is the approach that will be taken in the third session on epistemological approaches. But the next session will look instead at approaches to taking Hume's arguments seriously in the philosophy of science, approaches which, as we noted in the introduction to this chapter, are broadly methodological rather than epistemological in character.

Session 2 Philosophy of science responses to the problem of induction

Overview of the session

This session will discuss four responses from the philosophy of science that can be seen, in part, as responses to Hume's problem of induction. The first two are related. Both Sir Karl Popper (1902–94) and Imre Lakatos (1922–74) support forms of falsificationism. This is a position in the philosophy of science developed by Popper and then redeveloped (not entirely to the satisfaction of Popper) by Lakatos. It concentrates *not* on the positive use of evidence to support (by induction) generalizations and theories but rather on the refutation or falsification of theories by negative or disconfirming evidence. The underlying idea here is not so much to solve the problem of induction (despite what Popper says in the first case) but to bypass it. But it also aims to preserve a *rational* methodology for empirical science even without induction. The third and fourth responses differ in two respects. First, they argue that no such abstract rational methodology can be imposed by philosophical inquiry and instead argue that scientific method has to be investigated by local historical or sociological investigation. Secondly, however, they suggest that there is something much closer to an inductive practice albeit one that has to be investigated in a much more piecemeal empirical way.

What each of these four responses have in common is that they concern the attempt to characterize the general features of scientific method; they seek to chart the general relation between successive theories and evidence, to show how decisions are made as to which is the best or the better theory without concentrating on an unproblematic connection between evidence and a single theory.

As we will see in Session 3, this contrasts with responses that have been made to the problem of induction in the branch of philosophy called 'epistemology'. There, rather than attempting to characterize the relation between successive theories, philosophers have concentrated instead on the very idea or concept of knowledge and then applied their conclusions to the problem of whether inductive support can exist between evidence and theory.

In fact, as we anticipated in the introduction to this chapter, there is something to be said for both approaches. The readings in this session highlight the sort of structure presupposed by theory testing and thus undermine a naively inductivist picture of mere data gathering. To this extent, therefore, they deepen our understanding of how science actually works (we return to the implications of this for EBM at the end of this chapter). However, the arguments about scientific method in this session do nothing to disarm scepticism about induction as such. That is the goal of Session 3, which will in turn shed light on the nature of knowledge itself.

Falsificationism

The first response is by Sir Karl Popper, the philosopher of science (associated with although not a member of the Vienna Circle) who first developed falsificationism. We have already introduced Popper's work in Chapter 11. Perhaps the clearest statement of how falsificationism impacts on induction is given in: 'Conjectural knowledge: my solution to the problem of induction' in his *Objective Knowledge* (1972, chapter 1, pp. 1–31).

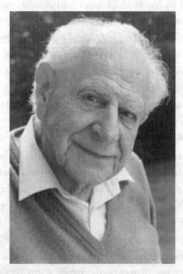

Fig. 16.1 Karl Popper

Induction and scientific rationality

Popper begins 'Conjectural knowledge' by qualifying how the problem of induction should be construed. He rejects both its key presuppositions: that the future resembles the past (unless this is construed so flexibly as to be vacuous), and that there are inductive inferences to be justified. He suggests that Hume responds to two different problems with two different and clashing answers. One concerns a logical problem of whether we are justified in reasoning from observed to unobserved instances. Hume responds that we are not. The other is the psychological problem of why we nevertheless have confidence in this form of reasoning. Hume's response to this is to invoke custom or habit. This response, Popper suggests, makes Hume an *irrationalist*. Popper flags early in the paper that his response, unlike Hume's, will not lead to a lack of rationality in scientific method.

Falsification not confirmation

The route to Popper's resolution of the problem of induction is to make a subtle change in the question that he thinks needs a positive answer. Instead of asking whether empirical reasons can be given to show that a universal theory (i.e. something that goes beyond observed facts) is true, one should ask whether such reasons can be given to show whether a theory is true *or false*. Theories can sometimes be shown to be false, he argues, and this is important because in general the question is asked within the context of science when there is more than one competing theory in play. He goes on to emphasize that this implies that 'we must regard all laws and theories as hypothetical or conjectural; that is, as guesses' (p. 9) and, later in the chapter, to suggest that his response remains within the domain of deduction rather than induction (p. 12).

This last point turns on a key distinction for falsification (more so on the more simple-minded versions; less so for more sophisticated versions as we will see). '[F]rom the point of view of deductive logic there is an asymmetry between verification and falsification by experience' (p. 12). The asymmetry is in the fact that, in principle, even a single observation can refute a universal claim—its falsity can be *deduced*—but no finite amount of observations can logically confirm such a claim. For this reason Popper stresses the role of severe tests of theories, or crucial experiments designed to disprove them. Nevertheless, as he points out later, this process of elimination of false theories by falsification is not a method of establishing truth because 'the number of *possibly* true theories remains infinite' (p. 15).

Given this focus on the negative side of theory testing, Popper emphasizes the intellectual virtue of theories that are, perhaps surprisingly, most easily falsified. Such theories, the boldest and most specific conjectures, are also the most informative and least vacuous. The reason for this is that they are true in the smallest number of possible worlds and thus if true, would more precisely specify the nature of the actual world. More probable theories are less informative because they rule out fewer alternative ways the world might be.

Practical theory choice

These logical conclusions leave open, however, the practical consequences for the guidance of action through beliefs arrived at by induction. Popper distinguishes between two such pragmatic issues:

- Pr1 Upon which theory should we *rely* for practical action, from a rational point of view?
- Pr2 Which theory should we *prefer* for practical action, from a rational point of view? (p. 21, emphases added)

He suggests as an answer to the first, that we should not rely on any theory 'for no theory has been shown to be true, or can be shown to be true' (p. 21). This reflects the fact that Popper does not so much solve the problem of induction—thus justifying inductive inferences—as side-step it. But this leaves no positive relation of support between evidence and theory and thus nothing to underpin reliance on theories.

Nevertheless, Popper argues that, while it is not rational actually to *rely* on any theory, it is entirely rational to *prefer* the best tested theories: theories that have so far survived rigorous attempts to falsify them. This last point is sensible advice from our normal induction-trusting perspective. It is consistent with the place of rigorously conducted research at the top of the evidence hierarchy in EBM (p. 436 above, this chapter). A study in which the researchers are 'blind' as to test and control results is more likely to detect a false theory (e.g. that a new medication is more effective than an established treatment) than a study in which the researchers know which is which and hence may (consciously or unconsciously) bias the results in favour of the theory they believe to be true. In this respect, then, Popper's observations on scientific methodology, are surely right. Science does proceed more by falsification than by confirmation. This is one powerful way in which we may genuinely learn from experience rather than being misled by our expectations.

It is worth asking, however, why, from the point of view of a purely falsificationist perspective, is it better to prefer a theory that has been severely tested and survived than any other theory that would have passed those tests? There will, after all, be an infinite number of these. Some can be generated by simply conjoining, with a previous theory, some additional claims about the future. Furthermore, this preference for specific theories can never amount to a justified reliance on them given the anti-inductivist stance of falsificationism. But how plausible an account of either science or our daily life is that? We do not merely *guess* that the roof will not collapse in the next few minutes. Much of clinical practice, for example, rests on lengthy trials where success in replication of results is as important as the elimination of false hypotheses. A Popperian can only explain the negative results of trials—showing that particular treatments do not work and can thus be rejected—but cannot offer an explanation of why repeated successful results should be taken as positive support for efficacy. On a strict falsificationist view of the matter, that is irrational.

Conjecture and refutation

As we discussed in Chapter 11, at the heart of falsificationism is the idea of conjecture and refutation. There are never *good reasons* to adopt or hold a theory. Reason works only negatively: pruning away at the bold conjectures that scientists advance. Once falsified by disconfirming evidence, theories should be rejected.

But as Popper himself realized things are more complicated than that in actual scientific practice. The observations that are to serve as tests of theories are themselves laden with theory. Successful theories often face disconfirming anomalies that take time to explain away. Theories are articulated within competing broader explanatory stances or programmes.

Consider that second point: theories are often born refuted but are not rejected for that reason. This is an important point in medical research. It is often very difficult to establish connections such as that between smoking and cancer. From a naïve falsificationist perspective a negative study falsifies or refutes a putative connection. However, that is not how good medical science progresses. Such results might themselves be scientific mistakes in hindsight. To be a realistic model of scientific practice, the falsificationist model of conjecture and refutation has to be augmented.

Lakatosian falsificationism

Such augmentation was provided in the work of the Hungarian philosopher of science, Imre Lakatos. Lakatos' model of scientific research programmes has been widely influential both in its own right and as an exemplar of the power of studying the history and philosophy of science as a combined discipline. The philosophical model was taken to provide the structure for a rational reconstruction of the history of science, demonstrating the rational methodology of science at play.

The key statement of Lakatos' position is given in his paper 'Falsificationism and the methodology of scientific research programmes' (Lakatos, 1970).

Three theories that presuppose hard data

Lakatos begins his discussion with three ways of understanding the relation of theory and evidence: justificationism, probabilism, and dogmatic falsificationism. These three are similar in their commitment to a class of hard data that can be used in one way or another as the basis for theories. In the first and second, observations are used either to confirm the theory (in the first) or at least to make the theory more probable (in the second). Dogmatic falsificationism is based on the logical point that Popper raised: that a no finite number of individual facts can logically or demonstratively confirm a universal claim (such as a statement of theory), but, in principle, a single fact can refute a universal claim. Thus falsification proposes that the purpose of evidence in theory testing is negative: the falsification by refutation of theories so as to eliminate false theories.

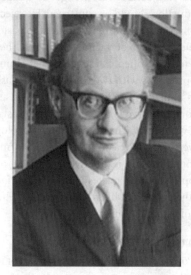

Fig. 16.2 Imre Lakatos

But are there any hard data?

But as Lakatos goes on to argue, this picture is too simplistic to characterize real science. The main problem is that rather than comprising an infallible class of foundational claims, observational claims are themselves fallible and theoretically charged, as we saw in Chapter 12. Lakatos argues for this by denying two claims that he suggests are implicit in dogmatic falsificationism:

1. there is a natural and psychological distinction between theoretical claims and observational claims, and

2. observational claims must be true.

His argument against (1) recapitulates some of the arguments from Chapter 12: observational claims presuppose the truth of theories about observational aids or psychology.

Can experience justify an observation statement?

The argument to deny the second claim is less convincing. The conclusion is that no factual proposition can ever be *proved* from an experiment. Lakatos's argument for it runs as follows: 'propositions can only be derived from other propositions, they cannot be derived from facts: one cannot prove statements from experiences—"no more than by thumping the table" ' (p. 99).

The underlying idea here is that if one wishes to prove a proposition, only other propositions have the right logical properties to stand in justificatory (or for that matter contradictory) relations to it. Events, such as a table being thumped, do not and neither, Lakatos suggests, do experiences. From this Lakatos concludes that factual propositions cannot be proved from an experiment (and neither could they be disproved).

The problem with such a line of reasoning is that it makes the contribution of experience to the justification of our beliefs completely mysterious. What is the point of our opening our eyes in the first place? The problem of explaining how experience can have a *rational* impact on our beliefs is the key issue in McDowell's *Mind and World* (1994), discussed in Chapter 12. McDowell, you will recall, argues that our conceptual abilities are always passively drawn into play in even the most basic cases of experience. Thus experiences can have the right logical 'shape' to confirm or undermine beliefs because they are always already conceptualized. But lacking any such account of how experience can rationally constrain beliefs, Lakatos can say the right thing about observation claims—that they are fallible—but for the wrong reason: namely that he can say nothing sensible about the *groundings* of observation claims in experience.

One can, however, deploy a different argument to Lakatos's conclusion based on his first point. If observational claims presuppose the truth of theories, and if the only evidence for theories are observational claims, then there can be no definitive test either of theory or of observational statements. The support for both will be provisional.

Lakatos goes on to argue that even if these objections to a distinction between theory and observation were not true, dogmatic falsificationism would still fail to take account of a different connection, which makes falsification much less clear-cut than simple examples (like those provided by Popper) suggest.

EXERCISE 5   (20 minutes)

Look at the extract below from

Lakatos, I. (1970). Falsification and the methodology of scientific research programmes. In *Criticism and the Growth of Knowledge* (ed. I. Lakatos and A. Musgrave). Cambridge: Cambridge University Press, pp. 91–195 (extract pp. 100–101)

Link with Reading 16.4

Here Lakatos tells a story about an imaginary 'misbehaving' planet and how scientists respond to it.

♦ What general conclusions can be drawn from the story?

A radical conclusion for refutation

Lakatos argues that the observed planetary 'misbehaviour' might be taken as a refutation of the existing Newtonian celestial mechanics but on the other hand it might be taken as evidence of the perturbing effect of another planet. Such a hypothesis suggests possible crucial observations of the postulated planet concerned. But if no such planet is observed, this still need not refute the theory that there is such a planet (itself deployed to defend existing celestial mechanics), which can in turn be resisted by

deploying the further hypothesis that there is opaque intervening material. And so on ad infinitum. In other words, *no apparently falsifying evidence is ever decisive*. Lakatos concludes that: 'Scientific theories are not only equally unprovable, and equally improbable, but they are also equally undisprovable.' (p. 103).

Rejecting dogmatic falsificationism, Lakatos goes on to consider two further revisions of falsificationism each of which provides insights into the nature of scientific methodology, though neither of which, he argues, sufficiently describes it. The two further versions are:

♦ Naive methodological falsificationism: this introduces the idea that observations and theory have to be considered holistically in science, i.e. as working together in groups rather than as isolated observation theory pairs.

♦ Sophisticated methodological falsificationism: the key idea here is of what Lakatos calls a 'research programme', i.e. groups of observations and theories operating over an extended period of time.

We will look briefly at each of these. Interestingly, Lakatos attributes all three versions of falsificationism (dogmatic, naive methodological, and sophisticated methodological) to Popper. His conclusion is that sophisticated methodological falsificationism gives the 'best fit' to what goes on in science. This conclusion, however, as we will see has been challenged by both historians and sociologists of science.

Naive methodological falsificationism...

Rejecting dogmatic falsificationism, Lakatos introduces the second of three pictures of science he discusses: naive methodological falsificationism. Lakatos attributes this position to some of the writings of Popper, although he later goes on to argue that Popper subsequently developed a yet more sophisticatedmethodological falsificationism (the third of Lakatos' pictures of science). Surprisingly (or perhaps not given the antecedent arguments), Lakatos reports that this is a form of *conventionalism*.

...is a form of conventionalism

This is a surprising concession because it appears to give up a key feature of empiricism: that scientific theories answer to the facts. Conventionalism in the philosophy of science is (in general) the label for a view of scientific theories in which they are taken to be adopted for their usefulness and convenience without any regard for their truth. Think of the convention that everyone should drive on the same side of the road. This is useful but in no sense answers to a Platonic 'fact' of motoring and is itself neither true nor false. Conventionalism is thus antirealist about scientific methodology. It is also (though again only in general) antirealist in the metaphysical sense: that is to say, conventionalism denies that it even makes sense to speak of scientific theories being true of the world.

Lakatos's subscription to conventionalism is not so radical, however. Conventionalism enters Lakatos's account of methodological falsificationism through two *decisions* that correspond to the two assumptions of dogmatic falsificationism discussed above. Some statements are deemed observational and thus themselves immune from falsification *by decision* (p. 106). This is a matter of using successful theories as extensions of our senses by allowing them to go unchallenged when they are used to challenge other theories. Thus, rather than relying on a decisive foundation (whether used to confirm or refute theories), methodological Falsificationism is based instead on 'piles driven into a swamp' (p. 108). The foundation of observation is only relatively stable rather than completely grounded. Thus even if 'falsified' by statements deemed observational, a theory may still be true. Lakatos mentions as an example of historical rashness the fact that Galileo and his disciples accepted 'Copernican heliocentric mechanics in spite of the abundance evidence against the rotation of the earth' (p. 115). In fact it turned out that that 'evidence' was misleading and Galileo was right to adopt the heliocentric view. Thus the rational advice—that falsified theories should be rejected—is fallible advice. It may result in the rejection of true theories.

Without a firm empirical basis of incontestable observation statements, the original falsificationist demarcation of science from non-science is undermined. However, Lakatos suggests that a conventionalist reworking of it is still acceptable. Theories will, however, only be 'falsifiable' in the light of methodological prescriptions about putting them to the test (cf. p. 111). A theory is scientific if it is 'falsifiable', but this now requires a kind of intellectual honesty from scientists to treat it as falsifiable and to test it accordingly as in principle the world can never decisively show that it is false.

Sophisticated methodological falsificationism

Despite the fact that naive methodological falsificationism is an improvement over dogmatic falsification in its attempt to come to terms with the holism implicit in theory testing, Lakatos suggests that it is still an implausible account of actual scientific practice. This leads him to suggest his third falsificationist model of scientific rationality, sophisticated methodological falsificationism.

The key development in moving from naive to sophisticated methodological falsificationism is to take the unit of assessment in science not as an individual theory standing in relation to evidence, but as a series of theories grouped within what Lakatos calls a research programme. A research programme (i.e. a series of theories) stands in relation both to the evidence and also to competing research programmes. Assessment is thus explicitly temporally extended.

Within a research programme, one theory can replace another if two conditions are satisfied:

1. the new theory predicts facts disallowed by the former theory while explaining the successes of the former theory, and

2. some of its 'excess content' (i.e. the additional facts predicted by the new theory) has passed empirical tests.

Within a research programme, therefore, theories are falsified *by other theories* in the light of evidence, rather than, as in Popper's original and simple formulation, by the evidence directly. A research programme, i.e. a series of theories, is said by Lakatos to be *progressive* if both the above conditions are met and to be *degenerating* if not. Crucial experiments are thus not just any experiments that produce results that are inconsistent with a research programme (Lakatos calls such results 'anomalies'), but only those that distinguish between competing theories in a series.

Research programmes: hard cores and protective belts, positive and negative heuristics

A research programme, as envisaged by Lakatos, comprises a hard core of central assumptions that are shared between different theories in a series; and also a 'protective belt' of further assumptions. The latter are those further theories and hypotheses that are needed to relate the hard core to observations.

For example, current research on changes in neurotransmitters in the brain in conditions such as depression is a research programme, in Lakatos' use of the term. There are many and competing particular theories of how this or that change in this or that neurotransmitter might be related to depression. But all these theories share, as one hard core of assumption, the belief that neurotransmitters and mood are related. This assumption is surrounded by a penumbra of other beliefs about, for example, neuroimaging techniques, particular brain chemistry and so on. This means that if, for example, a hypothesis about the connection between a particular mood and neurotransmitter were to fail to gain experimental support it could be explained as simply the wrong choice of mechanism, the failure of the imagining technique or whatever without being taken to cast doubt on the general idea that neurotransmitters and mood are related.

Lakatos then specifies two methodological rules: the positive and negative heuristic. The negative heuristic is the prescription that the hard core should be preserved even in the face of observational anomalies. The positive heuristic determines the kind of changes that should be made when there are anomalies. Thus the negative heuristic determines the continuity between different theories in a research programme in that it ensures constancy of the hard-core assumptions. This is deemed irrefutable by empirical evidence: a more or less conventionalist decision. The positive heuristic—which remains sketchier in Lakatos's account—concerns how potential anomalies are to be dealt with: what sort of auxiliary assumptions are built into the refutable 'protective belt'.

We can see both heuristics at work in our example (above) of the current research programme on neurotransmitters and depression. Thus, the negative heuristic protects the programme from evidence (such as that produced by Brown and Harris, see end of Chapter 15) that social factors have a role to play in depression: such factors, the negative heuristic specifics, must be understood as being mediated by neurotransmitters. The positive heuristic, in this case, concern, among other things, the general shape of mechanisms that might be appealed to. The idea, for example, that the mind has no physiological correlate and might float free of it will receive short shrift.

The history of science is, according to Lakatos, a history of the development of theories within a larger structure of competing research programmes. Research programmes are the units that progress or degenerate—according to how theories are developed in line with evidence—rather than the individual theories themselves.

Rational reconstructions and the history of science

Lakatos's approach is thus particularly interesting in the way it takes the simple logical point about the asymmetry of refutation and confirmation of universal claims by single instances, which Popper (1972) highlights, and shows that this does not by itself yield a plausible scientific methodology. In attempting to preserve Popper's emphasis on the negative use of evidence, Lakatos develops a model of a historically extended process in which groups of theories are assessed holistically, i.e. in relation to each other and to the data, which is itself regarded as fallible and to be assessed in the light of theoretical context. But as a result, the methodology cannot give decisive advice about when a theory should be accepted or rejected. In the main, it is better to support progressive rather than degenerating research programmes. However, exactly when it is appropriate to abandon a degenerating research programme is a matter of uncodifiable *judgement*. There are no settled criteria for this. A programme could be degenerating for any length of time before again making progress.

Lakatos's philosophical model gave rise in the 1970s to a project of writing rational reconstructions in the history of science. Effectively this was a way of viewing the history of science as exemplifying Lakatos's model of what is rational in the pursuit of science. Events that fitted the model of rational behaviour for scientists were thought to require no further explanation. Only events that did not fit that model called for further historical or sociological explanation. But as we will see below, this approach faces criticism.

Kuhn's account of the history of science

Thomas Kuhn's paradigms

Lakatos's (1970) methodology of scientific research programmes is an attempt in part to articulate a rational method of theory choice. Within a single research programme, theories are preferred if they meet the tests of sophisticated falsificationism while programmes as a whole are preferred if they are progressive.

But the view that there is any such clear rational method by which proceeds had already received sustained criticism from the historian of science Thomas Kuhn. Kuhn was originally a physicist who became interested in the history of science and wrote a very influential book, *The Structure of Scientific Revolutions* (1962), published shortly before Lakatos' definitive statement of

his own work described above. In it he sets out an account of normal scientific practice and occasional scientific revolution. Over the course of the next two decades a broadly Kuhnian view prevailed in the philosophy of science at least to the extent that conjoined history and philosophy of science departments carrying out Lakatosian 'rational reconstructions' has waned.

Kuhn argues that the kind of radical theory change emphasized in the starkest kind of falsificationism (if not so much in Lakatos's version) is the exception rather than the norm in the history of science. For most of their time, scientists engage not in the critical testing of current theories but in the gradual extension and application of them through 'puzzle solving'. Kuhn calls such activity 'normal science' and the taken-for-granted background of theory the dominant 'paradigm'. (In fact he uses this word in a number of different ways. One common effect of reading Kuhn is the subsequent indiscriminate use of the word 'paradigm'. Avoid it!)

In Chapter 14 we discussed Kuhn's account of the importance of *tacit* knowledge and agreement, which, according to Kuhn, partly constitute a shared paradigm. It is made up not only of explicit high-level theories but also implicit factors. These include metaphysical commitments about the kind of theoretical description of the world that is acceptable (in terms of particles or fields, for example) and implicit standards for what a satisfactory level of agreement is between theory and observation as well as tacit knowledge about how to solve theoretical puzzles. But it should be clear from this brief sketch that a Kuhnian paradigm is quite similar to a Lakatosian research programme with its hard-core of scientific and metaphysical claims.

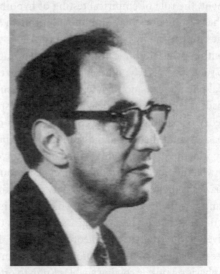

Fig. 16.3 Thomas Kuhn

Dominant paradigms can, however, be overturned in scientific revolutions. But although Kuhn gives a helpful account of the sorts of factors responsible for such revolutions—a growing number of unsolved puzzles, dissatisfaction among leading scientists with the paradigm, the development of alternatives, and so forth-the revolution itself, he suggests, is not subject to a rational methodology. Furthermore, and perhaps more contentiously, he argues that there are no rational measures by which to judge that science is cumulative or progressive to use Lakatos's phrase. The range and nature of puzzles after a revolution is merely different from that before and both are determined by the different paradigms operative at the time. Kuhn famously, or perhaps notoriously, even suggests that after a revolution scientists are effectively living in a different world.

EXERCISE 6   (15 minutes)

Read the extract from:

Kuhn, T.S. (1970). Logic of discovery or psychology of research? In *Criticism and the Growth of Knowledge* (ed. I. Lakatos and A. Musgrave). Cambridge: Cambridge University Press, pp. 1–23 (extract 4–6)

Link with Reading 16.5

Outline the key differences between Kuhn's approach and those of Popper and Lakatos. Is the difference merely one of emphasis?

The role of testing for Kuhn and Popper

In an introduction just before this extract, Kuhn (rather misleadingly) emphasizes the agreement between his view of science and that of Popper. Here, though, he takes as a first instance of their disagreement, the role of empirical testing of hypotheses. Kuhn suggests that testing does play an important role in science but not the one emphasized by falsificationism (p. 4).

Thus, within what Kuhn calls 'normal science', researchers attempt to solve 'puzzles'. Hypotheses are proposed to explain specific natural phenomena and then tested. However, such tests are not designed, as Popper supposed, to put 'maximum strain' on the overall theory or paradigm. To the contrary, within normal science the background theories and assumptions are presupposed in the very way the problems are defined and in the constraints placed on what an adequate solution or explanation would be. Solving puzzles is the most common activity of working research scientists and it is the method through which a dominant theory or paradigm is extended. The working assumption is that puzzles can be solved *within* the current theoretical setting. Failure is a mark of the inadequacy of the practitioner rather than the theory.

This emphasis on puzzle solving enables Kuhn to offer a rival to Popper's account of what is distractive about scientific method. Popper demarcates science from non-science by falsifiability of theories. Astrology, then, for Popper, is not scientific because it's

theories are not falsifiable. For Kuhn, by contrast, astrology is not scientific because the rules that constitute the paradigm of astrology do not determine any puzzles that could be solved. 'The occurrence of failures could be explained, but particular failures did not give rise to research puzzles, for no man, however skilled, could make use of them in a constructive attempt to revise the astrological tradition.' (p. 9).

Learning from one's mistakes

Kuhn then goes on to question the Popperian idea that a central aspect of scientific development is learning from one's mistakes. Kuhn argues that this idea makes sense within the context of normal science in which a mistake is a failure to follow the rules laid down by accepted theory and practice. But Popper attempts to apply that notion to *revolutions* in science and Kuhn argues that no sense can be attached to the idea that an abandoned theory— such as Ptolemaic astronomy—is mistaken. That would only make sense if there were an inductive logic by the rules of which theories could be shown to be good by induction from the data. But as there are no such rules, no theory is simply mistaken.

In addition to attacking the role of learning from mistakes, Kuhn also presses the point that has been discussed already in the context of Lakatos's work. Despite the attractions of naive falsificationism, the refutation of theories is not the straightforward business presupposed by that approach 'Rather than a logic', Kuhn suggests, 'Sir Karl has provided an ideology; rather than methodological rules, he has supplied procedural maxims' (p. 15).

How, then, if there is no such inductive logic, does science work? Kuhn's answer is to deploy an idea based on a different sense of the word 'paradigm'. Rather than thinking of science as turning on logically explicit theories, Kuhn suggests that it turns on implicit generalizations based on particular instances or 'paradigms'. This view, which emphasizes the importance of open-ended or open-textured concepts, also suggests that the response to anomalies is less determined than a view of scientific theories as strict universal generalizations would imply. Indeed, Kuhn goes so far as to suggest that some of the rhetoric of the Popperian account is an apt expression of the methodological imperatives that make up the tacit values of a paradigm. Such values, he concludes, should be understood through social psychology rather than through a logical methodology of theory change of the kind proposed by Popper.

Overview of Kuhn on theory and evidence

Kuhn's overall picture of science is clearly distinct in emphasis from that of Popper or even Lakatos. He suggests that the structure of science is one of stable normal research work interrupted by occasional radical revolutions. It is not a matter of constant revolution as described by falsificationism. He does, however, share with sophisticated forms of falsificationism a view that science comprises a complex structure of theory and observation against a background of taken for granted assumptions about the shape of any plausible theory. Empirical testing is thus not a matter of mere data gathering but involves much background theoretical presupposition. Without such a background, theory testing would be impossible. But for most of the time, the background itself is simply not called into question. Furthermore, much of this background is also tacit. Practitioners learn tacit skills in the practical manipulation of instruments, for example. They also learn to make assumptions about what factors do and do not matter in particular empirical contexts. In Kuhn's account, furthermore, as in Lakatos's, there is an important balance between loyalty to existing theory and a preparedness on occasion for radical revision when the data are in conflict with theory.

Kuhn's account of how science works is based on much historical analysis. Thus the burden of proof is carried by historical evidence rather than a priori reasoning. But Kuhn's views are shared and further developed in the work of contemporary sociologists of science. It is to the sociology of science, and the further debate it has stimulated about the role of rational methodology in the selection and testing of theory, that we turn in the last part of this session.

The sociology of science

The short extract (linked with Exercise 7 below) is part of a chapter from an influential textbook on the sociology of science written by David Bloor (1976). Although a sociologist, Bloor has also written philosophical papers on Wittgenstein. Unsurprisingly he argues for a reading of Wittgenstein that emphasizes the importance of *social* relations for understanding language and cognition (Bloor, 1997).

The main objective of Bloor's (1976) chapter is to set out a programme for the sociological investigation of science. It is thus concerned with rival models for the explanation of scientific development. But it also relates to the concerns of this chapter and session because it articulates a rival view of scientific rationality. Recall that Popper claimed for his 'solution' to the problem of induction the merit that it preserved a rational method for science. However, that claim was weakened in the modifications that Lakatos made to falsificationism, which were required to make it a plausible account of good but actual scientific practice. Bloor implicitly undermines the idea that there is *any* substantial universal model of scientific rationality. That is why science requires piecemeal and local sociological investigation.

EXERCISE 7 (15 minutes)

Read the extract from:

Bloor, D. (1976). *Knowledge and Social Imagery*. London: Routledge, (extract pp. 1–3).

Link with Reading 16.6

◆ What arguments does Bloor direct against Lakatos's ideas about the role of a philosophical model of scientific rationality?

◆ What relationship between a sociology of knowledge and a philosophy of science is suggested in Bloor's work?

Bloor's view of the role of sociology

Bloor sets out the challenge for sociology to explain the content of scientific knowledge. He argues that this is a natural extension of the area of competence of sociology and that it is merely a failure of nerve that has prevented sociologists from taking up this challenge in the past.

It is worth briefly reflecting on what is at issue here: Bloor thinks that there can be a sociological explanation not merely of the institutional context of scientific research, nor merely of the cultural impact of knowledge claims, but of those very claims themselves, of their very content.

This suggests (and this suggestion is borne out by subsequent sociological work) that a characteristically realist explanatory strategy is also being ruled out along with the more explicit attack on this reading on a form of a priori rationalism. The realist strategy is to explain the content of a knowledge claim in part at least by saying that it is true or that it is a fact. So in answer to the question: why did nineteenth century scientists accept such and such a claim, the realist replies that they accepted it because it was true. Bloor rejects this reply. He proposes instead a four-point characterization of what he calls the Strong Programme for the sociology of science, which is roughly:

1. It would be causal, that is, concerned with the conditions that bring about belief or states of knowledge.

2. It would be impartial with respect to truth and falsity, rationality or irrationality, success or failure. Both sides will require explanation.

3. It would be symmetrical in its style of explanation.

4. It would be reflexive. (cf. pp. 4–5)

Bloor goes on to contrast this view with the view of the relation of sociological or historical explanation and rationality that Lakatos develops. For Lakatos (1970), there is a sharp divide between 'internal' and 'external' history. The internal history of science is a demonstration of how scientific development accords with a philosophical model of scientific rationality—a model such as Lakatos's own methodological falsificationism. Sociological analysis is only needed as part of external history: the history of irrationality and failure. The underlying idea is that rationality is its own explanation. What needs concrete or substantial explanation is only deviation from this course.

Bloor characterizes Lakatos's view as a *teleological* view by contrast with his own *causal* view. The idea is that a teleological conception relies on the assumption that the rationality of an action or belief draws scientists on towards it. Such terminology needs some care, however, as most philosophers who subscribe to something like Lakatos's view here would also subscribe to a causal view in the philosophy of mind. And, again, most philosophers would agree that rationality plays a key and constitutive role in the explanation of behaviour. Bloor plays this down, but in fact nearly all sociological accounts help themselves to something like the everyday folk psychological pattern of rational action explanation. However, Bloor wants to distance himself from the idea, implicit in Lakatos, that nothing else needs to be said to explain action if it can also be said to be rational. This point is made even more clearly in the writing of another sociologist: Barry Barnes.

The Barnes view

Barry Barnes, like Bloor, a sociologist of science, wrote, at about the same time as Bloor, in support of more or less the same views (Barnes, 1974). Barnes, however, is more explicit about the connection between the problem of induction, the assumption among philosophers of science that there is a model of scientific rationality, and the rival sociological conception of scientific knowledge.

Barnes, like Bloor, contrasts causal analysis and rational explanation of action; however, in his case the underlying point of the contrast is clearer. The key problem of invoking the rationality of a belief or action in order to explain it, is not so much that such an explanation is false as that it begs the question. Barnes illustrates this point with the poison oracle among a tribe called the Azande. A chicken is given poison and a question is asked. If the chicken dies, the answer to the question is 'yes'. The irrationality of the oracle may seem obvious to twentieth century Western society. But Barnes asks us to consider how we would explain the actions of a member of that society who rejects the status of the oracle and subscribes to something more like Western thinking. Would that person's actions require no further explanation because his or her beliefs were (by twentieth century Western standards) rational? Barnes replies that precisely their deviance from (local) societal norms would, all the more, *require* explanation.

In other words, the problem with invoking a teleological conception of rationality is fleshing out what it involves. In a particular context, reasoning in a particular way that diverges markedly from our twentieth century views, may be rational. It may make sense to follow patterns of thought which we, initially at least, find alien. So the right conclusion to draw is not that sociological explanation flies in the face of rationality (as some sociologists of science sometimes appear to suggest), but rather that the content of acting or thinking rationally has to be unpacked in each context.

Bloor, Barnes, and delusion

As an aside, it is worth noting that neither Bloor nor Barnes, although sociologists, had, in the 1970s, anything more to say about the various forms of irrationality presented by psychopathology, than philosophers (see the quote from Anthony Quinton at the start of Chapter 2). Yet here, as in so many other contexts in philosophy, psychopathology, in all its diverse forms, presents, as Austin (see Chapter 5) and more recently Wilkes' (1988) have argued, a peculiarly sharp test of theory. Barnes (1974) might, perhaps, have pointed to delusions as an example of (extreme) departures from local norms of rationality. But as we saw in Chapter 3, it is very far from clear by precisely what standards such a departure is to be judged. Certainly, there is as

yet no causal story of the kind Bloor and Barnes envisaged, or indeed of any other kind, by which delusional and non-delusional beliefs are to be distinguished. Yet a distinction is made. Similarly, considerations will arise in the next section, when we consider in more detail the metaphysical claim that knowledge is justified true belief: the existence of delusions which are true and yet (in some deep but thus far unexplained sense) *un*justified beliefs (see Chapter 3), has simply not been recognized, still less engaged with, still less explained, by philosophers interested in the nature of knowledge.

Content and context and some preliminary conclusions for evidence-based medicine

In this session we have seen that Popper (1972) and Lakatos (1970) put forward a model of what a universal scientific rationality would amount to. Kuhn, as a historian as well as a philosopher of science, disagrees with Popper and Lakatos and argues that there is no such context-independent rational account of science to be had. Barnes (1974) and Bloor (1976) with their 'Strong Programme' go further and propose a causal, rather than a rational, account of science that seeks to explain, even-handedly, successful and unsuccessful outcomes of scientific research.

The debate does not show the model of scientific rationality has nothing to offer. Nor is it that a more detailed 'causal' explanation should eschew rational explanation. It is rather that the problem with any substantial but imposed model of scientific rationality is that it can fail to deliver the right results in context. There may be good reasons, for example, not to reject a theory in the face of refutation if it has accommodated similar anomalies in the past and is otherwise reliable. This is the sort of thing that Lakatos attempts to accommodate. But because he attempts to describe a rational method in a context-free manner it opens his model up to the charge that it is not substantial: its advice verges on 'Do the right thing!'. The sociologists' arguments are best interpreted as saying that the content of what is rational in any particular context has to be investigated piecemeal.

This is not to undermine the rationality of the best scientific practice. To some extent, scientific practice just is our model of rational decision making. But the attempt to codify what is rational in a universal a-historical and context-free manner has not proved successful. That provides an important lesson for EBM's more modest attempt to codify how best to learn from experience. Careful attention to the details of the traditional model of science suggests that it cannot give a detailed account of scientific practice. This does not undermine science, however, but show that we have a tendency to oversimplify its workings. The traditional model has to be made complicated especially in areas of science, which are themselves complex. Thus we should be wary of oversimplifying scientific practice in accounts of EBM.

Consideration of the philosophy of science has shown that whatever role induction from evidence does have in science—and if nothing else falsificationism shows the importance of refutation as well as confirmation—there is much more to the role of evidence and theory testing than a naively inductivist view would have us believe. Scientific research does not involve the harvesting of particular observations from which grow generalizations and eventually theories. As Chapter 12 already argued, evidence presupposes much theory. But as the historically informed accounts of science have plausibly shown in this session, the way that evidence is used is also subject to background theoretical considerations. The relation between theory and evidence is one of interdependence: both top-down and bottom-up.

Still, while Barnes (1974) explicitly discusses inductive inference as suitable for sociological investigation (as did Harry Collins discussed in Chapter 14) neither the sociology of knowledge, nor Kuhn's historical overview, nor falsificationism, provide a resolution of Hume's problem. One feature of the sociologists' rejection of a teleological construal of rationality is that they eschew a justificatory component in favour of description. Thus they provide no response to whether or why inductive inference is justified. For this reason, the next session will return to the problem of induction and responses to it made within philosophical epistemology. This will shed light on the nature of knowledge itself and its social dimension.

Reflection on the session and self-test questions

Write down your own reflections on the materials in this session drawing out any points that are particularly significant for you. Then write brief notes about the following:

1. What kind of response to Hume's problem of induction is suggested by the various readings in this session?

2. How does Popper address the problem?

3. What are the weaknesses of a naïve falsificationist model of scientific rationality?

4. What lessons are suggested by Kuhn's model of historical and other sociological approaches to scientific method described here?

Session 3 Epistemological responses to the problem of induction

Epistemology versus philosophy of science

In this session we will consider three responses to the problem of induction offered from within the perspective of epistemology rather than the more methodologically based philosophy of science. One difference in focus is that the approaches in this session attempt to resolve or dissolve the problem of induction rather than attempting merely to live with its sceptical consequences.

The discussion of philosophy of science responses in the previous session helped emphasize that the relation between theories and evidence is more complex than one might at first have thought. By considering Popper (1972), then Lakatos (1970), Kuhn (1970), and the Strong Programme (Barnes, 1974; Bloor, 1976), one theme emerged whatever the general conclusions one draws for the nature of scientific methodology. The relation of theories and evidence has to be understood in a broader context of scientific research whether one thinks of this as comprising research programmes or paradigms or historically situated forms of rationality. So equally citation of evidence in medicine turns on a similar background of higher and lower level scientific and metaphysical assumptions whether or not these are made explicit.

This session will consider lessons learnt from epistemology. One lesson in particular will be that knowledge can be transmitted from one individual to another without the second person being able to provide an argument to ensure that it is watertight. This is a lesson that we often forget when thinking about knowledge in a philosophical context—when we come over 'all philosophical'—and yet it informs our everyday use of the term. By examining the extent to which individuals are actively responsible for what they know we will shed light on what can reasonably be expected of EBM.

Again the route to these general views will start with a response to Hume's problem of induction. A good statement of a recent short response to Hume is given by a recent professor of philosophy: D.H. Mellor. His inaugural address aimed to defuse any lingering problem of induction. It is published as 'The warrant of induction' in his *Matters of Metaphysics* (1991).

Mellor's diagnosis of the problem of induction

EXERCISE 8 (15 minutes)

Read the two extracts from:

Mellor, D. H. (1991). The warrant of induction. *Matters of Metaphysics*. London: Routledge, (Extract sections 1 and 6)

Link with Reading 16.7

- What is Mellor's solution to the problem of induction?
- What view of knowledge does it presuppose?
- How does it differ from the views examined so far?
- Does it really solve the problem?

There can be knowledge by induction!

The most obvious contrast between Mellor's approach and those discussed in the previous session is that Mellor assumes that we can and do have positive knowledge. He says: 'This lecture will last for less than twenty-four hours. I know that and so do you.' (p. 254) The grounding of this knowledge is, according to Mellor, the directly observational or experiential knowledge we have that none, or almost none, of the previous lectures we have heard has lasted that long. We go on to form the further inductive belief—on the basis of the observational properties that identify an event as a lecture—that it will also have the as yet unobserved property of being shorter than a certain time. (This is reminiscent of Hume's talk of the connection between sensible powers and secret powers.)

The central question is *how* such past observations can warrant or justify claims about so far unobserved states of affairs. Mellor points out that such warrant is both weak enough to be overridden by observation—present observation can overturn a previous induction—and yet strong enough to trust one's life to (he gives the example of believing that the building will not shortly fall in). But how is this possible? The answer, Mellor suggests, lies in the Cambridge philosopher Frank Ramsey's (1903–30) suggestion that 'our conviction [in inductive arguments] is reasonable because the world is so constituted that inductive arguments lead on the whole to true opinions' (p. 254).

The structure of the paper

Mellor's paper then has the following structure. Having first introduced the problem and a thumbnail sketch of the solution, it goes on to explore an analogy with the warrant for beliefs that direct perception provides (so as to set an appropriate standard for induction to meet). Mellor suggests here a form of reliabilism: observation is a reliable method of arriving at true beliefs. We are causally disposed by observation to form beliefs that have a high probability of being true. Mellor then goes on to explain the objective construal of chance implicit in this claim and to reject the assumption that one needs to know that one is warranted in one's belief to be so warranted. Finally, he returns to the proposed solution to the problem of induction.

An analogy with observation

The analogy with observation is supposed to work like this. Observation is fallible. We can think that we see sparrows when we don't. To remind us of this, Mellor adopts the potentially confusing form of words that to 'observe' does not imply the truth of the object of that verb, although he does not himself use inverted commas. (In everyday life observing or seeing is a *success* concept—like knowing—if one sees that x is the case, then it is; and if one sees a y, there is a y to be seen.) Given this form of words, the fact that one 'observes' a sparrow does not entail, or logically imply, that there is a sparrow there. (To repeat, in everyday life this is an entailment, but Mellor does not want to assume that we see a sparrow when we seem to see a sparrow.) So if it is not a logical truth that when we 'observe' a sparrow there is a sparrow, what warrant or justification does 'observing' provide?

Mellor suggests the following approach. Think of the judgement that there is a sparrow present when we 'observe' one as an inferential disposition: a disposition to make that inference. Now dispositions are well known items in our causal picture of the world. The standing property of mass has further dispositional

properties such as being disposed to accelerate at a certain rate when acted upon by a specific force. Masses embody a causal link between forces and accelerations. Mellor suggests that just such a causal link underpins the warrant that 'observations' provide for perceptually based beliefs. The presence of sparrows causes the *belief* that sparrows are present.

In fact, he suggests that this causal link is probabilistic. The probability of there being sparrows when one 'observes' them is less than 1 but sufficiently close to it still to warrant the belief. This requires that Mellor construes probabilities or chances as objective indeterminacies, rather than as epistemic measures, to avoid the charge of circularity. Otherwise he would be guilty of explaining the warrant of our beliefs in terms of the warrant of our beliefs. On his preferred theory, chances can also themselves have causal effects. One such example is the pattern of radiation that results from the chances of decay of radioactive substances. Another, Mellor suggests, is the formation of beliefs as the causal effects of a probabilistic observational mechanism.

Knowledge and reliability

With these suggestions in place, Mellor (1991) is able to suggest more broadly that what it is for a belief to have a warrant is for it to have a high probability of being true. 'What better measure could there be of the prospects of truth which observation gives the beliefs it produces, and hence of how strongly it warrants them? (p. 261).

This is, in effect, a challenge for epistemology. Mellor suggests that the purpose of warranting or justifying beliefs is to provide good prospects for their truth. Nothing more is required.

You don't need to know that you know. The reliabilist account of knowledge . . .

This runs counter to a different, more traditional, assumption that a further necessary condition for justification or warrant is that it is self-intimating. That is, if one's belief is warranted, then one also knows that it is warranted. If one knows then one knows that one knows. Mellor raises two objections to this requirement. First, it leads to scepticism because the requirement escalates what one needs to know: one must know that one knows that one knows . . . ad infinitum. Secondly, given his own suggestion for the nature of warrants, the extra requirement would not increase the probability of truth of a belief already warranted.

It is worth pausing at this point. Mellor puts forward a view that has recently become much more popular in philosophy but can seem counter-intuitive. It is possible to know something even if one does not know that one knows it. Providing the source of one's beliefs is as a matter of fact reliable—again, whether or not one knows this—then one can acquire knowledge.

Thus a psychiatrist following the principles of EBM can make an appropriate search of sources of evidence. Providing that the resources invoked are as a matter of fact reliable then he or she can acquire knowledge whether or not he or she knows anything more about those sources of evidence. What matters is that they are reliable, presumably through the careful attention of other research workers.

The solution to the problem of induction?

Mellor is thus now in a position to set out his solution to the problem of induction. Forming beliefs by induction is itself an inferential disposition whose inputs are past observations and whose output is the inductive belief. How can these past observations warrant the subsequent belief when that belief is not true simply in virtue of those former beliefs? The proposal is that it can providing that the chance of the output belief being true given the input beliefs is sufficiently close to 1. Providing that there are laws linking observable properties then an inductive inference mechanism linking beliefs about one to the other will have a high probability of yielding true beliefs and thus it will be warranted. (By contrast counter-induction–see below–will not reliably yield true beliefs.) If on the other hand, there are no laws linking two observable properties then no inferential habit will reliably yield true beliefs (neither induction nor counter-induction will be reliable). Thus in a law-like world, induction unlike counter-induction is warranted. That is Mellor's solution to the problem of induction.

So to return to Mellor's initial example. Providing that we live in a world where the laws that govern social interaction, individual psychology and so on, which are applicable to the duration of lectures are stable then the fact that lectures have been shorter than 24 hours in the past warrants the belief that they will be in the future. The inductive leap from the past to the future is underpinned by the *de facto* regularity of nature.

One might now ask: but how do we know that the world behaves in this regular way? Is not that the real problem of induction? However, Mellor's point is that we do not need to know that in order to know that the lecture will last less than 24 hours. As long as the world is regular—whether or not we have taken a view on that—then we can have knowledge by induction.

Does it work?

Is this a satisfactory solution? It is worth returning to Mellor's first argument against the requirement that justifications or warrants should be self-intimating. As we saw in Session 1, the fires of Humean scepticism are fanned by just the requirement Mellor here rejects. If one needs to know that one knows in order to know, then the fact that one cannot know that induction is a reliable method of justifying beliefs implies that one cannot know anything by induction. Even if induction were reliable, the extra requirement rules out ground-level knowledge claims if one cannot—at the meta-level—vouch for induction. Mellor effectively blocks this swift route to scepticism. Even if we did not *know* that induction were reliable, providing that it were reliable, it would warrant our beliefs (even though unbeknown to us). And thus it may seem that scepticism is undermined.

Externalism

The denial that one needs to know that one knows marks a commitment to what is called in epistemology 'externalism'. Beware! This label is used in a variety of different philosophical contexts to mean different things. We will come across it again in Part V to refer to accounts of how meaning or intentionality come about. Here, it refers to the perspective from which knowledge is theorized about. Rather than thinking about the justifications that are *available to* a knowing subject, epistemological externalism characterizes the justificatory component of knowledge from a third person perspective. The article by McDowell discussed below is also written from this perspective, although it does not share Mellor's commitment to reliabilism. One of the motivations for epistemological externalism is that internalism seems to lead inexorably to inductive scepticism because of the regress of justifications for one's beliefs that one would need to know. But does externalism answer inductive scepticism?

Well one response is that it does not because the sceptic naturally ascends to a higher level with the question: 'Granted that you need not know that you know in order to know, but do you have inductive knowledge?' Mellor's solution is to say that providing induction is reliable, then we do have 'ground level' knowledge claims about the sun rising tomorrow, or bread nourishing, and we need not know that we know for this to be true. But Mellor admits that if induction is *not* reliable then we do *not* have ground level knowledge claims. So the sceptic can press the question: Which is it? Do we have ground level knowledge or not?

Mellor does not really answer this question. He can point out that even in worlds in which induction is not reliable, other strategies, including counter-induction—assuming that connections held in the past will *not* hold in the future—will also fail. So we may always be best off pragmatically by using induction. But that is not to say that we do have inductive knowledge. If we want a positive answer to this question, we want to know whether we know: to know that we know or know that we do not know. So although we need not first answer this question for us to have ground level knowledge, we do swiftly want to answer it when beset by inductive sceptical doubts. And it is not clear that reliabilism yields a positive answer here.

This is a potential problem for *any* epistemologically externalist account of knowledge. Although not knowing that one knows to the power n does not imply that one does not know that one knows to the power n-1, externalism by itself does not return a positive answer to the question of one's knowledge to the power n. And responding to inductive scepticism may make that the question we wish to be answered.

John McDowell offers a somewhat different response that aims to combine the virtues of an externalist approach while retaining the idea that knowledge has something to do with giving reasons. Looking to his account will provide a better way of thinking about knowledge and the extent to which one is responsible for one's own knowledge.

McDowell's diagnosis of the problem of induction

A different kind of externalism tied to the space of reasons

We have already come across McDowell's book *Mind and World* (1994) in earlier chapters (Chapters 12 and 15). Both those discussions emphasized the importance of the rational structure of reasons that McDowell, following the American philosopher Wilfrid Sellars (1912–89), calls the 'space of reasons' and which stands distinct from the 'realm of law'.

McDowell has also developed a sketch of knowledge that shares that emphasis on the role of reasons and that sheds light both on induction and the general context of learning from experience that applies to EBM.

McDowell's starting assumption

The key paper outlining McDowell's approach to knowledge is 'Knowledge and the internal' from *Meaning, Knowledge, and Reality* (1998 pp 395–413). It begins with an important, although gnomic comment. McDowell says that he will assume that knowledge is a 'sort of standing in the space of reasons' but will explore how that insight can be distorted in some philosophical accounts. It turns out that a key source of distortion is specific sceptical arguments and in particular, Descartes' argument from illusion (discussed below). Such arguments lead to the mistaken supposition that we ought to be able to achieve the standing in the space of reasons that amounts to knowledge 'without needing the world to do us any favours'. McDowell aims to give us a better picture of the nature of knowledge by diagnosing and rejecting Cartesian assumptions that are often made.

The distorting effect of the argument from illusion

Descartes' argument from illusion highlights the fact that sometimes when we take things in the world to be thus and so on the grounds of how they look, they are not thus and so. Sticks can look bent in water even when they are not. Thus if things are indeed as they seem then the world has done us a favour. Descartes used the ever present possibility of illusion to cast doubt on our ability to acquire knowledge. (This was a first step in his seminal epistemological enterprise that eventually sought to regain knowledge through a religious turn.). Even if we are not deceived in particular cases, is that not merely a matter of luck? And if so, does that not undermine the right to call any such perceptual beliefs 'knowledge' even if, as a matter of fact, they are true?

Responding to this worry we might try to build an account of knowledge restricted to epistemological states whose flawlessness we can ensure without this apparently problematic dependency on favours from the world. We might, in other words, commit ourselves no further than that it *looks* or *seems* to me as if things are thus and so. McDowell calls this philosophical move 'the interiorization of the space of reasons'.

The key assumption is that theorizing about knowledge should be carried out through description of states that do not depend on the world. Descartes and many epistemologists who have followed him hoped that the retreat to how things seem was only a temporary move. They hoped that there would be some way to regain the idea of knowledge claims about the world rather than just how it seemed. However, McDowell points out, this hope has generally proved futile.

If one adds to talk of how the world seems some further reasons or justifications of the fact that in specific kinds of circumstances such 'seemings' are reliable, then one will be able to say that the world is thus and so in a way that does not depend on the world doing us a favour. McDowell argues, however, that unless reason can equip us with policies that are utterly risk free, such a reconstruction will never add up to knowledge of the world: 'if one's method falls short of total freedom from risk of error, the appearance plus the appropriate circumstances for activating the method cannot ensure that things are as one takes them to be.' (p. 399).

Four responses to the argument from illusion

McDowell suggests that there are four responses to this problem. He himself advocates that we stop thinking about knowledge via the argument from illusion. But there are also three others:

1. Scepticism: we could simply conclude that the conditions for knowledge cannot be met for perception.

2. A form of a priori-ism: we could assume that there simply must be a priori risk-free policies for judging when appearances are reliable; however, this remains implausible.

3. A hybrid approach: we could retain the justificatory approach to knowledge implicit in talk of the 'space of reasons' still construed in an interiorized way but add a further component to it. On this approach knowledge has two ingredients: an epistemic standing or justification construed in the interiorized way as wholly under the subject's control plus another external condition not ensured by that: that the world does one a favour in being arranged as it seems to be. This further condition is truth. And the interiorized condition, the justification, concerns the 'reliability in a policy or habit of basing belief on appearance' (p. 400).

A contrast with Reliabilist Externalism

McDowell points out that, in the third approach, describing the reliability of one's policies as an internal matter goes against a standard view of reliabilism, as set out, for example, in the discussion of Mellor (1991) above. But McDowell rejects Mellor's sort of position because it fails to address the rational interconnected nature of our knowledge claims.

According to a full blown externalist approach, knowledge has nothing to do with positions in the space of reasons: knowledge is a state of the knower linked to the state of affairs known in such a way that the knower's being in that state is a reliable indicator that the state of affairs obtains. In the purest form of this approach, it is at most a matter of superficial idiom that we do not attribute knowledge to properly functioning thermometers.   (p. 401)

So McDowell regards the third hybrid option as more attractive than pure externalist reliabilism because it at least recognizes that we can have reasons for knowledge claims that fit into a rational structure. But just because reliability features in the pure externalist account as an external constraint, it does not do so in the hybrid conception because here it is supposed to capture the idea of a knowing subject raising questions about their policies of forming beliefs on the basis of appearances.

Two key problems with a hybrid approach

When so construed, however, internal reasons and the assessment of reliability of one's policies become divorced from the external constraint of truth. This leads to a problem. If the world actually being thus and so is not directly available to the resources of reason—if such facts are external to our reason—how can knowing subjects have the resources to assess the reliability of methods of basing beliefs on appearances? Some such facts would have to be taken for granted in order to test whether a method really was reliable, but that contradicts the assumption that having good reason is an internal matter and truth is external.

There is also a second objection to the hybrid conception. One of the points of the distinction between the concept of knowledge (as *justified* true belief) and mere true belief is that ascribing knowledge to someone is supposed to rule out the idea that they have a true belief as a mere matter of luck or accident. But if two people can achieve equally good standings in the space of reasons while only one of them is actually right about a matter, that extra external condition is merely a matter of luck or accident. In other words, the hybrid conception does not support the key distinction behind the concept of knowledge.

McDowell's alternative to the hybrid approach

McDowell suggests that the hybrid conception is often taken to be obvious. But he suggests that this stems merely from an apparent lack of other options. To counter this he suggests an alternative: one that rejects the argument from illusion as a good basis for thinking about knowledge. McDowell suggests that achieving a good standing in the space of reasons is itself dependent of the kindness of the world. This contrasts with the hybrid position, influenced by the argument from illusion. Even being justified requires a worldly contribution:

> But that the world does someone the necessary favour, on a given occasion, of being the way it appears to be is not extra to the person's standing in the space of reasons. Her coming to have an epistemically satisfactory standing in the space of reasons is not what the interiorized conception would require for it to count as her own unaided achievement; but then once she has achieved such a standing, she needs no extra help from the world to count as knowing.   (p. 406)

And again,

> Of course we are fallible in our judgements as to the shape of reasons as we find it, or—what comes to the same thing—as to the shape of the world as we find it. That is to say that we are vulnerable to the world's playing us false; and when the world does not play us false we are indebted to it. But that is something we must simply learn to live with, rather than recoiling into the fantasy of a sphere in which our control is total.   (pp. 407–408)

How can the space of reasons be 'external' to us?

There are two further clues as to McDowell's suggestion here. One is hinted at but not developed in a footnote. McDowell compares the idea of being justified with the idea of responsibility for one's actions, what one does. In this latter sphere, that of intervening in an objective world, one obviously does not have complete control over what happens. But in this case we do not think that what *we* actually achieve is somehow less than our final actual actions (which also require a favour from the world such as that our arms are not tied down or the door we are trying to open is not jammed shut). We are (for reasons he does not attempt to explain) less tempted in the case of action to postulate an internal realm (perhaps of pure willing) where we do have complete control over what happens. Similarly, he suggests, we should regard reason as requiring a favour from the world, while nevertheless not undermining the idea that this still comprises *our* epistemic standing.

Secondly, McDowell draws on an idea he has developed in the philosophy of thought and language and suggested in previous readings from *Mind and World*. One of the points of announcing that he would investigate having a standing in the space of reasons was to mark out the idea that thoughts stand in a network of rational relations. (This is the contrast with Mellor's (1991) externalism, which ignores this crucial feature of thought.) But what stand in these relations are thoughts about various different aspects of the world. Thoughts have (or simply are) 'contents' of the form: there is a door in front of me, that is a red patch, yellow is lighter than black. But if thought is construed as an internal contrast to the external world, if 'we set if off so radically from the objective world, we lose our right to think of moves within the space we are picturing as content-involving'. (p. 409)

So McDowell thinks that the underlying objection to the hybrid picture of our epistemological standing is more fundamental than just a question of epistemology: of the nature knowledge and justification construed narrowly. It is instead a broader or deeper problem of thinking of our mental states as world-involving at all.

In the case of beliefs based on perceptions, McDowell suggests that scepticism of the sort generated by the argument from illusion can be resisted by rejecting its grounding assumption: that in perceptual experience we always take in less than full facts and are restricted merely to appearances. In other papers, McDowell describes the philosophical account of perception that he rejects as a 'highest common factor' theory of perception. On such a theory, what the argument from illusion reveals is the *common* factor between illusory and veridical experience: an appearance that stops short of the facts. He argues instead for a 'disjunctive conception'. In veridical experience we take in the full facts: we see that there is a door before us, or whatever. Only in illusory experience do we take in a mere appearance, something that stops short of the facts.

Induction again

McDowell goes on to extend his argument from scepticism applied to perception to scepticism applied to induction. The idea that he wishes to reject in this context (analogous to rejecting that perceptions can be characterized as taking in appearances that stop short of facts, and thus do not require worldly favours) is that an epistemic position can be characterized prior to the application of risky inductive principles. If such a position can coherently be described then the further move to form inductive inferences may appear problematic and in need of further justification. Indeed this is what Hume presupposes when he says that he will ask what evidence there is to ground inferences about what lies 'beyond the present testimony of our senses, or the record of our memory'.

However, McDowell argues that if one takes seriously such talk of the *testimony* of our senses, then what the senses deliver must involve a characterization of the world, rather than simply a thin description of, for example, a 'wash of chromatic sensation'. But if so:

> there cannot be a predicament in which one is receiving testimony from one's senses but has not yet taken any inductive steps. To stay with the experience of colour ... colour experience's being testimony of the senses depends on the subject's already knowing a good deal about, for instance, the effect of different sorts of illumination on colour appearances ...   (p. 411)

> So the supposed predicament of the inductive sceptic is a fiction ... Hume's formulation can seem to describe a predicament only if one does not think through the idea that its subject already has the testimony of the senses and this means that scepticism about induction can seem gripping only in combination with a straightforwardly interiorizing epistemology for perception.   (p. 412).

The solution summarized

McDowell argues that it turns out that to have perceptual knowledge requires that one already has inductive knowledge. So scepticism about induction is not as localized as it might have seemed. It threatens to undermine perceptual knowledge as well. Furthermore, there is something unstable about thinking that one can talk about having reasons for beliefs if at the same time one construes those reasons as internal mental states that are cut off from the world. Coupled with the realization that a highest common factor account of perceptual experience can never account for the fact that knowledge concerns external worldly states, this helps undermine the attraction of a form of scepticism here.

In the case of perception, if one does not assume that perception stops short of taking in facts, then the question: 'how do we know that the appearances are reliable?' will not be pressing. Perception is reliable because it is a (fallible) but direct openness to the world. Similarly, in the case of induction, if one does not assume that one could characterize a state of trusting the testimony of the senses without induction, then one will not be drawn to ask whether that extra step is justified. McDowell's point here is that there is no such middle ground and thus no alternative to accepting induction alongside the reliability of perception.

Does it work?

But does this really block inductive scepticism? Like most forms of philosophical scepticism it seems that here again, once inductive scepticism is unleashed there is no way to *refute* it. The sceptic can continue to press the following point. While it may be necessary to *think* of induction as reliable in order to characterize the deliverances of the senses as world involving, why believe that it is actually reliable? Although we may have to think that tables and chairs will continue to exist into the next instant when we report seeing that they are there now, what assurance is there that they actually will?

On the other hand, such residual scepticism is strangely unmotivated. Without the thought that induction is a further and risky move beyond the secure base of perception (or that it is a further risk to construe the output of perception as anything more than mere appearances), what grounds are there for calling that 'further move' into question? Hume explicitly contrasts induction and perception when in fact they are interconnected and interdependent. McDowell's account does not make either an infallible method of arriving at beliefs but suggests that they stand or fall together.

The social articulation of the space of reasons and evidence-based medicine

McDowell's paper 'Knowledge and the internal' (1998 pp 395–413) was originally published with a reply from his colleague at Pittsburgh Robert Brandom called 'Knowledge and the social articulation of the space of reasons'. This contained in part an account of Brandom's particular views of the nature of meaning, which he argues depends on social practices. However, whether or not one follows that line of argument, McDowell's approach to knowledge dovetails particularly easily with a social approach.

One of the ways in which one's epistemic good standing can depend on a worldly favour is exemplified in asking for directions. Under favourable circumstances this is a way of getting knowledge of, for example, where the nearest station is. But typically when we ask for directions we cannot construct an argument from what we seem to hear, or whatever might be immune to Descartes argument from illusion, to a conclusion that the station has to be where we subsequently think it is. Reading Descartes, or when we 'come over philosophical', we may conclude that if we cannot do this then we cannot *know* where the station is. However, that is not how we normally use the concept of knowledge.

Asking for directions provides a model of, for example, inquiring about treatment options: a key aspect of EBM. To acquire medical knowledge we have to take responsible steps to acquire a good standing in the space of reasons. But we do not need to be able personally to vouch for every step in the process of validating medical evidence. McDowell thus begins to sketch out a model for thinking of the balance between personal and collective responsibility in EBM. Much of what we rely on is not explicitly articulated as evidence in the narrow sense but rather rubs off on us through a medical apprenticeship. But on the other hand, this need not make it any the less a matter of knowledge.

Note that two themes inter-relate here. One is the idea that there is a tacit dimension to knowledge even in the idea of being justified. This connects back to the more general discussion of tacit knowledge in Chapter 14. The suggestion that one can acquire justified beliefs by asking other reliable sources even if one cannot establish an argument oneself to show that the belief must be true is an application of idea of a tacit dimension to medical knowledge as well as practice. The second aspect is the social dimension. Knowledge can rub off on others. Taken together this is a powerful alternative view to the traditional Cartesian focus on an individual acquiring knowledge by him- or herself and being able to establish its credentials unaided. That Cartesian picture is very intuitive but provides an unrealistic picture of real knowledge.

Wittgenstein's picture of the inherited background to knowledge claims

Wittgenstein on knowledge versus certainty

The context for understanding EBM by thinking of McDowell's sketch of the nature of empirical knowledge generally and his attempt to dissolve inductive scepticism can be complemented by considering a more general account of the 'space of reasons' in which we frame knowledge claims. The importance of an inherited belief structure and the relation between knowledge and certainty were also explored in a fragmentary way by Wittgenstein in the last months of his life, subsequently published as *On Certainty* (1979). The work comprises a chronological arrangement of remarks which, unlike his *Philosophical Investigations* (1953), were not sorted into a rational order. They were working notes rather than remarks prepared for publication. The reading comprises a representative sample of the view developed throughout the book.

EXERCISE 9   (30 minutes)

Read the extracts from

   Wittgenstein, L. (1969). *On Certainty*. Oxford: Basil Blackwell

Link with Reading 16.8

◆ To what extent is Wittgenstein's account foundational?

Moore's attack on scepticism

Wittgenstein's remarks were prompted (possibly indirectly) by his fellow Cambridge philosopher G. E. Moore's defence of common sense realism against scepticism. Moore's argument was remarkably simple. He held one hand (his own) and claimed that he knew that it was a hand. As a hand, it was a material object. Thus he knew that there was at least one material object in the world. And thus philosophical arguments against the reality of the material world were refuted.

Wittgenstein rejects that argument by suggesting that a sceptic (or idealist as such scepticism is here characterized) will say that 'he was not dealing with the practical doubt that was being dismissed, but . . . a further doubt behind that one' §19. Moore mistakenly treats sceptical doubts as though they were practical doubts requiring practical justifications. Instead, Wittgenstein suggests a different response to scepticism, which turns on the point that: 'a doubt about existence only works in a language-game. Hence that we should first have to ask: what would such a doubt be like?, and don't understand this straight off.' (§24). Thus Wittgenstein's suggestion for how to respond to scepticism is to argue that any doubts, whether practical or sceptical, requires a context to give it its meaning.

Wittgenstein on ordinary doubts

In fact the main theme of *On Certainty* is not the problem of scepticism but charting the context of *ordinary* knowledge claims and expressions of doubt. Our knowledge claims and our doubts form a *system*. Without this context they would not have any clear meaning.

> All testing, all confirmation and disconfirmation of a hypothesis takes place already within a system. And this system is not a more of less arbitrary and doubtful point of departure for all our arguments: no, it belongs to the essence of what we call an argument. The system is not so much the point of departure, as the element in which arguments have their life.   (§105)

Wittgenstein also calls this system a 'picture of the world' that members of a community largely share. But we do not as individuals arrive at such a world picture by satisfying ourselves of its correctness. 'No: it is the inherited background against which I distinguish between true and false.' (§94). Thus the suggestion is that in order to test or check a claim just such a background is required to provide the ground rules for empirical inquiry. Thus the background itself cannot as a whole be checked for its truth.

Five other features of this background are important:

1. It comprises a motley of different sorts of 'claims'. Moore's example that 'this!' is a hand is one. Others include the claim that the earth existed long before my birth; that my name is such and such; that I have never been to the Moon. So if these claims are taken to express a kind of foundation for empirical inquiry, it is not a traditional view of foundations within philosophy. Traditionally, these have been construed as an

homogeneous class of claims about my own mental states, experiences, or appearings in my visual field.

2. There is some difficulty in characterizing our epistemic attitudes to the 'claims' that comprise the background. They are typically *not* claims we make. Contra Moore we do not *know* that 'this is a hand' because it not the sort of thing we could doubt or provide grounds for. Neither are they beliefs or assumptions. Rather they are certainties expressed by our *actions*. Thus for example, we do not *assume* that we have feet when we stand up, but our animal certainty here is expressed in our lack of tentativeness in standing. 'In the beginning was the deed' (§402).

3. As the point above suggests, Wittgenstein separates the concepts of knowledge (and doubt etc.) from that of certainty. He argues that there is symmetry between knowledge and doubt. We can only claim to know what it would also make sense to doubt. This is because both belong to a 'language-game' or linguistic practice of asking for and giving reasons. Certainty, by contrast, characterizes the necessary background for that practice. It is the mark of what lies at the edge of empirical inquiry and is not called into question. Certainties 'lie apart from the route travelled by enquiry' (§88).

4. Just as the background comprises a motley of different sorts of matters that are taken as certainties, so too the limits of reasonable empirical inquiry is taught by example. This is another case where the rationality comprising empirical inquiry resists codification as a theory. We do not have a theory about what can and cannot be doubted. 'We do not learn the practice of making empirical judgements by learning rules. We are taught *judgements* and their connexion with other judgements. A *totality* of judgements is made plausible to us.' (§140).

5. While the systematic background or picture of the world is a prerequisite for empirical testing, elements of it can be called into question. 'The mythology may change back into a state of flux, the river-bed of thoughts may shift. But I distinguish between the movement of the waters on the river bed and the shift of the bed itself; though there is not a sharp division of the one from the other.' (§97).

One application of Wittgenstein's account of knowledge and certainty in psychopathology has been the idea that delusions share many of the features of Moore propositions (their central role in reasoning; the fact they stand fast; their imperviousness to argument etc). (See, for example, Campbell, 2001.)

Wittgenstein on induction

More so than many of his works, the notes published in *On Certainty* are more descriptive than argumentative. Wittgenstein offers the account as a proposed description of our epistemic practices without providing a watertight case that it *must* be true. (There are some arguments: such as the argument that the giving

of reasons must terminate somewhere if inquiry is to be possible at all.) But it remains a plausible account to combine with McDowell's attempt to defuse scepticism discussed above. What, then, does Wittgenstein say about induction? Here are some (about half) of his explicit comments:

Have we in some way learnt a universal law of induction, and do we trust it here too?—But why should we have learnt one *universal* law first and not the special one straight away?   (§133)

But do we not simply follow the principle that what has happened will happen again (or something like it)? What does it mean to follow this principle? Do we really introduce it into our reasoning? Or is it merely a natural law which our inferring apparently follows? This latter it may be. It is not an item in our considerations.   (§145)

The squirrel does not infer by induction that it is going to need stores next winter as well. And no more do we need a law of induction to justify our actions or our predictions.   (§287)

I might also put it like this: the 'law of induction' can no more be *grounded* than certain particular propositions concerning the material of experience.   (§499)

Wittgenstein's suggestion is, in other words, that searching for a justification for a law of induction marks a misunderstanding of the role that induction plays in our epistemic practices. Reasoning from past experiences is taught by example in particular cases. We are not first taught a universal law as a piece of knowledge (for which reasons might thus be offered). Rather we are trained in drawing inferences from past experiences as a taken for granted, unquestioned and certain practice.

Furthermore, given practical certainty expressed in our reasoning from past experiences, nothing *could* be offered to ground the law of induction as it is as certain as anything that might be offered in support of it. 'When one says that such and such a proposition can't be proved, of course that does not mean it can't be derived from other propositions; any proposition can be derived from other ones. But they may be no more certain than it is itself.' (§1).

Endgame?

If Wittgenstein's account is correct then despite its fundamentally different aim and feel to the philosophy of science accounts in the previous session, it does reinforce a general moral. Empirical testing must take place against a background that is not simultaneously called into doubt. Of course, elements of that background can be called into question when the 'river-bed of thought' shifts. But any testing requires that some things are not called into question and are instead held certain. This view of science sometimes summarized in Otto Neurath's (1932) metaphor: a boat whose planks have to be replaced one by one even while it is afloat.

What Wittgenstein's discussion especially reinforces in Lakatos' (1970) and more especially Kuhn's (1970), Barnes' (1974), and Bloor's (1976) accounts is the practical and piecemeal character of what is held certain. This includes the way in which we learn from experience: both in the case of direct perception (to recapitulate the subject of Chapter 12) but also, the subject of this chapter, in the case of drawing general conclusions from finite past experience. What does and does not count as good evidence is not grounded on a general context-free method—as Hume suggests in setting up the challenge to justify a general method of induction—but in particular judgements we learn to make. This general claim will also apply to the evidence appealed to in EBM, as we will see in the next session.

Reflection on the session and self-test questions

Write down your own reflections on the materials in this session drawing out any points that are particularly significant for you. Then write brief notes about the following:

1. What is the main difference between philosophy of science responses to the problem of induction and epistemological responses?

2. How does Mellor attempt to defuse the problem?

3. How does McDowell's response differ from Mellor's?

4. What does Wittgenstein add to our understanding of knowledge?

Session 4 Evidence-based medicine and clinical trials

This chapter has so far examined conflicting responses to the problem of induction within two different philosophical traditions: the methodologically orientated philosophy of science and the more analytically orientated tradition of philosophical epistemology.

One key lesson from the philosophy of science was that there is at least debate about whether evidence is deployed in science to confirm or to refute theories. But more importantly, however evidence is used, any realistic account of scientific research has to stress a top-down influence of theory on evidence as well as a bottom-up dependence. Evidence is gathered in the context of broader theoretical structures—perhaps Lakatosian research programmes or Kuhnian paradigms—and these have a profound influence on the interpretation of evidence.

The key lesson from the branch of philosophy called epistemology was that the apparent profound difficulties with induction outlined by Hume stem from a particular intuitive but nevertheless misleading understanding of knowledge. More contemporary accounts suggest that knowledge is not a matter for one individual to ensure through a process of argument from scratch, as Descartes famously assumed. Instead to have knowledge depends on in part on factors outside an individual's control. An important example of this is the acquisition of knowledge

second hand through the testimony of others. This suggests that EBM should also not be assumed to be an individualistic project.

This final session will return to the concrete issue with which the chapter began: the growth of EBM in psychiatry.

Evidence-based medicine, science, and the philosophy of science

The key aim of EBM is to optimize learning from past experience so as to draw conclusions about future treatment options. It thus aspires to the practical codification of good inductive strategies. These centre on the use of research based on clinical trials. In this session we will look at how the philosophy discussed so far in this chapter and the topics discussed in previous chapters touch on the kind of evidence available for EBM.

The purpose of this discussion is not to criticize the application of EBM approaches to psychiatry in general. This reiterates the moral of this part of the book, which has examined what is involved in being a science. In so doing it has criticized intuitive but oversimple models of science, but it has not been antiscientific. The moral has been rather different: that the form of rationality exemplified by good scientific practice cannot be codified in simple models or mechanical principles. This is not to say that there is no place for general principles such as: 'favour simple explanations'; 'do not multiply entities needlessly'; 'favour generality'; 'pay attention to the evidence'; 'do not abandon a theory too soon in the face of anomalies'; etc. But the conflicting demands of these principles need to be weighed up together. They do not amount to an abstract model of scientific method.

In a similar way, then, the purpose of this session is not to criticize the very idea of EBM but to bring out the fact that behind simple formulations of it lurk principled complexities. These are especially important in the case of the application of EBM to psychiatry.

Trials and treatments: Mill's methods

Look again at a standard EBM hierarchy of evidence taken from Geddes and Harrison (1997).

1a Evidence from a meta-analysis of RCTs

1b Evidence from at least one RCT

2a Evidence from at least one controlled study without randomization

2b Evidence from at least one other quasi-experimental study

3 Evidence from non-experimental descriptive studies, such as comparative studies, correlation studies and case–control studies

4 Evidence from expert committee reports, or opinions and/or clinical experience of respected authorities.

EBM places considerable weight on research findings arrived at through clinical trials, in particular, through *randomized* clinical trials and meta-analyses of these trials. These are at the top of the list. At the bottom is a more traditional view of medicine: respect for authority. The list suggests that meta-analysis of RCTs provides a better way of learning from experience than consulting an authority. And this prompts a question: How do we know that the one is better than the other? More specifically why should we think that such trials are a reliable method of discovering causal connections between, for example, treatments and results.

There seem to be two possible answers to this question.

♦ *Either*, there is an a priori argument to show what method should be at the top of the list.

♦ *Or*, it is a matter of empirical discovery. But if so, how is the evidence for the issue marshalled?

To get a feel for this question we will consider a brief introduction to clinical trials set out in a typical textbook: S.J. Pocock, *Clinical Trials: a practical approach* (1983).

Clinical trials as experiments

Pocock states baldly that a clinical trial is a planned experiment (on patients with a medical condition). The further constraints that Pocock places on good clinical trials refine this thought, but the underlying connection between clinical trials and experiments remains. So a clinical trial is a particular type of experiment designed to provide evidence for some form of clinical hypothesis or theory.

The methodology of clinical trials

In a chapter of the reading called 'Controlled clinical trials and the scientific method' (p. 4) Pocock sets out a summary of the scientific rationale for a standard kind of clinical trial. These are comparative trials in which a (normally new) treatment is compared with other existing treatments in accordance to a specific and rigorous research method. (Pocock labels these 'phase III trials'.)

Pocock specifies a number of features of such trials:

1. They should be comparative. The experiences of patients on the treatment under trial are compared with a control group: the experiences of patients on other treatments (possibly including no treatment).

2. They should be randomized. This is supposed to prevent conclusions being drawn about the effects of drug treatments, for example, which are really the effects of some other uncontrolled for factor present in the sample.

3. They should, wherever possible, be double blind trials. Neither the patients nor the clinicians testing results should know whether they belong to the test group or control group.

Aside from these general features, Pocock claims that clinical trials should proceed through a predetermined series of steps 'if the principles of scientific method are to be followed' (p. 5). Those steps are:

1. Define the purpose of the trial: state specific hypotheses.

2. Design the trial: a written protocol.

3. Conduct the trial: a good organization.

4. Analyse the data: descriptive statistics, tests of hypotheses.

5. Draw conclusions: publish results.

Data gathering and theory

It is significant that neither the third step: 'conduct the trial' nor the fourth step 'analyse the data' make any reference to the further complexities involved in the idea of experimental data: direct theory free reports of how the world is found to be. As Chapter 12 argued, the very making of observations and forming of observation statements is itself charged with theory.

What is the foundation for randomized-controlled trials?

But there is a different question about the claim that these are just the steps that a clinical trial should follow if it is to be scientific. Consider, for example, whether the claim is *analytic*. Does it follow from the very meaning of the phrase 'scientific method'? And if it is not, what sort of claim is it? Is it a description of scientific method as it is usually carried out, or a prescription on how it *should* be carried out? If the latter, what argument or process of reflection leads to just these steps?

What should be obvious is that these steps could not have been arrived at purely by a priori reasoning. While, for example, anyone with experience of carrying out scientific research will be able to think of advantages in having a *written* protocol for experimental design, these reasons are founded in an understanding of human memory and communication. One can imagine other circumstances in which such written record would be unnecessary or even useless. Think of a culture with a strong aural tradition who were also plagued by dyslexia. So the steps identified are plausible rules for good conduct distilled from practical experience. But it would be rash to construe them as *the* Scientific Method, where that is construed as timeless, universal, and context-free.

(Recall in Chapter 13, Bernard Williams's invocation of scientific method as a way of making sense of his Absolute Conception of the world. McDowell argued that such an attempt was bound to fail because the very idea of the scientific method was either too vacuous (if it simply meant the best way to arrive at empirical truths) or itself too parochial to ground an absolute conception of the world, a view expressive of no particular perspective. If these rules governing clinical trials are construed as the scientific method, it is a very *local* construal of that method.)

This suggests that the author has based the list of steps on experience (his and others') of successful clinical trails rather than a priori reasoning. But if so this raises an interesting question akin to Hume's problem of induction. *How* should one learn from such experience? How can experience of the results of scientific methods themselves properly inform scientific method? This leads to an obvious suggestion: one should compare different methods of gathering data to determine the most reliable method. In other words, one should carry out a randomized control trial to determine the efficacy of just this sort of RCT. Clearly, however, this will beg a question because it will involve a prior assumption that RCTs are a reliable method of gathering data.

This line of thinking repeats an idea found in earlier readings in this chapter, especially those by Lakatos (1970), Kuhn (1970), and Wittgenstein (1969). Theory testing—in this case hypotheses about treatment efficacy or the aetiology of illnesses—can only take place against a background of other theories, hypothesis, and assumptions, which are not themselves simultaneously called into question. This background includes theories about the correct working of instruments. It involves methodological principles about how best and how often to take readings. But it also includes methodological assumptions about the efficacy of clinical trials. Now of course, this is not to say that the methodology of clinical trails in general could not itself be subject to testing. But it *is not* subject to testing in the course of routine medical trails. And testing it would require that other assumptions were held certain. This suggests that clinical trials are not so much the foundation of medical science but part of a fallible holistic and interdependent system that has no eternally fixed foundations.

We suggested earlier that there might be two approaches to the question: how should we determine what should lie at the top of the EBM evidence hierarchy? One answer is that we can find out from experience what the best of learning from experience is, which leads to a kind of circularity. The other approach is by developing a priori arguments. To see how such an argument might be begun at least consider the following intellectual tools drawn from the history of philosophy.

EXERCISE 10 (20 minutes)

Look at the statements of Mill's 'method of agreement' and 'method of difference' taken from J.S. Mill (1879) *A System of Logic*, chapter VIII, pp. 448–471:

The method of agreement

If two or more instances of the phenomenon under investigation have only one circumstance in common, the circumstance in which alone all the instances agree, is the cause (or effect) of the given phenomenon. (p. 451)

The method of difference

If an instance in which the phenomenon under investigation occurs, and an instance in which it does not occur, have every circumstance in common save one, that one occurring only in the former; the circumstances in which alone the two instances differ, is the effect, or the cause, or an indispensable part of the cause, of the phenomenon. (p. 452)

◆ What do they achieve?

◆ To your knowledge, how do they relate to clinical testing?

◆ What is their status and foundation (e.g. a priori or a posteriori) as methodological prescriptions?

The method of agreement and the cholera outbreak of 1854

Mill outlines five experimental methods, which he suggests underpin experimental inquiry. These are:

1. The method of agreement
2. The method of difference
3. The joint method of agreement and difference
4. The method of residues
5. The method of concomitant variations

It is worth reflecting on the applicability of these to clinical scientific research. We will pick out two. The method of agreement is stated: 'If two or more instances of the phenomenon under investigation have only one circumstance in common, the circumstance in which alone all the instances agree, is the cause (or effect) of the given phenomenon. (p. 451).

Now as a model of clinical research, the method of agreement is of limited use. One example that approximates to it was the work done by John Snow (1813–58) a member of the Royal College of Surgeons of England. After an outbreak of cholera in 1854, Snow investigated the spread of the disease by mapping its victims in London. He discovered that the key common element in each case was that the victims had drunk water from a particular well. After officials followed Snow's advice to remove the handle of the Broad Street Pump, the epidemic was contained.

But this is only an approximate application of the Method of Agreement. The method proper requires that the only condition that a variety of experimental cases have in common turns out to be the cause of the (controlled for) effect in question or, vice versa, is the effect of the cause in question. Clearly, the practical difficulties of picking a trial sample who were alike in only one respect would be enormous. But on further reflection this is really a principled problem because there is no limit to the number of (e.g. relational) properties that an individual (a human or simply a thing) has. All human subjects, for example, share the property of being in the earth's gravitational field, of being in this part of the galaxy, of being bigger than a pea, etc.

The method of difference

The method of difference, however, is a better model for clinical research. It is defined thus:

If an instance in which the phenomenon under investigation occurs, and an instance in which it does not occur, have every circumstance in common save one, that one occurring only in the former; the circumstances in which alone the two instances differ, is the effect, or the cause, or an indispensable part of the cause, of the phenomenon. (p. 452)

Mill suggests that the conditions for this method are rarely spontaneously met in nature as they require that two circumstances are exactly the same except for one feature. But they can be met experimentally. Mill suggests introducing a new phenomenon to a situation—perhaps by physically moving a substance—yields just this sort of pair of circumstances. Mill warns, however, that the method of bringing about a change might itself constitute an important difference from the initial circumstance.

The method of difference and clinical trials

The method of difference also forms a plausible model of much clinical research. As we have seen, clinical trials are generally contrastive. The effects of a drug on one trial group are compared with the effects of no such treatment (in fact generally a placebo) on another 'control' group. If the one group is treated in the same way as the other in all respects other than the administration of the drug, then the subsequent differences are the causal result of the drug treatment.

What the methods achieve

But what do these methods achieve? Mill describes them as methods of *eliminative* induction. This contrasts with the Humean idea of enumerative induction: building up generalizations from particular cases. Mill's methods are negative: they aim at eliminating conditions as irrelevant to cause–effect relations. They resemble falsificationism. Thus the method of agreement is a method of eliminating conditions from a list of conditions that are necessary for another condition, an effect, for example. (Any conditions that are *not* present when the effect in question occurs cannot be *necessary* conditions of that effect.) The method can also be used to determine sufficient conditions. In this case, one looks for those conditions that are *never* present when an effect is absent. (If a condition is present when an effect is absent then it cannot be sufficient for that effect.) Thus one slowly eliminates conditions from a list of potential sufficient conditions.

The method of difference provides a way of eliminating conditions that are not sufficient for an effect from some overall circumstance that is sufficient, i.e. when the effect is present. (Any factors that are present when an effect in question is not present cannot themselves be sufficient for that effect.) Now there may be many different sufficient conditions, but the method of difference is a way of paring down some complex combination, which is itself sufficient to find out which parts of it are not sufficient.

What the methods do not achieve

What should be clear is that these methods do not engage with Hume's problem. Mill assumes that there are law-like relations between conditions in nature such that some conditions are necessary and some sufficient for others. This assumption presupposes a positive response to Humean scepticism. But after the work of the last session, that is reasonable to make.

Mill's methods provide models for determining causal connections, models that can be arrived at a priori. But they are, however, overly simplified models of empirical research. They cannot provide an a priori argument for the EBM evidence hierarchy.

Think again of the criticism of the method of agreement above. It is impossible to ensure that different complex circumstances have nothing (except a condition under scrutiny) in common. Likewise in the case of the method of difference it is impossible to ensure that two different circumstances are identical in all but one respect. (If they are different, are they in different places, for example?) However, it is possible to ensure that nothing *causally relevant* is the same in the former case or different in the latter case. This suggests that Mill's methods cannot play a foundational role, a role that presupposes no other causal knowledge. Rather, in accordance with the argument drawn from the philosophy of science in the second session, the role of Mill's methods lies within a background of other fallible prior scientific beliefs about what causes what. They are a further constraint on our causal knowledge.

A further way of bringing this out is to consider Mill's use of letters to label different conditions (antecedent conditions A, B, C, etc. and succeeding conditions a, b, c, etc.). One of his critics, the philosopher of science William Whewell, wrote: 'Upon these methods, the obvious thing to remark is, that they take for granted the very thing which is most difficult to discover, the reduction of the phenomena to formulae such as are here presented to us.' (*Of Induction, With Especial Reference to Mr J Stuart Mill's System of Logic*, 1849, p. 44).

Mill simply assumes that we already possess, when searching for causal factors, a complete description that captures all the causally relevant factors. Given this, then elimination of irrelevant factors is comparatively easy. But from where did this vocabulary arise? As the readings in the second session above emphasized, it is a matter of much greater complexity than simply reading off inductive generalizations from the world.

Both of these points can be translated in to the context of mental health to raise yet further practical difficulties. Establishing conditions as the same in all but one respect (in the Method of Agreement) or different in all but one (Method of Difference) is difficult enough in the case of physical medicine, but establishing these cases for psychiatric conditions is even more difficult. To mention just one reason: psychiatric symptoms are rarely present in isolation but are combined in ways that are not exactly repeated between different patients. Weakening the requirement to that of causal relevance (as mentioned above) does not help. Likewise, the prospect of reducing a description of the state of individuals' mental lives to the letters illustratively used by Mill is grossly artificial.

The status of the evidence-based medicine evidence hierarchy

While some arguments can be given for the efficacy of clinical trials, experimental methods are themselves subject to scientific reasoning and experiment. They are thus subject to the same boot-strapping that has been an implicit theme of this part.

A proper understanding of scientific research and a better model of knowledge helps put the nature of EBM in context. We will finish this chapter with some reflections on the connections between EBM and other matters in this part and the next.

Evidence-based medicine and the theory dependence of observation

First, there is the application of the theory dependence of observation to the gathering of data in clinical trials. Chapter 12 discussed arguments to the effect that no principled separation of theoretical and observational claims was possible. Observation is always theoretically charged. In the context of this session this can be related to Whewell's (1849) criticism of Mill's methods. A clinical trial is only possible against a background of assumptions of what is and is not causally relevant, of what the best descriptions of effects are and so on. Not every feature of a trial can be attended to, controlled for or even described. And what is described, is described according to prevailing theory. Thus, to repeat a claim made earlier in this chapter, trials cannot be seen as methods of simply harvesting data for subsequent interpretation but instead have their role in a context already charged with theory.

Evidence-based medicine and natural classifications

Given that no principled separation of theory and observation is possible, there is no hope for thinking of descriptive psychotherapy as a purely descriptive enterprise that can escape assumptions about the underlying mental structures. Some such assumptions must form at the very least an implicit element of psychiatric classification and thus be presupposed in those clinical trails that pertain to mental health. This in turn raises a further question about the nature of evidence here. As we saw in Chapter 13, some clinicians and philosophers have argued both that there is an evaluative element to psychiatric diagnosis, which is found in neither physical science descriptions nor physical medicine and, further, that this implies that such classifications are not natural. They do not carve nature at its joints. As we saw in Chapter 13, there are arguments against the second, metaphysical, claim. But on the other hand, there is reason to be pessimistic in the assessment that classifications can be said to be natural.

Evidence-based medicine and tacit knowledge

This theme was further reinforced by consideration of psychiatric diagnosis in Chapter 14. Discussion of the nature of both explanation and replication in the physical sciences suggested an important role for tacit knowledge. It seems plausible, however, that a science of the mind must contain further elements of tacit or implicit knowledge. There are arguments that in this case diagnosis involves an overall judgement of a client's state of mind, which resists breaking down into component symptoms. These can only be identified in the context of the overall judgement. If this is so, then diagnosis is uncodifiable. It suggests in turn that the evidence available in EBM will turn on an important element of clinical judgement even though this is not explicit in bald reports of clinical data.

Evidence-based medicine, reasons and causes or laws

Why this might be so was explored further in Chapter 15. In addition to tracking down the causal aetiology of mental ill-health, psychiatry is also concerned to track meaningful relations among the causes and symptoms of conditions. But given arguments that the logical space of reasons and causes or, less question-beggingly, laws are not isomorphic, this suggests that the two aims are complementary rather different aspects of an underlying science.

Conclusions

The previous chapters have suggested that despite the attractions of a certain simple picture of science, which was further developed and given philosophical credibility by the Logical Empiricists, in reality, scientific method is necessarily more complex and resists simple codification as a recipe. In the context of EBM, the same general moral applies. There is no simple account of how evidence can be marshalled. But an awareness of the necessary complexities provides a vaccination against the dangers of assuming that there is.

In fairness, in the reading at the start of this chapter (linked with Exercise 1), Geddes and Harrison (1997) emphasize some of the complexities in the process of applying the results of clinical trails in practical clinical contexts. Thus although they argue that, ideally, treatment options should be based on evidence of effectiveness from a source as high up the list of favoured forms of evidence as possible, they also point out that the evidence of clinical trials has also to be *relevant* to the case at hand. So a further assessment has to be made of whether the subjects involved in the trial are a close enough match for the actual patient. Subjects in trials may be all of the same sex and they may be less likely to have only a single medical condition. However, what should also be pointed out is that complexities do not simply affect the practical application of such clinical findings, but also the scientific process of arriving at findings in the first place.

Thus a proper understanding of EBM plays up rather than plays down the need for critical judgement in assessing evidence. Here as throughout Part III there is a key role for the subjects engaged in scientific psychiatry to exercise skilled judgement in a way that is only ever partly codifiable.

To evidence-based medicine add values-based medicine

EBM, then, properly understood, is not a practical counterpart of the philosophers' logical positivism. It is an attempt to respond positively to the ever (and exponentially) expanding knowledge base of decision-making in health care by a reflective and methodologically formalized, approach to distilling the best available explicit evidence from the research literature.

EBM has of course been widely attacked by practitioners. Such attacks, to the extent that EBM claims, or has claimed for it by others, hegemony in health-care decision-making, are fully justified. But that there are problems with current EBM methodologies would be a poor reason to abandon the whole thing—no more should the 'problems' with (all) current scientific theories, indeed with the scientific method itself, suggest that we abandon science! Future EBMs like future sciences, informed by conceptual, methodological, statistical and other advances, and by growing experience, will be more sophisticated.

An even worse reason for abandoning the whole thing (EBM) would be that EBM itself, to the extent that it is concerned only with explicit knowledge, is an *incomplete* response to the growing complexities of the knowledge base of decision-making in health care. Our understanding of implicit knowledge, of the 'craft' knowledge of those with practical experience, is less well developed even than our understanding of explicit knowledge. However, developments in 'narrative-based-practice' (Greenhall & Hurwitz 1998), for example, and the potential resources of a wide rage of empirical (qualitative), philosophical (e.g. phenomenological, hermeneutic) and literary (e.g. thematic analysis) methods (Fulford *et al.*, 2002), are all available to supplement, not supplant, the resources of EBM.

The worse reason of all for abandoning EBM, would be that, even to the extent that it combines implicit with explicit knowledge, it misses out altogether the values base (as distinct from the evidence base) of health-care decision-making. Value-judgements, as R.M. Hare's account of their meanings so translucently shows (Part I, Chapter xx) are made on the basis of criteria that are *factual* (or descriptive) in nature. Value-judgements have an action-guiding (or 'prescriptive', in Hare's (1952) account) element as well, of course. This is why decision-making in health care, as in any other area, is always values based as well as evidence based. Evidence alone is not enough to determine decisions. Decisions are determined by evidence weighted by values: in deciding between treatments, for example, we weigh the (*desired*) effects against (*unwanted*) side-effects, and both against *cost*; and in any real life scenario, the different elements of the decision, factual, evaluative and other, will often be intimately woven together in an (apparently) seamless tapestry (Fulford, 1989, chapter 12). However, the point is that, to the extent that a decision *is* values-based, the factual criteria for the value-judgements in question should reflect, like any other factual question in medicine, the best available evidence—evidence, then, which in the model sketched here, is derived in part from craft knowledge, but also, when available, from the resources of EBM.

There is no clearer statement of the interdependence of explicit evidence, implicit (or craft) knowledge, and values, than in the introduction to one of the classics of EBM itself, David Sackett and colleagues' (2000) highly regarded 'Evidence-Based Medicine: How to Practice and Teach EBM'. In their introduction (p. 1), Sackett *et al.* define EBM as follows:

> Evidence based medicine is the integration of best research evidence with clinical expertise and patient values.

> By *best research evidence* we mean clinically relevant research... New evidence from clinical research and treatments both invalidates previously accepted diagnostic tests and treatments and replaces them with new ones that are more powerful, more accurate, more efficacious and safer.

> By *clinical expertise* we mean the ability to use our clinical skills and past experience to rapidly identify each patient's unique health state and diagnosis, their individual risks and benefits of potential interventions, and their personal values and expectations

> By *patient values* we mean the unique preferences, concerns and expectations each patient brings to a clinical encounter and which must be integrated into clinical decisions if they are to serve the patient.

Much of their book, reflecting the focus of EBM itself, is concerned with the first of these, research evidence. But this focus only underlines the need for equivalently sophisticated approaches to the roles of clinical expertise (implicit knowledge) and of values in health-care decision-making. For it is only when 'these 3 elements are integrated', Sackett and colleagues continue, that 'clinicians and patients form a diagnostic and therapeutic alliance which optimizes clinical outcomes and quality of life.' We have considered some aspects of both explicit and implicit knowledge in this part of the book. It is to values that we now turn in Part IV.

Reflection on the session and self-test questions

Write down your own reflections on the materials in this session drawing out any points that are particularly significant for you. Then, thinking back over the chapter as a whole, write brief notes about the following:

1. How does the broader discussion of responses to induction impact on EBM?

2. What is the connection between Mill's methods and EBM?

3. How should the EBM hierarchy itself be assessed?

Reading guide

A thorough practical introduction to EBM is provided by Sackett (2000) *Evidence based medicine: how to practice and teach EBM*. Specifically in relation to psychiatry, see Geddes and Harrison (1997) and Geddes and Carney (2001).

Hume and the problem of induction

◆ Hume's philosophy is described in a number of introductions, including David Pears (1990) *Hume's System*, and Barry Stroud (1977) *Hume*.

◆ The problem of induction is thoroughly set out and a particular solution suggested in Howson (2000) *Hume's Problem: induction and the justification of belief*.

Philosophy of science response to the problem of induction

◆ The following all contain accessible introductions to falsificationism in its Popperian and Lakatosian versions and Kuhn's philosophy of science: Bird (1998) *The Philosophy of Science* (chapters 5 and 8); Chalmers (1999) *What is this thing called science?* (chapters 4–8); and Ladyman (2002) *Understanding philosophy of science* (chapters 3 and 4).

◆ Book length introductions include: Corvi (1997) *An Introduction to the Thought of Karl Popper*; Larvor (1998) *Lakatos: an introduction*; Bird (2001) *Thomas Kuhn*.

◆ The sociology of the natural sciences is further explored in: Barnes (1974) *Scientific Knowledge and Sociological Theory*; Bloor (1991) *Knowledge and Social Imagery*; Collins (1985) *Changing Order*; Latour and Woolgar (1992) *Laboratory Life: construction of scientific facts*; Latour (1987) *Science in Action: how to follow scientists and engineers through society*.

Epistemology

◆ Two good introductions to epistemology are: Williams (2001) *Problems of Knowledge: a critical introduction to epistemology*; Dancy (1985) *An Introduction to Contemporary Epistemology*.

◆ McDowell's account of knowledge is discussed in Thornton (2004) *John McDowell* (chapter 5).

◆ The best of several discussions of Wittgenstein's *On Certainty* is: McGinn (1989) *Sense and Certainty*; Geddes and Carney (2001) 'Recent advances in evidence-based psychiatry'; Geddes and Harrison (1997) 'Evidence-based psychiatry: closing the gap between research and practice.'

References

Barnes, B. (1974). *Scientific Knowledge and Sociological Theory*. London: Routledge.

Bird, A. (1998). *The Philosophy of Science*. London: Routledge.

Bird, A. (2001). *Thomas Kuhn*. Chesham: Acumen.

Bloor, D. (1976). *Knowledge and Social Imagery*. London: Routledge.

Bloor, D. (1991). *Knowledge and Social Imagery*. Chicago: Chicago University Press.

Bloor, D. (1997). *Wittgenstein, Rules and Institutions*. London: Routledge.

Brandom, R. (1998). Knowledge and the social articulation of the space of reasons. Philosopy and Phenomenological Research 55: 895–908.

Campbell, J. (2001). Rationality, meaning, and the analysis of delusion. *Philosophy, Psychiatry, & Psychology*, 8/2 (3): 89–100.

Chalmers, A. (1999). *What is This Thing Called Science?* Buckingham: Open University Press.

Collins, H.M. (1985). *Changing Order*. London: Sage.

Corvi, R. (1997). *An Introduction to the Thought of Karl Popper*. London: Routledge.

Dancy, J. (1985). *An Introduction to Contemporary Epistemology*. Oxford: Blackwell.

Fulford *et al.* in "Many Voices: Human Values in Healthcare Ethics" pp 1–19.

Fulford. K.W.M., Dickenson, D.L., Murray, P.H. (eds) in (2002). *Healthcare Ethics and Human Valves: An introductory Text with Readings and Case Studies*. Oxford: Blackwell.

Fulford, K.W.M. (1989, paperback 1995). *Moral Theory and Medical Practice*. Cambridge: Cambridge University Press.

Geddes, J.R. and Carney, S.M. (2001). Recent advances in evidence-based psychiatry. *Canadian Journal of Psychiatry*, 46(5): 403–406.

Geddes, J.R. and Harrison, P.J. (1997). Evidence-based psychiatry: closing the gap between research and practice. *British Journal of Psychiatry*, 171: 220–225.

Greenhalgh, T. and Hurwitz, B. (1998). Narrative Based Medicine: Dialogue and Discourse in Clinical Practice. London: BMJ Books.

Hare, R.M. (1952). *The Language of Morals*. Oxford: Oxford University Press.

Howson, C. (2000). *Hume's Problem: induction and the justification of belief*. Oxford: Clarendon Press.

Hume, D. (1975). *Enquiries Concerning Human Understanding and Concerning the Principles of Morals*. Oxford: Oxford University Press.

Kuhn, T.S. (1962). *The Structure of Scientific Revolutions*. Chicago: Chicago University Press.

Kuhn, T.S. (1970). Logic of discovery or psychology of research? In *Criticism and the Growth of Knowledge* (ed. I. Lakatos and A. Musgrave). Cambridge: Cambridge University Press, pp. 1–93.

Ladyman, J. (2002). *Understanding Philosophy of Science*. London: Routledge.

Lakatos, I. (1970). Falsification and the methodology of scientific research programmes. In *Criticism and the Growth of Knowledge* (ed. I. Lakatos and A. Musgrave). Cambridge: Cambridge University Press, pp. 91–195.

Larvor, B. (1998). *Lakatos: an introduction* London: Routledge.

Latour, B. (1987). *Science in Action: how to follow scientists and engineers through society* Cambridge, MA: Harvard University Press.

Latour, B. and Woolgar, S. (1992). *Laboratory Life: construction of scientific facts*. Princeton: Princeton University Press.

McDowell, J. (1994). *Mind and World*. Cambridge, MA: Harvard University Press.

McDowell, J. (1998). *Meaning, Knowledge, and Reality*. Cambridge, MA: Harvard University Press.

McGinn, M. (1989). *Sense and Certainty*. Oxford: Blackwell.

Mellor, D.H. (1991). The warrant of induction. In *Matters of Metaphysics*. London: Routledge.

Mill, J.S. (1879). *A System of Logic*. London: Longman.

Neurath, O. (1932). Protokollsaetze. *Erkenntnis*, 3: 204–214.

Pears, D. (1990). *Hume's System*. Oxford: Oxford University Press.

Pocock, S.J. (1983). *Clinical Trials: a practical approach*. Chichester: Wiley.

Popper, K. (1972). Conjectural knowledge: my solution to the problem of induction. *Objective Knowledge*. Oxford, pp. 1–31.

Sackett, D.L., Straus, S.E., Scott Richardson, W., Rosenberg, W., and Haynes, R.B. (2000). *Evidence-Based Medicine: how to practice and teach EBM*, (2nd edn). London: Churchill Livingstone.

Stroud, B. (1977). *Hume*. London: Routledge and Kegan Paul.

Thornton, T. (2004). *John McDowell*. Chesham: Acumen.

Whewell, W. (1849). *Of Induction, With Especial Reference to Mr J Stuart Mill's System of Logic*. London: Parker.

Wilkes, K.V. (1988). *Real People: personal identity without thought experiments*. Oxford: Clarendon Press.

Williams, M. (2001). *Problems of Knowledge: a critical introduction to epistemology*, Oxford: Oxford University Press.

Williams, D.D.R and Garner, J. (2002). The case against 'the evidence': a different perspective in evidence-based medicine. *British Journal of Psychiatry*, 180: 8–12.

Wittgenstein, L. (1953). *Philosophical Investigations*. Oxford: Basil Blackwell.

Wittgenstein, L. (1979). *On Certainty*. Oxford: Basil Blackwell.

Conclusions to Part III

One central lesson of Part V as a whole has been this. Although scientific practice is, rightly, taken to be a paradigmatic form of rationality, it resists codification in any simple overarching and context-free account of scientific method. Such codifications (starting with a traditional model of scientific progress in Chapter 11, the more precise formulations offered by the Logical Empiricists introduced in Chapter 12, running through realist prescriptions for classification in Chapter 13, models of explanation in Chapter 14 and of causal explanation in Chapter 15, and to more recent accounts of the methodology of science in Chapter 16) are all useful in different ways for drawing attention to central aspects of scientific practice. Gathering data through observation, devising reliable and hopefully valid classifications, framing explanations that invoke natural laws, positing underlying causal entities, and testing theories against the data and against one another, are again all key aspects of scientific rationality.

Time and again, however, the traditional relatively simple and intuitive models of these different aspects of scientific rationality, have been shown to be inadequate. The traditional models have been shown to be inadequate *in principle* in all areas of science. However, they have been shown to be inadequate also *in practice* in those areas of science, like theoretical physics and psychiatry, in which the problems with which the science in question is concerned are as much conceptual as empirical in nature. Complex sciences such as these require more complex models.

To take two examples of this increased complexity: there is something powerful about the idea (1) that explanation involves a kind of logical argument for the explanandum (see Chapter 14), and (2) that the mark of scientific theory is that it is falsifiable (see Chapter 16). But while both ideas are most attractive when put at their simplest neither is completely plausible until refined and made more complex and less simple. That does not imply that there is nothing to the idea of comparing scientific explanations to deductive arguments or thinking of refutation as a central virtue of a scientific (by contrast with pseudo-scientific) claim. However, it does suggest that the underlying simple idea can only be an approximation of actual science and thus has to be considered to be one of many competing scientific 'virtues' rather than an element in an algorithmic method for generating uniquely scientific discoveries about the way the world is.

A further, and related, lesson from Part V as a whole is the irreducible role of individual judgement and science. Thus, the attempt to provide a logical algorithmic recipe for scientific progress is motivated in part by the (entirely proper) attempt to minimize bias. Science aims to avoid any dependence on a 'cult of personality', an aim that is well exemplified by EMB's emphasis, as in its hierarchy of knowledge, on controlled trials rather than expert judgement or individual experience (Chapter 16). However, while replication, reliability, and so on are (again rightly) central aspects of science's claim to objectivity, validity, and truth, nevertheless the skills and abilities and, centrally, the individual good judgement of practicing scientists, clinicians, and others, refuse to be eliminated from a realistic account of how science actually works in practice.

Good judgement plays a central role in the practical aspects of scientific know-how where, indeed, one would expect craft skills and tacit knowledge to be at work. However, good judgement is also, and equally irreducibly, at work in epistemic contexts: in deciding, for example, whether an observation is sufficiently independent of a theory to count as supporting it (as in Chapter 12); in choosing between classifications for use in different contexts and different purposes (as in Chapter 13); in formulating an explanation in terms of law-like regularities (as in Chapter 14); in postulating underlying causal entities (as in Chapter 15); and, above all perhaps, when it comes to what counts as progress, in knowing (as in Chapter 16) whether to move on an established theory, i.e. because the research programme to which it is attached is 'degenerating', or to stick with the theory in question in the face of accumulating evidence against it.

These two lessons from Part V as a whole, the lesson of 'added complexity' and the lesson of 'irreducible judgement', it is important repeatedly to remind ourselves, have been drawn from a philosophy of science that has been focused primarily, not on the human sciences, such as sociology and psychology, but on the natural sciences, notably physics. The human sciences, the considerations of Part II suggest, add to the first of these two lessons, the lesson of added complexity, a whole extra layer of difficulty characterized, variously in such terms as meaning, reasons, empathy, and understanding. The specifically *medical* human sciences, the consideration of Part I suggest, add to the second of the two lessons, the lesson of irreducible judgement, a whole further layer of extra difficulty characterized, as in Part I, in terms of values.

Debate, as we have seen in this part, continues about the role of values in the natural sciences. In the next part of the book we explore the role of values in the specifically *clinical* judgements; these are an irreducible element of the model of science that is needed when we add to the complexities of a natural science at the cutting edge, like theoretical physics, the further complexities of the science that, we have argued in this part, is at the cutting edge of the human medical sciences, psychiatry.

PART IV

Values, ethics, and mental health

Part contents

Introduction to Part IV

The aims of this part of the book are:

1. to outline some of the key ideas about bioethics and medical law currently around in the literature;

2. to examine the strengths and weaknesses of these ideas especially in relation to mental health; and

3. to introduce the concept of Values-Based Practice (VBP).

The storyline of Part IV

Chapter 17 explores the conceptual depth dimension of mental health ethics. It begins with the observation that, rich and varied as modern bioethics has become, it has so far largely failed to engage effectively with mental health. There are many possible reasons for this, as we will see. It is certainly not due to any shortage of ethical issues in mental health, however! For ethical issues are at least as pervasive in mental health as in any of the more high-tech areas of medicine on which bioethics has traditionally tended to focus.

Ethical issues in mental health, on the other hand, as we will see in Chapter 17, *are* more complex conceptually. Correspondingly, therefore, a conceptually sharper set of ethical tools is needed to support clinical work and research in this area. Both types of tool, we should say straight away, the blunter and the sharper, are important in health care. It is just that we need both—much as we need a sharper set of tools for eye surgery and a blunter set for orthopaedic surgery.

Chapter 18 starts the process of developing the required sharper sets of tools. After an initial introduction to bioethics, including its historical origins (Session 1), we review a number of the tools for working with ethical and other values in health care, as derived respectively from bioethics itself (Session 2), and from philosophy, including both substantive ethical theories (such as utilitarianism and deontology) and analytic ethical theory (Session 3).

It is from analytic ethical theory, of the kind introduced in Part I, that Values-Based Practice (VBP), as a distinctive contribution to the sharper set of tools required for mental health ethics, is derived. VBP, as we describe in the final session (Session 4) of Chapter 18, is a set of theoretical ideas and clinical skills designed to support health care decision making where (as is the case particularly in mental health) wide differences of values are in play.

Chapter 19, titled 'It's the law!' repeats the storyline of Chapters 17 and 18 but focusing now on law rather than ethics. We show how the tools of legal analysis, which, like those of ethical analysis have been developed primarily in respect of bodily disorders, need to be sharpened up if they are to be applied effectively to the move (evaluatively) complex cases arising in mental health.

We illustrate the need for sharper tools, including those of VBP, particularly in relation to concepts at the interface between medicine and law, such as capacity. Again, the particular diversity of values in mental health will emerge as one important reason why sharper legal tools are needed particularly in this area of health care.

Chapters 20 and 21, the final two chapters of this part, complete the story by showing the particular need for a sharper set of tools for working with values in that heartland of the traditional medical-scientific model, classification and diagnosis.

Chapter 20 starts with a case history, that of a man called Simon. Drawing on the theory and methods developed in Part I of this book, the pivotal importance of values in psychiatric diagnosis is shown by the very different diagnostic interpretations placed on Simon's story by psychiatry's two major classifications, the *International Classification of Diseases* (ICD) and the *Diagnostic and Statistical Manual* (DSM). The remainder of Chapter 20 and most of Chapter 21 is then taken up with exploring the wider implications of Simon's story, first from the (somewhat downbeat) perspective of traditional bioethics, and then from the (considerably more upbeat) perspective of VBP.

CHAPTER 17

Tools of the trade: an introduction to psychiatric ethics

Chapter contents

Outline

Following the use-before-definition approach of Austin's 'philosophical fieldwork', as developed in Part I, this chapter starts more or less straight in with practical case examples. We ask you to think about real situations, either from your general knowledge of mental health, or from your own experiences if you are a user or provider of services, and then to review the story of Mr AB, the man with depression treated on an involuntary basis introduced in Chapter 2.

Drawing on Mr AB's story:

◆ *Session 1* of the chapter outlines the scope of ethics in health care generally, focusing on the role of philosophy in ethics training and on what the objectives of such training should be.

◆ *Session 2* goes deeper into mental health territory, illustrating with two examples—capacity and confidentiality—the particular *conceptual* difficulties raised by ethical problems in mental health.

With these conceptual difficulties in mind, we then introduce a series of case vignettes, all of which, like the story of Mr AB, are about involuntary treatment. Our responses to these vignettes are then unpacked in:

◆ *Session 3*, which gives an introduction to the role of mental health law and how it connects with the role of bioethics.

Finally, in a brief *concluding session*, we review some of the reasons for the relative neglect of mental health by bioethics. Behind this neglect, we argue, is the influence of the traditional fact-centred medical model. Correspondingly, therefore, the more complete fact + value model to which we came at the end of Part I, provides a basis for developing the sharper set of tools required for mental health ethics. It is to these tools as provided by various kinds of ethical theory that we turn in Chapter 18. We return to mental health law in Chapter 19.

Session 1 Ethical and conceptual issues in psychiatry: aims and objectives

Getting started: the story of Mr AB

Ethics courses often start with an introduction to ethical theory. In this section we will be starting from the other end, as it were, from practical issues.

Starting from practical issues underlines the importance of ethics in everyday clinical care—even the most hard-nosed medical scientist recognizes the importance of ethical issues nowadays. However, starting from practice is also important for certain kinds of philosophical theory, notably linguistic analysis, as we saw in Part I, but also casuistry, as we will see later in this part, in Chapter 18.

EXERCISE 1 (30 minutes)

This first exercise is in three parts:

1. Think of a few examples of situations raising ethical issues in mental health. Try to think of (or imagine) one or more actual case examples rather than thinking abstractly in terms of general issues. Relevant case examples may be from your own experience, as a user or provider of services, or in both capacities; or they may be from your general knowledge of mental health. Then,

2. Write down a brief synopsis of the circumstances of your case(s) and of the ethical issues arising. Finally,

3. Think whether the issues can be grouped together or classified under more general headings.

After you have finished this for yourself, you may want to look at one or more of the overviews of ethical issues in mental health given in the Reading Guide. See how far your examples coincide with those of others. Do you think there is likely to be general agreement on what counts as an ethical issue in mental health?

Many people find that they struggle initially to think of ethics 'cases'. They can think of *issues* readily enough—after all, the newspapers, let alone professional journals, are nowadays full of them. When it comes to everyday experience, however, whether as providers or as users of services, for much of the time the ethical aspects of what we are doing are very much in the background.

The story of Mr AB

For our own example, we will give a rather more extended version of the story of Mr AB from Chapter 2[1]. We will be referring to Mr AB's story several times in this chapter and the next. This is how it ran.

Mr AB, a 48-year old bank manager, came to the casualty department of his local hospital complaining of burning pains in his face and head. He had a letter from his general practitioner saying that she believed Mr AB had become seriously depressed.

Mr AB admitted that he had had episodes of depression in the past, and that during one of these he had made a sudden and nearly fatal suicide attempt. Although appearing to be depressed, he denied any such feelings now. He refused to let the casualty officer call his wife. The casualty officer tried telephoning the GP but she was out 'on call'. He then got Mr AB's home number from 'directory enquiries' and telephoned his wife. Mrs AB was very concerned, being unaware that her husband had gone to see their GP. She confirmed what the GP's letter said, that over 3–4 weeks her husband had become gloomy and preoccupied and had lost interest in his work. But she added that on the last occasion, when he had complained similarly of head and facial pains, he had made a sudden and nearly fatal suicide attempt. Mrs AB was very

---

[1] As noted in Chapter 2, Mr AB's story is based on one described in chapter 10 (pp. 187–188) of Fulford (1989), which is in turn based on that of a real person, but with biographical and other details changed.

concerned that her husband should not be allowed to leave the hospital, at any rate before she could get there.

The casualty officer then called the duty psychiatrist to see Mr AB. Although initially guarded and suspicious, Mr AB eventually came out with what was really troubling him—he had 'advanced brain cancer'. After a careful neurological examination, the psychiatrist explained to Mr AB that there were no signs of this, but Mr AB remained adamant. All he wanted was something for the pains and to be allowed to go home.

Mrs AB (who had by now arrived) repeated to the psychiatrist that she was very much afraid her husband was planning to kill himself. He was behaving as he had done before his previous suicide attempt. For his part, however, Mr AB still insisted that he would not stay in hospital. It thus seemed to everyone that there was no option but to admit him as an involuntary patient. He accordingly came into the ward on a 'section', and, after further tests, made a full recovery on antidepressant therapy over a period of 8 weeks.

Mr AB's story: an ethical issue?

Mr AB's story is not unusual. It is not a high profile dramatic ethics 'case' of the kind that figures so often in the media. As already noted, most people find it is easier, first off, to think of 'big issues' than of individual stories like Mr AB's. The issue, in Mr AB's case, is involuntary treatment. But in this particular case, involuntary treatment (although always contestable in principle) appears to many people to be justified. This is why, in the terms of much ethics teaching, Mr AB's story is not an ethics 'case': on the face of it, there is nothing in Mr AB's story with which most people would want to take issue.

None the less, as a story of involuntary treatment, closer inspection will show that Mr AB's story does indeed raise ethical issues, issues that as we will see by the end of this part, run very deep: through the varieties of ethical theory in this chapter, to philosophical value theory in the next, to legal theory in Chapter 19 (including such contested areas as capacity, rationality, and best interests), and, in Chapters 20 and 21, to some of the worst abuses of psychiatry for purposes of political control, abuses arising (in part) from the (largely unrecognized) influence of a traditional medical model in which diagnosis is assumed to be a value-free area of medical science.

As with Mr AB's case, then, so with much else that happens in mental health, behind the everyday and the ordinary lie ethical issues many and deep.

Why, then, are we relatively blind to these issues? Why do so many people have such difficulty, first off, to think of particular 'ethics cases' from their own experience?

EXERCISE 2 (10 minutes)

What can we learn from this difficulty? What is the significance of the fact that we tend to be relatively blind to the ethical aspects of our day-to-day experience.

Write down your ideas on this before going on, thinking particularly about the work we did in Chapter 4 on 'definition and use'.

The main point of Exercise 1 was, straightforwardly, to *raise awareness* of the pervasiveness of ethical issues in mental health as a first step towards tackling them. We will be coming back to this in a moment. It is important to recognize, however, first, that our relative blindness to the ethical (and more broadly evaluative) aspects of everyday practice is closely similar to the relative blindness to conceptual issues that we looked at in Chapter 4 when we were thinking about philosophical methods.

Thus, recall that as with the concept of time, we remain largely unaware of the complex meanings of high-level organizing concepts, including (in medicine) the concepts of illness and disease, so long as we are able to *use* them (as by and large in bodily medicine we *have* been able to use them) without difficulty.

Much the same, then, is true of ethical aspects of practice: Mr AB's story, although raising a whole series of ethical issues, is not an obvious 'ethics case' because it is not, for most people, ethically contentious. As with conceptual issues in medicine, furthermore, so with ethical issues: it is appropriate that they should be ignored by practitioners so long as they are practically unproblematic. The danger, again with ethical as with conceptual issues, comes only when we are lulled into a sense of false security and fail to recognize the difficulties when they are there.

The two kinds of blindness, then, ethical and conceptual, are closely similar, and, as we will see by the end of this part, in mental health at least, they are indeed but two sides of the same 'use *versus* definition' coin.

Common kinds of ethical issue

For the moment, though, raising awareness of ethical issues is important primarily to get us started—unless we are at least aware of ethical issues, we cannot even get started on the task of finding ways of tackling them. And in mental health, once the process of raising awareness is started, the issues are not only evident but of familiar kinds.

The general issue raised by Mr AB is about *consent to treatment* and the highly contested role of compulsion. We will be considering this in detail later. Other issues that may have been raised by your own cases include *confidentiality, professional–client* (and *interprofessional*) relationships, and problems of *resource allocation*. Such topics are among the staples of bioethics and there is a voluminous literature on all of them (see Reading Guide at the end of this chapter).

This, however, raises a further question. If much that we do in mental health, and indeed in health care generally, although raising ethical issues in principle, is relatively uncontentious in practice, why is there this voluminous literature at all? After all, until the closing decades of the twentieth century, medicine got along fine with slimline codes, such as the Hippocratic Oath (to which we return later in this part). So why the disparity? Why the big literature when so much of practice is prima facie ethically straightforward?

We will return to this question in Chapter 18, with one kind of answer to it at the start of the chapter (an ethics-based answer) and another (values-based) answer at the end. Here, though, rather than answering the question directly, we will take it as a prompt to think carefully about what role, if any, there is specifically for *philosophy* in relation to ethical skills in health care.

A role for philosophy?

So why *think*? Why, more particularly, think *philosophically*? Religion, politics, our parents, our community, may give us ethical standards. But what can philosophy, by its nature abstract and impersonal, contribute?

Philosophers manic and philosophers depressive

We looked at the outputs from philosophy in general in Chapter 6. Philosophers themselves, we found, have had very different takes on this, some depressive, others more manic. Bernard Williams, you will recall, was among the depressives: while noting the important contributions of history, psychology, sociology, and a wide range of other disciplines to ethics, he thought that philosophy, or at any rate analytic philosophy, had got too big for its boots (Williams, 1985). In respect of medical ethics, R.M. Hare, although very far from overplaying the role of philosophy, had a less jaundiced view than Williams: the discursive skills of the philosopher, he argued, may have a critically important contribution to make in medicine (Hare, 1993).

Still other philosophers, coming closer perhaps to the *ethos* of philosophy and mental health, have pointed out that bringing theory and practice together in ethics has been helpful for *both* sides. In an article that has rightly become a classic of the early medical ethics literature, the American philosopher Stephen Toulmin (1982), argued that ethical issues in medicine came in the nick of time for an ethical philosophy that had run itself into what at the time looked like a blind alley.

Toulmin has made a number of important contributions at the interface between philosophy and practice. Later in this chapter we will come back to his work on the importance of casuistry as a method of ethical reasoning. He was also one of the first (in recent philosophy) to emphasize the importance of abnormal mental states for work in general philosophy on the nature of mind (Toulmin, 1980).

A 'full-field' picture

We summed up the view we finally came to in Chapter 6, about the outputs from philosophy, in terms of Gilbert Ryle's metaphor of a 'logical geography'. Philosophy, we concluded, finding a middle ground between manic and depressive extremes, gives us a *more complete* picture of the complex meanings of the higher-level organizing concepts by which the logical geography of a subject is defined.

We called the more complete picture of the health-care concepts to which we had come by the end of Part I, a 'full-field'

picture. This full-field picture, we suggested, could be regarded as a more complete picture of the logical geography at least of mental health, to the extent that it incorporated on an equal basis the values emphasized by antipsychiatry (left half-field) as well as the facts emphasized by psychiatry (right half-field). Similar full-field pictures were evident also in Part II, in the importance of meanings as well as causes in Jaspers' psychopathology; and in Part III, in the re-engagement, at various levels and in different ways, of observer with observed and the central importance of forms of non-algorithmic judgement in late twentieth century science. In Part V the objections to an easy reductionism of mind to brain and of the space of reasons to the realm of law make up another full-field picture.

Similarly, then, it is to a more complete, full-field, picture that we will arrive in this part. Medical ethics, as we will see, although developing in its modern form originally as a response to the challenges of scientific and technological advances in medicine, has, as one of has put it elsewhere (Fulford *et al.*, 2002, p. 5), "taken on the colours of its enemy." Medical ethics became *bio*ethics. And bioethics, as it is now called, like *bio*medicine and *bio*technology, has assumed (tacitly) what in the terminology of Chapter 6, is a right-field model of medicine, a model in which science is central and ethics peripheral. The tools of bioethics, correspondingly, have been largely right-field tools, helpful in responding to the problems arising in high-tech areas of medicine, but not always appropriately applied to the less dramatic if deeper and more pervasive issues arising in mental health.

Philosophy, then, in mental health ethics, could help to deliver a full-field set of ethical tools, not of course by abandoning the right-field tools of traditional bioethics, but by adding to them an equivalent set of left-field tools.

Four intermediate objectives for ethics training in health care

What does a 'full-field set of tools' amount to in practice? We hope to have developed at least a component of one kind of answer to this question by the end of this part of the book (with the theory and practice of Values-Based Practice (VBP)). This book is, however, first and foremost a textbook, a resource for learning and teaching. So, first things first: What, exactly, should the objectives of ethics *training* in health care be?

Back to our cases

In much ethics training, whatever theoretical model is adopted (rights based, utilitarian, etc., as described below, in Session 2), the practical objectives are usually left implicit. It is assumed that in some general warm-hearted way ethics teaching must be 'good' for practice. So, again, what should our objectives be? We can ground our consideration of this question in the needs of practice by returning to the cases we considered in Exercise 1 above.

EXERCISE 3   (60 minutes)

This is a two-stage exercise:

Stage 1 (10 minutes)

Go back to your cases and select one of them to look at in more detail. The case in question may raise a dilemma, i.e. where you are torn about what to do; or it might be a disagreement, i.e. where there is a difference of opinion about what ought to be done.

◆ What contribution do you think training in ethics might make to resolving or at least tackling such dilemmas and disagreements?

◆ How might this improve clinical decision-making?

Stage 2 (50 minutes)

In developing a course in practice skills for medical students in Oxford (described more fully below), Tony Hope and Bill Fulford defined four key objectives for medical ethics teaching: (1) raising awareness; (2) changing attitudes; (3) increasing knowledge; and (4) developing thinking skills.

◆ To what extent are these objectives relevant to your own cases?

◆ More generally, if training in medical ethics achieves these objectives, how would this help to improve the way we deal with things in everyday practice, whether as users of services or as mental health professionals?

Intermediate objectives for ethics training

As indicated in Stage 2 of Exercise 3, in developing their course in 'Practice Skills' for medical students in Oxford, Hope and Fulford defined four practical objectives for medical ethics education. The Practice Skills course, which is described in Hope *et al.* (1996), was aimed at medical students who, typically, are overwhelmed with an enormous syllabus of technical skills and scientific knowledge. Ethics training for medical students thus has to have a very clearly defined practical rationale.

As Hope and Fulford (1994) describe elsewhere, the overall guiding aim of the 'practice skills' approach was to improve clinical practice by improving the skills of *application* of medical knowledge. This indeed is what 'practice skills' are, according to this model. They are the ethical, legal, and communication skills, which together with technical skills and clinical experience, support the application of medical knowledge in a clinical problem-solving approach to day-to-day practice. This guiding aim, however, is rather too general and long term to serve as an objective for ethics education. Hence, drawing on work in the philosophy of education, by John Wilson (1979), a colleague at the time in the Oxford Department of Education, Hope and Fulford developed the four more narrowly defined objectives listed in Exercise 3, as 'intermediate objectives'.

Awareness, attitudes, knowledge, and thinking skills, then, in medical ethics education, are four intermediate objectives on the road to the ultimate objective of improving practice. But how, and if so in what ways and to what extent, are these intermediate objectives helpful? We will consider each of Hope and Fulford's intermediate objectives for medical ethics education in turn, referring as appropriate to Mr AB. (Obviously you should be testing out what we say by reference to your own cases.)

Objective 1—raising awareness: the first word, not the last

We have already seen that raising awareness of ethical aspects of practice is important if only to get things underway. Increased awareness *per se*, however, is not always or inevitably a good thing—it could lead to indecisiveness, for example. So raising awareness of ethical issues, as Austin (in Chapter 4) said of linguistic analysis as a method for raising awareness of conceptual issues, although sometimes the first word is certainly not the last word. In ethics a whole range of further clinical skills besides raised awareness are certainly needed.

Becoming aware of an ethical issue, none the less, *is* a necessary first step to doing something about it. And ethical issues, once we reflect on them, are often more or less readily visible. Sometimes they are not, however. What about your own cases, then, in the exercise above? Were all the issues up front? In Mr AB's case, the most obvious ethical issue was to do with consent: he didn't want treatment (for depression); everyone else thought he needed it (we return to consent in detail later on). But what about confidentiality? Most people would say that the casualty officer was right to telephone Mr AB's wife; he might have been negligent if he had not; but this *is* a breach of confidentiality (albeit justified in the circumstances).

On a wider front, raising awareness is important in respect of the role of values generally in health care. We return to this towards the end of Chapter 18 when we move from ethics, traditionally understood, to Values-Based Practice (VBP). In the VBP model, raised awareness of values, particularly through greater attention to language use, is the first of four key areas of clinical skills supporting balanced clinical decision-making where different values are in play. (Raising awareness falls under Principle 6 of VBP, see Box 18.1, Chapter 18.). As we will see in Chapter 18, the training methods developed for raising awareness of values in clinical contexts draw directly on philosophers, such as J.L. Austin and R.M. Hare (see Part I) working in the awareness-raising tradition of linguistic analytic philosophy. There is thus a particularly close link here between analytic philosophical theory and everyday clinical practice.

Objective 2—changing attitudes: (a) cross-cultural perspectives

As an educational objective, changing attitudes is more contentious—which attitudes should be encouraged is itself an ethical issue! In most ethics teaching in health care it is assumed that it is important to move people towards more open and patient-centred attitudes respectful of autonomy. This is not incompatible with holding strong personal views on matters such as abortion, for example. It is, however, not a value neutral attitude. It is a liberal ethic in its own right that requires a non-judgemental attitude to other peoples' values, even if, in some cases, respect for your own values may mean encouraging a patient to get help from someone else.

Dependency: a new 'top value'?

Yet even autonomy, although so widely taken for granted as a value in North America and western Europe, is very far from being a universally acknowledged principle of medical ethics. The theologian and philosopher, Alastair Campbell (1994), for example, in the next reading (linked with Exercise 4), argues for 'dependency' rather than 'autonomy' as the foundation value for medicine. He notes that autonomy fits fairly comfortably with the acute 'heroic' medical situations with which bioethics has been particularly preoccupied. He argues, though, that the scope of medical ethics should be widened to include the less dramatic but far more pervasive issues arising in chronic illness and disability, including the infirmities of old age. In the following extract Campbell starts to set out the conclusions that he believes we should draw from widening the scope of medical ethics in the way he proposes.

EXERCISE 4

Read the extract from:

Campbell A.V. (1994). Dependency: the foundational value in medical ethics. In *Medicine and Moral Reasoning* (ed. K.W.M. Fulford, G.R. Gillett, and J.M. Soskice). Cambridge: Cambridge University Press, p. 184

Link with Reading 17.1

Note that Campbell is not arguing for autonomy to be abandoned. His point is that in being set up as a foundational value, autonomy has become, and risks becoming further, unbalanced as a basis for health-care decision-making.

- However, do you think the answer to this is, as Campbell suggests, to set up a countervailing value as the foundation of medical ethics?

Campbell's concern in this article is that the dominance of autonomy in bioethics will result in unbalanced approaches to policy and practice in health care. Campbell's careful presentation of the case for making dependency the foundational value in medical ethics is anything but unbalanced. The danger, though, if Campbell's candidate for 'top value' (dependency) were to be successful, is of decision-making becoming unbalanced in the opposite direction. The danger here, indeed, as we will find later in this part, is a general one—making any

one value the top value, risks unbalanced decision-making. Values-Based Practice (VBP), we will see in Chapter 18, is premised on the need for balanced decision-making were complex and conflicting values are in play.

Cross-cultural perspectives and a balanced view

The limitations of autonomy have been particularly emphasized in cross-cultural ethics. It is not only in cross-cultural contexts that clashes of values arise, of course: the rationale for VBP, as we will see in Chapter 18, is precisely that differences rather than agreement on values are the norm in health care. Individually, furthermore, as we noted above, even in respect of such widely recognized values as autonomy, there will come a point beyond which any one person will not be prepared to go, a point at which, as we say, we 'draw the line' in respecting someone else's wishes.

A cross-cultural perspective, however, gives a sharp reminder of just how parochial the 'givens' of any one society at any one period may be. Autonomy is a case in point. As a distinctively 'Western' value, autonomy sits uncomfortably with the values of societies in which family ties and the integrity of communities rate ahead of individual self-fulfilment. An authoritative expression of this concern is to be found in the work of the Egyptian psychiatrist, Ahmed Okasha. As a former Chair of the World Psychiatric Association's Ethics Committee (and subsequently WPA President), and also Head of the WHO Coordinating Center at Ain Shams University in Cairo, he is well placed to appreciate the tensions to which cross-cultural clashes of values give rise. He spells this out succinctly in the following reading (linked with Exercise 5). Note, by the way, that this reading is not from a specialist ethical or indeed cross-cultural journal, but from a core psychiatric update journal aimed at the needs of everyday practical psychiatry .

EXERCISE 5

Read the following extract from:

Okasha, A. (2000). Ethics of psychiatric practice: consent, compulsion and confidentiality. *Current Opinion in Psychiatry*, 13: 693–698. (Extract p. 694.)

Link with Reading 17.2

- Are there wider lessons here?
- Are there lessons from Okasha's cross-cultural reminder of the parochial nature of autonomy for your own cases?

In Mr AB's case, the importance of families, and of the interests of carers, are clearly evident in the casualty officer's decision to call Mr AB's wife. In an autonomy dominated ethic this has to be 'justified' (the term we used above) as a breach of confidentiality. In an ethic that seeks to balance autonomy against family and communitarian values, any need for justification runs the other way. As the work of Okasha and others has shown, in cultures that value families and communities before individuals, it would be considered entirely natural and appropriate to make every effort to contact the relatives of Mr AB in circumstances of this kind.

Cross-cultural knowledge and understanding, which starts from mutual respect, can thus help to provide what we will argue in Chapter 18 is an essential balance of values in clinical decision making.

Objective 2—changing attitudes: (b) a role for virtue ethics

Changing attitudes as an educational objective is relevant particularly to what are called 'virtue ethics'. Credit for the late twentieth century renewal of interest in virtue ethics goes particularly to the British-born American philosopher, Alasdair MacIntyre, in his *After Virtue* (1982). The virtues are dispositions to act in certain ethically approved ways. Thus, William F. May, for example, of the Southern Methodist University at Galveston in the USA, has developed a detailed list of the virtues on which health-care ethics training should concentrate (May, 1994). Besides the more obvious virtues, such as respect, honesty, justice, and benevolence, May discusses fidelity, prudence, discretion, perseverance, and humility. The latter virtues may sound distinctly out of place as objectives of medical education. Drawing, however, on what again may seem an unlikely source, biblical scholarship, May shows how such virtues, properly interpreted and understood, may help to secure patterns of health-care decision making that are fully responsive to patients' real needs and concerns.

You can get a flavour of the rich mix of theoretical depth and practical relevance in May's approach from the following passage (linked with Exercise 6): this is concerned mainly with the virtue of prudence but finishes with a reference back to a related discussion of discretion.

EXERCISE 6

Read the extract from:

May, W.F. (1994). The virtues in a professional setting. ch 7 in *Medicine and Moral Reasoning* (ed. K.W.M. Fulford, G.R. Gillett, and J.M. Soskice). Cambridge: Cambridge University Press, (Extract pp. 85–86.)

Link with Reading 17.3

♦ What do you think of the three elements of prudence that May derives from the 'Medievalists'? Their unfamiliar Latin names aside, they read as rather precise learning outcomes!

♦ In the second extract, consider May's account of the virtues with Mr AB (or your own cases) particularly in mind.

Many of May's 'healthcare virtues' we nowadays take for granted, assuming that they will be acquired through apprenticeship learning as part of our training in the health-care professions—justice, beneficence, and so forth, might come within this category.

Other virtues proposed by May are less obvious, but, in mental health at least, they are clearly important. From May's list, perseverance and humility, for example, as characterized by him, were clearly important to the proper management of Mr AB's depression. The casualty officer concerned showed just these virtues in this case, but had he been less conscientious (showing less perseverance), or had he adopted a more high-handed attitude (showing less humility), things might have turned out very differently.

Objective 3: increasing knowledge—from fancy to fact

Knowledge is a neglected but increasingly important aspect of ethics, especially in mental health. Traditionally, ethicists have sometimes been openly cautious about the role of facts in ethics: what *ought* to be done, it is felt, should not be a function of what as a matter of fact *is* done (Gillon, 1996).

There is clearly much good sense in this. It is after all one consequence of the Humean 'no ought from an is' on which we drew so extensively in Part I. The downside, though, is that the facts have too often been ignored in ethical thinking in favour of fancies. Ethical reasoning, in particular, has too often been based on little more than taken-for-granted intuitions about what people want, feel, fear, and so forth, rather than on what they *actually* want, feel, fear, and so forth.

We can unpack the traditional intuition-led approach to facts in ethics into two closely related assumptions: the first assumption is that we can judge accurately what other people actually *want*; the second is that we can accurately judge what other people would regard as *satisfying* their wants. Neither of these assumptions are warranted. People in general and health-care practitioners in particular, perform rather badly on both counts (see, e.g. the reading below, linked with Exercise 8, from Peter Campbell, 1996). It is important, therefore, to use whatever means are available to find out what it is that people really *do* want.

This is not to say that, as a professional, it is always right to go along with what one's client or patient wants (we tackle the issues raised by this in the context of involuntary psychiatric treatment later). But at least we should try to be clear about the views of those concerned rather than just assuming that we know what they want.

From providers' fancies to users' facts

The readings in Exercises 7 and 8 illustrate two very different ways of getting information about the views of the users of mental health services. There are of course many other relevant methods for increasing knowledge of values, including a key role for good communication skills. We give further examples of the range of approaches that can be taken to increasing knowledge in the Reading Guides to chapters 4 and 18.

EXERCISE 7   (45 minutes)

Read the two extracts from:

Marshall, M. (1994). How should we measure need? Concept and practice in the development of a standardised assessment schedule. *Philosophy, Psychiatry, and Psychology*, 1: 29–31

Link with Reading 17.4

In these extracts Marshall shows that a standardized schedule developed by professionals to assess the needs of people with long-term mental health problems failed to take account of the perspectives of the client group (users and carers) concerned.

As you read these extracts, think about:

1. Why health-care professionals should be so bad at judging their clients' values and needs, and

2. Why, in particular, mental health-care professionals should be so bad at this.

We will be considering these two questions again in the next exercise. The 'values blindness' of professionals is a key observation under-pinning the move from traditional bioethics (in this chapter) to VBP (in Chapter 18).

Max Marshall's (1994) paper, which came out in the very first issue of *Philosophy, Psychiatry, and Psychology*, describes the conceptual work underpinning his research on the assessment of need in people with long-term mental health problems. At the time of writing his article, Marshall was a research psychiatrist working in the Department of Psychiatry in Oxford. He began by using the then current 'gold standard', the MRC Needs for Care Assessment Schedule. However, he soon found that, although claiming to replicate best clinical practice, the MRC schedule gave results that failed to match clinical assessments of need, and that, crucially, this was because it failed to incorporate the values of service users (as in the first extract, pp. 29–30) and carers (as in the second extract, pp. 30–31).

As Marshall describes in his paper, the MRC schedule failed in this respect essentially because it was guided by a flawed understanding of the *concept* of need. The MRC Schedule tacitly adopted, in the terminology of Chapter 6, a traditional right-field model (recall Aubrey Lewis on insight (chapter 3) as having a view that coincides with that of the physician). The MRC Schedule failed to recognize that in *best* clinical practice, professionals, contrary to the 'privileged access' model of professional knowledge implicit in the traditional medical model, were in practice taking close account of the views of their clients.

Combining empirical with philosophical methods

It is worth noting that Marshall's study began as a conventional empirical research project. It was in order to tackle the conceptual difficulties he ran into, that he had to turn to philosophy. In developing his new assessment schedule, therefore,

he collaborated with an Oxford philosopher, James Griffin, who had worked on the concept of need (see for example, Griffin, 1990). This is why, although publishing his new schedule and empirical research in main line journals, Marshall spelled out the key *conceptual* innovations guiding his work in his paper in *Philosophy, Psychiatry, and Psychology* (Marshall, 1994).

The commentaries to Marshall (1994), respectively by the philosopher Roger Crisp (1994) and by a consultant psychiatrist working in learning disability, John Morgan (1994), reflected the twin clinical and philosophical roots of his work.

Values blindness as a linguistic delusion

Returning, then, to the questions raised in Exercise 6 above, one reason for the values blindness of health-care professionals is a conceptual reason, namely, the influence of the traditional fact-centred medical model.

That it should take the brightest and best from both psychiatry and philosophy to break the stranglehold on our thinking of the traditional medical model, even in respect of an overtly evaluative concept such as that of 'need', is perhaps a sobering thought. Wittgenstein, you will recall from Part I (chapter 6), called similar strangleholds on thinking in philosophy, linguistic illusions, and aptly so, given that the strangleholds he had in mind arose from philosophers having an incomplete or otherwise distorted picture of the meanings of the concepts with which they were concerned. But the stranglehold of the traditional medical model is perhaps in some respects more like a *de*lusion, in that, judged at least by the growing volume of first-hand accounts from service users and carers, it has turned out to be so particularly hard to break.

User perspectives

Peter Campbell, whose work is illustrated in the next reading (linked with Exercise 8, Campbell, 1996), was an early contributor to the service user literature in mental health. He brings to this literature the perspective of someone who has experienced a series of manic-depressive episodes. While presenting well-balanced views on the role of medication and other contentious aspects of medical psychiatry, Campbell makes clear the extent to which professionals often simply fail to understand the real needs and wishes of the service users and carers who are their clients.

EXERCISE 8   (45 minutes)

Read the extract on what 'users' want from mental health crisis services from:

Campbell, P. (1996). What we want from crisis services. Pages 180–183 In *Speaking Our Minds: an anthology* (J. Read and J. Reynolds). Basingstoke: The Macmillan Press Ltd for The Open University, (Extract pages 182–183)

Link with Reading 17.5

In this article, Campbell describes some of the specific wishes and needs reported by people in crisis: to have more control of their own crisis situation, to gain understanding of and from their crisis situation, to be treated with respect and dignity, and to have access to 24-hour non-medical services.

Peter Campbell's work is very far from the polemics of the early 'antipsychiatry' movement. To the contrary, he is careful to point out that there is much (including as already noted the need sometimes for medication) on which professionals and service users can agree. All the same, far too often there are gaps between the values of service users and professionals, gaps of which professionals, for their part, seem all too often unaware.

Just how wide such gaps may be becomes clear particularly towards the end of the second extract when Peter Campbell records his own first mental health crisis. At this time, he says, none of the key issues from his point of view were in any conventional sense 'medical' issues at all.

User and provider perspectives: a resource

Is it really so surprising, though, that professionals should be relatively blind to the values of their clients? After all, to be a professional is (among other things) to have expert knowledge. But a professional's expert knowledge is, (1) *general* (where people's values are often highly individual), and (2) itself *driven by* particular values (i.e. of the individual professional, and of the profession as a whole). This combination means that professionals, just in being professionals, are at risk of drawing unwarranted conclusions about their client's values. And in the case of mental health, this risk is aggravated by the fact that, as we saw in Part I, mental health differs from other areas of health care precisely in that people's values in this area are *particularly* diverse. In mental health, then, the professional must become more aware, not only that the values of the client may be different from what he or she takes them to be, but that the values of any one client may be very different from the values of the next.

A particularly sharp difficulty, however, in the case of mental health, is the loss of insight by which some mental disorders are characterized (see Chapter 3). This is a particularly sharp difficulty, because, as the story of Mr AB illustrates, loss of insight is a characteristic particularly of psychotic disorders, which, as we saw in Chapter 3, may be among the most severe mental disorders. Hence it is just those who most *need* help who are most likely to *lack insight* into the fact that they need it. Peter Campbell, and many others, and not only in the user movement (e.g. Perkins and Moodley, 1993), have repeatedly warned of the hazards in the notion of insight; however, Mr AB illustrates the dilemma that 'loss of insight' raises. He lacked insight into his depression: what *he* wanted was pills, with which he was planning to kill himself before his (delusional) brain cancer got any worse; however, what *everyone else* thought he needed was treatment for depression.

In Mr AB's case, most people would agree that involuntary treatment was justified. The fact, however, that it may *sometimes* be right to act against patients' expressed wishes in situations in which their insight is psychotically disturbed, has led to a tendency among professionals to deny (usually tacitly) the validity of patients' values in the far more common situations in which their insight is *not* psychotically disturbed. As many of those with wide experience of training mental health professionals have often found, the most dangerous lack of insight in mental health is not service users' psychotic lack of insight but professionals' continuing lack of insight into service users' real needs (Perkins and Moodley, 1993)!

Again, we return to the practical implications of the differences between provider and user values, and indeed to the differences between the values of different health-care professions, in Chapter 18. As we will see, in a VBP model such differences of values cease to be merely a source of difficulty and become a positive resource for balanced health-care decision making.

Objective 4: improved thinking skills

We noted in chapter 6 of this book, and in our Preface, the role that philosophy may have in improving some of the generic thinking skills on which good practice depends. Yet the idea that it is possible to reason about ethical issues comes as a surprise to some people. They feel that 'ethics' is a matter of personal conviction. We could leave it at that, perhaps, if there were neither dilemmas nor disagreements for us to tackle; and it is certainly true that in reasoning about ethical issues we may eventually come to an impasse. Before we reach the point of impasse, however, there are a number of different ways in which we can try to think through ethical issues.

We start to examine some of the more important ways of reasoning about ethical issues in Session 2. First, though, we round off this session with a brief consideration of how training in ethics may contribute to clinical practice, starting with a word of warning!

Ethics training and ethical practice

The word of warning is that there are potential dangers even in the four eminently practical intermediate objectives for ethics education in health care outlined above.

The ethical downsides

Thus, increasing awareness could make practitioners *oversensitive* to ethical issues, paralysing action: changing attitudes can undermine peoples' established values and beliefs (this is especially important in cross-cultural work). Even knowledge can be misused if it is taken to imply that the expert necessarily 'knows best'.

Perhaps most important of all, too much discursive reasoning, 'thinking rather than doing', can come across in a situation demanding practical action at best as irrelevant 'waffling', at worst as yet a further exercise of professional power. The British social scientist, Patricia Alderson (1990), has described how the rise of ethical 'experts' in medicine has 'doubly disenfranchised' patients: they were already disenfranchised by specialist *technical* expertise; now they are disenfranchised by specialist *ethical* expertise.

Learning and doing

One way to minimize these dangers is to remind ourselves that, as with other areas of philosophy, ethics is as much a skill as a body of knowledge. We emphasised the skills acquisition objectives of this book in our Preface. It is with a view to skills acquisition that our materials are presented in an active rather than passive form, i.e. as a series of exercises linked by lines of argument with which the reader is encouraged to engage actively, disagreeing with, as well as sometimes being persuaded by, what is said.

With skills acquisition, then, in general as well as in ethics and philosophy, it is important to separate learning from doing, the development of a new skill from its deployment for real. If you come across a way of analysing ethical issues that you feel would be useful, whether in this book or elsewhere, try it out as an exercise when there is nothing practical hanging on the outcome and reflect on its success or failure. Repeating this process a couple of times will then allow you to use the new skill you have acquired in a natural and unselfconscious way when it is needed in practice. This is just like learning a new stroke in tennis by practising it before using it for real in a match.

Levels of ethical reasoning

R.M. Hare, to whose work we are indebted at several points in this book, has written about this aspect of the relationship between theory and practice in ethics in terms of different levels of moral reasoning. Hare (1981) distinguishes two levels of ethical reasoning. *Level 1* is the level of *everyday clinical practice*: at this level, we normally have to be decisive, and, to extend the above analogy with tennis, it is our ethical reflexes (or intuitions) by which we must be guided. *Level 2*, by contrast, is the level at which critical reflection on practice takes place. Level 2 thinking includes reflection both on the issues arising in particular practical situations and also on more abstract analyses of underlying concepts.

Hare's Level 1 (of more or less spontaneous responses in day-to-day practice) is closely related to the virtues (dispositions to act ethically); it is also the level at which training in ethics has a practical pay-off. Level 2 reasoning, on the other hand, as the level of reflection on practice, is the level at which practice skills and other practically oriented methods of ethics *training* operate. Training should not be on a 'one-off' basis, of course. It is essential to continue to reflect (sometimes) on practice if we are to continue to develop as practitioners.

Theoretical and applied ethics

Traditionally, applied ethics, concerned with the application of ethical theories to solving problems in practice, has been distinguished from theoretical ethics, concerned with the theories themselves. Theoretical ethics, in turn, has been divided into substantive theories, claiming to provide a theoretical basis for deriving answers to problems arising in practice, and analytic ethics, concerned with the meanings and implications of value terms and with other aspects of the conceptual structure of ethics.

Bioethics, as we will see in Chapter 18, has drawn particularly on substantive ethical theories (such as rights-based and utilitarian theories). With mental health, though, the particular *conceptual* difficulty of the subject means that in addition to substantive ethics, so defined, abstract analyses of concepts may also be crucial to Level 2 thinking. As we have seen in this chapter, and as we will be exploring in detail later in this part, a number of key ethical concepts (such as rationality, best interests, and so forth), which in many contexts in medicine and bioethics can be taken for granted, are often at the very heart of the ethical difficulties in mental health. As Dickenson and Fulford (2000) argue in their casebook, mental health ethics starts where general bioethics finishes.

Conceptual difficulties are at the heart of mental health ethics

It is in the analysis of concepts, therefore, drawing on the resources of general philosophy, that much of the work of mental health ethics must take place. This is why, as Fulford (1995) has argued, in mental health there is no real difference between pure and applied philosophy, pure and applied ethics. Certainly, we need to separate, as in tennis, learning from doing. Certainly, too, Hare's distinction between Level 1 (intuitive) and Level 2 (reflective) thinking is helpful in maintaining this separation. As to theoretical and applied ethics, though, it is analytic ethics, the least of theories in late twentieth century ethical theory, which as we will see, has the most direct practical applications in mental health ethics.

We return to analytic ethics as a resource for the toolkit of mental health ethics in Chapter 18. First, though, in Session 2 of this chapter, we need to look in more detail at some of the particular conceptual difficulties that are raised by mental health, and at how these are reflected in the special features of mental health ethics.

Reflection on the session and self-test questions

Write down your own reflections on the materials in this session drawing out any points that are particularly significant for you. Then write brief notes about the following:

1.   Thinking about Mr AB's story, ethical issues are not always transparent in mental health. What does this remind you of from Chapter 2?

2. What are the implications of the relative invisibility of ethical issues for the role of philosophy in mental health ethics?

3. List four intermediate objectives for training in mental health ethics: which of these is particularly important for strengthening the 'user voice'?

4. What are Hare's two 'levels' of ethical reasoning and how do they relate to the links between training and practice?

Session 2 Conceptual difficulties and mental health ethics

All areas of health care raise particular ethical issues. Transplantation is different from assisted reproduction, for example, and both are different from terminal care. There are some important common themes: we noted consent and confidentiality, for example, in the last session. However, each area of health care requires a degree of attention in its own right.

So, how does mental health fare?

EXERCISE 9   (15 minutes)

In this exercise we are going to consider how mental health has fared in bioethics, not directly, but indirectly, by way of a piece of Austinian 'philosophical fieldwork'.

Most bioethicists, if asked directly, will deny that mental health has been (until recently) relatively neglected. But what does the actual literature, the outputs of bioethics, show?

Look through the index of any large medical ethics textbook. Also look at the chapter headings. Notice:

1. how far the subjects covered correspond with the issues raised by your cases in Exercise 1 of this chapter, and

2. the prominence or otherwise of mental health ethics.

If you are working with Beauchamp and Childress (1989), look finally at the examples in their extensive appendix. Do you see any discrepancy between the topics covered in the book and the examples given in the appendix?

You will probably find that most of the issues raised by your cases (consent and confidentiality, for example, as noted in the last session) are in the subject index. Some of the subject headings may well have triggered further thoughts about your cases.

Neglect of conceptual difficulties

At one level, then, the issues raised by mental health are indeed generic, similar issues being raised by other areas of medicine. Notice, however, that whereas other areas of medicine often get a section in their own right, mental health tends not to.

Neglect of mental health

The contrast is especially sharp between mental health and areas of bodily medicine that involve high-tech or other dramatic interventions. In the index to the third edition of Beauchamp and Childress (1989), for example, aside from entries on general ethical concepts (such as autonomy), many of the most prominent entries are of this kind: 'Abortion', 'AIDS', 'Blood', 'Cancer', 'dialysis', 'experimentation', etc., all have prominent entries. Mental health, although represented, is by contrast relatively hard to find: these are short entries under 'addiction', 'depression' and 'dementia', but none for such mental health hot topics as schizophrenia or personality disorder.

Beauchamp and Childress, it is important to say straight away, are unusual among bioethical textbooks of this period, in paying considerable attention to mental health: we return in Chapter 18 to the detailed analysis they provide of the issues raised by involuntary psychiatric treatment. And in their appendix of examples, in contrast to the subject headings in their index, no less than eight of 38 cases are concerned with mental disorder (including mental impairment). Even so, the message of the relative invisibility of mental health in the index, is that, in bioethics as in biomedicine, mental health is an also-ran, a Cinderella discipline, to other more high-tech areas of medicine.

Neglect of conceptual issues

There are good historical reasons, to which we return at the end of this chapter, why bioethics has mirrored biomedicine in neglecting mental health. For the moment, though, we are concerned with the consequences of this neglect.

EXERCISE 10

Think about this for yourself before going on. Given our conclusions in earlier parts of this book, particularly in Part I, what consequences would you expect from bioethics' tendency to mirror biomedicine?

Our main conclusion in Part I was that mental health, although stigmatized in the twentieth century medical model as being deficient scientifically, was in fact conceptually more *difficult* than high-tech areas of bodily medicine.

The greater conceptual difficulty of mental health, furthermore, although evident in a number of different areas, includes one area of particular relevance to ethics, namely its more complex value structure. Values, as we found in Part I, although present in all areas of health care, are particularly prominent in mental health. This is not because mental health is less scientific. It is because people's values differ more widely in the areas with which mental health is concerned (emotion, desire, volition, sexuality, etc.) than in those with which (high-tech) areas of bodily medicine are concerned (severe bodily pain, imminent death, etc.).

Bioethics, then, to the extent that it has mirrored biomedicine, has failed to recognize the greater conceptual difficulty of mental health. Beauchamp and Childress (1989), as we will see in Chapter 18, are a partial exception to this: their detailed analysis of involuntary psychiatric treatment draws deeply on philosophical work on irrationality. All the same, even in Beauchamp and Childress, the relative neglect of conceptual difficulties is reflected in the absence of conceptual topics in their index: there are no entries for concepts of disorder, disease, dysfunction, illness, delusion, etc., nor even for values or value judgement.

We will see in Chapter 18, that this relative neglect of conceptual issues is a linguistic-analytic signal of the traditional medical model underlying Beauchamp and Childress' work, a model that is directly reflected in the conclusions they draw about involuntary psychiatric treatment.

But does it matter?

Bioethics, then, in neglecting mental health, has, like biomedicine, neglected conceptual issues, including those raised by diversity of values. In the case of biomedicine, its focus on empirical science is understandable, given medicine's huge successes in the twentieth century in meeting the challenge of major diseases. In respect of such diseases, values are present but unproblematic because they are largely shared (remember the example of a 'heart attack', in Chapter 6, which is a bad condition, in and of itself, in anyone's scale of values). In the case of bioethics, it is true, neglect of differences of values, and of related conceptual difficulties, is rather more surprising, ethics and values being closely related.

But does it matter than bioethics has mirrored biomedicine in neglecting conceptual issues? Anything approaching a full answer to this question will occupy us for the rest of this part of the book! In the remainder of this session, we will take a first step towards answering it by considering in more detail two examples of ethical difficulties, consent and confidentiality, generic in nature, but presenting particular problems in mental health. As we will see, in both cases, the particular difficulties arising in mental health are *conceptual* in nature. Our conclusion, then, will be that for mental health at least, it certainly *does* matter that bioethics has neglected conceptual issues.

Example 1: consent, capacity, and delusion

As before, we will start by considering actual case histories.

EXERCISE 11

This is another two-stage exercise. Again, it is important to do Stage 1, to think about the issues for yourself, before going on to the reading in Stage 2.

Stage 1 (45 minutes)
Consider any of your cases that involved consent (if none of them did, you might like to consider Mr AB). Consent is important in all areas of health care. But it can be especially problematic in mental health. Write short notes on:

1. what is required for genuine consent to a treatment, and

2. in what ways these requirements may be particularly difficult to fulfil in mental health.

Stage 2 (60 minutes)
Then look at any of the standard bioethical accounts of consent (for example Beauchamp and Childress). How far do your conclusions coincide with theirs?

Most authors agree with Beauchamp and Childress (1989) in defining two key conditions for consent: (1) *information*, and (2) *voluntariness (including freedom from coercion, which is sometimes treated as a distinct third condition)*.

Both conditions, information and voluntariness, raise many difficulties in any situation in medicine: how much information is appropriate? Is an apparently free choice covertly coerced, for example through an unequal power relationship between doctor and patient? And so on.

Mental disorder and the conditions for consent

Mental disorder shares with other areas of health care such difficulties. In addition, however, it is among those conditions that, in and of themselves, may impair the very *capacity* for consent. Other capacity impairing conditions include mental impairment, unconsciousness, or being a young child. Mental disorder, however, to complicate matters further, covers many different ways in which consent may be impaired, corresponding with the many different kinds of psychopathology. Some of these affect particularly the first condition for consent, others particularly the second. Here are a couple of examples.

* *Condition 1 (information)*: anxiety blocks the ability to retain and recall new information (we tend not to register names when first introduced to people in a crowd—the 'cocktail party' effect). Hence people suffering from the often extreme anxiety engendered by anxiety disorders will be *especially* incapacitated in this respect.

* *Condition 2 (voluntariness)*: choice is only truly voluntary where there is an equal power relationship. Mental disorder is often associated with feeling demoralized and powerless (as in depression). Hence mental disorder itself may often leave people feeling disempowered.

A consent Catch-22

Yet despite difficulties of this kind, involuntary treatment is used in mental health for situations in which it would never be considered in other areas of medicine. In the case of bodily disorders (as we will see in Chapter 19), it is now a cardinal principle of health-care law in many legislations around the world, that an adult patient who has the capacity to make the requisite choice may refuse even life-saving treatment if they so wish, provided that (as with some infectious diseases, for example) their condition carries no immediate risk of danger to others. A person may lack capacity in certain well defined circumstances—if they are unconscious, for example, as noted above, or are a minor (with different age thresholds being set for different kinds of decision), or have learning disability. In the absence of such capacity-impairing circumstances, however, consent to the treatment of bodily disorders is mandatory.

With a mental disorder, by contrast, and only with a mental disorder, treatment without consent may sometimes be considered appropriate for a *fully* conscious, *adult* patient of *normal* intelligence, not for the protection of others (though as we saw above involuntary psychiatric treatment is also used as in bodily medicine for the protection of others), but *in that person's own interests*. So here is a Catch-22 with a vengeance! In mental health, it may often be especially difficult to satisfy the *conditions* for consent (because of the effects of the mental disorder itself); yet it is also in mental health that the most radical *breaches* of consent occur!

The Catch-22 of involuntary psychiatric treatment is illustrated by Mr AB's case from the previous session. His treatment under the Mental Health Act was in direct conflict with his express wishes. Yet he was a fully conscious adult of normal intelligence. Further, treatment was needed (in the view of everyone except Mr AB) not to protect others but in his own interests. Mrs AB, among others, certainly did have an interest in her husband receiving treatment, just as she would have done if the threat to his life had been from a bodily illness (such as cancer). But the justification for involuntary treatment in Mr AB's case was the threat posed by his illness (depression) to, in the terms of condition 2 above, his own 'health or safety' (from suicide).

Capacity and mental disorder

The difference, of course, between Mr AB and someone with a bodily disorder (such as cancer), is that Mr AB's wishes were taken to be invalid: they were assumed to be, somehow, not his 'true wishes', a product rather of delusional beliefs arising in the context of a severe depressive illness; and Mr AB's refusal of treatment, correspondingly, was taken to be irrational. In other words Mr AB, consistently with health-care law generally, lacked the capacity to make decisions about his treatment. He lacked decision-making capacity, it is true, not for the reasons most often relevant to bodily disorders (impaired consciousness, for example, as immediately above), but he lacked capacity none the less. And he lacked capacity for a reason most often relevant to mental disorder, namely that he was suffering from delusions.

Delusions and the map of mental disorders

Delusions, you will recall from Chapter 2 in Part I, together with other functional psychotic symptoms, are at the centre of the map of psychopathology, our Rylean 'logical geography' of psychopathology, in part precisely because delusions represent

the paradigm case of a mental disorder rendering the person concerned not responsible for their actions. It will be worth dwelling for a moment on just how well established is the ethical intuition that delusion and other functional psychotic symptoms invalidate choice.

Thus, the basis of the intuition is, at first glance, evident enough. In some forms of mental illness, notably with delusions, people are 'irrational', and hence, as with other legal excuses (accident, inadvertence, duress, etc.), they are held to be 'not responsible' for their actions. It was this property of mental disorders, as just noted, that we highlighted as Feature 3 of our Rylean 'map' of psychopathology in Chapter 2. So widely acknowledged is the intuition that mental disorders excuse, it has been built into legislation in many different countries and right back to classical times. Aristotle, for example, included the 'mad' among those who could not be 'bad' (see his *Nichomachean Ethics*, Bk.3, Section 3; 1112^{a}11–31, 2000); and most legal systems since then have included madness as one form of legal excuse. We noted in Part II, Daniel Robinson's (1996) remarkable review of two and a half thousand years of the insanity defence (and its cognates) across a wide range of diverse cultures. In forensic psychiatry, the legal intuition that delusions excuse continues to be important in respect of serious crimes: and in jurisdictions that retain capital punishment, 'important' means, quite literally, that life or death may hang on the distinction between mad and bad.

Excusing conditions and invalidating conditions

Historically, the intuition that people who are suffering from delusions are not responsible for their actions has been more in evidence in relation to excusing conditions in criminal law than to incapacity as a condition justifying involuntary treatment. This is because consent itself, the need for explicit consent as a condition for medical treatment, is a relatively recent development in medical ethics—like autonomy in bioethics (as noted above), consent is relatively 'late and local'. But it is essentially the same intuition, of loss of responsibility for one's actions, that lies behind the more everyday, if less high profile, cases of involuntary treatment, like that of Mr AB. The importance of delusion as an invalidating condition, as it is called in this context, is evident in day to day clinical work: despite the wide definition of mental disorder in most mental health legislation (as in the UK, see above), involuntary treatment is in practice largely (though by no means exclusively) confined to psychotic disorders (see e.g. Sensky *et al.*, 1991).

Deep intuitions and deep divisions

'Mad or sad', then, as in Mr AB's case, is equivalent in this respect to 'mad or bad' in the insanity defence. As with the insanity defence, though, so also with involuntary treatment, while the general principle may be well established, that people with psychotic disorders may not be responsible for their actions, there may still be deep difficulties in particular cases about where to draw the line. There may be wide agreement, that is to say, on the principle that delusion is an excuse in law, and, correspondingly, an invalidating condition for treatment choice. There is, however, often considerable disagreement about whether the principle applies in a given case.

Even Mr AB's case, although introduced originally (by Fulford, 1989) as an example of a case in which all but the most radical of antipsychiatrists would agree involuntary treatment is justified, turned out, in a case vignette study (see below), to be a case over which opinion, for or against involuntary treatment, is split down the middle! In this case vignette study, as we will see, there were indeed other cases over which respondents were largely in agreement on whether or not involuntary treatment is justified. But Mr AB turned out not to be one of them! And the disagreement over cases such as Mr ABs, as we found when we first read Mr AB's story in Chapter 2, is not, or not primarily, as to the facts. The facts, as we saw in Chapter 2, may be all in, and yet there may still be disagreement as to how the facts should be interpreted. Such disagreements, then, as we concluded in Chapter 2, point to difficulties that are not empirical in nature but conceptual.

Bioethics, as we will find when we return to this topic in Chapter 18, has generally failed to recognize the particular conceptual difficulties underpinning involuntary treatment in psychiatry. Consistently with its mirroring of biomedicine, therefore, it has assumed that the tools it has developed to support decision-making in relation to involuntary treatment in bodily medicine, can be used essentially unchanged in mental health. The failure of this assumption leads directly to the sharper set of tools that are required for ethical issues generally in mental health.

Example 2: confidentiality and the concept of mental disorder

Compared with consent, confidentiality, although important generally as an ethical issue, has not been widely recognized to raise distinctively *conceptual* issues in mental health. As with consent, then, the tools for handling ethical issues around confidentiality developed in bodily medicine, have generally been applied essentially unchanged to mental health. But is this right? We will look briefly at this question before moving on to the role of mental health law.

EXERCISE 12 (20 minutes)

- Is the special conceptual trickiness of ethical issues in mental health limited to consent?
- What about confidentiality?

Think about this in relation to your cases (or Mr AB).

- What conceptual issues could lie behind the problems of confidentiality they raise?

Confidentiality and consent

The casualty officer in Mr AB's case, you will recall, breached confidentiality by letting Mrs AB know that her husband had turned up in casualty. This breach of confidence, we said, was justified in the circumstances.

But exactly how was it justified? One justification for breaching confidentiality is a 'clear and present' danger to an identified third party, as in the oft-cited Tarasoff case, described by Beauchamp and Childress (1989), in case 1 in their appendix. However, there was no such clear and present danger to a third party in this case. The commonest justification for breaching confidentiality is that it is done with the patient's consent. But Mr AB, we have suggested, lacked capacity to consent. So the justification in this case seems to go back to the condition from which he was suffering, a form of depression that, just as it invalidated his refusal of treatment, invalidated his refusal of permission for the casualty officer to contact his wife.

True, capacity is decision specific. Loss of capacity for one kind of decision does not in itself involve loss of capacity for a different kind of decision. In this case, however, the two decisions—to refuse treatment and to refuse permission to contact his wife—were both driven by Mr AB's delusion that he was dying from brain cancer.

Confidentiality and disorder as a distributed concept

With confidentiality, then, as for involuntary treatment, there may be particular ethical difficulties in mental health arising from establishing the proper boundary of the concept of mental disorder as an invalidating condition.

Confidentiality illustrates a further difficulty with the concept of mental disorder, however, namely that disorder itself may not be neatly located within any one individual. We noted earlier that the bioethical principle of autonomy runs into difficulties in societies that value family and social networks above individualism. In mental health, the problem may be that disorder itself is understood in family or social terms. In child and adolescent psychiatry, in particular, it is often within the dynamics of family relationships that disorders are located rather than within any one individual.

Confidentiality and sharing

In Chapter 6 we found that the diversity of values, which is integral to the concept of mental illness (insofar as it is distinct from the concept of bodily illness), is integral to good practice in mental health; in particular, it underscored the importance of the multidisciplinary team. If this is right, however, then in mental health practice, confidences *have* to be shared.

Again, there are problems throughout health care about when it is right to share information given in confidence. Such difficulties, in the case of mental health, are made particularly acute by the diversity of values by which the concept of mental disorder is characterized. In some cases, one value may indeed seem clearly to outweigh another: the lesson of the Tarasoff case, as noted above, is that where there is a 'clear and present' danger to an identified third party, the value of sharing information to protect that third party clearly outweighs the value of maintaining patient confidentiality. Even here, however, in Tarasoff-type cases, mental health presents particular difficulties. For one consequence of the value diversity of mental disorder is that balanced decision-making itself depends, *inter alia*, on a well-functioning multidisciplinary team. We return to this in Chapter 18, as a key feature of VBP. The problem here, however, in relation to confidentiality, is that it may not be possible to come to a balanced view about whether a third party is indeed in 'clear and present danger' without information being shared, not only within the members of a multidisciplinary team, but between a number of different agencies extending well beyond health and indeed social care (to include, e.g. the police). The British psychiatrist, George Szmukler, has estimated that over 30 different agencies are concerned with any one patient in community-based mental health services (Szmukler and Holloway, 2001).

With confidentiality, then, in mental health, the need for multidisciplinary and multi-agency working arising from the particular diversity of values by which the concept of mental disorder is characterized, leaves us with another Catch-22. A breach of confidentiality is justified if there is a clear and present danger to a third party. But establishing the presence of a clear and present danger depends on information being widely shared.

The conceptual depth dimension to mental health ethics

With confidentiality, therefore, as well as with consent, mental health ethics involves a depth dimension of conceptual difficulty that is lacking from the high-tech areas of bodily medicine on which bioethics has traditionally focused.

We should expect this, as we have seen, if the ideas about the concept of mental illness developed in Part I of this book are right. The bottom line of Part I was that mental health, contrary to the traditional medical model, is not a primitive or otherwise defective also-ran to bodily medicine, but an area of health care in which conceptual, as well as empirical, difficulties are writ large. We should expect particular conceptual difficulties in mental health ethics, then, and they are indeed there.

In Chapter 2, the conceptual difficulties embedded in Mr AB's case launched our discussion of the concept of mental illness, a discussion that, by the end of Chapter 6 led to our more complete or 'full-field' picture of the conceptual structure of health care. We pick up this discussion in Chapter 18, when we consider the implications of our 'full-field' picture for the sharper set of ethical tools required for mental health. First, though, in the final session of this chapter, we take a first look at the law as a resource for resolving ethical issues in mental health.

Reflection on the session and self-test questions

Write down your own reflections on the materials in this session drawing out any points that are particularly significant for you. Then write brief notes about the following:

1. In what respect is bioethics' attitude to mental health similar to that of biomedicine?

2. What are the conditions for consent (we noted two) and how are matters of consent made more difficult in mental health?

3. What particular kind of psychopathology is at the heart of the difficulties equally of consent and, in forensic contexts, of 'mad or bad'?

4. In addition to issues of consent, what further *conceptual* difficulties are involved with ethical problems of confidentiality in mental health?

5. What conflict of values is particularly associated with issues of confidentiality?

Session 3 Conceptual difficulties and mental health law

Thus far in this chapter, we have considered the nature of psychiatric ethics, its breadth, but also its conceptual depth. In Session 2, in particular, we noted how bioethics has tended to stop short just when things get interesting conceptually in mental health ethics. We considered two 'big issues' by way of illustration, consent and confidentiality, both generic issues, but both raising conceptual difficulties—about delusion and capacity, and about the wider concept of mental disorder, respectively. Difficulties of this kind, we argued, although legitimately left unspoken in other conceptually less complex areas of health care, are at the heart of the ethical difficulties in mental health.

In this session, we take a first look at medical law. As in Sessions 1 and 2 of this chapter, we start with some philosophical fieldwork, in this case by way of a series of case vignettes. In the next exercise, we will be asking you to respond to these case vignettes, not by way of philosophical analysis but as you would 'for real'. Unpacking our responses to these vignettes (initially in this session and then in more detail in Chapter 18), will show that health-care law, like bioethics, although providing a valuable general framework for the issues arising in mental health, needs to be combined with conceptually sharper tools for working with conflicting values if it is to be helpful to us practically, as users and providers of services, in mental health.

Philosophical fieldwork

We will start, then, with an exercise in 'philosophical fieldwork', in this case using a series of case vignettes (first published in Fulford and Hope, 1994).

Questionnaire

For instructions, please see Exercise13.

Time allowed: 5 MINUTES

CASES

(tick one box per case)

	YES	?	NO

1. Miss AN, age 21 student. Four-year history of intermittent anorexia. Currently seriously under weight, exercising and using laxatives; amenorrhoeic. Refusing admission on the grounds that she is 'too fat'. ☐ ☐ ☐

2. Mr OC, aged 27. Bank clerk. Three-year history of progressive slowness at work. Referred with depression and anxiety following suspension from work. Shows severe and progressive obsessional checking which he agrees 'is something wrong with him'. However, he drops out of treatment. ☐ ☐ ☐

3. Mr SD, aged 48. Bank manager. Presents in casualty with biological symptoms of depression and hypochondriacal delusions. History of attempted suicide. Asking for something to 'help him sleep'. He refuses to stay in hospital when he is told that he may be suffering from depression. ☐ ☐ ☐

4. Miss HM, aged 25. Novice nun. Brought by superiors for urgent outpatient appointment as they are unable to contain her bizarre and sexually disinhibited behaviour. Shows pressure of speech, grandiose delusions, and auditory hallucinations. Refusing to stay. ☐ ☐ ☐

5. Mr B, aged 16. School boy. Seen by GP at parents' request with failing vision in one eye. Despite progressively impaired vision refuses to accept that he is unable to see with that eye. Diagnosis of optic atrophy but refuses investigation through fear of hospitals. ☐ ☐ ☐

6. Mr A, aged 50. Doctor. Developed thickening of lips, hoarse voice, and enlargement of skull over several years. Refused to accept that these changes were anything other than age-related and rejected his colleagues' diagnosis of acromegaly. Refusing investigations. ☐ ☐ ☐

7. Miss HP, aged 30. Secretary. Admitted to neurology ward and transferred to psychiatry under protest. Unable to use right hand (patient right-handed). Paralysis 'non-anatomical'. History of self-injury. Rejecting psychological diagnosis and planning to discharge herself. ☐ ☐ ☐

8. Mrs CR, aged 47. Housewife. Refusing investigation of breast lump discovered on routine screening. Understands that she does not have to accept treatment if the lesion is found to be malignant. Normal mental state. ☐ ☐ ☐

9. Mr S, aged 18. Student. Emergency psychiatric admission from his College. Behaving oddly. Showed thought insertion (Mike Yardwood 'using his brain'). Complaining that people were talking about him. Refusing medication and planning to leave hospital. ☐ ☐ ☐

10. Mrs HF, aged 51. Shop worker. Complained to general practitioner of hot flushes and irregular periods. Had developed backache and X-rays showed osteoporotic change. Refusing HRT despite full explanation of the implications. ☐ ☐ ☐

11. Mrs AGP, aged 25. Housewife. Progressively housebound over 2 years with agoraphobic symptoms. Refusing behavioural treatment despite threat to job and marriage. ☐ ☐ ☐

12. Mrs M, aged 46. Nurse. Withdrawing from marital therapy because she resents the implication that their 'problems' are in their relationship. Says her husband is 'sick'. Her husband has been violent in the past and is now threatening to kill her. ☐ ☐ ☐

13. Mr PP, aged 23. Unemployed man. Seen in casualty by the duty psychiatrist. Brought in by a girlfriend because he is angry and threatening to kill a rival. Has been drinking. History of criminal assault. No other symptoms. Refusing to stay. ☐ ☐ ☐

14. Mr SC, aged 60. Retired. Recent diagnosis of bronchial carcinoma. Normal mental state. Wants repeat prescription of sleeping tablets. GP knows him to be a supporter of euthanasia and suspects he intends to kill himself. ☐ ☐ ☐

Fig. 17.1 Case vignette questionnaire.

EXERCISE 13 (4 minutes only!)

In this exercise you are asked to decide for yourself about involuntary treatment for a number of cases including bodily as well as mental disorders.

The cases are given in the questionnaire in Figure 17.1. As this shows, you have to decide for yourself what you would do in each case. If you are a health-care professional, imagine that the people described are your clients or patients; if not, imagine what you would want to happen if the person concerned were a close relative, your son, or your partner, say.

The time allowed for this exercise really is 4 minutes! The reason for this is that it is not a 'test' of theory but a way of bringing out what you would do, or want done, in practice. In J.L. Austin's terms, this is an exercise in using our concepts for real in the spirit of his 'philosophical fieldwork'. In R.M. Hare's terms (as in the last session), it is Level 1 moral thinking, acting on your intuitions in the heat of the moment.

Level 1 thinking, as Hare pointed out is how we all have to work if we are to remain effective. In practice, we simply do not have much time to think. We have to decide what to do and get on with it. Similarly, we often have to act on limited information, again as with these case vignettes.

Time yourself, then, and run quickly down the list of cases in Figure 17.1, relying on your intuitions to guide you. If you are working in a group, compare your responses (but don't change them!) before reading on.

Having done the case vignettes, we will be moving to Level 2 thinking, reflecting on what lies behind our intuitions as reflected in the 'real-life' choices we have made.

Well, how did you get on? Remember, there are no *definitive* right or wrong answers here. There are rules about involuntary treatment (we come to the legal rules in a moment). But the purpose of the exercise is to get your reactions as guided by your intuitions in the heat of the moment over choices of the kind that have to be made in everyday practice.

The responses people give to these cases are remarkably consistent. Table 17.1 shows the results from a typical group of respondents to the questionnaire. As this indicates, responses to the cases fall into three broad categories: for most cases, most people feel that involuntary treatment is *not* justified; but for two cases (4 and 9) almost everyone feels that involuntary treatment *is* justified; while for two further cases (1 and 3), opinion is sharply *divided*. Case 3, by the way, is of course based on Mr AB. As noted above, it was a surprise (for Fulford) to find (when he started using Mr AB's story in this questionnaire) that involuntary treatment in Mr AB's case was very far from being a foregone conclusion!

Table 17.1 Responses to the case vignette questionnaire

Cases	Respondents opting for involuntary treatment (%)
1 Anorexia	25
2 Obsessional disorder	10
3 Depression	50
4 Hypomania	≤100
5 Optic atrophy	1
6 Acromegaly	0
7 Hysteria	3
8 Breast lump	0
9 Schizophrenia	≤100
10 Osteoporosis	0
11 Agoraphobia	0
12 Marital problems	1
13 Personality disorder	1
14 Bronchial carcinoma	1

A consistent three-part pattern...

This overall three-part pattern, with responses falling into the three groups of a 'split vote' on involuntary treatment (cases 1 and 3), 'mainly yes' (cases 4 and 9), and 'mainly no' (the rest), has been replicated in teaching sessions with different groups of mental health-care professionals (psychiatric nurses, psychiatrists, social workers, etc.), with patient advocacy groups, and with groups in many different countries. It was even found with a group of former dissidents from one of the old Soviet block countries who had suffered politically motivated abusive uses of psychiatry (we return to this in Chapters 20 and 21).

There *are* differences, of course, in how people respond to the case vignette questionnaire. Between individuals the differences may be quite large. Your own responses may not have coincided with the three part pattern! We will see later (when we get to VBP in Chapter 18) that there are good reasons for such individual variation, reasons to do (in part) with the variation in human values. But the *overall* pattern of responses is none the less remarkably stable.

The pattern, furthermore, has a degree of face validity (see Part I, Chapter 2) to the extent that the cases actually picked out are all to a greater or lesser extent psychotic: the two clear 'yes' cases are overtly psychotic (case 4, with hypomania, and case 9, with schizophrenia), case 3 (one of the two with a split vote) has delusions, and case 1 (the other split vote) has anorexia, a condition that, although not among the classical psychotic disorders, may be associated in its more severe forms with psychotic disturbances of insight. Selecting these particular cases, then, is consistent with the literature cited above, showing the historically and cross-culturally stable association of psychosis with loss of responsibility for one's actions. It is also, as we noted in Session 1 above, consistent with current clinical practice.

...with differences

As a matter of Level 1 thinking, in Hare's terminology, these results thus indicate a high degree of consistency over our ethical intuitions about consent. The questionnaire, though, also, and crucially, shows inherent *differences* of view. This is shown in part by the (admittedly low) level of disagreement about all the cases. It is unusual with any group to get complete agreement on any of the cases.

The importance of differences of view, however, is also shown, more dramatically, by the split vote on cases 1 and 3. The fact that, even in the somewhat artificial context of a case vignette questionnaire, no less than two of 14 cases should regularly attract a vote that is split down the middle, shows clearly the depth of disagreement that there may be over issues of compulsion in mental health.

Such differences, with opinion split down the middle, are indeed clearly evident also in practice. In the polarized psychiatry versus antipsychiatry debate in the 1960s and 1970s that we explored in Part I, Szasz' antipsychiatry argument against the concept of mental illness was driven largely by his rejection of involuntary treatment. Pro-psychiatry arguments, on the other hand, are often driven equally strongly by endorsement of involuntary treatment, at least in cases like Mr AB's. John Wing, for example, the British social psychiatrist, whose foundational work in modern descriptive psychopathology we introduced in Chapter 3, described as 'morally repellent' the attitude of those (like Szasz) who would reject involuntary treatment for people (like Mr AB) who are suicidally depressed (Wing, 1978, p. 244). So we need to move to Hare's Level 2 thinking, to reflect on and to try to understand what lies behind our intuitive responses to cases such as these.

Interpreting the three-part pattern

Level 2 thinking about involuntary treatment, as illustrated by our case vignette questionnaire, could involve direct ethical debate about the contested cases: neither Szasz nor Wing, for example, would have been satisfied with the split vote over case 3 (see their contrasting views above about the ethics of involuntary treatment for suicidally depressed people noted immediately above). Direct ethical debate is important in health care. We will be introducing in Chapter 18 a range of ideas both from bioethics and from ethical theory that may contribute particularly to the thinking skills that are needed for ethical debate in health care.

Here, though, our approach, guided as it is by the observation that ethical problems in psychiatry are a product of deeper conceptual difficulties, has to be more circumspect. Our aim has to be, not to dispute but to explain. Drawing on the methods outlined in Part I, we will thus treat the three-part pattern of responses to the case vignette questionnaire as (in Gilbert Ryle's vivid metaphor) a 'logical geography' of consent, as a pattern reflecting the features of our ordinary (i.e. unreflective or intuitive) use of concepts in

relation to consent, and as a pattern therefore for which philosophical analysis has to account.

Linguistic analysis, you will recall from Part I, is not premissed on the correctness of this or that use of concepts: in the terms of Part I, therefore, interpreting the three part pattern of our responses to the case vignettes, means that we have either to *explain* or to explain it *away*. Either outcome will do. Either outcome, that is to say, will help to give us a more complete picture of the concepts guiding our intuitive responses to involuntary treatment as reflected in the three-part pattern.

Interpretation: (1) too much law, and too little

What, then, lies behind the three-part pattern of responses to our case vignette questionnaire. What account can we give of this pattern, and, hence, of the logical geography of consent?

EXERCISE 14   (10 minutes)

Think about this question yourself before going on. The idea at this stage is not so much to start thinking philosophically as simply to reflect on your own decisions, to consider what was influencing you for or against involuntary treatment in each of the cases.

Faced with this question, many people start by talking about the legal framework of health-care practice. If you are a mental health professional, and/or have had direct experience of mental illness, your understanding specifically of mental health law will probably have figured strongly in your decisions about the cases in the questionnaire.

A role for mental health law

The law is clearly relevant. Mental health law, indeed, as we noted earlier, directly reflects historically long-standing and cross-culturally stable intuitions about the loss of responsibility that goes with some kinds of mental disorder. Thus, modern mental health legislation requires (in one form or another) two conditions to be fulfilled for involuntary psychiatric treatment.

- *Condition 1 (mental disorder)*—the patient must be suffering from a mental disorder.
- *Condition 2 (risk)*—there must be a risk to the patient or others arising from the disorder.

These conditions vary in the detail of how they are defined in different legislations but they are always there in one form or another. In the UK, for example, Section 2 (Admission for Assessment) of the Mental Health Act 1983 (applicable in England and Wales), specifies (*Condition 1*) that the person concerned must be '...suffering from mental disorder...', mental disorder being defined earlier, in Section 1 of the Act, as 'mental illness, arrested or incomplete development of mind, psychopathic disorder and any other disorder or disability of mind'; and (*Condition 2*) that the patient '...ought to be so detained in the interests of his own health or safety or with a view to the protection of other persons'. So defined, then, these two conditions do indeed cover many of our cases. Many of our cases were suffering from a mental disorder (*Condition 1*) and they were also a risk to themselves or others (*Condition 2*).

To this extent, therefore, if you were thinking of mental health legislation in responding to the case vignette questionnaire, this would have been entirely in order. Indeed, if you are a mental health professional and had *not* been thinking of it, you would have been at risk of a negligence claim!

Too much law

So mental health law is relevant. Is it, however, sufficient to explain our responses (and thus to give us the required account of the logical geography of consent)? In other words, does applying the two legal criteria for consent to our cases reproduce the three-part pattern of our responses to them in the exercise above?

The answer, essentially, is 'no', because the two conditions, taken together, are considerably overinclusive. As defined in the legislation, the two conditions, although covering the cases in the vignette exercise for which involuntary treatment is widely felt to be justified, also covers many cases for which involuntary treatment is *not* widely felt to be justified.

This is illustrated by Table 17.2 (adapted from Fulford, 1992, p. 358), which shows what happens when we apply the two legal criteria for consent to the cases in our vignette questionnaire. The figure lists the vignette cases in the left-hand column with approximate percentage 'yes' votes next to them. The next column then gives a + sign for any case for which involuntary treatment would be allowed under mental health legislation incorporating the two conditions, of mental disorder and of risk.

Table 17.2 Responses to the case vignette questionnaire using the two key conditions for compulsion in the Mental Health Act 1983

Case vignettes	Respondents opting for involuntary treatment (%)	Possible basis of response Mental Health legislation—mental disorder + risk (self or others)
1 Anorexia	25	+
2 Obsessional disorder	10	+
3 Depression	50	+
4 Hypomania	≤100	+
5 Optic atrophy	1	
6 Acromegaly	0	
7 Hysteria	3	+
8 Breast lump	0	
9 Schizophrenia	≤100	+
10 Osteoporosis	0	
11 Agoraphobia	0	+
12 Marital problems	1	
13 Personality disorder	1	?
14 Bronchial carcinoma	1	

As the figure illustrates, the cases where many or most people's intuitions said 'yes' to involuntary treatment (cases 1, 3, 4, and 9) are well covered. But a great many more cases are covered as well!

There is room to argue about the details here. But the message is clear, that as a basis for explaining our intuitive ethical responses to these cases, mental health law, at least of this broadly drawn kind, is too inclusive.

Narrow excuses, wide invalidating conditions

Similar very wide criteria for involuntary psychiatric treatment are to be found in many other legislations (see Fulford and Hope, 1996). Such criteria, it is worth noting, stand in marked contrast with the corresponding legal criteria generally adopted for mental disorder as a legal excuse. As noted above, the 'insanity defence' has been based, centrally, on delusion. Other mental disorders may be put forward to a court in mitigation, in hope of a reduction in the severity of sentencing; but other mental disorders are not generally accepted as an excuse, i.e. as a condition removing the accused's responsibility for the crime altogether. In England and Wales, for example, a successful plea of 'insanity' must satisfy the very narrow constraints of the McNaughten rules, namely that the person concerned did not understand either the nature of the act (of killing someone) or that it was wrong. These rules are derived from a famous nineteenth century case in which Daniel McNaughton, after shooting and mortally wounding the Prime Minister, Sir Robert Peele's, private secretary, Edward Drummond (McNaughton thought his victim was the Prime Minister), was held to be not responsible for his actions because he was suffering from delusions (West and Walk, 1977).

Legislators, then, while restricting the insanity defence rather narrowly, and usually to delusion or other psychotic disorders, have tended to take a much more open-handed approach to involuntary treatment. This discrepancy points ahead to the bottom line of Chapter 19, namely that in law as in medicine, values, although not always recognized for what they are, may be crucially important not only to the way the law is interpreted but also to how it is drafted in the first place. With the insanity defence the primary concern (or value) of legislators is that the law should not be used inappropriately as an 'escape route' for those who have committed serious crimes (such as murder). With involuntary treatment, on the other hand, the primary concern (or value) of legislators is to ensure that the law is used appropriately to ensure that those who are in need of treatment receive it.

Too little law

The natural reaction to the overinclusiveness of the legal conditions for involuntary treatment, is to say: 'Ah, but it's not "mental disorder + risk" as such that explains our responses to the vignettes; it is "*serious* mental disorder and/or *serious* risk".' Take such legislation literally, this line of thought goes, and, yes, it is overinclusive with a vengeance; however, interpret it in a 'common sense' way, as being intended to be used only for serious cases, and it comes closer to our intuitive responses, surely.

The idea, then, is that legislation should be drawn widely, leaving professionals the room they need to apply it in appropriate, i.e. serious, cases. There are many points—legal, ethical, and practical—for and against such an approach. For our purposes, though, of explaining the logical geography of consent, the effectiveness or otherwise of stiffening up the legal criteria for consent with an implicit criterion of seriousness, depends on what meaning is given to 'serious'.

Interpretation: (2) law plus seriousness

What, then, is meant by 'serious' in the context of mental health legislation on consent? We will briefly consider two meanings of 'serious', a legal meaning attached to Criterion 1 (i.e. a legal definition of 'serious mental disorder'), and a bioethical meaning attached to Criterion 2 (i.e. a bioethical definition of 'serious risk'). Neither criterion, as we will see, and as is illustrated in Tables 17.3 and 17.4, sufficiently explains the three-part pattern of our responses to the case vignette questionnaire.

Psychopathology, by contrast, to anticipate the final part of this session, *does* provide an appropriate criterion of seriousness, in the concept of psychosis (introduced in Chapter 3). Psychosis, indeed, and the concept of psychosis furthermore as defined specifically for use in legal contexts by a group of lawyers and doctors (the 'Butler Committee') in the run up to the 1983 Act, fits the three-part pattern like a glove. If, then, use is indeed a guide to meaning (as Austin showed us in Part I), psychosis is closely relevant to the grounds of involuntary psychiatric treatment. The conceptual 'fit' between psychosis and involuntary treatment, however, begs the theoretical question of why some cases, at least, are controversial. It thus also begs the bottom line practical questions about how to improve decision-making in this area.

Legal 'serious' = 'warrants admission'

First, then, a legal criterion of seriousness. There is a measure of 'serious' built into the Mental Health Act 1983 in the notion that, in the words of Section 2 of the Act (Admission for Assessment), the required mental disorder should be '...of a nature or degree which warrants the detention of the patient in a hospital for assessment (or for assessment followed by medical treatment) for at least a limited period'.

There is much to commend this approach. First, it places the burden of decision firmly on those directly involved. It is not for lawyers to say who needs to be admitted to hospital. As a criterion of 'seriousness', furthermore, 'warrants admission' is responsive to changes in professional best practice. Since the 1983 Act was drafted, in the late 1970s and early 1980s, we have witnessed a radical shift in mental health from hospital-based to community-based services. This shift has been reflected in successive editions of the Code of Practice, a comprehensive guide to the use of the Act (in England and Wales, see chapter 19).

'Warrants admission' is thus a flexible criterion of seriousness, which, in principle, allows for relevant discretion in using what would otherwise be the very wide criteria for admission defined

Table 17.3 Responses to the case vignette questionnaire using the two legal criteria plus a further legal criterion of 'warrants admission' as a measure of seriousness

Case vignettes	Responses to vignettes—% 'yes' for involuntary treatment	Possible basis of response			
		Mental health legislation—mental disorder + risk (self or others)	Mental health legislation + criteria of seriousness		Severe mental disorder—by Butler criteria (= psychotic symptoms)
			Mental disorder warrants admission	Mental disorder + risk is life threatening	
1 Anorexia	25	+	?		
2 Obsessional disorder	10	+	?		
3 Depression	50	+	?		
4 Hypomania	≤100	+	?		
5 Optic atrophy	1				
6 Acromegaly	0				
7 Hysteria	3	+	?		
8 Breast lump	0				
9 Schizophrenia	≤100	+	?		
10 Osteoporosis	0				
11 Agoraphobia	0	+			
12 Marital problems	1				
13 Personality disorder	1	?	?		
14 Bronchial carcinoma	1				

Table 17.4 Response to the case vignette questionnaire using the two legal criteria plus a bioethical criterion of 'immediately life threatening' as a 'measure of seriousness'

Case vignettes	Responses to vignettes—% 'yes' for involuntary treatment	Possible basis of response			Severe mental disorder—by Butler criteria (= psychotic symptoms)
		Mental health legislation— mental disorder + risk (self or others)	Mental health legislation + criteria of seriousness		
			Mental disorder warrants admission	Mental disorder + risk is life threatening	
1 Anorexia	25	+		?	
2 Obsessional disorder	10	+			
3 Depression	50	+		+	
4 Hypomania	≤100	+			
5 Optic atrophy	1				
6 Acromegaly	0				
7 Hysteria	3	+			
8 Breast lump	0				
9 Schizophrenia	≤100	+			
10 Osteoporosis	0				
11 Agoraphobia	0	+			
12 Marital problems	1				
13 Personality disorder	1	?		+	
14 Bronchial carcinoma	1				

in the Act. If it is a helpful criterion, however, it is not (in itself) sufficient to focus the use of the Act appropriately. There are two reasons for this. First, as Table 17.3 shows, it begs the question. The '?' responses in Table 17.3 reflect the fact that 'warrants admission' is precisely what is at issue. Thus, mental disorders like obsessive-compulsive disorder (case 2) and agoraphobia (case 11) might well be treated on an out-patient basis nowadays. In the late 1970s and early 1980s, however, when the 1983 Act was in preparation, they were often thought to 'warrant admission' to hospital. Other cases on the list are actually described as already being in hospital (e.g. case 7, hysteria). The criterion of 'warrants admission' thus tracks, and tracks faithfully, our intuitive use of involuntary (hospital) treatment, but by the same token fails to provide guidance where it is the appropriateness of admission itself that is at issue.

The second reason why 'warrants admission' is not sufficient to focus the use of the Act, is that it has failed in practice. Thus, over the life of the 1983 Act, despite its in principle sensitivity to changes in clinical practice, it has failed to reflect the shift away from hospital-based services. The shift from hospital- to community-based services since 1983 means that, if 'warrants admission' were an effective constraint on the use of the Act, involuntary admissions should have fallen sharply. In fact, they have gone steadily up (MHAC, 2003).

There are many possible reasons for this, of course. It may be that, absent a criterion of 'warrants admission', use of the Act

would have increased over this period even more. The negative correlation between the use of the Act and the use of hospital admissions, however, is at least prima facie evidence that as a legal constraint, 'warrants admission' is not sufficient to guide decisions about the use of involuntary treatment in practice.

Bioethical 'serious' = 'immediately life-threatening'

In the bioethical literature, a general medical condition normally has to be immediately life-threatening before involuntary treatment is considered justifiable. This criterion, used as a criterion of 'seriousness' to strengthen the Mental Health Act Criterion 2, of risk to self or others, would certainly restrict the use of the Act. But if we apply *this* sense of 'serious' to our cases, we move from an overinclusive result to a result which is not inclusive enough! As Table 17.4 shows (adapted from Fulford, 1992), the criterion of 'immediately life threatening' excludes cases (e.g. cases 4 and 9) that most people *would* intuitively treat, and includes other cases (e.g. case 13) that most would *not* treat.

The Butler problem

The problem of finding an appropriate criterion of seriousness was very much in the minds of those involved in drafting the Mental Health Act 1983. In the run up to the Act, a government committee of enquiry was set up under Lord Butler to review the whole question of the treatment of the mentally disordered in law (Butler, 1975). Among many other issues, they considered in depth just how to provide a narrower criterion for mental illness as a legal excuse, and, correspondingly, for involuntary treatment. This is covered in Sections 18.26–18.36 of their report.

EXERCISE 15   (60 minutes)

Read the extract from:

Butler, Rt. Hon., the Lord. (1975). Chairman, Report of the Committee on Mentally Abnormal Offenders, Cmnd 6244. London: Her Majesty's Stationery Office. (Extract pp. 228–229)

Link with Reading 17.6

Although individual parts of the report are not attributed to particular members of the Committee, this section was written mainly by the British psychiatrist, Sir Denis Hill, at the time Professor of Psychiatry at the Institute of Psychiatry in London, and it provides an authoritative discussion of the issues.

How does the Butler Committee seek to define the particular kind of mental disorder which impairs rationality to the point that people are not responsible for their actions? Note the criteria they offer and then try applying these to our cases.

The Butler solution

The Butler Committee solution, then, as set out in the reading (linked with Exercise 15), was to define a category of 'severe mental disorder' corresponding broadly with the traditional psychopathological categories of 'psychotic disorder'. As the Committee noted, psychosis is difficult to define (we touched on this in Chapter 3, for example; see also Fulford, 1992) but at least we can identify certain particular psychotic symptoms. Hence, the Butler Committee concluded, 'severe mental disorder', for purposes of future mental health legislation, should be defined by reference to a number of widely recognized groups of psychotic symptoms of organic and functional disorders, specifically:

1. Lasting impairment of intellectual functions shown by failure of memory, orientation, comprehension, or learning capacity.

2. Lasting alteration of mood of such degree as to give rise to delusional appraisal of the patient's situation, his past or his future, or that of others, or to lack of any appraisal.

3. Delusional beliefs, persecutory, jealous, or grandiose.

4. Abnormal perceptions associated with delusional misinterpretation of events.

5. Thinking so disordered as to prevent reasonable appraisal of the patient's situation or reasonable communication with others.

This is a clear and distinct list. Each of the symptoms can be looked up in any medical textbook. Each of these symptoms,

moreover, can be identified with a high degree of reliability (see Chapter 3). Moreover, applying the Butler definition of 'severe mental disorder' to our cases fits the pattern of our responses like a glove. As Table 17.5 shows, the Butler definition picks out strongly cases 4 and 9, which had a more or less 100% 'vote' (both of these cases have two Butler symptoms each); case 3, with a 50% vote, less strongly (and case 3 has only one Butler symptom); and case 1, with only a 25% vote, rather weakly (anorexia nervosa displays Butler symptoms only to the extent that the extreme disorders of body image and beliefs about nutrition with which it is associated are regarded as psychotic). The remainder of the cases are firmly excluded by the Butler criteria.

Butler begs the question

So, problem solved? Well, at one level certainly. The Butler criteria 'fit' practice, not only with the case vignette exercise, but also in the empirical studies noted above, on the kind of cases actually treated on an involuntary basis, or regarded as legally not responsible (see, e.g. Sensky *et al.*, 1991, noted above; and Walker, 1967).

In the event, however, this was one of the few sections of the Butler report that failed to make it into the 1983 Act, the legislators employing instead the very wide definition of mental disorder cited above. In this the 1983 Act was following the norm. In Fulford and Hope's survey of European legislation, noted earlier, only Denmark defined its mental disorder criterion explicitly in terms of psychotic disorder—and even Denmark added a 'let out' rider to the effect that compulsion could also be used for 'any other similar condition' (Fulford and Hope, 1996).

The concern remained, therefore, at the time of the 1983 Act, that even though 'psychosis' might in general come near the mark as an appropriate criterion of 'serious mental disorder', as a definition it would prove too insensitive to the subtle judgements required of practitioners in particular cases.

The validity of this concern is reflected in the results of our case vignette questionnaire, in which, ironically, the very success of the Butler proposals in mirroring what we do in practice, also shows its limitations. The point is this: even in the artificially constrained circumstances of a questionnaire study, there were two cases (1 and 3) over which opinion was fundamentally divided. The Butler 'solution', as noted above, accurately reflects this division of opinion. But in itself the Butler Solution fails to explain just *why* opinion on these cases should be so divided. And if this is so under these ideal conditions, how much more so will it be 'in the field'?

Back to conceptual difficulties

The core difficulty, therefore, although indeed tracked by the Butler criteria for defining severe mental disorder, remains unresolved. The *nature* of the difficulty, on the other hand, is now clear. It is, as everything we have said in this chapter would lead you to anticipate, a *conceptual* difficulty, a difficulty, in this case, about the concept of irrationality.

Table 17.5 Responses to the case vignette questionnaire using the Butler criteria for defining serious mental disorder

Case vignettes	Responses to vignettes—% 'yes' for involuntary treatment	Possible basis of response			
		Mental health legislation— mental disorder + risk (self or others)	Mental health legislation + criteria of seriousness		Severe mental disorder—by Butler criteria (= psychotic symptoms)
			Mental disorder warrants admission	Mental disorder + risk is life threatening	
1 Anorexia	25	+	+	?	?
2 Obsessional disorder	10	+	+ (in 1983)		
3 Depression	50	+	+	+	+
4 Hypomania	≤100	+			++
5 Optic atrophy	1				
6 Acromegaly	0				
7 Hysteria	3	+	+		
8 Breast lump	0				
9 Schizophrenia	≤100	+	+		++
10 Osteoporosis	0				
11 Agoraphobia	0	+	+ (in 1983)		
12 Marital problems	1				
13 Personality disorder	1	?		+	
14 Bronchial carcinoma	1				

Thus, in our responses to the case vignette questionnaire we were picking out, if the analysis offered here is correct, serious mental disorders. The relevant sense of 'serious', however, the specific sense of 'serious' that guided our choices, was that the cases in question were 'psychotic'. The choices we made in Exercise 13, as we have several times noted, are consistent with a long historical and cross-culturally stable intuition that people with severe mental disorders are irrational in some particularly radical way that renders them not responsible for their actions. It is this intuition, traditionally reflected in the insanity defence, that re-emerges in a modern context in relation to involuntary psychiatric treatment. It is this same intuition that is reflected in our responses to the case vignette questionnaire in Exercise 13.

Back to the need for sharper conceptual tools

To identify the origin of the particular ethical difficulties associated with involuntary psychiatric treatment in this way, as being associated centrally with the concept of psychosis, is to focus attention appropriately on the key conceptual difficulties. As a step towards resolving the difficulties, this could be helpful. However, it is not, as such, to resolve them.

Our initial consideration of mental health law, then, in this session, like our initial consideration of bioethics in the last, leads back to the need for a sharper set of conceptual tools for tackling ethical and value issues in mental health. We return to the task of building the required tool kit in Chapter 18 when we look at one detailed account of irrationality in the bioethical literature, and again in Chapter 19 when we consider the current

front-runner in the UK for a legal criterion of seriousness, namely, incapacity.

Before coming directly to bioethics, though, we will take 'time out' to reflect briefly on why it is that, if the ethical problems raised by mental health are indeed deeper than in other areas of health care, they should have been relatively neglected in the bioethical literature.

Reflection on the session and self-test questions

Write down your own reflections on the materials in this session drawing out any points that are particularly significant for you. Then write brief notes about the following:

1. What was the 'philosophical fieldwork' on consent with which we started this session; and what was the overall result?

2. How consistent are the results of this fieldwork across different groups.

3. Are the results sufficiently explained by mental health law?

4. Are the results sufficiently explained by mental health law liberally interpreted to imply a standard bioethical criterion of 'seriousness', i.e. where a serious condition is one that is 'immediately life threatening'?

5. What are the 'Butler' criteria; and do they explain the pattern of responses in our philosophical fieldwork?

Conclusions: seven reasons for the neglect of mental health by bioethics

In this chapter, we have seen that the ethical issues arising in mental health, such as confidentiality and consent, although much the same kind of issues as those arising in other areas of health care, are conceptually trickier. This is why, we have argued, neither general bioethics nor law, although providing helpful guidance, has proven sufficient for tackling the conceptual difficulties at the heart of mental health ethics. This is why, we have further argued, a conceptually sharper set of tools may be needed to tackle them.

Given, however, the particularly acute challenges of mental health ethics, both practical and intellectual, its neglect by bioethics requires some explanation. Not, of course, by way of apology. Some explanation, however, *is* required here, if only as a basis for understanding how bioethics might now evolve to encompass, on an equal basis, mental health with other areas of health care.

Why, then, have these issues been relatively neglected until recently?

EXERCISE 16   (10 minutes)

◆ Given that ethical problems in mental health are both more pervasive and more difficult than in other areas of health care, why should they been relatively neglected?

◆ Why should mental health have been treated in this respect as a footnote to technological medicine?

If you are working in a group, discuss this together. Write down a few suggestions before going on.

This is a complex question, worthy of several good PhDs in the history of ideas! Here are a few possible answers:

1. *Mental health only appears ethically more problematic.* This is the kind of answer that is generated by the traditional medical model, as in Chapter 4, for example, with those who think that the concept of mental illness can be cleaned up evaluatively, and made to look more 'scientific', like the concept of bodily illness. Those who remain un-persuaded by the arguments of Part I will find this answer sufficient!

2. *Even if mental health is more ethically problematic, the problems are all solvable in a straightforwardly practical way without philosophical reflection.* We have argued in Session 1 of this chapter that, to the contrary, philosophical reflection is necessary. Philosophical reflection may not have been necessary in the past when there was little that medicine could do about *most* problems. But increasingly wide options about what *can* be done, opened up through scientific advances, have brought with them increasingly difficult problems about what *ought* to be done (see Fulford, 1989). Scientific advance, therefore, means a conceptually trickier medicine, and hence a conceptually

trickier medical ethics. We return to the science-led nature of the need for philosophy in medicine specifically in relation to philosophical value theory in the final session of Chapter 18 (on VBP).

3. *As a discipline, bioethics was started by philosophers who, being experts on rationality, were afraid of irrationality.* This is the point, made by the British philosopher Anthony Quinton in relation to philosophical work on rationality, with which we opened Chapter 2 (see Quinton, 1985). Again, though, this cannot be a sufficient explanation for the neglect of mental health by traditional bioethics, for key figures in the early bioethics movement were experienced in mental health issues. Will Galen, for example, one of the founders of the Hastings Centre, the first centre of excellence for bioethics in the USA, was actually a psychiatrist. So the subject was not neglected through ignorance.

4. *There is little money for research into the ethics of mental health.* This has certainly been a factor. Mental health, along with other areas of primary care, has been relatively starved of funding. Dan Callaghan, the founder of the Hastings Centre, has commented that of four projects for which they sought start-up funding for the centre, it was only the psychiatry project that failed to attract a grant (personal communication).

5. *The dominant medical model focused attention on high-tech areas of medicine.* Historically, this has been an important factor and we return to it at the start of Chapter 18. Bioethics came into existence as a response to the ethical problems raised by high-tech medicine and it was thus inevitable that its initial focus should have been on this area of health care. With this, however, came the standard 'medical model' according to which the 'high tech' of natural science is the hallmark of the medical. Even today, when in many countries the balance has shifted sharply towards primary care, issues raised by technological advance continue to dominate much of bioethics.

6. *The conceptual 'tools of the trade' developed by early bioethics worked straightforwardly with ethical problems in high-tech medicine, but were more difficult to apply in mental health.* This has probably been an important if largely unacknowledged reason for the relative neglect of mental health. In its early days, bioethics had to get results to survive and results were much harder to come by in mental health. Concentrating on the more straightforward (though still difficult enough) ethical problems of high-tech medicine was thus a legitimate strategy at this stage.

As an intellectual strategy, however, concentrating on the high-tech only worked because the *conceptual* problems implicit in ethical issues in technological medicine are relatively straightforward. In the ethics of euthanasia, for example, the rationality of the patient is assumed for bodily disorders, but is at the heart of the ethical issues raised by euthanasia for mental disorders (see Special Issue of *Philosophy, Psychiatry, and Psychology on Psychiatric Euthanasia*, 1998).

We will find later in this part that the utility of bioethics' early simplifications even in technological medicine is growing less all the time. Developing a conceptually sharper set of ethical tools will thus be important not only for mental health but for health care generally.

7. *We already have satisfactory bioethical tools that can be applied as required to mental health.* This implies that the ethical problems raised by involuntary *psychiatric* treatment, for example, notwithstanding the underlying conceptual issues explored in this chapter, are really no different from those raised by involuntary treatment in any other area of health care. In other words, to return to our case vignette examples, we really *do* have a satisfactory bioethical model of consent to which involuntary psychiatric treatment can be subsumed.

The idea that involuntary *psychiatric* treatment is a marginal note to an otherwise sound body of theory and practice about involuntary treatment generally, is implicit in many bioethics texts, in which, as we will see in Chapter 18, mental health is subsumed under a general topic of consent.

One conclusion from this part as a whole, however, will be that subsuming mental health ethics to other areas of healthcare ethics, is putting the cart before the horse. There is, certainly, no satisfactory bioethical account of consent in mental health. This is not, however, the result of a failure to apply a satisfactory general account of consent to an aberrant area of health care. To the contrary, the failure of bioethics to provide an adequate account of consent in mental health, we will argue, marks fault lines in bioethics' account of consent as a whole (Fulford, 1993). So this will turn out to be yet another example of the truth of what J.L. Austin (in Part I) called the negative concept wearing the trousers, i.e. of problems in mental health turning out to highlight and illuminate problems in healthcare generally.

Reading guide

Ethics teaching and ethics training

Resources for teaching psychiatric ethics

Bioethics is a growth industry and now offers a huge resource of books, journals, and electronic databases. As noted in the chapter, much of this is not specific to mental health ethics. None the less, these resources if searched carefully provide much useful material. Searchable literature databases useful for ethics training include those operated by the Kennedy Center, Bioethicsline, Medline, and Knowledge Finder. Philosophical literature (including books as well as peer-reviewed journals) are listed by Philosopher's Index.

There are also on-line discussion groups and list subscriber services such as that run by the Feminist Association of Bioethics. Among journals as resources for teaching and training, the *Bulletin of Medical Ethics* is a punchy newsletter-style update journal that covers developments internationally as well as in the UK. The journal *Philosophy, Psychiatry, & Psychology* focuses particularly on mental health and combines case studies with in-depth analysis of underlying conceptual and philosophical problems. Thematic issues, for example on psychiatric euthanasia (1998, Vol. 5(2)), are available to support training in particular topic areas. We list illustrative examples below and in later Reading Guides. *Philosophy, Psychiatry, & Psychology* is available on-line and these are also on-line versions of journals such as the Hastings Center Report.

A practical manual, including sample seminars, outlines of ethical theory, and a detailed Appendix covering literature sources, databases, and courses, all aimed at ethics education in medicine, is *The Oxford Practice Skills Course* (Hope, Fulford, and Yates, 1996). The development of this approach, and the main features of 'practice skills' as they apply to mental health, are described in a pair of chapters in Gillon and Lloyd's (1993) *Principles of Health Care Ethics* (Fulford and Hope, 1994, chapter 58; Hope and Fulford, 1994, chapter 59). Resources aimed specifically at psychiatry are less readily available. But Robert Michels and Kevin Kelly (1999), chapter 24 in Bloch, Chodoff, and Green's (1994) *Psychiatric Ethics*, describe a valuable topic-based approach.

Case books

Consistently with the 'philosophical fieldwork' approach of this book, case studies are particularly important in opening up the conceptual depth dimensions of mental health ethics.

An early case study drawing out the perspectives of all those involved in a vivid and highly readable way is *In That Case* (1982) by Alistair Campbell (a philosopher) and Roger Higgs (a general practitioner). The introductory chapter to Mike Parker and Donna Dickenson's (2000) *The Cambridge Workbook in Medical Ethics* includes a comparison of various approaches to reading cases in medical ethics. The workbook includes many mental health issues.

An early but still valuable source of cases in psychiatric ethics was published in America by the Group for the Advancement of Psychiatry (1990) *A Casebook for Psychiatric Ethics*. As the sister volume to Bloch, Chodoff, and Green's edited collection, *Psychiatric Ethics* (see above), Dickenson and Fulford's (2000) *In Two Minds: a casebook of psychiatric ethics* is a casebook with philosophical clout! The distinctive feature of 'In Two Minds' is the combination of detailed case histories illustrating a range of clinical-ethical problems in psychiatry, with in-depth philosophical treatment. *In Two*

Minds also includes detailed reading guides on many of the main topics in general medical ethics (as indicated below and in later Reading Guides in this part).

Involuntary psychiatric treatment, autonomy and consent

Roger Peele and Paul Chodoff (1999), chapter 20 in Bloch, Chodoff, and Green's (1999) *Psychiatric Ethics,* give a comprehensive overview of the ethical issues raised by involuntary psychiatric treatment particularly in the context of deinstitutionalization. The philosopher, Tom Beauchamp gives a clear account of autonomy, setting it in its philosophical-ethical context, in *The Philosophical Basis of Psychiatric Ethics* (see chapter 3 in Bloch *et al.*'s (1999) *Psychiatric Ethics*). Although not dealing specifically with psychiatry, Agich (1993) provides a highly relevant discussion of autonomy in *Autonomy and Long-term Care*. For an outline treatment of the ethical and conceptual issues underlying involuntary treatment in psychiatry, see Fulford (1995). Consent to psychiatric treatment in relation to children and young people is discussed from a legal, ethical, and practical viewpoint by Dickenson (1994) in a review article, 'Children's informed consent'. An analysis of the justification for involuntary treatment in terms of risk to others and self is given in the philosopher, Joel Feinberg's (1986) *Harm to Self: the moral limits of the criminal law*. Agich (1994) gives a succinct summary in a *Philosophy, Psychiatry, & Psychology* Key Concepts article on Autonomy. An early statement of the need for balanced decision making in involuntary treatment is Eastman and Hope (1988). Grisso and Appelbaum (1998) describe an influential and well validated model for assessing competence to consent to treatment. Culver and Gert (2004) provide an authoritative update and overview on competence.

Articles, with cross-disciplinary commentaries, exploring the conceptual underpinnings of consent and related ethical issues in psychiatry appear regularly in *Philosophy, Psychiatry, & Psychology*: see e.g. Moore, Hope, and Fulford (1994) on mania; Dickenson and Jones (1995) on children and developmental issues; Braude (1996) on multiple personality and moral responsibility; Charland (1998a) on the importance of emotion; Hinshelwood (1997a and b), with commentaries by Mace, 1997, Sturdee, 1997, and Thornton, 1997, on consent in psychotherapy; and Savulescu and Dickenson (1998) on advance directives. Other examples of the conceptually enriched nature of psychiatric ethics include Radden (1996) on multiple personality and other dissociative states; Charland (2004) on personality disorder, and Hinshelwood (1997c) on the distinction between psychotherapy and brainwashing. The special issue of *Philosophy, Psychiatry, & Psychology* on

psychiatric euthanasia (see Reading guide in Chapter 19) directly challenges the limitations of traditional bioethics when transferred from bodily health to mental health. As noted above, Dickenson and Fulford's (2000) *In Two Minds* combines detailed case histories with in-depth analysis of the conceptual and philosophical issues.

A growing number of authors (e.g. Okasha, 2000; Adshead, 2000), have pointed out that bioethicists have often conflated the very different approaches to issues of autonomy and consent that are taken by people in different parts of the world with different cultural traditions. Alternatives to the dominant principles-based approach include feminist ethics (e.g. Gilligan, 1993), narrative or hermeneutic ethics (Widdershoven, 2002), communitarian ethics (Parker, 1999), and Hegelian ethics (e.g. Dickenson, 1997). These approaches emphasize aspects of consent, such as relationship, emotion, and the social context, which are likely to be particularly important in psychiatry. Emotional aspects of competence to consent are explored in *Philosophy, Psychiatry, & Psychology* by Charland (1998a) in his article 'Is Mr Spock mentally competent? Competence to consent and emotion', with commentaries by Chadwick (1998), Elliott (1998), and Youngner (1998), and a response by Charland (1998b).

A more detailed reading guide on involuntary psychiatric treatment is given in chapter 2 of Dickenson and Fulford's (2000) *In Two Minds*. Reading guides on related topics in *In Two Minds*, include 'Abusive uses of psychiatry' (chapter 3), 'Responsibility and rationality' (chapter 4), 'Autonomy, capacity, competence and consent (chapter 6). Note also, 'Confidentiality' (chapter 7).

Confidentiality

All the large textbooks of medical ethics include sections on confidentiality: see for example, chapter 7 of Beauchamp and Childress' (1989) *Principles of Biomedical Ethics*. A recent collection of articles reviewing many important aspects of confidentiality in mental health is the forensic psychiatrist, Chris Cordess' (2001) *Confidentiality and Mental Health*. The ethical aspects of confidentiality in psychiatry are also reviewed by David Joseph and Joseph Orek (1999) in chapter 7 of *Psychiatric Ethics* (ed. Bloch, Chodoff, and Green).

Illustrative of the guidance issued by professional organizations is The Royal College of Psychiatrists' 'CR85', which covers issues raised by confidentiality in all areas of psychiatry, including research (Royal College of Psychiatrists, 2000).

Confidentiality is a growing issue in relation to publication. A valuable review of the practical, ethical and legal aspects of confidentiality in respect of case reports is provided by Wilkinson *et al.*'s (1995) in 'Case reports and confidentiality: opinion is sought, medical and legal'.

References

Adshead, G. (2000). Commentary on Case 7.1, 'Alan Masterson—clear and present danger'. In *In Two Minds: A casebook of psychiatric ethics* (ed. D. Dickenson and K.W.M. Fulford). Oxford: Oxford University Press, pp. 233–236.

Agich, G.J. (1993). *Autonomy and Long-term Care*. Oxford: Oxford University Press.

Agich, G.J. (1994). Key Concepts: autonomy. *Philosophy, Psychiatry, & Psychology*, 1(4): 267–270.

Alderson, P. (1990). *Choosing for Children: parents' consent to surgery*. Oxford: Oxford University Press.

Aristotle (2000) *Nicomachean Ethics* (ed Crisp, R.), Book 3, Section 3; 1112ª11–31. Cambridge: Cambridge University Press.

Beauchamp T. (1999). The philosophical basis of psychiatric ethics. In *Psychiatric Ethics* (ed. S. Bloch, P. Chodoff, and S.A. Green), (3rd edn). Oxford, Oxford University Press, Chapter 3.

Beauchamp, T.L. and Childress, J.F. (1989). *Principles of Biomedical Ethics*. Oxford: Oxford University Press.

Bloch, S., Chodoff, P., and Green, S. A. (1999). *Psychiatric ethics* (third edition). Oxford, Oxford University Press.

Braude, S.E. (1996). Multiple personality and moral responsibility. (Commentary by Clark, S.R.L., pp. 106–117 and Shuman, D.W., pp. 59–60) *Philosophy, Psychiatry, & Psychology*, 3/1: 37–54.

Butler, Rt. Hon., the Lord. (1975). Chairman, Report of the Committee on Mentally Abnormal Offenders, Cmnd., 6244. London: Her Majesty's Stationery Office.

Campbell, A.V. and Higgs, R. (1982). *In That Case: Medical Ethics in Everyday Practice*. London: Darton, Longman and Todd.

Campbell, A.V. (1994). Dependency: the foundational value in medical ethics. In *Medicine and Moral Reasoning* (ed. K.W.M. Fulford, G.R. Gillett, and J.M. Soskice). Cambridge: Cambridge University Press, p. 184.

Campbell, P. (1996). What we want from crisis services. In Read, J and Reynolds, J, Eds, Speaking Our Minds: An Anthology. Basingstoke, England: The Macmillan Press Ltd for The Open University pp. 180–183.

Chadwick, R. (1998). Commentary on 'Is Mr Spock mentally competent?'. (Commentary on Charland, 1998a) *Philosophy, Psychiatry, & Psychology*, 5/1: 83–86.

Charland, L.C. (1998a). Is Mr Spock mentally competent? Competence to consent and emotion. *Philosophy, Psychiatry, & Psychology*, 5/1: 67–82.

Charland, L.C. (1998b). Response to the Commentaries. *Philosophy, Psychiatry, & Psychology*, 5/1: 93–96.

Charland, L.C. (2004). Character: moral treatment and the personality disorders. In *The Philosophy of Psychiatry: a companion* (ed. J. Radden). New York: Oxford University Press, pp. 64–77.

Cordess, C. (ed.) (2001). *Confidentiality and Mental Health*. London, Jessica Kingsley Publishers.

Crisp, R. (1994). Commentary on 'how should we measure need?' *Philosophy, Psychiatry, and Psychology*, 1/1, 37–38.

Culver, C.M. and Gert, B. (2004). Competence. In *The Philosophy of Psychiatry: a companion* (ed. J. Radden). New York: Oxford University Press, pp. 258–270.

Dickenson, D. (1994). Children's Informed Consent to Treatment: Is the Law an Ass? (1994) Guest Editorial, *Journal of Medical Ethics*, vol. 20, no. 4, 205–206.

Dickenson, D. (1997). *Property, Women, and Politics: Subjects or Objects?* Cambridge: Polity Press.

Dickenson, D. and Fulford, K.W.M. (2000). *In Two Minds: a casebook of psychiatric ethics*. Oxford: Oxford University Press.

Dickenson, D. and Jones, D. (1995). True wishes: the philosophy and developmental psychology of children's informed consent. *Philosophy, Psychiatry, & Psychology*, 2(4): 287–303.

Eastman, N.L.G. and Hope, R.A. (1988). Ethics of enforced medical treatment: the balance model. *Journal of Applied Philosophy*, 5: 49–59.

Elliott, C. (1998). Commentary on 'Is Mr Spock mentally competent?'. (Commentary on Charland, 1998a) *Philosophy, Psychiatry, & Psychology*, 5/1: 87–88.

Feinberg, J. (1986). *Harm to Self: the moral limits of the criminal law*. Oxford: Oxford University Press.

Fulford, K.W.M. (1989). *Moral Theory and Medical Practice*. Cambridge: Cambridge University Press.

Fulford, K.W.M. (1992). Thought insertion and insight: disease and illness paradigms of psychotic disorder. In *Phenomenology, Language and Schizophrenia* (eds M. Spitzer, F. Vehlen, M.A. Schwartz, and C. Mund). New York: Springer-Verlag, p. 358.

Fulford, K.W.M. (1993). Bioethical Blind Spots: Four Flaws in the Field of View of Traditional Bioethics, *Health Care Analysis*, 1: 155–162.

Fulford, K.W.M. (1995). Psychiatry, compulsory treatment and the value-based model of mental health. In *Introductory Applied Ethics* (ed. B. Almond). Oxford: Blackwell, Chapter 10.

Fulford, K.W.M. and Hope, T. (1994). Psychiatric ethics: a bioethical ugly duckling? In *Principles of Health Care Ethics* (ed. R. Gillon and A. Lloyd). Chichester: John Wiley and Sons, pp. 681–695, chapter 58.

Fulford, K.W.M. and Hope, T. (1996). Informed consent in Psychiatry: Comparative Assessment of Section 5 of the National Reports—Control and Practical Experience.

Report for Biomed 1 project. Published as Control and Practical Experience, pp. 349—377, in Informed Consent in Psychiatry: European Perspectives on Ethics, Law and Clinical Practice, eds. H.-G. Koch, S. Reiter-Theil and H. Helmchen, Baden-Baden: Nomos Verlagsgesellschaft.]

Fulford, K.W.M., Dickenson, D.L. and Murray, T.H. (2002). Many voices: human values in healthcare ethics. Introduction, pp. 1–19. in K.W.M. Fulford, D.L. Dickenson and T.H. Murray, eds, *Healthcare Ethics and Human Values: an Introductory Text with Readings and Case Studies*. Malden, MA, USA, and Oxford, UK: Blackwell Publishers.

Gilligan, Carol, (1993). *In a Different Voice: Psychological Theory and Women's Development* (second edition). Cambridge, Massachusetts: Harvard University Press.

Gillon, R. (1996). Editorial to JME issue which included Robertson, D. Ethical theory, ethnography and differences between doctors and nurses in approaches to patient care. *Journal of Medical Ethics*, 22: 292–299.

Gillon, R. and Lloyd, A., (eds) (1994). *Principles of Health Care Ethics*. Chichester, England: John Wiley and Sons.

Griffin, J. (1990). *Well-being: its meaning, measurement and moral importance*. Oxford: Clarendon Press.

Grisso, T. and Appelbaum, P.S. (1998). *Assessing Competence to Consent to Treatment: a guide for clinicians and other health professionals*. New York: Oxford University Press.

Group for the Advancement of Psychiatry (1990). *A Casebook for Psychiatric Ethics*. New York: Brunner and Mazel.

Hare, R.M. (1981). *Moral Thinking: its Levels, Method and Point*. Oxford: Clarendon Press.

Hare, R.M. (1993). Medical ethics: can the moral philosopher help? In *Essays on Bioethics*. Oxford: Clarendon Press.

Hinshelwood, R.D. (1997a). Primitive mental processes: psychoanalysis and the ethics of integration. *Philosophy, Psychiatry, & Psychology*, 4(2): 121–144.

Hinshelwood, R.D. (1997b). Response to the Commentaries. *Philosophy, Psychiatry, & Psychology*, 4(2): 159–166.

Hinshelwood, R.D. (1997c). *Therapy or Coercion? Does Psychoanalysis Differ from Brainwashing?* London: H. Karnac (Books) Ltd.

Holmes, J. and Lindlay, R. (1989). *The Values of Psychotherapy*. Oxford: Oxford University Press.

Hope, T. and Fulford, K.W.M. (1994). Medical education: patients, principles and practice skills. Chapter 59 In *Principles of Health Care Ethics* (ed. R. Gillon). Chichester: John Wiley and Sons.

Hope, T., Fulford, K.W.M., and Yates, A. (1996). *The Oxford Practice Skills Course*. Oxford: Oxford University Press.

Joseph, D. and Orek, J. (1999). The ethical aspects of confidentiality in psychiatry. In *Psychiatric Ethics* (ed. S. Bloch, P. Chodoff, and S.A. Green), (3rd edn). Oxford, Oxford University Press, Chapter 7.

Mace, C. (1997). Primitive mental processes: psychoanalysis and the ethics of integration. (Commentary on Hinshelwood, 1997a) *Philosophy, Psychiatry, & Psychology*, 4(2): 145–150.

MacIntyre, A. (1982). *After Virtue*. London: Duckworth.

Marshall, M. (1994). How should we measure need? Concept and practice in the development of a standardised assessment schedule. (Commentaries by Crisp, R and Morgan, J., pp. 37–40) *Philosophy, Psychiatry, and Psychology*, 1/1: 27–36.

May, W.F. (1982). The virtues in a professional setting. Ch 7 In *After Virtue*. London: Duckworth.

May, W.F. (1994). The virtues in a professional setting. In *Medicine and Moral Reasoning* (ed. K.W.M. Fulford, G.R. Gillett, and J.M. Soskice). Cambridge: Cambridge University Press, Chapter 6.

Mental Health Act Commission (2003). *Placed Amongst Strangers. Tenth Biennial Report 2001–2003.* Twenty years of the Mental Health Act 1983 and the future for psychiatric compulsion.' London: TSO.

Michels, R. and Kelly, K. (1999). In *Psychiatric Ethics* (ed. S. Bloch, P. Chodoff, and S.A. Green), (3rd edn). Oxford, Oxford University Press, Chapter 24.

Moore, Hope, T., and Fulford, K.W.M. (1994). Mild Mania and Well-Being. *Philosophy, Psychiatry, & Psychology*, 1/3: 165–178.

Morgan, J. (1994). Commentary on 'How should we measure need?' *Philosophy, Psychiatry, and Psychology*, 1/1, 39–40.

Okasha, A. (2000). Ethics of psychiatric practice: consent, compulsion and confidentiality. *Current Opinion in Psychiatry*, 13: 693–698.

Parker, M. (1999). *Ethics and Community in the Health Care Professions*. London: Routledge.

Parker, M. and Dickenson, D. (2000). *The Cambridge Workbook in Medical Ethics*. Cambridge: Cambridge University Press.

Peele, R. and Chodoff, P. (1999). 'The ethics of involuntary treatment'. In *Psychiatric Ethics* (ed. S. Bloch, P. Chodoff, and S.A. Green), (3rd edn). Oxford, Oxford University Press, Chapter 20.

Perkins, R. and Moodley, P. (1993). The arrogance of insight. *Psychiatric Bulletin*, 17: 233–234.

Quinton, A. (1985). Madness. Ch 2 in *Philosophy and Practice* (ed. A. Phillips Griffiths). Cambridge: Cambridge University Press.

Radden, J. (1996). *Divided Minds and Successive Selves: ethical issues in disorders of identity and personality*. Cambridge, MA: MIT Press.

Robinson, D. (1996) *Wild Beasts and Idle Humours*. Cambridge, Mass: Harvard University Press.

Royal College of Psychiatrists (2000). *CR85. Good Practice Guidance on Confidentiality.* London: Royal College of Psychiatrists.

Savulescu and Dickenson, D. (1998). The Time Frame of Preferences, Dispositions, and the validity of Advance directives for the mentally ill. *Philosophy, Psychiatry, & Psychology,* 5/3: 225–246.

Sensky, T., Hughes, T., and Hirsch, S. (1991). Compulsory psychiatric treatment in the community, Part 1. A controlled a study of compulsory community treatment with extended leave under the Mental Health Act: and special characteristics of patients treated and impact of treatment. *British Journal of Psychiatry,* 158: 792.

Special Issue on Euthanasia (1998). *Philosophy, Psychiatry & Psychology,* 5(2).

Sturdee, P.G. (1997). Primitive mental processes: psychoanalysis and the ethics of integration. (Commentary on Hinshelwood, 1997a) *Philosophy, Psychiatry, & Psychology,* 4(2): 151–154.

Szmukler, G. and Holloway, F. (2001). Confidentiality in community psychiatry. In *Confidentiality and Mental Health* (ed. C. Cordess). London, Jessica Kingsley Publishers, Chapter 3.

Thornton, W.L. (1997). Primitive mental processes: psychoanalysis and the ethics of integration. (Commentary on Hinshelwood, 1997a) *Philosophy, Psychiatry, & Psychology,* 4(2): 155–158.

Toulmin, S. (1980). Agent and patient in psychiatry. *International Journal of Law and Psychiatry,* 3: 267–278.

Toulmin, S. (1982). How medicine saved the life of ethics. *Perspectives on Biology and Medicine,* 25 (4): 736–750.

Walker, N. (1967). *Crime and Insanity in England.* Edinburgh: Edinburgh University Press.

West, D.J. and Walk. A. (eds) (1977). *Daniel McNaughton: His Trial and the Aftermath.* London, The Royal College of Psychiatrists: Gaskell Books.

Widdershoven, G.A.M. (2002). Alternatives to principlism in Fulford, K.W.M., Dickenson, D., and Murray, T.H. (eds) *Healthcare Ethics and Human Values.* Oxford: Blackwell Science.

Wilkinson G, *et al.* (1995). Case reports and confidentiality: opinion is sought, medical and legal. *British Journal of Psychiatry,* 166: 555–558.

Williams, B. (1985). *Ethics and the Limits of Philosophy.* London: Fontana.

Wilson, J. (1979). *Preface to the Philosophy of Education.* London: Routledge.

Wing, J.K. (1978). *Reasoning about Madness.* Oxford: Oxford University Press.

Youngner, S.J. (1998). Commentary on 'Is Mr Spock mentally competent? (Commentary on Charland, 1998a) *Philosophy, Psychiatry, & Psychology,* 5/1: 89–92.

CHAPTER 18

From bioethics to values-based practice

Chapter contents

In this chapter we begin the process of building up the toolkit for tackling problems of values in mental health.

We start by outlining three important methods of ethical reasoning widely used in bioethics—principles, casuistry, and perspectives. We review the strengths and weaknesses of these methods, for health care generally in Session 1, and specifically for mental health in Session 2. Session 3 moves on to some of the main schools of general ethical theory—deontology, consequentialism, and analytic ethics—again looking at their strengths and weaknesses both generally and in relation to mental health. The last of these, analytic ethics, leads, finally, in Session 4, to the theory and skills base of values-based practice (VBP).

Session 1 Bioethics and health care

The main purpose of this session, then, is to introduce three approaches to ethical reasoning widely used in bioethics, principles, casuistry (or case-based reasoning), and perspectives, and to consider the pros and cons of these approaches as measured against the four practical objectives of training in ethics outlined in Chapter 17, awareness, attitudes, knowledge, and thinking skills.

In order to set what follows in context, however, we will start by considering three questions about bioethics itself: (1) What are its historical origins? (2) How should we understand its aims? (3) What have been its outcomes?

Bioethics: origins, aims, and outcome

Historical origins

Our first question, then, is what are the origins of bioethics? What historical factors have been important in driving concerns about ethical issues in medicine?

The modern discipline of bioethics grew out of traditional medical ethics over the 1960s and 1970s. Appearing first in North America, it has now become a growth industry all over the world.

Applied ethics, of which bioethics is an offshoot, is of course nothing new. In classical Greece, 'How should we live?' and 'What makes a life worth living?', were among the core questions with which philosophers were concerned. Ethical codes, too, have a long history: perhaps the most famous code of all is the medical 'Hippocratic Oath', written, probably by Hippocrates' students, in the fifth century BC. Even patient autonomy, the *summum bonum* of modern bioethics, has its origins, as the German doctor and historian of medicine, Ulrich Tröhler, has shown, in nineteenth and early twentieth century concerns about patient consent (Tröhler, 2002). So, just why did 'bioethics' spread so rapidly around the world in the last quarter of the twentieth century?

Think about this question for yourself before turning to the reading:

♦ List any factors that you believe may be behind the rapid growth of modern bioethics in the second half of the twentieth century.

♦ Then note the factors identified in the three extracts from:

Maehle, A-H. and Geyer-Kordesch, J. (ed.) (2002). Introduction, pages 1–9 in A-H. Maehle and J. Geyer-Kordesch (eds). *Historical and Philosophical Perspectives on Biomedical Ethics: from Paternalism to Autonomy?* Aldershot, England: Ashgate Publishing Limited. (Extracts pps 1–3).

Link with Reading 18.1

Maehle and Geyer-Kordesch are both historians of medicine. This edited collection, although not attempting an exhaustive treatment of the subject, provides many important historical insights into the growth of modern bioethics. History, as we noted in Chapter 7, is not futurology; but the perspectives of history on bioethics can help us to understand its emerging limitations as well as its evident successes.

Five historical factors

In these short extracts from their introduction, Maehle and Geyer-Kordesch (2002) touch on a number of factors widely regarded as being important to the growth of bioethics. There are no doubt other factors: and their list may be different from yours (in the first part of Exercise 1 above). Historically, each of the factors identified by Maehle and Geyer-Kordesch is worthy of a chapter in its own right. But briefly, these include:

1. *Mid-twentieth century atrocities.* The Nuremberg trials, noted in the second extract from Maehle and Geyer-Kordesch (pp. 1–2), shocked the world not just for the gross abuses of human rights they revealed, but for the complicity of doctors in those abuses in the name of medical research.

2. *Rapid advances in medical science and technology.* Maehle and Geyer-Kordesch open their Introduction with this factor. 'New technologies', they say (first extract, p. 1), create new ethical dilemmas'. This has been true in the past as well as today: a little later (p. 2), Maehle and Geyer-Kordesch pair Mary Shelley's nineteenth century cautionary tale of *Frankenstein* in the same paragraph with Dolly the Sheep (Dolly was the first successful sheep clone). From the 1960s onwards we have witnessed medical science and technology advancing at an unprecedented pace. Combined with the loss of trust in medicine arising from a recognition of the abuses to which medical science can be harnessed, technological advance has been a major factor in the growth of corresponding ethical

concerns. The bottom line of Chapter 17 was that *bio*ethics, or *bio*medical ethics as Maehle and Geyer-Kordesch call it in the introduction to their book, is aptly named as a response predominantly to *bio*medicine.

3. *Opening up the doctor–patient relationship.* In part because of a loss of trust in medicine, the hitherto privileged status of the doctor–patient relationship was challenged by other professionals, notably, as Maehle and Geyer-Kordesch indicate, 'lawyers, moral philosophers, theologians, and sociologists.' Although only touched on by Maehle and Geyer-Kordesch (at this point in their Introduction), the shift from trusting relationship to legal contract in the doctor–patient relationship has been a major factor shaping modern bioethics. The founder of the first modern centre for bioethics in the UK was a lawyer, Ian Kennedy. Kennedy's landmark publication on the subject was called evocatively *The Unmasking of Medicine* (Kennedy, 1981, emphasis added as underline).

4. *Wider social changes: the Civil Rights Movement.* An important factor in the United States was the 1960s rise of civil rights. As Maehle and Geyer-Kordesch put it, the momentum created by the movement for 'equality of ethnic minorities, and women's liberation paved the way for patients' rights and a new approach to ethics in medicine' (p. 3). From North America, then, as the birthplace of 'bioethics', this 'new approach' spread to western Europe and around the world.

5. *The Four Principles.* Maehle and Geyer-Kordesch are perhaps unusual in emphasizing the importance of Tom Beauchamp and James Childress' (1989) book on the *Principles of Biomedical Ethics*.

We return to the four principles (autonomy, beneficence, non-maleficence, and justice) below. We will see that they have been subject to wide-ranging criticisms. As historians, though, Maehle and Geyer-Kordesch are perhaps better placed than many to recognize the significance of this book, first published in 1979, in the development of bioethics. Coming as it did when the new movement was expanding rapidly, it provided a comprehensive framework for tackling ethical problems, philosophically well-grounded (Beauchamp is a philosopher; Childress a theologian), and yet directly practical in application. As such, it gave expression to, and consolidated, what has become perhaps the defining feature of the new bioethics, patient autonomy. Since the publication of this book, Maehle and Geyer-Kordesch say (third extract, p. 3), 'It has … become customary to view modern biomedical ethics as being guided by the principle of patient autonomy. The older medical ethics, by contrast, are usually seen as an expression of the beneficent paternalism of doctors.'

From origins to aims

The origins of bioethics, as a modern offshoot of applied ethics, can be summarized thus: bioethics developed in response to medicine's complicity in mid-twentieth century abuses of human rights, which, combined with Frankenstein fears of rapidly advancing medical science and technology, led lawyers and others to open up the previously sacrosanct relationship between doctor and patient, putting patients' rights in place of trust in doctors, and patient autonomy in place of medical paternalism.

The corresponding aims of bioethics can be summarized similarly: bioethics aims to empower patients, giving them autonomy in how they are treated, by codifying their legal rights to self-determination, thus breaking the power of the 'doctor-knows-best' assumption of medical paternalism, and controlling the uses to which advances in medical sciences and technology are put, all with the ultimate aim of ensuring that abuses, such as those witnessed in mid-twentieth century Europe, never happen again.

Bioethical outcomes

But how have things worked out? There is little doubt that doctors are more conscious of the need to get patients' consent to treatment. And as Maehle and Geyer-Kordesch (2002) note, in terms of outputs, the proliferation of ethical codes and legal sanctions is a matter of historical fact.

But, again, how have things worked out? Have these developments led to improvements in health care? It is perhaps little short of heresy in the current climate to suggest that bioethics might be in some respects *bad* for our health! However, we noted in Chapter 17 the relatively 'late and local' nature of bioethics' guiding principle of autonomy: it is a late comer to medical ethics, historically speaking; and it is a local, not universal, principle, being recognized only in those cultures that value individuals ahead of families and the wider community. So what about bioethics as a whole? *Has* it been good for our health?

EXERCISE 2

Think about this question before going on. Concentrate here on bioethics as a whole rather than this or that 'school' or approach. And focus on the way bioethics has actually *worked out in practice* rather than on its nature as an academic discipline.

Write down any 'downsides' of the practical impact of bioethics that you can think of.

As an academic discipline bioethics has developed a rich tradition of scholarship spanning not only history and philosophy but also such disciplines as politics, economics, psychology, and social theory. It has an expanding research base, too, encompassing a range of empirical as well as legal and ethical methodologies (Fulford *et al.*, 2002a).

As a practical discipline, by contrast, bioethics has developed largely as an extension of medical law. We can understand this in terms of its origins and aims: the perceived need was for medical science and technology to be regulated by laws strengthening patients' rights. Bioethics has thus sought to give these laws 'teeth' by detailing their implications in codes and guidelines, supported, where necessary, by quasi-legal regulatory bodies with powers of interpretation and enforcement.

Three bioethical downsides

It is predominantly by way of quasi-legal 'rules and regulation', then, that bioethics has interacted with practice. This 'quasi-legal' approach has important strengths (see below). Paradoxically, though, it has also had a number of 'downsides' (Fulford, 2001).

Different groups, different individuals, identify different downsides to the growth of quasi-legal bioethics in health care. We will see later that these differences reflect different value perspectives. The downsides identified by a group of senior health-care providers—mainly voluntary and statutory sector chief executives—are given in Table 18.1. Your lists may of course be different. Summing across different groups, though, the downsides to quasi-legal bioethics can be thought of as falling into three broad areas that we will call, code inflation, practitioner deflation, and problem conflation.

1. *Code inflation: the growth of rules and regulation.* Maehle and Geyer-Kordesch (2002), in the reading linked with Exercise 1, touch on the growing tide of codes and other regulatory documents. The British Medical Association, whose guidance on ethics for doctors 50 years ago was a slim-line leaflet, has just published its latest advice in an 800-page *magnum opus*.

   Such code inflation would be acceptable if it were having its intended effects. But as Maehle and Geyer-Kordesch note, at the end of the second extract (pp. 1–2) from their Introduction, in volume and complexity alone, modern ethical codes are becoming counter-productive; and as they signal at the end of the third extract (p. 3), it is far from clear that, even as a way of securing patient autonomy, the rules and regulations approach is proving effective.

2. *Practitioner deflation: defensive (and other bad) practices.* The original mainspring of bioethics, as noted above, was a desire to prevent abusive misuses of medical science and technology: 'never again' was the watchword after Nuremberg. But no set of rules and regulations can ever be foolproof. There is always an 'again'. There is always another 'scandal' when the

rules and regulations are breached. So there is always a perceived need to tighten up the rules and regulations still further. A vicious cycle, of which code inflation is the main symptom, is the inevitable result.

Again, practitioner deflation might be acceptable if it were effective. But the rules and regulations to which health-care practitioners are subject, have become increasingly divorced from the realities of practice, to the extent that far from preventing bad practice they are in some cases actually promoting it. The most direct effect of this has been the growth of 'defensive practice': health-care decisions increasingly being taken, not in the best interests of clients or patients but on the basis of least risk of being hauled up before an ethics tribunal, or, indeed, finding oneself in court (Fulford, 2001).

Other adverse effects on practitioners noted in Table 18.1 include 'burn out', a culture of mutual suspicion rather than of collaboration, and the squandering of health-care resources on litigation.

3. *Problem conflation: disadvantaging patients.* Less well recognized, perhaps, but certainly the most significant downside of the quasi-legal form in which bioethics has interacted with

Table 18.1 'Downsides' to quasi-legal bioethics identified by one group of senior health-care service providers

- Cross-culturally insensitive
- Makes doctor–patient relationship impersonal
- Leads to hostility
- Risk phobic
- Rights obsessed
- Too many guidelines
- Contradictory guidelines
- 'Burn out'
- Defensive practice
- Cost of litigation rising
- Conflicts with individual needs/wishes

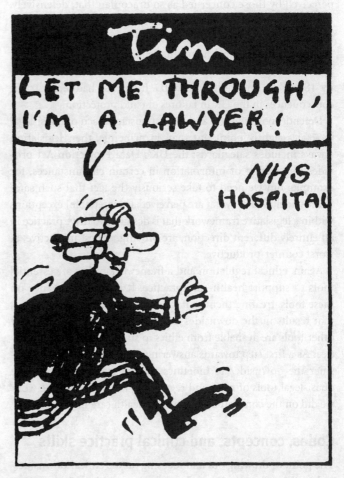

Fig. 18.1

practice, has been the extent to which it has had the opposite of its intended effects.

As noted above, and as we will consider in more detail below, rules and regulations have an important place in health care. But the *extent* to which they have been taken has resulted in patients actually being *dis*empowered, rather than, as intended, *em*powered. The British social scientist, Patricia Alderson, was among the first to point out this paradoxical effect of the new 'profession' of bioethics: patients, she pointed out, once disenfranchised by the specialist knowledge of the medical profession, are now doubly disenfranchised by the growing specialist knowledge of the new professional ethicist (Alderson, 1990, 1994). Similar concerns are beginning to be raised about the growing bureaucracy of research ethics committees (Gennery, 2005; Osborn, 1999; Savulescu, 2001; Warlow, 2005). In place of the traditional hegemony of 'doctor knows best', then, as one of us has put it elsewhere, we are at risk of a new hegemony of 'ethicist knows best' (Fulford *et al.*, 2002a, p. 4).

There is of course a growing and ever more powerful 'patient voice' in health care, a voice that is increasingly well able to take on the ethical as any other professional mafia! The effects of over-regulation, though, will continue to be felt most acutely by vulnerable groups. In the UK, for example, a Data Protection Act, designed to secure patients' rights to confidentiality, has been perceived by those concerned as so draconian that, defensively, they have sometimes failed to communicate information when this was essential to good clinical care. This has become a generic concern in mental health with its reliance on multidisciplinary and multiagency team working for effective 'care in the community' (Szmukler and Holloway, 2001). It has also had recent tragic consequences in the UK in failures of child protection.

Defenders of the rules and regulations approach of quasi-legal bioethics rightly point out that, in principle, their legislation always includes safeguards: the UK's Data Protection Act provides for sharing of information in certain circumstances, for example. But we need to take seriously the fact that such safeguards, included as (what are perceived as regrettable) exceptions within a legislative framework that is designed to drive practice in an entirely different direction, are proving, at best ineffective, at worst counter-productive.

Again, ethical regulation and a framework of law are essential tools to support health-care practice. It is an *over*-reliance on these tools, treating them as if they were the only tools we need, that results in the downsides outlined in this section. So, what other tools are available from ethics to support health-care practice? As a first step towards answering this question, we will consider the downsides to bioethics, arising from overuse of the quasi-legal tools of rules and regulation, in the light of the work we did on the conceptual structure of health care in Part I.

Codes, concepts, and clinical practice skills

The point of drawing out and focusing on the ethical 'downsides' to bioethics, then, in its predominantly quasi-legal interactions with practice, is not to suggest that we can do without codes of practice, still less a framework of law, altogether. On the contrary, as tools in the toolkit, as we put it above, they are essential. Clear statements of rights, indeed, backed with legal action, have been important in rolling back embedded prejudices. They remain important, as we will see later, in providing a framework for practice. But the point is that if these tools are the *only* tools in the toolkit, and if therefore they are used for the wrong task, or for the right task in the wrong way, they can become counter-productive: like using a hammer to tighten a screw, or a screwdriver to hammer in a nail!

So, what has gone wrong? The historical origins of bioethics, in gross abuses of human rights, explains its over-reliance on quasi-legal tools. But what, exactly, is the *right* use of such tools? Why, exactly, are they no *panacea*? And what *other* tools do we need?

EXERCISE 3

Think about these three questions. There are a number of ways they might be approached—through jurisprudence, for example, or political theory.

But think about them with the work we have done in earlier parts of this book in mind. In particular,

1. Part I generally, on concepts: What kind of answer might Austin have given to these questions in terms of his key methodological distinction between definition and use?

2. Part III, in particular the second half of Chapter 14, on implicit (or craft) knowledge: are the decisions that quasi-legal ethics seeks to control simple or complex? If complex, what does this imply about the ways in which they might be guided?

Code inflation: definition and use

Austin's ideas, in Part I, about philosophical fieldwork, started from a recognition of the limitations of explicit definitions: remember St Augustine's complaint that he knew what he meant by time until somebody asked him!

Lawyers, like doctors, believe in starting by defining their terms. As we saw in Part I, this can be helpful. But there are also situations in which language use is more helpful than definition as a guide to meaning. Hence one way to understand the downsides to over-reliance on the tools of quasi-legal bioethics, is that they could be a result of an over-reliance on explicit definition. 'Code inflation', in particular, as we called the first downside to quasi-legal ethics, could arise when we try to define the indefinable. Attempts to anticipate and to close down all 'loopholes' could fail essentially because the key concepts expressed in our codes are higher-level concepts, concepts of the kind, like time, that we are better able to use than to define. We explore this possibility further in the next reading.

EXERCISE 4

Read the following version of the Hippocratic Oath from:

Dorland's American Illustrated Medical Dictionary, (25th edn). (1974). Philadelphia, PA: Saunders.

Link with Reading 18.2

◆ List the main prescriptions of the Oath.

◆ What 'higher-level' concepts can you identify?

◆ How does the Oath avoid the limitations of explicit definition?

As the most famous of medical codes, the Hippocratic Oath avoids the problem of defining the indefinable by taking the form of an overall framework of general principles reflecting higher-level concepts, and, rather than seeking to define these sufficiently to cover all contingencies, it provides a number of concrete specific examples.

A framework of general principles

The power of this approach is reflected in the fact that many of the 'framework principles' in the Hippocratic Oath sound surprisingly modern! Thus the principles of beneficence and non-maleficence are directly reflected in the Hippocratic injunction that 'I will prescribe regimen for the good of my patients according to my ability and my judgement and never do harm to anyone.' The opening clauses of the Oath, about professional solidarity and peer education, are perhaps less significant nowadays—but many perceive a clear need to move them back up the agenda! Confidentiality, much in the news at present, is mentioned towards the end. There is a familiar injunction against seducing one's patients or members of their households. There is also a clear reference to working within one's area of professional expertise (not to 'cut for stone'). True, there is no mention of 'autonomy'. But autonomy, as we have several times noted, is a 'late and local' value in health care.

Some of the many higher-level concepts shaping these principles are evident enough: 'beneficence' and 'non-malevolence', noted above, are higher-level ethical concepts. Other such concepts are less evident but no less important to the structure of the Oath. Thus, in the opening clauses the very scope of application of the Oath is defined by a brief reference to 'this art'. Well, what art? The Oath is assumed to be a *medical* oath; and Hippocrates was a physician; but there is no attempt directly to define the 'art' in respect of which the Oath is taken. And wisely so, perhaps, given that any definition of 'medicine' would turn (in part) on definitions of such contested concepts as 'illness' and 'disease'.

'Confidentiality' may seem more straightforward, but it turns out to be highly complex conceptually (Fulford, 2001). Correspondingly, therefore, the Hippocratic Oath neatly side-steps any difficulties of definition with a tautology: physicians,

the Oath enjoins, are to keep confidential only that 'which ought not to be spread abroad.'

Same principles, different examples

The Hippocratic Oath, then, specifies, but does not seek to define, its own key concepts. It does, however, moving in Austin's terms from definition to use, illustrate its key concepts with specific examples. And whereas the general principles often seem familiar by modern standards, some of the examples, by contrast, seem distinctly odd.

Avoiding harm, for instance, for most doctors, certainly does not extend to refusing abortion; and even the prohibition against administering a deadly poison is being actively challenged by a growing pro-euthanasia lobby. Similarly with professional solidarity, few if any of the health-care professions would recognize this as extending to living 'in common' with one's teachers, still less to sharing one's worldly goods with them; and neither teacher nor pupil, nowadays, would welcome the relationship of parent and child! 'Cutting for stone', again, *is* now a properly *medical* activity, surgeons being part of the profession. The ban on 'pleasures of love', although still applicable to one's patients, does not extend to their family members, servants, and friends (providing always that these fall outside one's professional relationships). And keeping secret the 'precepts and instruction' of medicine would be considered positively *un*ethical nowadays: the emphasis today is all on openness and sharing of medical information.

The currency of the Hippocratic Oath is thus to be found primarily in its general principles rather than in the specifics of how these principles are applied. But the specifics, we have suggested, are, in Austin's terms, the higher-level concepts in *use*. And use, we learned in Part I, is a better guide to meaning than explicit definition. So the variations between Hippocrates' time and our own in the specifics of the Oath reflect variations in values that are *considerably wider* than is apparent from the shared higher-level concepts—solidarity, beneficence, etc.—in terms of which the Oath's general principles are defined. We share the same 'framework' principles, certainly, principles such as beneficence and solidarity. But those same principles, if the examples given by Hippocrates are any guide, meant something very different when the Oath was written from what they mean today.

Codes as a framework of shared values

This J.L. Austin-led interpretation of the Hippocratic Oath suggests that one proper role for codes, as a tool in the ethical toolkit, is to give expression to those values that are shared within a given group. That the particular meaning attached to these 'framework values' as we might call them, changes, from time to time, from culture to culture, from person to person, and so on, may seem, to the moral absolutist, to undermine the cogency of such values. But understood as higher-level concepts, such variations are no more than we should expect: to revert to our example in Part I, interpretations of the meaning of 'time' vary while time remains none the less an essential higher-level concept for physics.

As to practical utility, we noted above the effectiveness of 'codes' in highlighting and pushing back against abuses. A currently important example, highlighted by the Hippocratic Oath, is the value of professional solidarity. Currently lost in the glare of the new value of patient autonomy, the value of professional solidarity is perhaps overdue for a come back. One factor in the current demoralization of health-care professionals is their loss, severally and together, of professional collegiality. We need to rethink what professional solidarity means in the twenty-first century. We should not wish to return to the medical cartel. But the Hippocratic Oath, in prompting such a rethink, would be prompting us to think precisely what the value of professional solidarity means for our particular time, for our particular place, for our particular culture. The results of such a rethink would be specific examples, different from those of cohabiting and sharing of goods in the original Hippocratic code, but relevant to professional practice today.

A proper use of codes, then, in answer to our first question above, is to give expression to the framework values shared by a given group. Such frameworks, to the extent that they rely on higher-level concepts, should be cast in general terms rather than attempting to define specific rules to cover all contingencies. If further guidance is needed, then specific examples, rather than more detailed rules and further regulation, are appropriate.

A paradigm of this approach, balancing general principles and specific examples, is the Code of Practice of the Royal Australian and New Zealand College of Psychiatrists (1998): this gives general principles applicable across the college as a whole with annotations specific to each subspecialty.

Codes are no panacea

This J.L. Austin led interpretation also gives one kind of answer to the second of our three questions immediately preceding Exercise 3 above, namely, why, exactly, codes, although in some respects practically effective, are no panacea. Thus, the specific meanings attached to shared values, we have suggested, vary not only across historical periods but also from culture to culture, and even from individual to individual. Hence, the more energetically a code seeks not only to express shared values but also to pin down the specific meanings to be attached to those shared values, the greater will be the opportunities for conflict between the values expressed by the code and the values of those to whom the code is intended to apply. Pinning the specifics down in one way may be consistent with the values of *some* individuals within the group; but given the variation in human values, it will be inconsistent with the values of *others*.

Code inflation, then, arises from the (understandable) attempt to close loop-holes by writing ever-more detailed rules to cover all contingencies. Codes, though, if the Hippocratic Oath is any guide, rely on higher-level concepts, that, we found in Part I, are beyond the reach of complete definition. Code inflation, in consequence, is (1) mistaken in principle, in that it involves, as we put it above, defining the indefinable, and (2) unhelpful in

practice to the extent that, in moving beyond general statements of the shared framework values with which codes are properly concerned to detailed rules of application, they will necessarily be in conflict with the values of many of those to whom the codes in question are intended to apply.

Professional deflation: explicit and implicit knowledge

Code inflation, and the conflicts of values to which this gives rise, is itself one reason for 'professional deflation', the second of the downsides to overuse of quasi-legal ethics noted above. Confidentiality in mental health, as we noted above, provides a current case in point. Quasi-legal ethical, and indeed legal rules, in seeking to pin down confidentiality of patient information, have squeezed professional practice to the point that the sharing on information on which good practice in mental health depends, is at risk of increasingly being squeezed out. Professionals are thus left in a 'damned if you do, damned if you don't' double bind, a recipe for defensive practice, demoralization and burnout if ever there was one.

A second reason for professional deflation is to be found in the nature of the decisions by which professional practice itself is characterized. We will look at this briefly in the next exercise.

EXERCISE 5

In the above example, we used the conflict between the values of confidentiality and sharing of information. Both values, at least in mental health, are important. They are, then, in the sense outlined above, shared framework values. Yet they are in conflict.

Now go back to the Hippocratic Oath. What has it to say about this?

As you reread the Hippocratic Oath, think particularly about the nature of the kind of knowledge on which you would draw in balancing confidentiality and sharing of information in the concrete circumstances of a particular case. In the terms of Part III (Chapter 14) of this book, is this explicit or implicit knowledge? If the latter, what does this say about the overuse of quasi-legal ethics and 'professional deflation'?

As noted above, confidentiality is one of the higher-level shared values expressed by the Hippocratic Oath. It is worth looking at the relevant passage in detail, though. In the first place, it differs from modern codes in calling for confidentiality of 'All that may come to my knowledge in the exercise of my profession or outside of my profession or in daily commerce with men . . .'. So it is a good deal broader than, merely, professional ethics. But this otherwise impossibly high standard is then, in the next passage, sharply restricted to such knowledge as 'ought not to be spread abroad'.

A tautological principle, then, as we noted above! And unlike other principles in the Oath, we are given no specifics. So we have no direct guidance on precisely what information, at Hippocrates' time, 'ought not to be spread abroad'. We can make educated guesses, though, by taking this principle along with others. The principle of professional solidarity would preclude spreading abroad the 'precepts and instruction' of the art, at any rate beyond the family of the physician's teacher and properly signed up pupils. As noted above, this directly conflicts with modern views on what counts as 'sensitive' information.

Suppose, on the other hand, it comes to your attention, as a physician in Hippocrates' time, that someone from a different 'college' is planning, in the words of the Oath, to 'give a woman a pessary to secure an abortion': presumably that *should* be spread abroad. But what if the person giving the pessary is a colleague? How does professional solidarity square with the prohibition on abortion when it comes to confidentiality? Or what if the woman is your sister and is pregnant through rape? Ought your knowledge that a colleague is about to give her a pessary to secure an abortion, be spread abroad; or would the resulting harm, to both your colleague and sister, outweigh the demands of the anti-abortion principle? Note here that the injunction against doing harm is general, it is 'never do harm to *anyone*', not just to patients through the exercise of the art.

Balancing framework values

The problems of balancing confidentiality, as one framework value in the Hippocratic Oath, against others, are thus evident enough. Similar problems are familiar enough in present-day discussions of ethical issues. However ready we are to sign up to any one of the values expressed by a code, there will always be difficulties arising from trading one value against another in the concrete particulars of everyday practical situations. 'Particularism', as it is sometimes called, the extent to which moral judgements are particular or can be subsumed under general rules, has been widely discussed in ethical theory (see, e.g. Hooker and Little, 2000). In relation to codes, though, and the 'professional deflation' downside of the overuse of quasi-legal ethics, it is helpfully understood in terms of a distinction more familiar in the philosophy of science, between explicit and implicit, or craft, knowledge.

Thus, the trade-offs required in practice between the different values expressed in a given code, suggest that the decisions required of professionals are necessarily highly complex. Even, therefore, granted excessive zeal on the part of code makers, there will be barriers of principle to full codification of the rules for successful trade-offs. In other words, rather like riding a bicycle, no set of explicit rules will ever be sufficient for successful performance of the required trade-offs between values. Such trade-offs, to the contrary, will rely on implicit knowledge, knowledge of the kind that professionals, after training, characteristically display; knowledge that is acquired through experience rather than from 'book learning'; knowledge that is aptly called 'craft' knowledge. (Hence the reference in the above Exercise 5 to implicit knowledge in Part III, chapter 14.)

Professional judgement

It may be no coincidence, then, that in the Hippocratic Oath, the physician is required to practise his art 'according to my ability

and my judgement' (emphasis added). Certainly, the distinction between explicit knowledge and craft skills was well understood in Classical Greece: the distinction, you will recall from Part III, was made explicitly about a hundred years after Hippocrates, by Aristotle, who distinguished logic and other forms of discursive reasoning, from what he called in *The Nicomachean Ethics* ('Ethics') (2000), 'practical reasoning'. At all events, the implications for practice are clear. Attempts to apply ethical codes, not for their proper purpose of giving expression to the high-level values shared within a profession, but for the purpose of specifying in detail how these values are to be balanced in particular circumstances, will end up, as it were, cutting the craft from under the feet of the professionals concerned. Small wonder, then, that when codes are used to pin professionals down ever more tightly in their day-to-day practice, they are demoralizing in their effects. They are, literally, de-professionalizing.

There is a middle path to be struck here, of cause. *Some* guidance is required, indeed helpful, if only because professions progress and new kinds of decision are constantly arising. But writing ever more detailed codes is not the answer. And there *are* alternatives. One alternative, the most directly indicated by the 'craft knowledge' model of values trade-offs, is wider use of case examples, as in the Hippocratic Oath itself. Such examples tap directly into the well of implicit knowledge and they translate readily into practice. Law, indeed, where it relies on cases, works well in this respect. There are new questions here, arising from the changing role of patients, about *whose* experience should guide decision-making. Balanced decisions can no longer rely on the experience, merely, of the professional. We must find ways of incorporating also the experiences of patients (Fulford, 2001). All the same, implicit as well as explicit knowledge, is irreducible if the trade-offs required between the different values expressed by codes are to be successfully negotiated in the values-complex environment of everyday practice.

From right outcomes to good process

As tools in the ethical toolkit, codes of practice, and the regulatory bodies responsible for interpreting and enforcing them, are outcome focused: they prescribe 'right outcomes' by which clinical (and managerial) decisions should be guided.

This is the strength of quasi-legal bioethics. Like a rights-based legal framework, prescribed right outcomes set clear limits, defined, as we have seen, by shared values. It is also its focus on 'right outcomes', however, that leads to some of the downsides of quasi-legal bioethics if it is the only tool in the toolkit. It is *over-*specification of outcomes that leads to the vicious cycle of code inflation. It is *over-*regulation of the trade-offs between rules, leaving insufficient space for professional discretion reflecting implicit knowledge gained through experience, that leads to professional deflation.

This brings us to the third question raised at the start of this section, namely, what further tools are needed for the ethical toolkit. For if the tools of quasi-legal ethics focus on outcomes, and if it is this focus that makes them counterproductive if over-used, then there is a clear case for a switch from outcomes to process—not, of course, to throw out the tools of right outcomes, but to add to them tools of good process.

Advocates and adversarial 'good process'

One tool of good process, of which excellent use has been made in law, is advocacy. Due process in many court proceedings is secured by both sides appointing advocates who then argue their respective corners in front of an impartial judge, and, in serious cases, a jury. The outcome of this process, within wide limits, is not pre-judged but depends on the case advanced by each side operating within a broad set of rules of procedure designed to ensure fair play. Such rules, it is important to emphasize, are essential. But they are aimed at securing good process rather than this or that particular prescribed 'right' outcome.

Problem conflation: adversarial and other 'tools'

Advocacy, as a tool of good process, has an important place in health-care ethics when we come to the third downside of the overuse of quasi-legal bioethics, problem conflation. Problem conflation, you will recall, was the paradoxical result that rules and regulations, designed to secure the rights of vulnerable groups, if taken to an extreme can have the opposite effect. They can put at risk just those vulnerable groups they were designed to protect.

Problem conflation is a clear consequence of the outcomes focus of quasi-legal ethics. The values of vulnerable groups are as diverse as those of any other group. If outcomes are *over* speci-fied, therefore, the necessary conflicts of values noted above, between the outcomes specified and the values of those falling under the rules and regulations in question, will arise for vulner-able as for any other groups. Vulnerable groups, though, by def-inition, will be less able to fight their corner than non-vulnerable groups. Vulnerable groups, therefore, more than non-vulnerable, are at risk of what we called earlier, 'ethicist knows best'.

Advocacy, as a tool of good process, can be helpful, therefore, in securing a balanced approach to clinical decision-making. The difficulty, though, with advocacy is that it so readily becomes adversarial, a contest in which those with the resources to pay the most effective advocates come out top of the league. Advocacy alone, therefore, although a further useful tool in the toolkit, will never be sufficient to avoid problem conflation. So long as we rely on an essentially adversarial process for resolving questions of value, whoever is at the time disadvantaged, inherently or through lack of support, will lose out.

Three tools of bioethical reasoning

The tool of adversarial exchange, then, like outcome-based codes, is important in its place but not sufficient (in itself) to support good process in clinical decision-making where, as in health care, 'good' is measured from the perspective of vulnerable groups. So, what other tools are available? In the final section of this session we introduce three such tools derived from modern bioethics—principles,

casuistry, and perspectives. As we will see, these are three methods of ethical reasoning, or reasoning about values, that, in the values-complex environment of modern health-care decision-making, are rapidly becoming recognized as essential clinical practice skills. We consider the strengths and weaknesses of these three tools specifi-cally for mental health ethics in Session 2 of this chapter.

Principles, causitry, and perspectives

There are two main approaches to practical ethical reasoning in the bioethical literature, *principles* and *causitry*. To these, the psychi-atrists and Professor of Medical Ethics in Oxford, Tony Hope, has added a third approach, *perspectives* (Hope *et al.*, 1996). In this sec-tion we will first outline each of these approaches and then consider their strengths and weaknessess generally in health care. As just noted, we turn to their applications to mental health in Session 2.

The four principles

As indicated above, the principles approach was developed origi-nally in America at Georgetown University by Tom Beauchamp and James Childress in their *Principles of Biomedical Ethics* (1989). In the UK the approach has been taken up and extended by the first Professor of Medical Ethics at Imperial College in London, Raanon Gillon. His *Philosophical Medical Ethics* (1985, and subsequent reprints) helped to introduce bioethics into British medicine and remains a valuable introduction to the sub-ject. In his monumental *Principles of Health-care Ethics* (Gillon and Lloyd, 1994), original articles were gathered together on every aspect of bioethics exploring the strengths and weaknesses of the four principles approach.

Gillon, although openly an enthusiast for the four principles as a framework for ethical reasoning, has been careful to spell out the limitations of the approach: they can provide a common moral framework, but within this framework people may none the less disagree (they may 'weigh' the principles differently, for example). Moreover, there are important issues raised by the *scope of application* of the principles (Gillon, 1994). The scope of the principles was largely taken for granted in Beauchamp and Childress' (1989) original book but it becomes important when we move from the clear-cut dilemmas of technological medicine to the more heterogeneous difficulties raised by primary care. As well as being a leading medical ethicist, and at the time of writ-ing his 1994 article, editor of *The Journal of Medical Ethics*, Gillon was indeed a primary care physician (working as a family doctor).

Turning to the four principles themselves, then, they are:

1. *Autonomy*: respecting the patient's wishes
2. *Beneficence*: doing good
3. *Non-maleficence*: avoiding harm
4. *Justice*: in particular, fairness in the provision of care

These are prima facie principles (Beauchamp and Childress' term). That is, they are all prima facie relevant to ethical issues in health care and have to be balanced one against another in particular cases. There are no general rules for balancing principles. This has to follow intuition.

It is often said against the principles approach that it is too algorithmic—you feed in the problem, crank through the principles, and get out an answer. Gillon makes it clear that such mechanical uses of the principles approach would be quite wrong; and in their book, Beauchamp and Childress (1989) themselves carefully spell out that this would be a gross misuse of principles reasoning.

Casuistry or case-based reasoning

The principles approach is top down. It tackles ethical problems by applying general principles to particular cases. The casuistic approach is bottom-up. It starts from particular cases. Where there is a dilemma or disagreement, casuistry asks two questions,

1. what *changes* to the case can you imagine that would make it clearer what to do, and

2. what *related* cases would be either more or less problematic ethically.

Historically, casuistry has had a bad reputation. It became associated with the practice of moulding cases to fit ones own beliefs and wishes. The term was rehabilitated recently by two American scholars, Stephen Toulmin (you will recall his article 'How Medicine Saved the Life of Ethics' in the last session), and A.R. Jonsen, in their seminal book, *The Abuse of Casuistry* (1988). In this they describe their experience on an American government committee, the President's Commission on Bioethics. They noted that on many ethical issues, most people on the Commission agreed what ought to be done, but they disagreed about why. This, they argued, showed the irrelevance of theory. The way to reason about ethical issues is not to apply general theories but to look carefully at the details of particular cases.

A valuable introduction to casuistry is the article, 'Medical ethics, moral philosophy and moral tradition', by the American philosopher Tom Murray (1994). Tom Murray, at the time Director of the Center for Biomedical Ethics at Case Western Reserve University, Cleveland, Ohio, went on to become Director of the Hastings Centre and President of the Society for Health and Human Values. In this article he contrasts casuistry with principles reasoning (he calls this deductivism, i.e. deducing moral conclusions from general principles), and sets it in the context of recent work on moral tradition.

Casuistry has sometimes been viewed by ethicists as a competitor to the four principles, even as a more 'advanced' ethical method. There is something of this in Murray's article. He distinguishes two sense of casuistry (though noting that it has many meanings):

1. immersion in the particulars of a case, and

2. the claim that moral judgement rooted in moral tradition (as against philosophical and other moral 'theories') may be a source of moral knowledge, or at any rate guidance.

In the detail and complexity of real life cases, Murray argues, immersion in and interpretation of moral theory are inescapably linked. In real life, moreover, the moral traditions of a culture are an essential resource of moral guidance. In both the above senses, then, ethical reasoning in health care must look to case-based, bottom-up approaches, rather than principle-led, top-down approaches. But is this a recipe for rigid conservatism, for the perpetuation of received values? No, Murray argues, for cultures have a power of dynamic change.

We will return to the importance of the dangers of rigid conservatism in mental health in Session 2. In this respect (and in others), as we will see, the two approaches—casuistry and principles—are complementary in mental health ethics.

Perspectives

The perspectives approach emphasizes the importance in ethical reasoning of the different points of view (ie perspectives) of those concerned (Hope *et al.*, 1996). Perspectives are important to both principles and casuistry. How, for example, can the principle of beneficence be applied if we do not understand what someone wants? How, on the other hand, in reasoning casuistically, can the circumstances of a case be varied in an ethically meaningful way without understanding what is relevant from a particular person's point of view?

Perspectives is a relative newcomer on the bioethical scene, essentially because it was always assumed that what people want is more or less transparent. In some cases this may be true—for example, with abortion, or transplant surgery, many of the ethical issues arise from clear *conflicts* of perspectives. However, perspectives may be misunderstood: for example, contrary to the usual expectations of hospital staff, clinical experience suggests that the relatives of young people killed in accidents may sometimes welcome the idea of organ transplantation as a way of allowing something good to come out of something bad.

Misunderstandings about perspectives are especially common in primary care and mental health. This is because, as we saw earlier, people's values are inherently more diverse in this area.

Perspectives are particularly well brought out through the literary and other resources of what are often called narrative ethics. An early case study in narrative ethics that draws out the perspectives of all those involved in a vivid and highly readable way is by Alastair Campbell (a philosopher) and Roger Higgs (a family doctor) (1982), in their book 'In that care'.

Strengths and weaknesses

In practice, especially in mental health, these three approaches—principles, casuistry, and perspectives—are often usefully combined. However, in order to get clearer about the approaches themselves, and to think about their strengths and weaknesses, we will now try using them separately in connection with the cases that we considered at the start of Chapter 17.

EXERCISE 6   (30 minutes)

Go back to your initial cases in Chapter 17 and think about how you might use the above three approaches, principles, casuistry, and perspectives, to help resolve the dilemmas or disagreements they raise.

If you are working in a group, a good approach is to agree on a case that you would like to examine in detail (one involving consent always works well); then divide up into three subgroups, each examining the case using one of the above approaches to ethical reasoning.

As you do this, write down your reasoning, noting any advantages/disadvantages of the method that you are working with, and thinking particularly about the four intermediate objectives of training in ethical reasoning we examined in Chapter 17.

Some advantages and disadvantages of the three approaches are listed in Table 18.2. You may have found some extra advantages or disadvantages; and you may agree or disagree with some of those we have listed. But some important general points that often come up include the following:

♦ The *principles approach* is intuitively straightforward. It has also been shown to reflect many of the ideas that people fall back on naturally when faced with ethical issues in health care: this was shown clearly, for example, by the (at the time) medical student, David Roberston's (1996), empirical and conceptual study of ethical decision making in old age psychiatry.

The principles approach can be especially helpful in broadening our understanding of a case. In terms of our four intermediate objectives, principles reasoning may: (1) increase awareness (by forcing us to think about more than one aspect of a case); (2) change attitudes (by showing that a particular approach may be biased towards, say, beneficence at the expense of patient autonomy); (3) point to knowledge that

may be lacking (this ties in with perspectives especially); and (4) it can improve thinking skills (by giving us a well-structured way of analysing the pros and cons in a given case).

The main danger with the principles approach is that it can suggest that ethical issues may be solved, like mathematical or scientific problems, in a clear-cut way. In fact, as we noted above, this would be to misunderstand the approach (remember that prima facie principles have to be weighed intuitively); but it is a danger, none the less, especially when the principles approach is used on its own.

♦ *Casuistry* was developed in part as a response to the misuse of 'principlism'. Based as it is on cases, it has the great advantage of being directly relevant practically. Reasoning about cases is something that all practitioners are familiar with in other clinical contexts, and this kind of reasoning can often lead to agreement.

One problem with casuistry is that it can be very unstructured. A more significant difficulty, however, especially with the importance of different value perspectives in mental health, is the danger of reinforcing prejudices. Casuistic reasoning only 'goes through' to agreement where the value perspectives of those concerned are in fact shared. But in the case of mental health, as has repeatedly been noted in earlier sections, values are often *not* shared.

♦ *Perspectives* is the most patient-centred of the three approaches. It is especially important as the basis of good communication, an essential requirement for good practice in health care (Hope *et al.*, 1996).

There are no significant disadvantages to being sensitive to people's perspectives (to their values and beliefs). But unlike principles and casuistry, the perspectives approach, in itself, gives us no method of *reasoning* ethically. Simply being aware of people's perspectives, crucially important as it is, gives us no way of deciding what ought to be done. The perspectives approach provides essential *data* for ethical and other aspects of clinical decision-making; but it has to be linked up to a substantive theory of *some* kind if it is to give grounds for action.

A related theoretical danger with the perspectives approach is relativism, an underlying assumption that 'anything goes'. But it is of the essence of the professional relationship that, as against simple consumerism, there has to be a *balance* of values. (We return to the need for a balance of perspectives below, in Session 4, on Values-Based Practice. See also, Fulford, 1995.). So perspectives are essential (especially in mental health, because of the variety of people's values in this area) but they are not sufficient.

Each of the three main methods of bioethical reasoning thus offers strengths and weaknesses. In the next session we consider the roles of these methods specifically in relation to mental health.

Table 18.2 Advantages and disadvantages of three main approaches to ethical reasoning in bioethics

Main approaches	Advantages	Disadvantages
Principles	Increases awareness Changes attitudes Points to relevant facts Improves thinking skills	Algorithmic approach Professional-centred
Casuistry	Based on real life links with case method Often leads to agreement in practice	Agreement can mean bias, prejudice, and hence abuse Professional-centred
Perspectives	Patient-centred Knowledge-based	No reasoning method Relativism

Reflection on the session and self-test questions

Write down your own reflections on the materials in this session drawing out any points that are particularly significant for you. Then write brief notes about the following:

1. By what developments in medicine was the modern emergence of 'bioethics' prompted?

2. Have there been 'downsides' to bioethics? We listed three; what are they?

3. How are these 'downsides' related to the conceptual difficulties of mental health?

4. What three methods of ethical reasoning may be particularly helpful in practice?

5. Are these mutually exclusive or complementary?

Session 2 Bioethics and mental health

In this session, we consider how the three main bioethical approaches to reasoning about values—principles, casuistry, and perspectives—work out in mental health.

We will be considering this question, not in a general way but by reference to involuntary treatment and our responses to the case vignette questionnaire introduced in Chapter 17. You will recall that the Mental Health Act failed to map on to, or fit, our intuitive responses to these cases. The notion of 'psychotic disorder', by contrast, as a particular interpretation of 'serious mental disorder' gave a good fit. But it left open the question of how psychotic disorder itself was to be understood. As such, therefore, it took us little further towards a clearer understanding of the issues involved in those cases (1 and 3) in which, even in the relatively artificial circumstances of a case vignette questionnaire, opinion was deeply split over whether involuntary treatment was justified.

We now take this story a step further with the tools of modern bioethics. As we will see, these provide further clarification but still fail on the central point for mental health ethics of explaining the ethically relevant features of 'psychotic disorder'. We will start with the four principles.

Four principles (top-down reasoning)

An important strength of the principles approach is that it provides an open framework within which to explore the ethical aspects of treatment decisions. It thus looks promising as a way of explicating involuntary psychiatric treatment. It is

important to think about this for yourself before taking up the next reading. Hence the next exercise is in two stages.

EXERCISE 7   (60 minutes)

This exercise is in two stages:

Stage 1

Think for yourself about how you would analyse involuntary psychiatric treatment in terms of Beauchamp and Childress' four principles. Try applying the four principles to each of the cases in the case vignette questionnaire from Chapter 17. How well do they 'fit'?

Stage 2

Now read the extract from:

Fulford, K.W.M. and Hope, R.A. (1994). Psychiatric ethics: a bioethical ugly duckling? Chapter 58 In *Principles of Healthcare ethics* (ed. R. Gillon and A. Lloyd). Chichester, England: John Wiley and Sons, (Extract pp. 684–686.)

Link with Reading 18.3

This reading summarizes Beauchamp and Childress' (1989, chapter 3) detailed and carefully worked out analysis of the ethical issues raised by involuntary treatment as these arise in medicine generally, though with psychiatry being taken as a case in point.

As you read through this, think particularly about:

1. how Beauchamp and Childress analyse involuntary treatment in terms of their four principles,

2. the model of autonomy and voluntariness they describe as lying behind and underpinning the application of the four principles to involuntary treatment, and, finally,

3. whether or to what extent their model is consistent with the intuitive responses we made to the case vignette questionnaire in Chapter 17.

That Beauchamp and Childress should in effect take involuntary *psychiatric* treatment to be a subcase of involuntary *medical* treatment is a clear illustration of the point made earlier (in chapter 17), that much of traditional medical ethics reflects an essentially medical model of the conceptual structure of health care. We will see the importance of this in a moment. However, the case example they discuss (Beauchamp and Childress, 1989, p. 80), consistently with the prominence they give to psychiatric cases in their appendix (also in chaptr 17), is about a patient with *dementia*. This underscores the point that Beauchamp and Childress, unlike many in traditional bioethics, take fully seriously the particular difficulties of psychiatric ethics.

Balancing autonomy and beneficence

Essentially, then, Beauchamp and Childress (1989) take the key ethical issue in involuntary treatment to involve balancing (primarily) two principles: the principle of autonomy (respecting the patient's wishes) and the principle of beneficence (the professional's responsibility to act in the patient's best interests).

Normally, the best guide to anyone's best interests is their express wishes. In the past, however, in a 'doctor knows best' model, professionals have been assumed to be experts to *patients'* best interests. More recently, this 'paternalistic' approach has given way to a recognition of the importance of patient autonomy. But most people recognize cases, even so, where a person's express wishes are not the most reliable guide to their best interests (young children, for example). Hence we cannot simply substitute a 'patient knows best' principle for the old 'doctor knows best' approach. There will always be cases where 'best interests' and 'express wishes' are in conflict, and it is this conflict, interpreted by Beauchamp and Childress in terms of beneficence and autonomy, which is at the heart of the ethical dilemmas and difficulties presented by involuntary treatment.

This then leads naturally into an account of involuntary psychiatric treatment. For mental illness, as we noted in Session 3 of Chapter 17, to the extent that it involves people becoming irrational, impairs their capacity for *rational*, and hence fully *autonomous*, choice. Hence, this is one of the situations in which beneficence may be in conflict with autonomy. Of course, not *all* irrationality impairs autonomous choice sufficiently, or in the relevant way, to justify involuntary treatment. After all, we are all irrational at times! In Chapter 17, we noted that in the case of mental illness at least, it is psychotic irrationality that is (intuitively) required to justify involuntary treatment, but that this begged the question of precisely why. Beauchamp and Childress, correspondingly, turn to philosophical literature on the nature of rationality to draw out the criteria that must be satisfied if a choice is to be considered genuinely autonomous.

The criteria derived by Beauchamp and Childress can be summarized thus. For a choice to be autonomous, it must be: (1) intentional; (2) made with understanding; (3) free from external controlling influence (i.e. uncoerced); and (4) a product of intact cognitive capacities, in particular the capacities for coherent thought and deliberation. Correspondingly therefore, if these criteria are *not* satisfied, a person's choices may not be fully autonomous and involuntary psychiatric treatment may be justified on grounds of beneficence (and/or non-maleficence).

Balancing autonomy and beneficence in mental health

But, and this is a crucial 'but', do these criteria really fit what actually happens? In Exercise 7 (see part 3 of the second stage) you should have tried this for yourself. Beauchamp and Childress' (1989) case example of dementia fits the criteria rather well. But in our case vignette questionnaire, what about the young man with schizophrenia (case 9), say?

You may want to go through the cases again, checking them against the Beauchamp and Childress' criteria, before going on.

But the conclusion that Fulford and Hope (1994) reach is that, sophisticated as Beauchamp and Childress' approach is, and successful as it is in explaining *some* cases of involuntary treatment (including their own example of dementia), it fails to explain a large number of other cases of involuntary psychiatric treatment as they arise in everyday practice in mental health.

A further failure of fit

One indication of the failure of Beauchamp and Childress' (1989) account to explain many cases of involuntary psychiatric treatment, is a failure of fit, as described by Fulford and Hope (1994), between the principles approach and most people's responses to the case vignette questionnaire we introduced in Chapter 17. This 'failure of fit', between our responses to the questionnaire and the Beauchamp and Childress criteria, is illustrated in Table 18.3 (which is based on figure 58.2, p. 687 in Fulford and Hope, 1994). You may well disagree with some of the details, but the overall conclusion is clear, that the criteria proposed by Beauchamp and Childress, like the legal criteria in chapter 17, simply fail to fit our intuitive responses to most of these cases.

Three points are important to emphasize before going on:

1. This further 'failure of fit' does not, in itself, either validate or invalidate our intuitive responses. This goes back to a point made in Chapter 4, in the discussion of the implications of philosophical work on the concepts of mental illness: a good philosophical theory of mental illness must explain the features of the logical geography of the concept, either why it *has* the features it has, or why it only *appears* to have these features. In Chapter 4, it was the overall 'map' of psychiatry we had in mind; here, it is the pattern of involuntary psychiatric treatment. The Beauchamp and Childress criteria fail to account for this pattern either as reflecting *justified* involuntary treatment or as reflecting involuntary treatment that only *appears* to be justified.

2. The failure of fit does not, in itself, show that the principles approach, as such, is wrong. The underlying analysis of rationality is, perhaps, wrong (at least in part). But involuntary treatment is, none the less, appropriately analysed, among other ways, in terms of a balancing act between beneficence and autonomy.

3. Neither does the failure of fit, in itself, show that the underlying analysis of rationality is, as such, wrong. On the contrary, the analysis really *does* fit many cases of involuntary treatment, in general medicine, and even in psychiatry. It fits some cases very well, notably Beauchamp and Childress' own case of dementia. The point is that the analysis fails to fit the *full range* of diverse cases represented by involuntary *psychiatric* treatment. This is the full-field/half-field point again, then, to revert to the summary diagram at the end of Chapter 6. Beauchamp and Childress offer us a half-field view, sufficient for most areas of bodily medicine, but not the full-field view that is required for a satisfactory analysis of the conceptual and ethical issues raised by mental health.

Table 18.3 Correlation between results of the case-vignette study (column 2) and the principles of beneficence and autonomy (Adapted from: Fulford, K.W.M. and Hope, T. (1994). Psychiatric ethics: a bioethical ugly duckling? In *Principles of Health Care Ethics* (ed. R. Gillon and A. Lloyd). Chichester: John Wiley and Sons, pp. 681–695) (cases re-ordered in descending order of likelihood of involuntary treatment.)

	Likelihood of involuntary treatment (%) in case study	Beneficence	Autonomy					Psychotic symptoms
			Not intentional	Lacks understanding	Controlling influences	Competence		
						Lacks deliberative capacity	Incoherence	
4 hypomania	100			+		+	+	++
9 schizophrenia	100						+	++
3 depression	50	+						+
1 anorexia	25	+						?
2 obsessional disorder	10							
7 hysteria	<5		?	+				
5 optic atrophy	<5		+	+				
12 marital problems	<5							
13 personality disorder (drunk)	<5	+	+			+	+	
14 bronchial carcinoma	<5	+						
6 acromegaly	0			+				
8 breast lump	0							
10 osteoporosis	0							
11 agoraphobia	0							
Dementia (Beauchamp and Childress)		+	+	+		+	+	+

Values-free diagnosis?

Fulford and Hope (1994), in their article, offer a series of linguistic indications (i.e. J.L. Austin-type indications) that the half-field view of the Beauchamp and Childress approach is none other than the half-field of the *medical* model. These are summarized in the next reading.

EXERCISE 8   (30 minutes)

Read the second extract from:

> Fulford, K.W.M. and Hope, T. (1994). Psychiatric ethics: a bioethical ugly duckling? Chapter 58 In *Principles of Health-care ethics* (ed. R. Gillon and A. Lloyd). Chichester, England: John Wiley and Sons, (Extract pp. 688–689.)

Link with Reading 8.4

Note:

- the several linguistic indications that Fulford and Hope find in Beauchamp and Childress' account of an implicit medical model; and

- the further indication that this model, as implicit in Beauchamp and Childress' thinking, specifically excludes values from psychiatric diagnostic assessment.

Beauchamp and Childress, then, Fulford and Hope point out, despite noting the value-laden nature of judgements of rationality, draw an explicit contrast between such judgements and 'medical' diagnoses: value judgements, to repeat Beauchamp and Childress' (1989) key phrase, bring in 'moral *rather than* medical considerations' (p. 84, emphasis added).

Beauchamp and Childress's model is thus essentially Boorse's version of the medical model (Chapter 4, above), with facts at the centre, and values, although recognized to be important, marginalized, pushed out to the edge of the picture. Like Boorse, therefore, Beauchamp and Childress seek to exclude values from medical diagnosis, conceiving diagnosis to be a matter of scientific value-free fact. To the extent, therefore, that judgements of rationality are (as Beauchamp and Childress note) value-laden, such judgements have no place (according to their view) in *medical* diagnosis. We rejected this view in Part I, arguing on linguistic analytic grounds that value judgements are important in all areas of medicine, including diagnosis. The failure of fit between Beauchamp and Childress' criteria and many cases of mental disorder, taken together with their (implicit) adoption of the traditional value-excluding medical model, provides further evidence that values may indeed be important in diagnosis.

Casuistry (case-based reasoning)

We return to the role of values in psychiatric diagnosis below, in Session 4 of this chapter on Values-Based Practice, and then in detail in Chapters 20 and 21. For now, though, we need to pursue the implications of the conclusion that values are integral to judgements of rationality and hence to decisions about involuntary psychiatric treatment.

At first glance, this would seem to suggest that casuistry will give us a better basis for analysing the ethical issues in this area; however, casuistry brings with it its own values-related dangers.

EXERCISE 9 (45 minutes)

Read the extract from an article by the American philosopher, Loretta Kopelman:

Kopelman, L.M. (1994). Case method and casuistry: the problem of bias. *Theoretical Medicine*, 15: 21–37. (Extract pp. 25–27.)

Link with Reading 18.5

Think particularly about two questions:

1. just why does casuistry work as a method for reaching agreement (you may want to refer back to our discussion of this in Chapter 17)?, and

2. given Kopelman's observations about bias, why does the very power of casuistry make it potentially dangerous in mental health?

Kopelman's (1994) discussion, steering as it does a careful path between supporters and opponents of casuistry, provides a number of important insights into the nature of this approach to ethical reasoning. A key point that she brings out is the extent to which casuistry (along with other methods of ethical and indeed scientific reasoning) is biased by values.

In the case study in this extract, an initially plausible casuistic conclusion (in case A) is reversed when further information, shifting the point of salience, is introduced (in case B). In case B, the values of the family are seen to be salient in a way that, as presented in case A, they were not. In case C, again, yet another conclusion is reached from a third perspective.

Casuistry and a common value system

We noted when we were looking at the objectives of training in ethics that, contrary to the common presupposition, no approach to ethical reasoning can be value-free; even the (important) principle of autonomy reflects a value base (in liberal democracy). And in the case of casuistry, the very *power* of the method, what makes it 'go through', is a *shared value system*. The reason why the members of the President's Commission on Bioethics, in Jonsen and Toulmin's original observation, agreed on *what* ought to be done, is that (despite their different theories about *why* it should be done), they shared a common value system. In Kopelman's

terms, then, as in this extract, they shared a common (implicit) understanding of what the cases in question consisted in and what the (ethically) salient features of these cases were.

Casuistry and the case vignette questionnaire

But this is also why casuistry, if used in isolation, is potentially dangerous in mental health. For in mental health, as we have repeatedly emphasized, people's values are characteristically not shred but divergent.

The central importance of differences of values in mental health is well illustrated by the case vignette questionnaire. There is a clear sense in which the very problem of involuntary treatment is a problem of conflicting values. In the extreme, the conflict is between a patient whose central value is (or involves) *not* being treated, and everyone else (doctors, social workers, relatives, etc.) whose shared central value is that the patient *ought* to be treated. A casuistic approach, therefore, operating in isolation, cannot but fail to impose the values of the majority on the minority (the patient). In this situation, therefore, the Jonsen and Toulmin observation of everyone agreeing on what ought to be done, is, at best, hazardously extended to mental health.

In mental health, then, casuistry, although a powerful method of ethical reasoning, needs to be used in conjunction with other, more transparent and discursive, methods. To rely, exclusively, on casuistic reasoning, is as likely to endorse as to prevent abusive practices in mental health, to the extent that such practices consist in the imposition of one group's or one person's values on others.

Perspectives

Both the principles approach and casuistry, applied to involuntary psychiatric treatment, have brought out for us the central place of values in mental health. The principles approach, useful as it is for some kinds of mental disorder (e.g. dementia) fails to help with major areas of functional disorder (as in the case vignette questionnaire), essentially because, in adopting a medical model, a 'right-half-field' view of the conceptual structure of medicine, it excludes (diagnostic) values. Casuistry includes values, its very power, as a method of ethical reasoning, being derived from shared value systems. But this means that, given the essentially divergent values characteristic of mental health, casuistry carries with it serious risks of abuse through the imposition of majority values on minorities.

Perspectives and involuntary psychiatric treatment

If, then, values are central, this brings us directly to the importance of perspectives in mental health ethics. Even perspectives, though, are no sinecure! (Notice, by the way, how mental health ethics is already emerging as the trickiest and intellectually most challenging area of health-care ethics.) One problem with perspectives, you will recall, was a danger of relativism, of 'anything goes'. We have seen earlier in the book, that 'anything goes' is not what follows from acknowledging the central place of values in the conceptual structure of medicine, and we will return to this at several points later on. But in the case of involuntary psychiatric treatment, where casuistry carries a risk of the values of the majority being imposed on the patient, perspectives carries the opposite risk, of the patient's values being imposed on the majority.

The tension here, between the values of the patient and the values of others, has, and continues to be, played out in an often tragic way in mental health (Robinson, 2003). We return to this in Session 3, in a discussion of rights and responsibilities, and at several points later in the book. But it is important at this stage to understand exactly why the perspectives approach, if unsupported by other methods of ethical reasoning, fails on the centrally important issue of involuntary psychiatric treatment.

Perspectives, insight, and psychosis

The essential difficulty with the perspectives approach in relation to the ethics of involuntary psychiatric treatment, is precisely that, from the patient's perspective, there is nothing psychologically wrong with them. This is captured in the core psychopathological notion of 'loss of insight'. In psychotic disorders, as we saw in Chapter 3, there is 'loss of insight'. That is to say, in psychotic disorders, insight is lost in the specific sense that from the patient's perspective, what is wrong is not that they are ill but that something is being done to them (e.g. with persecutory delusions) or that they have done something (e.g. with delusions of guilt).

We may, with the antipsychiatrists, see this as sufficient justification for avoiding involuntary psychiatric treatment altogether. But this simply denies (rather than giving an account of) the widespread intuition that in some cases involuntary treatment is not only justified but ethically obligatory.

A balanced perspective

Perspectives, then, lead us back to the key ethical significance of the concept of psychosis. Before leaving perspectives, though, it is important to see just how much this approach can contribute. This is brought out in what has justly become a classic in the developing tide of research and narrative reports on user experience, Ann Rogers, David Pilgrim and Ron Lacey's (1993) *Experiencing Psychiatry*. In this book the authors describe the results of a survey carried out on behalf of the patients' advocacy group MIND (now called the National Association for Mental Health). Chapter 5 is concerned with users' views of treatment. On an antipsychiatry model of the relationship between professionals and patients, we might expect rejection of drug therapy out of hand, especially where this is part of involuntary treatment. And there is certainly much evidence of failures of professional-led research to recognize the adverse effects of many commonly prescribed medications. But the chapter evidences a point that has been made repeatedly by those who use services

about values in mental health care. The point is not whether to accept a particular treatment, a particular medication, say. It is not, even, whether involuntary treatment may or may not be justified. It is, rather, the extent to which the values of the individual concerned are built into the way in which decisions about these important issues are made.

Most users of services, though certainly not all, do not reject drug treatment as such. But there are vitally important issues from the user's perspective as an individual with a unique set of values which are (often needlessly) neglected in the way decisions about such issues are actually made (the importance of side-effects, in particular, is often largely neglected).

Conclusions

In this session, we have looked at some of the applications to mental health of the three main methods of ethical reasoning employed in bioethics as it has developed as a relatively distinct discipline, principles, casuistry, and perspectives.

All three methods, although carrying risks particularly if used in isolation, are important in mental health: principles for the open framework of discursive argument they supply; casuistry for the power of case-based reasoning to attach ethical arguments to the realities of day-to-day care; and perspectives for the focus they give to the (logically) essential place of the values of the individuals concerned. In the next session, we look at the role of general ethical theory, in which bioethical reasoning has its origins, for mental health.

Reflection on the session and self-test questions

Write down your own reflections on the materials in this session drawing out any points that are particularly significant for you. Then write brief notes about the following:

1. What are the 'four principles'?

2. How is treatment without consent justified by the 'four principles'?

3. How well do the four principles explain the response pattern for the case vignette philosophical fieldwork exercise in Chapter 17?

4. Why does casuistry 'work' as a method for resolving ethical difficulties?

5. Why does the way casuistry works make it a potentially dangerous tool for ethical problem solving in mental health (if used unreflectingly)?

6. Why are 'perspectives' not a panacea in mental health ethics?

Session 3 Philosophical ethical theory

The three forms of ethical reasoning examined in the last two sessions—principles, casuistry, and perspectives—have not been invented out of the blue. They reflect long-standing traditions in general ethics.

It is important to be aware of these traditions. First, although further from the coal-face of practice, they offer a range and depth of argument that underpins the more pragmatic tools of bioethics. Second, and following on from this, the more abstract philosophical approaches can help to extend the tools of bioethical reasoning from the relatively straightforward problems raised by technological medicine, for which they were invented, to the more complex questions raised by primary care and mental health.

Substantive and analytic theories

Philosophical ethical theory has been of two main kinds, which we can call substantive and analytic. Substantive theories are concerned with the most general kinds of consideration that are relevant to establishing ethical conclusions. Analytic philosophical ethics is concerned with the meanings and implications of value terms and the general logical form of ethical argument. In this section we will be looking first at substantive theories, and then going on to consider the role of analytic ethics, in both cases with a particular eye to mental health.

EXERCISE 10   (20 minutes)

Before going on, go back to the cases and the arguments that we considered in the last session, where we used the three bioethical approaches of principles, casuistry, and perspectives.

   Think about how these approaches could themselves be justified by reference to more general ethical ideas. What is 'good' about the principle of autonomy, for instance? Or why, thinking casuistically, is the suicide risk in Mr AB's case, for example, ethically relevant? (i.e. why would it be relevant to imagine his case without this risk). Again, what is important ethically about recognizing the values inherent in Mr AB's perspective, even though, clinically, he 'lacked insight'?

   As before, write down your thoughts about these questions before going on. Remember that it is the general kinds of ethical consideration with which we are concerned here, not the particulars of individual cases.

Substantive ethical theories: deontology and consequentialism

In discussions of the questions raised in Exercise 10, two rather different kinds of consideration usually emerge, corresponding broadly with two major traditions in philosophical ethics—duties and consequences.

Duties and consequences

Duty-based ethics and consequentialist ethics are the two main kinds of substantive ethical theory. They have been variously named (duty-based ethics is sometimes called 'deontological' ethics, for example), but broadly speaking they can be characterized thus:

◆ *Duty-based ethics*. Duty-based ethical theories, as the name implies, seek to define duties that are incumbent upon people no matter what the consequences might be. Duties are closely linked with rights and responsibilities, and also with law.

   Thus, in Mr AB's case, the professionals could be said to have a duty to treat him under the Mental Health Act. This duty arises from the rights of the patient (and others) to protection, and the responsibility of the professionals to provide such protection. If they fail in this they could be held negligent in law, and so on.

◆ *Consequentialist ethics* seek to base ethical conclusions on the consequences of the various possible courses of action. The best-known consequentialist ethic is utilitarianism, the slogan for which is the well known 'the greatest good of the greatest number'.

In Mr AB's case, consequentialist arguments for treating him under the Mental Health Act could include his future happiness, avoiding the tragedy for his family of suicide, and so forth.

   Both kinds of substantive theory lie behind and underpin bioethical reasoning.

All for one and one for all

At first glance the principles approach is closest to duty-based ethics. Mr AB had a 'right' to treatment, which the professionals had a 'duty' to give—hence the principle of beneficence. Equally, though, Mr AB's right to 'bodily integrity' would normally stand in the way of medical treatment against his wishes—hence the principle of autonomy.

   Consequences, on the other hand, seem at first glance more closely relevant to casuistry and to perspectives. Reasoning casuistically, for instance, it is relevant to imagine Mr AB's case without suicide risk because suicide, to the extent that it is a consequence of failing to treat him on an involuntary basis, is so disastrous an outcome that it outweighs the adverse effects of treating him against his wishes. Similarly, though, even if such treatment is ethically right, the best action (as the article by Rogers *et al.*, 1993, in the last session showed) will be determined by whether or not it is carried through with an understanding of Mr AB's particular perspective.

   Closer inspection shows, however, that the ethical territory is not so sharply divided between duties and consequences as all that. Autonomy, as a principle, is justified not only deontologically but also by the good outcomes of respecting people's wishes (the principle of non-maleficence is *primarily* justified by the importance in medicine of avoiding *bad* outcomes). Conversely, casuistic reasoning must have regard to duties; and the duties that individuals recognize are crucial to their perspectives.

Duties, consequences, and bioethics

So, both kinds of substantive ethical theory are important to the underpinning of all three main approaches to ethical reasoning in bioethics. And the two substantive theories are not, of course, incompatible. Indeed, they are often complementary. The Oxford philosopher, R.M. Hare, on whose work we drew in Part I, makes this point specifically in relation to medical ethics, in his 'Medical ethics, can the moral philosopher help?' (Hare, 1993a, pp. 1–14). As Hare nicely puts it in this article, if the moral philosopher cannot help with medical ethical difficulties, he or she ought to 'shut up shop'. This is because medical ethical difficulties are so typical of the kind of problems with which moral philosophers have traditionally claimed particular expertise.

Moral philosophy, moreover, as we have noted, offers two powerful approaches to reasoning about ethical problems, duty based and consequentialist. These might, perhaps, sometimes be seen as competing ethical theories. But this, Hare says, is certainly not so in medicine. For the two kinds of theory are applicable, respectively, at two different levels of ethical reasoning, the *intuitive* and the *critical*. We noted these two levels in Chapter 17 (where we used Hare's terminology of Level 1 and Level 2 reasoning). His point, here, is that duty-based theories are particularly relevant to the intuitive 'guts feel' response which must guide us in the hurly-burly of day-to-day practice, whereas consequentialist theories are particularly helpful when we stand back and reflect critically on what ought to be done.

Duties, consequences, and analytic ethics

Hare (1993a) also argues in this paper that, with a proper understanding of the meanings of moral words, duty-based and consequentialist theories can be effectively combined in medical ethical reasoning. We touched on his theory that moral judgements are 'universal prescriptions' in Part I (in the discussion of descriptivism and non-descriptivism).

This part of his article is thus concerned with analytic ethical theory. We will return to analytic ethics shortly in relation to psychiatric ethics. First, though, we need to think briefly about the advantages and disadvantages of the two kinds of substantive ethical theory in mental health.

Duties and mental health

There are advantages and disadvantages of both kinds of substantive ethical theory for mental health ethics. The deontological approach is valuable especially where it is necessary to protect the rights of vulnerable groups (such as the mentally ill). However, the legalistic tendencies of deontology, can often make it excessively bureaucratic and rule-bound in practice.

Thus, Jonathan Montgomery, a British lawyer who has worked particularly on the role of rights in medicine and psychiatry, has examined the strengths and weaknesses of rights-based thinking for the development of patient-centred care in his 'Patients first:

the role of rights' (1996). In this article, Montgomery notes that rights (with their corresponding duties) can provide important protections against other people's vested interests and, indeed, their well-intentioned interference. But rights talk is not enough. Too often rights are prescribed, particularly by politicians, as a substitute for providing what people really need—Montgomery cites the UK's Patients' Charter as a case in point. Rights, therefore, need legal teeth. But the danger of this, as Montgomery goes on to describe, is that genuine care can all too easily become tied up in bureaucratic knots. So, patient-centredness in health care requires rights with teeth but a balance must be maintained with the professional's freedom of right action.

Consequences and mental health

Consequences are not without their problems either, though. Consequences do force us to look squarely at the facts. But they leave us exposed to the ever-present danger of the 'abuse of casuistry', of the facts being fitted to suit what one would *like* to be done rather than what *ought* to be done!

An interesting attempt to use utilitarianism in health-care ethics is the QALY approach to resource allocation. This approach aims to make the balance of utilities more objective by basing it on the expressed utilities of the parties to the decision-making process. A QALY is a 'Quality-Adjusted Life-Year'. The idea is simple enough. Ask a number of people to rank different kinds of disease and disability in terms of seriousness, weight them for duration, and you have a basis for equating the relative costs of the implied utilities.

The Oxford philosopher, Roger Crisp, was among the first to point out some of the adverse consequences of what he calls in the next reading this 'Totting-up conception' for mental health.

EXERCISE 11   (45 minutes)

Read the extract from:

Crisp, R. (1994). Quality of life and health care. Chapter 13 In *Medicine and Moral Reasoning* (ed. K.W.M. Fulford, G.R. Gillett, and J.M. Soskice). Cambridge: Cambridge University Press. (Extract p. 181.)

Link with Reading 18.6

◆ What can go wrong when the (prima facie eminently reasonable) QALY approach is applied to mental health, according to Crisp?

Crisp (1994) reviews in this article a number of unacceptable consequences of balancing utilities in the way required by the QALY approach. The particular unacceptable consequence outlined in this extract is that, despite its promise of fairness, the QALY approach leads to consequences that, applied in the mathematical way it requires, *excludes* considerations of fairness. Even accepting that the 'severely mentally defective' have a very low quality of life (a point that those concerned with caring for this group would contest), considerations of fairness would normally imply that we increase, rather than as the QALY approach requires, withdraw resources from this group.

QALYs as a utilitarian calculus

Mental disorder is also unglamorous, in the public image at any rate. It is much easier to raise 'votes' for eye disease, for example, or cancer research. Hence, the mentally ill, already disadvantaged, are further disadvantaged in any 'one-QALY, one-vote' system.

But perhaps the most serious difficulty with the QALY approach is a difficulty behind all utilitarian calculations, that of imaginative identification with other people's (or our own future) states. As noted above, there may be many different views about the quality of life of a person with severe learning difficulties. Here the problem is compounded by the difficulty they may have in speaking for themselves. But the utility of a year with, say, cancer, as measured by someone suffering from the disease, may be very different from what anyone without the disease would imagine. Indeed, as we will see in the last session in this chapter, we have every reason (from philosophical and sociological work on values) to believe that the actual and imagined utilities will be very different.

This is not to say that QALY thinking is all wrong. After all, squaring health service budgets, balancing needs with resources across a wide spectrum of very different conditions, is impossibly difficult. We need all the help we can get with health economics, which is what QALYs were designed for. But QALY thinking, without the balancing of rights expressing the needs especially of the disadvantaged, leads to serious injustices.

Duties, consequences, and mental health

The importance of balancing duty-based and consequentialist thinking in mental health is nicely illustrated by recent developments in mental health legislation in Europe. This was the subject of a comparative study carried out by one of us (KWMF) with Tony Hope in Oxford, in a research programme led by the German psychiatrist, Professor Dr Hanfred Helmchen, within the European Community (Fulford and Hope, 1996).

As Fulford and Hope showed, the driving motivation behind recent developments in mental health law in Europe has been to protect people with mental illness (conceived as a vulnerable group), from the misuse of the psychiatrist's powers of involuntary restraint and treatment. This, in itself, is vitally important. There is a clear imbalance of power between doctor and patient which, as recent experience in France, discussed in Fulford and Hope's study, shows, is not always adequately redressed merely through the assertion of a voluntary code of ethics.

As the study also showed, however, in protecting rights through legal powers, there is a danger of an excessively bureaucratic and legalistic approach to clinical work emerging, in which the patient, as the holder of 'legal rights', nevertheless fails to get satisfactory treatment. The French philosopher, Ann Fagot-Largeault's phrase, cited by Fulford and Hope (1996), sums this up. Patients, she notes, can now literally run away before the legal process is completed. So the *consequences* of an excessively legalistic approach, designed as it is to protect patient's rights, may be to impair the professionals' powers of action to the point where they are unable to carry out their *duties* adequately.

This is not to say that in any given situation this or that approach is right—perhaps it is a good thing that patients can 'run away'! But as we will see in Chapter 20, the unbalanced hegemony of any one perspective, however well-intentioned, is ever at risk of leading to abusive practices. One way to avoid such imbalances is by weighing up duty-based and consequentialist ethical considerations, rather then treating either as primary. Another, complementary, way, is to recognize the importance of analytic considerations in ethical reasoning.

Analytic ethical theory

Analytic ethics

Analytic ethics, concerned with the meanings of moral and other value words, has been given a hard time recently in philosophy (recall Bernard Williams in his *Ethics and the Limits of Philosophy*, 1985, in Part I). Philosophers, concerned to be seen to be contributing directly to practical issues, have turned away from questions of meaning to questions of substance. But were they right to do this?

EXERCISE 12	(15 minutes)

Go back to the cases we have been considering. How far do either the tools of bioethics or those of substantive philosophical ethics resolve the issues they raised?

We noted in Chapter 17 that it is in the nature of ethical questions that at some point we may reach an impasse. But do the approaches we have considered thus far even bring us to the core of the ethical difficulties and dilemmas that arise in mental health? Is there something important missing?

The missing factor is the meanings of the terms in which the dilemmas and disagreements are couched. Analytic ethics has focused traditionally on the most general of *ethical* terms, like good, duty, responsibility, and so forth. In the case of mental health, crucially important also are the most general of *clinical* terms, disease, disorder, and, not least, mental illness.

The concept of mental illness and bioethics

This brings us back to the importance of conceptual difficulties in mental health ethics, as spelled out in Chapter 17. Mr AB's involuntary treatment, for example, to the extent that it was justified ethically, turned on him being, not merely at risk, nor merely at risk as a result of being sad, nor even at risk as a result of being sad on the basis of a false belief (that he had brain cancer). The critical ethical consideration was that he was at risk as a result of a psychotic mental illness.

Similarly in the case vignette study, involuntary treatment as an option mapped, not on to the Mental Health Act as such, nor on to the bioethical principles of autonomy and beneficence as such, but on to these only as and in so far as they incorporated the notion of psychosis. Just how 'psychosis' should be understood, moreover, turned out to be highly problematic—even the sophisticated analysis of irrationality offered by Beauchamp and Childress (1989) was consistent only with certain types of psychotic mental disorder (such as dementia).

The concept of mental illness: from substantive to analytic ethics

As we noted a moment ago, analytic ethical theory has traditionally been concerned with the meanings of the most general value words, 'good', 'duty', and so forth. (Of course, analytic philosophy as a whole has ranged far more widely, see Chapter 6.)

The general moral words were very much the focus of R.M. Hare's work, as one of the leading analytic ethical philosophers of the twentieth century. In the next reading, we come to the second of two articles he wrote applying his theory (that moral value judgements are universal prescriptions) to ethical problems in health care. In Exercise 8, earlier in this session, we looked at the first of these articles. In this he argued that his 'universal prescription' theory reconciled duty-based and consequentialist approaches to medical ethical problems. In the next reading, Hare extends this approach to psychiatric ethics, taking involuntary psychiatric treatment as a case in point.

EXERCISE 13   (60 minutes)

Read the extract from:

Hare, R.M. (1993b). The philosophical basis of psychiatric ethics. Pages 15–30 In *Essays on Bioethics*. Oxford: Clarendon Press. (Extract pp. 28–29.)

Link with Reading 18.7

Think carefully about Hare's argument for excluding analytic considerations, other than those concerned with the moral words. Thus, he argues earlier in the article that the concept of 'person' is irrelevant, or certainly not critical, to the ethical issues raised by abortion; and in this extract, similarly, that the concept of 'disease' is not critical to the ethical issues raised by involuntary psychiatric treatment. But is he right?

In this extract, Hare (1993b) turns to the topic that will occupy us in detail in Chapters 20 and 21, namely the diagnostic problem, the problem of whether this or that medical condition is properly understood as a disease. Unlike the many authors reviewed in Part I of this book, Hare takes it as self-evident that disease is an evaluative concept. It comes as something of a surprise, then, given the importance to us of Hare's conceptual work in Part I, that in this extract he dismisses the relevance of analytic philosophy to settling questions about the disease status of particular conditions. He has, he implies, settled the relevant analytic

question (that disease is an evaluative concept), and he believes that the work of analytic philosophy, in psychiatric as in other areas of medical ethics, is to be done exclusively in terms of the general moral words (good, ought, etc.).

Right answers from philosophy?

Elsewhere in this article, and in other publications from his later output (e.g. Hare, 1981), Hare (1993b) shows how an understanding of the logic of the moral words (derived from analytic philosophy), combined with plausible assumptions about people's values, can provide a rational basis for debate about moral problems. Applying this approach, however, as he does in this extract, to the diagnostic problem in mental health, risks abusive consequences. It will be worth pausing on why this is so. As an analytic philosopher, and one for whom the evaluative element in the meaning of disease and related concepts is self-evident, understanding precisely why Hare's restriction of analytic methods to the general moral words risks abusive consequences in mental health, will provide an important link to the rather different use of analytic philosophy that we will be making in the last session of this chapter, as the basis of Values-Based Practice.

Thus, the crucial question, Hare says in the extract linked with Exercise 13, in coming to a conclusion about whether this or that condition is a disease, is whether the condition in question (homosexuality and political revisionism are his two examples) is a condition of which we 'approve' (p. 29). Whether we *should* approve of a given condition in turn depends, according to Hare's method of reasoning, on whether those concerned consider that 'treatment to remove [their condition] will on the whole be for the best for [them] and others' (p. 29). As to involuntary treatment, he continues, this 'can only be justified by large countervailing gains (e.g. in the protection of the public from dangerous mental patients)'. And '. . . It is hard to see what those gains could be . . . [for homosexuality and political revisionism]' (all p. 29).

Up to a point, then, Hare's account must be right. If, as he says, disease is an evaluative concept, what we take to be a disease necessarily involves (in part) value judgements. But the risks of abusive consequences become clear when we consider the particular way in which Hare suggests the relevant value judgements are to be made, i.e. by relying on societal consensus. True, he refers, first, in respect of voluntary treatment, to the values of those concerned. But even here, the relevant value judgement is whether treatment to remove their condition will '*on the whole be for the best for* [them] *and others*' (p. 29, emphases added). So, it is by the values of people in general that we should be guided as to whether voluntary treatment should be given (and hence disease status ascribed). The role of societal consensus is still more explicit in respect of involuntary treatment. For in this case, the 'large countervaluing gains' by which, in Hare's approach, involuntary treatment is justified, are illustrated by 'protection *of the public* from *dangerous* mental patients' (p. 29, emphases added); and who, in Hare's account, is in a better position to judge what is 'dangerous' to the public than the 'public' themselves?

We can understand Hare's reliance on societal consensus as being driven by his (perceived) need to derive substantive conclusions from his analytic moral philosophy. You will recall from Part I that analytic philosophy came under attack over the period in which Hare was writing, for being practically impotent. Hare himself, analytic philosopher though he was, felt obliged to argue that an understanding of the logic of the moral words (derived from analytic philosophy), combined with information about the values that people actually hold, leads to conclusions that are to all intents and purposes definitive 'right answers' to moral problems. In the Introduction to his 1981 book, for example, on 'Moral thinking: its levels, method, and point', he makes this explicit: '. . . I shall be maintaining', he writes, 'that, if we assumed a perfect command of logic and of the facts, they would constrain so severely the moral evaluations that we can make, that in practice we would be bound all to agree to the same ones' (Hare, 1981, p. 6).

From right answers to good process

Yet it is precisely this assumption of 'right answers', of values to which everyone is 'bound' to agree, that is challenged by the diversity of values in mental health. In Session 4 (and again in Chapters 20 and 21), we will be looking at the practical consequences of taking seriously the *analytic* tools of analytic philosophy in the form of Values-Based Practice. The idea behind Values-Based Practice is to provide a toolkit for reasoning about values in health care in circumstances in which, far from there being a consensus, values are highly diverse. In developing this toolkit, analytic philosophy, as we will see, shifts our attention from 'right answers' to 'good process'. And 'good process', we will argue, far from being practically impotent, is highly effective practically where values conflict. And good process is effective, furthermore, while avoiding, or at any rate limiting, the risks of abuses arising from the imposition of one individual's or group's 'right values' on those whose values are different.

The importance of 'good process' rather than 'right values' in mental health will already be clear: mental health, as Hare's analytic work in particular (on the general moral or value words) helped us to see in Part I, is an area of health care in which human values are highly diverse. Hence mental health is an area in which societal consensus, if the sole basis on which judgements of health and disease are made, is at risk of abusive consequences. This is why Hare's initially plausible analysis is at risk of generating just the abusive consequences he would have been at pains to prevent.

But are these abusive consequences merely theoretical? Or do they occur in practice? We will look briefly at this question (we return to it in Chapters 20 and 21) before turning to an introduction to Values-Based Practice in Session 4 of this chapter.

Analytic ethics: from theory into practice

Hare was not alone in failing to recognize the importance of the concept of mental illness in psychiatric ethics. Indeed, the divorce between ethical and conceptual issues in mental health is

well-illustrated by an extraordinary divide that there has been in the literature generally between, on the one hand, bioethics (as covered in this part of the book), and, on the other, the debate about the concept of mental illness (as covered in Part I).

This divide, into ethical and conceptual strands, is a good example of the pervasive influence of a (generally implicit) biomedical model. We saw in Chapters 2, 4, and 6 that the medical model was highly influential on the form of the debate about mental illness, restricting its terms of reference to whether or not mental illness could be directly mapped on to what was assumed to be a paradigmatically value-free concept of bodily illness. In this chapter, similarly, we have found that essentially the same model has been operating in bioethics (in Beauchamp and Childress, 1989, for example).

Practical consequences

Just how deeply mistaken the divorce of ethical and conceptual issues may be from a practical point of view, is illustrated by the next reading (Fulford *et al.*, 1993).

This article was the result of a collaboration between one of us (Fulford), a Russian psychiatrist (Smirnoff), and a Russian-speaking social worker (Snow). These three authors set out to examine the extent to which the concepts of disorder current in the former USSR over a period when abusive uses of psychiatric diagnosis became widespread, differed from those prevalent in the 'West'. As the article describes, the analysis was based on a survey of the literature on concepts of disease in Russian-language academic journals.

EXERCISE 14   (60 minutes)

Read the two extracts from:

Fulford, K.W.M., Smirnov, A.Y.U., and Snow, E. (1993). Concepts of disease and the abuse of psychiatry in the USSR. *British Journal of Psychiatry*, 162: 802–803

Link with Reading 18.8

The readings describe the findings from the authors' review of Russian-language journals:

◆ What strikes you about the Soviet literature on concepts of disease from this period?

◆ What model does it reflect?

The institutionalized abuse of psychiatry in the former USSR provoked a considerable literature at the time in the West, much of it overtly ethical. This literature, however, was, in effect, concerned with the factors that allowed abusive practices to become widespread (unbalanced political power, poor standards of training, and so forth). It thus failed to consider why psychiatry, rather than, say, surgery, should be vulnerable to abuse in the first place. Insofar as this was considered at all, it had been assumed that it was due to diagnoses of mental disorder being made on the basis of inadequate clinical examination and/or defective science.

This of course is a reasonable assumption given a scientific medical model of disorder. As the authors of this paper show, however, Soviet psychiatry was operating with a model of disorder which was if anything *a more hard-wired scientific medical model* than those being employed at the time in western Europe and America. The themes of the Soviet literature, as described particularly in the second extract, are very similar to those around the 'medical' model even today. I.V. Davidovskii, in particular, whose ideas dominated this period (from his first major publication in 1962), was a pathologist. His strongly biological concept of disease directly influenced ideas on schizophrenia as a 'biological' disorder. He published a joint paper with the originator of the Soviet concept of 'sluggish schizophrenia', A.V. Snezhnevsky (Davidovskii and Snezhnevsky, 1972).

The authors explore a number of interpretations of this finding and conclude that, far from an unscientific model of mental disorder being the origin of Soviet psychiatric abuse, a spurious scientific authority was given to diagnoses of severe mental disorder made on the basis, merely, of political deviance as judged by the dominant Soviet values of the day.

As has several times been noted, findings of this kind do not undermine the place of science in mental health. To the contrary, such findings graphically illustrate the need for a full-field view of the conceptual structure of the subject, incorporating facts, but also values, on an equal basis, as outlined in Chapter 6. It is to the practical consequences of this full-field view, drawing on the resources particularly of analytic ethical theory, that we turn in the concluding session of this chapter. We return to the role of values in psychiatric diagnosis in Chapters 20 and 21.

Reflection on the session and self-test questions

Write down your own reflections on the materials in this session drawing out any points that are particularly significant for you. Then write brief notes about the following:

1. What is deontology? And where is it used in practice?

2. What is consequentialism? And where is it used in practice?

3. What is analytic ethics?

4. Why is analytic ethics important especially in mental health? What extra 'tools' does it deliver?

5. What is the key shift of thinking about ethical issues that is required if we are to draw equally on analytic as on substantive ethical theory to derive 'tools' for ethical reasoning in practice?

Session 4 Values-based practice

In this session we outline the 10 principles of Values-Based Practice, or VBP, as a contribution to the values toolkit of health care.

VBP is a response to the growing complexity of health-care decision-making. In this respect it is like evidence-based practice, or EBP. VBP and EBP, as we will see, are complementary: EBP is a response to the growing complexity of the facts bearing on health-care decision-making, VBP is a response to the growing complexity of the corresponding values. VBP, then, is the theory and skills base for effective health-care decision-making where different, and hence potentially conflicting, values are in play.

Aim: extending the toolkit

VBP, although (as we noted in the last session) derived from the somewhat abstract concerns of analytic philosophical value theory, has primarily practical aims. As such, we will be emphasizing in this session the many ways in which the practical tools of VBP, derived from philosophical value theory, differ from the predominantly quasi-legal practical tools derived from bioethics.

VBP might in consequence be thought to be anti-ethics! VBP is certainly anti the overuse of the tools of quasi-legal ethics—as we saw earlier in this chapter, overuse of such tools leads to untoward consequences for health care (remember the three '-flations', code inflation, practitioner deflation, and problem conflation). But it is no part of VBP to suggest that we can do without a framework of law and codes of practice altogether. To the contrary, the tools of quasi-legal ethics, used where they are 'fit for purpose', are essential: and the theory of VBP, as we will see, helps to define where and how the tools of quasi-legal ethics are indeed fit for purpose.

VBP, then, is about supplementing, not supplanting, quasi-legal ethics. VBP is not about throwing out the tools of quasi-legal ethics from the values toolkit of health care. VBP is about adding new tools.

Structure of the session

This is a long session but it is divided into five sections covering, respectively, the premiss and 10 key principles of VBP, the latter as summarized in Box 18.1. Briefly, then, the sections run thus:

1. *Ethics, values, and mental health* draws on earlier parts of the book to derive the distinctive premiss of VBP. Traditional ethics starts from a presumption of 'right' values, VBP starts from the 'democratic' premiss of respect for differences of values. Consistently with its democratic premiss, VBP relies of 'good process' rather than prescribed 'right outcomes' for its effectiveness as a contribution to the decision-making toolkit of health care. Good process in VBP is summarized in the 10 principles shown in Box 18.1 and described in the rest of the chapter.

2. *VBP and EBP* (principles 1–3) defines three key principles of the strongly interdependent relationship between VBP and EBP as decision support tools for health care.

3. *VBP and new models of service delivery* (principles 4 and 5). Like ethics, VBP starts from patients' values (Principle 4); but

it adds to these the values of others, including professionals, seeking a balance of values, in particular through multidisciplinary models of service delivery (Principle 5).

4. *Training initiatives* (principles 6–9): this section shows how the effective application of Principles 4 and 5 in turn depends on four key areas of clinical skill, awareness (Principle 6), knowledge (Principle 7), reasoning skills (Principle 8), and communications skills (Principle 9).

5. *VBP, EBP, and a new alliance in health-care decision-making* (principle 10): the final section returns to the relationship between values and evidence in clinical decision-making. Principle 10 of VBP is about 'who decides?' It shifts the locus of control in health-care decision-making from external experts (such as lawyers and ethicists) to those directly concerned in a given decision—patients, carers, health professionals, voluntary workers, managers, policy makers, etc. Combined with EBP, this VBP shift is the basis for a new and more positive alliance between users and providers of services.

Box 18.1 **Ten principles of values-based practice**

Values-based practice and evidence-based practice

1st Principle of VBP: the two feet principle

All decisions stand on two feet, on values as well as on facts, including decisions about diagnosis

2nd Principle of VBP: the squeaky wheel principle

We tend to notice values only when they are diverse or conflicting and hence are likely to be problematic

3rd Principle of VBP: the science driven principle

Scientific progress, in opening up choices, is increasingly bringing the full diversity of human values into play in all areas of healthcare

Values-based practice and service delivery

4th Principle of VBP: the patient-centred principle

VBP's 'first call' for information is the perspective of the patient or patient group concerned in a given decision

5th Principle of VBP: the multidisciplinary principle

In VBP, conflicts of values are resolved primarily, not by reference to a rule prescribing a 'right' outcome, but by processes designed to support a balance of legitimately different perspectives

Values-based practice and clinical practice skills

6th Principle of VBP: raising awareness

Careful attention to language use in a given context is one of a range of powerful methods for raising awareness of values

7th Principle of VBP: knowledge

A rich resource of both empirical and philosophical methods is available for improving our knowledge of other people's values

8th Principle of VBP: reasoning

Ethical Reasoning is employed in VBP primarily to explore differences of values, not, as in quasi-legal bioethics, to determine 'what is right'

9th Principle of VBP: communication

Communication skills have a substantive rather than (as in quasi-legal ethics) a merely executive role in VBP

Values-based practice, evidence-based practice, and a New Alliance

10th Principle of VBP: who decides

VBP, although involving a partnership with ethicists and lawyers (equivalent to the partnership with scientists in EBP), puts decision-making back where it belongs, with users and providers at the clinical coal-face

1) Ethics, values, and mental health

In health care, values are generally equated with ethics. Why, then, is this session called 'Values-Based Practice' not 'Ethics-Based Practice'? Values and ethics are related in *some* way. But how? How are they similar? How are they different?

For values read ethics?

These are questions we might have raised in Part I, in our work on values and their roles in shaping the core concepts of health care—illness, disease, dysfunction, and so forth. We drew in Part I on certain general logical properties of value terms as teased out by Hare, Warnock, and others, working in a tradition of philosophical value theory, the so-called 'is-ought' debate, running from Hume's dictum 'no ought from an is'.

Yet philosophical value theory, although concerned in principle with the meanings and implications of *value terms in general*, has in practice focused mainly on *ethics*. Even Hare (1952), who sets up an expressly analytic philosophical agenda in his *The Language of Morals*, is mainly concerned to define specifically ethical (or moral) values (as *universal* prescriptions). And in Hare's subsequent work, the examples he uses, the problems he tackles, and the conclusions he draws, are all largely concerned with ethics.

The 'is-ought' debate, it is true, has recently been extended to economics: recall Roger Crisp's (1994) analysis of QALYs earlier in this chapter; and in economics generally, note the work of the Nobel prize-winning economist, Amartya Sen (1987). Again, though, the concern has been with essentially ethical questions of justice rather than with wider issues of the roles and functioning of values in general in economics. Aesthetics, similarly, has been pursued largely as a philosophical tradition distinct from ethics. While as to values in science, even as recently as the start of the new millennium, the American philosopher, Hilary Putnam, felt it necessary to emphasize that 'epistemic values are values too' (Putnam, 2002, p. 30)!

Small wonder, then, that in health care, following philosophy, we tend to assume 'for values read ethics.' Why, then, the need for 'VBP'? Why not the more familiar-sounding 'ethics-based practice'? In the next exercise we start to unpack these questions by reflecting on the differences between ethics and values.

EXERCISE 15 (20 minutes)

What are the differences between ethics and values? Write down a few words or short phrases that you associate (1) with 'ethics', and (2) with 'values'.

Don't think too deeply about your two lists. This is not an exercise in philosophical depth analysis! It is a 'word association' exercise intended, in the spirit of Austin's 'philosophical fieldwork', to draw out some of the features of our ordinary uses of these two concepts.

Table 18.4 gives two lists as produced by a small group, some with a background in philosophy, others coming from health care (with both user and practitioner experience). Your two lists may of course be very different. But these are typical. For most groups, two broad themes stand out:

1. *Values are wider than ethics.* As noted above, values includes not only ethics but also aesthetics, economics, and the epistemic values guiding science. To these we might add, values in risk assessment (and 'games theory' generally), prudential values, and so on.

2. *Values are open, ethics closed.* Most people think of values as being 'personal', 'acquired', and 'variable', while ethics are 'impersonal', 'given', and 'invariant'. Thus, in religion, ethical values, although personal in the sense of being owned by an adherent of a given religion, are perceived as being derived from an external authority. In (some) philosophies they are part of a Platonic realm of ideals; they may be fixed by reason (Kant's categorical imperative), or by logic (Hare's 'universal prescriptions').

The premiss of Values-Based Practice: respect for diversity

The above is only an approximate characterization, of course, of the different associations of ethics and values. As such, though, the

Table 18.4 One group's responses to Exercise 15 on the differences between ethics and values

Values	Ethics
◆ Personal Emotive Meaningful	◆ Rules Doing the right thing Biomedical dilemmas
◆ Taste Choice Preferences	◆ Something to rely on Rules—certainty Absolutes
◆ Wide range Culture specific Preferences	◆ Professional guidelines Rules Respect for *rights*
◆ Anything important Things Places People	◆ Right and wrong Value-based Guide good decision-making
◆ Subjective Personal judgement Ideals Emotional judgement Worth	◆ Morals Integrity Conduct—'taking a stand'
◆ Social conditioning Emotional judgement Worth	◆ Prescriptions Religion Social coherence
◆ Standards Principles Estimation	◆ Structured study of values Code of conduct Institutional rules

two broad themes explain the importance of *values*-based rather than *ethics*-based practice in health care. As already noted, bioethics is a rich and open-minded discipline at the level of theory. As an academic discipline, therefore, we could say in terms of our two word-association lists, that bioethics is concerned as much with values as with ethics. But the tools derived from bioethics to support decision-making in practice, the quasi-legal tools of codes, regulatory bodies and so forth, reflect the narrower and prescriptive associations of ethics rather than values.

VBP, then, really is about values rather than ethics. It is about values, broadly and inclusively understood, not just about ethical values. It is also open, rather than closed, in the sense that, as noted at the start of this session, it is premissed not on 'right values' but on respect for differences of values.

For our purposes, here, of adding to the decision-making toolkit of health care, the premiss of VBP is sufficiently grounded contingently, i.e. in the given diversity of human values noted in Part I. The premiss has also, though more contentiously, an analytic basis in the distinction between description and evaluation (Fulford, 2004). As we saw in Part I, the 'is-ought' divide is best understood as a distinction rather than a dichotomy. As such, though, the essence of Hume's 'law' is preserved, that from a mere description (however complete), no evaluative conclusion can be drawn. To this extent, then, values, as it were, 'float free' from determination by facts.

A democracy of values

It is important to recognize that the premise of VBP, in respect for differences of values, is very far from being empty of practical implications. The justification for a closed impersonal ethic is that without this, we will have no defence against the 'anything goes' chaos of ethical relativism. Well, we saw in Part I that recognizing a role for values is not, in itself, a recipe for chaos because human values, if diverse, are not chaotic. Conversely, we will see in Chapter 21, that it is absolutism, not relativism, that, historically, has been the greater menace in mental health. As the Italian philosopher and historian of science, Paolo Rossi has argued, drawing on the lessons of Renaissance science, we should be ever on our guard against obscurantism (Rossi, 2003). But values as such, and an acknowledgement of the diversity of human values, is not a recipe for chaos in health care decision-making.

One way to understand the move from ethics-based (quasi-legal ethics-based) to values-based decision-making in health care is by analogy with the move from totalitarian to democratic politics. A totalitarian regime—centrally led, top-down, with prescribed values enforced by a secular or religious authority—might seem a stronger system than a democracy in which, by definition, all voices count equally. And a totalitarian regime may indeed be appropriate where overwhelming shared values are at stake—even in a democracy, martial law is declared where survival itself is at stake! But in practice, at least in the complex values-rich environment of industrial and post-industrial societies, it is democracy that has proved the more robust.

From premiss to principles

The move from quasi-legal ethics to VBP is thus in some respects like the move from a totalitarian to a democratic political regime. Like a political democracy, VBP, as a democracy of values, relies, as we noted at the start of this session, on good process rather than on right outcomes to support decision-making in health care.

The 10 principles of VBP, set out in Box 18.1, summarize the key elements of good process in VBP as these relate to health-care decision-making. As Box 18.1 shows, these fall into four groups defining, respectively,

◆ the relationship between VBP and EBP (Principles 1–3)

◆ a VBP model of service delivery (Principles 4 and 5)

◆ four key clinical skills underpinning VBP (Principles 6–9), and

◆ a shift in the 'locus of control' leading to a new alliance between users and providers of services in health-care decision-making (Principle 10).

We will consider each of these four groups of principles separately in the remainder of this session.

2) Values-Based Practice and Evidence-Based Practice

A central feature of the good process on which VBP relies for its effectiveness in health-care decision-making, is a particularly strong model of the relationship between values and evidence.

This relationship, which is the basis of a new and more positive alliance between stakeholders in health-care decision-making (see Principle 10, below), is defined by the first three principles of VBP.

Principle 1 of Values-Based Practice: the 'two feet' principle

The first principle of VBP—the 'two feet' principle—is that all decisions stand on two feet, on values as well as on facts. So far, so good. To the extent that decisions are based on reasons, they are based on what Aristotle first called 'practical reasoning'. Such reasoning combines, as Aristotle put it, desires (values) as well as beliefs (facts). And modern 'decision theory', similarly, combines utilities (values) with probabilities (facts) (see, eg, Hunink and Glasziou, 2001).

The 'two feet' principle of VBP, however, goes on to make the more contentious claim that fact and value are woven together in *all* decisions, including decisions about *diagnosis*. Here, then, VBP is at variance with the traditional medical model in which, as we saw in Part I, diagnosis is reserved to 'value-free' science. We will be returning to values in psychiatric diagnosis in Chapter 21. But it will be worthwhile reviewing here, briefly, the grounds for VBP's challenge to the traditional medical model on this key point.

EXERCISE 16	(10 minutes)

Skim through earlier chapters of this book and pick out arguments supporting Principle 1 on its claim that even decisions about diagnosis stand on a values-foot as well as the better recognized fact-foot.

Values in diagnosis: an Ariadnean thread

The role of evaluation, alongside description, in diagnostic assessment in health care, runs like Ariadne's golden thread through earlier chapters of this book.[1] It was central to the work we did on concepts of illness and disease in Part I; it emerged again in Part II in the tension in Jaspers' work between value-laden and value-free understandings of psychopathological concepts; and in Part III, on the philosophy of science, it was implicit in the perspectival nature of observation, and explicit in the epistemic values guiding theory choice.

The distinction on which the 'two feet' principle of VBP rests, between fact and value (or, more exactly, description and evaluation), has of course been subject to recent philosophical critiques. As we noted in Part I, these critiques can be understood as the latest moves in the 'is-ought' debate, a debate about the logical relationship between description and evaluation. Such critiques are widely taken to show that the fact-value distinction is illusory, a distinction without a difference. What they actually show, however, is that the distinction cannot be driven all the way back. In Putnam's (2002) helpful terminology, introduced in Part I, the *dichotomy* has collapsed but the *distinction* remains useful.

---

[1] In classical Greek legend Ariadne escaped from the Labyrinth by following a golden thread that she spun out behind her as she was taken by her captors to be sacrificed to the bull-headed Minotaur monster.

Putnam's (2002) way of conceptualizing the relationship between description and evaluation, by (loose) analogy with entanglement in quantum physics, is indeed a helpful pointer to Principle 1 of VBP. We summed up Putnam's model in Part I as 'no ought without an is, and vice versa'. Putnam joins with Amartya Sen (1982) in attacking positivist economic models for their illusory assumption of 'is without ought'. Similarly, then, the thrust of earlier parts of this book may be understood as an attack on positivist medical models for their illusory 'is without ought' diagnostic categories.

Principle 2 of Values-Based Practice: The 'squeaky wheel' principle

Principle 2 of VBP is derived from the work we did in Part I about values becoming visible when they are diverse and, hence, may cause trouble. The 'squeaky wheel', as they say, 'gets the grease'. So it is the values that cause trouble that we notice.

We looked in Chapter 6 at R.M. Hare's work on this—remember his example of 'good picture' (values visible) versus 'good strawberry' (values invisible) and how this parallels 'mental illness' (values visible) versus 'bodily illness' (values invisible). We will see in Chapter 21 that similar differences in the extent to which values are agreed upon, underpin the difference between the apparently value-free diagnostic concepts of bodily illness and the overtly value-laden diagnostic concepts of mental illness.

Principle 3 of Values-Based Practice: the 'science driven' principle

A corollary of the standard 'fact-only' medical model is that with future advances in the neurosciences, values will become less prominent in psychiatry, the discipline coming increasingly to look like bodily illness in this respect—remember from Part I that this was a welcome expectation in the minds of those, like R.E. Kendell, who argued that mental illness is essentially no different from bodily illness. VBP has contrary implications.

EXERCISE 17   (20 minutes)

Think about these contrary implications for yourself before going on. In particular,

1. Why should science increase, rather than as the traditional medical model would suggest, decrease, the value-ladenness of medicine?

2. Why should we welcome a future increase in the value-ladenness of medicine rather than joining with Kendell in welcoming a future decrease in the value-ladenness of psychiatry?

One way of approaching these questions is to consider recent developments in an area of bodily medicine, such as reproductive medicine, which has seen dramatic advances in its scientific basis. Has this gone with an increase or a decrease in values-related issues? And why?

The example of reproductive medicine makes the point here. Far from becoming less value-laden, recent dramatic advances in

this area—in assisted reproduction, foetal selection, and so forth—have greatly increased the value-ladenness of the discipline. Why? Well, because scientific advances open up a widened range of *choices*, with choices go *values* (Principle 1), and with a widened range of choices goes *diversity* of values, and, hence, greater *prominence* of values (Principle 2).

We should welcome the increasingly value-laden nature of bodily medicine, therefore, as a reflection of increasing patient choice. Whereas, correspondingly, if psychiatry were to become *less* value-laden, as Kendell anticipated, this would reflect *reduced* patient choice.

A Kendell-type outcome, it is worth adding, an outcome in which scientific advance is associated with *reduced* value-ladenness, is always possible in principle. But it is only possible through the results of scientific advance being, somehow, hijacked by one particular interest group. In such circumstances the uses to which the results of scientific advances are put will reflect the values only of that particular group; and the diversity of human values, which is a key aspect of our individuality as unique human beings, will in consequence be squeezed out of the decision-making process.

3) Values-Based Practice and new models of service delivery

In a political democracy good process depends, *inter alia*, on appropriate institutional structures and an open electoral franchise. In VBP, good process depends, *inter alia*, on appropriate models of service delivery developed within an international 'open society' in mental health.

An open society in mental health

VBP, as you might expect, does not prescribe any *particular* model of service delivery! To the contrary, as in a political democracy, the values-democracy of VBP depends crucially on an open and dynamic exchange of ideas and experience at local, national, and international levels.

Good process in VBP, then, depends on what the British psychiatrist, Jim (J.L.T.) Birley, recalling the open society advocated by the philosopher of science, Sir Karl Popper (1962), called an international 'open society' in mental health. Such an international open society, Birley said (drawing on his experience as the founder President of the human rights organization, the Geneva Initiative for Psychiatry), is a defence against the repeated collapse of psychiatric services into abusive practices (Birley, 2000).

In such an open society, then, there is no place for a pre-set centre, a dominant model assuming the moral high ground. To the contrary, in VBP different models of service delivery, adapted to different circumstances and to different times, responsive to local needs, and building on local skills and resources, are a positive resource, a mutual 'learning set' providing checks and balances in a 'continuous evolution' approach to service development.

The NSF model of service delivery

An understandable fear with this open democratic approach, as we noted above, is that in giving up on right answers (or 'right outcomes' as we called them), we risk 'anything goes'. But substituting good process for right outcomes is no more likely to lead to 'anything goes' in the values democracy of VBP than it is in a political democracy. Box 18.2 illustrates how, through one particular model of service delivery, developed in the UK, the values democracy of VBP may work out in practice.

Box 18.2 The NIMHE Values Framework

The National Framework of Values for Mental Health

The work of the National Institute for Mental Health in England (NIMHE) on values in mental health care is guided by three principles of Values-Based Practice:

1. *Recognition*—NIMHE recognizes the role of values alongside evidence in all areas of mental health policy and practice.

2. *Raising awareness*—NIMHE is committed to raising awareness of the values involved in different contexts, the role/s they play and their impact on practice in mental health.

3. *Respect*—NIMHE respects diversity of values and will support ways of working with such diversity that makes the principle of service-user centrality a unifying focus for practice. This means that the values of each individual service user/client and their communities must be the starting point and key determinant for all actions by professionals.

Respect for diversity of values encompasses a number of specific policies and principles concerned with equality of citizenship. In particular, it is anti-discriminatory because discrimination in all its forms is intolerant of diversity. Thus respect for diversity of values has the consequence that it is unacceptable (and unlawful in some instances) to discriminate on grounds such as gender, sexual orientation, class, age, abilities, religion, race, culture or language.

Respect for diversity within mental health is also:

♦ *user-centred*—it puts respect for the values of individual users at the centre of policy and practice;

♦ *recovery oriented*—it recognizes that building on the personal strengths and resiliencies of individual users, and on their cultural and racial characteristics, there are many diverse routes to recovery;

♦ *multidisciplinary*—it requires that respect be reciprocal, at a personal level (between service users, their family members, friends, communities and providers), between different provider disciplines (such as nursing, psychology, psychiatry, medicine, social work), and between different organizations (including health, social care, local authority housing, voluntary organizations, community groups, faith communities and other social support services);

♦ *dynamic*—it is open and responsive to change;

♦ *reflective*—it combines self monitoring and self management with positive self regard;

♦ *balanced*—it emphasises positive as well as negative values;

♦ *relational*—it puts positive working relationships supported by good communication skills at the heart of practice.

NIMHE will encourage educational and research initiatives aimed at developing the capabilities (the awareness, attitudes, knowledge, and skills) needed to deliver mental health services that will give effect to the principles of Values-Based Practice.

Box 18.2, gives a National Framework of Values for Mental Health. As you will see, it is very different in form and content from the lists of aspirational values that such 'frameworks' generally consist of.

It was developed by NIMHE (the National Institute for Mental Health in England), the section of the UK's National Health Service responsible for implementing government policy on mental health in England and Wales, as set out in the UK government's National Service Framework for Mental Health (Department of Health, 1999), the National Health Service Plan (Department of Health, 2000), and the Priorities and Planning Framework (Department of Health, 2002).

NIMHE's first action, established by ministerial announcement at its launch conference in 2001, was to launch a Values Project Group, chaired by Piers Allott, an expert in recovery (see e.g. Allott *et al.*, 2002), and reporting directly to NIMHE's Chief Executive, Anthony Sheehan. Over about 1 year, the Group developed the Values Framework and piloted it with potential stakeholders from both user and provider communities. The Framework was published initially in an on-line conference organized by the Group with Toby Williamson and Bernard Fleming of the Mental Health Foundation, a mental health NGO, on behalf of NIMHE, the Sainsbury Centre for Mental Health (see below) and Warwick University (http://www.connects.org.uk/conferences). The framework has subsequently been published on NIMHE's website (see Useful Websites, below) and in hard copy (e.g. National Institute for Mental Health England, The Sainsbury Centre for Mental Health and the NHSU, 2004; Woodbridge and Fulford, 2004).

In the next exercise we look at the VBP features of the Framework. We consider some of the risks it carries with it and how these are reduced or avoided, including in particular the risk of 'anything goes'.

EXERCISE 18

Read through the Framework shown in Box 18.2. It is explicitly a Framework for VBP. As you read through the Framework, therefore, mark:

1. any VBP principles you can identify, referring particularly to the model of service delivery defined by Principle 4 (patient-centred practice) and Principle 5 (multidisciplinary working);

2. the practical corollaries of VBP that are identified in the Framework; and

3. any indications there are in the Framework itself of how it will be implemented.

Referring, then, to Box 18.2, you will see that the first part of the Framework refers to 'three principles' of VBP, summarized as 3 R's, Recognition, Raising Awareness, and Respect. Clearly, the first two R's correspond closely with two particular VBP principles as shown in Box 18.1: Recognition corresponds with Principle 1, the first of the principles of VBP theory, and Raising Awareness corresponds with Principle 6, the first, and as we will see below, key area of VBP clinical skills.

Principle 4 of Values-Based Practice: the user-centred principle

Respect, the third R, refers mainly to Principle 4 of VBP, namely the 'patient-centred' principle. As in a political democracy, although VBP starts from equality of respect, there are particular contexts, defined by particular relationships, in which particular prominence is given to a particular individual or group. The parent–child relationship is special, for example: it is consistent with democratic processes that parents give particular weight to the interests of their own children. Similarly in health care, then, service user centrality is, as the third R puts it, '. . . a unifying focus for practice'. And '. . . the values of each individual service user/client and their communities must be the starting point and key determinant for all actions by professionals.'

At first glance, this might look like one or another familiar rhetoric: the rhetoric of the politicized 'user movement'; or the rhetoric of bioethical 'autonomy'; or the rhetoric of 'consumerism' in health care. But the wording of the third R, which was drafted by Simon Allard, a user of services who led a major field study of users' values in London before joining the NIMHE Values Project Group, is very precise.

Thus, the third R is not about a hypothetical set of generic service users' values defining a political 'platform' statement. As rhetorical devices, such statements have been important in empowering users. But the wording here, consistently with the VBP premise of respect for diversity, is about the 'values of each *individual* service user/client and their communities' (emphasis added). Similarly for the rhetoric of bioethics: the third R is not about autonomy, at least as a bioethical principle. An individual's

values, on this VBP model, could equally be about *dependence* (as in Alistair Campbell's article, see reading 17.1). As to the rhetoric of 'consumerism', while the third R is indeed user-centred, the wording makes clear that the values of others, including professionals, are important as well. The values of the user are 'a unifying focus', but not an *exclusive* focus; they are a 'starting point', but not an *end* point; and they are a 'key determinant', but not the *only* determinant.

Principle 5 of Values-Based Practice: the multidisciplinary principle

The principle of service user centrality comes in again as the first of the bullet points that appear in the second half of the Framework (see Box 18.2). These bullets, to come to the second question in Exercise 18, spell out some of the specific corollaries for policy and practice of VBP. Here, then, besides user centrality (bullet point 1), the importance of other voices is made fully explicit in the commitment to multidisciplinary working, spelled out in bullet 3. Bullet 3 makes clear that in VBP the premise of respect is a premise of *mutual* respect, between users, carers and providers, between different health care disciplines, between statutory and voluntary organizations, and so forth.

This is all very different from the approach of quasi-legal ethics, then: VBP places an onus of respect on users as well as providers of services; it gives weight to the values of providers as well as those of users; and, as we will see in more detail under Principle 10 below, it replaces regulatory control of medicine and science with a partnership model of service delivery.

No 'anything goes' in the NSF

User-centred policy and practice and multidisciplinary models of service delivery are both central to the model of service delivery defined by the UK's National Service Framework (NSF). The NSF, as we noted above, together with various updates, define current government policy on mental health in England and Wales. To the extent, therefore, that these NSF principles correspond directly with two key principles of VBP, respect for diversity is very far from the feared 'anything goes'.

A number of other VBP constraints on policy and practice are spelled out in the Framework. Some of these are negative. Thus, the final unnumbered paragraph in the top half of the Framework spells out that VBP is 'anti-discriminatory': racism, for example, is inconsistent with democratic respect for difference. Other constraints are positive. Being 'open and responsive to change' (bullet 4) is a direct reference to the 'open society' of VBP noted above. Again, VBP emphasizes *positive* self-regard (it is reflective, bullet 5), it is concerned with *positive* as well as negative values (it is 'balanced', bullet 6), and with *positive* working relationships supported by good communication skills (it is 'relational', bullet 7). VBP, then, in a word, is 'recovery' oriented: it builds on the 'strengths and resiliencies of *individual* users', recognizing that 'there are many *diverse* routes to recovery' (bullet 2, emphasis added).

Implementation

VBP thus has a rich set of practical corollaries as identified in the Framework. But the Framework, coming now to the last question in Exercise 18, also gives a number of clear indications of how policy is to be converted into practical action. Some of these are implicit: the last three bullet points, specifying that VBP is reflective, balanced, and relational, cover attitudes that are essential to effective working where values conflict. The Framework, though, also makes explicit in its final unnumbered paragraph, that implementation will depend on future 'educational and research initiatives'.

VBP, then, is very far from a recipe for 'anything goes'. It has the potential, at least, to be practically effective. But what risks are there of taking VBP into policy and practice in mental health? What are the possible downsides?

Dangerous downsides

In piloting the Values Framework, many respondents joked about 'lists of worthy values that get stuck up on the wall in the Chief Executive's office and are then promptly forgotten'! The NIMHE Values Framework is not such a list. To the contrary, it is a framework for *action*. But could its very potency have downsides?

EXERCISE 19 (10 minutes)

Think about this question. What are the risks of having a 'National Framework of Values for Mental Health' that, far from being a list of aspirational values mouldering on the Chief Executive's wall, has the potential, in the final words of the Framework, to 'give effect to the principles of Values-Based Practice'?

In piloting the Values Framework, members of the Values Project Group received much positive support for the approach (also reflected in 'hits' on the 'connects' website noted above since publication).

Two equal and opposite dangers in implementation were identified, however. On the one side was the danger already noted, of the Framework remaining, like the all-too-familiar lists of values, merely aspirational. On the other side, though, was the danger of the Framework being used, not to free up the resources of diversity, but as a weapon that allows one group of stakeholders to impose their values on other stakeholders.

Avoiding these twin dangers, the equal and opposite dangers of ineffectiveness and of all-too-effective partisan take-overs, will depend on the training and research initiatives signalled in the last paragraph of the Framework. We describe recent training initiatives in VBP in the next section. We return to research in Chapter 21.

4) Values-Based Practice and clinical practice skills

The skills underpinning VBP cover four areas, defined by Principles 6–9 of VBP, awareness, knowledge, reasoning skills, and communication skills.

Training in ethics and in Values-Based Practice

The skill areas of VBP correspond broadly with the aims of ethics teaching in health care outlined in the first section of Chapter 17. There are differences, however, as we should expect, given that the overall aim of VBP is to add new tools to the values toolkit of health care.

Thus, 'change of attitudes', one of the aims of ethics teaching, does not appear as a training objective in VBP at all. This is because, unlike ethics, at least in the quasi-legal form in which it impacts on practice, VBP does not seek to prescribe 'right' attitudes to the development of which training should be directed (unless respect for difference, as the premiss of VBP, is considered an attitude). The remaining skills areas, although important in both kinds of training, are important in different ways and for different reasons. We will consider each of these briefly.

Principle 6 of Values-Based Practice: raising awareness

Raising awareness is the first skills area emphasized both in ethics training and in VBP. As an area that is fundamental to VBP, it has been the subject of an extensive process of development and piloting of training materials in what we believe is a unique joint programme, initiated by Matt Muijen, as Director of a major mental health NGO, The Sainsbury Centre for Mental Health (SCMH), and the Philosophy and Ethics of Mental Health (PEMH) programme at Warwick University. In the next exercise, we look at how this works out in practice.

EXERCISE 20

Box 18.3 gives an extract from a training workbook in VBP, including all four VBP skills areas, developed by the SCMH programme lead for VBP, Kim Woodbridge, and Bill Fulford (Woodbridge and Fulford, 2004). As you will see, this is an exercise that aims to raise awareness of values.

1. Can you identify the philosophical origin of the exercise?, and

2. How does this differ from a corresponding exercise in raising awareness in traditional ethics?

The workbook in VBP was developed and piloted by Woodbridge and Fulford with mental health professionals and users of services in such challenging areas as assertive outreach teams and crisis intervention. The objectives of the workbook could thus not be more practical. The exercise, though, is directly based on J.L. Austin's 'ordinary' language approach to philosophical method. Thus the reader is encouraged to review a piece of text drawn from practice—a letter, or care plan, etc.—and to focus, not on the message, but on the words actually used.

In Chapter 4, we adopted Austin's approach as a research method: it was one way of gaining clearer (or more complete) understanding of the meanings of concepts—illness, disease, mental illness, etc.—that are important in mental health. Here,

Box 18.3 Activity 8: Raising awareness through language

Please read through the following extract, which is an example of the sort of text that can be found in many policy documents, and then answer the questions below:

This Trust is supporting the change and reconfiguration of services to best meet NSF and other guidance for both adult and older mental health service users. There are some common themes for services throughout the Trust. These include:

• Developing effective management structures to lead and support change.

• Developing organisational structures in each area to support clinical governance, risk management and health and safety requirements.

• Implementing financial structures to ensure balanced budgets.

• Establishing cross area development groups to take forward required service developments in adult, older people, child and adolescent, and drug and alcohol services.

• Ensuring services provide fully integrated health and social care teams.

• Providing single points of access to services to ensure effective referral pathways and to support the targeting of resources.

• Reconfiguring where required to organise adult services to support functional models, to target skills and resources against standard and enhanced CPA [Care Planning Approach] levels of care.

• Developing minimum standards for CPA.

• Progressing approaches to provide a workforce fit for purpose, concentrating on training, modernising roles and responsibilities and supporting staff at work (including compliance with NHS Plan 'Improving Working Lives' standards).

• Influencing workforce planning Trust-wide with direct access of senior Trust representatives into workforce planning decision making, where previously local services have been isolated and with little influence on the mental health agenda.

• Establishing joint commissioning approaches and reaffirming Local Implementation Teams as the key commissioning groups for each area.

• Progressing service developments and/or monitoring arrangements to maximise the repatriation of expensive out-of-area private placements and minimise the use of private sector services.

• An acceptance that resources currently available are significantly insufficient, but a key objective that services will be targeted and arranged to be as effective as possible within those limited resources.

• The argument for additional resources will be best made once services are configured, as far as possible, to match best-practice models, NSF and performance targets.

• Limited resources should mean the targeting of services and not the arrested development of skills, training, roles and supporting information technology systems.

Question 1

Underline any value judgements (for example: effective, limited, best).

Question 2

What values are apparent throughout the extract? What is seen as desired, important or a priority?'

Question 3

Whose are these overall values? What are the implications for the values identified? Do they conflict in any way?

Question 4

Are there any values missing or that you would like to be emphasized?

essentially the same approach is used as a training method: attention to language use highlights and allows trainees to recognize the values—some explicit, others implicit—shaping their practice. In pilot programmes this has proved highly effective with service providers in both voluntary and statutory sectors (Fulford et al., 2002a; Woodbridge and Fulford, 2003).

The workbook in VBP (Woodbridge and Fulford, 2004) was launched by the Minister of State with responsibility for mental health, Rosie Winterton, at a conference in London in July 2004. In its own right, and as one of the two sources for a national training programme in generic skills for mental health and social care (the other source being EBP), the workbook will support a rollout of training in both voluntary and statutory sectors in the UK from 2005 (National Institute for Mental Health England, et al., 2004), and there are similar initiatives in a number of other countries (Fulford et al., 2004). This is clearly an area, then, in which analytic philosophy, far from being as its critics in the 1980s and 1990s suggested, practically impotent, is proving highly effective in some of the most challenging areas of mental health practice.

Many variations of this awareness raising theme have been developed by the SCMH/PEMH partnership. Their shared origin, though, is in the linguistic analytic methods pioneered by Austin. Correspondingly, therefore, their objectives are very different from the objectives of awareness raising methods in ethics. In ethics, dilemmas—difficult or contentious cases—are used to raise awareness of ethical issues: dramatic rather than everyday cases serve this purpose best; and there is often someone who has 'got it wrong' (failing to respect autonomy, for example–see, e.g. Kushner and Thomasma, 2001). In VBP, attention to language use helps to raise awareness of values generally; everyday rather than dramatic texts serve this purpose best; and the intention is to raise awareness as such, not to highlight 'good' and 'bad' values.

Principles 7–9 of Values-Based Practice

Similar contrasts can be drawn between VBP and ethics training for the remaining skills areas.

◆ *Increasing knowledge* (Principle 7) is of secondary importance, even somewhat suspect (Gillon, 1996), in ethics. Recently, there has been a growing recognition of the importance of basing ethical decision-making on fact not fancy (Widdershoven *et al.*, forthcoming). In VBP, any method for gaining knowledge of values, qualitative or quantitative, narrative, evidence-based, or whatever, is fundamental. It is fundamental theoretically because, as in Hare's analysis of value terms (Hare, 1952), the criteria for value judgements are descriptive (or factual) criteria. It is fundamental practically because our intuitions about other people's values are demonstrably unreliable (Fulford *et al.*, 2002b).

◆ *Reasoning skills* (Principle 8). Any of the methods of ethical reasoning described earlier in this chapter have a place equally in VBP as in traditional ethics. Their role is different, though. In ethics, reasoning skills are used to decide what is 'right'. In VBP their role is to help us explore the values likely to be operative in a given context. VBP is in this respect closer to theoretical bioethics than to the dominant quasi-legal regulatory approach of ethics in practice. In their original description of the use of principles in bioethics, Beauchamp and Childress (1989), as noted above, make clear that prima facie principles, as they call their four principles, should be used to open up our thinking about an ethical issue, not, as they have often been misrepresented, to generate answers.

◆ *Communication skills* (Principle 9) have an executive role in quasi-legal ethics but a substantive role in VBP. In quasi-legal ethics communication skills are used to explore a situation in order to decide what rules apply and then to help make the rules 'stick'! Their role is thus secondary. In VBP, by contrast, communications skills have a primary role. In VBP a 'good decision' is defined as much by 'how' as by 'what': that is to say, in VBP a good decision is defined as much by *how* the decision is arrived at, and *how* it is implemented, as by *what* decision is taken and *what* is actually done.

6) Values-Based Practice, Evidenced-Based Practice, and a new alliance between users and providers in health-care decision-making

The 10th principle of VBP, described in Box 18.1 as the 'who decides' principle, has the effect, as we will see, of building a new alliance in health-care decision-making.

Principle 10 of Values-Based Practice: 'who decides'

In shifting the 'locus of control' in health-care decision-making, Principle 10 of VBP marks a further and perhaps crucial

difference between VBP and quasi-legal ethics. In quasi-legal ethics, it is ethicists, lawyers, members of ethics committees, and others external to the decision in question, who decide what ought to be done. Ethicists and lawyers write the rules: regulatory bodies interpret and enforce them. In VBP, by contrast, it is those directly concerned in a given decision who decide. VBP, in the words of Principle 10, 'puts decision-making back where it belongs, with users and providers' (and, we might add, with managers and policy makers) 'at the clinical coal-face'.

Principle 10 as a summary of Values-Based Practice

Principle 10 captures many of the important features of VBP understood as a new set of tools to support health-care decision-making, a set that extends, without displacing, the tools of quasi-legal ethics.

Thus, Principle 10, in transferring the locus of control in health-care decision-making from ethicists/lawyers to users/providers, also transfers responsibility. The buck, as they say, stops with the decision-maker. One consequence of this is the new and more substantive roles for the four areas of clinical skills defined by Principles 6–9, awareness, knowledge, reasoning skills, and communication skills.

The 'decision-maker' in VBP, however, is an alliance of user and provider. VBP is 'patient-centred', certainly (Principle 4); in a democracy of values, *health-care decisions*, to repeat the crucial phrase from the third R of the NIMHE Framework, should start from 'the values of each individual service user/client and their communities'. But VBP is premised on *reciprocal* respect (the key word used in bullet point 2 of the NIMHE Framework). VBP, therefore besides being patient-centred, is also multidisciplinary (Principle 5).

This is not a matter, merely, as it might be even in quasi-legal ethics, of fairness. The different values represented by the many different professional and voluntary groups involved in multidisciplinary service provision, supply the 'balance of legitimately different values' (Principle 5 again), to which good process in VBP is directed, and on which effective health-care decision-making, whether about diagnostic assessment or treatment (Principle 1), whether explicitly value-laden or not (Principle 2), and whether in mental health or, increasingly, in other areas of health care (Principle 3), critically depends.

Principle 10 and the parallels between Values-Based Practice and Evidence-Based Practice

Principle 10 of VBP, if highlighting and drawing together some of the differences between VBP and quasi-legal ethics, also brings us back to the parallels between VBP and EBP. Again, we should not be surprised by the extent of these parallels, VBP being a product of the same philosophical value theory, that, in Part I (chapter 6), led to our 'full-field' fact + value model of the conceptual structure of medicine. Thus,

◆ *Principle 1* of VBP, the two-feet principle, directly corresponds with the equal and complementary roles of fact and value, or more exactly, description and evaluation, in the full-field theoretical model of Part I.

- *Principle 2* of VBP, the 'squeaky wheel' principle, applies equally to both sides: health-care decision-making has always been based jointly on facts and values; but we need EBP as we need VBP, nowadays, because of the growing complexity of both factual and evaluative sides of the decision-making equation.

- *Principle 3* of VBP, the 'science driven' principle, also applies to both sides: the growing complexity of health-care decision-making is driven by advances in science and technology, directly on the fact side, indirectly on the value side, i.e. as described above, by way of the extended choices in health care opened up by science and technology.

Principle 10 and the anti-parallels between Values-Based Practice and Evidence-Based Practice

The tools of VBP, of course, fashioned as they are to deal with different aspects of the growing complexity of health-care decision-making, are different from the tools of EBP. In EBP, as we saw in Part III, the focus is on information that is as *perspective-free* as possible. At the top of EBP's 'evidence hierarchy', then, are the results of meta-analyses of high quality research. The tools of such meta-analyses, statistical and IT-based, are designed to approximate to the traditional scientific ideal of what Thomas Nagel characterized as a 'view from nowhere' (Nagel, 1986). The outputs from EBP, correspondingly, the clinical practice guidelines that support health-care decision-making, are derived by consensual closure through progressive reduction of differences of view.

In VBP, by contrast, the need is for information that is as *close as possible* to the perspectives of those involved in a given decision. At the top of the 'values hierarchy' of VBP, then, is *perspectival* information about values. The tools of VBP, correspondingly, the tools to deliver perspectival information, are the practice skills defined by Principles 6–9 of VBP, combined with the models of service organization defined by Principle 4 (the Patient-Centred Principle) and Principle 5 (the Multidisciplinary Principle). Practice skills deliver high-quality information about values, which, combined with appropriate models of service organization, support what one of us has called elsewhere a 'dissensual' approach to health-care decision-making, i.e. an approach to health-care decision-making that is based, not on consensual closure through reduction of differences, but on an open balance of legitimately different value perspectives (Fulford, 1998).

Principle 10 and the interdependence of Values-Based Practice and Evidence-Based Practice

VBP and EBP, then, as we noted at the start of this section, being responses to different aspects of the growing complexity of health-care decision-making, are complementary. They are complementary in their parallels. They are complementary in their antiparallels. They are also, although presented here as distinct sets of decision-support tools, strongly interdependent. The tools of EBP, for example, are important in VBP under Principle 7, the 'knowledge' principle, in helping to supply high-quality generalizable evidence about values (Fulford *et al.*, 2002b). Similarly, the tools of VBP are the basis for a more balanced and positive approach to the 'ethics' of research and the role and functioning of research ethics committees (Dickenson and Fulford, 2000, chapter 10).

There are also deeper theoretical links between VBP and EBP. Value judgements, you will recall from Part I, are, in Hare's clear formulation, based on descriptive criteria: so, EBP, where relevant, will supply evidence about whether or not a given criterion is satisfied. Conversely, work in the philosophy of science, as we saw in Part III, has shown the extent to which epistemic and other values permeate all aspects of the scientific process, from observation, through the selection and design of research programmes, to the interpretation of results, and the adoption of theories. To the extent, therefore, that legitimately different values are in play, the tools of VBP have a potential role in science no less important than their role in health-care decision-making.

Principle 10 and a new user-provider alliance in health care

It is the complementary and interdependent natures of EBP and VBP which is the basis for a new alliance between users and providers in health-care decision-making. As noted in the last section, overuse of the tools of quasi-legal ethics has a number of downsides. Among the most serious of these has been a progressive alienation of users from providers of services. This is inevitable where ethics, as in its current dominantly quasi-legal interactions with practice, adopts the role primarily of guardian, 'protecting' users of services from what are portrayed as essentially predatory providers.

The justification for this approach is that providers sometimes deliberately exploit their positions of power to the disadvantage of users. It is a proper function of law and ethical regulation, therefore, as we noted above, to provide a framework of principles, procedures, and sanctions, aimed at protecting users from such betrayals of the central health care value of patient-centred practice.

Extend this proper 'framework' function of law, however, to the 'code inflation' of quasi-legal ethics, and the danger, faced equally by users as by providers of services, is of a wedge of mutual fear and resentment increasingly being driven between them. Principle 10 of VBP, in restoring the 'locus of control' to the users and providers involved in a particular decision, aims to reverse this process, replacing alienation with alliance. In this, surely most urgent of aims, VBP and EBP, as the final reading in this section makes clear, are indeed both complementary and interdependent.

Read the extract from the Introduction to a widely read and respected textbook on EBP:

Sackett, D.L. Straus, S.E., Scott Richardson, W., Rosenberg, W., and Haynes, R.B. (2000). *Evidence-Based Medicine: how to practice and teach EBM*, (2nd edn). Edinburgh: Churchill Livingstone

Link with Reading 18.9 (on disk already)

◆ What model of health care is reflected in this definition of EBP?

EBP is widely thought to be concerned only with applying the results of research to practice. In this reading, however, Sackett *et al.* (2000) define evidence-based medicine as involving three key elements, best research evidence, clinical experience, and patients' values. There could surely be no clearer statement of the full-field, fact+value, model to which we came at the end of Part I, and from which, in this session, we have derived the principles of VBP.

Reflection on the session and self-test questions

Write down your own reflections on the materials in this session drawing out any points that are particularly significant for you. Then write brief notes about the following:

1. What is Values-Based Practice?

2. Where does Values-Based Practice start from (what is its premiss)? And how does it differ from substantive ethics.

3. What three principles link Evidence-Based with Values-Based approaches to health-care decision-making?

4. What model of service delivery is required to support 'good process' in Values-Based Practice?

5. What particular clinical skills are required to support good process in Values-Based Practice? (We noted four.)

6. What is the aim of combining Values-Based with Evidence-Based approaches to decision-making in health care?

Conclusions: combining law and ethics with Values-Based Practice

Complementary tools in the toolkit

In this chapter we have considered a range of tools for working with values in mental health derived respectively from bioethics (principles, casuistry, and perspectives), general ethical theory (deontological and utilitarian), and analytic ethical theory (VBP).

Mental health, we have argued, requires a sharper set of tools because of the additional depth dimension of conceptual difficulty underlying ethical problems in this area, as outlined in Chapter 17. VBP, we have further argued, offers a set of tools for dealing with a particular aspect of this complexity, namely, the greater diversity of values in mental health compared with other areas of health care, particularly the high-tech areas on which bioethics, at least in the strongly regulative form it has taken in practice, has traditionally concentrated.

The relationship between regulative ethics, or quasi-legal ethics as we have called it, and VBP, understood as different sets of tools in the toolkit for working with values in health care, is shown diagrammatically in Figure 18.2.

In this figure regulative ethics is shown as being properly concerned with the 'framework' values that are widely shared for a given group. These shared framework values include, for current health-care practice, autonomy and beneficence, as discussed earlier in this chapter. Other shared values, as shown in the figure, include confidentiality and sharing of information, and acting in the patient's best interests. So understood, then, as being concerned with the values that (for a given group at a given period) are widely shared, quasi-legal ethics is

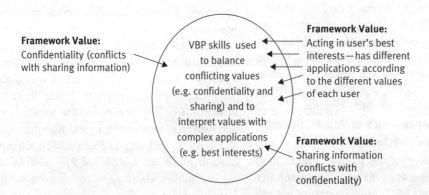

Framework Value: Confidentiality (conflicts with sharing information)

VBP skills used to balance conflicting values (e.g. confidentiality and sharing) and to interpret values with complex applications (e.g. best interests)

Framework Value: Acting in user's best interests—has different applications according to the different values of each user

Framework Value: Sharing information (conflicts with confidentiality)

Fig. 18.2 The complementary relationship between quasi-legal ethics and Values-Based Practice.

an extension of what the Oxford philosopher of law, H.L.A. Hart, described as the proper function of law itself, to provide a choosing framework (Hart, 1968).

Such a framework, of shared ethical values filling out health care law, is, as we have several times emphasized, essential for health-care decision-making that seeks to maximize choice. As the diagram in Figure 18.2 shows, however, there are two reasons why the framework of ethics and law cannot, in itself, be sufficient. First, framework values conflict: autonomy is in tension with beneficence, as Beauchamp and Childress (1989) argued; and confidentiality is in tension with the sharing of information (Fulford, 2001). Second, framework values have complex interpretations: 'best interests', for example, will mean very different things according to the often very different values of those concerned in a given decision.

It is where framework values conflict, then, and/or have complex interpretations, that the good process model of VBP complements and extends the tools of quasi-legal ethics. In the next chapter we turn to law itself, and to its role in supporting health-care decision-making especially in the values-complex environment of mental health. We return to VBP, and to its role particularly in relation to diagnosis, in chapter 21.

Useful websites

- http://www.basw.co.uk/articles.php?articleId=2&page=6 Values and principles of social work.

- http://www.doh.gov.uk/mentalhealth/implementationguide.htm For the extract on values underpinning the Mental Health National Service Framework.

- http://www.nice.org.uk National Institute for Clinical Excellence (NICE). Schizophrenia guidelines and other information.

- http://wwwnimhe.org.uk National Institute for Mental Health England. For information regarding implementation guides and mental health policy.

- http://www.nmc-uk.org Code of professional conduct for nursing and midwifery.

- http://www.rcpsych.ac.uk/publications/cr/council/cr83.pdf The duties of a doctor registered with the General Medical Council.

- http://www.scmh.org.uk For further useful information in general about practice and policy issues.

- http://www.scie.org.uk Social Care Institute for Excellence. For information regarding social models of care and other general social care information.

- http://www.warwick.ac.uk The University of Warwick.

- http://www2.warwick.ac.uk/fac/med Warwick Medical School.

Reading guide

Ethics and bioethics

Detailed reading guides on general ethical theory and on bioethics are given in chapter 2 of Dickenson and Fulford's (2000) *In Two Minds*. Among introductions to ethics, a modern classic is James Rachels' (2003) *The Elements of Moral Philosophy*. D.D. Raphael's (1994) *Moral Philosophy* includes a guide to further reading for both classic and modern sources. Mary Warnock's *Ethics since 1900* (1978) remains an exceptionally clear introduction to each of the main ethical theories noted in this chapter. R.M. Hare's (1997) *Sorting Out Ethics* offers a brief but authoritative introduction to each of the main philosophical theories of ethics. A clear summary of Kantian, consequentialist and virtue ethics, organized as an extended debate, is given in Marcia W. Baron, Philip Petit, and Michael Slote (1997) *Three Methods of Ethics*.

Mental health and mental illness are among the subjects covered in Michael Parker and Donna Dickenson's (2000) *The Cambridge Workbook in Medical Ethics*. The Cambridge Workbook also introduces new approaches beyond principlism and casuistry, particularly from the European tradition. Grant Gillett's (1989) *Reasonable Care* is an entertainingly written introduction drawing on much case material.

Principles

The classic of the principles approach is Tom Beauchamp and James Childress' (1989) *Principles of Biomedical Ethics*. Raanon Gillon's (1985) *Philosophical Medical Ethics* offers a brief and practically focused introduction to the principles approach. Gillon's edited collection on the principles approach, his *Principles of Health Care Ethics* (Gillon and Lloyd, 1994), includes Fulford and Hope's (1994) 'Psychiatric ethics: a bioethical ugly duckling', which discusses the strengths and limitations of the principles approach in psychiatry.

Casuistry

Al Jonsen (a theologian) and Stephen Toulmin (a philosopher) (1988) wrote their now classic book on casuistry *The Abuse of Casuistry* after serving on a Presidential Commission on Bioethics (see text).

Principles and casuistry are compared as approaches to ethical issues of consent in psychiatry in Fulford and Hope's (1994) chapter in Gillon and Lloyd's *Principles of Health Care Ethics*. Priscilla Alderson's (1990) *Choosing for Children* shows the value of qualitative research.

Perspectives

The Oxford psychiatrist and Professor of Medical Ethics, Tony Hope, was among the first to emphasize the importance of perspectives in ethical reasoning in medicine; see his *Medical*

Ethics: a very short introduction (2004). Narrative ethics has recently come into prominence as part of narrative-based (in contrast to evidence-based) medicine: see Anne Hudson Jones' (1999) article, *Narrative in Medical ethics*, which was published as part of a series on narrative approaches to medicine in the *BMJ*. Carl Elliott's (1999) collection of essays, *A Philosophical Disease* illustrates the value of storytelling in biomedical ethics. The *Declaration of Madrid*, the first code to spell out the importance of the 'user' voice in clinical decision-making, was published by the World Psychiatric Association, Geneva (1996).

Professional ethics and the role of codes

Authoritative introductions to these two areas specifically for psychiatry are Allen Dyer's 'Psychiatry as a profession' and Sidney Bloch and Russell Porgiter's 'Codes of ethics in psychiatry' (chapters 5 and 6, respectively, of *Psychiatric Ethics*, Bloch, Chodoff, and Green, 1999). See also Ruth Chadwick's (1994) edited collection *Ethics and the Professions* for an excellent overview. The practical and theoretical links between ethical codes, concepts of disorder, and communication skills in psychiatric ethics, is described in Fulford and Bloch's (2000) chapter in the *New Oxford Textbook of Psychiatry*, on 'Codes, concepts and clinical practice skills'. Chapter 11, on 'Inter-professional relations', of the BMA's (1993) *Medical Ethics Today* is a helpful review of the ethical issues arising in multidisciplinary team working. The ethics of teamwork between professionals is also explored in Perkins and Repper (1998) *Dilemmas in Community Mental Health Practice*.

Psychiatric ethics

As noted in the text, the first edition of Sidney Bloch and Paul Chodoff's, *Psychiatric Ethics*, was one of the trail blazers for the otherwise relatively neglected area of psychiatric ethics (Bloch and Chodoff, 1981). The third edition (Bloch, Chodoff, and Green, 1999), together with complementary case studies and guides to further reading in its sister volume, Dickenson and Fulford's *In Two Minds*, includes chapters on each of the main areas of ethical concern in psychiatry as noted in this and other reading guides. Rem B. Edward's (1982) *Psychiatry and Ethics* is a valuable edited collection of classic articles. Also important among early publications were Michael Moore's (1984) *Law and Psychiatry: rethinking the relationships*, and Alan Stone's (1984) *Law, Psychiatry and Morality*. Early reviews defining the subject include those by Kopelman (1989), Hope (1990), and Anzia and Puma (1991). Potter's (2004) explores gender issues.

A number of both psychiatric and bioethics journals have included special issues on psychiatric ethics, for example (Fulford and Radden, 2002) 'Bioethics: Special Issue on psychiatric ethics'). The update journal, *Current Opinion in Psychiatry*, includes regular articles on ethical issues both in specific clinical topic areas and in the *History and Philosophy Section*.

Philosophy, Psychiatry, & Psychology publishes articles that explore the conceptual issues underpinning problems in psychiatric ethics: see, e.g. by Pat Bracken (1995) and Eric Mathews (1995) on Michel Foucault and critical psychiatry; Hinshelwood (1995) on personal identity (see also Part V), and on the ethics of psychotherapy (Hinshelwood, 1997a), with commentaries by Mace (1997), Sturdee (1997a), and Thornton (1997), and a detailed response (Hinshelwood, 1997b; also Hinshelwood, 1997c). *Philosophy, Psychiatry, & Psychology* has had a special issue on suicide and psychiatric euthanasia (1998; volume 5/2).

Other topics explored have included Dickenson and Jones (1995) on developmental issues (in their 'True wishes: the philosophy and developmental psychology of children's informed consent'), with commentaries by Eekelar (1995), McCormick (1995), Murray (1995), Parker (1995), and Wells (1995); Stocker's (1997) 'Aristotelian akrasia and psychoanalytic regression', with a commentary by Sturdee (1997b); Putnam (1997) on 'Psychological courage' with a commentary by Moore (1997); Gillett (1998a) on 'Relativism and the social constructivist paradigm' with commentaries by Fourcher (1998) and Phillips (1998), and a response by Gillett (1998b); on feminism, Burman's (2001) 'Feminist contributions' to reframing current controversies around memory, Potter's (2001) 'Feminism', and Richmond's (2001a) 'Psychoanalysis and feminism: anorexia, the social world, and the internal world', with commentaries by Adshead, 2001, Mitchell (2001) and Hinshelwood (2001), and responses by Burman, (2001b) and Richmond (2001b); on race, Nissim-Sabat's (2001) 'Psychiatry, psychoanalysis and race'; and on power relations, Lilleleht's (2002a) 'Progress and power: exploring the disciplinary connections between moral treatment and psychiatric rehabilitation' with commentaries by Charland (2002) and Bracken (2002), and a response by Lilleleht (2002b).

The particular problems raised by psychiatric research ethics are discussed in Fulford and Howse (1993) 'Ethics of research with psychiatric patients: principles, problems and the primary responsibilities of researchers'. Chapter 10 of *In Two Minds* gives a worked case example of psychiatric research ethics.

Values-based practice: (1) The theory

The theory and skills base of VBP are set out in Fulford's (2004) chapter in Radden's *Companion*. The chapter includes a case history done as a series of vignettes illustrating how each of the 10 principles work out in the story of a particular person, Diane Abbot, an artist who found she could not 'see colours'. Holmes and Lindley's (1989) *The Values of Psychotherapy*, and Marina's (1999) 'The problem of values in psychiatry', set out the issues from which VBP starts; and Perkins (2001) and Campbell (2002) make explicit the service user perspective. As described in the text, VBP is derived from philosophical value theory as in the work particularly of Hare (1952), Geoffrey Warnock (1971), and others in the Oxford analytic tradition, applied to health-care contexts in Fulford (1989, *Moral Theory and Medical Practice*), and combined with substantive work on value diversity using both analytic methods, notably Sadler (2002, *Descriptions & Prescriptions: values, mental disorders, and the DSMs*), phenomenology, notably Stanghellini (2004, *Deanimated Bodies and Disembodied Spirits*), and empirical research, notably Colombo (1997, *Understanding Mentally Disordered Offenders: a multi-agency perspective*), Colombo *et al.* (2003, 'Evaluating the influence of implicit models of mental disorder on processes of shared decision making within community-based multi-disciplinary teams'), and Tan *et al.* (2003, 'Anorexia nervosa and personal identity: The accounts of patients and their parents').

The theory of VBP is further developed in relation to:

1. Child and adolescent mental health services, in Fulford and Williams (2003) 'Values-based child and adolescent mental health services?'. This is a review article setting VBP in a policy context for the UK and illustrating each of the ten principles with examples from child and adolescent mental health.

2. The relationship between clinicians and managers, in Fulford and Bennington's (2005) 'VBM²: A collaborative values-based model of health care decision making combining medical and management perspectives' (in Williams (ed.) *Medical and Management Perspectives in Child and Adolescent Psychiatry*). This article illustrates the resources of VBP for bringing together medical (K.W.M.F.) and management (J.B.) perspectives. The VBM² of the title captures the idea that differences of values, which are a 'problem' to be solved in traditional quasi-legal ethics, become a positive resource for health-care decision-making in VBP.

In a discussion of Colombo and Fulford's work on models of disorder (see Part I) in *Philosophy, Psychiatry, & Psychology*, Bendelow (2004), Williams (2004), Williamson (2004), and Heginbotham (2004), provide important critiques of developments in VBP, respectively from the perspectives of the social sciences, for professional training and regulation, for multiagency organization of services, and for policies that are capable of delivering genuinely user-centred care.

Articles on aspects of ethics and value theory relevant to different areas of psychopathology have been published in *Philosophy, Psychiatry, & Psychology*, for example: (1) Moore *et al.*'s (1994) 'Mild mania and well-being', with commentaries by Nordenfelt (1994) and Seedhouse (1994); (2) Potter's (1996) article on false memory syndrome ('Loopholes, gaps, and what is held fast: democratic epistemology and claims to recovered memories'), with a commentary by Code (1996); (3) Mitchell's (1998a) 'Neurosis and the historic quest for security: a social-role analysis', with a commentary by Schwartz and Wiggins (1998) and a response by Mitchell (1998b); (4) Ward's (2002a) article on the nature of evil, 'Explaining evil behavior: using Kant and M. Scott Peck to solve the puzzle of understanding the moral psychology of evil people', with commentaries by Sverdlik (2002), Adshead (2002), and Mullen (2002), and a response by Ward (2002b); (5) on depression, Radden's (2003a) 'Is this Dame Melancholy? Equating today's depression and past melancholia', with commentaries by Brendel (2003) and Hansen (2003), and a response (Radden, 2003b); and (6) Clegg and Lansdall-Welfare (2003a), on 'Death, disability and dogma', with commentaries by Colman (2003), Casenave (2003), and Reinders (2003), and a response by Clegg and Lansdall-Welfare (2003b).

References

Adshead, G. (2001). Commentary on 'Impossible things before breakfast': A Commentary on Burman (2001) and Richmond (2001). *Philosophy, Psychiatry, & Psychology*, 8/1: 33–38.

Adshead, G. (2002). Through a glass, darkly: Commentary on Ward. (Commentary on Ward, 2002a). *Philosophy, Psychiatry, & Psychology*, 9/1: 15–18.

Alderson, P. (1990). *Choosing for Children: parents' consent to surgery*. Oxford: Oxford University Press.

Alderson, P. (1994). *Children's Consent to Surgery*. Buckingham: Open University Press.

Allott, P., Loganathan, L., and Fulford, K.W.M. (2002, in press). Discovering hope for recovery from a British perspective. In *International Innovations In Community Mental Health* (ed. S. Lurie, M. McCubbin, and B. Dallaire) (Special Issue). *Canadian Journal of Community Mental Health*, 21(2).

Anzia, D.J. and La Puma, J. (1991). An annotated bibliography of psychiatric medical ethics. *Academic Psychiatry*, 15: 1–7.

Aristotle (2000). *The Nicomachean Ethics*. (ed. Crisp, R.) Cambridge: Cambridge University Press.

Baron, M.W., Petit, P., and Slote, M. (1997). *Three Methods of Ethics*. Oxford: Blackwell.

Beauchamp, T.L. and Childress, J.F. (1989; 4th edn 1994). *Principles of Biomedical Ethics*. Oxford: Oxford University Press.

Bendelow, G. (2004). Sociology and concepts of mental illness. (Commentary on Fulford and Colombo, 2004). *Philosophy, Psychiatry and Psychology*, 11/2, 145–146.

Birley, J. (2000). Psychiatric ethics: an international open society. In *In Two Minds: a casebook of psychiatric ethics* (ed. D. Dickenson and K.W.M. Fulford). Oxford: Oxford University Press, pp. 327–335.

Bloch, S. and Porgiter, R. (1999). Codes of ethics in psychiatry. In *Psychiatric Ethics* (ed. S. Bloch, P. Chodoff, and S.A. Green). Oxford: Oxford University Press, Chapter 6.

Bloch, S. and Chodoff, P. (1981) *Psychiatric ethics* (first edition). Oxford: Oxford University Press.

534 CHAPTER 18 FROM BIOETHICS TO VALUES-BASED PRACTICE

Bloch, S., Chodoff, P., and Green, S.A. (1999). *Psychiatric Ethics*. Oxford: Oxford University Press.

BMA (1993). Inter-professional relations. *Medical Ethics Today*, Chapter 11.

Bracken, P.J., (1995). Beyond Liberation: Michael Foucault and the Notion of a Critical Psychiatry. *Philosophy, Psychiatry, & Psychology*, 2/1, 1–14.

Bracken, P. (2002). Commentary 'Listening to Foucault'. (Commentary on Lilleleht, 2002a). *Philosophy, Psychiatry, & Psychology*, 9(2): 187–188.

Brendel, D.H. (2003). A pragmatic consideration of depression and melancholia. (Commentary on Radden, 2003a). *Philosophy, Psychiatry, & Psychology*, 10/1: 53–56.

Burman, E. (2001a). Reframing current controversies around memory: feminist contributions. *Philosophy, Psychiatry, & Psychology*, 8/1: 21–32.

Burman, E. (2001b). Remembering feminisms: a response to the commentary. *Philosophy, Psychiatry, & Psychology*, 8/1: 39–40.

Campbell, A.B. and Higgs, R. (1982). *In That Case: medical ethics in everyday practice*. London: Darton, Longman and Todd.

Campbell, P. (2002). What we want from crisis services. In *Healthcare Ethics and Human Values* (ed. K.W.M. Fulford, D. Dickenson, and T.H. Murray). Oxford: Blackwell Science.

Casenave, G. (2003). Death, disability, and dialogue. (Commentary on Clegg and Lansdall-Welfare, 2003a). *Philosophy, Psychiatry, & Psychology*, 10/1: 87–90.

Chadwick, R. (ed.) (1994). *Ethics and the Professions*. Aldershot, England: Avebury Press.

Charland, L. (2002). Commentary Tuke's healing discipline. (Commentary on Lilleleht, 2002a). *Philosophy, Psychiatry, & Psychology*, 9(2): 183–186.

Clegg, J. and Lansdall-Welfare, R. (2003a). Death, disability, and dogma. *Philosophy, Psychiatry, & Psychology*, 10/1: 67–80.

Clegg, J. and Lansdall-Welfare, R. (2003b). Commentary on 'Living with contested knowledge and partial authority'. *Philosophy, Psychiatry, & Psychology*, 10/1: 99–102.

Code, L. (1996). Loopholes, gaps, and what is held fast. (Commentary on Potter, 1996). *Philosophy, Psychiatry, & Psychology*, 3(4): 255–260.

Colman, S. (2003). What's in the box then, Mum?—death, disability and dogma. (Commentary on Clegg and Lansdall-Welfare, 2003a). *Philosophy, Psychiatry, & Psychology*, 10/1: 81–86.

Colombo, A. (1997). *Understanding Mentally Disordered Offenders: a multi-agency perspective*. Aldershot, UK: Ashgate.

Colombo, A., Bendelow, G., Fulford, K.W.M., and Williams, S. (2003). Evaluating the influence of implicit models of mental disorder on processes of shared decision making within community-based multi-disciplinary teams. *Social Science & Medicine*, 56: 1557–1570.

Crisp, R. (1994). Quality of life and health care. Chapter 13 In *Medicine and Moral Reasoning* (ed. K.W.M. Fulford, G.R. Gillett, and J.M. Soskice). Cambridge: Cambridge University Press.

Davidovskii, I.V. (1962). *Problems of Causality in Medicine*. Moscow: The State Medical Publisher.

Davidovskii, I.V. and Snezhnevsky, A.V. (1972) *Schizophrenia*. Moscow: News of the Academy of Medical Science.

Department of Health (1999). *National Service Framework for Mental Heath, Modern Standards and Service Models*. London: HMSO.

Department of Health (2000). *The NHS Plan, A plan for investment, A plan for reform*. London: HMSO.

Department of Health (2002). Improvement, Expansion and Reform: the next 3 years. Priorities and Planning Framework, 2003–06. London: Department of Health.

Dickenson, D. and Fulford, K.W.M. (ed.) (2000). *In Two Minds: a casebook of psychiatric ethics*. Oxford: Oxford University Press.

Dickenson, D. and Jones, D. (1995). True wishes: the philosophy and developmental psychology of children's informed consent. *Philosophy, Psychiatry, & Psychology*, 2(4): 287–304.

Dorland's American Illustrated Medical Dictionary, (25th edn). (1974). Philadelphia, PA: Saunders.

Dyer, A. (1999). Psychiatry as a profession. In *Psychiatric Ethics* (ed. S. Bloch, P. Chodoff, and S.A. Green), (3rd edn). Oxford: Oxford University Press, Chapter 5.

Edwards, R.B. (Ed) (1982). *Psychiatry and ethics: insanity, rational autonomy, and mental health care*. New York: Prometheus Books.

Eekelaar, J. (1995). True wishes. (Commentary on Dickenson and Jones, 1995). *Philosophy, Psychiatry, & Psychology*, 2(4): 305–308.

Elliott, C. (1996). Key concepts: criminal responsibility. *Philosophy, Psychiatry, & Psychology*, 3(4): 305–308.

Elliott, C. (1999). *A Philosophical Disease: bioethics, culture and identity*. Routledge.

Fourcher, L.A. (1998). Relativism and the social-constructivist paradigm. (Commentary on Gillett, 1998). *Philosophy, Psychiatry, & Psychology*, 5/1: 49–54.

Fulford, K.W.M. (1989, reprinted 1995 and 1999). *Moral Theory and Medical Practice*. Cambridge: Cambridge University Press.

Fulford, K.W.M. (1995). The concept of disease and the meaning of patient-centred care. In *Essential Practice in Patient-Centred Care* (ed. K.W.M. Fulford, S. Ersser, and T. Hope). Oxford: Blackwell Science.

Fulford, K.W.M. (1998). Dissent and dissensus: the limits of consensus formation in psychiatry. In *Consensus Formation in Health Care Ethics* (ed. H.A.M.J. ten Have and H.-M. Saas). Philosophy and Medicine Series. Place: Kluwer, pp. 175–192.

Fulford, K.W.M. (2001). The paradoxes of confidentiality: a philosophical introduction. In *Confidentiality and Mental Health* (ed. C. Cordess). London: Jessica Kingsley Publishers, pp. 7–23.

Fulford, K.W.M. (2004). Ten principles of values-based medicine. In *The Philosophy of Psychiatry: a companion* (ed. J. Radden). New York: Oxford University Press.

Fulford, K.W.M. and Benington, J. (2005). VBM²: a collaborative values-based model of health care decision making combining medical and management perspectives. In *Medical and Management Perspectives in Child and Adolescent Psychiatry* (ed. G. Williams). Oxford: Oxford University Press.

Fulford, K.W.M. and Bloch, S. (2000). Psychiatric ethics: codes, concepts, and clinical practice skills. In *New Oxford Textbook of Psychiatry* (ed. M. Gelder, J.J. Lopez-Ibor, and N. Andreasen). Oxford: Oxford University Press, pp. 27–32.

Fulford, K.W.M. and Hope, R.A. (1994). Psychiatric ethics: a bioethical ugly duckling? In *Principles of Health Care Ethics* (ed. R. Gillon and A. Lloyd). Chichester: John Wiley, pp. 681–695.

Fulford, K.W.M. and Hope, T. (1996). Control and practical experience. In *Informed Consent in Psychiatry: European perspectives of ethics, law and clinical practice* (ed. H.G. Koch, S. Reiter-Theil, and H. Helmchen). Baden-Baden: Nomos Verlagsgesellschaft, pp. 348–379.

Fulford, K.W.M. and Howse, K. (1993). Ethics of research with psychiatric patients: principles, problems and the primary responsibilities of researchers. *Journal of Medical Ethics*, 19: 85–91.

Fulford, K.W.M. and Radden, J. (ed.) (2002). Bioethics: Special Issue on psychiatric ethics. *Bioethics*, 16: 5.

Fulford, K.W.M. and Williams, R. (2003). Values-based child and adolescent mental health services? *Current Opinion in Psychiatry*, 16: 369–376.

Fulford, K.W.M., Smirnoff, A.Y.U., and Snow, E. (1993). Concepts of disease and the abuse of psychiatry in the USSR. *British Journal of Psychiatry*, 162: 801–810.

Fulford, K.W.M., Dickenson, D., and Murray, T.H. (2002a). Human values in healthcare ethics. Introduction. Many voices: human values in healthcare ethics. In *Healthcare Ethics and Human Values: an introductory text with readings and case studies* (ed. K.W.M. Fulford, D. Dickenson, and T.H. Murray). Malden, MA: Blackwell Publishers, pp. 1–19.

Fulford, K.W.M., Williamson, T., and Woodbridge, K. (2002b). Values-added practice (a values-awareness workshop). *Mental Health Today*, October: 25–27.

Fulford, K.W.M., Stanghellini, G. and Broome, M. (2004). What can philosophy do for psychiatry? Special Article for *World Psychiatry (WPA)*, Oct 2004, pps. 130–135.

Gennery, B. (2005). Academic clinical research in the new regulatory environment. *Clinical Medicine: Journal of the Royal College of Physicians of London*. Vol 5: 39–41.

Gillett, E. (1998a). Relativism and the social-constructivist paradigm. *Philosophy, Psychiatry, & Psychology*, 5/1: 37–48.

Gillett, E. (1998b). Response to the Commentaries. *Philosophy, Psychiatry, & Psychology*, 5/1: 61–66.

Gillett, G. (1989). *Reasonable Care*. Bristol, England: The Bristol Press.

Gillon, R. (1985). *Philosophical Medical Ethics*. Chichester: Wiley.

Gillon, R. (1994). Preface: Medical Ethics and the Four Principles, pages xxi–xxi, in in Gillon, R. and Lloyd, A., (eds) *Principles of Health Care Ethics*, Chichester, England: John Wiley and Sons.

Gillon, R. (1996). Editorial to JME issue which included Robertson, D. (1996). Ethical theory, ethnography and differences between doctors and nurses in approaches to patient care. *Journal of Medical Ethics*, 22: 292–299.

Gillon, R. and Lloyd, A. (ed.) (1994). *Principles of Health Care Ethics*. Chichester: Wiley.

Hansen, J. (2003). Listening to people or listening to prozac? Another consideration of causal classifications. (Commentary on Radden, 2003a). *Philosophy, Psychiatry, & Psychology*, 10/1: 57–62.

Hare, R.M. (1952). *The Language of Morals*. Oxford: Oxford University Press.

Hare, R.M. (1981). *Moral Thinking: its levels, method, and point*. Oxford: Clarendon Press.

Hare, R.M. (1993a). Medical ethics, can the moral philosopher help? In *Essays on Bioethics*. Oxford: Clarendon Press, pp. 1–14.

Hare, R.M. (1993b). The philosophical basis of psychiatric ethics pp. 15–30. In *Essays on Bioethics*. Oxford: Clarendon Press.

Hare, R.M. (1997). *Sorting Out Ethics*. Oxford: Oxford University Press.

Hart, H.L.A. (1968). *Punishment and responsibility: essays in the philosophy of law*. Oxford University Press.

Heginbotham, C. (2004). 'Psychiatric Dasein' (Commentary on Fulford and Colombo, 2004). *Philosophy, Psychiatry, & Psychology*, 11/2, 147–150

Hinshelwood, R.D., (1995). Commentary on "Psychoanalysis. Science, and Commonsense". *Philosophy, Psychiatry, and Psychology*, 2/2, 115–118.

Hinshelwood, R.D. (1997a). Primitive mental processes: psychoanalysis and the ethics of integration (With commentaries by Mace (1997), Sturdee (1997a), and Thornton (1997), and a detailed response (Hinshelwood, 1997b) *Philosophy, Psychiatry, & Psychology* 4(2): 121–144.

Hinshelwood, R.D. (1997b). Response to the Commentaries. *Philosophy, Psychiatry, & Psychology*, 4(2): 159–166.

Hinshelwood, R.D. (1997c). *Therapy or Coercion? Does psychoanalysis differ from brainwashing?* London: Karnac Books Ltd.

Hinshelwood, R.D. (2001). A Kleinian contribution to the external world. (Commentary on Richmond, 2001a). *Philosophy, Psychiatry, & Psychology*, 8/1: 17–20.

Holmes, J. and Lindley, R. (1989). *The Values of Psychotherapy*. Oxford: Oxford University Press.

Hooker, B. and Little, M.O. (ed.). (2000). *Moral Particularism*. Oxford: Clarendon Press.

Hope, R.A. (1990). Ethical philosophy as applied to psychiatry. *Current Opinion in Psychiatry*, 3: 673–676.

Hope, T. (2004). *Medical Ethics: a very short introduction*. Oxford: Oxford University Press.

Hope, T., Fulford, K. W. M. and Yates, A. (1996). *The Oxford Practice Skills Course: Ethics, Law and Communication Skills in Health Care Education*. Oxford: The Oxford University Press.

Hudson Jones, A. (1999). Narrative in medical ethics. *British Journal of Medicine*.

Hunink, M.G.M. and Glasziou, P.P. (2001). *Decision making in health and medicine: Integrating evidence and values*. Cambridge: Cambridge University Press.

Jonsen, A.R. and Toulmin, S. (1988). *The Abuse of Casuistry: a history of moral reasoning*. University of California Press.

Kennedy, I. (1981). *The Unmasking of Medicine*. London: George Allen and Unwin.

Kopelman, L.M. (1989). Moral problems in psychiatry. In *Medical Ethics* (ed. R. Veatch). London: Jones and Bartlett.

Kopelman, L.M. (1994). Case method and casuistry: the problem of bias. *Theoretical Medicine*, 15: 21–37.

Kushner, T.K. and Thomasma, D.C. (2001). *Ward ethics: dilemmas for medical students and doctors in training*. Cambridge: Cambridge University Press.

Lilleleht, E. (2002a). Progress and power: exploring the disciplinary connections between moral treatment and psychiatric rehabilitation. *Philosophy, Psychiatry, & Psychology*, 9(2): 167–182.

Lilleleht, E. (2002b). Listening, acting, and the quest for alternatives: a response to Charland and Bracken. *Philosophy, Psychiatry, & Psychology*, 9(2): 189–192.

Mace, C. (1997). Primitive mental processes: psychoanalysis and the ethics of integration. (Commentary on Hinshelwood, 1997a). *Philosophy, Psychiatry, & Psychology*, 4(2): 145–150.

Maehle, A-H. and Geyer-Kordesch, J. (ed.) (2002). Historical and philosophical perspectives on biomedical ethics. *Historical and Philosophical Perspectives on Biomedical Ethics: from Paternalism to Autonomy?* Aldershot, England: Ashgate Publishing Limited.

Marina, J.A. (1999). The problem of values in psychiatry. In *Archivos de Psiquiatria: Introduccion al Proyecto: Hechos y Valores en Psiquiatria. Suplemento 3*. (Facts and Values in Psychiatry: an introduction) (ed. J. Ortega y Gasset, G.R. Lafora, and J.M. Sacristan). Madrid: Editorial Triacastela, 3: 55–68.

Matthews, E. (1995). Moralist or Therapist? Foucault and the Critique of Psychiatry. *Philosophy, Psychiatry, and Psychology*, 2, 19–30

McCormick, S. (1995). True wishes. (Commentary on Dickenson and Jones, 1995). *Philosophy, Psychiatry, & Psychology*, 2(4): 309–310.

Mitchell, J. (1998a). Neurosis and the historic quest for security: a social-role analysis. *Philosophy, Psychiatry, & Psychology*, 5(4): 317–328.

Mitchell, J. (1998b). Response to the Commentary. *Philosophy, Psychiatry, & Psychology*, 5(4): 333–336.

Mitchell, J. (2001). Anorexia: social world and the internal woman. (Commentary on Richmond, 2001a). *Philosophy, Psychiatry, & Psychology*, 8/1: 13–16.

Mongomery, J. (1996). Patients first: the role of rights. In *Essential Practice in Patient-centred Care* (ed. K.W.M. Fulford, S. Ersser, and T. Hope). Oxford: Blackwell Science, Chapter 9.

Moore, A. (1997). Psychological courage. (Commentary on Putnam, 1997). *Philosophy, Psychiatry, & Psychology*, 4/1: 13–14.

Moore, A., Hope, T., and Fulford, K.W.M. (1994). Mild mania and well-being. *Philosophy, Psychiatry, & Psychology*, 1(3): 165–178.

Moore, M.S. (1984). *Law and Psychiatry: rethinking the relationship*. Cambridge: Cambridge University Press.

Mullen, P.E. (2002). Moral principles don't signify. (Commentary on Ward, 2002a). *Philosophy, Psychiatry, & Psychology*, 9/1: 19–22.

Murray, T.H. (1994). Medical ethics, moral philosophy and moral tradition. In *Medicine and Moral Reasoning* (ed. K.W.M. Fulford, G. Gillett, and J.M. Soskice). Cambridge: Cambridge University Press, pp. 91–105.

Murray, T.H. (1995). Commentary on true wishes. (Commentary on Dickenson and Jones, 1995). *Philosophy, Psychiatry, & Psychology*, 2(4): 311–312.

Nagel, T. (1986). *The View from Nowhere*. Oxford: Oxford University Press.

National Institute for Mental Health England, The Sainsbury Centre for Mental Health and the NHSU (2004). *The Ten Essential Shared Capabilities for Mental Health Practice*. London: Sainsbury Centre for Mental Health.

Nissim-Sabat, M. (2001). Psychiatry, psychoanalysis, and race. *Philosophy, Psychiatry, & Psychology*, 8/1: 45–60.

Nordenfelt, L. (1994). Mild mania and theory of health. (Commentary on Moore et al., 1994). *Philosophy, Psychiatry, & Psychology*, 1(3): 179–184.

Osborn, D. P. J. (1999). Research and ethics: leaving exclusion behind. *Current Opinion in Psychiatry*, 12: 601–604.

Parker, M. (1995). True wishes. (Commentary on Dickenson and Jones, 1995). *Philosophy, Psychiatry, & Psychology*, 2(4): 313–314.

Parker, M. and Dickenson, D. (2000). *The Cambridge Workbook in Medical Ethics*. Cambridge: Cambridge University Press.

Perkins, R. (2001). What constitutes success? The relative priority of service users' and clinicians' views of mental health services. *British Journal of Psychiatry*, 179: 9–10.

Perkins, R., and Repper, J., (1998). *Dilemmas in Community Mental Health Practice: Choice or Control*. Aberdeen, England: Radcliffe Medical Press.

Phillips, J. (1998). Commentary on 'Relativism and the social-constructivist paradigm'. *Philosophy, Psychiatry, & Psychology*, 5/1: 55–60.

Popper, K. (1962). *Open Society and Its Enemies*, Vol. 1. USA: Princeton.

Potter, N.N. (1996). Loopholes, gaps, and what is held fast: democratic epistemology and claims to recovered memories. *Philosophy, Psychiatry, & Psychology*, 3(4): 237–254.

Potter, N.N. (2001). Feminism. *Philosophy, Psychiatry, & Psychology*, 8/1: 61–72.

Potter, N.N. (2004). Gender. In *The Philosophy of Psychiatry: a companion* (ed. J. Radden). New York: Oxford University Press, pp. 237–243.

Putnam, D. (1997). Psychological courage. *Philosophy, Psychiatry, & Psychology*, 4/1: 1–12.

Putnam, H. (2002). *The Collapse of the Fact/Value Dichotomy and other Essays*. Cambridge, MA: Harvard University Press.

Rachels, J. (2003). *The Elements of Moral Philosophy*, 4th Edition. McGraw-Hill.

Radden, J. (2003a). Is this Dame Melancholy? Equating today's depression and past melancholia. *Philosophy, Psychiatry, & Psychology*, 10/1: 37–52.

Radden, J. (2003b). The pragmatics of psychiatry, and the psychiatry of cross-cultural suffering. (Response to the commentaries on Radden, 2003a). *Philosophy, Psychiatry, & Psychology*, 10/1: 63–66.

Raphael, D.D. (1994). (Second Edition). *Moral Philosophy*. Oxford, Oxford University Press.

Reinders, H. (2003). The ambiguities of 'meaning'. (Commentary on Clegg and Lansdall-Welfare, 2003a). *Philosophy, Psychiatry, & Psychology*, 10/1: 91–98.

Richmond, S. (2001a). Psychoanalysis and feminism: anorexia, the social world, and the internal world. *Philosophy, Psychiatry, & Psychology*, 8/1: 1–12.

Richmond, S. (2001b). A Response to Mitchell (2001), Hinshelwood (2001), and Adshead (2001). *Philosophy, Psychiatry, & Psychology*, 8/1: 41–44.

Robertson, D. (1996). Ethical theory, ethnography and differences between doctors and nurses in approaches to patient care. *Journal of Medical Ethics*, 22: 292–299.

Robinson, D.N. (2003). Psychiatry and law. In *Nature and Narrative: An Introduction to the New Philosophy of Psychiatry* (eds K.W.M. Fulford, K.J. Morris, J.Z. Sadler, and G. Stanghellini). Oxford: Oxford University Press.

Rogers, A., Pilgrim, D., and Lacey, R. (1993). Getting the treatment. In *Experiencing Psychiatry: Users' Views of Services*. London: Macmillan, in association with Mind Publications.

Rossi, P. (2003). Magic, science, and equality of human wits. In *Nature and Narrative: An Introduction to the New Philosophy of Psychiatry* (eds K.W.M. Fulford, K.J. Morris, J.Z. Sadler, and G. Stanghellini). Oxford: Oxford University Press, Chapter 17.

Royal Australian and New Zealand College of Psychiatrists (1998). *Code of Ethics* (2nd edn). Melbourne: Royal Australian and New Zealand College of Psychiatrists.

Sackett, D.L., Straus, S.E., Scott Richardson, W., Rosenberg, W., and Haynes, R.B. (2000). *Evidence-Based Medicine: how to practice and teach EBM*, (2nd edn). Edinburgh: Churchill Livingstone.

Sadler, J.Z. (ed.) (2002). *Descriptions and Prescriptions: values, mental disorders, and the DSMs*. Baltimore: The Johns Hopkins University Press.

Savulescu, J. (2001). Taking the plunge. *New Scientist* 3 March, pp. 50–51.

Schwartz, M.A. and Wiggins, O.P. (1998). Neurosis and the historic quest for security. (Commentary on Mitchell, 1998a). *Philosophy, Psychiatry, & Psychology*, 5(4): 329–332.

Seedhouse, D. (1994). The trouble with well-being: a response to mild mania and well-being. *Philosophy, Psychiatry, & Psychology*, 1/3, 185–192.

Sen A. (1987). *On Ethics and Economics*. Oxford: Blackwell.

Stanghellini, G. (2004). *Deanimated bodies and Disembodied Spirits. Essays on the psychopathology of common sense*. Oxford: Oxford University Press.

Stocker, M. (1997). Aristotelian akrasia and psychoanalytic regression. *Philosophy, Psychiatry, & Psychology*, 4(3): 231–242.

Stone, A.A. (1984). *Law, Psychiatry and Morality*. Washington, American Psychiatric Press.

Sturdee, P.G. (1997a). Primitive mental processes: psychoanalysis and the ethics of integration. (Commentary on Hinshelwood, 1997a). *Philosophy, Psychiatry, & Psychology*, 4(2): 151–154.

Sturdee, P.G. (1997b). Aristotelian akrasia and psychoanalytic regression. (Commentary on Stocker, 1997). *Philosophy, Psychiatry, & Psychology*, 4(3): 243–246.

Sverdlik, S. (2002). Unconscious evil principles. (Commentary on Ward, 2002a). *Philosophy, Psychiatry, & Psychology*, 9/1: 13–14.

Szmukler, G. and Holloway, F. (2001). Confidentiality in community psychiatry. In *Confidentiality and Mental Health* (ed. C. Cordess). London: Jessica Kingsley Publishers, Chapter 3.

Tan, J.O.A., Hope, T., and Stewart, A. (2003). Anorexia nervosa and personal identity: the accounts of patients and their parents. *International Journal of Law and Psychiatry*, 26: 533–548.

Thornton, W.L. (1997). Primitive mental processes: psychoanalysis and the ethics of integration. (Commentary on Hinshelwood, 1997a). *Philosophy, Psychiatry, & Psychology*, 4(2): 155–158.

Toulmin, S. and Jonsen, A.R. (1988). *The Abuse of Casuistry*. Berkeley, CA: University of California Press.

Tröhler, U. (2002). Human research: from ethics to law, from national to international regulations. In *Historical and Philosophical Perspectives in Biomedical Ethics: from Paternalism to Autonomy?* (ed. A.-H. Maehle and J. Geyer-Kordesch). Aldershot, England: Ashgate Publishing Ltd, pp. 95–117.

Ward, D.E. (2002a). Explaining evil behavior: using Kant and M. Scott Peck to solve the puzzle of understanding the moral psychology of evil people. *Philosophy, Psychiatry, & Psychology*, 9/1: 1–12.

Ward, D.E. (2002b). Commentary on 'The complexity of evil behavior'. *Philosophy, Psychiatry, & Psychology*, 9/1: 23–26.

Warlow, C. (2005). Over-regulation of clinical research: a threat to public health. *Clinical Medicine: Journal of the Royal College of Physicians of London*, Vol 5: 33–8.

Warnock, G.J. (1971). *The Object of Morality*. London: Methuen and Co Ltd.

Warnock, M. (1978). *Ethics Since 1900* (third edition). Oxford: Oxford University Press.

Wells, L.A. (1995). True wishes. (Commentary on Dickenson and Jones, 1995). *Philosophy, Psychiatry, & Psychology*, 2(4): 315–318.

Widdershoven, G.A.M., Hope, T., van der Scheer, L. and McMillan, J. (Forthcoming). (Eds.) Empirical ethics in Psychiatry. Oxford: Oxford University Press.

Williams, R. (2004). Finding the Way Forward in Professional Practice. (Commentary on Fulford and Colombo, 2004.) *Philosophy, Psychiatry, & Psychology*, 11/2, 151–158.

Williamson, T. (2004). "Can Two Wrongs Make a Right?". (Commentary on Fulford and Colombo, 2004.) *Philosophy, Psychiatry, & Psychology*, 11/2, 159–164.

Woodbridge, K. and Fulford, K.W.M. (2003). Good practice? Values-based practice in mental health. *Mental Health Practice*, 7(2): 30–34.

Woodbridge, K. and Fulford, K.W.M. (2004). *Whose Values? A workbook for values-based practice in mental health care*. London: Sainsbury Centre for Mental Health.

World Psychiatric Association (1996). *Declaration of Madrid*. Geneva: World Psychiatric Association.

CHAPTER 19

It's the law! Rationality and consent as a case study in values and mental health law

Chapter contents

In this chapter we shall be examining the concepts of rationality and consent from a medico-legal viewpoint. These concepts have been central to the way the English courts have tried to reconcile the perception that the patient has a right to decide what happens to him with the perception that the doctor has a duty to try her best to heal her patient.

The tension between these two perceptions, as we have seen in Chapters 17 and 18, is central to the ethical issues raised specifically by involuntary psychiatric treatment. In common law the English courts, like most courts around the world, have repeatedly affirmed that an adult patient of 'sound' mind has an absolute right to accept or reject medical treatment. Correspondingly, therefore, the courts will sometimes override this right where the patient is of 'unsound' mind. The Mental Health Act, as we saw in Chapter 17, gives statutory authority to this autonomy override in respect of mental disorders, albeit not on the same incapacity basis applied by common law. Other legislation covers contexts, such as the patient being a child, or where the welfare of a viable foetus is at stake.

From the 'man of science' to legal value judgements

In all these cases, to anticipate a little, whether in common law or under the Mental Health Act, the model with which the courts work is essentially our, by now familiar, medical model. In considering a given case, it is assumed that the soundness or otherwise of a person's mind, or the 'appropriateness' of treatment, is a matter for 'expert evidence', the expert in question being, in the words of the well-worn legal aphorism, a 'man of science.' On closer inspection, however, we will find that, in some cases, the courts have been hesitant to inquire too closely into a patient's state of mind where it has felt compelled to intervene to protect the patient's medical *best interests*. Judgements of rationality in these cases have in practice turned on how 'sympathetic' the court is to the patient's point of view. These judgments do not reflect value-neutral concerns, therefore. Rather, they are value-laden judgements, judgements that is to say, in which the court's values are crucial to the medical and judicial determination of a patient's 'soundness' of mind.

It turns out, furthermore, that this 'value ladenness' is especially pertinent in the context of mental disorder, where, as we will see, evaluative issues enter into assessments of rationality and competence to a significant extent. We should *expect* this, given everything that has been said in earlier chapters about the inherent diversity of values in the areas of human experience and behaviour encompassed by mental disorders. And when we review these legal determinations with our now 'J.L. Austin-sharpened eye', it is clear that it *is* so.

Aims of the chapter

As in previous chapters our aim in exploring these legal cases, general medical and psychiatric, will not be to suggest that court procedures, to the extent that they involve value judgements, are somehow inherently flawed. Our aim, rather, will be to highlight, in the light of earlier chapters, the value judgements in question,

and to recognize their significance particularly in respect of mental disorders, as a step towards improving the validity of the procedures themselves.

Our focus, consistent with the case study approach of this book, will be mainly on a particular legislative framework (that of England and Wales) rather than attempting a general review. The issues, of course, are generic; but we shall be exploring them in, as it were, the particular. Similarly, even within the particular case (of the law in England and Wales), our aim will not be to provide a comprehensive review of mental health law, but to draw out the particular themes noted above, as themes of growing *practical* importance to which philosophy has a distinctive contribution to make.

The chapter also has the secondary aim of filling out an understanding of how value judgements come into the assessment of mental disorders generally. You will recall J.L. Austin's methodological point, in 'A plea for excuses' (1956/7), that legal cases make good (linguistic analytic) philosophy, because legal cases *have* to be resolved one way or another (Chapter 4). Examining the role of value judgements in legal cases involving mental disorders will thus help to pave the way for our more detailed examination of values in psychiatric diagnosis in Chapters 20 and 21.

Topics to be covered

These are the aims, then. We will start, though, by going back to basics. Hence in this chapter, we will:

- Look at the ethical basis of the doctrine of consent, placing it in the context of the concept of 'human rights'.

- Note the various ways a patient can give consent to medical treatment

- Identify the legal basis of the doctrine of consent.

- Distinguish the meanings of the terms 'rationality', 'capacity', and 'competence'.

- Define 'capacity'.

- Examine the meaning of 'informed consent' in English law.

- Consider the legal remedies available to patients who are treated against their wishes.

- Explain the '*Bolam*' test as it relates to standards in negligence in relation to assessing capacity and gaining consent.

- Uncover the hidden evaluative assessments behind recent so-called enforced Caesarean cases.

- Comment on recent proposals in England and Wales to introduce generic incapacity legislation, which will have the effect of further distinguishing the law relating to the treatment of mental disorders under statutory mental health legislation from the law relating to the treatment of bodily disorders.

- Apply the ethical and legal principles explored in this section to a hypothetical case of 'rational suicide'.

We introduce a number of key legal terms and concepts from English Law along the way. For ease of cross-reference, we list these here in the order in which they are introduced: tort (p. 542), statute and common law (p. 542), estoppel (p. 543), status test (p. 544), cause of action (p. 549), civil and criminal law (p. 549), battery (p. 550), and negligence (p. 550).

Three sessions (and a focus on philosophy)

The chapter is divided into three sessions. *Session 1* sets out some of the key features of the law on consent (as it has been developed in England and Wales). *Session 2* takes a closer look at the legal concepts of capacity (including its links with rationality) and information. As we will see, what counts as sufficient information for valid consent in law draws out some of the hidden values driving legal determinations of capacity for consent. Finally, in *Session 3*, the importance of values becomes explicit in the legal concept of 'best interests' at the heart of legislation covering those who lack the capacity for consent.

Clearly, all of the topics covered in this chapter could occupy several legal tomes! We will thus not be attempting to provide a detailed legal commentary on them as they relate to mental health, still less to health care in general. Rather, our approach will be to tease out the underlying principles, as they are currently understood and illustrated by the law (mainly) of England and Wales. This will provide a basis for understanding the specifically philosophical contributions, i.e. by way of conceptual insights, to resolving the legal and practical problems in the area as they arise in mental health.

Session 1 The legal basis of consent

In this first session we lay the foundations for understanding the legal concept of consent by considering, briefly, its moral and cultural background, and then examining how the law (mainly in England and Wales) has developed. From this discussion, the rationale for the three key legal elements of consent will emerge. As noted above, we will be considering mainly the first of these, capacity, in this session, the second session will extend the discussion to information, and the third to voluntariness.

First, then, the background moral and cultural tradition.

The moral and cultural tradition

Difficulties with consent in health care normally (though not always) arise where a patient disagrees with the doctor's treatment proposal. The issue then arising is: should the doctor's or the patient's point-of-view prevail? This issue becomes especially serious where the patient's refusal puts that patient's life and health at risk. As we saw earlier in this part, a tension then arises between two ethical principles:

◆ The principle of *patient autonomy*.
◆ The principle of *medical beneficence*.

Both principles have deep roots, which it will be worth exploring briefly before coming to their instantiations in law. Thus the principle of *autonomy* is an important concept in modern liberal political philosophy. According to this philosophy, part of what it is to be a free individual is to have the liberty to make choices affecting one's own person. This principle of individual liberty can be extended to the doctor–patient relationship in which the patient is normally in a vulnerable condition and potentially subject to procedures that affect him or her intimately. According to this way of looking at things, human dignity is closely associated with the patient's ability to make decisions about what happens to their own body. Correspondingly, a doctor does not have the right to compromise that dignity by treating that patient without that patient's consent, even if it is in that patient's therapeutic best interests.

The principle of medical *beneficence*, on the other hand, is associated with a venerable tradition within the history of the practice of medicine. This tradition enjoins a doctor, as a fundamental duty, to do all that he or she can to heal his or her patient, even if the patient does not agree with what the doctor has proposed. The underlying assumption of this tradition is that the patient is not in a position to decide what is best for him precisely because that patient is ill and vulnerable. This assumption has been criticized by modern academic commentators, perhaps rather pejoratively, as representing an attitude of medical *paternalism*.

Medical paternalism and the Hippocratic Oath

The seeds of this attitude of medical paternalism can perhaps be identified in the Hippocratic Oath (introduced in chapter 18), which stipulates that the doctor shall:

> Perform these duties calmly and adroitly, concealing most things from the patient while you are attending to him. Give necessary orders with cheerfulness and sincerity, turning his attention away from what is being done to him; sometimes reproving sharply and emphatically, and sometimes comforting with solicitude and attention, revealing nothing of the patients' future condition.

The relevant point of note here is that the doctor–patient relationship is assumed to be an uneven power relationship, with the doctor holding most of the power. This model of the doctor–patient relationship assumes the reality of this power imbalance. The model of doctor–patient interaction envisaged in the Hippocratic Oath could be characterized as one of *entrustment*. The reality of this trust relationship gives rise to a corresponding 'trust duty' on the part of the doctor. Lawyers call this kind of duty a *fiduciary* duty. The word 'fiduciary' is related to the Latin word *fides* broadly meaning, faith, trust, or belief. Other examples of fiduciary relationships are the parent–child relationship, the teacher–pupil relationship, or the priest's relationship with one for whom he is providing pastoral care. So the question arises, should there be 'power equality' in the doctor–patient relationship? If so, why? If not, why not? And how can the law help?

Legal frameworks

These questions are explored in the first reading in this chapter, which is by the British lawyer, Ian Kennedy, in terms of rights. Kennedy sprang to fame in the 1980s, with a book provocatively entitled *The Unmasking of Medicine* (Kennedy, 1981). In this, he lifted the lid on what were increasingly seen as misuses of medical power, and he went on to set up the first major centre for medical ethics and law in England, at King's College in London. As a lawyer, Kennedy has wide experience of medical issues, and he has written many detailed and insightful legal commentaries on cases involving consent. The following reading provides a more general introduction to his views.

EXERCISE 1   (30 minutes)

Read the three short extracts from:

Kennedy, I. (1996). Patients, doctors and human rights. In *Treat Me Right: Essays in Medical Law and Ethics*. Oxford: Clarendon Press, (Extract pp. 385–390.)

Link with Reading 19.1

◆ What is Kennedy's line on medical paternalism here?

◆ What is his lawyer's answer to promoting patient self-determination?

Consent and human rights

Kennedy (1996) contends that trust between the doctor and patient cannot be taken for granted. Rather, the doctor has to earn the patient's trust in the context of a relationship that is already established on the ethical and legal foundations of 'human rights'. He (anticipating recent developments) argues that English medical law needs a much more highly developed concept of human rights in order to ensure that the courts respect the principle of self-determination. In his view, the English law of consent as it has hitherto developed, is more concerned with protecting doctors than patients. A human rights analysis would be advantageous in two respects:

1. It would force the courts to hold the patient's interests as being of primary importance and at the same time challenge medical paternalism.

2. It would provide the courts with a theoretical framework within which to develop the law more consistently and systematically.

The Human Rights Act

In this article, Kennedy (1996) was anticipating, by over 10 years, the incorporation of the European Convention on Human Rights into UK domestic law in the form of the Human Rights Act 1998. The result, as Kennedy anticipated, is that the courts have been forced to take on a new set of international

ethical and legal obligations. This is significant when we consider that the concept of human rights lies at the heart of the European Convention and that a number of Articles in the Convention have been used to assert the rights of patients. It is likely that the courts will be compelled to envisage the doctor–patient relationship as one involving fundamental issues of human freedom, which will need to be expounded in keeping with reasoned moral analysis. This may involve the need for a significant change in the way the courts approach the law of consent. This in turn brings us to a technical legal concept, referred to several times by Kennedy in this article, to the 'law of tort' or 'tort law'.

So, just what is tort law?

Tort law

Tort law is essentially the law of civil 'wrongs', the word 'tort' being derived from the French word for 'wrong'. The law of negligence is the largest part of the law of tort. The aim of tort law is to compensate a person for an injury wrongfully suffered at the hands of the other, e.g. because of a negligent act or omission. The aim, in terms of compensation, is to put the claimant back into the position he would have been in had he not been injured. Thus, if you suffer an injury through the act of a negligent driver, then that driver, or his insurers, will have to compensate you for all the damage that he could reasonably have foreseen would result from his negligent act, e.g. hospital bills (if any), loss of earnings, etc. From a legal point of view, it is to avoid an action in negligence that patients are nowadays normally required to give their consent to a medical procedure.

The difference between statute law and common law

A second terminology point that is worth noting at this stage is the difference between statute law and common law.

There are (apart from European Community Law) two main sources of jurisdiction in the English legal system:

1. Parliament.

2. The Courts/Judges.

Parliament-made law is known as statute law. A statute is 'enacted' by Parliament in an Act of Parliament. Before it is enacted it is known as a 'Bill'. For example, the Human Rights Bill became the Human Rights Act on 2 October 2000.

Judge-made law is also known as the 'common law'. However (and this can seem confusing), 'common law' has a number of meanings. It can refer to the existing body of 'case law' (a static meaning). It can also refer to the power judges have to interpret and develop the law (a dynamic meaning), including by interpreting statutes. Moreover, the term 'common law' is sometimes distinguished technically from the term 'equity', which relates to a jurisdiction that had a separate existence before the late nineteenth century, before merging with the common law.

Varieties of legal consent

Back, now, to consent.

EXERCISE 2 (10 minutes)

This reading is a typical NHS consent form reprinted in:

McHale, J. Fox, M., and Murphy, J. (1999). *Health Care Law: text and materials* London: Sweet and Maxwell, p. 335

Link with Reading 19.2

◆ What kind of consent is envisaged here?

◆ What is the role of the consent form in consent?

◆ In particular, do you think that such forms can be designed to cover everything that a patient in reality agrees to in the context of a particular medical procedure, e.g. heart surgery?

In practice, a patient can give consent in one of three ways. Consent can be:

◆ express

◆ implied, or by

◆ estoppel.

1. *Express consent.* A patient gives express consent when she states in clear, direct terms what she is agreeing to. Express consent can take one of two forms:

   ◆ *Written*—e.g. by signing a consent form like the one in Exercise 2 above produced by the NHS that stipulates what is being agreed to. It should be noted, however, that the signed form is not itself 'the consent', but rather evidence of what the patient has agreed to. A court will be concerned with 'the reality' of what has been consented to, including the way in which consent was 'obtained', which may or may not be adequately reflected in the contents of the form. Patients usually sign a consent form when they are about to undergo surgery in a hospital, perhaps not the best time for processing complete information! (We return to information in Session 2.)

   ◆ *Oral*—patients normally consent to most forms of medical treatment by word of mouth. A patient can either agree with what the doctor has proposed, or stipulate what he or she has agreed to.

2. *Implied consent.* If a patient has not signed a form or given oral consent, then that patient's consent may be implied from the circumstances. For example, in one legal case, the court held that a patient who presented her arm to a nurse in a line of people who were receiving a vaccination prior to disembarking from an ocean liner had implicitly given consent to that procedure (O'Brien v Cunard SS (1891) 28 NE 266 (Mass Sup Jud Ct), see Kennedy and Grubb, 2000, p. 90).

3. *Estoppel.* This is not so much a way of giving consent, as of overcoming a patient's denial that he has given consent. In some circumstances, the notion of an 'implied' consent can seem rather artificial. For example, you cannot impute consent to someone who is unable to give it because they are unconscious or otherwise without capacity (e.g. the patient is too young or suffering from a mental disorder). Instead, you can argue that implied consent is in fact a form of 'estoppel'.

What this perhaps somewhat archaic legal word means in practice is that a patient cannot deny that he has given his consent if a reasonable person would conclude that the patient had given consent, looking at the situation in the light of all the circumstances. This may be relevant for example to decisions about whether a patient who has consented to routine blood tests in a hospital has also, by implication, consented to an HIV test undertaken without her knowledge. There is nothing in her conduct, unlike the ocean liner case, to indicate that she has agreed to that extra procedure. The doctrine of estoppel may help capture the reality of the situation better than the notion of implied consent. You can look at the situation and ask, what would the reasonable person have concluded in the circumstances in the light of all the facts?

The legal basis of consent

We have looked at the argument that the concept of human rights in the context of the doctor–patient relationship is underpinned by the ethical principle of self-determination. But how does this ethical principle translate into law?

Kennedy (1996, p 389) defines the doctrine of consent in human-rights terms as 'the legal and ethical expression of the human right for autonomy and self-determination'. In the medical context, the ethical notion of self-determination has found classic expression in the widely cited statement of Justice Cardozo in the case of *Schloendorff v Society of New York Hospital* 211 NY 125 (1914): 'Every human being of adult years and sound mind has a right to determine what shall be done with his own body; and a surgeon [or any doctor] who performs an operation without his patient's consent commits an assault, for which he is liable in damages.'

Although Justice Cardozo's statement can be read as a ringing affirmation of the ethical and legal principle of self-determination, notice that there are two important conditions of eligibility:

◆ adult years

◆ sound mind.

Thus, according to Justice Cardozo, the principle of self-determination is not absolute. The principle is qualified by considerations of age and mental health. But what is the justification for qualifying the principle of patient autonomy on these grounds? To explain this question, we turn first to the meaning of legal *competence*.

Legal competence to consent

In the legal context, the term 'competence' has a technical meaning that aims to fix limits to those expressions of the patient's will that should be legally guaranteed. Legal competence, which relates to the patient's ability to make valid treatment choices, must be distinguished from the popular meaning of 'competence', which can be understood much more widely.

As in any other area of technical expertise, authorities vary as to precisely how the legal concept of consent should be defined. A widely respected authority on all aspects of medical law in the UK, and a valuable textbook, is Kennedy and Grubb (2000). Kennedy and Grubb reflect the prevailing approach of the courts in most administrations in regarding a patient as 'competent' to make a treatment choice, and effecting consent, if that patient has:

1. the *capacity* to make a decision that warrants a legal guarantee;

2. sufficient *information* about the treatment proposed to give a true consent; and

3. made a decision *voluntarily*.

For ease of recall, we could frame the ingredients of a legally valid consent in question form (let us assume that the questioner is the patient):

1. Is *this* (i.e. medical treatment) what I want?

2. Do I *know* enough to decide that this is what I want?

3. Is this what *I* want?

Here, then, we have the three key conditions of competency for legal consent, as widely understood. They seem straightforward enough! But the rest of this chapter will be taken up with spelling out some of the complications with them, starting, in the rest of this session, with capacity.

Competence, capacity, rationality, and status

First, we need to draw some tricky distinctions. In the legal literature, the words, 'competence', 'capacity', and 'rationality' are often used interchangeably, but in fact they bear subtle differences of meaning, and all three have to be distinguished from the legal 'status'. The terms competence and capacity, furthermore, are used with different meanings in different administrations. Current usage in England and Wales, however, makes the following distinctions:

◆ *Competence* is a composite term containing the three ingredients noted above: capacity, information, and voluntariness. All of these must be present to warrant the legal protection of the patient's right of self-determination.

◆ *Capacity* is one ingredient in the composite definition of competence. A patient must be *capable* of making a true treatment

choice. We will look at the legal test for capacity in greater detail below. Capacity must be distinguished from *actual* understanding, which may turn on how much information a doctor is prepared to disclose to a patient. There is thus a subtle conceptual distinction separating the first ingredient from the second ingredient of the composite legal test of competence.

◆ *Rationality* is perhaps most widely understood as referring to the patient's actual cognitive decision-making abilities, but could be understood in other ways. We will return to the legal concept of rationality later.

◆ *Status*. The legal test of capacity may take into account 'status' factors such as age and mental disorder. We will look at these 'status tests' next. They are particularly material to recent discussions (in the UK) about replacing the Mental Health Act, 1983 (which relies on the status test of mental disorder, albeit not as a trigger for applying an incapacity test) with a generic incapacity test as the legal basis of involuntary psychiatric treatment.

Status tests

A 'status' test of competence is one that attributes capacity to a patient on the basis of their status, e.g. a child or a mental health patient. A number of cases have rejected status tests regarding children, and patients suffering from a *mental* disorder who are treated for their *physical* disorders. However, the law in this area is very far from being clear and definite.

A patient suffering from a mental disorder who needs treatment for that mental disorder is liable to be compulsorily detained under the provisions of the Mental Health Act 1983 for the purposes of assessment and treatment. The Mental Health Act makes provision then for the compulsory treatment of 'detained' patients. However, the basis for this, as we saw in Chapter 18, is the status test of 'mental disorder' (plus 'appropriateness' of admission to hospital and 'risk', to self or others) rather than competence. Hence this constitutes an important exception to the common law principle that a competent patient has an absolute right to decide what happens to him, i.e. because a patient may satisfy the criteria of legal competence, and yet, if diagnosed with a mental disorder and if satisfying other 'secondary' criteria, be treated on an involuntary basis against his or her wishes. Hence, in turn, current discussion about abandoning the status test of mental disorder in favour of a generic incapacity test, both because of the 'inequity' of the distinction and because the distinction *per se* between 'treatment for mental disorder' and 'treatment for physical disorder' is not a robust one (Matthews, 1999).

The basic legal principles underlying consent

We will now take a closer look at the legal principles underlying consent, staring with an important case, Re T.

Read the extract from the case of Re T [1992] 4 All ER 649 reprinted in:

McHale, J. Fox, M., and Murphy, J. (1999). *Health Care Law: text and materials* London: Sweet and Maxwell, pp. 269–271

Link with Reading 19.3

♦ Did T consent or refuse to consent to treatment?

♦ Can a doctor treat a competent patient without their consent? What might happen if the doctor does?

♦ What happens when a patient needing treatment can't make a treatment decision?

♦ What test of capacity does Lord Donaldson lay down?

♦ Does a patient's decision have to be rational?

♦ Does the judge say how informed the patient's choice must be?

This case, together with a second case, *Airedale NHS Trust v Bland* [1993] 1 All ER 821, has clarified the basic legal principles applying to the English law of consent. The principles defined in these cases are usefully supplemented by those set out in the case of *F v West Berkshire Authority* [1989] 2 All ER 545, which deals with the circumstances in which a patient can be treated without consent in her best interests. Taken together, these cases provide us with a useful analytical framework for tackling the law of consent. The basic legal position on consent can thus be summarized as follows.

1. The law will presume that all adult patients have the right and *capacity* to consent or refuse consent to medical treatment, even if it is life-saving and life-sustaining treatment. The doctor's fundamental duty to do all that she can to heal her patient must give way to a competent patient's right to decide what happens to him, whatever the cost to that patient. In other words, the competent patient's point of view prevails over that of the doctor.

2. However, there are exceptions, in particular the presumption of capacity (and therefore of competence) can be overridden if there is evidence to show that the patient in question does not have the capacity to make a legally valid consent. Establishing lack of capacity is, in practice, commonly arrived at as a *medical* judgement but subject to legally established capacity criteria (to which we will return shortly); although the ultimate arbiter of capacity is always potentially the court.

3. If the patient's doctor concludes that her patient is 'incompetent', then that doctor has a duty to treat that patient in his 'best interests'. The meaning of 'best interests' was perhaps initially restricted to refer to the patient's medical or 'therapeutic' interests. But the courts have recently broadened 'best interest' to refer to the patient's 'welfare' interests which includes both

medical factors—which doctors are clearly competent to determine—and non-medical factors—which they may not be competent to determine (see espically R. (on the application of Oliver Leslie Burke) v. the GMC-[2004] EWHC 1879).

The basic legal position, then, in English law (and in most other jurisdictions currently), is 'patient choice with exceptions'. So, what about these exceptions? In what circumstances can patients be treated without consent?

Exceptions (for adults)

An adult patient can be treated without consent in the following circumstances. In each case, the doctor is obliged to treat the patient in his or her 'best interests':

♦ *Incompetence*: where the patient lacks the capacity to make a true treatment choice, e.g. due to age or mental illness.

♦ *Emergency*: e.g. where a patient is unconscious following an accident needing emergency surgery. Though the doctor has a fundamental duty to act in his patient's best interests, he must do no more than is reasonably necessary in the circumstances.

♦ *Necessity*: the principle of necessity is especially applicable to states of affairs that are permanent or semi-permanent, e.g. in the case of mentally disordered or mentally handicapped persons. The sterilization of mentally handicapped women in order to prevent conception, under the doctrine of necessity, has stretched the definition of 'best interests' in a controversial direction. Are such sterilizations 'therapeutic'?

The scope of what is genuinely medical treatment is likely to be a matter of particular concern in coming years in new mental health legislation in the UK and elsewhere.

♦ *Mental Health Act 1983*: the Act allows otherwise competent patients to be treated without their consent in certain circumstances (see below).

Children

The legal position is more complicated where children (i.e. persons under 18 years of age) are concerned.

1. Under Section 8 of the Family Law Reform Act 1969, children under 18 years of age, but over 16, are treated as if they were adults for the purposes of surgical, medical, and dental diagnosis and treatment. However, the Act is unclear in three respects, namely whether it extends to:

♦ clinical advice, over and above diagnosis and treatment;

♦ 'therapeutic' treatment, over and above the cosmetic treatment (e.g. teeth-straightening);

♦ a parental or judicial right to consent on the child's behalf.

2. Children under 16 are presumed to be incompetent unless they have a sufficiently full and mature understanding of the treatment proposed. In the House of Lords case *of*

Gillick v West Norfolk and Wisbech AHA [1985] 3 All ER 402. Lord Scarman held that:

> ... the parental right to determine whether or not their minor child below the age of 16 will have medical treatment terminates if and when the child achieves a sufficient understanding and intelligence to enable him or her to understand fully what is proposed. It will be a question of fact whether a child seeking advice has sufficient understanding of what is involved to give a valid consent in law.

Thus, children under 16 are not by definition unable to consent to medical treatment. The law will recognize the right and capacity of a child to decide what happens to them if they are so-called 'mature minors' or 'Gillick competent'.

3. A treatment refusal by a 'Gillick' competent child, whether under or over the age of 16, may currently be overridden by proxy consent in certain limited circumstances (*Re R (A Minor) (Wardship: Medical Treatment)* [1991] 4 All ER177; *Re W (A Minor) (Medical Treatment: Court's Jurisdiction)* [1992] 4 All ER 627). However, it is questionable whether a parental or judicial veto of a mature minor's treatment decision is consistent with the ethics and law of consent. A capacity to consent to treatment must surely entail a right to *refuse* treatment (a position strongly implied in the *Gillick* case).

4. A limited class of people have the legal power to make treatment choices as proxies on behalf of children until (subject to 3 above) they are 'Gillick competent' (e.g. parents and the courts).

   It should be noted that currently no similar power now exists (although it did at one time) to make proxy decisions on behalf of incompetent *adults*. This is an important respect in which mental health law in England and Wales differs from that in most other administrations. Australian courts, for example, have retained this jurisdiction and, in addition, have enacted specific laws that allow third parties other than doctors to make treatment choices on behalf of incompetent adults. Although doctors will usually take the views of close relatives and friends of incompetent adults into account, they are not obliged to do so, and such views are merely informative towards establishing best interest. In cases of adult incompetence, and in the absence of proxy consent for an immature minor, the 'best interests' test applies.

The Mental Health Act 1983

Under Section 63 of Part IV of the 1983 Act, a patient who is detained under the act may be treated without consent: 'The consent of a patient shall not be required for any medical treatment given to him for the mental disorder for which he is suffering, not being treatment falling within Section 57 or 58 above, if the treatment is given by or under the direction of the responsible medical officer.'

Sections 57 and 58 contain safeguards requiring the patient's consent and/or a second opinion before certain treatments can be given (currently electroconvulsive therapy, the administration of medicines for more than 3 months, psychosurgery, and the surgical implantation of hormones for the reduction of the male sexual drive).

A number of conditions must be met before a patient can be treated without consent under the Act:

1. The patient must be detained under the Act. The patient can be detained for treatment under Section 3 if that patient is 'suffering from mental illness, severe mental impairment, psychopathic disorder or mental impairment and his mental disorder is of a nature or degree which makes it appropriate for him to receive medical treatment in a hospital.'

2. What is proposed must count as 'medical treatment'.

3. The treatment proposed must constitute treatment *for* the mental disorder, albeit this includes treatment for consequences of the mental disorder (*B v Croydon Health Authority (1994) 22 BMLR 13*).

Mental disorder is defined very widely in Section 1 of the Act. It means 'mental illness, arrested or incomplete development of mind, psychopathic disorder, and any other disorder or disability of mind'. A psychopathic disorder is defined as a persistent disorder or disability of the mind, which results in abnormally aggressive or seriously irresponsible conduct. Mental illness is not defined by the Act.

The courts, in a line of recent cases, have interpreted the meaning of 'treatment' for mental disorder within the terms of the Act expansively, such that it amounts essentially to any intervention carried out under the authority or auspices of the 'Responsible Medical Officer' (*Reid v Secretary of State for Scotland [1999] 2 AC 513*). The *Code of Practice* for the Mental Health Act, 1983, requires (though it is not as such a strict *legal* requirement) that staff should seek to secure the agreement of the patient first (Department Health and the Welsh Office, 1993).

Summary of the law of consent

Let us sum up the law of consent in the medical context:

1. According to English medical law, doctors have a fundamental duty to treat their patients in their 'best interests'. This is the legal expression of the ethical duty of beneficence.

2. This duty, however, gives way to the right of a legally competent adult patient to decide what happens to him or her. This is the legal expression of the ethical right of self-determination.

3. Where, in the case of a competent adult, the relevant provisions of the Mental Health Act apply, or where for some reason an adult is unable to consent to treatment, perhaps because of an emergency or because he is suffering from a serious mental disorder, the best interests test continues to apply.

4. Where children are too young (and/or immature) to decide for themselves, it falls to a legally authorised proxy, usually parents, to decide on the child's behalf. This authority may, in certain circumstances, include the right to override a 'Gillick-competent' child's treatment refusal. The law presumes parents to be the best arbiters of the child's best interests, although, in rare cases,

the demands of public policy may override parental values (e.g. in certain cases involving blood transfusions and Jehovah's Witnesses).

5. Currently, there is no legal basis in England and Wales for proxy decision-making on behalf of adult patients.

Reflection on the session and self-test questions

Write down your own reflections on the materials in this session drawing out any points that are particularly significant for you. Then write brief notes about the following:

1. What two principles lie behind the law on consent in health care? From what particular aspect of the moral and cultural traditions of medicine are they derived.

2. In what distinctively legal form are these two principles often cast?

3. What varieties of legal consent are commonly recognized? (We noted three.)

4. What are the three legal components of valid consent?

5. What is a 'status' test? Give two examples.

Session 2 Capacity, information, and causes of action

Having set out the basic legal principles that apply to the issue of consent, it is now time to look more closely at the meaning of capacity, particularly its link with rationality, before going on to look at the other components of competence, information, and, in the next session, voluntariness.

In this session we will also be considering what, in legal terms, is called 'causes of action', essentially the routes to redress open to someone who believes they have been wrongly treated without consent. But we will start with a further look at capacity.

EXERCISE 4   (30 minutes)

Read the brief extracts from:

(1) Roth, L., Meisel, A., and Lidz, C. (1977). Tests of competency to consent to treatment. *American Journal of Psychiatry* 134: 279 (extracted in Kennedy, I. and Grubb, A. (2000). *Medical Law: text with materials*, (3rd edn). London: Butterworths, pp. 124–129), and (2) the case of Re C (Adult: Refusal of Treatment) [1994] 1 All ER 819. pp. 819–825

Link with Reading 19.4

◆ What do you understand by the term 'rationality'?

◆ Which of the tests of competence noted by Roth *et al.*, best fits your understanding of rationality?

◆ Do you think that C was 'rational'? If so, in what sense?

◆ What were C's values? Did the court take them into account?

◆ What if C had been a cult member with extreme religious views?

◆ What does Re C add to the case of Re T (in the last session)?

Capacity and rationality

The concepts of capacity and rationality, although used with different meanings in different legislations, and in different areas of the Law within a given legislation, are closely connected in practice. We will look first at capacity and then come back to its links with rationality in relation to concept to treatment.

Capacity

The legal test for capacity in England and Waler was set out in the High Court case of *Re C*, subsequently endorsed by the Court of Appeal in *Re MB* (*Medical Treatment*) [1997] 3 Med. LR 217. In *Re MB*, Lady Justice Butler-Sloss (at 224) held that:

A person lacks capacity if some impairment or disturbance of mental functioning renders the person unable to make a decision whether to consent to, or to refuse treatment. The inability to make a decision will occur when: (a) the patient is unable to comprehend and retain the information which is material to the decision, especially as to the likely consequence of having, or not having, the treatment in question; (b) the patient is unable to use the information and weigh it in the balance as part of the process of arriving at a decision.

The capacity criteria set out by *Re C* and *Re MB*, taken together, can be summarised thus:

1. *Understanding* and *retaining* information relevant to the treatment decision.

2. *Believing* it.

3. *Weighing up* the relative risks and benefits of treatment.

4. *Arriving* at a clear choice.

As the extract from Roth *et al.*, shows, there are many other definitions of capacity. But we will consider the case of Re C in detail by way of exploring the key legal concepts involved in all attempts to define capacity, and their links to values.

The case of Re C: the facts

'C' was a 68-year-old patient in Broadmoor Hospital with a diagnosis of paranoid schizophrenia. He developed gangrene in his left foot, which left him with an 85% likelihood of death unless he agreed to have his leg amputated immediately below the knee. He refused, arguing that 'he would rather die with two feet than survive with one' and 'because he had complete faith in God and, subject to one reservation, the Bible.' He trusted that with good medical care from his care team, he would survive. Moreover, he believed that his foot, if he did die, would not cause his death. C also expressed grandiose delusions of an international career in medicine during the course of which he had never lost a patient and a persecutory delusion that whatever treatment was offered was calculated to destroy his body. Notwithstanding, the hospital refused to give C's solicitor an undertaking that it would not amputate C's leg without his express written consent. As a result, C's solicitor applied to the High Court for an injunction restraining the hospital from carrying out an amputation without that consent. In the event, C survived with conservative surgery and antibiotics.

The judgment

Mr Justice Thorpe held that C was, despite his delusions, capable of understanding the 'nature, purpose and effects' of the treatment proposed. Although C's capacity was impaired by his mental disorder, he still had sufficient 'understanding' for the purposes of giving a legally valid consent. He could understand and retain the relevant information, believe it, weigh up the risks and benefits and arrive at a clear choice. The court was therefore affirming the principle that a person with a diagnosed *mental disorder* could still be competent to refuse treatment for *a physical disorder*. It thus represents, in the context of physical disorder, a rejection of a '*status*' test for individuals suffering from a mental disorder where what is proposed is treatment for an unrelated physical condition. As we shall see below, a UK Government 'Green Paper' has endorsed a Law Commission proposal to introduce statutory incapacity criteria within an Incapacity Act, which are essentially based on this case, reaffirmed by the Court of Appeal in *Re MB, while still maintaining a separate Mental Health Act for* treatments for *mental disorder administered under the latter Act.* Mr Justice Thorpe's decision also reaffirmed a principle laid down in an earlier case, *Re T (Adult: Refusal of Treatment)* [1992] 4 All ER 649) that linked capacity with 'understanding', albeit decisions in subsequent cases have adopted an approach that seems to go somewhat beyond simply the capacity rationally to 'weigh information in the balance' and to incorporate 'the content of the weighing' into those factors that can overturn capacity—see, for example, *Brady v Hopper 751 F 2d 329 (1984)*]), thereby perhaps allowing the values of the person doing the weighing up into the court's assessment of their capacity. But what did Mr Justice Thorpe understand by 'understanding'?

Analysis

In his judgment, Mr Justice Thorpe worked within the framework of the basic legal principles applying to the law of consent. He needed to determine whether C had the capacity to decide what was to happen to him. In order to do that, he needed to satisfy himself that C *sufficiently* understood the broad nature, purpose and effects of the treatment proposed, i.e. the amputation. The word 'sufficiently' is significant. Mr Justice Thorpe did not suggest that C needed a complete and full understanding of the proposed surgery, but enough to demonstrate that he could make a true choice in the context of this particular medical procedure at the time that it was proposed.

Mr Justice Thorpe was not deciding anything new here. His decision was consistent with Lord Donaldson's 'sliding scale' approach, in *Re T*, i.e. a greater level of understanding is required for a more serious medical procedure. This suggests rather more than the 'evidencing a choice' test expounded in Roth *et al*'s article. Though it is likely that, in non-serious cases, the courts will not feel the need to inquire too closely into the patient's state of mind. In C's case, a mere verbal or behavioural expression of will was not enough to demonstrate genuine understanding. The court needed some evidence that he grasped the reality of his predicament.

Understanding, 'rational reasoning' and values

Mr Justice Thorpe did not make his working concept of 'understanding' explicit in the judgment. It has to be inferred from the contents of his decision. Clearly, he rejected mental illness as a barrier to capacity (i.e. a status test). Rather, C's capacity for autonomy turns on a set of general capacity criteria, i.e. that he could understand the information he was given, believe it, weigh it up, and arrive at a clear choice. Must C be able to engage in *rational reasoning* to satisfy the test of capacity, i.e. the ability to reason to a conclusion from a set of premises? This will depend on what is meant by an ability to reason.

English law does not require a patient's treatment refusal to be 'rational, sensible and well considered' (see *Re T*, per Lady Justice Butler-Sloss). However, the law probably does draw a distinction between somebody who is deluded about the world (e.g. the belief that blood is poison) and somebody who is able to reason to a conclusion from premises that few people share, e.g. Jehovah's Witnesses who refuse blood transfusions on religious grounds.

The law does seem, then, in this case at least, implicitly to recognize that sometimes very diverse values can legitimately inform treatment decisions. On the one hand C's treatment refusal could be understood as a perfectly intelligible expression of his theological commitments and his faith in the competence of his care team. On the other hand, C's grandiose delusions may have suggested that he was losing touch with reality. Mr Justice Thorpe was prepared, perhaps, to find C competent because his delusions did not appear to be directly relevant to his treatment decision.

'Reasonable outcome': objective test or value judgement?

To what extent is Mr Justice Thorpe's decision explicable in terms of the '*reasonable outcome*' test, the second level of 'competence' or, as some would put it, 'rationality' described in Roth *et al*'s article?

The capacity criteria appear to give a degree of objectivity to the way a doctor or a court determines capacity. But there may be a hidden evaluative dimension to the assessment. For example, might Mr Justice Thorpe have come to a different conclusion if C had been a member of an extreme sect with unpopular views rather than a patient expressing a largely orthodox Christian position? While a judge may not doubt a patient's ability to use, process, and evaluate the information he is given, he may not like the way in which the patient does it. A judge could, without detection, and perhaps without even realizing it, penalize a patient for holding values he does not share.

As Roth *et al*'s article puts it, 'if patients do not decide the "wrong way", the issue of competency will not arise'. And the notion of being able to 'weigh' information opens up the 'way' for this: what is involved in assessing 'weighing' may include consideration both of which factors are properly to be included in the weighing, and of the 'weights' to be attached to each.

Capable of understanding or actual understanding?

The 'capable of understanding' test, the fourth one described in Roth *et al*'s article, perhaps best reflects the position in English law. This test seems to be consistent with the legal view that the patient is free not to make a sensible, rational or well-considered decision (although it must be rational in the sense of being based on rational manipulation of relevant information). As it happens, 'C's' decision was, arguably, perfectly sensible given his presuppositions and his reading of his situation.

The 'actual understanding' test (the fifth one described) probably goes too far and, if it did apply in English law, would, rather ironically, underscore medical paternalism. Doctors could, in theory at least, find a perfectly capable patient 'incompetent' by withholding from him the amount of information he would need to 'actually understand'. The test of patient competence would therefore turn on what the doctor would choose to tell the patient, rather than on the patient's decision-making capacity. The 'actual understanding' test, which should represent the highest view of patient autonomy, would, in practice, place in doctors' hands even greater power to determine competence.

Kennedy and Grubb (2000) have argued that:

> Competence or incompetence is a state inherent in the individual patient which cannot depend on how much the doctor tells the patient. It must, therefore, be the law that competence is determined by reference to the unvarying conceptual standard of capacity or ability to understand. Whether, thereafter a patient who is judged competent because she has the capacity or ability to understand, in fact consented, is a distinct question turning on the reality of the consent based upon legally adequate information.

It is to this issue of the standard of legally adequate information that we now turn.

Information

We learned earlier in this chapter that the legal test of competence was a composite test with three ingredients: capacity, information, and voluntariness. We have already considered the issue of capacity. The legal test of capacity is set out in the case of *Re C* and requires a patient to be able to understand and retain the information he is given about his treatment proposal; be able to believe it;

and be capable of weighing up the information so as to arrive at a true choice. Thus, it is clear that the test of capacity itself implies that the patient's consent must be 'informed' to a certain degree. However, the requirement that consent be 'informed' begs the question, how informed is informed? The second ingredient of the composite test is associated with this question.

It should be noted that the requirement that consent be informed is not equivalent to the doctrine of 'informed consent' that many American jurisdictions have adopted. This doctrine relies on the language of individual rights and pays especial attention to the particular circumstances of the patient. Contrary to popular belief, the doctrine of 'informed consent' in that sense, is not a requirement of English law, and there is little evidence that the English courts will adopt that doctrine in the near future.

How much must a doctor tell the patient in order for that patient to give a legally valid consent? In English law, a doctor must tell the patient whatever is necessary to avoid civil actions in battery or negligence. Accordingly, the English law of consent is essentially *defensive*, i.e. it is designed to protect the doctor from civil litigation rather than to promote individual patient rights. For this reason, the English law of consent is criticized (Brazier, 1992, p. 92) for its continuing contribution to a culture of medical paternalism.

To explore this point, it will be helpful to consider, first, the ingredients of the law of battery and that of negligence. This will involve a brief excursion into a number of additional legal concepts before we return to the question of how much a patient needs to know in order to consent to medical treatment. First, we need to understand the legal concept of a 'cause of action'.

Causes of action

What happens when the doctor treats a patient without first having obtained that patient's consent? What redress is open to the patient? In legal terms, what are that patient's possible 'causes of action'?

In a nutshell, the doctor may be liable to criminal and/or civil proceedings:

- *criminal law* for the crime of battery (known as criminal battery), and/or

- *civil law* for:
  - trespass to the person (known as civil battery), and/or
  - negligence.

You should note that both civil battery and negligence are causes of action to fall under the legal 'head' of tort law (see above, Session 1 of this chapter)

Thus, there are three main contexts in which the issue of consent in the doctor–patient relationship arises:

1. in the *crime* of battery

2. in the *tort* of battery

3. in the *tort* of negligence.

These causes of action apply to doctors who *do* things to patients without consent; they do not apply to the failure to obtain consent in itself, albeit a doctor can be negligent in the manner in which she purports to gain consent (for example, in the information that she gives to the patient during the process).

Criminal law

The word 'battery' refers both to the criminal offence or the civil action of trespass to the person.

However, a doctor will very rarely, if ever, be prosecuted for the crime of battery. A doctor who fails to obtain his patient's consent 'in the ordinary practice of medicine in good faith' will, in almost all cases, be liable to a civil action in battery or negligence. However, a criminal prosecution might follow a misrepresentation or fraud to secure consent to treatment, e.g. obtaining a patient's consent to sexual intercourse by presenting it as a legitimate medical examination.

For our purposes, therefore, when we refer to 'battery', it will be to the civil action rather than the criminal offence, unless otherwise stated. It should be noted that both criminal and civil battery actions share the same ingredients.

Civil law: the ingredients of battery

There are three ingredients to a civil battery action:

* touching

* damage

* proximity and foreseeability (non-remoteness) of damage.

We will deal with each of these in turn:

1. *Touching*. There must be physical contact between the doctor and the patient. A doctor may be liable if, for example, he injects a patient with a drug without his consent. But he will not be liable in battery if, without that patient's consent, he gives him a pill to take. In the latter case, there has been no physical contact and, therefore, no battery. The patient would be left to pursue any claim he had against the doctor in negligence.

2. *Damage*. It is *not* necessary for a patient to show that the damage occurred as a result of any touching. The patient need only prove that the doctor touched him without first obtaining his consent. Indeed, a patient could succeed even if the doctor's treatment actually benefited him. In a negligence action, by contrast, the patient must show that it was the doctor's negligent conduct that caused the damage.

3. *Remoteness of damage*. A doctor, if damage does occur, is responsible for all damage that results from the touching. Indeed, punitive damages may be awarded if the doctor's conduct was particularly disgraceful. In negligence, by contrast, the doctor is responsible only for damage that he could have reasonably foreseen might result from his negligent act or *omission*. Note that in negligence a doctor can be found negligent both for his positive acts and also for *failure to act* where he ought to have acted. Unforeseen damage will not be compensated. Note also that damages in negligence are awarded to compensate the plaintiff for his loss, not to punish the defendant.

Civil law: negligence

There are three ingredients to a negligence action. All three must be present if the patient is to succeed in his action against the doctor. These are:

* owing a duty of care

* breach of standard of care

* causation.

Again, we will consider each of these ingredients in turn:

1. *Duty of care*. The patient must establish that the doctor treating him/her owed him/her a duty of care. Normally, this will not be difficult to prove. However, complications can arise within the interdisciplinary context of an enlarged NHS community, e.g. in the context of a 'team' with collective responsibility for the patient's care. In order to establish the presence of a duty of care, the patient must demonstrate all of the following:

   * *Reasonable forseeability*. The patient must establish that the doctor could have reasonably foreseen that his act or omission would harm the patient.

   * *Proximity*. There must be a sufficiently close relationship between the doctor and the patient to warrant legal redress. The doctor must have some role in the care of the patient. For example, it is not enough to show that the doctor was merely present in a busy hospital building when the patient was brought in for treatment.

   * *Public policy*. It must be just and reasonable to find the doctor liable in the circumstances. In some circumstances, the courts on public policy grounds will disallow a claim in negligence even though the injury in question was reasonably foreseeable and a relationship of proximity existed between the doctor and patient, for example so-called 'wrongful life' claims premised on the view that it would, for some, have been better never to have been born at all.

2. *Standard of care*. The patient must show that the doctor fell below the medical standard of care applicable to someone exercising his particular medical art. It is not enough to show that the doctor made an error of judgement. The medical standard of care is unique in that the medical profession itself under the so-called *Bolam* test, determines it. We shall look at this test in greater detail later.

3. *Causation*. The patient must prove that the doctor's negligent act or omission *caused* the damage the patient suffered. In other words, the patient must show that 'but for' the defendant's allegedly negligent conduct, no damage would have resulted (the so-called 'but for' test). This must be proved on the balance of probabilities (i.e. more than 50% chance). It can be, and often is, extremely difficult to prove causation, e.g. in 'lost chance' cases. For example, the House of Lords (the highest court in England and Wales) rejected a claim for damages, which reflected a percentage of a lost chance of recovery

resulting from an earlier misdiagnosis. A boy who fell out of a tree would have had a 25% chance of recovering from his injuries had his doctor's properly diagnosed and treated him the first time. The House of Lords held that the claimant had failed to prove on a 'balance of probabilities' that the defendants had 'caused' his injuries. He could not recover an amount corresponding to his 'lost chance', i.e. 25% of the amount of a full award. It was all (over 50% probability) or nothing (under 50% probability).

'Nature and purpose' (for battery)

A doctor who 'touches' his patient without that patient's consent will be liable to an action in battery, even if that touching benefited the patient. Therefore, it is of great importance for the doctor that he ensures that he has secured the patient's agreement to treatment. Of course, if there is no physical contact between the doctor and the patient, then no action in battery will arise and the patient will be left to pursue a claim against the doctor in negligence. In order to succeed, the patient will then have to show that the doctor owed the patient a duty of care, that the doctor fell below the medical standard of care and that the doctor caused damage to the patient.

But when will a patient be taken to have given a 'real' consent? The legal position is that a patient can be taken to have given a real consent when that patient understands in broad terms the nature and purpose of the treatment proposed (*Chatteron v. Gerson* [1981] 3 WLR 1003). Thus, a doctor will be liable in battery where he misrepresents to the patient the nature of what is being done. An action in battery will clearly lie in cases of fraud where, as in the example above, a doctor 'dupes' a patient into agreeing to 'therapeutic' sexual intercourse. Actions in battery have also succeeded where a doctor has misrepresented to the patient the nature of what is being undertaken.

However, in some cases, the line between battery and no-battery may not be clear and distinct. Suppose you go into hospital and agree to a series of routine blood tests preparatory for surgery. Unknown to you, an extra HIV test is 'thrown in' that you would have refused if asked. You understood that several tests would be carried out on your blood, though not necessarily which ones. Yet, you might have wanted to avoid the risk altogether of the stigma, discrimination, and personal anxiety that a positive result would entail. It is suggested that you would not have given a real consent to the test because the HIV test is one for which, on policy grounds, your express consent should have been sought.

'Effects' (for negligence)

The courts have shied away from finding doctors liable in battery where the issue is not the nature and purpose of the treatment proposed, but the effects, i.e. where the risks of the procedure were not explained. For example, in the case of *Chatterton v Gerson*, a woman, Mrs Chatterton, failed in her action in battery for her doctor's alleged failure to inform her of the possible side-effects of her postoperative medication, i.e. pain and numbness.

The High Court rejected her claim arguing that the appropriate cause of action was in negligence, not in battery. Mr Justice Bristow stated:

> In my judgment once the patient is informed in broad terms of the nature of the procedure which is intended, and gives her consent, that consent is real, and the cause on which to base a claim for failure to go into the risks and implications is negligence, not trespass [i.e. *trespass* to the person or civil *battery*]. Of course, if information is withheld in bad faith, the consent will be vitiated by fraud.

The House of Lords has subsequently endorsed this view in the case of *Sidaway v Board of Governors of the Bethlem Royal and the Maudsley Hospital* [1894] 2 WLR 788 at 790. The Canadian courts have also adopted a similar position. Thus, apart from claims involving fraudulent misrepresentation of risks, the tort of battery probably now has a vestigial role in the law of consent.

Difficulties in winning negligence actions

By making negligence the appropriate cause of action for a doctor's failure to inform the patient of any risks inherent in an operation, the courts may arguably have compounded the pro-doctor character of the English law of consent. This is because it is more difficult to prove that a doctor is negligent than it is to prove that he 'touched' the patient without consent. Also, the test of negligence is itself based on essentially a medical standard, incorporating therefore medical and not patient values (see below).

As we outlined above, in order to succeed in negligence, a patient must prove that the doctor in question owed a duty of care, fell below the medical standard of care, and caused the damage that ensued. This is quite difficult to achieve. Medical negligence actions are notoriously slow moving, frequently lasting more than 10 years. Doctors and health authorities also have the advantage of powerful medical defence unions to handle their litigation. Patients often feel intimidated in the face of such institutional strength. Perhaps the greatest obstacle to patient success in negligence litigation lies in the nature of negligence action itself, namely the medical standard of care. This is unique in that, as noted above, the professional standard for doctors is largely set by the medical profession itself, rather than according to a judicially determined standard of 'reasonableness'.

In the last part of this session we will turn to an important legal test for negligence cases: the Bolam test, and its recent interpretation.

The 'Bolam' test

The *Bolam* test is so-called because it derives from a leading English case relating to the medical standard of care, i.e. *Bolam v Friern HMC* [1957] 2 All ER. In the *Bolam* case, a doctor will not be liable in negligence if he can establish that his conduct was: '...in accordance with a practice accepted as proper by a responsible body of medical men skilled in that particular area'.

There is continuing debate about what, precisely, the Bolam Test means: the judge in Bolam also used the term 'reasonable body' of opinion; in other judgements it becomes 'respectable body'.

Broadly, though, all agree that Bolam establishes that in English Law medical standards of care are subject to what has become know as a 'reputable minority' defence. This means that surgeons will be judged by the standards proper to surgeons, physicians to physicians, etc. Provided that a doctor can establish a reputable minority of relevant colleagues would have done what he or she did, the doctor will escape liability. His conduct will be deemed proper even if the majority of doctors practising in his area of medicine would have conducted themselves differently, provided that a 'responsible' minority of doctors would have endorsed his conduct. Whether such a reputable minority of doctors exists will be a matter of medical expert evidence. Despite more recent intimations to the contrary, the court has no discretion to substitute a judicially constructed 'reasonable doctor' test, although any 'accepted practice' must satisfy a basic test of being 'logically based' (see *Bolitho* below). As a result, many believe that *Bolam* is a charter for medical paternalism, reinforcing the assumption in the English courts that 'doctor knows best'. As we will see in the next reading, the Bolam test has found application particularly in relation to the information component of consent.

EXERCISE 5   (30 minutes)

Read Sidaway v Bethlem RHG [1985] 1 ALL ER 643, extracted in:

> McHale, J. Fox, M., and Murphy, J. (1999). *Health Care Law: text and materials* London: Sweet and Maxwell, pp. 341–51

Link with Reading 19.5

Read each judgment carefully.

◆ How does each judge apply the Bolam test (if at all)?

◆ How much must a doctor disclose to his patient to avoid an action in negligence?

The 'Sidaway' case: the facts

The House of Lords case of *Sidaway v Board of Governors of the Bethlem Royal Hospital* [1985] 1 All ER 643 represents a major challenge to the view that the medical profession ultimately determines the scope of its obligation to the patient, at least in the context of information disclosure.

Mrs Sidaway underwent surgery to relieve severe pain in her neck, right shoulders and arms. As a result, she was left paralysed. She sued the surgeon and the hospital for the surgeon's failure to disclose the inherent risks of the operation, i.e. that there was a 1–2% risk of damage to the nerve roots and spinal cord. She argued that 'but for' this failure, she would not have consented to surgery and thus avoided paralysis. The surgeon's death prior to the trial complicated the issue of causation, which turned on what precisely he had told Mrs Sidaway. The Lord's decided the legal issue (i.e. how much should a doctor tell the patient) on the factual premiss that the surgeon (Mr Falconer) had not disclosed these risks.

The decision, the patient, and the patient's values

Mrs Sidaway lost her case. There was evidence to suggest that there was a reputable minority of neurosurgeons who would have chosen not to disclose the small risks inherent in the operation. All the judges agreed that Mrs Sidaway could not prove what was said in the consulting room. They unanimously agreed that a doctor was obliged to answer all the patient's specific inquiries. To this extent then, the patient's values should determine the extent of the information required in consent.

But the judges also agreed to reject a totally subjective test, i.e. what this particular patient wanted to know in this patient's particular circumstances, assuming that the patient has not made specific inquiries. The Bolam test was thus upheld against the patient's values, though the status of the *Bolam* test itself was left in doubt. Perhaps this is because the law still construes the doctrine of consent defensively, rather than as an expression of the patient's human rights. In other words, it is concerned with the question, what does it take to, as it were, get the doctor off the hook, legally speaking?, rather than 'what should we tell the patient in order to honour her dignity as a decision maker?' It is significant that the strongest critic of the Bolam test, Lord Scarman, was the Law Lord with the reputation of being most attentive to the concept of 'human rights'. In addition, the moment that a degree of judicial objectivity is allowed to qualify the medically determined standard of care relating to information, there is no reason in principle why a degree of judicial scrutiny should not also apply to questions of treatment and diagnosis. The range of views expressed by the judges in this case reflects the range of positions in English law at the present time on the balance to be struck between patients' values and those of professionals (usually taken by the courts to mean doctors). We will look at each of these in turn.

Lord Scarman: patients' values

Lord Scarman wanted to substitute the 'prudent patient' test, adopted in America, Canada, and Australia, for the *Bolam* test. This test, if adopted, would apply in the absence of a specific enquiry by the patient (which would otherwise need to be answered in full). The prudent patient test asks what the 'prudent' or 'reasonable' patient would want to know in the circumstances. This would include the obligation to disclose 'material' risks, which Lord Scarman defines as the risks the patient could reasonably expect to be informed of in the circumstances (a rather circular test, perhaps).

The prudent patient test is therefore distinguishable from a totally 'subjective' test, which is concerned with what a particular patient, who has not made a specific enquiry, actually wants to know. This, of course, assumes that there are ways of telling what a patient wants to know in the absence of putting specific questions to the doctor. However, Lord Scarman accepted that there were circumstances when it would be right for a doctor to withhold information from the patient on the basis of 'therapeutic privilege'. In other words, a doctor would be permitted to withhold information from the patient if it could be shown that 'a reasonable assessment of the patient would have indicated to the doctor that disclosure would have posed a serious threat of psychological detriment to the patient'. Again, then, we have an approach that amounts to 'patient choice with exceptions'.

Lord Diplock: doctors' values

Lord Diplock advocated the direct application of the *Bolam* test. He was therefore endorsing the *status quo*, i.e. an unabridged medical standard of care. Lord Diplock argued that to alter the *Bolam* test in the context of information disclosure would result in different standards of obligation across the clinical process. The *Bolam* standard would apply to diagnosis and treatment, but not to information disclosure. Lord Diplock thought that there was no warrant for varying the standard of care in this way.

The majority: doctors' values within limits

The majority (Lords Bridge, Keith (who concurred with the Lord Bridge) and Templeman) argued that the *Bolam* standard would apply in most cases. However, the courts remained the ultimate arbiters of the scope of the doctor's obligation. According to Lord Bridge, how much the doctor should tell a patient was not exclusively a matter of expert testimony, although great weight would always be given to the views of the experts.

Lord Templeman argued that doctors were obliged to act 'rightly' (Note the explicit value term here) and could be impugned for not doing so, even if a 'reputable minority' of doctors endorsed their conduct. According to both judges, doctors were obliged to disclose inherent risks in treatment in certain circumstances, even in the face of medical opinion. Lord Bridge argued that doctors should disclose 'substantial risk(s) of adverse consequence(s)', e.g. a 10% risk of a stroke. Lord Templeman argued that doctors should disclose 'special' as opposed to 'general' risks. Again, we can understand this is an attempt (implicit, no doubt) to give certainty in the face of potentially different evaluations of what, by this or that person's values, should count as a *substantial* risk of *adverse* consequences.

Post-Sidaway

As you can see, there was a broad spectrum of opinion in the Sidaway case. Lord Diplock delivered the most conservative judgment endorsing the traditional interpretation of the medical standard of care. In other words, it is up to the medical profession to determine how much information doctors should give their patients. Lord Scarman delivered the most radical judgment, endorsing the transatlantic 'prudent patient' test. In other words, doctors should tell their patients what the 'prudent' or 'reasonable' patient would want to know in the circumstances. The majority adopted a middle position in the form of a qualified version of the *Bolam* standard.

Subsequent 'information' cases have interpreted Sidaway both conservatively and liberally. For example, in a number of cases,

patients have taken doctors to court for failing to inform them of the inherent risks of sterilization procedures. In two Court of Appeal cases, the court applied the traditional *Bolam* standard to aspects of the doctor–patient relationship that *Sidaway* supposedly excluded. For example, in *Blyth v Bloomsbury Health Authority* [1993] Med LR 151, the court held that it was up to doctors to decide how much to tell their patients, even in response to specific enquiries. In *Gold v Haringay Health Authority* [1987] 2 All ER 888, the court perversely adopted Lord Diplock's judgment as the centre of the *Sidaway* decision (see the judgment of Lloyd LJ). Academic critics have impugned these two cases as overprotective of the medical profession. According to one, to read *Gold* 'is to imagine that *Sidaway* had not happened'. (Kennedy, 1996, p. 210).

Whose values?

However, a number of very recent information cases have reaffirmed the courts' role in setting limits to medical judgment. In the House of Lords case of *Bolitho v City and Hackney Health Authority* [1997] 4 All ER 771, the court argued that medical opinion must have a logical basis to it, even if it satisfies the 'reputable minority' standard. Medical opinion must be reasonable, responsible, and respectable. This is in keeping with the *Bolam* judgment itself, which refers to a *responsible* body of medical practitioners exercising a particular medical art. But the essential spirit of the test remains, that, at least within very wide limits, it is the values of the profession (as expressed in at least a minority of its members), rather than of the patient (or even a composite 'prudent patient') that determines the extent of the information required for consent.

Reflection on the session and self-test questions

Write down your own reflections on the materials in this session drawing out any points that are particularly significant for you. Then write brief notes about the following:

1. What are the four key elements in the legal test of decision-making capacity defined by the case of ReC in the English courts?

2. Where (if at all) might values come into this test?

3. If a doctor treats someone without consent unlawfully, what 'causes of action' may a patient have under English law, in criminal law, and in civil law?

4. What are the elements of battery?

5. What are the elements of negligence?

6. What is the 'Bolam' test?

7. What is a prudent patient test?

8. Who 'sets the tests' and what are they really about?

Session 3   Consent, voluntariness, and best interests

The *third* ingredient of consent is voluntariness. In order to give valid consent, a patient must have the functional ability to understand the nature, purpose, and effects of the proposed treatment and arrive at a clear choice *without duress or undue influence*.

For example, in the case of *Re T*, the Court of Appeal upheld the lawfulness of an emergency Caesarean section on a supposedly non-compliant 34-year-old woman. The court held that the patient's mother—a Jehovah's Witness—had pressurized the patient into refusing potentially life-saving blood transfusion. The court also held that the mother's pressure had prevented the patient from making an independent decision and, therefore, a 'true choice'. As a result, the doctors were free in the ensuing emergency to act in the patient's best interests in the absence of a real refusal of consent.

The courts will perhaps be readier to find involuntariness where the patient has appeared to refuse than appeared to consent. For the doctor may be liable in battery where the patient appears to consent but later claims the consent was involuntary. Where the patient appears to refuse, doctors will be harder pushed to examine the state of the patient's mind, and to justify supposedly non-consensual treatment.

Medical paternalism, patient autonomy, and judicial values

While the courts have often affirmed the principle of patient self-determination, they have not always acted consistently with that affirmation. Kennedy (1996, p. 386) argues that the courts have traditionally analysed the doctor–patient relationship within the framework of doctor's duties rather than patient rights. It seems that the courts will hold back from too closely enquiring into the patient's state of mind in order to expand the scope of the doctor's clinical discretion. The principle of patient self-determination becomes a concession to the patient rather than a legitimate right.

The essentially defensive character of English consent law is evident in the longevity of the *Bolam* standard, the anomalous responses to treatment refusals by children and the expansive use of mental health legislation to overcome treatment refusals by clearly competent adults. Thus, the courts, arguably, have used the concepts of 'rationality', 'capacity', and 'competence' as levers to achieve what they think are reasonable outcomes. There can be few clearer examples of the operation of (implicit) judicial values!

Perhaps the most conspicuous examples of this kind of judicial leverage reflecting implicit judicial values are a number of controversial 'enforced Caesarean cases'.

Enforced Caesareans

The English courts have stated repeatedly that an adult patient who suffers from no mental incapacity has an absolute right to make a treatment decision. The only possible exception to this principle cited in English law is where a treatment refusal might lead to the death of a viable foetus, i.e. a foetus that is sufficiently developed to survive outside the womb, albeit with medical help. This presumed exception to the legal capacity of a woman was perhaps always a dubious legal proposition, but the courts have taken advantage of the loophole on several occasions, especially in the mental health context.

Take two High Court cases, for example:

1. In *Tameside and Glossop Acute Services v CH (A Patient)* [1996] 1 FCR 753, the court declared that Caesarean section could constitute necessary treatment for a non-compliant woman's schizophrenia under Section 63 of the Mental Health Act 1983.

2. In *St George's Health Care National Health Service Trust v S (No. 2); R v Collins, exp S (No. 2)* [1998] 3 All ER 673, a non-compliant woman suffering from pre-eclampsia was sectioned under Section 3 of the Mental Health Act. She knew that she was putting herself and her foetus at risk, but she wanted her child to be born naturally. Although she was treated for her mental disorder, nevertheless a declaration was sought authorizing a Caesarean section, premissed presumably on the assumption that the woman in question was incompetent.

The Court of Appeal has castigated the use of mental health legislation as a lever for treating otherwise competent women against their will. In the case of *Re MB (a Caesarean section)* [1997] 8 Med LR 217, the court held that: 'The Act cannot be deployed to achieve the detention of an individual against her will merely because her thinking process is unusual, even apparently bizarre and irrational, and contrary to the views of the overwhelming majority of the community at large.'

However, the court none the less allowed the Caesarian section on the perhaps even more unlikely ground that, in this case, fear (of needles) had 'paralysed the [woman's] will'.

There is other evidence of the judicial reluctance to examine closely the patient's state of mind before authorizing treatment on non-compliant women. The courts have acted on incoherent legal grounds (*Re S* [1992] 4 All ER 671), and on untested hearsay evidence (*Norfolk and Norwich (NHS) Trust v W* [1996] 2 FLR.

Clashes of values (and a role for Values-Based Practice?)

The enforced Caesarean section cases are significant because they show how the concepts of rationality, capacity, and competence, may operate in a 'gendered' fashion. In other words, most judges, being male, do not tend to identify with the values or beliefs of prospective mothers when they put themselves in danger of their lives and of the lives of their unborn children. Justice Cardozo might have added to his two conditions of eligibility (Adults and Sound Mind), a third (Not Very Pregnant).

These cases, however, illustrate a broader problem about the role of values and beliefs in assessments of rationality and capacity. We raised this issue above in the case of *Re C* and considered the possibility that the judge might have declared C competent because he identified with C's values. Similarly, it could be argued in the St George's Healthcare NHS Trust case (see above, previous page) that the woman was declared incompetent because the court did not identify with her reasons for refusing potentially life-saving treatment, i.e. because she wanted to bear her child naturally. The three-part competence test in *Re C* could easily be driven by unacknowledged medical and judicial value judgements. A woman might be capable of understanding and retaining the information, believing it, and arriving at a clear choice. But if she failed to weigh up the information in the way the judge thought right, then that judge could easily find her incompetent.

The problem, it seems, with the established competence test is its almost exclusive focus on the 'functional approach' to assessments of capacity. The medical profession and the courts have not, perhaps, adequately acknowledged that assessments of rationality and competence do not occur in an evaluative vacuum. This is not especially problematic in the context of most bodily disorders, where, as we saw in Part I, there is a greater likelihood of an identity of values between doctor, patient, and judge. However, differences of values become more problematic even in the context of bodily disorders, where the life of the patient or her viable foetus is put at risk.

You may think that the expansive use by the courts of mental health legislation to overturn a patient's 'wrong' treatment decision is a worrying development in that it could be a step towards abusive uses of psychiatry for coercive social purposes rather than for treating mental health problems. We return to the abusive uses of psychiatry later in this part. The essential point that will emerge is that the most serious abuses arise, not from deliberate ill will, but from a failure to recognize the operation of value judgements in assessments of rationality (and, correlatively, related concepts of competence, capacity, and so forth). Such failures, as we will see, are compounded by a naive medical model in which diagnostic assessments are assumed to be objective and, hence, value-free.

The English courts, then, in falling back on mental health legislation, in their (wholly understandable) attempt to hang on to an objective test of capacity, are at risk of just this form of abusive misuse of psychiatry. It is an open question whether, in legal as in health-care practice, values-based approaches may usefully complement court procedure in such cases. But as we argued in Chapter 18, the first and necessary step is to recognize the difficulty for what it is, a difficulty arising from (largely implicit) conflicts between (legitimately) different value perspectives, rather than a failure to find a 'golden bullet' in the form of a value-free, exclusively objective, test.

A generic incapacity act?

One response to the concerns about abusive uses of psychiatry is to put mental health on the same basis as bodily health when it comes to patient autonomy and consent to treatment.

Thet Mental Capacity Act, 2005, for England and Wales seeks to put on a statutory footing many of the common law principles that we have been discussing. We will not consider the Act in detail (it is not due to come into force until April, 2007) but will highlight some of the salient points. Section 2(1) of the Act provides: 'For the purposes of this Act, a person lacks capacity in relation to a matter if at the material time he is unable to make a decision for himself in relation to the matter because of an impairment or disturbance in the functioning of the mind or brain.'

Section 1(2) transmutes into statutory form, with small modifications and elucidations, the presumption against lack of capacity in adults (i.e. people over 16 years of age) the incapacity criteria developed at common law and the 'best interests' test. Section 1(4) lays down a detailed checklist of things that must be done in order to determine 'best interests'. Nothing in the draft Bill will, if enacted, affect those provisions in existing mental health legislation, which allow compulsory treatment for mental disorder of otherwise (according to the draft Bill and common law) 'competent' people.

The provisions of the Bill represent a qualified transmutation of the contents of an earlier Government 'Green Paper', *Who Decides? Making Decisions on Behalf of Mentally Incapacitated Adults* (Lord Chancellor's Department, 1997). Interestingly, the terms of reference of the original Law Commission work (on which the Green Paper proposals were based) excluded consideration of 'treatment for mental disorder', which was to remain under a separate Mental Health Act. This has been seen by many as reinforcing the stigma that has traditionally attached to a diagnosis of mental disorder, via continued 'discriminatory' legislation, which was based not on the (autonomy driven) principle of incapacity but on the (paternalistic) pragmatism of 'appropriateness' of medical treatment (Szmukler and Holloway, 1998, see reading linked with Exercise 6, below). However, others have argued that, even if incapacity had been extended to treatment for mental disorder, that might in reality have obscured yet further the value judgements that lie at the heart of all medical diagnoses, in the context of physical disorder, but with practical importance especially in the area of mental disorder (see readings linked with Exercise 6).

In the next set of readings we look at a section from the original discussion paper, *Who Decides*, together with three views on the role of generic incapacity legislation in mental health.

EXERCISE 6	(90 minutes)

Read the extracts from:

a) Lord Chancellor's Department (1997). The key principles: capacity, best interests, and the general authority to act reasonably. In: *Who Decides? Making Decisions on Behalf of Mentally Incapacitated Adults*. Cmnd 3803. London: The Stationary Office Ltd, pp. 11–13 (Chapter 3)

b) Szmukler, G. and Holloway, F. (1998). Mental health legislation is now a harmful anachronism. *Psychiatric Bulletin*, 22: 663, 664

c) Fulford, K.W.M. (1998). Replacing the Mental Health Act 1983? How to change the game without losing the baby with the bath water or shooting ourselves in the foot. *Psychiatric Bulletin*, 22: 666, 667, 668

d) Sayce, L. (1998). Transcending mental health law. *Psychiatric Bulletin*, 22: 669

Link with Reading 19.6

◆ What are the advantages and disadvantages of applying a Re C type competence test to treatment decisions relating to a patient's mental disorder?

This discussion speaks for itself! There are clear arguments, based on issues of equality and non-stigmatising treatment, for generic incapacity legislation to include mental disorder. But if the capacity test employed is insensitive to the greater conceptual and evaluative complications of mental disorder, this could prove abusive.

The point, as we have repeatedly emphasised in this book, is that diagnoses of mental disorder are complicated by particular conceptual difficulties not shared in the diagnosis of most bodily disorders. In the context of mental disorder, the principle of self-determination thus acquires a deeper dimension of conceptual difficulty. For patient autonomy is expressed not simply through the articulation of a treatment decision but by indicating to doctor and judge alike how the patient's condition is to be understood. This, again, requires a greater commitment by doctor and judge alike not only to examine the state of the patient's mind, but also to be guided in part by the patient to a proper understanding of his/her condition. Judicial past practice, e.g. in the enforced Caesarean cases, shows that this acknowledgement of the patient's role in determining their own diagnosis (rather than just their treatment), will require as significant a shift in legal as in medical thinking.

Rational suicide, psychiatric euthanasia, and best interests

The conceptual difficulties raised by consent in the context of mental health are brought to a particularly sharp focus by end of life issues.

The difficulties are illustrated by the following case, which raises important issues with respect to voluntariness in the context of mental health care.

EXERCISE 7   (10 minutes)

Read the extract from the case of Martin McKendrick, Case 4.1 in

Dickenson, D. and Fulford, K.W.M. (2000). *In Two Minds: a casebook of psychiatric ethics*. Oxford: Oxford University Press, p. 91–97 (Extract pp. 91–92.)

Link with Reading 19.7

Dickenson and Fulford discuss this case mainly from an ethical and philosophical point of view.

◆ What issues do you think it raises in mental health law?

◆ Is Martin's death wish rational? Is he of 'sound mind'?

◆ Could it ever be in his 'best interests' to die?

◆ who decides (and who should decide) what is truly in someone's 'best interests'?

'Rational suicide' and the Mental Health Act 1983

Martin had been detained under the Mental Health Act on several occasions. On the basis of the information we have, he was probably a candidate for admission under Section 3 (treatment) of the Act. Under Section 63 of the Act, Martin's doctors could lawfully have treated him without his consent, although as a matter of good practice, they should have sought to obtain his consent first. However, Martin's doctors must have obtained Martin's consent first before giving him electroconvulsive therapy (being a treatment falling under Section 58). All treatment proposed and carried out must constitute treatment for Martin's 'mental disorder'. The Act does not define 'mental illness' or 'mental disorder' (to the extent that this incorporates 'mental illness') but there is little doubt that Martin was suffering from depression with delusions.

However, whether Martin's desire to die was a symptom of mental illness is a moot point. Can we simply assume that Martin is mentally ill because he wants to die? If Martin's desire for death is a consequence, or aspect of mental illness, then he can be treated under the provisions of the 1983 Act for that mental illness. If it is not, then his request for suicide falls to be considered under the common law.

A few preliminary comments about the criminal law and suicide need to be made.

Criminal law

It is no longer unlawful in Britain to commit suicide (Suicide Act 1961). But it remains an imprisonable offence to assist the suicide or attempted suicide of another (Section 2). Under English criminal law, therefore, there is no scope for acceding to Martin's death wish. With one exception, no jurisdiction in the world has yet successfully legislated for a law of assisted suicide and/or euthanasia, except briefly in the Northern Territories of Australia. The one exception is the enactment in the United States of The Oregon Death With Dignity Act 1994. In the Netherlands, doctors who assist suicide or euthanatize their patients enjoy immunity from prosecution provided they conform to legally prescribed guidelines and statutory reporting procedures. The criminal law aside, then, what would Martin's position be under common law in the UK?

Sound mind and Self-determination

Under common law Martin has a legally protected right of self-determination provided he is an adult, of sound mind (and of course not heavily pregnant), even if it means refusing life-sustaining treatment. However, the question arises, is Martin of 'sound mind'? Does his suicide request, by definition, reverse the presumption of capacity? This would depend on how related his death wish was to his other symptoms of mental disorder (delusion and depression), which, collectively, indicated that he had lost touch with reality. If we recall, the court, in the case of 'Re C', was prepared to disaggregate C's delusions, which suggested that 'C' had lost touch with reality, from his reasons for refusing the amputation. In other words, his irrationality was not all-pervasive.

In Martin's case, the court would have to decide whether Martin's symptoms indicated that he had lost his grip on reality or represented an intelligible existential commitment (i.e. life has no meaning therefore death is the only option). Moreover, the court would have to be satisfied that Martin's decision for death was unequivocal. Perhaps it was C's unequivocal decision for death that distinguishes the case of *Re C* from many of the enforced Caesarean cases (e.g. *Re T*), where the courts were not satisfied that there was a clear death wish.

The legal position in Martin's case is, however, distinguishable from the case of *Re C* in a significant respect. Martin is not refusing treatment but making a request for active 'treatment' in the form of assisted suicide or euthanasia. While doctors cannot treat competent patients against their wishes, they are not obliged to accede to treatment requests, especially if they involve the death of the patient. Such requests, if acceded to, would represent a fundamental abridgement of the Hippocratic tradition that lies at the basis of medicine in the West. Perhaps the best way of expressing the legal position is to say that the doctor has a fundamental duty to act in his patients 'best interests' qualified only by the patient's right to self-determination. Thus, Martin's doctor is not obliged to *do* anything that is not in Martin's 'best interests'. As we have seen, in the United Kingdom treatment is lawful provided that a responsible body of professional opinion would regard it as in the patient's best interests (*F v West Berkshire Health Authority* [1989] 2 All ER 545.). This is basically the *Bolam* test as applied to the meaning of 'best interests'.

'Best interests'

But this begs perhaps the fundamental question. What are Martins' 'best interests'? And who is best qualified to determine those interests? Can it ever be in Martin's 'best interests' to die? All these questions, of course, central as they are to the legal issues, are questions of value. A relevant case, that brings out the clearly value-laden nature of judgments 'best interests', is that of Tony Blond.

The 'Tony Bland' case

The courts have decided, in the case of permanently insensate patients, that it may sometimes lie in the patient's best interests to die (*Airedale NHS Trust v Bland* [1993] 1 All ER 821). In the 'Tony Bland' case, a young man, Tony Bland, suffered hypoxic brain damage when he was crushed during the Hillsborough disaster (a football match crowd disaster). His injuries caused the cessation of all his higher brain functions leading to an eventual diagnosis of 'persistent vegetative state', from which he would almost certainly never recover. Tony Bland was fed and hydrated through a tube in order to keep him alive. He was able to breathe unaided and digest his food. The hospital sought a court declaration allowing them to discontinue his 'treatment', i.e. his feeding and watering, which would lead to his almost inevitable death.

The case eventually reached the House of Lords. Here, the Law Lords were keen to detach the issue of 'best interests' from the eventuality of Tony Bland's inevitable death and relate it rather to the issue of his 'treatment'.

Thus three of the Law Lords (Lords Goff, Browne-Wilkinson, and Lowrie) argued (in what is clearly a process of balancing different values) that the burdens outweighed the benefits of continued treatment, thus rendering it 'futile' (another clearly evaluative judgment) and, therefore, not in Tony Bland's 'best interests'. Two others (Lords Mustill and Keith) argued that Tony Bland's injuries had deprived him of his interests entirely, thus there was nothing to weigh in the balance. Their Lordships were not clear about whether Tony Bland's doctors had a duty or discretion to discontinue 'futile' treatment. Their Lordships were clear, however, that the patient's interests were a matter of clinical judgment (following *F v West Berkshire*). Whether their Lordships were right to translate the *Bolam* test for the medical standard of care into the critical legal justification for the withdrawal of treatment remains a moot point.

Living wills (or advance directives)

Martin's case can be distinguished from Tony Bland's case in one obvious respect, namely that Tony Bland was not in a position to make his wishes known. Patients can give advance indications of treatment refusal, in the form of what now in the UK amounts to a legally binding 'living will' (in the case of refusal of specific interventions in clearly defined circumstances) *or* can indicate their wishes, either in favour or against types of treatment, through an 'advance statement' (in relation to less clearly defined circumstances and treatment). Both advance refusals and advance statements become applicable in the event of subsequent incompetence. The current draft Mental Health Bill, however, will continue the current exclusion of treatment for mental disorder under the Act from the terms of advance refusals, although looser and non-binding advance statements may have some role to play. The Mental Capacity Act, 2005 dealing with treatment for physical conditions, as well as mental conditions not treated under the Mental Health Act, puts advance decisions to refuse treatment in the event of incapacity on a statutory footing where the patient is suffering 'because of an impairment of or a disturbance in the functioning of the brain.' Where advance refusals are unambiguous and unequivocal (in writing, signed and witnessed), both doctors and the courts will be required to honour them, even if refusal of life-saving treatment is stipulated.

However, would it ever be possible to indicate a desire for assisted suicide or euthanasia in advance? This brings us back to the crux of the issue of rational suicide, i.e. the inescapable role of values, and of balancing different values, in ethical and legal determinations of best interests.

True values?

If 'best interests' are constituted by the values of the patient, then it is difficult to see how the patient could not be best placed to determine them. Martin sincerely believes that there is no meaning or value in his life. Who are we to disagree? Martin's mental anguish might be so extreme that he no longer has a worthwhile life. In other words the burdens of his continued existence outweighs the benefits, thus rendering his continuing existence 'futile'. If Martin's death wish is unequivocal, then does the court not have a legal obligation to endorse his wish to be treated (as he is the best judge) in his 'best interests'?

We could argue, on the other hand, that the issues of a worthwhile life and worthwhile treatment need to be distinguished, as they were in the Tony Bland case. This line of reasoning is based on the doctrine of *double effect*, a principle that seeks to resolve tension between some kinds of conflicting values by stipulating that it is good to intend the good even though bad will inevitably result. In the Tony Bland context, it was right to discontinue futile treatment (good) even though his death would inevitably result (bad).

This is quite different, however, from being asked to endorse a patient's self-assessment as a mark of respect for patient self-determination. In other words, Martin can kill himself if he wants to, but don't make us a part of it. Because, by helping him, we will be endorsing implicitly the value proposition that some lives can be worthless. It could be argued that doctors are not required to identify with their patient's values, but merely to help him live or die in a manner that is consistent with those values. However, should things be that simple? Doctors have never been automatons responding mechanically to patient treatment requests. Doctors have to set criteria to distinguish hopeless cases from those for whom there is still hope. Yet this perhaps suggests, with a return to the desire for the 'golden bullet' of an objective test, some 'true values' standard against which the patient's values must be judged.

Reflection on the session and self-test questions

Write down your own reflections on the materials in this Session drawing out any points that are particularly significant for you. Then write brief notes about the following:

1. What do legal cases involving enforced Caesarian sections show in terms of judicial values?

2. Why might judicial values be problematic?

3. What does generic capacity legislation seek to achieve?

4. Does the concept of 'best interests', widely used as it is in legal contexts, make legal judgments objective?

Conclusions: diagnostic values in law and medicine

We have aimed in this chapter to examine the concepts of rationality and consent from a medico-legal viewpoint with particular reference to the (irreducable) role of (often conflicting) values and hence the (potential) importance of values-based approaches.

In relation to consent, we have argued that the law of consent reflects the ethical principle of self-determination. The law has sought to give a legal guarantee to those expressions of will that demonstrate that the patient has made a true choice. The theory is that a patient will be deemed competent if he can prove that he is capable of understanding the nature, purpose, and effects of the treatment proposed. The courts will regard a patient as competent if he can demonstrate to the court that he has the requisite cognitive decision-making powers to make a genuine treatment decision. This decision-making capacity, in adults, will be presumed, but, in children under 16, and perhaps between 16 and 18, will require evidence. The courts have strongly indicated that they are prepared to apply largely cognitive criteria in the cases of children (*Gillick*) and those adults suffering from mental disorders (*Re C* and the moves towards generic incapacity criteria).

Values visible!

However, the courts have been prepared to abridge the principle of self-determination in certain cases and this is where values start to become visible.

Thus, the courts have extended their protection where the life of the patient is in danger, or where non-intervention would have grave and adverse effects on the patient's health. With children, this has involved a dubiously defensive interpretation of the 'common law' of consent, and, with heavily pregnant women, rather an expansive use of mental health legislation. With both, the courts have revealed a reluctance to inquire too closely into the state of the patient's mind, perhaps for fear of finding the patient's cognitive decision-making powers intact. In these cases, arguably, hidden or acknowledged values are driving the courts to push the law of consent away from autonomy (self-determination) and towards beneficence (protective interventions).

Values invisible (and dangerous)

From the perspective of mental health, it is a particular concern that the unacknowledged legal values at work in these cases are *diagnostically related* values, i.e. values operating through such legal concepts as 'soundness of mind' and 'rationality'. To the extent that these concepts are assumed to be matters for expert testimony, hence matters of value-free medical evidence (from a 'man of science', you will recall, in the legal aphorism), the courts are working with the same incomplete conceptual model of medicine, the half-field view, that we explored in detail in Part I, and that, in Chapter 18, we identified as being at the root of the vulnerability of psychiatry to abusive misuses of its diagnostic categories (as in the former USSR).

Diagnostic determinations, legal and medical

This is not to say that such abuses are a feature of current legal determinations. But the risk is there so long as the courts operate, and as we have argued medicine itself continues to operate, with an incomplete—fact-only and values-free—model of its diagnostic concepts. The risk, furthermore, as we saw in Part III, is compounded so long as psychiatry, in particular, as the most 'medical' of the mental health professional disciplines, continues to work within an oversimplistic model of its own scientific infra-structure, a model embracing only one side (the 'causal' side) of the much richer, if conceptually more challenging, twin-stranded (causes + meanings) model, the origins of which, in Jaspers' psychopathology, we traced in Part II to the *Methodenstreit* of nineteenth century philosophy and psychology, and that, in Part V we will find reflected in a major debate in modern philosophy of mind about the relationship between *reasons* and causes or, more precisely, reasons and (causal) laws.

A key item, then, on the agenda of mental health in the twenty-first century, will be to clarify the role of value judgements in the assessment of mental health problems in general, and in medical diagnostic assessments in particular. It is to the contribution par-ticularly of linguistic analytic philosophy to this agenda that we turn in Chapters 20 and 21.

Reading guide

Introduction to medical law

A lively and readable introduction to key issues in medical law is Margot Brazier's (1992) *Medicine, Patients and the Law*. 'Kennedy and Grubb' (Kennedy, I. & Grubb, A., 2000) *Medical Law: text with materials*, (3rd end) has become known as 'the Bible of UK medical law'. It contains extracts from legal cases, legislation, and scholarly articles. Eastman and Peay's (1999) *Law Without Enforcement*, analyses the interface between the-ories of justice and mental health.

Other useful sources include:

- Moore (1984) *Law and Psychiatry: rethinking the relationship*;

- Davies (1996) *Textbook on Medical Law*: chapters 6 (Ethical and legal basis of consent), and 7 (Informed consent to medical treatment);

- Mason and McCall Smith (1999) *Law and Medical Ethics*: chapters 10 (Consent to treatment), 21–22 (Psychiatry and the law);

- McHale, Fox, and Murphy (1999) *Health Care Law: text and materials*: chapters 5 (Capacity), 6 (Consent), 7 (Children), 9 (Mental health), and 12 (Reproductive choice II: abortion);

- Montgomery (1997) *Health Care Law*: chapters 10 (Consent to treatment), and 12 (Care for children).

If you are interested in following through the some of the cases qualifying the traditional medical standard of care, have a look at:

- Maynard v West Midlands RHA [1984] 1 WL-1-R 643 (House of Lords) (pre-Sidaway) Smith v Tunbridge Wells Health Authority [1994] 5 Med LR (High Court), and Joyce v Merton, Sutton and Wandsworth Health Authority [1996] 7 Med LR 1 (Court of Appeal)

An important exemplar of the value of comparative empirical studies of decision-making by lawyers and others is Jill Peay's (2003) *Decisions and Dilemmoy*.

Rationality, responsibility and mental illness as an excuse in law

Detailed reading guides on rationality and responsibility in medical ethics and law are included in chapter 4 of Dickenson and Fulford's *In Two Minds*.

Rationality, responsibility and psychopathology

Although there is a large philosophical literature on rationality and irrationality (to which we return later, especially in Part V), the rich variety of different forms of irrationality represented by psychopathology has been largely ignored. Among important exceptions are Bermudez (2001) on delusion, and Gardner's (1993) *Irrationality and the Philosophy of Psychoanalysis*. As noted in chapter 18, Beauchamp and Childress' (1989) *Principles of Biomedical Ethics* is one of the few bioethical accounts to take seriously the problem of judgements of rationality specifically in psychiatry. As also noted in Chapter 18, Fulford and Hope (1993) have argued that Beauchamp and Childress' competen-cies approach works well for organic conditions such as demen-tia but fails to account for the kinds of irrationality exhibited by the functional disorders. A detailed treatment of the failure of traditional accounts of rationality to explain the ethical and legal status of delusion and other psychotic symptoms is given in chapter 10 of Fulford's (1989) *Moral Theory and Medical Practice*; this is developed further in his *Value, Action, Mental Illness, and the Law* (1993). See also the classic, Fingarette's (1972) *Insanity and Responsibility*, and among more recent accounts, Bermudez, 2001.

A feminist reconstruction of rationality, exploring the tradi-tional philosophical links between agency and rationality, can be found in Donna Dickenson's (1997) *Property, Women and Politics: Subjects or Objects?*, in the section 'Rationality and its discontents' (pp. 148–152). The significance of self-injurious behaviour is explored in Potter (2003a), with commentaries by Kruger (2003), Morris (2003), Sargent (2003), Woolfolk (2003), and a response by Potter (2003b).

Mental illness as a legal excuse

Mental illness as an excusing condition and, correspondingly, as a condition invalidating choice, is explored in *Philosophy*,

Psychiatry, & Psychology in Lavin's (1995) 'Who should be committable?' with a commentary by Brazier (1995). The issues of responsibility raised by dissociative states are discussed by Braude (1996) in his 'Multiple personality and moral responsibility' with commentaries by Clarke (1996) and Shuman (1996). Both Wilson's (1996) 'Sanity and responsibility', with commentaries by Fields (1996c) and Elliott (1996), and Robinson's (2000a) 'Madness, badness and fitness: law and psychiatry (again)', with a commentary by Broekman (2000) and a response (Robinson, 2000b), examine wider issues of mental disorder and responsibility.

A clear introduction to legal responsibility from the perspective of philosophy of law is H.L.A. Hart's (1968) *Punishment and Responsibility*. Anthony Flew's (1973) *Crime or Disease?* is a classic philosophical treatment of the issues. Lucas (1993) *Responsibility* is a clear analysis of the philosophical issues. McMillan (2003) provides an excellent recent update.

The role of mental illness as an excuse in law has been widely debated particularly in relation to the 'insanity defence' and related legal pleas. We noted in Part I, Daniel Robinson's (1996) scholarly historical *tour de force* on this topic, in his *Wild Beasts and Idle Humours*. Classic treatments include Nigel Walker's (1968) *Crime and Insanity in England* and the philosopher Anthony Flew's (1973) *Crime or Disease?*. The first chapter of R.A. Duff's (1986) *Trials and Punishments* offers a careful philosophical treatment. Lawrie Reznek's (1997) *Evil or Ill?* includes a valuable review of the issues. Henry Tam's (1996) *Punishment, Excuses and Moral Development* is a useful edited collection covering issues of responsibility from a number of perspectives, legal, bioethical, sociological, etc.

A clear introduction to the philosophical deep waters of determinism and responsibility is Mary Warnock's (1998a) 'Freedom, responsibility and determinism' (chapter 5 in her *An Intelligent Person's Guide to Ethics*). Jonathan Glover's (1970) *Responsibility* includes detailed analyses of the ways in which different forms of psychopathology may undermine responsibility.

Philosophy, Psychiatry, & Psychology has published a number of articles on responsibility and personality disorder: see, for example, Elliott's (1994) 'Puppetmasters and personality disorders: Wittgenstein, mechanism, and moral responsibility' with a commentary by Grant Gillett (1994); Fields' (1996a) 'Other-regarding moral beliefs, and responsibility' with commentaries by Adshead (1996), Duff (1996), Radden (1996), and a response by the author (Fields, 1996b); Benn's (1999a) 'Freedom, resentment, and the psychopath' with commentaries by Adshead (1999), Harold and Elliott (1999), Gillett (1999), and Slovenko (1999), and a response by Benn (1999b); and Ciocchetti's (2003a) 'The responsibility of the psychopathic offender' with commentaries by Adshead (2003), Benn (2003), and Shuman (2003), and a response by Ciocchetti (2003b). Woodbridge's (2003) *The Forgotten Self: training mental health and social care workers to work with service users*

shows the continuities between so-called borderline personality disorder and everyday responses to trauma, that can be explored in training.

Court-ordered Caesarian sections

The phenomenon of court-ordered Caesareans has caused much controversy and debate. See, for example Rhoden (1986) 'The Judge in the delivery room: the emergence of court ordered caesareans', and Stern (1993) 'Court-ordered Caesarian sections: in whose interests?'.

Psychiatric euthanasia

Jonathan Glover's (1977, second edition 1992) *Causing Death and Saving Lives* is a readable and thought-provoking pioneering work, written from a broadly utilitarian viewpoint. Many aspects of the rationality (or otherwise) of suicide are explored in a thematic issue of *Philosophy, Psychiatry & Psychology* on Suicide and Psychiatric Euthanasia (Volume 5 (2), 1998). This issue is based around a series of case studies by the Oxford psychiatrists, Sally Burgess and Keith Hawton (1998a), with commentaries by Warnock (1998b), Berghmans (a perspective from the Netherlands) (1998), Heginbotham (1998), Burnside (1998), Kelleher (1998), and the author's response (Burgess and Hawton, 1998b). Fairbairn explores the linguistic-analytic issues in his (1998a) 'Suicide, language, and clinical practice', with commentaries by Harré (1998) and Sadler (1998) and a response (Fairbairn, 1998b). Matthews' (1998) provides a philosophical overview, 'Choosing death: philosophical observations on suicide and euthanasia', and Montgomery (1998) a detailed legal 'footnote' in 'Suicide, euthanasia, and the psychiatrist'. Advance Directives in psychiatry and the importance of 'time frames' are explored in Savulescu and Dickenson's (1998a) 'The time frame of preferences, dispositions, and the validity of advance directives for the mentally ill', with commentaries by Dresser (1998), Brock (1998), Burgess (1998), and Eastman (1998), and a response (Savulescu and Dickenson, 1998b).

References

Adshead, G. (1996). Psychopathy, other-regarding moral beliefs, and responsibility. (Commentary on Fields, 1996a). *Philosophy, Psychiatry, & Psychology*, 3(4): 279–282.

Adshead, G. (1999). Psychopaths and other-regarding beliefs. (Commentary on Benn, 1999a). *Philosophy, Psychiatry, & Psychology*, 6/1: 41–44.

Adshead, G. (2003). Measuring moral identities: psychopaths and responsibility. (Commentary on Ciocchetti, 2003a). *Philosophy, Psychiatry, & Psychology*, 10(2): 185–188.

Austin, J.L. (1956–7) A plea for excuses. Proceedings of the Aristotelian Society 57:1–30. Reprinted in White, A.R., ed. (1968) *The Philosophy of Action.* Oxford: Oxford University Press, pps 19–42.

Beauchamp, T.L. and Childress, J.F. (1989). *Principles of Biomedical Ethics.* Oxford: Oxford University Press.

Benn, P. (1999a). Freedom, resentment, and the psychopath. *Philosophy, Psychiatry, & Psychology*, 6/1: 29–40.

Benn, P. (1999b). Response to the Commentaries. *Philosophy, Psychiatry, & Psychology*, 6/1: 57–58.

Benn, P. (2003). The responsibility of the psychopathic offender: a comment on Ciocchetti. (Commentary on Ciocchetti, 2003a). *Philosophy, Psychiatry, & Psychology*, 10(2): 189–192.

Berghmans, R. (1998). Suicide, euthanasia, and the psychiatrist (Commentary on Burgess and Hawton, 1998a). *Philosophy, Psychiatry, & Psychology*, 5(2): 131–136.

Bermudez, J.L. (2001). Normativity and rationality in delusional psychiatric disorders. *Mind & Language*, 16(5): 457–493.

Braude, S.E. (1996). Multiple personality and moral responsibility. *Philosophy, Psychiatry, & Psychology*, 3/1: 37–54.

Brazier, M. (1992). *Medicine, Patients and the Law.* London: Penguin.

Brazier, M. (1995). Who should be committable? (Commentary on Lavin, 1995). *Philosophy, Psychiatry, & Psychology*, 21: 49–50.

Brock, D.W. (1998). Time frame of preferences, dispositions, and advance directives.(Commentary on Savulescu and Dickenson, 1998a). *Philosophy, Psychiatry, & Psychology*, 5(3): 251–254.

Broekman, J. (2000). Unordered lives. (Commentary on Robinson, 2000a). *Philosophy, Psychiatry, & Psychology*, 7(3): 223–228.

Burgess, S. (1998). Time frame of preferences, dispositions, and advance directives. (Commentary on Savulescu and Dickenson, 1998a). *Philosophy, Psychiatry, & Psychology*, 5(3): 255–258.

Burgess, S. and Hawton, K. (1998a). Suicide, euthanasia, and the psychiatrist. *Philosophy, Psychiatry, & Psychology*, 5(2): 113–126.

Burgess, S. and Hawton, K. (1998b). Response to the Commentaries. *Philosophy, Psychiatry, & Psychology*, 5(2): 151–152.

Burnside, J.W. (1998). Suicide, euthanasia, and the psychiatrist (Commentary on Burgess and Hawton, 1998a). *Philosophy, Psychiatry, & Psychology*, 5(2): 141–144.

Ciocchetti, C. (2003a). The responsibility of the psychopathic offender. *Philosophy, Psychiatry, & Psychology*, 10(2): 175–184.

Ciocchetti, C. (2003b). Some thoughts on diverse psychopathic offenders and legal responsibility. (Response to commentaries). *Philosophy, Psychiatry, & Psychology*, 10(2): 195–198.

Clark, S.R.L. (1996). Multiple personality and moral responsibility. (Commentary on Braude, 1996). *Philosophy, Psychiatry, & Psychology*, 3/1: 55–58.

Davies, M. (1996). *Textbook on Medical Law.* London: Blackwell.

Department of Health and Welsh Office (1993) *Code of Practice: Mental Health Act 1983.* London: HMSO.

Dickenson, D. (1997). Rationality and its discontents. In *Property, Women and Politics: subjects or objects?* Cambridge: Polity Press, pp. 148–152.

Dickenson, D. and Fulford, K.W.M. (ed.) (2000). *In Two Minds: a casebook of psychiatric ethics.* Oxford: Oxford University Press.

Dresser, R. (1998). Time frame of preferences, dispositions, and advance directives. (Commentary on Savulescu and Dickenson, 1998a). *Philosophy, Psychiatry, & Psychology*, 5(3): 247–250.

Duff, R.A. (1986). *Trials and Punishments.* Cambridge: Cambridge University Press.

Duff, R.A. (1996). Psychopathy, other-regarding moral beliefs, and responsibility. (Commentary on Fields, 1996a). *Philosophy, Psychiatry, & Psychology*, 3(4): 283–286.

Eastman, N.L.G. (1998). Time frame of preferences, dispositions, and advance directives. (Commentary on Savulescu and Dickenson, 1998a). *Philosophy, Psychiatry, & Psychology*, 5(3): 259–262.

Eastman, N., and Peay, J., (1999) (Eds) *Law without enforcement: Integrating mental health and justice.* Oxford and Portland, Oregon: Hart Publishing.

Elliott, C. (1996). Key Concepts: Criminal Responsibility. *Philosophy, Psychiatry, & Psychology*, 3/4: 305–308.

Elliott, C. (1994). Puppetmasters and personality disorders: Wittgenstein, mechanism, and moral responsibility. *Philosophy, Psychiatry, & Psychology*, 1(2): 91–100.

Fairbairn, G.J. (1998a). Suicide, language, and clinical practice. *Philosophy, Psychiatry, & Psychology*, 5(2): 157–170.

Fairbairn, G.J. (1998b). Response to the Commentaries. *Philosophy, Psychiatry, & Psychology*, 5(2): 179–180.

Fields, L. (1996a). Psychopathy, other-regarding moral beliefs, and responsibility. *Philosophy, Psychiatry, & Psychology*, 3(4): 261–278.

Fields, L. (1996b). Response to the Commentaries. *Philosophy, Psychiatry, & Psychology*, 3(4): 291–292.

Fields, L., (1996c) Commentary on Wilson (1996) "Sanity and Irresponsibility". *Philosophy, Psychiatry, & Psychology*, 3/4, 303–304.

Fingarette, H. (1972). Insanity and responsibility. *Inquiry*, 15: 6–29.

Flew, A. (1973). *Crime or Disease?* New York: Barnes and Noble.

Fulford, K.W.M. (1989). *Moral Theory and Medical Practice*. Cambridge: Cambridge University Press.

Fulford, K.W.M. (1993). Value, Action, Mental Illness and the Law. In Shute S., Gardner J., and Horder, J., eds. *Action and Value in Criminal Law*. Oxford: Oxford University Press, pps 279–310.

Fulford, K.W.M. (1998). Replacing the Mental Health Act 1983? How to change the game without losing the baby with the bath water or shooting ourselves in the foot. *Psychiatric Bulletin*, 22: 666–668.

Fulford, K.W.M. and Hope, T. (1993). Psychiatric ethics: a bioethical ugly duckling? In *Principles of Health Care Ethics* (ed. R. Gillon and A. Lloyd). Chichester: John Wiley and Sons, Chapter 58.

Gardner, S. (1993). *Irrationality and the Philosophy of Psychoanalysis*. Cambridge: Cambridge University Press.

Gillett, G. (1994). Puppetmasters and personality disorders. (Commentary on Elliott, 1994). *Philosophy, Psychiatry, & Psychology*, 1(2): 101–104.

Gillett, G. (1999). Benn-ding the rules of resentment. (Commentary on Benn, 1999a). *Philosophy, Psychiatry, & Psychology*, 6/1: 49–52.

Glover, J. (1970). *Responsibility*. London: Routledge & Kegan Paul.

Glover, J. (1977). *Causing Death and Saving Lives*. England: Penguin Books Ltd (2nd edn 1992).

Harold, J. and Elliott, C. (1999). Travelers, mercenaries, and psychopaths. (Commentary on Benn, 1999a). *Philosophy, Psychiatry, & Psychology*, 61: 45–48.

Harré, R. (1998). Suicide, language, and clinical practice. (Commentary on Fairbairn, 1998a). *Philosophy, Psychiatry, & Psychology*, 5(2): 171–174.

Hart, H.L.A. (1968). *Punishment and responsibility: essays in the philosophy of law*. Oxford: Oxford University Press.

Heginbotham, C. (1998). Suicide, euthanasia, and the psychiatrist (Commentary on Burgess and Hawton, 1998a). *Philosophy, Psychiatry, & Psychology*, 5(2): 137–140.

Kelleher, M.J. (1998). Suicide, euthanasia, and the psychiatrist (Commentary on Burgess and Hawton, 1998a). *Philosophy, Psychiatry, & Psychology*, 5(2): 145–150.

Kennedy, I. (1981). *The Unmasking of Medicine*. London: George Allen and Unwin.

Kennedy, I. (1996[1988]). Patients, doctors and human rights. In *Treat Me Right: essays in medical law and ethics*. Oxford: Clarendon Press.

Kennedy, I. and Grubb, A. (2000). *Medical Law: text with materials*, (3rd edn). London: Butterworths.

Kruger, C. (2003). Self-injury: symbolic sacrifice/self-assertion renders clinicians helpless. (Commentary on Potter, 2003a). *Philosophy, Psychiatry, & Psychology*, 10/1: 17–22.

Lavin, M. (1995). Who should be committable? *Philosophy, Psychiatry, & Psychology*, 21: 35–48.

Lord Chancellor's Department (1997). *Who Decides? Making Decisions on Behalf of Mentally Incapacitated Adults*, CM 3803, London: The Stationary Office Ltd.

Lucas, F.R. (1993). *Responsibility*. Oxford: Clarendon Press.

Mason, J.K. and McCall Smith, R.A. (1999). *Law and Medical Ethics*. London: Butterworths.

Matthews, E. (1998). Choosing death: philosophical observations on suicide and euthanasia. *Philosophy, Psychiatry, & Psychology*, 5(2): 107–112.

Matthews, E. (1999). Mental and Physical Illness: An Unsustainable Separation? In Eastman, N. and Peay, J. (eds). *Law without Enforcement: Integrating mental health and justice*. Oxford and Portland, Oregan: Hart Publishing.

McHale, J., Fox, M., and Murphy, J. (1999). *Health Care Law: text and materials*. London: Sweet and Maxwell.

McMillan, J. (2003). Dangerousness, mental disorder, and responsibility. *Journal Medical Ethics*, 0: 232–235.

Montgomery, J. (1997). *Health Care Law*. Oxford: Oxford University Press.

Montgomery, J. (1998). Suicide, euthanasia, and the psychiatrist: a legal footnote. *Philosophy, Psychiatry, & Psychology*, 5(2): 153–156.

Moore, M.S. (1984). *Law and Psychiatry: rethinking the relationship*. Cambridge: Cambridge University Press.

Morris, K. (2003). Commentary on 'Did you hurt yourself?' (Commentary on Potter, 2003a). *Philosophy, Psychiatry, & Psychology*, 10/1: 23–24.

Peay, J. (2003). *Decisions and Dilemmas: Working with Mental Health Law*. Portland, Oregon: Hart Publishing.

Potter, N.N. (2003a). Commodity/body/sign: borderline personality disorder and the signification of self-injurious behavior. *Philosophy, Psychiatry, & Psychology*, 101: 1–16.

Potter, N.N. (2003b). In the spirit of giving uptake. Response to the commentaries. *Philosophy, Psychiatry, & Psychology*, 101: 33–36.

Radden, J. (1996). Psychopathy, other-regarding moral beliefs, and responsibility. (Commentary on Fields, 1996a). *Philosophy, Psychiatry, & Psychology*, 3(4): 287–290.

Reznek, L. (1997). *Evil or Ill?*. London: Routledge.

Rhoden, N, (1986). The Judge in the delivery room: the emergence of court ordered caesareans, *California Law Review*, 74: 1951.

Robinson, D. (1996). *Wild Beasts and Idle Humours*. Cambridge, MA: Harvard University Press.

Robinson, D.N. (2000a). Madness, badness, and fitness: law and psychiatry (again). *Philosophy, Psychiatry, & Psychology*, 7(3): 209–222.

Robinson, D.N. (2000b). Stories as tales and as histories: A response to the commentary. (Commentary on Robinson, 2000a). *Philosophy, Psychiatry, & Psychology*, 7(3): 229–230.

Sadler, J.Z. (1998). Suicide, language, and clinical practice. (Commentary on Fairbairn, 1998a). *Philosophy, Psychiatry, & Psychology*, 5(2): 175–178.

Sargent, C. (2003). Gender, body, meaning: anthropological perspectives on self-injury and borderline personality disorder. (Commentary on Potter, 2003a). *Philosophy, Psychiatry, & Psychology*, 10/1: 25–28.

Savulescu, J. and Dickenson, D. (1998a). The time frame of preferences, dispositions, and the validity of advance directives for the mentally ill. *Philosophy, Psychiatry, & Psychology*, 5(3): 225–246.

Savulescu, J. and Dickenson, D. (1998b). Response to the Commentaries. *Philosophy, Psychiatry, & Psychology*, 5(3): 263–266.

Sayce, L. (1998). Transcending mental health law. *Psychiatric Bulletin*, 22: 666–670.

Shuman, D.W. (1996). Multiple personality and moral responsibility. (Commentary on Braude, 1996). *Philosophy, Psychiatry, & Psychology*, 3/1: 59–60.

Shuman, D.W. (2003). A Comment on Christopher Ciocchetti: The responsibility of the psychopathic offender.

(Commentary on Ciocchetti, 2003a). *Philosophy, Psychiatry, & Psychology*, 10(2): 193–194.

Slovenko, R. (1999). Responsibility of the psychopath. (Commentary on Benn, 1999a). *Philosophy, Psychiatry, & Psychology*, 6: 53–56.

Stern, K (1993). Court-ordered Caesarian sections: in whose interests? Modern Law Review, 56: 238–243.

Szmukler, G. and Holloway, F. (1998). Mental health legislation is now a harmful anachronism. *Psychiatric Bulletin*, 22: 662–665.

Tam, H. (1996). *Punishment, Excuses and Moral Development*. Aldershot: Avebury Press.

Walker, N. (1968). *Crime and Insanity in England*. Volume one: The Historical Perspective. Edinburgh: University Press.

Warnock, M. (1998a). Freedom, responsibility and determinism. In *An Intelligent Person's Guide to Ethics*, Chapter 5.

Warnock, The Baroness M. (1998b). Suicide, euthanasia, and the psychiatrist (Commentary on Burgess and Hawton, 1998a). *Philosophy, Psychiatry, & Psychology*, 5(2): 127–130.

Wilson, P.E. (1996). Sanity and irresponsibility. *Philosophy, Psychiatry, & Psychology*, 3(4): 293–302.

Woodbridge (2003). *The Forgotten Self: training mental health and social care workers to work with service users*. Philosophy, Psychiatry, & Psychology, 10/4: 373–378

Woolfolk, R. (2003). On the border: reflections on the meaning of self-injury in borderline personality disorder. (Commentary on Potter, 2003a). *Philosophy, Psychiatry, & Psychology*, 10/11: 29–32.

CHAPTER 20

Values in psychiatric diagnosis

Chapter contents

In this chapter we will follow through the key point to emerge from earlier chapters in this part, i.e. that in psychiatric ethics, at least, we need to move on from the increasingly quasi-legal form that bioethics is taking in its connections with practice, to what we have called Values-Based Practice (VBP).

The essence of this move, as we indicated at the end of Chapter 18, is to start, not from prescribed values (encoded in the rules and regulations of quasi-legal bioethics), but from respect for the often very different values of the particular individuals and groups involved in particular clinical contexts. VBP, as we called the approach resulting from this move, is not a recipe for relativism and ethical chaos: to the contrary, it places strong constraints on practice, illustrated in Chapter 18 with the NIMHE Values Framework (Figure 18.6). VBP, furthermore, builds on and extends the tools for clinical decision-making provided by the framework of law within which health care operates. We outlined some of these legal tools in Chapter 19. We found that, in the context of mental health at least, the use of these legal tools in practice, no less than the quasi-legal tools of mainstream bioethics, involved value judgements.

Background: the medical model of diagnosis

What all this amounts to, then, on the ground as it were, is that health-care decision-making, although based firmly on evidence (broadly understood as including implicit as well as explicit knowledge), necessarily also involves making value judgements.

It is relatively easy to see that values as well as evidence are important in connection with issues of treatment choice. What we will find in this chapter is that in the area of *mental* health at least, values (as well as evidence) are important also to *diagnosis*.

From the perspective of the traditional science-based 'medical' model, the claim that values are important in diagnosis as well as treatment, may seem to involve a radical, even subversive, departure from the aspirations to scientific 'objectivity' on which the authority of health-care professionals has traditionally been taken to rest. Thus, we have encountered the medical (fact only) model of diagnosis at several points:

- it was implicit in the psychiatry versus antipsychiatry debate from which we started in the first chapter of Part I;

- it was made explicit in the conceptual work of Christopher Boorse, in his distinction between disease (as covering the science-based theoretical core of medicine) and illness (as bringing in values to medical practice, see Chapter 4);

- earlier in this part, the same medical model was shown to lie behind the focus in traditional bioethics on issues of treatment choice (recall Beauchamp and Childress' conclusion, that values are indeed involved in judgements of rationality but that this makes such judgements a matter of morals *not* medicine).

- and it is essentially the medical model of diagnosis, too, which lies at the heart of some of the particular difficulties of application of health-care law in mental health (Chapter 19).

Fact and value in psychiatric diagnosis

The traditional medical model, then, rests on the idea that, however crucial values may be in other areas of health care, diagnosis is a 'purely' scientific exercise. In psychiatry this amounts to the claim that *psychopathology* (symptoms) and the *classification* (of disorders), on which the *process of diagnosis* depends, must all be value-free.

It is with this claim that we will be concerned in this chapter and the next. Our conclusion, as already noted, will be that the traditional medical model, and the claim to value-free diagnosis on which it rests, is unsupportable; and that, to the contrary, diagnosis, although properly grounded on facts is also, and essentially, grounded on values. This conclusion, we will further indicate, set within the framework of VBP introduced at the end of Chapter 18, although currently of practical importance mainly for psychiatry, will become, under the pressure of twenty-first century medical-scientific advances, increasingly important in bodily medicine as well.

The conclusion that values are important in diagnosis, involving as it does 'adding values' rather than 'subtracting facts', is consistent with the additive nature of the full-field model of the conceptual structure of medicine to which we came at the end of Part I; it is consistent also with, and indeed spells out one element of, Jaspers' attempt to build a twin-track meanings + causes model of psychopathology (recall the values in/values out tension in his work that we traced in Chapter 10 at the end of Part II); and it is consistent with late twentieth century work in the philosophy of science, touched on at various points in Part III, showing the extent to which the scientific process, from observation and classification to explanation and theory construction, does not depend on merely passively recording data, but is instead actively shaped in complex judgements that resist full codification. It is also consistent, finally, with the view of psychiatric understanding in Chapter 15 and the subject matter of that understanding (to be explored throughout Part V), which resists assimilation to a model of science that stresses only subsumption of events under natural laws and construes mental states as reducible to brain states. Instead, as we will see in Part V, whatever the close dependence of mental states on brain states, psychiatry trades in the normatively structured space of reasons as well as the realm of natural law.

All the same, the conclusion that values are important in diagnosis, *is* a radical conclusion, at least from the perspective of the traditional medical model. It is a conclusion, furthermore, as we indicate in the final session of Chapter 21, which, however well founded theoretically, is in part promissory on future R&D. As with most other parts of this book, therefore, in reading this chapter and the next, it will be important to engage actively with the arguments rather than approaching them passively, as the presentation of a settled *corpus*.

Plan of Chapters 20 and 21

Chapters 20 and 21 should be read as a pair. Chapter 20 sets up the problem: it shows that values (although not always recognized as such) are present, and in some (central) cases diagnostically determinate, in the 'best of the best' diagnostic tools of modern medical-scientific psychiatry.

Chapter 21 then goes on to tackle the problem: it shows that the shift, outlined in Chapters 17 and 18 of this part, from quasi-legal bioethics to VBP, turns what would have traditionally been seen as the 'problem' of values in diagnosis, into an asset for balanced clinical decision-making.

The sessional structure of Chapters 20 and 21

The storyline of the two chapters runs thus:

- *Chapter 20, Session 1: the central place of values in psychiatric diagnosis—the case of Simon.* This session opens up the issues with a case study, involving a man called Simon, about delusion and religious experience. The differential diagnosis in this case suggests that, whatever the theoretical issues, values come into psychiatric diagnosis in its own scientific heartland, at the centre of the most scientific of modern classifications of mental disorder, the American DSM-IV.

- *Chapter 20, Session 2: generalization—the pervasiveness and importance of values in psychiatric diagnosis.* This session explores, (1) the pervasiveness of values in psychiatric psychopathology and classification, and (2) reviews key theoretical points from earlier chapters.

    The key message here will be the 'bottom line' of both Part I (concepts) and earlier chapters in this part of the book, namely, that values are important practically in psychiatric diagnosis, not because psychiatry is a primitive science, but because human values, in the areas with which psychiatry is concerned, are highly diverse.

- *Chapter 20, Session 3: bioethics and values in psychiatric diagnosis.* Unlike general bioethics, some of those working in psychiatric ethics have recognized the ethical importance of diagnosis. We look in detail at a key paper by Walter Reich from Sidney Bloch, Paul Chodoff and Stephen A. Green's ground-breaking *Psychiatric Ethics* (1999). We analyse the positive and negative points made by Reich about the ethics of psychiatric diagnosis.

- *Chapter 21, Session 1: philosophy, values, and psychiatric diagnosis.* This sets the contribution of philosophical value theory in context with other philosophical work on classification and diagnosis in psychiatry.

- *Chapter 21, Session 2: from fact-only to a fact + value model of psychiatric diagnosis.* Session 2 continues the analysis of Reich's paper (from chapter 20) but with an important new twist. Session 1 ended by identifying the origin of Reich's attitude to psychiatry (it is a mainly negative attitude) in the standard biomedical model. Session 2 moves 'beyond bioethics' to look at the way Reich's argument would run if we adopt the fact + value model developed in Part I of this book in place of the fact-only biomedical model.

- *Chapter 21, Session 3: reversing Reich.* This session applies the fact + value model to Reich's arguments against psychiatric diagnosis and shows, to the extent that they are indeed arguments *against* anything, they apply equally to diagnosis in bodily medicine.

- *Chapter 21, Session 4: practical applications—Values-Based Practice and psychiatric diagnosis.* The final session of Chapter 21 brings us to the practical applications of the recognition of the importance of values in psychiatric diagnosis. The approach here, again as anticipated earlier in this part, is of VBP, i.e. of values, as a key component of clinical decision-making, working alongside and inextricably linked to facts. This involves, in relation to diagnosis, communication skills and the 'user's' values, the role of different implicit models of disorder held by different members of multidisciplinary teams, and the importance of an 'open society' in psychiatry.

The last session of Chapter 21 is a 'blue skies' session, looking at the clinical and research agendas that are opened up by recognizing and taking seriously the importance of values in psychiatric diagnosis. It includes a sneak preview of a report, dated 2010, and commissioned by the (imaginary) future Chair of the Taskforce charged with producing DSM-VI. We leave it to you to decide whether this will turn out to be science fiction or what the British science-fiction writer, Arthur C. Clarke, calls 'science faction'!

Do the exercises!

A final 'scene setting' point is to note is that recognizing and understanding the importance of values in diagnosis requires a considerable shift of mindset from the traditional medical model. The idea that diagnosis is, somehow, a value-free scientific aspect of medical expertise is so deep rooted, in all of us (not just doctors and lawyers), that, even if it is mistaken, a considerable effort is required to displace it. And not only to displace it but to work through the implications, positive and negative, of giving up the fact-only model and replacing it with a fact + value model.

There will be new ideas to tackle, therefore, as well as some new literature (although we will also be drawing on and taking a fresh look at materials from earlier chapters). Grasping new ideas requires practice. Hence many of the exercises in this and Chapter 21, starting with the case history of Simon (below, Exercise 1), are 'thinking exercises', not just readings. As we have several times emphasized, you will get much more out of these exercises if you take the time to do them for yourself. Remember that 'short cuts make long routes home'.

Session 1 The central place of values in psychiatric diagnosis: the case of Simon

The first reading in this session is a practical exercise in what is called in medicine 'differential diagnosis'. The idea is to read the case history of Simon and to write down your interpretation of what is going on. In the rest of the session we will be looking at the two very different interpretations of Simon's case offered by the two major psychiatric classifications of mental disorder, the ICD and DSM.

The case of Simon

The exercise is not a philosophical or indeed medical 'test'. Simon's story, exactly as reproduced here, is used by one of us (K.W.M.F.) in routine teaching sessions on diagnosis for trainee psychiatrists. So if you are a 'medic' or other health-care professional, imagine that you are seeing Simon in the context of your everyday clinical work. If you are not a health-care professional, imagine that he is a friend, colleague, or relative. Either way, the idea is to think *for real* about how you would understand his story and hence what you would do, or would want done, *in practice*.

EXERCISE 1 (20 minutes)

Read Simon Greer's case history (case 4.3) from:

> Dickenson, D. and Fulford, K.W.M. (2000). *Rationality, responsibility and values*. Chapter 4, *In Two Minds: a casebook of psychiatric ethics*. Oxford: Oxford University Press. (Extract, p. 109–111.)

Link with Reading 20.1

Then write down:

1. your differential diagnosis, i.e. a list, in descending order of probability, of what you think could be going on, and

2. a few brief notes on your diagnostic reasoning, i.e. a few lines, again in note form, on the grounds for your interpretation(s) of Simon's case.

(This is based on a case described in Jackson and Fulford, 1997a.)

Note: there is a temptation here to jump straight to the 'answers' given below! But you will get much more out of this session, whether or not you are a health-care professional, if you spend some time thinking about Simon's story for yourself, and writing down your own views, before going on.

A differential diagnosis of Simon's case

Most psychiatrists reading Simon's story come up with a list of possible diagnoses along the following lines:

- schizophrenia
- hypomania (or bipolar disorder)
- schizoaffective disorder
- organic disorder (? drug induced)
- hysteria
- stress-induced disorder.

Similar lists are produced by other groups of health-care professionals (e.g. psychiatric nurses, social workers, etc.) and by lay or non-professional groups (with one exception, see below!).

Simon's experiences and the Present State Examination

Your own list may be different from the above but it is important to start from the fact that this is an entirely respectable set of possibilities, medically speaking. Indeed if a doctor, faced with Simon's story, failed to think of schizophrenia (top of the list) or some other psychotic condition (everything on the list except hysteria), he/she would justifiably be at risk for an action in negligence!

We looked at psychiatry's standard diagnostic reasoning, its two-step process from symptoms to syndromes, in Chapter 3. Applied to Simon's case, this two-step process runs roughly thus.

Step 1: identification of symptoms

Most psychiatrists pick out a clear symptom of schizophrenia (a 'first rank' symptom, as they are called) in Simon's account of his experiences of the 'wax seals' or 'suns'—this is what is called 'delusional perception', i.e. a set of delusional beliefs triggered by a normal perception. Psychiatrists also identify a possible further first rank symptom in Simon's account of his mind 'going on the fritz'. This could be 'thought insertion', the strange phenomenon we encountered in Chapter 3, the phenomenon of experiences that you are thinking and yet you experience as the thoughts of someone else.

Simon's account of his experiences have been 'rated' by people trained in the use of a research version of the standard psychiatric examination, the PSE (Present State Examination; Wing *et al.*, 1974). Such ratings consistently identify delusional perception, and, though less consistently, thought insertion.

The glossary to the PSE, as we noted in Chapter 3, defines over a hundred key psychiatric symptoms (and is thus a very useful source book for clear definitions of these symptoms). The PSE definitions of 'delusional perception' and 'thought insertion' show just how well Simon's experiences fit.

- *delusional perception*: PSE symptom 82 describes this as being 'based on sensory experiences' and involving 'suddenly becoming convinced that a particular set of events has a special meaning'.

- *thought insertion*: PSE symptom 55 describes this as 'the essence of the symptom is that the subject experiences thoughts which are not his own *intruding into his mind*' (emphasis in original).

Simon thus has one and possibly two clear 'first rank' symptoms, as defined by one of the gold standards of modern descriptive psychopathology. So what does this mean diagnostically?

Step 2: from symptoms to syndrome

The 'first rank' symptoms were originally thought to be diagnostic of schizophrenia but are now known to occur also in other psychotic conditions. The differential diagnosis thus depends on associated symptoms: Simon's somewhat grandiose self-references suggest 'hypomania' or the hybrid 'schizoaffective disorder'; its late onset, in a middle-aged man, raises the possibility of organic disorder (i.e. of gross pathology, such as Alzheimer's disease, affecting the brain, or drug use); hysteria, psychotic symptoms that are unconsciously motivated, is suggested (to some) by the rather dramatic 'style' of Simon's presentation; and stress-induced disorder is suggested by the close temporal link to his highly adverse life situation at the time (acute stress not uncommonly induces brief psychotic episodes).

Simon: the ICD diagnosis

One gold standard for the second step in psychiatric diagnosis is the World Health Organization's ICD-10. As we saw in Part III (Chapter 13), a key stage in the development of modern classifications of mental disorders was the move, inspired by the advice to the WHO of the philosopher of science, Carl Hempel, from aetiology-based to symptom-based classifications of mental disorder. Hence the criteria for most of the diagnoses in these classifications are based on symptoms or clusters of symptoms.

The ICD-10 criteria for schizophrenia are given in Box 20.1. As you can see, leaving aside the other differential diagnostic possibilities, these criteria leave us in no doubt that Simon's most likely diagnosis is schizophrenia. The diagnosis requires the presence of at least one 'first rank' symptom, and Simon has two! (He also satisfies the other criteria of more than 1 month's duration, etc.).

So, the diagnostic bottom line, according to two gold standards of psychiatric diagnosis, the PSE and ICD, is schizophrenia (or some related psychotic disorder).

Box 20.1

Extract from: WHO (1992). *The ICD-10 Classification of Mental and Behavioural Disorders*. Geneva: World Health Organization, Geneva.

Although no strictly pathognomonic symptoms can be identified, for practical purposes it is useful to divide the above symptoms into groups that have special importance for the diagnosis (of schizophrenia) and often occur together, such as:

(a) thought echo, thought insertion or withdrawal, and thought broadcasting;

(b) delusions of control, influence, or passivity, clearly referred to body or limb movements or specific thoughts, actions, or sensations; delusional perception;

(c) hallucinatory voices giving a running commentary on the patient's behaviour, or discussing the patient among themselves, or other types of hallucinatory voices coming from some part of the body;

(d) persistent delusions of other kinds that are culturally inappropriate and completely impossible, such as religious

or political identity, or superhuman powers and abilities (e.g. being able to control the weather, or being in communication with aliens from another world);

(e) persistent hallucinations in any modality, when accompanied either by fleeting or half-formed delusions without clear affective content, or by persistent over-valued ideas, or when occurring every day for weeks or months on end;

(f) breaks or interpolations in the train of thought, resulting in incoherence or irrelevant speech, or neologisms;

(g) catatonic behaviour, such as excitement, posturing, or waxy flexibility, negativism, mutism, and stupor;

(h) 'negative' symptoms such as marked apathy, paucity of speech, and blunting or incongruity of emotional responses, usually resulting in social withdrawal and lowering of social performance; it must be clear that these are not due to depression or to neuroleptic medication;

(i) a significant and consistent change in the overall quality of some aspects of personal behaviour, manifest as loss of interest, aimlessness, idleness, a self-absorbed attitude, and social withdrawal.

Diagnostic guidelines

The normal requirement for a diagnosis of schizophrenia is that a minimum of one very clear symptom (and usually two or more if less clear-cut) belonging to any one of the groups listed as (a) to (d) above, or symptoms from at least two of the groups referred to as (e) to (h), should have been clearly present for most of the time during a period of 1 month or more. Conditions meeting such symptomatic requirements but of duration less than 1 month (whether treated or not) should be diagnosed in the first instance as acute schizophrenia-like psychotic disorder and are classified as schizophrenia if the symptoms persist for longer periods.

Viewed retrospectively, it may be clear that a prodromal phase in which symptoms and behaviour, such as loss of interest in work, social activities, and personal appearance and hygiene, together with generalized anxiety and mild degrees of depression and preoccupation, preceded the onset of psychotic symptoms by weeks or even months. Because of the difficulty in timing onset, the 1-month duration criterion applies only to the specific symptoms listed above and not to any prodromal nonpsychotic phase.

The diagnosis of schizophrenia should not be made in the presence of extensive depressive or manic symptoms unless it is clear that schizophrenic symptoms antedated the affective disturbance. If both schizophrenic and affective symptoms develop together and are evenly balanced, the diagnosis of schizoaffective disorder should be made, even if the schizophrenic symptoms by themselves would have justified the diagnosis of schizophrenia. Schizophrenia should not be diagnosed in the presence of overt brain disease or during states of drug intoxication or withdrawal.

Simon's case history: outcome

The outlook, then, for Simon is not good. Schizophrenia of late onset, particularly associated with affective symptoms (suggested by his somewhat grandiose style), has a better prognosis than some. But schizophrenia is a severe illness, subject to relapse, and often associated with long-term loss of drive (the so-called 'negative' symptoms). So, what happened to Simon

---

EXERCISE 2   (10 minutes)

Read the second extract of Simon's story from:
Dickenson, D. and Fulford, K.W.M. (2000). Rationality, responsibility and values. Chapter 4, *In Two Minds: a casebook of psychiatric ethics*. Oxford: Oxford University Press. (Extract, p. 112.)

Link with Reading 20.2

◆ How does Simon's 'outcome' influence your diagnostic thinking?

◆ Does he really have schizophrenia?

The good outcome of Simon's story generally produces a split vote among mental health professionals. One reaction, perhaps the most common, is to say that he had a 'benign form' of schizophrenia. The counter to this is that he was not ill, after all, but undergoing a religious experience. Either way, the positive outcome of Simon's story comes as a shock to psychiatry. After all, the whole point of the careful description of symptoms and delineation of syndromes, on which modern psychiatric diagnosis is based, was to differentiate pathology from other, perhaps odd and unusual, but none the less non-pathological, states. This careful descriptive approach has been aimed precisely at clarifying the boundary between medicine and morals, here crucially instantiated in the difference between delusion and religious experience.

Simon's case, therefore, presenting with unequivocal symptoms of severe mental illness (as defined by the PSE and ICD), yet issuing in a highly adaptive rather than pathological outcome, prompts us to look more carefully at the diagnosis, and in particular at how we differentiate between spiritual experience and psychosis. The similarities between them have been recognized for many years. William James, the philosopher-psychologist who was one of the founding fathers of cultural anthropology, described 'delusional insanity' as 'religious mysticism turned upside down' (James, 1902). But how, then, are they to be differentiated?

Distinguishing delusion from religious experience

One approach is to rely on the general features distinguishing normal from pathological experience. We covered these in Chapter 4. The point was that all experiences occur in both normal and pathological forms—pain, nausea, etc. may all be normal as well as symptoms of illness. Psychologists, sociologists, and others, have studied the features that mark out the pathological: they

include severity and duration, for example. Such features, however, are not sufficient to distinguish delusion from religious experience here, for Simon's experiences are extreme (in this sense, severe) and they continued for at least 18 months.

A further marker of pathology, again considered in detail in Part I, is maladaptiveness. Here we seem closer to Simon's case, something along these lines being reflected in phenomenological approaches to the distinction (Jackson and Fulford, 1997a, p. 62, list a variety of such approaches in a summary table). Maladaptiveness, furthermore, has been incorporated as a distinct criterion in another gold standard of psychiatric classification, the American DSM.

Simon: the DSM diagnosis

The ICD and DSM, although in many respects closely similar, differ in an important respect in the criteria by which they define psychotic disorders. The ICD, as we have seen, sticks with the traditional first rank symptoms (together with secondary criteria such as a minimum duration).

Box 20.2 DSM IV, summary diagnostic criteria for schizophrenia

Diagnostic criteria for schizophrenia

A. Characteristic symptoms: Two (or more) of the following, each present for a significant portion of time during a 1-month period (or less if successfully treated):

(1) delusions

(2) hallucinations

(3) disorganized speech (e.g., frequent derailment or incoherence)

(4) grossly disorganized or catatonic behavior

(5) negative symptoms, i.e., affective flattening, alogia, or avolition

Note: Only one Criterion A symptom is required if delusions are bizarre or hallucinations consist of a voice keeping up a running commentary on the person's behavior or thoughts, or two or more voices conversing with each other.

B. Social/occupational dysfunction: For a significant portion of the time since the onset of the disturbance, one or more major areas of functioning such as work, interpersonal relations, or self-care are markedly below the level achieved prior to the onset (or when the onset is in childhood or adolescence, failure to achieve expected levels of interpersonal, academic, or occupational achievement).

C. Duration: Continuous signs of the disturbance persist for at least 6 months. This 6-month period must include at least 1 month of symptoms (or less if successfully treated) that meet Criterion A (i.e., active-phase symptoms) and may include periods of prodromal or residual symptoms.

During these prodromal or residual periods, the signs of the disturbance may be manifested by only negative symptoms or two or more symptoms listed in Criterion A present in an attenuated form (e.g., odd beliefs, unusual perceptual experiences).

D. Schizoaffective and Mood Disorder exclusion: Schizoaffective Disorder and Mood Disorder with Psychotic Features have been ruled out because either (1) no Major Depressive, Manic, or Mixed Episodes have occurred concurrently with the active-phase symptoms; or (2) if mood episodes have occurred during active-phase symptoms, their total duration has been brief relative to the duration of the active and residual periods.

E. Substance/general medical condition exclusion: The disturbance is not due to the direct physiological effects of a substance (e.g., a drug of abuse, a medication) or a general medical condition.

F. Relationship to a Pervasive Developmental Disorder: If there is a history of Autistic Disorder or another Pervasive Developmental Disorder, the additional diagnosis of Schizophrenia is made only if prominent delusions or hallucinations are also present for at least a month (or less if successfully treated).

The DSM's criteria are given in Box 20.2. This is taken from DSM-IV. The DSM gives detailed descriptions of all the conditions it covers together with boxes summarizing key diagnostic criteria (it is thus an excellent textbook in its own right).

Box 20.2 gives the summary box for schizophrenia. As you will see, besides the traditional first rank symptoms (defined more synoptically but in essentially the same way in DSM's Criterion A), DSM now includes a new criterion, Criterion B. This criterion, of 'social/occupational dysfunction' covers the 'maladaptation' element in the meaning of pathology and it is prima facie directly relevant to Simon's case.

EXERCISE 3   (10 minutes)

Read the criteria for schizophrenia in the DSM (look particularly at Criterion B) from Box 20.2.

♦ How does Criterion B affect your thinking about Simon?

♦ Does he have schizophrenia as defined in DSM?

Most people reading Criterion B in connection with Simon's case conclude that, by this criterion, Simon does *not* have schizophrenia. In so far as our information goes, far from showing a deterioration in social/occupational functioning, he was empowered!

DSM versus ICD

In the USA, then, as against the rest of the world, the gold standard tools of psychiatric diagnosis do not force us down the route of a diagnosis of schizophrenia (or other psychotic illness). In the USA we can say, consistently with the positive and empowering effects of Simon's experiences, that, idiosyncratic as they were, they are more appropriately understood in terms of religious or spiritual experience than in terms of pathology.

At first glance, this might seem to be very much 'one up' to evidence-based medicine. The justification for the American Psychiatric Association's determination to go their own way, and to develop a classification of mental disorders independently from the World Health Organization, was that it gave them the freedom to base their categories directly on best scientific evidence. Whereas the ICD, on this view, is in part a product of the compromises required for wide international acceptance.

The opening paragraphs of the Introduction to the DSM, as the next reading shows, reflect its overt commitment to a strongly evidence-based approach.

EXERCISE 4   (10 minutes)

Read the short extract from the Introduction to:

American Psychiatric Association (1994). *Diagnostic and Statistical Manual of Mental Disorders* (4th edn). Washington, DC: American Psychiatric Association. (Extract, p. xv.)

(We looked at a longer extract from the Introduction to DSM-IV in Reading 11.2.)

Link with Reading 20.3

♦ How many references (explicit or implicit) to evidence-based medicine can you spot?

In this paragraph alone there are two explicit references ('breadth of available evidence' and 'formal evidence-based process') and a number of implicit references (e.g. 'experts' twice; a 'wide range of perspectives', and 'consensus scholars') to an evidence-based approach in the DSM.

Values and Simon's diagnosis

This explanation, however, that the DSM has greater face validity in Simon's case than the ICD because ie is more evidence-based, fails to hold up when we look more carefully at Criterion B, the critical diagnostic criterion in Simon's case.

EXERCISE 5   (5 minutes)

Reread Criterion B from the DSM criteria for schizophrenia in Box 20.2 above. Is this an exclusively evidence-based criterion? If not, what else besides evidence (facts) is required to decide if Criterion B is satisfied in a given case?

Reading Criterion B with an eye sharpened philosophically by Part I of this book, it is manifestly an *evaluative* (rather than purely descriptive or factual) criterion: 'social/occupational *dysfunction*' (rather than merely different functioning), which is 'markedly *below* the level previously achieved', or, in the case of children, they '*fail* to achieve' their expected levels.

Fact and value in Criterion B

The conclusion, then, seems inescapable that Criterion B, notwithstanding the strongly evidence-based ambitions of the DSM, involves a series of value judgements. As with all value judgements, the facts are crucial (we covered this in general in Part I and return to it in this context in Session 2). But the facts are only part of the diagnostic story. The differential diagnosis in Simon's case also turns, and turns crucially, on a series of value judgements.

Into the (values) maelstrom?

Psychiatrists are often resistant to the idea that Criterion B introduces a series of value judgements into psychiatric diagnosis. By the standards of the fact-only medical model, they have every reason to be! DSM, as we saw in Part III (in Chapter 11 and Chapter 13), is self-styled as the pinnacle of scientific psychiatric diagnostic classification. Rumour has it that Criterion B was excluded from the World Health Organization's ICD-10, despite every effort being made to harmonize the two classifications, precisely because those concerned believed that it would undermine the scientific credentials of psychiatry! The WHO instead produced a separate classification of functioning, the ICF, or International Classification of Functioning, Disability and Health (WHO, 2001). In the ICD, of course, if the arguments of Part I are correct, an evaluative criterion is present by implication. But in DSM, with Criterion B, it is made explicit. And Criterion B, as in Simon's case, is at the centre of the diagnosis of a condition—schizophrenia—which itself is at the centre of traditional psychopathology (see Chapter 2 for the philosophical map of psychiatry). This is why schizophrenia, in Thomas Szasz's phrase, is the 'sacred symbol' of psychiatry (Szasz, 1960).

If, therefore, even schizophrenia cannot be diagnosed without making value judgements, what hope is there for the rest of psychiatry? With schizophrenia, then, according to the standard fact-only medical model, go the hopes of psychiatry for elevation to full membership of the scientific medicine club.

EXERCISE 6   (10 minutes)

In the final exercise in this session, review for yourself the implications of the conclusion that Criterion B imports values into the centre of psychiatric diagnosis. Write down a few notes in particular on,

1. What escape routes there might be for the standard medical model? If there are no actual escape routes, what are the possibilities for 'damage limitation'? (Think here about the different approaches to description and evaluation in the debate about mental disorder, as we explored them in Part I.)

2. If there is no escape, if value judgements are irreducibly part of psychiatric diagnosis, what are the implications for psychiatric practice, in clinical work and research?

These are large questions! The answers (or some elements of some possible answers) to them will occupy us for the rest of this chapter and Chapter 21.

All the same, please think about them for yourself at this stage. We have recommended that you spend just a few minutes on each. But write down your own ideas, brainstorming as widely as you can, and only then move on to the next session.

Reflection on the session and self-test questions

Write down your own reflections on the materials in this session drawing out any points that are particularly significant for you. Then write brief notes about the following:

1. Does a values-based model of medical diagnosis add values or subtract facts?

2. What is a delusional perception (as defined for example in the PSE)?

3. What is the diagnostic significance of a delusional perception (as in ICD-10)?

4. What is the key difference between the ICD and DSM diagnostic manuals in their criteria for schizophrenia?

5. Is the DSM evidence-based, values-based, or both?

Session 2 Generalization: the pervasiveness and importance of values in psychiatric diagnosis

At the end of the last session we raised two questions, (1) whether there were any escape routes for the 'medical model' of psychiatric diagnosis, including damage limitation exercises, once values are recognized to be at the heart of its scientific classifications (in Criterion B), and (2) what the significance of these values is in practice, in clinical work and research in psychiatry.

Review of the gameplan

In this session we will be dealing with the first question, the 'escape routes': we will find that there is no escape for the medical model, essentially because the importance of values in psychiatric diagnosis brings it firmly within the brief of ethics (or at any rate values) as well as of science.

In the third session of the chapter we will review some of the established ethical literature on psychiatric diagnosis. The conclusion of the present session, though, that psychiatric diagnosis is value laden because human values in the areas with which psychiatry is concerned are diverse, will give this literature a rather different interpretation from that of conventional ethics, an interpretation that is closer to the concept of VBP introduced in Chapter 18. This VBP interpretation will lead us, finally, in Chapter 21, back to the second question raised at the end of the last session, namely, to the practical implications of the importance of values in psychiatric diagnosis.

The great escape?

First, then, in this session, the possible escape routes for the medical model. We will explore two kinds of possible escape route, (1) via damage limitation, and (2) via philosophical value theory. Damage limitation, as we will see, amounts to arguing that values, if present in psychiatric classification and diagnosis, have only a limited scope of application. Philosophical value theory, as an escape route, amounts to drawing on descriptivist and other theories, to show that values, if present, can (or will be) reduced to scientific facts, and hence are (or will be) unimportant.

We will consider damage limitation first and then come back to possible escape routes based on the philosophical theories of description and evaluation introduced in Part I. We will find that, either way, there is no escape for the medical model! Values are both pervasive and important in psychiatric classification and diagnosis.

The pervasiveness of values in psychiatric diagnosis

Damage limitation, from the perspective of the medical model, means accepting that values come into psychiatric diagnosis but limiting as far as possible their scope of application.

What this amounts to, by the lights of the value-free model of science guiding the medical model, is the claim that psychiatric diagnosis is in principle as exclusively scientific as diagnosis in any other branch of medicine: and this claim is often combined, consciously or unconsciously, with the belief that as the brain sciences become more sophisticated, so the pervasiveness of values in psychiatric diagnosis will diminish, the end-point being that psychiatric diagnosis will eventually look no different from the 'scientific' diagnoses characteristic of the rest of medicine.

We will return to this line of thought in a moment. But one straightforward damage limitation exercise along these lines is to regard Criterion B, and its entailed value judgements, as a one-off, a (value-laden) exception which proves the (normally factual) rule of diagnosis.

Values and the DSM's evidence-based agenda

We have already seen (in Exercise 4) that the Introductory section of DSM-IV sets a strongly evidence-based agenda for its classification. In our full-field fact + value model, evidence is of course important. Our understanding of mental distress and disorder should be as evidence-based as possible. The point of Exercise 4 was to spell out the lengths to which the DSM-IV Taskforce went to adopt an evidence-based process to support the development of the new classification: we noted such phrases as 'breadth of available evidence', 'consensus scholarship', and 'formal evidence-based

process'. And in the fact-only traditional medical-scientific model, being evidence-based means being values-free.

Values in or values out?

But what happens later, deeper into the body of the DSM classification? Are values in or out? Has the Taskforce been successful in excluding values from the DSM? Of course, we have already noted the values in Criterion B. And we consider the theoretical implications of these later in this session. But what about other categories of mental disorder in the DSM? Are these value-free? What about the classification as a whole? As a classification of mental *disorders* is DSM, as well as being evidence-based, value-free?

EXERCISE 7   (10 minutes)

Read the further short extracts (Introduction, pp. xxi–xxii; Personality disorders, p. 630; Paraphilias, p. 523) from:

> American Psychiatric Association (1994). *Diagnostic and Statistical Manual of Mental Disorders* (4th edn). Washington, DC: American Psychiatric Association

---

Link with Readings 20.4, 20.5 (2 short extracts) and 20.6

The first extract is the DSM's definition of mental disorder. The second and third extracts are from the DSM's definitions of personality disorder and paraphilia, respectively. (Essentially similar passages in DSM-IV TR occur, respectively, at pps xxx/xxxi, 689 and 566.)

Can you identify any inconsistencies:

1. between the DSM's definition of disorder and its scientific self-image, and/or

2. between the DSM's definition of the general category of disorder, and its definitions of the particular conditions, personality disorder and paraphilia?

In both cases think particularly about the way DSM treats values. Is this satisfactory?

This double exercise has a direct message and an indirect message. The direct message is that DSM is inconsistent in the way it treats values, both upwards from its definition of disorder (to its scientific self-image) and downwards (to particular diagnostic categories).

An upward inconsistency

Thus, the definition in the first extract from Exercise 7 includes a caveat—that a diagnosis of mental disorder should not be made on the basis of social values alone, it 'must not be merely an expectable and culturally sanctioned response' (p. xxi). Well, fair enough: we come later in the chapter to the abuses to which psychiatry is subject once it is made a means of controlling social dissidence. But the point here is that this wording itself actually implies the importance of social values as a component of the definition of mental disorder in general and hence of particular mental disorders.

It is the word 'merely' that gives this away. If DSM were true to its fact-only scientific aspirations (as expressed in the first extract), it would have been sufficient to say, straightforwardly, that mental disorder should not be diagnosed on the basis of social values—finito. The categories of mental disorder, this wording would unequivocally say, like botanical categories (e.g. 'dog rose'), or chemical categories (e.g. 'oxygen'), are not social constructs.

Downward inconsistencies

The downward inconsistencies in these extracts are even more transparent. Thus, as just noted, the DSM definition of disorder says that mental disorder should not be diagnosed merely on the basis of social values. Yet in the second reading (the criteria for personality disorders) we read that '... impairment in social, occupational or other important area of functioning (Criterion C).' (first extract, 'Introduction', pp. xxi, xxii) ... '... may not be considered problematic by the individual ...' (second extract, 'Personality disorders', pp. 630). Similarly, in the third extract (the criteria for paraphilia, p. 523), we read that 'These individuals are rarely self-referred and usually come to the attention of mental health professionals only when their behaviour has brought them into conflict with sexual partners or society'.

Notwithstanding, therefore, its general restriction on diagnosing mental disorder on the basis of social values alone, DSM, in effect though of course not in intent, does just this for both these categories. True, they can both be diagnosed on other grounds: but they *can* be diagnosed, by DSM criteria, on the basis of social values alone.

True, also, DSM, in its definition of mental disorder (first extract, pp. xxi, xxii), adds an overarching general constraint on psychiatric diagnosis in the form of a criterion of 'clinical significance'. This constraint, in the second extract (p. 630), also appears in the first clause of Criterion C for personality disorder. But this further constraint, on closer inspection, amounts to no more than the tautological definition of mental disorder (considered in Part I), that mental disorder is what doctors treat. For the DSM gives no definition of clinical significance other than saying that it is 'an inherently difficult *clinical* judgement' (American Psychiatric Association, 1994, p. 7, emphasis added). To the extent, furthermore, that clinical significance is connected in DSM to 'distress or impairment in social, occupational, or other important areas of functioning...', p. 7), the implication (though, again, not the intention) is that the clinical judgements in question are (at least in part) *value* judgements.

Two messages

The direct message, then, of this double exercise is that DSM is, at best, inconsistent in the way it treats values. The indirect message is that these inconsistencies reflect a failure of awareness, namely a failure to recognize the pervasiveness of values in psychiatric diagnosis.

In this respect, then, the inconsistencies in DSM are the counterpart of similar inconsistencies that we found earlier in the book in the literature on concepts of disorder. In the latter literature we found that authors such as Boorse (1975), and more recently Wakefield (2000), had been inconsistent in arguing for a *value-free* scientific core to medical theory (respectively in the concepts of 'disease' and of 'dysfunction'), while, at the same time using these terms with clear *evaluative* connotations (see Part I; also Fulford, 1989, ch 3 on Boorse, and 2000 on Wakefield).

Values in or values out again

In the debate about concepts of disorder, as we saw in chapter 4, inconsistencies of this kind pointed to the importance of values in the meanings of ostensibly 'scientific' concepts such as disease and dysfunction. Boorse, Wakefield, and others, so the (linguistic analytical) argument went, might stipulate value-free definitions of these terms for theoretical purposes; however, they were unable to use them value-free in practice because the evaluative element in their meanings was essential to the (linguistic) work that the terms do.

A similar situation arises in DSM, then. The authors of DSM strive after a value-free, and hence in their terms scientific, classification of mental disorders. But the importance of the evaluative element in the definition of mental disorder, hence in the definitions of particular disorders, and hence in psychiatric diagnosis, makes it inevitable that values slip back in. Values, then, are 'in' psychiatric classification; and they are 'outed' (shown for what they are) by the very language of DSM (see Fulford, 1994, for a more extended discussion of this analytic point; and Sadler, 2004, for a comprehensive review of values in all areas of psychiatric diagnosis).

No damage limitation

There is little scope, then, for damage limitation. Values, it seems, contrary to the fact-only medical model, are not limited to Criterion B in DSM. They are pervasive throughout the classification and, it would seem, logically important (they are doing important linguistic work for us, as the prongs of a garden fork do important gardening work for us).

We should not be surprised at this conclusion, given our findings in the first session of the chapter, that Criterion B imports values into psychiatric diagnosis. As we noted above, Criterion B is at the heart of the diagnosis of a disorder (schizophrenia), which is at the heart of the broader category of psychotic disorder, which in turn is at the heart of psychiatry's descriptive psychopathology as a whole.

The map of mental disorders, introduced in Chapter 2, makes this clear. A key feature of the map, as we saw, is that it illustrates how mental disorders provide a bridge (a conceptual bridge, of course) between medicine and morals.

In Chapter 2, we noted that conditions on the edge of the map of psychopathology are more overtly value laden than those at the centre. This property of these 'marginal disorders' has been reflected here in the overtly evaluative criteria in DSM for personality disorders and paraphilias. But what Session 1 of this chapter has shown us is that, when we look carefully, with a philosophically sharpened eye, at the criteria by which the central conditions (such as schizophrenia) are defined in DSM, these too, by virtue of Criterion B, include evaluative criteria. Add to this the overtly evaluative language with which the agenda of DSM is set up, and we are back with the conclusion of Part I, that values are indeed pervasive and important throughout all areas of psychiatry's psychopathology, hence in psychiatry's nosology (disease classification), and hence in psychiatric diagnosis.

DSM and ICD

DSM, it is important to add, is not in this respect less satisfactory than ICD. Precisely similar arguments apply to ICD. The evaluative element is more difficult to identify in ICD because of ICD's more synoptic treatment of psychiatric classification. The less said, as it were, the less chance of inconsistency! This is why, as noted in Session 1, the authors of ICD resisted the inclusion of a Criterion B. The authors of DSM, on the other hand, in seeking to make the basis of psychiatric classification and diagnosis as transparent as possible, have gone part way to exposing the evaluative element of meaning, which is there, albeit more deeply hidden, in ICD. (As noted above, the WHO has a separate classification of functioning, the ICF (World Health Organization, 2001).

The importance of values in psychiatric diagnosis

We return later in the chapter to the implications of making this evaluative element fully overt, of 'outing' it. First, though, we need to consider the other escape route. If values are there, and if they are pervasive in psychiatric classification, is there a way of eliminating them?

This will occupy us for the remainder of this session. In effect, we will be reviewing arguments about the concept of mental disorder covered in detail in Part I. We will not need the details of those arguments, however. We will be reviewing them briefly, therefore, and with an eye specifically to whether they offer escape routes for the medical model in respect of psychiatric diagnosis.

We will tackle this initially by way of a further case history, that of Elizabeth Orton. The ethical and philosophical aspects of Elizabeth Orton's case are discussed in detail in one of the sister volumes to this book, Dickenson and Fulford's (2000) *In Two Minds: a case book of psychiatric ethics*.

A suitable case for treatment

Elizabeth Orton was a 35-year-old lawyer with a 10-month-old baby, Anthony. She had called her Health Visitor for help after finding herself shaking Anthony. The Health Visitor had reported the incident to Social Services and the child protection machinery had been put into action. Anthony was placed on the Child Protection Register, and Elizabeth was obliged by Social Services

to see a psychiatrist, Daniel Isaacson, on pain of Anthony being taken into care.

The background to the incident was that Elizabeth had felt trapped: she did not want Anthony and would have had him adopted if her husband, Tim, had not objected. Elizabeth had been depressed in the postnatal period but now appeared, and felt, normal. Tim, who was 50, was semi-retired. He normally took most of the responsibility for looking after Anthony but had been away for a few days before the 'shaking' incident.

In the next exercise we pick up Elizabeth's story at the point where a case conference has been convened between Health and Social Services.

EXERCISE 8   (25 minutes)

Read the extract from the case of Elizabeth Orton (case 3.1) in:

Dickenson, D. and Fulford, K.W.M. (2000). Basic concepts: your myth or mine. Chapter 3, *In Two Minds: a casebook of psychiatric ethics*. Oxford: Oxford University Press. (Extract, pp. 59–60.)

Link with Reading 20.7

This is a short extract but we have suggested 25 minutes for the exercise to allow you to think in detail about how and in what ways values are driving this case. Think, in particular, about the medical model of mental disorder. Who is influenced by it here? What would Thomas Szasz, from an antimedical model perspective, and R.E. Kendell, from a pro-medical model perspective, have made of this case? (You may like to refer back to Chapter 4 here.)

Models and values

In their casebook, Dickenson and Fulford discuss Elizabeth Orton's story as an example of the overuse of the medical model: by the lights of this model, her problem of lack of feeling for her baby is pathologized and a mental disorder requiring the intervention of a medical psychiatrist. Dickenson and Fulford contrast Elizabeth Orton's case with a second case (3.2, Sam Benbow) in which there is, on the face of it, *under*use of the medical model (Sam is a learning disabled man with a paranoid psychosis who needs treatment for a bodily condition).

As Dickenson and Fulford point out, getting the balance right, between over- and underuse of the medical model, involves a number of related concepts—autonomy, capacity, rationality, and so forth. Values, though, both in their own right and as elements in these related concepts, are crucially important.

There are certainly values aplenty washing about in this case. Elizabeth Orton's wish to offload Anthony; her husband, Tim's, equally strong determination to hang on to him (did he take early retirement to facilitate this?); Dr Isaacson's concern for the proper role of psychiatry; Social Services' over-riding concern with 'child protection issues'. We will see later in the chapter that these values, and the conflicts between them, are crucially important practically. But the point for now is the way in which they are driving the model of Elizabeth's problem as a 'mental disorder'. The feeling, not of course expressly stated, is that for a woman to fail to 'bond' with her baby is such a negative condition that 'she must be mad.' This gender bias is clear, for example, in the Social Worker 'chair's' acknowledgement to Dr Isaacson that if the roles in the Orton family were reversed, if it had been Tim who had shaken the baby and Elizabeth who was available to look after him, he (Tim) would not have been referred to a psychiatrist!

Disease and dissent

Having just read the first part of this session, the value-ladenness of the issues in Elizabeth Orton's case will not come as a surprise. We will see in Session 3 that they are also no surprise when we consider the abusive use of psychiatry as a means of social control. Political dissenters in the former USSR were 'diagnosed' as suffering from delusions of reformism! There, as we will see, the dominant political values drove the pathologizing of political dissent. Dickenson and Fulford give the example of 'spermatorrhoea', a 'disease' of excessive sexual activity in Victorian England. In the Southern States of the USA before the abolition of slavery, running away was the disease of 'drapetomania'.

In each of these cases, then, dissent from a dominant value system (political, moral, and commercial, respectively), we might well conclude, was pathologized as disease. Small wonder, therefore, that Elizabeth Orton's dissent from 'family values' was pathologized similarly!

Szasz versus Kendell

But what would the two sides in the antipsychiatry versus psychiatry debate have made of this? As we saw in Part I, this debate was essentially between those who believed mental disorder to be no different (other than perhaps in the sophistication of its science) from bodily disorders, and those who believed mental disorders to be crucially different in some way from bodily disorders. A key component in this debate was how the two sides treated values.

Thus, both sides recognized that mental disorder is more value laden than bodily disorder. We have seen this in various ways in this part (the value-laden Criterion B, the many ways in which values come into DSM, etc., all have no counterpart in the classification of bodily disorders). But the protagonists differed radically over what they made of this. Those 'for' psychiatry, like R.E. Kendell (1975), believed that closer inspection showed the values in question to be epiphenomenal: Kendell argued for an evolutionary understanding of disorder according to which mental and bodily disorders were both defined by reduced life and/or reproductive expectations. Those against psychiatry, on the other hand, such as Thomas Szasz (1960) argued that the value ladenness of mental disorder showed it to be, in reality, not a matter for medicine at all but for morals. Bodily disorders, he said, were defined by factual norms of anatomy and physiology. Mental disorders, by contrast, were defined by 'psycho-social, ethical, and legal' norms. Mental disorders, so

called, were therefore 'problems of living' in Szasz' view, no different from any other moral or life problem.

In Part I we found that, despite appearances, the key difference between Szasz and Kendell was not over mental disorder but over bodily disorder (they wrote about illness, in fact). It was because they adopted different definitions of bodily disorder that they came to different conclusions about mental disorder. This limits the practical utility of the debate. In Elizabeth Orton's case we can imagine the argument running thus:

Szasz: 'we are judging Elizabeth Orton by ethical and social norms; there are no anatomical or physiological abnormalities here. Therefore she is not ill.'

Kendell: 'but "failure to bond" between mother and baby will result in reduced numbers of offspring; hence this is a case of biological disadvantage; hence she *is* ill.'

From disorder to disease

There is simply no point of contact here, then, there is no shared frame of reference within which issues of the proper scope of application of the medical concepts can be resolved. In practice, of course, the debate would continue.

Kendell: '...And there is little doubt that in a few years we will understand the bodily changes (in brain, endocrines, etc.) underlying failure to bond. We will then have the anatomical and physiological norms required by your theory.'

Szasz: 'In which case, I will accept "failure to bond" as a disorder. But it will be a disorder as in *brain disease*, not a *mental illness*.'

(Szasz has said something similar of schizophrenia in a debate some years ago on BBC Channel 4 with Jonathan Miller.)

EXERCISE 9 (10 minutes)

Think about this last comment of (our fictional) Thomas Szasz. Is there something disturbing about his willingness to shift positions over Elizabeth Orton on the basis of, say, a brain scan finding?

This is a disturbing move for both theoretical and practical reasons. We examined the theoretical reason in Part I: to the extent that it relies on the demonstration of causation, it implies that an understanding of the bodily changes underlying *successful* maternal–foetal bonding (as opposed to *failure* to bond) will make that a brain disease too!

The point is that, absent a 'ghost in the machine', *all* human experience and behaviour must have a basis 'in the brain'. Yet all too often the discovery of a brain basis for some particular aspect of experience or behaviour is taken to be equivalent to proving that it is a disease. In Part I we considered this as a theoretical point. But it is also an increasingly practical point as the new neurosciences are extending our knowledge of brain functioning. The spectacle of barristers waving brain scans around in court to prove that their client was 'not responsible' is more and more a reality. In Part V, we will encounter an example of this with the newspaper headline announcing the discovery of a change in the anatomy of the brain in women with anorexia—'It's a *real* disease, after all!' was the storyline (see Chapter 22). We will also be considering the case of 'Mrs Lazy,' whose brain tumour presented with the 'symptom' of giving up housework! (This case is also described in Fulford, 2000a.)

An evolutionary escape route? Boorse and Wakefield

Szasz's willingness to move from (moral) problems of living to (medical) brain diseases on the basis of findings 'in the brain', as we saw in Part I, points to the need for bringing in some way of distinguishing good from bad departures from the norms of anatomy and physiology. Rather as with Criterion B, in Session 1 above, it is not enough that there should be, merely, a *difference* in anatomy and physiology for us to talk of disease. The difference must be for the *worse*.

> *Kendell*: '... and the relevant direction of change, what 'for the *worse*' means in terms of anatomy and physiology, is defined by the evolutionary norms of survival and reproduction. *Failure* of maternal–foetal bonding is nothing if not "evolutionarily dysfunctional", by these criteria.'

> *Szasz*: 'Is it, though? Surely this depends on the way a particular society operates. It would be true if there were few women wanting to have babies. But in our over-crowded world, it may be adaptive for the maternal instinct to be in short supply! And as to the division of labour between the sexes, paternal-foetal bonding, in our world of equality of the sexes, may be even more adaptive. At the very least, then, your criteria, applied to human beings, are socially relative. Elizabeth Orton, far from being "evolutionarily dysfunctional" could be ahead of her evolutionary time!'

An evolutionary blind alley

This (again, entirely fictional) further exchange brings out one kind of difficulty with evolutionary arguments, that they are better *post hoc* than *propter hoc*, better at explaining what has been than at predicting what will be. It also points to their limited utility when applied to human beings. This is because, perhaps uniquely in our case, 'natural' selection is something we can to an extent take or leave alone. Culture, perhaps, is a product of evolution. But its effect has been to allow us to circumvent many of the checks and balances which, in a natural environment, defined 'fitness'.

A more radical critique of evolutionary arguments, though, at least as providing an escape route for the medical model in respect of psychiatric diagnosis, is that, in practice, they fail in their objective of excluding values. We looked at this point in respect of Boorse's version of the evolutionary approach to defining dysfunction in value-free terms in Part I. One of us (K.W.M.F.) has also set it out fully in his *Moral Theory and Medical Practice* (1989, chapter 3). What it comes down to is the gap, noted above, between the stipulative definition of disorder in value-free terms and its continued use, even by those concerned, with clear evaluative force. Boorse (1975), to repeat our example from chapter 4, defines disease value-free (*inter alia*) as a 'departure

from functional norms' and then uses the term to mean the evaluative 'failure of functional efficiency'.

Wakefield (2000) is among the latest to explore the evolutionary approach. His line (on disorder) is to define function, and hence dysfunction, by reference to a particular kind of causal process characteristic of evolutionary systems, one in which an effect is part of its own causal explanation. This is a powerful approach. It suggests, for example, contrary to the (fictional) Szasz argument offered above, that Elizabeth Orton's failure to bond should be regarded as a disorder, whatever the virtues of her position in our particular culture, provided only that maternal–foetal bonding (as a product or effect of evolutionary causal processes) is itself part of the evolutionary causal process by which maternal– foetal bonding evolved. Given the survival value of maternal–foetal bonding in a 'natural' environment, this seems not unlikely! Yet Wakefield's definition (of dysfunction), even more transparently than Boorse's, incorporates the very evaluative element of meaning it aims to exclude. This element was implicit in earlier statements of Wakefield's views (see Fulford, 1999). It becomes explicit in a later version, his 'new black box essentialism'; in this version, for example, the relevant 'effects' are derived by Wakefield from those which are, he says, using an explicitly evaluative term, 'beneficial' to the organism concerned (Wakefield, 2000; see also discussion in Fulford, 2000b).

Evolutionary theory, then, turns out to be, not an escape route for the medical model, but a blind alley. Boorse and Wakefield seek to exclude values (at least from the core of medical scientific theory—both recognize that values come into medicine elsewhere); but their own continued use of evaluative language shows that, stipulate as they may, the value terms will just not go away!

A moral descriptivist escape route? G.J. Warnock

A further escape route is by way of moral descriptivism. Again, this is covered in detail in Part I but is worth summarizing here, if only to bring us back to the practical implications of these arguments for psychiatric diagnosis, as in Elizabeth Orton's case.

An important modern exemplar of moral descriptivism is the Oxford philosopher, the late G.J. Warnock. Warnock never worked on the medical concepts (he died a few years ago). Had he done so, the difference between his position and the Boorse/Wakefield position might have been characterized thus: Boorse and Wakefield seek to *exclude* values, thus distilling out a purely factual medical concept (of disease or of dysfunction, respectively); Warnock sought rather to *redefine* (some kinds of values) in terms of facts (strictly, evaluations in terms of descriptions, hence 'descriptivism').

Descriptivism of the G.J. Warnock brand thus allows us to have our cake and to eat it. In so far as the relevant value terms are definable in terms of facts, it allows us to regard them as matters for value-free science; but because the values are redefined (not excluded) the terms can still be used with clear evaluative force. 'Disease', then, and 'dysfunction', if expressing the relevant kind of value, can properly be regarded as scientific terms (defined by facts) while still being used to express values (implied by the same facts). Hence in a moral descriptivist medical model there is no contradiction between defining disease (with Boorse) or dysfunction (with Wakefield) value-free, while continuing to use these terms (as both do use them) to express evaluative meaning.

A non-descriptivist model: R.M. Hare

Whether or not one can 'have one's cake and eat it', logically speaking, in this way, depends on whether moral descriptivism, the analytic ethics basis for a descriptivist medical model, is right. This in turn depends on the view one takes of a long tradition of argument in analytic ethics, the so-called 'is–ought' debate, stretching back at least to David Hume. Again, we outlined this debate in Part I but we will review the key points briefly here.

Thus, the 'is–ought' debate is concerned with the logical relationship, the relationship of meaning between description and evaluation. Warnock, as just noted, is among those who have concluded that it is at least sometimes possible to get an evaluation from a set of descriptions, an 'ought from an is'. Others, though, including David Hume, have argued that, however persuasive the psychological connection between a given description of a situation and an evaluation of that situation, there is always a logical gap between them.

A modern exemplar of the latter, non-descriptivist, position is another Oxford philosopher, R.M. Hare (see references in Part I and Reading Guide). Hare's position is sometimes called prescriptivism because he emphasized the prescriptive, or action guiding, meaning of value terms. Thus, to take a non-medical example (described fully in Part I), an eating apple may be sweet, crisp, and clean-skinned. Most people would commend such an eating apple, they would judge it to be a 'good eating apple'. But, Hare argued, the move from the description 'sweet, crisp, and clean-skinned' to the evaluative 'good eating apple' is a psychological not a logical move. The move is driven by our psychology: it just is the case that for most people a good eating apple is one that is sweet, crisp, and clean-skinned. These descriptions, then, for most people, are the (descriptive) criteria by which they judge an eating apple to be good. But 'good eating apple,' here, does not mean simply 'an apple that is sweet, crisp, and clean-skinned.' 'Good eating apple' means an apple that, in being sweet, crisp, and clean-skinned, is good for eating.

A watershed in models: from (negative) escape routes to (positive) assets

The difference here, between psychologically and logically connected meanings, may seem a rather fine one! But it has profound consequences for psychiatric ethics in general, and in particular for our understanding of the role of values in the areas of psychopathology, classification, and diagnosis. In the remainder of this session we will look briefly at its theoretical consequences, the kind of 'medical model' to which it leads. We will return to its practical consequences (psychiatric abuse) in Session 3.

A non-descriptivist model: the theory

A full account of the model of the medical concepts to which non-descriptivist value theory leads would take us well beyond the scope of this session. Such an account has been developed by Fulford in

his *Moral Theory and Medical Practice* (1989, especially chapters 2–5) together with a recent article in *Philosophy, Psychiatry, & Psychology* (Fulford, 2000b). It is also covered in some detail in Part I.

So far as psychiatry is concerned, though, we can get a handle on a key advantage of non-descriptivism over descriptivism by thinking through the connection between descriptive and evaluative meaning, as we have just done for 'apple', for a second non-medical example, 'picture'.

> **EXERCISE 10**   (20 minutes)
>
> In this exercise we want you to try writing down a set of descriptive criteria for a good picture. To limit the exercise, think of yourself in a concrete situation, for example as a member of a committee choosing the pictures for a hospital ward or an academic common room. If you are working in a group, write your lists separately and then compare them. Don't spend too long on this exercise. Limit yourself to the suggested 20 minutes!
>
> (If you have done Part I you may want to skip this exercise.)

Most people trying this exercise find it very difficult—hence the suggested 20-minute time limit! There are various kinds of difficulties involved: imaginative identification, the variety of scenarios, etc. But what they all come down to is a profound difficulty over deciding what the criteria for a 'good picture' should be.

In the case of eating apples, most people (more or less) readily agree on a (fairly) limited list of (quite) well-defined criteria (usually including the criteria 'sweet, crisp, and clean skinned' as above). In the case of pictures, by contrast, there is nothing approaching this level of agreement. Over what is a good apple, people agree. Over what is a good picture, people disagree. In other words, in the case of what is good or bad in pictures, there is nothing corresponding with the agreed descriptive criteria of 'sweet, crisp, and clean skinned' for good eating apples. A given individual at any one time may be able to point to some feature of a particular picture, some description of it, which leads him or her to judge it good or bad ('I like landscapes', 'what photographic detail!', 'its by so-and-so', etc.). But unlike apples, the descriptive criteria for value judgements of pictures vary widely, between individuals, between cultures, and for a given individual between different occasions.

With the contrast between apples and pictures in mind, we can now come back to bodily medicine and psychiatry.

Apples and pictures, bodily medicine and psychiatry

The quick, but key, point here is that in respect of diversity of values, medicine (or at any rate high-tech bodily medicine) is like apples, while psychiatry is like pictures. Again, this is covered in detail in Part I. Think of, say, a 'heart attack'. Involving as this does, pain, collapse, and imminent death, it amounts to a condition that is a bad condition for anyone. It may have good consequences, e.g. escape from a protracted and even more painful death from cancer. But in itself the condition is one which nearly everyone would judge a bad condition to be in. In psychiatry, by contrast, the conditions with which we are concerned are defined by emotions, desires, volition, beliefs, and other areas of human experience and behaviour in which our values are widely diverse.

Diversity of values feeds through as one clear source of the difficulty of psychiatric diagnosis. In the traditional medical model, psychiatric diagnosis is difficult only because psychiatry's science is primitive. On this model, while the scientific difficulties are real enough, we have differences of values to deal with as well. Of course, the values are there (on this model) in all areas of medical diagnosis. But they can be ignored for practical purposes in bodily medicine to the extent that they are widely agreed upon and hence unproblematic in practice.

The dangers of descriptivism

Taking this point the other way shows up the dangers of a descriptivist medical model for psychiatry. Descriptivism works for practical purposes where human values are, as a matter of psychological fact, shared. Thus in the case of apples, it may (if Hume and Hare are right) be theoretically true that there is a gap between 'is and ought', but this makes little difference practically. The fact is that people tend not to disagree over whether a 'sweet, crisp, clean-skinned eating' apple is good. The danger, though, is in extrapolating the apple case to cases where people disagree. There is not much risk of this with pictures. They are just so different anyway. But there is a real danger of extrapolation from bodily illness (cases such as heart attacks) to mental illness (cases such as Simon's, in Session 1). The danger is of one group's or individual's values being imposed on another's. The danger, in short, is of an abusive imposition of values.

This was one aspect of the problem in Elizabeth Orton's case. As we will see later, her case is merely one of a range of similar cases driven by differences in gender and cultural values. These in turn are but an extreme form of abuses arising from neglect of values, which, the growing first-hand literature from the user movement makes clear, is generic to psychiatry.

We will be examining some of these abuses of psychiatric diagnosis in the next session and returning to what can be done about them in Chapter 21.

Reflection on the session and self-test questions

Write down your own reflections on the materials in this session drawing out any points that are particularly significant for you. Then write brief notes about the following:

1. Is there an escape route for the fact-only medical model by way of circumscribing the role of values in psychiatric diagnosis? or are values pervasive?

2. Is there an escape route for the fact-only medical model by way of an (express or implied) generic criterion of clinical significance?

3. Is there an escape route for the fact-only medical model in positing (actual or hypothetical) underlying bodily causes?

4. What is moral descriptivism?

5. Is there an escape route for the fact-only medical model in moral descriptivism.

6. Are there dangers in moral descriptivism for psychiatry?

7. Is there an alternative?

Session 3 Bioethics and values in psychiatric diagnosis

We noted at the start of this part, in Chapter 17, that psychiatry has been relatively neglected by mainstream bioethics. Like biomedicine, bioethics has focused on the more high-profile problems of high-tech medicine. This, we noted there, is something of a paradox, psychiatry being more not less ethically problematic than these high-tech areas. And one of the key ways in which it is more ethically problematic, is that ethical issues are raised by diagnosis in psychiatry as well as by the areas, mainly of treatment choice, on which traditional bioethics has focused.

The outcome of this story, in Chapter 18, was that, once the origin of the ethically problematic nature of psychiatric diagnosis had been correctly identified, not in psychiatry's (supposedly) primitive science but in the (legitimate) diversity of human values, then psychiatric ethics, far from being the poor relation of bioethics, becomes (to switch metaphors) a window on good practice in medicine as a whole. In yet another metaphor, psychiatric ethics is bioethics' ugly duckling (Fulford and Hope, 1993), relatively neglected by mainstream bioethicists but with the potential to emerge as the swan of the flock!

Psychiatric diagnosis as an ethical problem

The question that we need to consider now, though, is whether traditional bioethics, in considering psychiatric diagnosis, has been able to break away from the traditional fact-only medical model sufficiently to recognize the origin of the ethically-laden nature of psychiatric diagnosis in the diversity of human values. It is this question that will occupy us (along with a number of related questions) in the next reading. This is a classic paper by one of the key figures in bioethics responsible for putting psychiatric ethics, and the ethical problems of diagnosis in particular, on the map. It is by the American lawyer and human rights campaigner, Walter Reich. Reich was among those who first brought to the world's attention the abusive use of psychiatry for the control of political dissent in the former Soviet Union. His article picks out and generalizes the ethical lessons that he believes psychiatry should learn from this episode in its history.

We are going to spend some time on Reich's article because it has a number of important lessons for us, some positive, others negative. This first exercise involves reading it right through quickly and as a whole. In later exercises, we are going to return to it for more detailed study of key passages.

EXERCISE 11   (60 minutes)

Read:

Reich, W. (1999). Psychiatric diagnosis as an ethical problem. In *Psychiatric Ethics* (ed. S. Bloch, P. Chodoff, and S. Green) (3rd edn). Oxford: Oxford University Press, pp. 193–224

Link with Reading 20.8

As just noted, you should read the article through as a whole. As you read it, make two checklists:

1. a list of positive points, i.e. of points made by Reich about the ethical aspects of psychiatric diagnosis that strike you as being true; and

2. a list of negative points, i.e. of points which Reich makes that are critical of psychiatry (explicitly or implicitly) and that strike you as not being true (because misdirected, inconsistent, stigmatizing, or for any other reason).

Note: The article is a scholarly tour de force and you could spend a week on these two lists! But we have suggested 60 minutes on the basis that you should read the article right through to get the 'feel' of the positive and negative points rather than trying to think through all Reich's arguments at this stage. We will be returning to particular sections of the article in more detail later on.

As with all our exercises, there is a temptation to 'cheat' here, to jump straight to the lists given below rather than reading the article yourself! Given the 'skills development' nature of philosophy outlined at the start of this book, we hope you won't do this! Also, in particular for this exercise, you may well come up with different lists from ours, and indeed with a different conclusion. So don't take our observations for granted!

A list of positives

Reich's article pulls together a series of crucially important points about psychiatric ethics. Some of these we have covered already in the book, some are still to come. It is a reflection of the importance of diagnosis in psychiatric ethics that it should act, in the hands of a skilled commentator, as a centre of gravity for the whole subject! Positive points from Reich's article include:

1. *Psychiatry is ethically laden*: Reich emphasizes the ethically-laden nature of all aspects of psychiatry from its emergence as a separate discipline up to the present day (p. 193).

2. *Diagnosis is ethically central*: he gives a clear statement not just of the pervasiveness of ethical issues in psychiatry, but of the *central place in all these issues* of psychiatric diagnosis—he writes 'common to all these activities is one psychiatric act: diagnosis' (p. 193).

3. *A classification of misdiagnoses*: he provides a useful *summary and categorization* of the different ways in which psychiatric misdiagnosis may be ethically problematic; abstracting from pp. 194–195, we can list these as:

   • *'honest' errors*—mistakes despite observing good practice;

   • *culpable errors*—mistakes due to inattention, lack of training, etc.;

   • *purposeful misuse*—deliberate false diagnosis in full knowledge of what one is doing;

   • *non-purposeful misuse*—the 'issuing' (Reich's term) of an incorrect diagnosis without being aware of what one is doing;

   • *intermediate cases* (not his term)—a spectrum of cases falling between purposeful and non-purposeful.

4. *Non-purposeful misdiagnosis ethically central*: he spells out the perhaps surprising fact that *non*-purposeful misdiagnoses are the most ethically significant ... '... though purposeful misdiagnosis should be a serious concern, it is the *other* kind—misdiagnosis that results not from the wilful misapplication of psychiatric categories, but from primarily *non-purposeful* causes—that deserve the greatest scrutiny' (p. 194, emphasis in original).

5. *Many empirical difficulties*: his account provides what amounts to a useful summary of the empirical *difficulties* of psychiatric diagnosis. These, as set out in his sections on 'The inherent limitations of the diagnostic process' (pp. 195–196) and 'The power of diagnostic theory to shape psychiatric vision' (pp. 196–205), include many of the issues we considered in Part III. They include reliability (agreement between observers and on different occasions), reliance on symptoms and subjective assessments, different 'schools' of thought on classification, cultural diversity, the influence of social factors, and the 'theory-laden' nature of diagnosis.

6. *The lessons of Soviet psychiatry*: he makes clear that the experience of Soviet psychiatry is a *cautionary tale* for the subject (this occupies most of pp. 196–205, his section on 'diagnostic theory' influencing 'psychiatric vision')

7. *Implications of psychiatric diagnosis*: he spells out the wide range of crucially important *implications* of psychiatric diagnosis. The subheadings in Reich's section on 'The beauty of diagnosis as a solution to human problems' (pp. 205–217) make up a valuable checklist: diagnosis is: (1) explanation, mitigation, exculpation (this is one of the areas we covered particularly in Chapter 19, on legal aspects); (2) reassurance; and (3) the humane transformation of social deviance into medical illness. Psychiatric diagnosis is also (though it is less clear what is 'beautiful' about the rest of Reich's list): (4) a means of exclusion and dehumanization; (5) a self-confirming hypothesis; and (6) a vehicle of discreditation and punishment.

   Reich sums up the positive attributes of psychiatric diagnosis at the start of his 'beauty' section (p. 205) thus '... [psychiatric diagnosis] can turn the fright of chaos into the pleasure of certainty; the shame of hurting others into the pride of helping them; and the dilemma of moral judgement into the clarity of medical truth'.

8. *Origin of ethical problems in human nature*: Reich locates the origin of the ethical problems with psychiatric diagnosis in the nature of human beings. In the concluding section of his chapter (p. 218, penultimate para), he writes 'Psychiatrists have to understand that... all abuses of diagnoses are a psychiatric problem in considerable measure because they are a *human* problem...' (emphasis in original).

A list of negatives

The second half of this exercise was to develop a checklist of negative points made by Reich against psychiatry. One reason that we suggested you made the lists in parallel, and while reading the whole article through quickly, is because most people find it easier (on first reading) to identify negatives than positives.

Taken at first blush, indeed, Reich is negative about psychiatry *full stop*. We could find only one overtly positive comment in the whole article, the suggestion (in the second paragraph of his opening section, p. 194) that psychiatry has '... the potential for causing good as well as harm.' But the rest of the chapter is all about harm. We return later to just why Reich should adopt this highly critical tone.

Parallel lists

The negative 'set' of Reich's article ties in with the second reason for asking you to make the lists in parallel, namely that they are parallel lists. Everything that we have included in our list of positives is also capable of being read, and indeed is presented by Reich as, a negative. Actually, there are a great many more negative points! You will probably have found your own list of negatives to be a long one. But the (Reichean) negative of (our) positive list runs roughly thus:

1. *Psychiatry is ethically-laden*. Reich presents the ethically laden nature of psychiatry as a matter of ethical criticism... 'it is *criticised* for ethical abuses in every sphere of its activity.' (p. 193, emphasis added).

2. *Diagnosis is ethically central*. Having clearly identified the ethically central place of psychiatric diagnosis (as in our list of positives), Reich continues in terms that, although capable of being read neutrally (though not positively), invite negative connotations; 'It is the *prerogative* to diagnose that enables psychiatrists to *commit patients against their wills*', he writes, 'that delineates the populations *subjected* to their care, and that *sets in motion* the *methods* they will use for treatment' (p. 193, emphases added). The image this phraseology conjures up is not of the caring doctor seeking to the best of her ability to use her skills to help people in trouble! It is of a powerful figure wielding authority over an unwilling population that is 'subjected' to methods of treatment following

mechanically on ('set in motion' by) a divine right ('prerogative') of diagnosis.

3. *A classification of misdiagnoses*. Again, read neutrally, Reich's classification of misdiagnoses is a 'positive' in his paper. But in this section his negative set against psychiatry is made fully explicit. The section starts (top of p. 194) with 'of course, the ethical problem of diagnosis stems from its capacity for misuse—that is, the knowing misapplication of diagnostic categories...'. This puts people '... at risk for the harmful effects of psychiatric diagnosis.' The (relatively) neutral list of the consequences of psychiatric diagnosis is now converted into an overt list of harms—'loss of personal freedom', 'subjection to noxious psychiatric environments and treatments', the possibility of 'lifelong labelling', etc.

4. *Non-purposeful misdiagnosis ethically central*. For Reich, then, the 'ethical problem' of psychiatric diagnosis is the knowing exposure of people who are not ill to unpleasant treatments. The implication is that psychiatric treatments (like other medical treatments) have harmful side-effects, and that it is unethical to expose people to these side-effects vicariously. This is no different in principle from, say, a surgeon 'non-purposefully' carrying out an abdominal operation on someone who doesn't need it. This, one must hope, does not happen very often. Yet, as we noted in our positive list, Reich continues by suggesting that it is misdiagnoses that are 'primarily *non-purposeful* that deserve the greatest scrutiny' (p. 194, his emphasis).

There is an apparent conflict here, then. Reich starts by claiming the ethical problem of diagnosis stems from 'the *knowing* misapplication of diagnostic categories' (p. 194, as cited above, but with emphasis now added). But he goes on to say that the bigger problem is non-purposeful misdiagnoses, i.e. misdiagnoses of which the psychiatrist is *unaware*.

A new diagnostic entity?

Reich resolves this conflict, however, a couple of paragraphs later (p. 195), with a psychoanalytic idiom of dissociation.... Sometimes he writes (p. 195) 'such awareness (that the psychiatrist in question is issuing an incorrect diagnosis) is altogether absent... sometimes, however, awareness would be present were it not for the efforts of the psychiatrist, through the use of various techniques of denial and self-delusion, to escape the moral self-condemnation that would result from such awareness.'

The bottom line, then, is that the ethical problem of diagnosis is the misapplication of diagnostic categories by psychiatrists who, but for dissociative splitting, would be well aware of what they are doing. The ethical problem of psychiatric diagnosis is, in psychiatric diagnostic terms, a problem of what we might call 'dissociative misdiagnosis'. (Recall the example of hysterical paralysis, in Chapter 3, a paralysis caused by motivations that, like those hypothesized by Reich in the case of psychiatric misdiagnosis, are split off from awareness (dissociated) because they are too painful to tolerate consciously.)

This is not, as they say, a pretty picture! It is a picture, it is important to add, with which many in the user/survivor movement would identify. But right or wrong, it is a picture that demands some explanation. Why should psychiatrists, particularly, need the 'use of various techniques of denial and self-delusion'? Why not surgeons? Why not lawyers? Why not human rights campaigners? We return to this question in a moment. But Reich offers a detailed explanation of his own. There are, he says, 'three sources' of non-purposeful misdiagnoses (p. 195)—empirical problems, theory-ladenness, and 'beauties'. We can 'map' these respectively on to points 5–7 of our list.

5. *Many empirical difficulties.* The first of Reich's 'sources' of non-purposeful misdiagnoses is the empirical difficulties presented by psychiatric diagnosis. These, as we noted in our positive list, are well recognized, not least by psychiatrists. Properly understood they are one aspect of the particular *difficulty* of clinical work and research in psychiatry (the factual aspect). As we saw in Part III, these difficulties are the basis of the need for a more sophisticated understanding of science in psychiatry than in other, conceptually simpler, areas of medicine (such as abdominal surgery). They are also why, as we will see in the first part of the next chapter, the American philosopher, Jennifer Radden, devotes so much of her detailed review of philosophical aspects of psychiatric nosology to the philosophy of science.

But in Reich's account, these difficulties are transformed into *deficiencies*. The pejorative language is unremitting. Psychiatric diagnosis shows '*vulnerability* to error', its reliability is '*poor or questionable*', it 'may *suffer from* bias', and so on (p. 195, emphases added). 'At best', Reich concludes this section, 'psychiatrists are no better than their tools; and they must acknowledge the *limitations* of these tools as the starting point of their own (limitations)' (p. 195, emphases added).

6. *The lessons of Soviet psychiatry.* Reich's second source of non-purposeful psychiatric misdiagnoses is 'the power of diagnostic theory to shape psychiatric vision' (the title of this section of his chapter, p. 196). As we noted above (in our positive list), and as we will see in Chapter 21, the institutionalized abuse of psychiatric diagnosis in the former Soviet Union is a cautionary lesson for psychiatry. But the lesson drawn by Reich, is not the positive lesson that there is more to good diagnostic practice in psychiatry than good science. The lesson drawn by Reich is the negative lesson that psychiatrists are poor scientists.

There are, he says, 'yet other vulnerabilities (i.e. other than problems of reliability) that are even more subtle, more pervasive, and more difficult to recognize....' He then reminds us of his guiding theme that the essence of the ethical problem of diagnosis in psychiatry is the misfeasance of psychiatrists. 'Again', he continues, 'the danger is misdiagnosis—non-purposeful but still damaging—and the ethical problem is the degree to which psychiatrists *allow themselves* to ignore the forces and circumstances that lead to, and make use of, such misdiagnoses' (p. 196, emphasis added).

What, then, are these 'forces and circumstances' to which psychiatric diagnosis is so vulnerable? One factor is plain social bias; however, psychiatrists are 'at least dimly aware of these problems' (p. 196). The rest of the section follows with discussions of the 'reification' of categories, the influence of dominant paradigms (the 'Moscow school' in the Soviet case), and so forth. All, then, fair comment so far as it goes. But entirely begging the question of why psychiatry should be more 'vulnerable' in these respects than doctors in other areas of medicine (or indeed other sciences); and why indeed Soviet psychiatry should have been more vulnerable than psychiatry in other countries. Again, we return to this 'why?' question in a moment.

7. *Implications of psychiatric diagnosis.* This is the third of Reich's sources of the ethical problem of psychiatric diagnosis. It is the least and also the most contentious part of Reich's chapter. It is the least contentious in that it spells out, forcefully, some of the non-medical implications of psychiatric diagnosis. Psychiatrists, influenced as they (rightly) are by the medical model, need reminding of these.

It is the most contentious section, though, because the 'beauties' of psychiatric diagnosis, as Reich calls them, are presented by him as false beauties. They are indeed the most powerful of the sources of psychiatrists' tendencies to 'denial and self-delusion'. There is no doubt that the 'medical model' is overused by psychiatrists (no doubt, from the evidence of the user literature, for example). But there is an equal and opposite danger from the critics of psychiatry of underuse of the medical model. The importance of this balance is underlined in Dickenson and Fulford's casebook (2000), with the balancing cases of Elizabeth Orton (overuse of the medical model) and Tom Benbow (underuse of the medical model.)

Like any other area of medicine, then, fine judgements have to be made in psychiatry between the goods and harms involved in a given clinical situation. If, as Reich suggests, psychiatrists are more vulnerable to getting such judgements wrong, it is not enough to catalogue the harms involved. We have to explain *why* they are more vulnerable.

8. *Origins of ethical problems in human nature.* This recurring question, why psychiatry should be so peculiarly vulnerable to the abuses Reich so fully (and accurately) documents, comes to an explicit focus in the concluding section of his chapter.

We can see this by completing the quote given earlier in our positive list. That quote ran 'Psychiatrists have to understand that...all abuses of diagnoses are a psychiatric problem in considerable measure because they are a *human* problem, ...' (p. 218, emphasis in origin). The passage continues '...and probably stem less from the *corruption* of the profession than from the needs and vulnerabilities of us all.' (emphasis added).

For Reich, then, identifying the origins of the ethical problems raised by psychiatric diagnosis in human nature, means identifying them in our *fallen* nature—the 'needs and vulnerabilities of *us all*' (p. 218, emphasis added). We will suggest in a moment that this (now bleakly negative!) interpretation is wrong. But even if it were right it would still beg the question of why psychiatric diagnosis should be more ethically laden than diagnosis in other areas of medicine. Is Reich suggesting that psychiatrists are more 'corrupt' than other doctors? If so, why? Why, in Reich's terminology, do psychiatrists misdiagnose purposefully more than other doctors? Or is Reich suggesting rather that psychiatrists have the same 'needs and vulnerabilities' as everyone else? If so, why do they misdiagnose *non*-purposefully more than other doctors?

Reflection on the session and self-test questions

Write down your own reflections on the materials in this session drawing out any points that are particularly significant for you. Then write brief notes about the following:

1. Note four positive points about psychiatric diagnosis in Walter Reich's article? (We listed eight.)

2. From Reich's own perspective, are these points positive or negative points about psychiatry.

Conclusions: new tools from Values-Based Practice?

In this chapter we have illustrated the central place of values in psychiatric diagnosis drawing particularly on psychiatry's own scientific classifications, the ICD and DSM. In the final session we focused particularly on Walter Reich's work because he is one of the few, in the bioethical literature, to take seriously the ethical, or more broadly evaluative, issues raised by the diagnosis of mental disorders.

Reich's essentially negative 'take' on psychiatric diagnosis, we will argue in the next chapter, arises from his implicit adoption of a traditional fact-centred medical model. In adopting this model, Reich is in line with similar fact-centred medical models adopted not only in biomedicine (as we saw in Part I), but also in bioethics itself (Chapter 17) and in medical law (Chapter 19). Such a model, we have repeatedly emphasized, is appropriate, up to a point, for values-simple areas of health care, i.e. areas of health care (notably in high-tech acute medicine) where the operative values are largely shared. But *mental* health, as we have seen, is above all a values-*complex* area of health care, an area in which human values far from being largely shared are highly diverse.

Psychiatric ethics, then, we argued in Chapter 18, requires, in addition to the tools of traditional bioethics, a further set of tools, a set of tools developed as a response to the complexity of values in mental health, the tools of VBP. It is to the application of the tools of VBP to psychiatric diagnosis that we turn in Chapter 21.

Reading guide

Delusion and spiritual experience

The story of Simon was first described by the British psychologist, Mike Jackson, in his DPhil with Gordon Claridge at Magdalen College, Oxford, and subsequently published in Jackson (1997) 'Benign schizotypy? The case of spiritual experience' (in *Schizotypy: relations to illness and health* edited by G.S. Claridge). The role of values in distinguishing delusion from spiritual experience was explored, with several case studies (including that of Simon described here) by Jackson and Fulford (1997a) in their article in *Philosophy, Psychiatry, & Psychology* on 'Spiritual experience and psychosis', with commentaries by Littlewood (1997), Lu *et al.* (1997), Sims (1997), Storr (1997), and the authors' response (Jackson and Fulford, 1997b); also, in a shortened from in Jackson and Fulford, 2002a. The significance of Simon's case for our understanding of the role of values in diagnosis particularly in cross-cultural psychiatry is explored in Fulford's article *From Culturally Sensitive to Culturally Competent Mental Health Care: a seminar in philosophy and practice skills* (1999). For a valuable edited collection on the relationship between psychiatry and religion, see Bhugra (1996) *Psychiatry and Religion*.

The issues were developed further in a special issue of *Philosophy, Psychiatry, & Psychology* (Volume 9(4), December 2002), with articles and cross commentaries critiquing Jackson and Fulford's original paper, respectively, by Caroline Brett (2002a) from the perspective of the mystical tradition, and by Marek Marzanski and Mark Bratton (2002a) from that of the theological tradition. Brett (2002b) commented on Marzanski and Bratton, while Marzanski and Bratton (2002b) commented on Brett. An additional commentary on Brett was given by the philosopher Michael McGhee (2002) and on Marzanski and Bratton by the theologian, Stephen Sykes (2002). Both main authors responded to the commentaries (Brett, 2002c; Marzanski and Bratton, 2002c). Jackson and Fulford (2002b) wrote a short paper giving an overview response to the issues raised by both sets of papers.

Abuses of psychiatric diagnostic concepts

For a detailed reading guide on ethical and conceptual aspects of the abusive uses of psychiatry, see chapter 3 of Dickenson and Fulford's (2000) *In Two Minds: a casebook of psychiatric ethics*. *Psychiatric Ethics* (edited by Bloch, Chodoff and Green, 1999) includes a number of relevant chapters: in particular, Paul Chodoff (chapter 4) reviews a number of high profile abuses of psychiatry in Nazi Germany, Japan, and in the USSR. More detailed accounts of each of these are to be found in chapters 22 (by Benno Mueller-Hill), 23 (by Timothy Harding), and 24 (by Sidney Bloch) of the second edition of *Psychiatric Ethics* (Bloch and Chodoff, 1991). Alan Stone's *Law, Psychiatry, and Morality* (1984) explores legal implications of the abuse of psychiatry.

That psychiatry remains vulnerable to abusive manipulation is graphically illustrated by the American psychiatrists

Alfred Freedman and Abraham Halpern's (1999) description of the growing involvement of psychiatrists in executions in some parts of the USA, and by ongoing concerns about potential misuses of psychiatric diagnostic concepts in widely different cultural and political systems: see, for example, (1) in the UK recent debate about new mental health legislation (e.g. Szmukler and Holloway, 1998; Bindman *et al.*, 2003), and (2) concerns about the possible political uses of psychiatry in China (see Human Rights Watch, 2002). The need for a dynamic 'open society' in mental health to reduce the risks of such abuses is noted by Birley (2000).

Values in diagnosis: (1) The ethics literature

As already noted, Bloch and Chodoff's trail-blazing edited collection on *Psychiatric Ethics* has been unusual in the ethical and bioethical literature in tackling head-on and explicitly the importance of values in psychiatric diagnosis. The casebook sister volume, Dickenson and Fulford's *In Two Minds*, includes the story of Simon (chapter 4, though first published in Jackson and Fulford, 1997), and, in chapter 3, cases illustrating both overuse and underuse of the medical model, the values-aspects of which are explored here in chapter 20.

The *Philosophy and Medicine* book series published by Kluwer under the general editorship of Tris Engelhardt and Stuart Spicker has included a number of important volumes on philosophical and ethical aspects of classification and diagnosis, in particular Volume 40, *The Ethics of Diagnosis* (edited by José Luis Reset and Diego Gracia, 1992), which includes historical, anthropological, and sociological perspectives. Volume 15 of the *Episteme* book series (also from Kluwer), on *Diagnosis: philosophical and medical perspectives* (Laor and Agassi, 1990) includes a number of relevant chapters, in particular chapter 4, 'Ethics of diagnostic systems', which examines the issues from the novel perspective of systems analysis. A further useful collection is an issue of *The Journal of Medicine and Philosophy*, edited by Kopelman (1992), on 'Philosophical issues concerning psychiatric diagnosis' (Volume 17, number 2).

Bill Fulford, Tom Murray, and Donna Dickenson's (2002) *Many Voices* (the introduction to their edited collection on healthcare ethics and human values) provides a bridge between ethics and Values-Based Practice. The collection is of classic texts, newly commissioned articles and patient narratives, structured around the stages of the clinical encounter, and illustrating the diversity of human values involved in all aspects of health care. The introductory chapter discusses how respect for different values complements and extends the resources of traditional 'ethics' for clinical decision-making.

References

American Psychiatric Association (1994). *Diagnostic and Statistical Manual of Mental Disorders* (4th edn). Washington, DC: American Psychiatric Association.

Bhugra, D. (1996). *Psychiatry and Religion.* London and New York: Routledge

Bindman, J., Maingay, S., and Szmukler, G. (2003). The Human Rights Act and mental health legislation. *British Journal of Psychiatry*, 182: 91–94.

Birley, J. (2000). Psychiatric Ethics: an International Open Society. Chapter 11, pages 327–335 in Dickenson, D. and Fulford, K.W.M. *In Two Minds: A Casebook of Psychiatric Ethics.* Oxford: Oxford University Press.

Bloch, S. & Chodoff, P. (1991). *Psychiatric ethics* (second edition). Oxford: Oxford University Press.

Bloch, S., Chodoff, P., and Green, S. A., (1999) *Psychiatric ethics* (third edition). Oxford: Oxford University Press.

Boorse, C. (1975). On the distinction between disease and illness. *Philosophy and Public Affairs*, 5: 49–68.

Brett, C. (2002a). Psychotic and mystical states of being: connections and distinctions. (Commentary on Brettford, 2002a). *Philosophy, Psychiatry, & Psychology*, 9(4): 321–342.

Brett, C. (2002b). Spiritual experience and psychopathology: dichotomy or interaction? (Commentary on Marzanski and Bratton, 2002a). *Philosophy, Psychiatry, & Psychology*, 9(4): 373–380.

Brett, C. (2002c). Response to the commentaries. The application of nondual epistemology to anomalous experience in psychosis. *Philosophy, Psychiatry, & Psychology*, 9(4): 353–358.

Dickenson, D. and Fulford, K.W.M. (2000). *In Two Minds: a casebook of psychiatric ethics.* Oxford: Oxford University Press.

Freedman, A.M. and Halpern, A.L. (1999). The Psychiatrists Dilemma: a Conflict of Roles in Executions. *Australian and New Zealand Journal of Psychiatry*, 33, 629–635.

Fulford, K.W.M. (1989). *Moral Theory and Medical Practice.* Cambridge: Cambridge University Press.

Fulford, K.W.M. (1994). Closet logics: hidden conceptual elements in the DSM and ICD classifications of mental disorders. pps 211–232, ch 9 In Sadler, J.Z., Wiggins, O.P., Schwartz, M.A., (eds) *Philosophical Perspectives on Psychiatric Diagnostic Classification.* Baltimore: Johns Hopkins University Press.

Fulford, K W M, (1999). From Culturally Sensitive to Culturally Competent: A Seminar in Philosophy and Practice Skills. Ch 3 in Bhui, K. and Olajide, D. eds. *Mental Health Service Provision for a Multi-cultural Society.* pp 21–42. London: W.B. Saunders Company Ltd.

Fulford. K.W.M. (2000a) Disordered Minds, Diseased Brains and Real People. Chapter 4, in *Philosophy, Psychiatry and Psychopathy: Personal identity in mental disorder.* (ed. C. Heginbotham). Avebury Series in Philosophy in association with The Society for Applied Philosophy. Aldershot (England): Ashgate Publishing Ltd, pps 47–73.

Fulford, K.W.M. (2000b) Teleology without Tears: Naturalism, Neo-Naturalism and Evaluationism in the Analysis of

Function Statements in Biology (and a Bet on the Twenty-first Century). *Philosophy, Psychiatry, & Psychology* 7/1: 77–94.

Fulford, K.W.M. and Hope, T. (1993). Psychiatric ethics: a bioethical ugly duckling? In *Principles of Health Care Ethics* (ed. R. Gillon and A. Lloyd). Chichester: John Wiley and Sons, pp. 681–695.

Fulford, K.W.M., Murray, T.H., and Dickenson, D. (ed.) (2002). *Many Voices. Introduction to Healthcare Ethics and Human Values: an introductory text with readings and case studies.* Malden, MA: Blackwell Publishers.

Human Rights Watch/Geneva Initiative on Psychiatry (2002). *Dangerous Minds: political psychiatry in China today and its origins in the Mao era.* New York: Human Rights Watch.

Jackson, M.C. (1997). Benign schizotypy? The case of spiritual experience. In *Schizotypy: relations to illness and health* (ed. G.S. Claridge). Oxford: Oxford University Press.

Jackson, M. and Fulford, K.W.M. (1997a). Spiritual experience and psychopathology. *Philosophy, Psychiatry, & Psychology*, 4/1: 41–66.

Jackson, M. and Fulford K.W.M. (1997b). Response to the Commentaries. *Philosophy, Psychiatry, & Psychology*, 4/1: 87–90.

Jackson, M.C. and Fulford, K.W.M. (2002a). Spiritual Experience and Psychopathology. Chapter 20 pps 141–149 in Fulford. K.W.M., Dickenson, D. and Murry, T.H. (eds) *Healthcare Ethics and Human Values: An Introductory Text with Reading and Case Studies.* Malden, USA, and Oxford, UK: Blackwell Publishers.

Jackson, M.C. and Fulford, K.W.M. (2002b). Psychosis good and bad: values-based practice and the distinction between pathological and nonpathological forms of psychotic experience. (Response to Brett, 2002a, and Marzanski and Bratton, 2002a). *Philosophy, Psychiatry, & Psychology*, 9(4): 387–394.

James, W. (1902). *The varieties of religious experience.* New York: Longmans.

Kendell, R.E. (1975). *The Role of Diagnosis in Psychiatry.* Oxford: Blackwell Scientific Publications.

Kopelman, L.M. (ed.) (1992) Philosophical Issues Concerning Psychiatric Diagnosis. *The Journal of Medicine and Philosophy*, 17 (2).

Laor, N. and Agassi, J. (1990). Ethics of diagnostic systems. In *Diagnosis: philosophical and medical perspectives.* Episteme Book Series, Vol. 15. Kluwer Academic Publishers.

Littlewood, R. (1997). Spiritual experience and psychopathology. (Commentary on Jackson and Fulford, 1997a). *Philosophy, Psychiatry, & Psychology*, 4/1: 67–74.

Lu, F.G., Lukoff, D., and Turner, R.P. (1997). Spiritual experience and psychopathology. (Commentary on Jackson and Fulford, 1997a). *Philosophy, Psychiatry, & Psychology*, 4/1: 75–78.

Marzanski, M. and Bratton, M. (2002a). Psychopathological symptoms and religious experience. A critique of Jackson and Fulford. *Philosophy, Psychiatry, & Psychology*, 9(4): 359–372.

Marzanski, M. and Bratton, M. (2002b). Response to the commentaries. Minding your language: a response to Caroline Brett and Stephen Sykes. *Philosophy, Psychiatry, & Psychology*, 9(4): 383–386.

Marzanski, M. and Bratton, M. (2002c). Commentary on 'Mystical states or mystical life? Buddhist, Christian, and Hindu perspectives. *Philosophy, Psychiatry, & Psychology*, 9(4): 349–352.

McGhee, M. (2002). Commentary on 'Mysticism and psychosis: descriptions and distinctions.' (Commentary on Brett, 2002a). *Philosophy, Psychiatry, & Psychology*, 9(4): 343–348.

Reich, W. (1999). Psychiatric diagnosis as an ethical problem. *Psychiatric Ethics* (3rd edn), (ed. S. Bloch, P. Chodoff, and S. Green). Oxford: Oxford University Press, pp. 193–224.

Reset, J.L. and Gracia, D. (ed.) (1992). *The Ethics of Diagnosis.* Philosophy and Medicine Book Series, Vol. 40 (series ed. T. Engelhardt and S. Spicker). Kluwer.

Sadler, J.Z. (2004) *Values and Psychiatric Diagnosis.* Oxford: Oxford University Press.

Sims, A. (1997). Spiritual experience and psychopathology. (Commentary on Jackson and Fulford, 1997a). *Philosophy, Psychiatry, & Psychology*, 4/1: 79–82.

Stone, A. (1984). *Law, Psychiatry, and Morality.* Washington, DC: American Psychiatric Press.

Storr, A. (1997). Spiritual experience and psychopathology. (Commentary on Jackson and Fulford, 1997a). *Philosophy, Psychiatry, & Psychology*, 4: 83–86.

Sykes, S. (2002). The borderlands of psychiatry and theology. (Commentary on Marzanski and Bratton, 2002a). *Philosophy, Psychiatry, & Psychology*, 9(4): 381–382.

Szasz, T. (1960). The myth of mental illness. *American Psychologist*, 15: 113–118.

Szasz, T.S. (1960[/1976]) *Schizophrenia: The Sacred Symbol of Psychiatry.* New York: Basic Books.

Szmukler, G. and Holloway, F. (1998). Mental health legislation is now a harmful anachronism. *Psychiatric Bulletin*, 22: 662–665.

Wakefield, J.C. (2000). Aristotle as sociobiologist: the 'function of a human being' argument, black box essentialism, and the concept of mental disorder. *Philosophy, Psychiatry, & Psychology*, 7/1: 17–44.

Wing, J.K., Cooper, J.E., and Sartorius, N. (1974). *Measurement and Classification of Psychiatric Symptoms.* Cambridge: Cambridge University Press.

World Health Organization (1992). *The ICD-10 Classification of Mental and Behavioural Disorders.* Geneva: World Health Organization.

World Health Organization (2001) *International Classification of Functioning, Disability and Health.* Geneva: World Health Organization.

CHAPTER 21

From bioethics to values-based practice in psychiatric diagnosis

Chapter contents

Before tackling the bioethical literature on psychiatric diagnosis in detail, we will briefly summarize the story so far as set out in the last chapter.

In Chapter 20

In Session 1 of Chapter 20, the case of Simon showed that values are inherent in psychiatric diagnosis, not peripherally but at the very heart of traditional psychopathology, in the differential diagnosis of schizophrenia. That value judgements are involved in this differential diagnosis is implicit in ICD. It is explicit in DSM, in the DSM's additional Criterion B of 'social/occupational dysfunction'.

The long Session 2 in Chapter 20 then showed that there is no escape for the traditional fact-only medical model. Simon, still less Criterion B itself, is not an 'exception that proves the rule'. To the contrary, (1) values are pervasive throughout psychiatric classifications, such as ICD and DSM, and, (2) in-depth philosophical analysis (covered in more detail in Part I), showed that the values concerned cannot be defined away. Even the most promising of medical models (based on moral descriptivism) founders on the diversity of human values involved in psychiatric diagnosis; and for similar reasons, (3) advances in neuroscience, leading to better understanding of the brain basis of human experience and behaviour, will make it more, not less, important to take seriously the evaluative (as well as factual) elements in psychiatric diagnosis.

In this chapter

Psychiatric diagnosis, then, is a matter for ethics (values) as well as science (facts). It was with the ethical literature on psychiatric diagnosis, and the work particularly of Walter Reich, that we were concerned in the final Session 3 of Chapter 20.

That literature, we will argue in this chapter, has been deeply influenced by the traditional fact-only medical model. This is consistent with one of our key conclusions earlier in this part about the bioethical literature in general, in so far as it has been concerned with psychiatry. In this chapter we will find that it is true also of the bioethical literature as it has been concerned specifically with psychiatric diagnosis. The challenge, though, is to work out in practical terms the implications of substituting a fact + value model of diagnosis for the fact-only traditional medical model.

It is this challenge that provides the storyline of this chapter. We start, in *Session 1*, with a brief review of philosophical issues generally in psychiatric classification and diagnosis (covered also in detail in Part III (Chapters 13 and 14) and how work in philosophical value theory in particular fits with these. *Session 2* then returns to Reich's observations on psychiatric diagnosis from Chapter 20 but with a view to adding values to (what we will argue is) Reich's fact-only bioethical medical model. Moving, then, from bioethics (fact-only) to values-based practice (VBP) (fact + value), reverses Reich's arguments. *Session 3* shows that instead of the value-laden nature of psychiatric diagnosis being

grounds for criticism, it is grounds for a positive approach to working effectively with values, as well as science, in psychiatric diagnosis. This leads, finally, in *Session 4*, to the practical applications of VBP (many of them still promissory) to clinical work and research on psychiatric classification and diagnosis.

Session 1 Philosophy, values, and psychiatric diagnosis

A brief review and notes from Parts I and III

We will start with a review article by the American philosopher, Jennifer Radden. Radden is one of the founding members and a past Chair of the American Group, the Association for the Advancement of Philosophy and Psychiatry. This article, published in *Philosophy, Psychiatry, & Psychology* in 1994, appeared not long after DSM-IV (APA, 1994). The issues reviewed were 'hot' then and they are 'hot' now!

EXERCISE 1   (20 minutes)

Read the two short extracts from this review article:

> Radden, J. (1994). Recent criticism of psychiatric nosology: a review. *Philosophy, Psychiatry, & Psychology*, 1(3): 194, 197

Link with Reading 21.1

It is well worth studying this article as a whole. It is short but very clear and provides an authoritative overview of the philosophical issues surrounding psychiatric classification in the wake of the publication of DSM-IV. It thus sets the ethical literature in context with other philosophical aspects of psychiatric diagnosis

Two points to think about are:

1. The overall links suggested by these extracts between this part (on ethics) and Part III (on science)

2. Looking to the future, do you agree with Radden's prediction about homosexuality?

Other philosophical areas

An important feature of Radden's review is that, besides values, she covers a wide range of other areas of philosophy relevant to psychiatric diagnosis. Indeed values as such have only a limited place! Thus, if you read the article as a whole, you will find, *inter alia*, philosophy of science, the mind–body problem, the philosophy of action, phenomenology, and, not least, conceptual analysis.

Remarkable by its absence, on the other hand, is traditional ethics (as distinct from philosophical value theory, concerned with concepts). This is a further reflection of the divide between ethics and science in medicine. We will follow up various aspects of this divide later in this session.

Links to other chapters

If, however, values (as dealt with in philosophical value theory) have a limited place in this review, pride of place goes to philosophy of science; and much of what Radden says here concerns, by way of developments in the subject in recent years, the significance and importance in science of value judgements.

This of course connects directly with the storyline of Part III on the philosophy of science, namely that a more sophisticated understanding of science is necessary to underpin clinical work and research in psychiatry. It also reflects the way in which, in all areas of psychiatry, including diagnosis, science and ethics, properly understood, are complementary. Both: (1) are expressions of human values and interests (Chapter 13); (2) depend on the same kind of complex judgement that cannot be completely captured in a codification or algorithm (Chapter 14); (3) are underpinned by an ineliminable element of tacit knowledge (Chapter 14); and (4) involve normative elements (Chapter 15).

Besides values, Radden touches on rationality, in her comments on psychosis. We explored legal concepts of rationality in Chapter 19; and the related ethical concepts of autonomy and capacity, in relation to involuntary treatment, in Chapters 17 and 18. Values turned out to be important in both contexts, legal and ethical. Rationality is also impatant to understanding the particular *kind* of negative evaluation by which the medical categories of disorder are defined: i.e. illness is distinct from ugliness, foolishness, wickedness, etc.

We covered this question, of the particular kind of value expressed by the medical concepts, at a conceptual level in detail in Part I. Although not the express focus of this chapter on psychiatric diagnosis, the range of issues it raises is clearly highly relevant to the implications of diagnostic assessment for the overtly ethical issues (involuntary treatment, mental illness as an excuse in law, civil capacity, and so forth) that we have covered in earlier chapters. It is also the basis of an enriched model of the internal structure of psychiatric classifications (Fulford, 1989, chapters 4, 9 and 10). We return to rationality in Part V where it plays an important role—throughout the part—in the debate about whether mental states can be reduced to brain states and whether meanings can be subsumed under the realm of scientific laws.

From bioethics to values-based practice

Radden's (1994) article, as we noted above, in reviewing the philosophical problems raised by psychiatric classification and diagnosis, has (rightly) as much to say about the philosophy of science and other areas of philosophy, as about ethics. There is, none the less, an ethical literature on psychiatric diagnosis. Indeed an important characteristic of the specifically psychiatric ethical literature is that, unlike other areas of bioethics, it has recognized the ethically laden nature of diagnosis.

We ended the last chapter with a detailed discussion of an article by an exemplar of the psychiatric ethical literature on diagnosis, Walter Reich (1999). This article illustrated the largely negative stance towards psychiatric diagnosis that the bioethical literature has tended to share with the biomedical literature (as in Part I). In the rest of this session we are going to continue our examination of Reich's account of psychiatric diagnosis. This, as we will see, will lead us from the negative stance of bioethics to the more positive stance of Values-Based Practice.

The best of bioethics?

Before returning to Reich's (1999) paper, though, it is worth reminding ourselves why we are spending so much time on it. The last session of Chapter 20 may have seemed critical of Reich. In a sense it was: it was critical of Reich's antipsychiatric mind-set. However, we have focused on his article because it is a closely argued and exemplary statement of one clear position on psychiatric diagnosis. It has been the same with other articles that we have looked at in detail. We have focused on them because they present a strong position clearly and with authority. We may disagree with that position (you may not!). But our aim is to engage with the *best* statement of the position in question.

Reich, as we noted earlier, is among the few, and perhaps the best, of traditional bioethicists to have clearly identified and sought to analyse the central ethical significance of psychiatric diagnosis. He is not one of those who, in the image adopted by one of us elsewhere, has a blind spot for this crucial aspect of psychiatric ethics (Fulford, 1993).

But Reich puts a largely negative spin on this. His account, broadly, is that psychiatrists are vulnerable to self-deception. This in turn is partly due to the limitations of psychiatric science, partly to the theory-ladenness of psychiatric classification, and partly to the seductions (the 'beauties' as Reich called them) of psychiatric diagnosis. However, psychiatric science (although as we saw in Part III, certainly harder) is no more limited than any other area of science. It is also no more and no less theory-laden. And Reich offers no explanation for why psychiatrists more than any other group of doctors should be seduced by the 'beauties' of diagnosis. So what is his model of psychiatric abuse? Why does he think psychiatrists make unethical diagnoses, in general (Reich claims) and particularly in the Soviet case?

EXERCISE 2 (20 minutes)

Re-read the short section in:

Reich, W. (1999). The inherent limitations of the diagnostic process. *Psychiatric Ethics* (3rd edn), (ed. S. Bloch, P. Chodoff, and S. Green). Oxford: Oxford University Press, pp. 195–196

Link with Reading 21.2

How far does this reflect a standard fact-only medical model? If you have read Part I, think in particular about the assumptions we found lying equally behind pro- and antipsychiatry positions in the debate about mental illness.

The biomedical model in biomedical ethics

This short section captures the nub of Reich's assumptions about psychiatry and its ethically problematic nature. There are various ways of thinking about this. The essence of it, though, is the traditional medical model, a model built on such paradigms as cardiology and gastroenterology, in which medicine is assumed to be based on value-free scientific theory with ethics coming in only in the 'appliance of science', with treatment. This is reflected in the literature on concepts in the two assumptions we identified in Part I in the debate about mental illness.

◆ *Assumption 1*: that mental illness is *the* problem

◆ *Assumption 2*: that physical illness, relatively speaking, is *not* a problem.

Thus, Reich, although he calls this section the limitations of 'the diagnostic process', actually writes exclusively about the limitations of the *psychiatric* diagnostic process. The first paragraph reviews literature on the unreliability of psychiatric diagnosis. The second tells a story of 'these limitations being eased' by the introduction of 'relatively objective criteria' but with the warning that 'In the absence of clear, conclusive, and universally accepted criteria, such as physical evidence for the presence of, say, one or other type of schizophrenia or affective disorder, such diagnostic approaches... provide important, though by no means certain, safeguards against diagnostic error.' (p. 196). In other words, when psychiatry has brain diseases on a par with physical medicine, this source at least of diagnostic error, will disappear. Reich is very close, then, in this passage, to Szasz's position: show me the brain cause of schizophrenia, Szasz says, and I will accept it as a disease; but it will be a *brain* disease not a mental illness.

In the next session, we continue our analysis of Reich's paper by looking at how his assumption of the standard fact-only medical model of diagnosis has shaped his attitude to psychiatry. This will lead to the different 'spin' on the bioethics literature, anticipated in the introduction to this chapter, which is generated by a fact + value model, a model that adds values rather than subtracting facts, as developed in Part I.

Reflection on the session and self-test questions

Write down your own reflections on the materials in this session drawing out any points that are particularly significant for you. Then write brief notes about the following:

1. On what area of philosophy does Radden particularly focus in her review of philosophical issues in psychiatric classification and diagnosis?

2. What assumptions about psychiatric diagnosis does Reich share with both Szasz and Kendells in the debate about mental illness?

3. Does a values-based understanding of psychiatric classification and diagnosis, add values or subtract facts?

Session 2 From fact-only to fact + value model of psychiatric diagnosis

At the end of Chapter 20 we identified the origin of Reich's antipsychiatry mind set in his assumption, which he shares with a majority of bioethicists, of the standard fact-only medical model of diagnosis. By the time we get to the end of this session we will have moved beyond bioethics, from a fact-only to a fact + value model.

Our route from fact-only to fact + value model will be by way of the list of points (positive for us, negative for Reich) that we examined in the last session of Chapter 20. Reich's assumption of a fact-only model, we will suggest, has led him (and with him, bioethicists in general) to look the wrong way for an explanation of the vulnerability of psychiatric diagnosis to abusive misuses. It is not the 'fact' side of diagnosis that is the origin of this vulnerability. It is the 'value' side. Recognizing this will lead, in Session 3 of this chapter, to a very different agenda for avoiding (or at any rate limiting the scope for) abusive misuses of psychiatric diagnoses, and, in Session 4, to the practical applications of this agenda in terms of Values-Based Practice.

The fact-only medical model: converting positives into negatives

In the first exercise in this session, then, we will start by looking through Reich's arguments again, this time looking for direct evidence of the fact-only biomedical model at work in his ethical thinking.

EXERCISE 3   (30 minutes)

In the next exercise on this important article, run through the positive and negative lists again, that we produced in Chapter 20. Review Reich's position. How far is it driven by a traditional fact-only medical model of diagnosis? How does a fact + value model convert his negative points into positives? This is another potentially open-ended exercise. But again, don't spend too long on it. Just try to pick out a few examples of the medical model at work.

Then think about a further question. If the medical model is at work here, why might it lead us, in psychiatric ethics, dangerously astray? You might like to refer here to the reading by Fulford *et al.* (1994) linked with Exercise 14 in Chapter 18.

Once the 'medical model' lying behind Reich's article is identified, the many ways in which he converts potential positives about psychiatry into negatives, fall into place. We will review these briefly using the same list (up to point 7) as in the last session. They illustrate a number of important points about psychiatric ethics and the need to break away from the traditional (fact only) to a more comprehensive (fact + value) model of diagnosis in medicine.

1 *Psychiatry as ethically laden.* In a model that emphasizes science, the pervasiveness of ethical issues in psychiatry is necessarily (as Reich finds it) suspect. Psychiatry just doesn't 'look' scientific. It's a problem! In a fact + value model, on the other hand, psychiatry, in displaying these ethical issues so prominently, points lessons for medicine as a whole. The prominence of ethical issues in psychiatry, in a fact + value model, thus ceases to be a problem and becomes an asset (see Chapter 18, especially final session).

2 *Diagnosis as ethically central.* The value-ladenness particularly of psychiatric *diagnosis* is (as, again, Reich finds it) a *particular* problem for the fact-only medical model. As we saw in chapter 4 (notably in the work of Christopher Boorse), the more sophisticated versions of this model are fact-*centred* rather than fact-only. They make medical theory—Boorse's 'disease theory'—a matter of value-free science, and they recognize ethical issues but only as arising in the practical fringe.

In such models, therefore, diagnosis (above all) should be value-free. Whereas in a fact + value model, we should positively expect values as well as facts to be operative in diagnosis.

3 *A classification of misdiagnoses.* The difficulty for the medical model with the value-ladenness of psychiatric diagnosis, is clearly evident in Reich's notion of what we called above, dissociative misdiagnosis. Guided by a fact-centred medical model, ethical issues have to arise for Reich in the *application* of theory in practice, in this case the application of disease concepts in the diagnostic process. The paradigm of unethical practice, on Reich's medical model, is deliberate misapplication (what he calls purposeful misdiagnosis).

Reich, like most antipsychiatrists, draws the line at openly accusing psychiatrists as a profession of wilful misdiagnosis. Yet, on his model of the ethical issues, he is unable to let psychiatrists off the hook altogether—they are not completely or innocently unaware of what they are doing. Hence he ends up with the half-way house of the dissociative model, with psychiatrists using '… various techniques of denial and self-delusion…' (p. 195, as quoted above—and well worth a repeat quote!).

4 *Non-purposeful misdiagnosis ethically central.* A fact + value model, on the other hand, puts an entirely different interpretation on the ethically central place of non-purposeful misdiagnoses. The fact-only (or fact-centred) model, as in Reich's article, has to contrive a compromise between the paradigm of unethical practice as *purposeful misdiagnosis* (with malice aforethought, as it were) and the *non*-purposeful misdiagnoses that Reich rightly identifies as the focus of ethical concern in psychiatry.

In a fact + value model, on the other hand, non-purposeful misdiagnoses arise, directly, from a failure to attend equally to the evaluative as to the factual elements in diagnosis. Psychiatrists do not intentionally neglect the values involved in psychiatric diagnosis, nor do they 'use techniques of denial and self-delusion'. They are simply unaware of the relevant values (at least for what they are). Our opening session in Chapter 20, concerned with the story of Simon, illustrated this in detail. It showed that the relevant values, in psychiatric diagnosis, are there (overtly so, in the case of Criterion B), but tend to be neglected (for the reasons derived, mainly, from R.M. Hare's work in philosophical value theory, in Part I).

This in turn is not a matter of dissociative thinking. It is, on this model, a reflection of the dominance of the fact-only model of medicine. If there is a 'weakness' (Reich's word) here, among psychiatrists, it is not a moral weakness. It is an inattention to a key aspect (the evaluative aspect) of the medical concepts. If this is a weakness, it is a *conceptual* weakness. And it is a 'weakness', as we have several times noted, which is shared by bioethics as much as by biomedicine!

5 *Many empirical difficulties.* In a fact + value model, however, there is really no weakness among psychiatrists. Or rather, psychiatrists are no 'weaker' conceptually than anyone else. As we saw in Part I, it is a general characteristic of us all that we are better at using concepts than at defining them; this is because our powers of direct conceptual introspection are limited and we thus tend to focus on limited aspects of the full meanings of complex high-level concepts; we suffer Wittgenstein's 'delusions of language' (*illusions*, really, as we called them in Part I, i.e. distorted or one-sided understandings of our high-level concepts); and the fact-only medical model, we argued in Part I, is simply this—a one-sided understanding of the high-level *medical* concepts (disease, illness, etc.).

The fact-only medical model, as a one-sided understanding of the medical concepts, has two consequences, one negative, one positive. The negative consequence is the point noted earlier, that in explaining the value-ladenness of psychiatric diagnosis, there is a tendency to look the wrong way. It is assumed that, as medical theory (on this model) is essentially value-free scientific theory, the 'problem' must be inadequate science. More values equals less science, is the equation suggested by this view.

Reich on psychiatric science

Reich (1999), as we noted in the last exercise, makes the equation of 'more values equals less science' explicit in his brief section on the limitations of diagnosis. Reich's 'limitations' are *scientific* limitations. His 'diagnosis' is *psychiatric* diagnosis. The cure, then, of psychiatry's ethical problems with diagnosis, is better science. And better science, for Reich, means the introduction of 'objective criteria…' (like those in bodily medicine), 'clear, conclusive, and universally accepted criteria, such as physical evidence…' (p. 196, again well worth a repeat quote).

Reich, along with many others, casts the difficulties of psychiatric science as *deficiencies*. He thus regards these scientific deficiencies (limitations, he calls them) as an important source of psychiatry's tendency to (dissociatively) misdiagnose. Hence, on his view, Soviet psychiatric science must have been a good deal more 'limited' than psychiatric science elsewhere in the world.

Reich's negative view of Soviet psychiatric science

But *was* Soviet psychiatric science really any different from psychiatric science generally in the 1950s and 1960s? In their article on Soviet abuses (in Chapter 18, linked with Exercise 14), Fulford et al. (1993) showed that the psychopathological concepts involved were no different from those employed in 'the West' at the time. Notably, the notorious Soviet 'sluggish schizophrenia' was equivalent to the 'Western' 'latent' or 'simple schizophrenia'. This indeed was born out by the international collaborative study of schizophrenia, the International Pilot Study of Schizophrenia (the IPSS), which is cited at length by Reich, but which actually treats these diagnostic concepts, the Soviet sluggish schizophrenia and Western simple schizophrenia, as equivalent.

There is a clear suspicion of implicit bias, therefore, in Reich's account, mediated through a distorting pair of (fact only) retrospective spectacles! This bias becomes overt in point 6, in Reich's critical account of Soviet psychiatric science.

> 6 *The lessons of Soviet psychiatry*. Reich, like many others in Britain and America (and indeed in many other countries outside the former Soviet Union) looks to poor science for the origin of the abuse of psychiatric diagnostic concepts. As we saw in Chapter 18 (linked with Exercise 14, the reading on Soviet disease concepts by Fulford et al., 1993), a variety of factors, including, though not limited to, poor standards of applied or clinical science, were involved in these abusive misdiagnoses becoming widespread in the final (and fading) decades of the Soviet empire. But the development of psychiatric science, as such, was no more and no less 'sound' than in non-Soviet countries at the time, notably in Reich's own USA.

This comes through clearly in Reich's (1999) account (p. 198) of the career of the chief 'conspirator', Andrei Snezhnevsky. This reads as the career of a man gaining power and influence for some (unstated) reason of his own. Well, maybe he did. But Snezhnevsky's career parallels that of many other influential figures in the history of medicine. Indeed Reich's account would fit that of a correspondingly powerful leader of research over a similar period at the Institute of Psychiatry in London, Professor Sir Aubrey Lewis. (We looked in detail at Lewis important on clasification in chapter 13.).

EXERCISE 4   (10 minutes)

This is a 'fun' exercise, though with a serious point. Go back to the description of Snezhnevsky's career in Reich's (1999) article, i.e. the para starting 'This Soviet diagnostic system...', p. 198.

See how much of it you can translate directly into Aubrey Lewis' career. If you are not familiar with Aubrey Lewis' career, just imagine how it might have been.

A powerful way to do this exercise is to print out the page from Reich's article and then do a direct translation of the key words: i.e. translate 'Snezhnevsky' into 'Lewis', 'Soviet' into 'British', and 'Moscow' into 'London', etc.

Reich on Aubrey Lewis

The following are some of the passages in Reich's account of Snezhnevsky's career that we believe can be transposed directly to an account of the career of Aubrey Lewis. We have shown substitutions of Aubrey Lewis' career for that of Snezhnevsky by square brackets.

Thus, Reich writes, [Aubrey Lewis] was '... head of the Institute of Psychiatry [of the UK],... the central psychiatric research institution in that country...' and 'chairman of... probably the most prestigious institute [in the UK] for advanced and training degrees.' '[He] dedicated [its] resources [*inter alia*] to the problem of schizophrenia'... [he and his staff] doing 'clinical research designed to elaborate its details'. 'By the early 1970s many of his former students and trainees were in charge of the nation's academic psychiatric centres...' and so 'The pattern of psychiatric teaching and research in centres far from [London] felt the effects of his guidance and views, exerted through his role as an influential member of review committees for government committees responsible for the approval of research and training grants'. The result was that 'By the middle and late 1970s the hegemony of the [London School] in the realm of psychiatric theory and practice, particularly diagnostic theory and practice, was almost complete: it was clearly the dominant force in [British] psychiatry, and its diagnostic system was the standard [British] approach to the diagnosis of mental illness'.

We should not be surprised by the parallels here. As we saw in Part III especially in the outline of Kuhn's work, and of the sociology of science in Chapter 16, it is in the nature of science that, like any other area of human activity, it is subject to political and professional power structures, to the influence of scientific 'top dogs'—remember Max Planck's quip that 'new scientific theories are not born, old scientists just die'! In more recent psychiatric history, many perceive the American Psychiatric Association (the APA), and the DSM in particular, playing just the role of power broker in which Reich castes Snezhnevsky.

New York and Moscow

Reich's account of Soviet psychiatric science, then, although certainly shared by many in 'the West', is biased, in the sense that much of what he says by way of criticism of Soviet psychiatric science applies, *mutatis mutandis*, to Western psychiatric science too. This comes through particularly clearly in the criticisms Reich makes specifically of Soviet psychiatry's diagnostic system.

Thus, Reich argues that '... its (Soviet psychiatry's diagnostic system's) definitions of the schizophrenic disorders... employed such broad and loose criteria that it permitted the diagnosis of schizophrenia in cases in which, in the West, there would be no finding of any mental illness'. Well, it is true that Soviet criteria were broad; but no broader than many systems 'in the West'. Indeed, although not cited by Reich, the first clear evidence that different apparent prevalences of schizophrenia around the world reflected different diagnostic criteria came from the US–UK Diagnostic Project. This showed that much broader criteria were being used in America (New York) than in England (London). It was this that led to the IPSS (as above), which compared diagnostic concepts in nine countries.

The IPSS is actually cited by Reich. But he uses its findings to further criticize Soviet science. He suggests that Moscow emerges as a deviant centre, whereas, in fact, the most deviant centre (in terms of rates of diagnosis) was Washington. Moreover, as to the concept of schizophrenia, the IPSS showed

- that a core condition, defined by the particular symptoms, which now figure in both ICD and DSM, and which symptoms were also the basis of the classical Schneiderian definition of schizophrenia, could be clearly identified in *all nine centres*;

- that Washington, as well as Moscow, had adopted relatively broad criteria for schizophrenia, as compared with the narrower criteria used not only in London but in Columbia, Czechoslovakia, Denmark, India, Nigeria, and Taiwan;

- that the concept of 'sluggish schizophrenia', which Reich criticizes, is the direct counterpart of comparable subtypes of schizophrenia (called 'simple' or 'latent') in other systems. As noted above, these categories (sluggish, simple, latent) were treated as equivalent by the IPSS. Indeed, the only difference (so far as the IPSS is concerned) between Washington and Moscow was that this category of schizophrenia (sluggish/simple/latent) when put through a computer diagnostic algorithm, was reclassified mainly as paranoid and manic psychoses in Washington, and as personality disorder in Moscow. (Remember that we are concerned here only with the *vulnerablility* of psychiatry to abusive practices as these may arise from its scientific basis. Other factors—poor training, etc—may well have been involved in abuses becoming widespread—see Fulford *et al.*, 1993.)

7 *Implications of psychiatric diagnosis*. As we saw earlier, the extent of the 'non-medical' implications of psychiatric diagnosis, from the perspective of a traditional bioethics working within the (tacit) assumptions of the fact-only medical model, is, merely, the other side of the coin of psychiatry's (supposedly) limited science.

One side of this coin, on this view, is that psychiatric diagnosis lacks the objective certainties provided to bodily medicine by (cardiological, gastroenterological, etc.) science. *Wobbly* psychiatric science makes for *wobbly* diagnoses, which in turn leave room for *unethical* diagnoses. This is the nub of Reich's treatment of the role of psychiatric science in the former Soviet Union—it is incompetence-mediated conspiracy!

The other side of the coin, then, is that less science in psychiatric diagnosis, on this fact-only model of medicine, means more non-medical implications, and it is these, that in Reich's section on the 'beauty of diagnosis as a solution to human problems,' generates his catalogue of ethical, legal, and social implications of diagnosis.

Adding value to fact

As we noted earlier, Reich's catalogue of the 'beauties' of psychiatric diagnosis is a valuable feature of his article. The ethical,

legal, and social implications he describes are certainly there in psychiatric diagnosis. Moreover, influenced as psychiatrists themselves are by the fact-only medical model, they are insufficiently aware of these implications.

Among the 'beauties' of diagnosis, however, Reich fails to include curing illness. Curing illness is remarkable by its absence from his catalogue. Surely curing illness (or as a step towards curing illness) is at the heart of what is important and attractive (beautiful) about medical diagnosis. But of course it is absent from Reich's catalogue because Reich is concerned with what he regards as *false* beauties—non-scientific, and hence, on this fact-only model, non-medical implications of diagnosis, implications that, those wedded to this model believe, find their way into the space left vacant by the lack of an adequate psychiatric science.

Diversity of human values

In a fact + value model, by contrast, the 'beauties' are real beauties; or rather, the values implied by Reich's use of the word 'beauty' are part of, rather than external to, diagnosis. In a fact-only model, the values (and hence the implications catalogued by Reich), are contingent on the lack of an adequate science. But in a fact + value model, they are (partly) *constitutive* of the diagnostic process itself.

Diversity of human values: theory and practice

This brings us back then, to the point on which we have settled so many times in this book—that the difference between psychiatry and bodily medicine (as two ends of a spectrum) is not in scientific adequacy but in diversity of human values. This difference is important theoretically: it gives us the 'psychiatry first' message of Part I, that psychiatry is at the cutting edge intellectually in medicine, rather than, as it is perceived to be in the standard fact-only medical model, scientifically backward.

This in turn makes the difference between fact-only and fact + value models important practically. On Reich's model, the practical point of emphasizing what he regards as the 'non-medical' implications of psychiatric diagnosis, is to warn psychiatrists against being led astray by non-scientific will-o'-the-wisps. The practical point of these same 'non-medical' implications in a fact + value model, by contrast, is to make us face up to and take seriously the diversity of human values as they bear on the process of diagnosis in psychiatry.

Reflection on the session and self-test questions

Write down your own reflections on the materials in this session drawing out any points that are particularly significant for you. Then write brief notes about the following:

1. What model of medicine lies behind Reich's essentially negative take on psychiatric diagnosis?

2. What dangers might there be in adopting this model?

3. What view does Reich take of Soviet psychiatric science?

4. Could his view of Soviet psychiatric science apply equally to British and North American psychiatric sciences?

5. Why does Reich seek to subtract values from, rather than to add values to, psychiatric diagnosis?

6. What alternative is there if we are concerned, like Reich, to reduce the risks of abusive uses of psychiatric diagnostic concepts?

Session 3 Reversing Reich

In the final two sessions of this chapter we are going to fill out the key point made at the end of the last session, about taking seriously the diversity of human values as it bears on psychiatric diagnosis, in two way. First, in this session, by reversing Reich's arguments, i.e. by seeing how far Reich's criticisms of psychiatric diagnosis apply to bodily medicine as well. Then, in the final session of this chapter, we will return to the practical implications of taking the values involved in psychiatric diagnosis seriously within the framework of values-based practice.

Reich's argument applied to bodily medicine

First, then, reversing Reich's argument. Reich takes what he calls the non-medical implications of psychiatric diagnosis (i.e. ethical, legal, and social implications) to be substitutes for the (scientific) implications of (genuinely) medical diagnosis.

If Reich is wrong, therefore, if his *non*-medical implications are in fact (partly) constitutive of the diagnostic process itself, then they should be present to some degree at least in diagnosis in bodily medicine as well as psychiatry.

EXERCISE 5   (15 minutes)

In this exercise, we want you to flick though Reich's list of 'beauties' and to see whether you can think of situations in bodily medicine in which diagnosis has the same implications as those attributed by Reich to psychiatric diagnosis, albeit not necessarily to the same degree.

As with other exercises in this session, you could write a whole essay on this! Don't spend too long on it, though; skim through Reich's psychiatric list and come up with a few bodily medicine counterparts.

Here are a few examples we have come up with:

◆ *Diagnosis as explanation, mitigation, and exculpation* (Reich, 1999, pp. 205–207)—well, what about an 'off-work' certificate from the family doctor for a bad back?

◆ *Diagnosis as reassurance* (pp. 208–209)—this depends, presumably, on what is diagnosed! But diagnosis does indeed 'reassure' to the extent that knowing 'what is wrong' reassures in bodily medicine no less than in psychiatry.

◆ *Diagnosis as the humane transformation of social deviance into medical illness* (pp. 209–210)—a tougher one this. But it follows from 'mitigation and exculpation' above; so, what about epileptic automatism in cases of violent murder? This is a well-established legal excuse.

◆ *Diagnosis as exclusion and dehumanization* (p. 210)—in a word, AIDS.

◆ *Diagnosis as a self-confirming hypothesis* (pp. 213–215)—but isn't it always, to some extent? People with physical disabilities are increasingly pointing to the way in which their disability operates as a self-fulfilling prophecy: 'poor old so-and-so, he can't manage that'; so he *doesn't* manage it; so it becomes *true* that he can't manage it!

(Reich's case history, p. 214, by the way, is an example of the self-fulfilling nature of psychiatric diagnostic labels that rivals Rosenhan's classic study! See in Part I, Rosenhan, 1973.)

◆ *Diagnosis as discreditation and punishment*—as Reich rightly identifies, calling someone 'mad' is a powerful way of discrediting them. Any label, though, can discredit whether it is bodily or psychological: try 'obese' for size here! Or 'midget'; even 'asthmatic'; not to mention 'syphilitic'; or 'the liver in bed 3', as hospital staff sometimes refer to their patients.

As to punishment, this takes us into the area of what Reich calls purposeful misdiagnosis. Purposeful misdiagnosis is clearly unethical if it is done for reasons not connected with the patient's best interests. Purposeful misdiagnosis may be ethical, of course, or arguably so, if well motivated. But, again, this is true equally of bodily medicine as of psychiatry. Thus, a false diagnosis of schizophrenia in Soviet Russia may have been well motivated, e.g. saving the person concerned from a slow death in Siberia: Bloch and Reddaway in their seminal work on the abuse of psychiatry in the USSR (1997) noted such cases. But this is no different in principle from a false diagnosis of heart disease saving the person concerned from, say, the military draft. Conversely, either false diagnosis, whether of schizophrenia or of heart disease, could be ill motivated; and among ill motivations a desire to punish the person concerned would be ill indeed.

◆ *Diagnosis as the reflection of social trends.* Reich's highly pertinent example here, of false memory syndrome, illustrates the 'witch hunts' that can result when, as he puts it '. . . diagnostic procedures (are) distorted . . .' (p. 217).

But is that not just the point? Reich's example is indeed an example of *distortion* of the diagnostic process. The hysterical over-reaction of psychologists, therapists, and others, as well as psychiatrists, described by Reich, was a distortion driven by the fashions of the time. Psychiatrists, in fact, as Reich records, although like every other group including some followers of fashion, were also among the most forward in *condemning* the over-reaction. And the history of medicine is full of over-reactions in other areas, bodily as well as mental. How many of us, over 50, lack tonsils because of a fashion for tonsillectomy in the 1940s and 50s; many think we are over the top on vaccinations nowadays, etc., etc.

Reich, right or wrong?

8 *The origins of ethical problems in psychiatry*. Fashions, then, as we saw in Part III, are as influential in science, including medical science, as in any other area of human activity.

So does this mean that Reich, to return to the eighth point on our list, is right after all to identify the origin of the ethically problematic nature of psychiatric diagnosis in the frailty of the flesh, in the 'needs and vulnerabilities of us all' (p. 218), the 'needs and vulnerabilities' in question being, on this interpretation, fashions?

EXERCISE 6   (20 minutes)

Think about this question for a few minutes before going on.

In thinking about this, it may be helpful to refer back briefly to, (1) the opening paragraph of Reich's (1999) conclusions (p. 217), and (2) Session 1 of this chapter.

One way to do this exercise is in the form of a diagnostic formulation. If you are a psychiatrist, or have read Chapter 2 (Part I), you will be familiar with this way of unpacking a medical problem into four main points: (1) diagnosis (i.e. an accurate description of the problem); (2) aetiology (origins of the problem); (3) treatment (what to do about it); and (4) prognosis (likely outcome).

Reich's diagnosis of the problem

In our view, there is a sense in which Reich's diagnosis of the problem is right, and a sense in which it is wrong. Reich is right, in our view, to emphasize that the Soviet experience is not unique: it is an experience that has a key lesson for us all—diagnosis in psychiatry *is* peculiarly vulnerable to abuse. This is a vulnerability that is shared by psychiatrists as a whole. To this extent, then, to the extent of his diagnosis of the problem, we can agree with Reich.

We can agree with Reich further, when it comes to his account of the origin (or aetiology) of the problem, to the extent that (in this passage at least) he identifies this, not in some aberrant property of psychiatric diagnosis, still less in Soviet psychiatric diagnosis, but in human nature.

Where Reich is wrong, however, again in our view, is, as we suggested earlier, in identifying the origins of the vulnerability of psychiatric diagnosis in our *fallen* human nature. This identification runs as a key theme through his chapter and it surfaces explicitly in his conclusions. We have quoted some of this before but it is worth quoting again.

Thus he opens his conclusions (p. 217) with examples of people coming to psychiatrists to circumvent the law... 'they have sought (psychiatric) diagnosis to help them get abortions or evade the military draft'. Seeking a psychiatric diagnosis is

an effective strategy, we find later in the paragraph, in part because '...the law itself has a certain weakness for diagnosis... (it is)...partial to its charms...' (p. 217). And the paragraph finishes, as we noted a moment ago, with an overt reference to corruption—the ethical problems of psychiatric diagnosis, Reich concludes, '...probably stem less from the corruption of the (psychiatric) profession than from the needs and vulnerabilities of us all.' (p. 218).

Reich's aetiology

To continue the 'diagnostic formulation' approach, then, while we share Reich's descriptive diagnosis, we disagree with his proposed aetiology. We agree with Reich's description of psychiatric diagnosis as being more ethically-laden (or at any rate more values-laden) than diagnosis in other areas of medicine; we agree, too, that the Soviet experience of abusive uses of psychiatric diagnosis for coercive purposes of social control, is a signal (writ large) of its more ethically-laden nature. But we believe Reich's aetiology, his theory of the origins of such abuses, in the frailty of human nature, is wrong.

This is essentially because, as we saw in the preceding session, his proposed aetiological factors fail to explain why psychiatrists in general *are*, and Soviet psychiatrists in particular *were*, more liable to make socially-coercive uses of diagnosis than any other group of doctors. Reich's three (proposed) aetiological factors—diagnostic process, diagnostic theory, and diagnostic 'beauties'—fail to stack up: (1) the supposed deficiencies of psychiatric science are not deficiencies but *difficulties* (and Soviet psychiatry was no less 'scientific' than psychiatry in the USA at the material time); (2) the theory-ladenness of psychiatric 'vision', similarly, is not unique to psychiatry (as we saw in Part III, there is no such thing as theory-free data); and (3) the 'beauties' of psychiatric diagnosis, in so far as they *are* beauties (recall that three of Reich's 'beauties' were not beautiful at all!), are beauties of diagnosis in *all* areas of medicine.

Reich's treatment

We will return in a moment to what we believe is the correct aetiology. But before coming to this, it is important to consider the extent to which Reich's formulation of the problem of psychiatric diagnosis, if it is wrong at the level of aetiology, leads to the wrong treatment and indeed to the wrong prognosis.

EXERCISE 7   (20 minutes)

What has Reich (1999) to say (explicitly or implicitly) about the treatment for and prognosis of, the ethical problems of diagnosis? We have covered this already, at least in principle. But spend a few minutes drawing together your own thoughts on this. Concentrate on Reich's conclusions. Could his views on treatment and prognosis be counter-productive?

If the aetiology of the ethically-laden nature of psychiatric diagnosis is, essentially, human frailty, then the cure, essentially, is to stiffen up standards. This is Reich's 'treatment'. Of the three aetiological factors he proposes, two demand scientific stiffening (diagnostic process and diagnostic theory) and the third ethical stiffening (diagnostic 'beauties'). Thus the cure, on Reich's view, for the abuse of psychiatric diagnosis is: (1) to work towards a less defective scientific base for psychiatry; (2) to be less easily influenced by psychiatric theory; and (3) to stiffen our moral resolve in the face of the seductive 'charms' of psychiatric diagnosis.

There is much here with which, transposed from negative to positive, we can agree, both scientifically and ethically. Certainly, we need better science; and greater awareness of the theory-ladenness of science, from observation through to theory choice, will contribute to this. Similarly, a balanced ethical approach to the use of psychiatric diagnostic labels is also essential: recall here, again, Elizabeth Orton's case from Dickenson and Fulford's (2000) 'In Two Minds' (above), in which, consistently with Reich's concern with the false beauties of diagnosis, the psychiatrist (it was the psychiatrist, note) felt that a *medical* understanding of her problem was *in*appropriate; but also the balancing case of Tom Benbow, in which a failure to use the medical model was abusive (case 3/2 in Dickenson and Fulford, 2000).

The devil, though, is in the detail, scientific and ethical. Better science, for Reich, means a psychiatric science that is closer to the paradigm of physical medicine—recall his references to the need for 'clear, physical criteria'. Reich sees these as providing greater 'objectivity' (his term quoted above), which, in turn, is the antidote required to stop our vision being shaped by theory. Better ethics, on the other hand, for Reich, means more moral fibre—strengthening the role of law, reinforcing ethical rules, and reducing the occasions of sin. As Reich puts it, in his concluding section, 'only the most stringent efforts on the part of psychiatrists, and the most serious attention on the part of their teachers, will keep them from yielding unknowingly to those beauties—indeed, will keep psychiatrists from failing to recognise that they even exist' (p. 218).

Reich's prognosis

Reich, as we have several times noted, is not alone in this negative formulation of the ethically-laden nature of psychiatric diagnosis. And the dangers, scientific and ethical, are indeed very real. But they are the dangers, to which we have returned many times, of a fact-only (or fact-centred) medical model. We can summarize these under prognosis (likely outcomes):

◆ *Scientific dangers.* The danger arising from psychiatry modelling itself on physical medicine is that it could actually hold back the development of psychiatric science (the paradigm of liver disease is not necessarily transferable to the brain, see Part III).

◆ *Ethical dangers.* Ethically, the danger of the (unreconstructed) medical model is, as we put it earlier, that it looks the wrong way. In looking solely to value-free science for psychiatric diagnostic theory, it fails to recognize that the ethical difficulties arise from its evaluative (ethical) rather than the descriptive

(scientific) element in diagnosis. Aside from the inherently pejorative attitude to psychiatric science implied by this, it thus has the consequence that ethicists (lawyers, psychiatrists, and lay people) end up 'waiting for Godot', waiting for an illusory 'bodily medicine' of psychiatry that will, somehow, resolve the ethical (or more broadly, evaluative) problem of psychiatric diagnosis. While, in the meantime, all that ethicists and lawyers can do is to thump the ethical drum, exhorting psychiatrists to greater moral endeavours, hedging them around with ever more detailed rules, and subjecting them to ever more radical external regulations.

The ineffectiveness of the fact-centred medical model was evident, in the reading from Fulford *et al.*'s (1993) study of Soviet psychiatry (see the reading linked with Exercise 14 in Chapter 18). The key lesson of this study, as we saw in Chapter 18, is that Soviet psychiatry in general, and the work of Snezhnesky and others on schizophrenia in particular, was guided by a hard-line biological medical model, a model no different, other than in the extra hardness of their hard-line, from the medical model prevalent in the West—prevalent then, and, as we have suggested, prevalent now!

Adding values to science in psychiatric diagnosis

The lesson of Soviet psychiatry, then, is that a more hard-line 'scientific' approach to diagnosis in psychiatry, far from being a protective factor in relation to the abuse of psychiatric diagnostic concepts, may actually be a risk factor, a factor that increases rather than decreases the risks of abuse, a factor that makes the prognosis for psychiatric abuse *worse*.

Science as a factor making the prognosis worse?

The idea that science makes matters worse is counter-intuitive from the perspective of the traditional fact-only medical model, whether in biomedicine or (as in Reich's case) in bioethics. It is entirely consistent, though, with a fact + value model. For, as we have suggested in this chapter, and as Fulford *et al.* (1993) argue in their paper, the fact-only medical model excludes what is essential to an understanding of the abuse of psychiatric diagnosis, the evaluative element in the meaning of the medical concepts. The medical model is indeed 'looking the wrong way'. It is looking to the factual element in diagnosis when it should be looking to the evaluative element.

Why? Because, if everything we have said in this chapter and the last on diagnosis, and in earlier sections of the book both on concepts (Part I) and on psychiatric ethics in general (in Chapters 17 and 18), if all this is right, then the vulnerability of psychiatric diagnostic concepts to abuse arises, not from the (supposed) scientific weakness of psychiatry, nor from the (supposed) ethical weakness of its practitioners, but from a failure to recognize, and hence take seriously, the diversity of values in the areas of human experience and behaviour with which psychiatry, as a medical discipline, is concerned.

Ethics as a factor making the prognosis worse?

So far as the science side of Reich's treatment is concerned, then, there is evidence (as well as an a priori expectation) that a reliance on science, or science at least as conceived in the traditional fact-only medical model of diagnosis, could well make the prognosis for abuses of psychiatric diagnosis worse. What about the ethics side of Reich's treatment, though? What about stiffening up the ethical rules and regulations governing psychiatry? Surely, you may say, this couldn't be ethically counter-productive? Or could it?

EXERCISE 8 (5 minutes)

Can you think of any examples of bioethics being perceived as counter-productive by practitioners (i.e. any 'practitioner', whether as a professional or user, concerned with mental distress and disorder in practice)?

This is a brief 'brainstorm' exercise only! Think about psychiatry in general, not just diagnosis, and write down your answers.

Two examples of traditional bioethics being seen by many practitioners as increasingly counter productive, are confidentiality and research. These are both areas in which many practitioners, users and professionals, increasingly feel that ethicists, in demanding ever tighter regulation, have gone, as one of us has put it elsewhere, a 'rule too far' (Fulford, 2001). The 'rule too far' for Fulford is over confidentiality. The British psychiatrist, David Osborn, has made a similar point in relation to standards of consent in psychiatric research (Osborn, 1999).

What Fulford and Osborn both have in mind is partly a matter of the rules and regulations in question becoming, merely, impractical. The French bioethicist, Ann Fagot-Largeault, gives an example of this in connection with involuntary psychiatric treatment. French mental health law, as Fagot-Largeault describes, came late to the 'autonomy' party. But it then went to such lengths to protect patient autonomy that, as Fagot-Largeault puts it, patients 'escaped' before they could even be assessed (cited in Fulford and Hope, 1996).

But there is also a deeper reason why ethics, of the quasi-legal 'rules and regulation' variety, may be counter-productive, a reason connected with the diversity of human values, as to why we should be concerned about the growing hegemony in bioethics of rules and regulations, at least in psychiatry.

EXERCISE 9 (10 minutes)

Think about this 'deeper reason' for yourself before going on. What is it? The point we are after here follows from the fact that bioethics itself, at least to the extent that in practice it takes the form of rules and regulations, is driven by values.

This is one of those points that ought to be obvious but is not. We have asked you to think about it to bring out the fact that it is not obvious. The fact that it is not obvious is itself an important

observation, important for all psychiatric ethics, not just diagnostic ethics.

No value-free ethics

To cut to the quick, then, the point (the 'obvious when you think about it' point) is that rules and regulations themselves *express particular values*. This is unproblematic in many areas of bodily medicine in which, as we have seen at several points in this book, the values guiding practice are widely agreed upon. This is one reason, then, why a 'rules and regulation' approach from traditional bioethics has been effective in bodily medicine. The rules and regulations in question express shared values.

But it is also the reason why we should be chary of the rules and regulation approach in psychiatry. For psychiatry, if what we have suggested in Part I of this book is right, lacks the value uniformity that is a necessary precondition for the rules and regulation approach to be effective practically. In psychiatry, values, far from being shared are characteristically diverse. Hence in psychiatry, the more tightly the rules are drawn, the more encompassing the regulations are made, the more abusive they will become. For in psychiatry, a rule or regulation expressing a *given* value, will necessarily be at variance with the very *different* values of many of those to whom the rule or regulation is intended to apply.

The paradox of unethical ethics

In psychiatry, then, there is a built-in mismatch between the 'rules and regulation' approach, dependent as it is on uniformity of values, and the diversity of values by which psychiatry is characterized.

In bodily medicine, to put the point metaphorically, what is sauce for the goose is (by and large) sauce for the gander. Whereas in psychiatry, to switch metaphors, one person's meat is (not uncommonly) another person's poison. Hence, to extend these metaphors, rules and regulations in attempting to specify and to enforce a particular set of values, may well be providing sauce for the goose and gander alike in bodily medicine (i.e. because the operative values are largely shared); however, in psychiatry, just in that a rule or regulation is providing meat for one person, it may well be providing poison for another (because in psychiatry our values are often *not* shared).

This apparently paradoxical result, of an ethically motivated approach being responsible for abusive outcomes, as noted immediately above, follows directly from the diversity of human values operative in psychiatry. But is it, really, so paradoxical? To explore this idea we will return to a consideration of bodily medicine.

EXERCISE 10 (10 minutes)

This is another thinking exercise! Can you think of examples, not necessarily in medicine, where ethically motivated actions have led to abusive outcomes?

With any examples you come up with, ask yourself 'why?', why did they have this result? And how does this help to explain why bioethics is increasingly being perceived in some contexts as being in certain respects counterproductive.

Ideology in ethics

The examples we have in mind are of ideologically motivated actions, political, religious, etc. Missionaries, of whatever persuasion, can do a great deal of good. But they can also do a great deal of harm: classic examples are the effects of Christian missionaries, particularly in the Victorian and Edwardian eras, on so-called 'primitive' cultures; think also about the Inquisition, and witch trials (see Chapter 7, History of Mental Disorder).

As to the 'why?' the common factor, surely, is blind conviction, the belief that one's own values, whether political or religious, are in some absolute sense, right. A degree of conviction is motivating, of course. But having the 'courage of your convictions' can all too easily slide into bigotry.

Faced with the legitimate diversity of human values, the fear, in respect of psychiatric ethics in general (Chapter 18), and in respect of psychiatric diagnosis in particular (earlier in this chapter), is of relativism. The fear, as we put it chapter 18, is that we will be precipitated into the 'maelstrom', at best subject to chaos, at worst paralysed by uncertainty. But the lesson of history, in medicine and psychiatry as in politics and religion, is that it is from absolutism, not relativism, that we have most to fear (Fulford 1998, 2000 and 2000c).

From good idea to bad ideology?

It is this lesson, too, that bioethics is at risk of forgetting. In the early days of bioethics, it was appropriate that a tough line was taken in facing down the dominant medical ideology of paternalism, of 'doctor knows best'. 'Doctor knows best' may have been an appropriate ideology when there was not much that doctors could do, for better or worse, other than to give hope through the reassurance of authority. But as technology advanced, especially in the middle years of the twentieth century, extending the range of resources available, and with it the possible goods and harms of different treatment choices, so the values of the patient became increasingly pertinent. Hence it was important that medical paternalism was increasingly balanced with patient autonomy. Bioethics, in its early days, helped to promote that balance. But what we are now faced with is an ideological over-reaction; bioethicists telling everyone else, patients and professionals alike, what to do. We are faced, in other words, with a new ideology, an ideology not of 'doctor knows best' but of 'ethicist knows best'.

It is not only in psychiatry that bioethics is perceived by many to be getting, as it were, too big for its boots. As we noted in Chapter 18, one of the first to point this out was the social scientist, Priscilla Alderson, from her work on the way children and parents were involved in consent issues in surgery: as she put it, patients increasingly find themselves 'doubly disenfranchised', originally by the expertise of the health-care professional, and now by the expertise of an increasingly professionalized bioethics (Alderson, 1990).

Ideology in diagnosis

This is one of the areas, then, in which psychiatry, through its intrinsic diversity of values, could lead the way in medicine. But what way should we go? How do we avoid the equal and opposite extremes of value relativism (anything goes) and value absolutism (what I say goes)?

One way to avoid these extremes, a way increasingly adopted by health-care professionals and users alike, is to 'get round the rules'. High profile cases regularly hit the headlines (e.g. the case in the UK of a woman denied a baby by AID from her dead husband by the Human Fertilization and Embryology Authority). But these cases are the tip of an iceberg of dissent. Social workers, for example, as the British forensic psychiatrist, Christopher Cordess (2001) notes, faced with what they see as rules on confidentiality that prevent them doing their job properly, put their job before the rules. Researchers, similarly, are increasingly rebelling against unrealistic regulations on consent (Osborn, 1999, see above). There is indeed a particularly urgent need for research ethics committees to become partners in promoting good research rather than seeing themselves primarily as protecting patients from bad research (Dickenson and Fulford, 2000, chapter 10).

The counterpart for psychiatric diagnosis of these negative ethical strategies, is adapting one's diagnostic assessment to the 'rules and regulations' defined by the categories in the official classifications. In countries (such as the USA) in which access to health care (for example through insurance) is dependent on a recognized diagnosis, this may be a positive counterpart of the negative abuses illustrated by the Soviet case. But is there a better way? It is to this question that we turn in the last session of this chapter.

Reflection on the session and self-test questions

Write down your own reflections on the materials in this session drawing out any points that are particularly significant for you. Then write brief notes about the following:

1. How many of Reich's negative points about the 'beauties' of psychiatric diagnosis could be applied, appropriately modified but essentially unchanged, to diagnosis in bodily medicine?

2. What is Reich's 'diagnosis, aetiology and treatment' for the misuses of psychiatric diagnosis as guided by the Soviet experience?

3. Could stiffening up scientific standards make matters worse?

4. Could stiffening up ethical 'rules and regulation' make matters worse?

Session 4 Practical applications: values-based practice and psychiatric diagnosis

As we have seen, one important consequence of recognizing the diversity of human values in psychiatry, is the need for improved clinical skills. This is embodied in the model of Values-Based Practice (VBP) in two key principles (which in turn relate to the four skills areas and the 'alliance' model of service delivery (summarized in Box 18.1, Chapter 18). Thus, the two key principles are:

♦ *the patient's values*: to take seriously and to identify the values of each individual patient (Principle 4 of VBP)

♦ *the multidisciplinary team*: as providing a balance of values (Principle 5 of VBP).

To these we should add a third implication, namely, the need for:

♦ *an open society* as the basis of service delivery, national and international, in psychiatry, to ensure a dynamic of effective checks and balances.

We will now consider how these consequences work out in psychiatry in relation to diagnosis, (1) in clinical work, and then, (2) in research.

Values-based diagnosis in clinical work

The three consequences of taking the diversity of values in psychiatry seriously are self-evident enough, at least once they have been worked through (as in Chapter 18 and our earlier materials in Part I). Applying them to diagnosis, though, rather than to the better recognized ethical issues raised by treatment choice (the area of traditional bioethics, see Chapter 17), takes us into the 'blue skies' of new research and of work that is still (largely) waiting to be done. None the less, some general points, anticipating the results of this further research, can be made.

1. *Patient's values in psychiatric diagnosis*. If the values operative in psychiatry are diverse (if they vary from person to person, from culture to culture, and from time to time), and if values come into diagnosis, then it is clear that coming to an understanding of the values of individual patients should be part of the process of diagnostic assessment.

Asking about values

Easily said, not so easily done! For a start, there are generic practical difficulties, i.e. difficulties standing in the way of *any* advance in practice—vested interests, lack of resources, time pressures, and so forth.

But there are also difficulties specific to diagnosis. In the first place, there are difficulties of communication. It is one thing to recognize the principle of starting from an understanding of a patient's values in diagnosis. It is quite another to know how we should go about this in practice.

As with values in any other area, however, we have two main sources of information, the person concerned, and background knowledge and experience of similar people in similar situations.

EXERCISE 11 (20 minutes)

Think about the first of these sources of information, the person concerned. Write down a few questions that you might ask in exploring the values of, say, Simon (in Session 1 of the last chapter), in the context of a diagnostic assessment.

You don't have to be a health-care professional to do this! Write down your own ideas verbatim, i.e. the words you would actually use.

It is surprisingly difficult to ask people directly about their 'values'. We rarely do this, in fact, our values being implicit in and shaping everything we do and say. But here are a few suggestions...

♦ 'Sometimes with [experiences of this kind], as well as being frightened/anxious about it, people find it helpful in some ways. Are there any good/positive aspects to your experiences (as well as bad/negative aspects)?'

♦ 'Do you find that [your experiences] stop you doing things you want to do, or are they sometimes helpful to you?'

♦ 'Is [the experience] comforting or supportive in some ways?'

♦ 'Do you have any ideas about where [the experience] comes from?'

These are, though, just suggestions. This is an area in which there is no research evidence on which to base practice. Our suggestions may make sense; yours may make better sense. But there is as yet no body of evidence on the effectiveness of methods for assessing the evaluative aspects of diagnosis, comparable with the twentieth century evidence available on the effectiveness of methods for assessing the descriptive aspects of diagnosis. And as we saw in Part III (Chapter 13) the lesson of the research leading up to the development of such diagnostic 'tools' as the PSE (a structured interview schedule) and the ICD and DSM (modern classifications of mental disorder), is that the 'obvious' is often far from obvious. It required considerable research effort to establish which aspects of the descriptive elements in diagnosis were reliably identifiable; and this has left us with unresolved questions of validity, not to mention practical utility.

So, this is one area in which research is urgently needed. Exactly what form such research should take is itself an open question. We return to some early initiatives in this area in the next section.

Other sources of information about values

Clinically, however, we have to start somewhere, and in the absence of research on the evaluative aspects of diagnosis comparable with that available on its descriptive aspects, something along the lines suggested above might reasonably become part of routine diagnostic assessment.

Questions of value, furthermore, in the individual case, can now be backed up with a large and growing body of information on the values of users of services in general. We reviewed some of the sources of this information in Chapter 18. It includes official reports, social science research, epidemiological studies, and, above all, first-hand narrative accounts. Additional examples are given in the guide to further reading at the end of this chapter.

Problems with value differences

2. *The multiagency team and psychiatric diagnosis.* Individual patient's values, as we have seen, are important especially in psychiatric diagnosis, because of the inherent diversity of values relevant particularly to *psycho*pathology. There is an aspect, though, specifically of *psycho*pathology, which makes the diversity of values in psychiatry a two-edged sword, and particularly in diagnosis.

EXERCISE 12   (10 minutes)

What do you think we have in mind here? Think back to Chapters 17 and 18, in which we explored the aspects of involuntary psychiatric treatment which make it so uniquely difficult ethically.

A key difficulty turned on an aspect of psychopathology that is central to the categories of mental disorder most often involved in involuntary treatment. What aspect was this? And how does it connect through value diversity to the role (a new role, as we will see) for the multidisciplinary team?

The relevant aspect of psychopathology, in a word, is 'insight'—or rather, 'loss of insight'. Loss of insight as we saw in Chapter 3, is the defining feature of that range of psychotic symptoms—delusion, hallucination, and thought disorder—by which such central categories of mental disorder as schizophrenia, are defined.

It is the psychotic disorders, furthermore, as we found in Chapter 18, that are most often involved in involuntary psychiatric treatment. This is essentially because loss of insight involves a very radical disturbance of rationality in which the person concerned is taken to lose their ability to make autonomous choices. Much the same considerations, as we saw, lie behind the corresponding place of psychotic disorders as the central case of mental disorder as a legal excuse ('not guilty by reason of insanity').

Values and other diagnostic concepts

That easy formula, 'not guilty by reason of insanity', relies on a series of difficult concepts—rationality, capacity, responsibility—that we explored in Chapters 18 and 19, and all of which are central to psychiatric diagnosis. As we saw in Part I, values are necessary but not sufficient to define diagnostic and psychopathological concepts. A disease, illness, or disability, is not just a *bad* condition to be in (other things being equal), it is a bad condition in *the specifically medical sense of bad*, a sense different from, e.g. ugliness, wickedness, foolishness, etc.

It is important to remind ourselves of this periodically as many of the most difficult ethical issues in psychiatry turn not just on questions of value but on questions of the particular kind of value expressed by the medical concepts. With mental disorder as a legal excuse, for example, the issue is not (just) 'good or bad?', but '*mad* or bad?'; and in involuntary treatment (for depression, say), it is not (just) 'good or bad?' but '*mental disorder* or sad?' (see generally, Part I and earlier in this part).

That said, though, all these diagnostic concepts (rationality, capacity, etc.), in so far at least as they are part of psychiatric diagnosis, do involve questions of value. They are not *sufficiently*, but they are *necessarily in part*, defined by values. And the rub is this. Value diversity in psychiatry means that, above all in psychiatry, a key aspect of diagnostic assessment (loss of insight and its related set of concepts) will involve *conflict* of values. In the case of involuntary treatment, for example in Mr AB's case at the start of Chapter 17, the problem is precisely that the patient wants one thing and everyone else wants the opposite.

A balance of evaluative perspectives

So, what to do? Again, there is no magic formula. Good communication is a key, and it is increasingly recognized that with time and care, a stand-off can often be avoided. But there will always be cases where, when everything is understood, there are still irreconcilable differences.

Our options, when conflicts of values arise in diagnosis, are exactly as Dickenson and Fulford (2000) discuss for psychiatry and health care in general. What is required, Dickenson and Fulford argued, to limit the scope for abuses, is a *balance of evaluative perspectives*.

This is where, as Principle 5 of VBP emphasizes (see Box 18.1), a well functioning multiagency team may be helpful. In the traditional fact-only model, in which diagnosis is an exclusively scientific process reserved to doctors, the multiagency team provides a range of skills relevant to treatment. In a fact + value model, the multiagency team retains this role but takes on, in addition, a new role, to provide *a balance of evaluative perspectives in diagnostic assessment*.

The 'multiagency team', it is worth adding, should be broadly understood in this context. It should include, subject to issues of confidentiality, people from backgrounds that are similar to those of the person concerned. There is a growing recognition of the importance in psychiatry of a culture (and gender) de-centred approach to diagnosis, a key component of which is the balance of values provided by a well-functioning multi-agency team (Colombo *et al.*, 2003a and b).

Values and the organization of psychiatry

3. *The 'open society' and psychiatric diagnosis.* With patient-centredness, then, and a balance of evaluative perspectives (combined, remember, with all the descriptive aspects of diagnosis emphasized in the traditional fact-only approach), are we out of the woods? Why, as Dickenson and Fulford (2000) suggest, do we need the third element, their 'open society'?

In a short but important chapter in Dickenson and Fulford (2000) J.L.T. (Jim) Birley, draws on a lifetime of experience of psychiatry in an international context. In particular, he was the founder President of the *Geneva Initiative for Psychiatry*, an organization set up by a Dutch social scientist, Robert van Voren, originally to oppose the abusive uses of psychiatry in the former USSR, and now to promote initiatives aimed at restoring clinical standards in post-Soviet psychiatry.

Dangers of consensus

Jim Birley's (2000) bottom line is that an 'open society' in psychiatry is necessary if we are to avoid the closed systems, institutional or political, in which abuses are so likely to arise. Translating this into terms of values, the 'open society' provides a dynamic of mutual checks and balances as the basis of what one of us has called elsewhere, "dissensus" (Fulford, 1998). It was the closed nature of a totalitarian society that, as we saw, allowed a political value system to become (largely unawares) dominant in psychiatric diagnostic assessment in the former Soviet Union. But there is the same danger at all levels in psychiatry, through national organizations, to local institutions, and of course, on into multiagency teams. (Note that in Simon's case (Exercise 1, chapter 20), his cultural peers did not endorse his experiences.)

At all levels, then, the danger is consensus, the hegemony of the values of the many over the values of the few or indeed the one. An 'open society' is not an absolute barrier to such abuses. But the lesson of history is that it is a necessary if not sufficient protection all the same.

Values-based diagnosis in research

In addition to the growing body of theoretical work on values in psychiatric classification and diagnosis, outlined in this and earlier parts of the book, a number of early initiatives have been taken in applied research. Central to applied research will be the development of research methods equal in reliability and validity to those developed in the twentieth century to support work on the descriptive elements in diagnosis (described in Part III). Just what reliability and validity mean in this context is itself a moot point. Thus, in Chapter 13 we discussed the relationship between reliability, validity, and the very idea of natural classification. While there are fairly agreed practical tests of reliability, there is disagreement and debate in the philosophy of science about how to assess the validity of a scientific taxonomy. This will again find an echo in the field of values.

Research methods

A research methods meeting in London in 2003, funded by a section of the Modernisastion Agency in the UK's National Health Service, the National Institute for Mental Health in England (NIMHE), brought together stakeholders, including users of services, with researchers (some of whom had been directly involved in the research on the descriptive aspects of diagnosis). Building on a wider meeting organized by John Sadler in 1997 in Dallas (Sadler, 2002), the London meeting focused directly on candidate

methodologies for clinical and research work on the role of values in diagnostic assessment. Exemplars of such methods include:

1. phenomenology (Stanghellini, 2000, 2004)
2. formal survey methods (Schwartz, in press)
3. semistructured interviews (Tan *et al.*, 2003)
4. surveys (Jackson, 1997)
5. combined linguistic-analytic and social science methods (Fulford and Colombo, 2004)
6. hermeneutics (Widdershoven and Widdershoren-Heerding, 2003)
7. discursive analysis (Sabat and Harré, 1997; Sabat, 2001).

The London meeting established an informal network of researchers and stakeholders and agreed a 'platform statement' for research in this area (reproduced in Fulford, 2005).

In addition to the work of individual members of the network (see Reading Guide), ongoing research on values in psychiatric diagnosis has included a further NIMHE-funded meeting on values in the diagnostic assessment of decision-making capacity, drama-based approaches to improving cross-cultural understanding, extensions of the combined philosophical and social science work on models of disorder, educational research, and an initial appraisal of a new interview schedule for general clinical use.

A research agenda

Besides research directly on the evaluative element in psychiatric diagnosis, balancing earlier work on the descriptive element, what other lines of research are opened up by the recognition of the diversity of values in psychiatric diagnostic concepts?

The research agenda opened up by the recognition of values in psychiatric diagnosis is discussed in the final section of Jackson and Fulford's article in *Philosophy, Psychiatry, & Psychology* (1997). This is the article in which Simon's story (set out earlier in this part) was first described, and it includes other similar cases.

A wide research agenda

In the final section of their paper, then, Jackson and Fulford (1997) look briefly at the research agenda opened up by cases like Simon's. The essential point for future research made by Jackson and Fulford, is that once the place of values in psychiatric diagnosis is recognized, *values themselves become a key variable*. In many areas of bodily medicine, the values 'variable' is for practical purposes a constant (i.e. because, and to the extent that, the human values operative in bodily medicine are shared values). But wherever values are diverse they become a variable in the research design, and in some cases a key variable. Jackson and Fulford's list of research areas in which values may be a key variable includes

- psychopathology
- epidemiology
- cognitive-behavioural therapy
- neuroscience

From the point of view of research, neuroscience illustrates the 'values is a key variable' point particularly clearly. Brain imaging research that fails to distinguish people like Simon from people with schizophrenia (because they both have psychotic experiences) conflates two very different syndromes. Such research is also missing a methodological trick, namely the opportunity to compare psychotic experiences as they arise in normal as well as in pathological contexts.

Cognitive-behavioural therapy is particularly interesting clinically as the basis of a 'cognitive problem solving' model of psychotic experience. According to this model, psychotic experience as such is not pathological. As in Simon's case, and others described by Jackson and Fulford, it may be a mechanism for *resolving* problems. This mechanism can go wrong, of course, and where it goes seriously wrong, psychotic experience (like any other kind of experience) may be pathological. But the cognitive problem-solving approach aims to move people from the pathological to the adaptive end of this spectrum. And the point for diagnosis, is that exactly how a given individual's psychotic experience develops may be critically determined by how people react to it on first presentation. Some people are indeed ill (and on this model, they may indeed be helped by neuroleptics and other medical treatment). But an *assumption* of pathology, as the fact-only medical model requires, may be, as Reich argues above (see his 'beauties' of diagnosis), a self-fulfilling prophecy.

Futures perfect and imperfect in psychiatric diagnosis

Persuasive as the arguments, theoretical and practical, might be for recognizing the importance of values in psychiatric diagnosis, it is important to recognize how radical a departure this is from the traditional fact-only medical model.

Future imperfect

Richard Bentall, a professor of psychology, brought this point home to psychiatry a few years ago with an article provocatively titled 'A proposal to classify happiness as a disease' (1992).

EXERCISE 13   (15 minutes)

Read the two extracts from this short article:

Bentall, R.P. (1992). A proposal to classify happiness as a psychiatric disorder. *Journal of Medical Ethics*, 18: 94–98

Link with Reading 21.3

Bentall writes in the great tradition of the psychiatry/ antipsychiatry debate. But what do you make of his concluding point about the implications of values in psychiatric classifications?

Bentall wrote this article as a dig at psychiatry. In fact, it caused quite a stir (it made the National Press!) and the *British Journal of Psychiatry* published a number of commentaries on it. What is eye-catching about it (besides being very well written) is the central claim that happiness should be a disease. Of course, mania is pathological happiness. But what Bentall claims is that by the criteria of medical psychiatry, happiness *as such*, no less than depression, should be classified as a disease.

His point then is the antipsychiatry point from Part I, that the scientific criteria adopted by medical psychiatry (including evolutionary criteria, as in Kendell's (1975) pro-psychiatry position, are incapable of distinguishing happiness (normal, every-day happiness) from disease. The point that he *could* have made is the linguistic-analytic point that, if these criteria fail to mark this distinction, it must be marked by something else ('must' in the sense that the distinction is there, it is part of the 'logical geography' of ordinary usage, and hence has to be explained or explained away; it can't simply be denied—see generally, Part I on ordinary language philosophy). If the distinction is not marked by facts, then, why not by values? This indeed is the burden of Bentall's concluding comment that '. . . only a psychopathology that openly *declares* the relevance of values to classification could persist in *excluding* happiness from the psychiatric disorders.' (p. 97, emphases added).

The implication of Bentall's concluding point is that psychiatric diagnostic classification is either absurd (because making happiness a disease) or unscientific (because value-laden). Behind his ingenious arguments, then, is the 'medical' model, an exclusively 'scientific' model of genuinely *medical* disorder, which, as we found in Part I, was behind both Szasz (as representing antipsychiatry) and Kendell (representing pro-psychiatry).

But if values are the relevant criterion for distinguishing between non-pathological happiness and happiness as a disease, this has the further consequence that happiness could, after all, be a disease! This is essentially because of the open-endedness of the possibilities (logical possibilities) for evaluation. Recall from Chapter 6, that non-reductive theories of the relationship between fact and value (description and evaluation) allow the possibility (the logical though not the psychological possibility) that anything may be evaluated positively or negatively. Hence, just as homosexuality, partly in response to changes in social values, has disappeared from DSM, so it is possible that it could once again, in the future, reappear! This is repugnant to *us*. But that reflects *our* values. And if homosexuality can reappear in DSM, why not heterosexuality too. And, by extension, happiness.

Future imperfect in the UK

These examples may seem fanciful. But there was an example of the risk of just such a shift in the boundary between medicine and morals in a recent proposal by the UK government to make psychiatrists responsible for people perceived to be dangerous. An early draft of this proposal was framed in such a way as to risk making dangerousness *per se* a disease (Department of Health, 2002). This was not the intention of the proposals and it is not the effect of subsequent draft legislaion (Department of Health, 2002). But there were many parallels between the 2002 proposals and the Soviet case—a 'no nonsense' medical-scientific model, and an over-riding political value (to protect the public from dangerous 'psychopaths'). Like the Soviet case, too, it was well-intentioned. There *is* a real need for public protection in some cases. But pathologizing dangerous behaviour carries all the potential for abuse that pathologizing political dissent had in the USSR.

Planning for dissensus

The boundary between mental disorder and mental difference, then, as we found in Part I, is variable. And it is variable partly because human values are variable. The way to avoid abusive misdiagnosis, then, is not to deny this variability but to acknowledge its origin and to establish processes, both in the evolution of psychiatric diagnostic concepts and in day-to-day clinical diagnostic practice, which seek as far as possible to track and to respond to the values involved.

The 'mistake', then, to return to Radden's (1994) term in the first exercise in this chapter, was not the original inclusion of homosexuality in DSM, nor indeed its subsequent removal. The mistake is not, as such, to include or exclude this or that category. The mistake is the failure to recognize the diversity of human values and their relevance to the validity of a given diagnostic category in a given (personal and social) context. Rather than seeking to exclude values, therefore, our response, as we have several times noted, should be to improve the processes—the clinical skills and forms of service delivery—which will support what might be called in the language of VBP, dissensual diagnosis, an approach that combines meticulous attention to the facts with a balanced approach to the diagnostic values relevant in individual cases.

Future perfect?

The idea that values are present in medical diagnosis, and substantively so in psychiatric diagnosis, is, from the perspective of the traditional medical model, radical—*dangerously* radical, some may think! (See, for example Robert Spitzer's (2005) carefully argued concerns: as the chair of the DSM-III Taskforce, Spitzer was a key figure in the twentieth century scientific development of psychiatric classification—see chapter 13). Yet the incorporation of an explicitly evaluative element into psychiatric diagnosis would not, as such, alter it radically. There are other reasons for thinking that future classifications of mental disorders might look rather different from our current ICD and DSM. But these have to do with other conceptually problematic elements of psychiatric diagnosis (capacity and rationality, as noted above; see also Fulford, 1989, chapters 4 and 9). But the incorporation of values as such would leave our classifications in many respects more or less unchanged.

EXERCISE 14   (20 minutes)

This is a short two-part exercise.

1. Go back to Box 20.2 in Chapter 20, the summary diagnostic criteria for schizophrenia in DSM. Try rewriting these criteria to make the evaluative element fully explicit.

2. Then look at the extract from Fulford's (2002a) futuristic 'Report to the Chair of the DSM-VI Task Force'.

The figure in the extract from Fulford's article is an imaginary version (in a future DSM-VI) of the diagnostic criteria in Box 20.2 in Chapter 20 (from the current DSM-IV). Two key points to note are,

1. *Descriptive*: the DSM-VI criteria are identical to those in DSM-IV in so far as the criteria are descriptive. This emphasizes the fact that there is nothing 'antiscience' in a fact + value view. Everything that is genuinely factual remains intact and indeed is clarified.

2. *Evaluative*: the (imaginary) changes in the DSM-VI criteria are in the 'value added' component of the fact + value view. The DSM-VI criteria spell out explicitly what is implicit in DSM-IV, that value judgements are involved in applying Criterion B. The summary box also includes indications of possible steps involved in a diagnostic process leading to a balanced judgement on the relevant values.

Fulford's article (2002a) is of course largely an exercise in futurology. As we have noted, much of the research programme implied by the recognition of the place of values in diagnosis is waiting to be done. By casting his article in this form, however, Fulford sought to emphasise that such research, far from being dangerously radical, would be in important respects no more than a twenty-first century continuation of the development of psychiatry in the twentieth century.

Reflection on the session and self-test questions

Write down your own reflections on the materials in this session drawing out any points that are particularly significant for you. Then write brief notes about the following:

1. What three principles of values-based practice are particularly important for psychiatric diagnosis in clinical practice; and why?

2. What further principles are important in research contexts; and why?

3. In what areas of research are values-based (as well as evidence-based) approaches relevant?

4. In what way would the criteria in classifications like the ICD and DSM differ in a values-based as well as evidence-based classification?

Session 5 Conclusions: values-based diagnostic assessment and user empowerment

This chapter has been something of a Star Trek expedition. We have set out 'to boldly go' into new territory about the role of values in psychiatric diagnosis. This is above all an area, as we have several times emphasized, in which there is no settled view, no party line.

An ongoing debate

Nor, if everything we have looked at in earlier chapters is right, should there be a settled view. In the debate about the concept of mental disorder (of which the questions explored in this chapter are a part), there is mature opinion on both sides, both for and against the view that values are ineliminable. These views reflect, consciously or unconsciously, deep lines of research both in philosophical value theory (the 'is-ought' debate, about the logical relationship between description and evaluation, see Chapters 4 and 6) and in the philosophy of science (the debate about the relationship between normatively based understanding in the social sciences and the subsumption under natural laws exemplified in the natural science: the space of reasons versus the realm of law as described in Chapter 15). These debates, in turn, as debates in the philosophy of psychiatry, are but the latest manifestations of a tension running through the history of psychiatry, between medical and moral interpretations of mental disorder, going back over 2000 years (see Chapter 7).

The role of philosophy

We should not have expected 'answers', then, in the sense of conclusions to which everyone of 'good sense' will subscribe. This is an area in which, rather, the role of philosophy is, as we put it in Chapter 6, to avoid premature closure. The role of philosophy is to say 'hang on a minute', to prevent us settling for wrong answers, answers that, although easy to understand and comfortable to cling to, are, at best, incomplete: the extremes of the psychiatry versus antipsychiatry debate, we argued in Chapter 6, offered answers of this kind—out and out assimilations of mental disorders respectively to bodily disorders on the one hand, or to morals on the other.

Two caveats

Two points, though, made in earlier chapters, bear repetition. They amount to final caveats:

Caveat 1: value added not science substracted. The model of mental health practice guiding this book is of an enriched health-care discipline in which values are added to facts (or more formally, evaluations to descriptions) rather than values ousting facts (or vice versa). There is nothing in this 'full-field' view, as we called it in Chapter 6, which is antiscience.

True, our model of science may have to be more sophisticated if it is to incorporate evaluation alongside description. But that is because human beings are a more complex 'object of study' than, say, plants or rocks. Hence as we said at the end of Chapter 6, everything that is genuinely descriptive in psychiatry is no less important in a 'full-field' view than in the traditional medical model.

There is a sense indeed in which the descriptive element is even more important in a full-field model. For as we saw in Part I, and again in Part III, in a full-field model, the descriptive criteria for mental disorders serve two roles. In a full-field model,

descriptions, (1) define particular conditions, and (2) serve as criteria for the value judgements involved in taking a given condition to be a *bad* condition, a *disorder*.

Caveat 2: user empowerment not practical paralysis. The danger with 'value added', as perceived within a traditional fact-only model of diagnosis, is 'relativism', replacing the certainties of science with the paralysis of uncertainty in the minds of professionals. In a fact + value model, by contrast, 'value-added' brings with it empowerment of those on the receiving end of diagnosis, those who use rather than provide services.

Concerns about relativism, as we have seen, although understandable enough, reflect a mistaken view of the way values work in practice (see above, Chapter 4, R.M. Hare's work); and in psychiatry, at any rate, the greater danger is not relativism but absolutism (see above with regard to the USSR). So far as diagnostic agreement is concerned, bringing values explicitly into the frame could well increase the scope for agreement. At the very least, bringing the 'user's' values explicitly into the frame brings him or her back to centre stage in diagnosis as the defining step in the clinical encounter.

Having a say in how your problems are understood

Dr V.Y. Allison-Bolger, a consultant psychiatrist in England with wide experience of the psychopathology of psychotic conditions, has made this key point about user empowerment in values-based diagnosis by analogy with the move in traditional bioethics from paternalism to autonomy.

'In bioethics', she has pointed out, 'we have got used to the idea of users of services 'having a say' in how they are treated. We call this patient autonomy. Recognizing the importance of values in diagnosis means that, as professionals, we have got to get used to the idea of users of services 'having a say' also in how their problems are understood.'

Allison-Bolger (personal communication)

Reading guide

Values in diagnosis: (2) The philosophy literature

A valuable edited collection covering most of the key conceptual issues in psychiatric diagnosis and classification is the American psychiatrist and philosopher, John Sadler et al's (1994) *Philosophical Perspectives on Psychiatric Diagnostic Classification*. Edited jointly with two leading figures in the early years of the new philosophy of psychiatry, the psychiatrist Michael Schwartz and the philosopher Osborne Wiggins, this book was published to coincide with the appearance of DSM-IV. It has a foreword by Allen Frances, the Chair of the DSM-IV task force. Sadler has subsequently published two major books specifically on values in psychiatric diagnosis: (1) an edited collection, including contributions from users of services and carers as well as clinicians, philosophers and neuroscientists, *Descriptions and Prescriptions* (Sadler, 2002), and (2) an extended monograph with detailed studies of the values impacting on each of the main classes of psychiatric disorder *Values and Psychiatric Diagnosis* (Sadler, 2004).

The potential impact of Fulford's (1989 and 1994) analytic and Sadler's substantive work on the form and content of future editions of psychiatric classification such as the ICD and DSM is explored in Fulford's (2002a) futuristic *Report to the Chair of the DSM-VI Task Force*, and (2002b) *Executive Summary*. The role of users of services and families in the development of these classifications is argued for in Sadler and Fulford, 2004. A discussion of the issues from widely different viewpoints has been presented in *World Psychiatry*—see Fulford *et al.* (2005). 'Looking with both eyes open: fact *and* value in psychiatric diagnosis?' with commentaries by Sadler, First, Wakefield, Spitzer, Sartorius, Banzato and Pereira, Mezzich, Tan, Kitamura, Van Staden and King (all 2005).

As detailed in Part I, Fulford (1989), draws on linguistic-analytic philosophy to show how values help to define diagnostic concepts in all areas of medicine, but are especially important practically in psychiatry because of the diversity of human values in the areas of experience and behaviour with which psychiatry is concerned. The possible relevance of this diversity to the diagnosis of bipolar disorder is noted by Goodwin, 2002.

Articles on the importance of values in all areas of psychopathology appear regularly in the international journal, *Philosophy, Psychiatry, & Psychology*. Besides Jackson and Fulford (as above, chapter 20), examples include Kopelman (1994) 'Normal grief: Good or bad? Health or disease?'; Moore *et al.* (1994) 'Mild mania and well-being'; Sadler (1996) 'Epistemic value commitments in the debate over categorical vs. dimensional personality diagnosis'; Sadler and Agich (1995) on 'Diseases, Functions, Values, and Psychiatric Classifications', with a reply by Wakefield (1995).

Values-based practice: (2) Resources

Resources to support VBP are now well developed through a number of initiatives in the UK and internationally in policy, training and research.

Policy

The National Framework for Values-Based Practice (reproduced in 18.2, chapter 18) has been developed by the National Institute for Mental Health in England (NIMHE) to support policy, training, and research within the UK Government's policies for mental health as defined by the National Service Framework for Mental Health (Department of Health, 1999). As a policy implementation body, the NIMHE Values Framework reflects early recognition of the need for a new user-led approach to service development. It has implications for a number of workstreams,

including 'experts by experience' (user-led service developments), recovery practice, spirituality, social inclusion, and black and minority ethnic initiatives. The NIMHE Values Framework is available at www.connects.org.uk/conferences. (See also, Woodbridge and Fulford, 2004a; and Department of Health, 2004).

A detailed discussion paper exploring some of the key issues about values for the Experts by Experience programme, one of the work programmes of the NIMHE, is Wallcraft (2003) *Values in Mental Health—the role of experts by experience* (available at www.connects.org.uk/conferences). Jan Wallcraft is the NIMHE's National Fellow for 'Experts by Experience'. The links between VBP and recovery are described in Allott *et al.* (2002) 'Discovering hope for recovery.' (Special issue of the *Canadian Journal of Community Mental Health*). The role of VBP in providing links between policy and user-led service developments are explored in Williamson (2004) 'Commentary "Can Two Wrongs Make a Right?"' (*Philosophy, Psychiatry, & Psychology*).

Training

There are two sources of VBP training in the UK

- A training manual for Values-Based Practice, 'Whose values?', developed jointly by the Sainsbury Centre for Mental Health in London and the Department of Philosophy and the Medical School at Warwick University (Woodbridge and Fulford, 2004b). It was launched by Rosie Winterton, Minister of State in the Department of Health with responsibility for mental health, at a conference in London in July 2004.

- A detailed manual developed by the West Midlands Mental Health Partnership to support training in values for mental health and to provide an informal audit tool to monitor their implementation, is West Midlands Mental Health Partnership is *Values in Action: developing a values based practice in mental health* (West Midlands Mental Health Partnership, 2003.)

These resources will support a UK training initiative in the generic skills required for working in mental health, the Ten Essential Shared Capabilities (10 ESCs, see Department of Health (2004b). The 10 ESCs are built on values-based and evidence-based sources aimed at developing the skills-base for the new roles and ways of working for professionals (Department of Health, 2004c) that are required to support the National Workforce strategy (Department of Health, 2004a).

Papers describing early work on the development of training methods for VBP include:

1. Fulford *et al.* (2002) 'Values-Added Practice (a Values-Awareness Workshop)'. This paper describes the first of the series of training workshops that Kim Woodbridge, Toby Williamson, and Bill Fulford developed and on which the workbook is based.

2. Woodbridge and Fulford (2003) 'Good practice? Values-based practice in mental health'. This paper covers similar material to reading 5 but in the form of an interactive workshop suitable for self-study.

3. Woodbridge, and Fulford (2004) 'Right, wrong and respect.' (*Mental Health Today*).

There is a large social science literature on values and value diversity. A classic textbook exploring the impact of diversity in a wide variety of health-care settings, including cross-cultural perspectives on the human life cycle, the social effects of medical technology, and cultural aspects of pain, stress, physical disability, and impairment, is Helman (2000) *Culture, Health and Illness: an introduction for health professionals*, (4th edn). A resource of literature and patient narratives illustrating the importance of differences of values in all areas of health care, is Fulford et al., (2002) 'Introduction. Many voices: human values in health care ethics (in ed. Fulford, Dickenson, and Murray, *Healthcare Ethics and Human Values: an introductory text with readings and case studies*).

Sessions on VBP are included in a number of training programmes, for example those run by the Sainsbury Centre for Mental Health (see website below); in Piers Allott's Masters Programme in Recovery at Wolverhampton University in the UK; in the medical school programmes at Pretoria Medical School, South Africa and Warwick Medical School, UK; and at workshops organized by the philosophy and Humanities and Psychopathology Section of the WPA and AEP, and the Philosophy Special Interest Group in the Royal College of Psychiatrists.

Research

As described in the text, work in the analytic philosophical tradition on values in psychiatric diagnosis is relatively recent. There is, however, a rich tradition of phenomenological scholarship in this area. A recent exemplar, in English, is Giovanni Stanghellini's (2004) exploration, drawing on extensive clinical experience, of values in the experience of people with schizophrenia.

Recent empirical work on values and value diversity specifically in relation to classification and psychiatric diagnosis, includes the Oxford psychiatrist, Jacinta Tan's studies of the assessment of decision-making capacity in anorexia nervosa (Tan et al., 2003) 'Anorexia nervosa and personal identity: The accounts of patients and their parents.' Juan Mezzich's proposals (Mezzich, 2002; and Mezzich et al., 2003) for an idiographic classification, to stand alongside current symptom-based classification, noted in chapter 13, accommodates personal values as a key aspect of the individuality of responses to mental distress and disorder.

Colombo et al.'s (2003a) work on models of disorder, in 'Evaluating the influence of implicit models of mental disorder on processes of shared decision making within community-based multidisciplinary teams', gives the results of work combining philosophical-analytic and empirical social science methods to elicit implicit models (values and beliefs) of mental disorder. As described in Part I, the groups studied—psychiatrists, approved social workers, community psychiatric nurses, people who use services and informal carers—all had very different implicit models. Colombo et al.'s (2003b) 'Model behaviour' gives the main findings from the study and describes its importance for user-centred practice. (*Openmind* is the journal of one of the main voluntary sector mental health advocacy groups in the UK.) Fulford and Colombo (2004) 'Six models of mental disorder: a study combining linguistic-analytic and empirical methods' discuss the methodological implications of combining philosophical-analytic and empirical social science methods.

The NIMHE-funded conferences described in the text are available at the Mental Health Foundation website (see below). The proceedings from John Sadler's foundational conference in 1997 in Dallas are the basis of Sadler's (2002) (ed.) *Descriptions & Prescriptions: Values, Mental Disorders, and the DSMs*. Updates on developments in this area include Fulford's 2002a and b, 2005. The issues are discussed in a Forum Issue of *World Psychiatry* based around a target article by Fulford, Broome, Stanghellini, and Thornton (2005) on 'Looking with both eyes open' with responses from a range of perspectives expressing widely different views about the merits or otherwise of recognizing a role for values in psychiatric diagnosis.

Web-based resources

◆ A good starting point is the Mental Health Foundation Website, http://www.connects.org.uk. This website hosts two on-line standing conferences, including extensive discussions by users and carers, of values in psychiatric diagnosis and in the assessment of decision-making capacity.

◆ http://wwwnimhe.org.uk The National Institute for Mental Health England. As noted above, NIMHE is responsible for mental health policy implementation in the UK. The website includes information regarding implementation guides and mental health policy. Search on "values" for all relevant entries.

◆ http://www.doh.gov.uk/mentalhealth/implementationguide.htm gives an extract on the values underpinning the Mental Health National Service Framework.

◆ http://www.scmh.org.uk This website for the Sainsbury Centre for mental Health, which spearheaded with Warwick

University the development of VBP training materials, see above. This gives much useful information in general about practice and policy issues. The training workbook in Values-Based Practice, 'Whose Values?' (Woodbridge and Fulford, 2004b) can be ordered on-line from this site.

♦ http://www.warwick.ac.uk *and* http://www2.warwick.ac.uk/fac/med, are the websites, respectively, for The University of Warwick, with links to the Philosophy Department, and for the Warwick Medical School, SCMH's partners in the development of VBP training materials.

♦ http://www.skillsforhealth.org.uk The Health Functional Map and other curriculum support tools published by Skills for Health.

Other useful websites includes

♦ http://www.basw.co.uk/article.php?articleId = 2&page = 6 Sets out the values and principles of social work.

♦ http://www.nice.org.uk The National Institute for Clinical Excellence (NICE). Schizophrenia guidelines and other information.

♦ http://www.nmc-uk.org This gives the code of professional conduct for nursing and midwifery in the UK.

♦ http://www.rcpsych.ac.uk/publications/cr/council/cr83.pdf Sets out the duties of a doctor registered with the General Medical Council, the professional body responsible for the regulation of medical practice in the UK.

♦ http://www.scie.org.uk Social Care Institute for Excellence. SCIE is the equivalent for social care of the NICE for health care. The website includes information on social models of care and other general social care information.

International initiatives can be viewed through: (1) the World Psychiatric Association website: see especially, the Home Pages for the Philosophy and Humanities and the History sections, the *WPA Bulletin* for announcements, and the on-line version of the journal, *World Psychiatry*; and (2) the website for the International Network for Philosophy and Psychiatry (http://www.inpponline.org), for conferences, national, and subject-based groups, and information about publishing and training opportunities.

Information about relevant books in the Oxford University Press series, International Perspectives in the Philosophy of Psychiatry is available at http://www.oup.co.uk, and for articles in *Philosophy, Psychiatry, & Psychology* see the on-line resources at Project Muse in the Johns Hopkins University Press website at http://muse.jhu.edu.

References

Alderson, P. (1990). *Choosing for Children: parents' consent to surgery*. Oxford: Oxford University Press.

Allott, P., Loganathan, L., and Fulford, K.W.M. (2002). Discovering hope for recovery. In: innovation in community mental health: international perspectives. Special Issue. *Canadian Journal of Community Mental Health*, 21(2): 13–33.

American Psychiatric Association (1994). *Diagnostic and statistical manual of mental disorders* (fourth edition). Washington, DC: American Psychiatric Association.

Bentall, R.P. (1992). A proposal to classify happiness as a psychiatric disorder. *Journal of Medical Ethics*, 18: 94–98.

Birley, J.L.T. (2000). Psychiatric ethics: an international open society. Chapter 11, In *In Two Minds: A Casebook of Psychiatric Ethics* (eds D. Dickenson and K.W.M. Fulford). Oxford: Oxford University Press.

Bloch, S. and Reddaway, P. (1977). *Russia's Political Hospitals: the abuse of psychiatry in the Soviet Union*. Southampton: The Camelot Press.

Colombo, A., Bendelow, G., Fulford, K.W.M., and Williams, S. (2003a). Evaluating the influence of implicit models of mental disorder on processes of shared decision making within community-based multidisciplinary teams. *Social Science & Medicine*, 56: 1557–1570.

Colombo, A., Bendelow, G., Fulford, K.W.M., and Williams, S. (2003b). Model behaviour. *Openmind* 125: 10–12.

Cordess, C. (2001). *Confidentiality and mental health*. London: Jessica Kingsley Publishers.

Department of Health (1999). *National Service Framework for Mental Health—modern standards and service models*. London: Department of Health.

Department of Health (2002). *Draft Mental Health Bill*. Cm5538-I. London HMSO.

Department of Health (2004). *NIMHE Guiding Statement on Recovery*. London: Department of Health.

Department of Health (2004a). *Mental Health Care Group Workforce Team: national mental health workforce strategy*. London: National Institute for Mental Health England.

Department of Health (2004b). *The Ten Essential Shared Capabilities: a framework for the whole of the mental health workforce*. London: The Sainsbury Centre for Mental Health, the NHSU (National Health Service University), and the NIMHE (National Institute for Mental Health England).

Department of Health (2004c). Interim Report of the National Steering Group: guidance on new ways of working for psychiatrists in a multi-disciplinary and multi-agency context. London: The Royal College of Psychiatrists; National Institute of Mental Health in

England, and the Modernisation Agency—Changing Workforce Programme.

Dickenson, D. and Fulford, K.W.M. (2000). *In Two Minds: a casebook of psychiatric ethics*. Oxford: Oxford University Press.

Fulford, K.W.M. (1989). *Moral Theory and Medical Practice*. Cambridge: Cambridge University Press.

Fulford, K.W.M. (1993). Bioethical blind spots: four flaws in the field of view of traditional bioethics. *Health Care Analysis*, 1: 155–162.

Fulford, K.W.M. (1994). Closet logics: hidden conceptual elements in the DSM and ICD classifications of Mental disorders, pps 211–232, ch 9 In Sadler, J.Z., Wiggins, O.P., Schwartz, M.A., (eds) *Philosophical Perspectives on Psychiatric Diagnostic Classification*. Baltimore: Johns Hopkins University Press.

Fulford, K.W.M. (1998). Dissent and dissensus: the limits of consensus formation in psychiatry. In ten Have, H.A.M.J. and Saas, H-M. (eds) *Consensus Formation in Health Care Ethics*, pps 175–192. Kluwer: Philosophy and Medicine Series.

Fulford, K. W. M. (2001). The paradoxes of confidentiality. pps 7–23 in *Confidentiality and mental health* (ed. C. Cordess). London: Jessica Kingsley Publishers.

Fulford, K.W.M. (2002a). Report to the Chair of the DSM-VI Task Force from the Editors of *Philosophy, Psychiatry, & Psychology* on 'Contentious and noncontentious evaluative language in psychiatric diagnosis' (Dateline 2010). In *Descriptions & Prescriptions: Values, Mental Disorders, and the DSMs* (ed. J.Z. Sadler). Baltimore, MD: The Johns Hopkins University Press, Chapter 21.

Fulford, K.W.M. (2002b). Values in psychiatric diagnosis: Executive Summary of a Report to the Chair of the ICD-12/DSM-VI Coordination Task Force (Dateline 2010). *Psychopathology*, 35: 132–138.

Fulford, K.W.M. (2005) Values in Psychiatric Diagnosis: Developments in Policy, Training and Research. *Psychopathology*, 38: 4: 05, 171–176.

Fulford, K.W.M. and Colombo, A. (2004). Six Models of Mental Disorder: A Study Combining Linguistic-Analytic and Empirical Methods. *Philosophy, Psychiatry, & Psychology*, 11/2: 129–144.

Fulford, K.W.M., Dickenson, D. and Murray, T.H. (eds) (2002) *Healthcare Ethics and Human Values: An Introductory Text with Readings and Case Studies*. Malden, USA, and Oxford, UK: Blackwell Publishers.

Fulford, K.W.M. and Hope, T., (1996). Control and practical experience. In *Informed Consent in Psychiatry: European perspectives on ethics, law and clinical practice* (ed. H.-G. Koch,

S. Reiter-Theil, and H. Helmchen). Baden-Baden: Nomos Verlagsgesellschaft, pp. 349–377.

Fulford, K.W.M., Smirnoff, A.Y.U., and Snow, E. (1993). Concepts of disease and the abuse of psychiatry in the USSR. *British Journal of Psychiatry*, 162: 801–810.

Fulford, K.W.M., Williamson, T., and Woodbridge, K. (2002). Values-added practice (a values-awareness workshop). *Mental Health Today*, October: 25–27.

Fulford, K.W.M., Broome, M., Stanghellini, G., and Thornton, T. (2005). Looking With Both Eyes Open: Fact *and* Value in Psychiatric Diagnosis? *World Psychiatry*, 4: 2,78–86.

Commentaries (on Fulford et al 2005):

Sadler, J.Z. (2005). Bug-eyed and breathless: emerging crises involving values. *World Psychiatry*, 4: 2, p87.

First, M.B. (2005). Keeping an eye on clinical utility. *World Psychiatry*, 4: 2, p87.

Wakefield, J.C. (2005). On winking at the facts, and losing one's Hare: value pluralism and the harmful dysfunction analysis. *World Psychiatry*, 4: 2, p88.

Spitzer, R.L. (2005). Recipe for disaster: professional and patient equally sharing responsibility for developing psychiatric diagnosis. *World Psychiatry*, 4: 2, p89.

Sartorius, N. (2005). Recognizing that values matter. *World Psychiatry*, 4: 2, p90.

Banzato, C.E.M., Pereira, M.E.C. (2005). Eyes and ears wide open: values in the clinical setting. *World Psychiatry*, 4: 2, p90.

Mezzich, J.E. (2005). Values and comprehensive diagnosis. *World Psychiatry*, 4: 2, p91

Tan, J. (2005). Bridging the gap between fact and values. *World Psychiatry*, 4: 2, p92

Kitamura, T. (2005). Looking with both the eyes and heart open: the meaning of life in psychiatric diagnosis. *World Psychiatry*, 4: 2, p93.

Van Staden, C.W. (2005). The need for trained eyes to see facts and values in psychiatric diagnosis. *World Psychiatry*, 4: 2, p94

King, C. (2005). Coloring our eyes. *World Psychiatry*, 4: 2, p95.

Goodwin, G. (2002). Hypomania: what's in a name? *The British Journal of Psychiatry*. Vol 181: 94–95

Helman, C (2000). *Culture, Health and Illness: an introduction for health professionals* (4th edn). Oxford: Butterworth-Heinemann.

Jackson, M.C. (1997). Benign schizotypy? The Case of Spiritual Experience. In *Schizotypy: relations to illness and health*, ed. G. S. Claridge. Oxford, Oxford University Press.

Jackson, M. and Fulford, K.W.M. (1997). Spiritual experience and psychopathology. *Philosophy, Psychiatry, & Psychology*, 4/1: 41–66.

Kendall, R.E. (1975). The concept of disease and its implications for psychiatry. *British journal of Psychiatry*. 127: 305–315.

Kopelman, L.M. (1994). Normal grief: good or bad? Health or disease? (Commentaries by Dominian, J. and Wise, T.N. pp. 221–224; response by Kopelman, pp. 226–227.) *Philosophy, Psychiatry, & Psychology*, 1/4: 209–220.

Mezzich, J. E. (2002). Comprehensive diagnosis: a conceptual basis for future diagnostic systems. *Psychopathology*, Mar–Jun; 35(2–3): 162–5.

Mezzich, J.E., Berganza, C.E., Von Cranach, M., Jorge, M.R., Kastrup, M.C., Murthy, R.S., Okasha, A., Pull, C., Sartorius, N., Skodol, A., Zaudig, M. (2003.) IGDA. 8: Idiographic (personalised) diagnostic formulation. In Essentials of the World Psychiatric Association's International Guidelines for Diagnostic Assessment (IGD), *The British Journal of Psychiatry*, Vol 182/Supplement 45: 55–57.

Moore, A., Hope, T., and Fulford, K.W.M. (1994). Mild mania and well-being. (with commentaries by Nordenfelt, L., and Seedhouse, D.) *Philosophy, Psychiatry, & Psychology*, 1/3: 165–192.

Osborn, D. (1999). Research and ethics: leaving exclusion behind. *Current Opinion in Psychiatry*, 12(5): 601–604.

Radden, J. (1994). Recent criticism of psychiatric nosology: a review. *Philosophy, Psychiatry, & Psychology*, 1(3): 193–200.

Reich, W. (1999). Psychiatric diagnosis as an ethical problem. *Psychiatric Ethics* (3rd edn), (ed. S. Bloch, P. Chodoff, and S. Green). Oxford: Oxford University Press, pp. 193–224.

Rosenhan, D. (1973). On being sane in insane places. Science, 179: 250–258.

Sabat, S.R. (2001). *The Experience of Alzheimer's Disease: Life Through a Tangled Veil*. Oxford: Blackwell Publishers.

Sabat, S.R. and Harré, R. (1997). The Alzheimer's disease sufferer as semiotic subject. *Philosophy, Psychiatry, & Psychology*, 4(2): 145–160.

Sadler, J.Z. (1996). Epistemic value commitments in the debate over categorical vs. dimensional personality diagnosis. (Commentaries by Livesley W.J., and Luntley, M., pp. 223–230.) *Philosophy, Psychiatry, & Psychology*, 3/3: 203–222.

Sadler, J.Z. (ed.) (2002). *Descriptions & Prescriptions: values, mental disorders, and the DSMs*. Baltimore, MD: The Johns Hopkins University Press.

Sadler, J.Z. (2004). *Values and Psychiatric Diagnosis*. Oxford: Oxford University Press.

Sadler, J.Z. and Agich, G.J. (1995). Diseases, Functions, Values, and Psychiatric Classifications. *Philosophy, Psychiatry and Psychology*, 2(3), 219–232.

Sadler, J.Z. and Fulford, K.W.M. (2004). Should Patients and Families Contribute to the DSM-V Process? *Psychiatric Services*, Vol 55, No 2: 133–138.

Sadler, J., Wiggins O.P., and Schwartz, M.A. (ed.) (1994). *Philosophical Perspectives on Psychiatric Diagnostic Classification*. Baltimore, MD: The Johns Hopkins University Press.

Schwartz, S.H. (in press). Basic human values: their content and structure across countries. In *Valores e trabalho* [Values and work] (ed. A. Tamayo, A. and J. Porto). Brazil: Universidade de Brasilia.

Stanghellini, G. (2000). At issue: vulnerability to schizophrenia and lack of common sense. *Schizophrenia Bulletin*, 26(4): 775–787.

Stanghellini, G. (2004). *Deanimated Bodies and Disembodied Spirits. Essays on the psychopathology of common sense*. Oxford: Oxford University Press.

Spitzer, R.L. (2005). Recipe for disaster: professional and patient equally sharing responsibility for developing psychiatric diagnosis. *World Psychiatry*, 4:2, p89.

Tan, J.O.A., Hope, T. and Stewart, A. (2003). Anorexia nervosa and personal identity: The accounts of patients and their parents. *International Journal of Law and Psychiatry*, 26: 533–548.

Wakefield, J.C. (1995). Dysfunction as a value-free concept: a Reply to Sadler and Agich. *Philosophy, Psychiatry, & Psychology*, 2(3): 233–246.

Wallcraft, J. (2003). *Values in Mental Health—the role of experts by experience*. (Available at www.connects.org.uk/conferences).

West Midlands Mental Health Partnership (2003). *Values in Action: Developing a Values Based Practice in Mental Health* (available from West Midlands Mental Health Partnership).

Widdershoven, G.A.M. and Widdershoven-Heerding, I. (2003). Understanding dementia: a hermeneutic perspective. In *Nature and Narrative: an introduction to the new philosophy of psychiatry* (ed. K.W.M. Fulford, K.J. Morris, J.Z. Sadler, and G. Stanghellini). Oxford: Oxford University Press, Chapter 6.

Williamson, T. (2004). Can two wrongs make a right? (Commentary on Fulford and Colombo, 2004a.) *Philosophy, Psychiatry, & Psychology*, 11(2): 159–164.

Woodbridge, K. and Fulford, K.W.M. (2003). Good practice? Values-based practice in mental health. *Mental Health Practice*, 7(2): 30–34.

Woodbridge, K. and Fulford, K.W.M. (2004a). Right, wrong and respect. *Mental Health Today*, September: 28–30.

Woodbridge, K. and Fulford, K.W.M. (2004b). *Whose values? A workbook for values-based practice in mental health care*. London: Sainsbury Centre for Mental Health.

PART V

Philosophy of mind and mental health

Part contents

Introduction to Part V

Introduction: philosophy of mind is a central discipline of philosophy as a whole

The philosophy of mind is the area of philosophy that has the closest connections to mental health care. Much of what gives psychiatry its character turns on the fact that human minds are its main focus and thus the philosophy of mind is a central aspect of its philosophy.

Philosophy of mind has also been a growth area over the twentieth century. Much detailed work has been done on central aspects of our understanding of mind. A wide variety of models of the general relation of mind and body have been articulated and assessed. Theories of how mental states can possess intentionality or aboutness have developed. Competing accounts of how we can have knowledge of other minds have been assessed in the light of empirical evidence. Specific work has been carried out on action, free will, and consciousness.

Some of the key debates in philosophy as a whole can be found echoed in debates about the mind. The general debate between reductionists and antireductionists is reflected, for example, in the opposition of those who think that the mind, meaning, and consciousness can be understood in, for example, causal relational terms and those who think that it has necessarily special experiential and intrinsic qualities that cannot be explained in other terms. In Louis Armstrong's phrase (about jazz): if you have to ask what it is you'll never know. This latter group of philosophers have been called the 'New Mysterians' because they take consciousness to hold an essential mystery. Thus philosophy of mind is, currently, a central and influential part of philosophy as a whole.

The growth of philosophy of psychiatry

During the last two decades there has also been a growth in philosophy of mind influenced philosophy of psychiatry. Psychopathology presents a challenging set of test cases for philosophical understanding. Thus there have been sustained attempts to shed light on the general nature of delusions, drawing on different broader approaches to meaning. More specific cases such as thought insertion or Cotard's delusion have been the subject of more specific interpretations. One view of such philosophical interpretation is provided by the Warwick-based philosopher of mind Johannes Roessler: '[T]he philosopher takes the part of an explorer charting certain remote regions of the "space of reasons". For example, John Campbell has argued that reports of thought insertion "show that there is some structure in our ordinary notion of the ownership of a thought which we might not otherwise have suspected".' (Roessler, 2001, p. 178).

The selection of material for this part and its overall aim

Consistently with the general approach of this book, we will not attempt to give an overview of this rich field. We will not, for example, summarize the recent philosophical work on the nature of delusion. (In Chapter 3, by contrast we have summarized key philosophical work in a number of areas of psychopathology.) Rather than attempting to summarize the many, detailed debates on specific topics in philosophy of mind and its application to psychiatry and psychopathology, the chapter instead gives a broader overview of some important higher-level themes in the philosophy of mind that have a clear connection to the conceptual structures that underpin practice.

Briefly then the chapters run as follows. The first two chapters (Chapters 22 and 23) examine models of the relation between mind and body and the significance of the mind for ascriptions of responsibility, experience, etc. in mental health care.

The next two chapters (Chapters 24 and 25) examine the place of meaning and intentionality in our scientifically informed picture of the world in general. This is again a return to one of the central themes of this book as a whole: the relation of reasons and causes. That theme returns again in the discussion of freedom and action in Chapter 26. Can reasons play a causal role in free action?

The final chapters (Chapters 27 and 28) examine knowledge of other minds and autism and then personal identity and schizophrenia.

The part thus serves as an intellectual primer to the more specific debates that grow from these broad themes. (Reading Guides are provided to specific issues.)

The central role of rationality

A theme that will recur throughout the part is the central role of rationality both in our understanding of minds and mental states and in marking off the mind as different from other aspects of the natural world.

Rationality is most apparent in arguments about the ascription of meaning and mental states based on the work of Daniel Dennett and Donald Davidson. Such arguments emphasize the constitutive role of rationality for the possession of a mind. However, if sound, those arguments also suggest an argument against the reduction of mental states to brain states, which does not turn on the intrinsic feel of experiences and such like. This suggests that the distinction between the space of reasons and the realm of law, introduced in Part III Chapter 15, also plays a part in understanding the subject matter of this part.

More detailed chapter summary

- *Chapter 22 Mind, brain, and mental illness: an introduction to the philosophy of mind.* This chapter looks at the connection between mental descriptions in psychiatry and the role of experience, subjectivity, and values. While psychiatric practice and broader scientific discovery emphasizes the importance of descriptions of physiological and neurological processes, the mind cannot be eliminated without the loss of what is valued in psychiatric care.

- *Chapter 23 The mind–body problem and mental health, a philosophical update.* This chapter brings the discussion of the relation of mind and body up to date. Starting with the question of what is shown in brain imaging, the chapter looks at two influential models of mind and body (functionalism and Davidson's anomalous monism) and at some more general relations that might hold (supervenience, type, and token identity). The analysis suggests that no model successfully accords with all our intuitions about mind and body.

- *Chapter 24 Reasons and the content of mental states: 1. Reductionist theories.* Starting with a conventional textbook account of different pathways through the mind postulated to explain our understanding of speech, this chapter digs deeper into what kind of explanation can be given of meaning or intentionality in the mind. It looks at two influential philosophical models of how meaning might be underpinned by mechanisms and the grave difficulties they still face.

- *Chapter 25 Reasons and the content of mental states: 2. Antireductionism and discursive psychology.* This chapter looks at a very different approach to meaning found in discursive psychological work. Again it explores philosophical models that might underpin a discursive approach and argues that the claim that both meaning and minds are necessarily public should be distinguished from the claim that meanings are socially constructed.

- *Chapter 26 Agency, causation, and freedom.* This chapter starts with a recent work on Libet's empirical arguments against the possibility of free will. By looking both at philosophical models of action explanation and at an influential paper by Strawson on our reactive attitudes it aims to sketch a reconciliation between increasingly deterministic neurological understanding and our standing assumption that we possess free will.

- *Chapter 27 Knowledge of other minds.* Mental health care is premised on our ability to understand other minds. However, there has been a long-standing puzzle about how this is possible. The chapter outlines both the recent history of the Problem of Other Minds and three proposed solutions, and looks to how empirical evidence from autism bears on the issue.

- *Chapter 28 Personal identity and schizophrenia.* This chapter examines the connection between philosophical models of personal identity, including philosophical doubts that identity is a real feature of the human mind, and the psychopathology of schizophrenia.

References

Roessler, J., (2001). Understanding Delusions of Alien Control. *Philosophy, Psychiatry, & Psychology*, 8/2/3, 177–188.

CHAPTER 22

Mind, brain, and mental illness: an introduction to the philosophy of mind

Chapter contents

Madness is a subject that ought to interest philosophers; but they have had surprisingly little to say about it

Anthony Quinton (1985)

Introduction

Mental health practitioners—users of services and carers, nurses, general practitioners, psychiatrists, psychologists, etc.—claim a special expertise in the mental. The philosophy of mind should thus be, uniquely, *their* philosophy. Conversely, mental health practice, given the remarkable range of abnormal mental phenomena with which it is concerned, should be uniquely interesting to philosophers of mind. Yet for much of the twentieth century, the two sides, philosophers and practitioners, have studiously avoided each other.

It was ever so! Historically, philosophy and *general* psychology were not sharply distinct (Wilhelm Wundt, for example, who founded the first experimental psychology laboratory at Leipzig in 1879, was a professor of philosophy). However, abnormal psychology, madness, has nearly always been very much at the fringes of philosophical interest. The oddity of this, as we noted at the start of Part I of this book, was pointed out by the Oxford philosopher, Anthony Quinton, in an article, reviewing philosophical work on madness, from which the above quote was taken (1985, pp. 17–41). Most of the great philosophers touched on the subject; a few explored it in more detail, though usually aside from their main philosophical work (Locke and Kant, for example). But we have to go back to classical sources, such as Plato and the Stoics or forward to the end of the nineteenth century (with the work of such founding figures as the philosopher-psychiatrist Karl Jaspers) for examples of substantive philosophical work in this area. (For discussions of Plato and the Stoics see Kenny (1969, pp. 229–253), and Nordenfelt (1997a, pp. 286–291; with commentaries by Ivy-Marie Blackburn, Stanley A. Leavy, Emilio Mordini, and Rosamund Rhodes, all 1997, with a response from Lennart Nordenfelt, 1997b, from *Philosophy, Psychiatry, & Psychology*, pp. 293–306).)

Interglacial or global warming

Historically, then, the overall pattern of the relationship between philosophy and *abnormal* psychology, has been, like recent geological history, that of a long ice age punctuated by brief interglacials. At the start of the twenty-first century, philosophy, psychiatry and abnormal psychology, are coming together again. Whether this is another brief interglacial, or the start of a permanent change of intellectual climate, it is too early to say (Fulford *et al.*, 2003). But, as we will see in this and subsequent chapters, it is above all in the philosophy of *mind* that there are deep points of contact between philosophical theory and mental health practice and research.

Many points of contact

One of the deepest of these points of contact is a topic that, in the popular imagination at least, is the mother of philosophical problems, the mind–body problem. It is with this that we are mainly concerned in the first two chapters in this part. The philosophy of mind, though, covers a number of other topics critically important in mental health that are already becoming known, collectively, as 'philosophical psychopathology' (see, in particular, George Graham and G. Lynn Stephen's (1994) book of that title, and John Cutting's recent *Principles of Psychopathology*, 1977). The philosophy of mind, moreover, overlaps with, and in part underpins, topics in the philosophy and ethics of mental health covered in earlier chapters of this book: for example, 'folk' psychology, the unconscious, and the status of psychoanalysis, rationality and practical reasoning, and the core notions of action and agency underpinning our very concepts of disorder.

In all these areas, then, from the central metaphysical deeps of the mind–body problem, through the diversity of philosophical psychopathology, to the underpinnings of key topics in the philosophy of science, ethics, and conceptual analysis, the philosophy of mind is crucially important for mental health practice and research. But in all these areas, too, mental health practice and research are also crucially important to philosophy. Here, above all, it is the 'real people' of Kathleen Wilkes' (1988) ground-breaking book of that title, who are crucial to philosophical theory. Here, above all, echoing J.L. Austin (from Part I), it is the 'negative concept which wears the trousers'. It is the *disorders* of mind to which real people are subject that provide the sharpest philosophical probes into the nature of *mind*.

The structure of this chapter

This chapter is divided into four sessions. Sessions 1 and 2 identify the main elements of the mind–body problem as they bear on mental health practice and research. Sessions 3 and 4 begin the process of outlining philosophical responses to the problem. Thus,

- *Session 1* looks at the mind–body problem in ordinary usage, drawing on a number of short articles from journals and newspapers, which reveal tensions in our everyday understanding of the relation of mind and brain.

- *Session 2* looks at a case history, the story of 'Mrs Lazy', which displays these tensions as they are reflected in clinical practice.

- *Session 3* then traces some of the philosophical history of work on mind and body from Descartes.

- *Session 4* examines a more recent attempt to side-step the Cartesian framework.

This prepares the way for an examination of contemporary responses to the mind–body problem and how they relate to the growing science of brain imaging in Chapter 23.

Session 1 The mind–body problem in ordinary use

If psychology in general is concerned with the mind, psychiatry, and related mental health disciplines, work especially at the interface between mind and body. Psychologists may, perhaps by definition must, ignore the body. Doctors concerned with the body (cardiologists, rheumatologists, etc.) may, though with less justification, ignore the mind. But psychiatrists, mental health nurses, and those in related disciplines, *necessarily* work with mind *and* body.

Being concerned with mind *and* body has had, however, a whole series of adverse consequences. The *intellectual* difficulty of the mind–body problem means that professionals in this area may appear confused, their research slower to get going, their authority less absolute. *Practically*, this makes them vulnerable (antipsychiatry exploited this), and, hence, defensive; there is a tendency, then, to *retreat*, to get off the fence. Psychoanalysis has tended to retreat to a purely 'mental' model, medical psychiatry to a purely 'biological' model. And in such retreats, it is users of services, treated thereby as *less* than persons, who are the losers.

Mind–body and ordinary usage

There is no easy way with the mind–body problem. Indeed, a function of philosophy for mental health practitioners, is to show just *how* difficult—intellectually and practically—the problem is. In this first session, then, we need to get a clearer picture of the mind–body problem: to identify the features of the mind, and its relationship with the body, that make it problematic, and the difficulties which, inherent as they are in psychiatric as well as in lay thinking, leave mental health practitioners, on the one hand open to spurious criticism, and on the other to avoidable errors in practice and research.

True to J.L. Austin's linguistic analytic principle, of putting 'use' before 'definition', we will start with a series of short readings taken from everyday, non-philosophical, sources (i.e. from what Austin called 'ordinary' as distinct from philosophical usage).

EXERCISE 1 (30 minutes)

Read the extract from the review by the British historian, Roy Porter:

Porter, R. (1997). Edward Shorter's *A History of Psychiatry*. Evening Standard Review

Link with Reading 22.1

This is a very short review aimed at the general public (it appeared in a daily newspaper, the *London Evening Standard*). However, it carries a whole series of important messages about the mind–body problem in mental heath practice.

As you read this, make a note of anything at all to do with mind and body that you can identify. Think particularly about: (1) antipsychiatry; (2) concepts of illness and disease; and (3) the reflection of mind–body dualism in (a) psychiatric categories of disorder, (b) psychiatric treatments, and (c) psychiatric research. Finally, (4) what model of mind and body do you think lies behind Shorter's book, and (5) is it one that as a mental health practitioner (as a professional or as a user of services) you would like to see adopted?

Reminder: Don't forget—philosophy is a skill, not a body of knowledge. So it is essential to do the exercise for yourself before going on. This is why a full 30 minutes has been allowed for a reading of only about 300 words.

Roy Porter was a Professor of the History of Medicine at the prestigious Wellcome Institute in London. He has often been identified by psychiatrists as a member of the opposition, as an antipsychiatrist. He made a number of trenchant criticisms of psychiatry, based on important work on the history of the subject (we drew on his work in Part II), and this comes through in the tone of his review (the opening rhetoric is not psychiatry friendly!). In this reading, he is careful, though, not to identify directly with Shorter's equally (though on different grounds) antipsychiatric message. This is because, as he says at the end, history teaches us to take with a 'pinch of salt' the exclusively brain-based, or 'biological', approach that Shorter advocates.

Five signals of the mind–body problem

Porter thus recognizes the importance of science (of this brain-based kind) but is also well aware of its limitations. We need to do something about the released 'psychopaths' (in his opening line); and if psychiatry's traditional models are as inept as he implies, neuroscience looks an attractive option; but the lesson of history is that a 'monoculture' approach, focusing exclusively on either brain-based or mind-based solutions, will fail.

Behind Porter's review, therefore, there is an unresolved tension between mind and body. In a larger, more discursive, review, this tension would be more deeply hidden. But in this short, punchy, piece it shows through as a series of signals of the mind–body problem. Here are some of these signals as they relate to the topics in the exercise (you may have identified others as well):

1. *Antipsychiatry.* We have already noted that a broadly antipsychiatry position is shared by Porter and Shorter. Its links to the mind–body problem are clear at a number of points, e.g. in paragraph 2 we are asked whether mental illness is '*real* like smallpox or cancer' (Porter's emphasis), or 'all in the mind'. By linking psychiatry with the mind, then, antipsychiatry implies that psychiatry is dealing with something that is not real (in Szasz's famous dismissal, a 'myth'–see Parts I and III).

2. *Concepts of illness and disease.* This contrast ('mind' = not real; 'body' = real) is embodied in a medical/psychiatric context in the distinction between illness and disease. In paragraph 2 for example, Porter says it is 'clear what physical *disease*' is, but, he continues, 'what of mental *illness*?' (our emphasis). As we saw in Part I of this book, illness and disease are often conflated, and much (though not all) of the debate about the validity of 'mental illness' turns on this. Here we get a clear signal that part of the rhetorical power of this conflation stems from an implicit reference to body (= disease = real) and mind (= illness = unreal).

3. *Diagnosis, treatment, and research.* This is one clear signal, then, of the mind–body problem. Others include

    (a) psychiatric *categories of disorder*—Porter suggests, again in paragraph 2, that psychiatry split 'into two camps, the organic and psychogenic';

    (b) *treatments*—in paragraph 4, Shorter is said to describe psychiatry as developing in two directions, with physical treatments (lobotomy, electroconvulsive therapy, etc.), and psychoanalysis; and

    (c) *research*—Shorter sees, in paragraph 6, a new biological psychiatry, 'based on *hard* science', as an '*alternative*' (Porter's word, but not his emphasis) to talking therapies.

4. *Shorter's eliminativism.* Behind each of these aspects of Shorter's account, then, at least as interpreted by Porter, there lies a model of mind and body. Yet if we were to ask Shorter *what his own model is*, he would have to say 'eliminative materialism', or words to that effect. The 'hard science', which is his alternative to talking therapies, is 'neurophysiology and chemistry'. All that is important in psychiatry, then, concerned as it is with mental disorders, is to be had from studies of the brain (and of the rest of the body). Talk of the mind, then, can be eliminated once we have an adequate account of the brain. Hence, *eliminative* materialism. Porter makes this explicit. He takes Shorter to be claiming that 'Investigating the brain will bare the mysteries of the mind'.

5. *Practical significance.* But is this really as 'hopeful' a message for mental health practitioners as Shorter suggests (paragraph 7)? Porter has his doubts, as we have seen. History warns us against such retreats to any one overarching approach in psychiatry. But there are clear *philosophical* warnings, too, i.e. in the language used. Where physical treatments failed, they were 'bizarre' (paragraph 4); that they were based on the 'hard science' of the day is conveniently forgotten. Psychoanalysis, similarly, although conceived by Freud, at least in his early work, as a preliminary to neuroscience, is dismissed as 'aimless chat'. Even, therefore, within a body-only solution to the mind–body problem, it is, merely, *today's* neuroscience that is acceptable to Shorter. A view as narrow as this, promoted, as Porter notes, in an 'upbeat, even euphoric' tone, signals dogma. And as we saw particularly in Part IV, dogma, from whatever perspective, is the basis of much abusive practice in mental health.

Packed into this short review, then, we find a whole series of signals of the importance of the mind–body problem in mental health practice and research. The tone of the article, as we have seen, is by and large adverse to the mind; Shorter's very programme is to eliminate mind in favour of brain. There are, though, two key properties of mind, which, though not signalled in this first reading, are, on the face of it, incompatible even in principle with Shorter's approach.

Mind and consciousness

These two key properties are (1) consciousness, and (2) freedom. These are closely linked: we normally take only conscious activity to reflect free choice (though not all conscious activities are in this sense free). Both have been subject to endless philosophical scrutiny. Both must be accommodated (if only by elimination) to any theory of mind. Both, moreover, are important in ordinary conceptions of the mind and, hence, in mental health practice and research. The reading linked with the following exercise is an example of the 'ordinary use' of consciousness.

EXERCISE 2   (30 minutes)

Read the *New Scientist* editorial:

   Editorial (1997a). A comet at heaven's gate. *New Scientist*, 5 April: 3

Link with Reading 22.2

Think particularly about, (1) the model of mind and brain the article is 'debunking', and (2) what is put in its place. Is the latter a sufficient account of consciousness, though? If not, what is the real philosophical value of the abnormal states of consciousness to which the article refers? As before, make brief notes on these points before going on.

This editorial is redolent of anti-mind sentiments: consciousness (or at any rate conscious control) is an 'illusion' to be assimilated to mass delusions; minds are 'souls' (ghosts? theological? superstition?), and so on. Specifically, the article aims to 'debunk' the 'common illusion that our conscious self sits inside us, looking out on the world and controlling our actions'. This model, attributed to the seventeenth century French philosopher, René Descartes, is said to be 'like the Wizard of Oz'.

Dissolving the mind–body problem

Well, fair enough, this may be a false picture of the mind. But in its place we are offered the brain, in the form now of modern neuroscience. This, certainly, has come up with some challenging findings, for example that brain activity may precede awareness of that activity (the tennis ball being back over the net before the player is aware of hitting it). And a series of 'deficit states' show that our conscious awareness is not as indivisible as we normally suppose (blindsight, in which subjects can identify objects correctly even though they have no conscious visual awareness, is a dramatic example of this).

The article is at this point touching on hugely important and exciting advances in neuroscience. We will be returning to these later, in particular in connection with developments in cross-disciplinary work between philosophers, neuroscientists, psychologists, and psychiatrists, on consciousness and its disorders (including the remarkable disorders of *self*-consciousness in schizophrenia).

Deepening the mind–body problem

But this work *deepens*, rather than dissolves, the problem of consciousness (as a key aspect of the mind–body problem). It shows that consciousness is far more *complex* than had been appreciated (from ordinary introspection); and that the *causal* role of consciousness (usually thought of as concerned in some way with planning and/or monitoring activity) is not as self-evident as it had appeared.

Deeper still, though, substituting brain (or neurosciences) for mind fails wholly to account for the central mystery of plain *awareness*, what is sometimes called phenomenal consciousness. Neurophysiology may give us an increasingly sophisticated picture of how the brain works, including those aspects of brain activity that are associated with conscious awareness. Could this, however, as an explanation merely of the *mechanisms* subserving consciousness, cut to the problem of how anything that is material can be aware? How can matter, however subtly organized, have a point of view? Or to put the point differently, how could any account of someone's brain (even if we knew enough to say *what* they were experiencing) be the same thing as an account *of* their experience?

Mind, freedom, and responsibility

Note, again, that these are deep questions, to which we will return. But the point at this stage is to be suspicious of triumphalists claims for neuroscience, for a rhetoric that seeks to assimilate the problem of consciousness to an illusory belief in flying saucers. This is important in general (it is important for good science, if in no other ways). And it is crucially important for mental health because of the link between consciousness and the second key property of the mind, freedom.

We have already encountered this link in the form of the undermining of responsibility by severe mental illness. It was a feature of the conceptual map of psychiatry introduced in Chapter 2: 'mad or bad?' was the key question in criminal law, you will recall, 'mad or sad?' the corresponding key question in civil procedures involving involuntary treatment (for depression). Not all severe mental illness undermines responsibility, however. Indeed a key feature of the conceptual map of psychiatry was the way that mental disorders span between the deterministic world of bodily disease categories (on the right) and the moral world of free-to-be-responsible people (on the left).

There is a tension here, then, which we can now see was an aspect of the tension between mind and body. An action that is performed unconsciously is perceived as brain-driven and hence one for which the person concerned is clearly not responsible: for example, an act of violence arising in the course of an epileptic automatism. However, with mental illness matters are less clear cut. In some cases, paradigmatically with delusions, there is a strong intuition that the person concerned is not responsible. But, disturbed as their consciousness may be, they are not, as such, unconscious. We may have theories about unconscious sources of behaviour, of course, but such theories, insofar as they

are accepted at all (in their specifics), have the same implications for the freedom of our *non*-pathological as of our *pathological* actions. Hence we need some other explanation for the undermining of responsibility by severe mental illness. The brain looks a good candidate, and brain scans an attractive way of evidencing the origins of someone's action *in* their brain, rather than (this approach implies) in their own free (and hence responsible) choices.

This clutch of everyday ideas is illustrated by the two readings linked with the next exercise.

EXERCISE 3 (30 minutes)

In this exercise we are going to read two short articles both of which illustrate, again through ordinary usage rather than philosophical analysis (we come to this later), the importance of freedom as a characteristic of mind:

Editorial (1997b). Inadmissible evidence. *New Scientist*, 22 March: 3

Link with Reading 22.3

Anon (1997). Anorexia trigger found in the brain. *Sunday Times*, 13 April

Link with Reading 22.4

These articles reflect different ways in which people react to the implications of research on the brain for responsibility. Try to characterize the difference and suggest what might be motivating it. Also, think more generally about the significance of this difference in response for the eliminativist programme. Finally, why should advances in brain science seem to undermine free choice?

These two articles are both concerned with responsibility. Being responsible usually means that you were free to have behaved differently ('ought' implies 'can' is the well-worn philosophical slogan). This is the human world of free agents, then, morally responsible and responsible in law. But brain science is all about the *causes* of behaviour, and causation (scientific determinism) seems to be incompatible with free choice. Hence, advances in brain science, giving us more detailed knowledge of the brain basis of behaviour, appear to move us out of the moral world of free agents into the scientific world of deterministic objects.

Freedom of the will, neuroscience, and mental illness

This of course is the traditional philosophical problem of 'freedom of the will'. But the traditional problem has been given an extra edge by developments in neuroscience, which, for the first time, are giving us credible models of the 'higher' mental functions concerned with responsibility, such as volition, desire, and belief. And this is critically important in mental health because of the strong intuitive link between severe mental illness and loss of responsibility.

Equal and opposite reactions

How, then, are we to take developments in the brain sciences? The two articles linked with Exercise 3 take not only different but diametrically opposed views. The *New Scientist* editorial castigates the use of brain scans in criminal trials as 'Inadmissible evidence': this is a device used by unscrupulous lawyers to get morally and legally responsible crooks 'off the hook'. The *Sunday Times* article, on the other hand, welcomes the finding of an abnormality in the brain of some teenagers with anorexia, as a sign that the condition is, after all, a real disease, for which, therefore, neither the patient nor her parents need feel 'guilty'. In the last column, the psychiatrist says he is glad he will be able to say 'There is a major biological factor happening in your daughter's brain and causing her to behave this way. It is not your fault'.

At one level, the difference in reaction, here, is driven by how we feel towards the people concerned. The criminals we perceive as wicked—hence we want to deny the significance of 'brain findings' and keep them in the moral world of people with freedom of choice who are thus responsible legally. Towards young women with anorexia, on the other hand, we feel protective. We thus want to remove them from the moral world of guilt into a medical-scientific world of care and cure.

Emphasizing the tractable

This may seem naive. But as with consciousness, there is no quick way with freedom and responsibility as features of the mind. The problem of freedom of the will, like the closely related problem of consciousness, is among the deep problems of general metaphysics.

So deep, indeed, are these problems that in recent years, philosophers, taking their cue from the natural sciences, have tended to shy away from them and focus on less fundamental but more tractable issues. Instead of the traditional problem of phenomenal awareness, much philosophical work focuses on the *structure* of consciousness, on its parts. Instead of the traditional problem of freedom of the will, much philosophical work focuses on the *components* of agency (Austin's 'machinery of action').

Denying the intractable

This is a sound strategy. It is yielding high-quality results that are the basis of the increasingly fruitful co-operation between philosophers, neuroscientists, artificial intelligence experts, psychologists, and, more recently, psychiatrists.

Yet such work, as we have seen, cannot dissolve, and tends, if anything, to deepen the traditional problems. Philosophers, under pressure like everyone else to 'get results', have sometimes denied this. Daniel Dennett, a master of memorable titles, called his book on the *structure* of consciousness (1993), 'Consciousness *Explained*'! (We return to his important work on the intentional stance in chapter 25.) However, the proper function of philosophy here is rather to deepen our understanding of such problems by avoiding premature closure, the quick fix, the short cut, whether this is to a mind-only solution or to a brain-only solution.

Brain-only and mind-only solutions

If, then, even philosophers have been tempted to give up on the mind–body problem, it is no surprise to find non-philosophers adopting similar strategies. And this is what lies behind the equal and opposite reactions to the findings of brain research illustrated by the two readings linked with Exercise 3.

The *Sunday Times*, describing the discovery of a 'trigger' for anorexia in the brain, opts in effect for a brain-only solution. This makes anorexia a 'real' disease, caused by something wrong in the brain, and, hence, outside the moral world of persons. Anorexia is 'all in the brain'.

The *New Scientist* editorial, jumping the other way, opts in effect, for a mind-only solution. This is less obvious because the moral (mind-only) view of crime is hidden behind much reassuring brain-talk. It is, the editorial claims (thunders?), 'blindingly obvious' that 'impaired judgement goes hand in hand with most violent crime'. *Brain* scans, it implies, can reveal this. But, continuing the *brain*-talk theme, 'we' knew it all along because 'alcohol is involved in more than 90% of murders'. Yet, switching only a few lines later to a mind-only account of crime, we are told, equally firmly, that 'there isn't a brain-imaging technique in the world that can establish'.... 'whether he (the defendant) was oblivious to the difference between right and wrong'.

The brain-only talk then returns with references to 'the illusion of moral judgement and free will' and a corresponding acknowledgement that 'violent crime does have some connection with involuntary, disturbed patterns of brain activity in the frontal lobes'. Like Shorter in the first reading, then, and their own editorial in the second ('A comet at heaven's gate'), this is the *New Scientist* casting off the myth of mind. This is neuroscience, in Porter's phrase, laying 'bare the mysteries of the mind'. And yet, once again, a mind-only account of crime finally breaks through. This time it is in the contrast in which the *New Scientist* couches its final conclusion. Brain scans, it says, should be used only for 'diagnosing *medical* conditions, not *moral* ones' (our emphasis).

We are minds

Again, there is no easy way with these issues. The *New Scientist* is tackling a problem that has taxed the best minds for over two thousand years. But the concluding phrase in their editorial shows how even those most committed to brain-only solutions (those for whom consciousness and free will are 'illusions') *cannot avoid mind-talk* when they are speaking of people.

This is a nice case of Austin's 'use' of concepts speaking louder than 'definition', then. Earlier in this book we had an example of this in the work of Christopher Boorse on the concept of disease. Boorse stipulated a value-free definition of disease, yet could not avoid evaluative language in his use of the concept. This suggested that values are essential, logically essential, essential by virtue of the very meaning of 'disease'. Similarly, then, the way mind-talk breaks through in people-talk even in an editorial from the stipulatively eliminativist *New Scientist*, suggests that mind is essential to the concept of *person*. The Oxford philospher,

Peter Strawson (1977), in a now classic text on personal identity, indeed argued that the concept of person is 'primitive', logically speaking: that is to say, the very meanings of mind-concepts and body-concepts are *derived* from the more basic concept of 'person'.

We are brains

It is, then, because the *New Scientist* editorial is not about brains but about persons, in a moral world of crime and responsibility, that mind-talk is inevitable, i.e. because of the very *meaning* of what it is to be a person.

Which is, though, not to say that we can avoid brain-talk. In other contexts (as in certain theological treatments of free will) attempts are made to float the (moral) mind free of the (deterministic) brain. This is the mind-only solution, then. Both dogmas are widespread in everyday thinking, brain-only and mind-only. Yet both deny the twin aspects of what it is to be a person. And both are, thereby, in different ways, equally abusive.

This is true in general. It is true in particular in the case of the equivocally placed, the stretched between mind and brain, concept of mental illness. It is thus to a case example that we turn in the next session.

Reflection on the session and self-test questions

Write down your own reflections on the materials in this session drawing out any points that are particularly significant for you. Then write brief notes about the following:

1. Name two adverse effects on mental health of the difficulty of the mind–body problem. (We noted five.)

2. What implications have people drawn from (putative) neuroscientific discoveries of the brain basis of behaviour for responsibility and freedom of choice?

3. What central concept links both mind-talk and brain-talk in ordinary usage? What did Strawson say about this concept?

Session 2 The mind–body problem: the case of Mrs Lazy

In the last session, we used the J.L. Austin method for 'getting started', exploring some of the intuitive features of mind and body through ordinary usage. This showed us: (1) the richness of the connections between the mind–body problem and mental health practice and research (the Roy Porter review of Shorter); (2) the significance of consciousness as a feature of the mind ('A comet at heaven's gate'); and (3) the link between minds, brains, freedom, and responsibility (the two different ways in which people take the significance of brain research for responsibility represented by the *New Scientist*'s 'Inadmissible evidence', and the *Sunday Times*' 'Anorexia trigger' article). This led us to a conclusion about the essentially mind *plus* body nature of persons.

In this session, we continue the J.L. Austin way of getting started by thinking about a case history reported in the London *Times* newspaper. This report, which we can call the 'Case of Mrs Lazy', draws together many of the points made above about the mind–body problem in mental health. It will also help us to see just how much can be done with something *less* than mind and body, i.e. with *brain* and body; and, by contrast, what is left out when we leave out the mind. We will then be ready to start on philosophical accounts of mind and body in the next session.

EXERCISE 4	(30 minutes)

Read the extract from the newspaper report of the 'Lazy wife':

> Anon (1996). Lazy wife has her head examined. *The Times*, 2 September (1), page 7 (Report identified by Paul Sturdee; discussion, Fulford, 2000.)

Link with Reading 22.5

This is just the first two paragraphs. We will come to the rest of the story, in two bites, in a few minutes. With this first extract, (1) write down any mind–body points you can think of which it illustrates, and (2) also note your clinical thoughts, i.e. what do you think could be wrong, if anything, and what would you do (as 'Mrs Lazy's' GP, say, or as her husband)? Finally, (3) think how the two sets of points, the mind–body points and the clinical points, relate to each other.

Mind or brain

As a case report, this article is a rich source of observations about the 'ordinary use' of mind–body concepts in relation to questions of health, illness, and disease. Indeed, with just these first two paragraphs we go right to the heart of the mind–body problem. Mrs Lazy is introduced as a free agent who 'decided' she was fed up with housework. Antipsychiatry, therefore, would identify closely with the phrase that follows, she 'had to defend herself' against doctors, who, with what could reasonably be regarded as an unwarranted extension of the concept of illness, 'feared that she was ill'. The case against the doctors would seem strengthened by the fact that her 'defense' does indeed look reasonable—many women, after decades of housework, decide it is time to put their feet up, or to branch out in some other direction.

On the other hand, clinically, once we view this as a 'personality change', the shift in Mrs Lazy's behaviour, from a conscientious to unconscientious pattern, would be consistent with damage to the frontal lobes of her brain: a key feature of the 'frontal lobe syndrome' is just this loss of responsibility.

Moreover, Mrs Lazy's husband's concerns are highly relevant in this respect. On an antipsychiatry model, he would be viewed as motivated by the need to control his wife: her decision is medicalized and therefore invalidated, making her subject to interventions designed to control her deviance, to bring her back into line. But relatives are often sensitive to pathology that doctors, who may not know the patient so well, may miss (parents, as any family doctor will tell you, are often very good at knowing when their children are really ill even if, at the time, there are no obvious or well-defined symptoms).

A practical compromise

So, how do we pull this together? One practical course is to get Mrs Lazy's agreement to a brain scan, as a non-invasive procedure, and one that is likely to show if there is anything wrong (such as a tumour) about which something can be done (tumours in the frontal lobes of the brain are often 'silent' clinically, i.e. they show no signs or symptoms, apart sometimes from loss of the sense of smell in one nostril, due to pressure in the brain on the nerves from that side of the nose). This is what was done.

EXERCISE 5   (15 minutes)

Now read the second extract from the 'Case of the lazy wife'. Where does this take us, with the mind–body problem, and clinically?

Anon (1996). Lazy wife has her head examined. *The Times*, 2 September (2)

Link with Reading 22.6

Clinically, the discovery of a large tumour, and its successful removal, vindicated the surgeon's and Mrs Lazy's husband's concerns. In relation to the mind–body problem, moreover, this case illustrates some of the *mis*uses of mind in antipsychiatry.

Antipsychiatry got it wrong?

You will recall from the first reading (Porter's review of Shorter linked with Exercise 1), much denigratory talk of psychiatry being split into 'heroic (physical) interventions' (including brain surgery) and the 'aimless chat' of the talking therapies. This case shows, on the contrary, that psychiatry, no less indeed than neurosurgery or any other branch of medicine, needs both. It needs to attend to mind *and* body, in diagnosis and in treatment.

In this case, talking would indeed have been 'aimless chat' but surgery was appropriate. In many cases of mental disorder, surgery is not currently an option. But this is for technical reasons. There is no objection of principle to physical treatments, any more than, in principle, talking therapies should be inappropriate in principle. Talk, we must suppose, changes how the brain functions! Much of antipsychiatry, therefore, no less than much of psychiatry, is prone to a *false* separation of mind and brain.

Psychosomatic medicine

The extent of this false separation is well illustrated by the history of psychosomatic concepts in medicine. It is not so long ago that biologically minded doctors were inclined to deny that a patient's state of mind could influence the state of their body. How, it was argued, could feeling sad for example, possibly alter the blood supply to the heart (increasing the risk of a 'heart attack'), or affect the healing of a surgical wound.

Nowadays this seems positively antediluvian! Not only do we have a well-established concept of psychosomatic medicine but there is a whole subdiscipline of psychiatry specializing in the links between mind and body, called liaison psychiatry (liaison psychiatrists liase with general physicians, surgeons and other 'body-doctors'). Even at the time, the denial of mind–body links reflected a number of unjustified empirical presuppositions, namely

- that (relatively) distinct anatomical entities (hearts, livers, a leg, the skin, etc.) could be, or were even likely to be, functionally independent of each other and of the body as a whole (including the brain); or, at any rate, that everything we needed to *know* about these anatomical entities could be discovered by considering them in isolation

- that because causal connections between psychological states and bodily organs had not been identified, there were *no* such connections; or at any rate that the prevailing disease paradigms or research models precluded such connections.

In the present state of our knowledge, not only is the intimate connection between mind and body in questions of health taken for granted, but some of the causal pathways connecting them are beginning to be well understood.

The origins of the philosophical problem of mind and body

Descartes, the first liaison psychiatrist?

Interestingly, one of these causal pathways is the pineal gland. This was the organ by way of which the seventeenth century French philosopher, René Descartes, the man responsible for the mind–body problem in its present form, speculated that mind and body might interact. This is often treated as a philosophical joke. But it was a reasonable hypothesis. The pineal is a pea-sized organ situated more or less in the centre of the head with a cord or stalk of nervous tissue connecting it directly with the deep parts of the brain. In Descartes' time it had no obvious function and to all appearances it could well have been a mind–body transceiver.

We return to Descartes in Session 3. It is worth noting, however, that this construal would require qualifying the nature of Descartes' mind–body dualism. Descartes' arguments, as we will see, aimed to show the distinction between mind and brain. But it is arguable that if they interacted in the way he suggested, this would make the mental turn out to be in one sense *physical*.

There is a general problem of defining what is meant by 'physical' in non-question-begging terms, to which we return later. But it is plausible that anything that is causally interactive with items within the physical realm is itself *part of that realm*. This would still be different from arguing that mental states are really states of the body. The mind, for example, perhaps like the signal arriving at a TV set, could be a distinct field interacting with the body through the brain (see McGinn, 1993, for discussion of this possibility).

All the same, there is a clinically important sense in which Descartes' hypothesis about the pineal has turned out to be right.

The pineal is now known to be an important conduit between the *brain* and the rest of the body (there are others, e.g. the autonomic nervous system). Thus, the pineal secretes a wide variety of hormones that influence the state of the body; these secretions are under the control of higher centres in the brain that mediate emotional and other psychological functions (including the reception of signals from the outside world); these psychological functions, in turn, are influenced by the hormones stimulated (directly or indirectly, i.e. via the bodily changes they produce) by the pineal. And all this falls firmly within the remit of liaison psychiatry.

Brain–body dualism and psychiatric disease classification

Descartes' hypothesis about the pineal, reinterpreted as mediating *brain*–body dualism, thus anticipated the development of liaison psychiatry and, indeed, a range of modern biomedical disease categories such as 'psychosomatic disorder', 'endogenous depression', 'psychogenic pain', and 'organic psychosis'.

Such categories are often taken to reflect mind–body dualism. Yet they need not be taken to express anything more mysterious than the idea that the *brain* interacts with the rest of the body. We can reconstruct these categories, in terms of brain–body dualism, as follows.

- '*Psychosomatic disorders*' become bodily diseases caused, or made worse, by those states of the brain that mediate psychological functions (e.g. ulcerative colitis, a severe bowel disease, is often aggravated by long-term anxiety); in this sense, then, psychosomatic disorders are no more mysterious than what we might call 'dermatohepatic' disorders—i.e. skin disorders caused by states of the liver (e.g. jaundice).

- '*Endogenous depression*' becomes depression that appears to arise from an internal influence on the (putative) parts of the brain mediating sadness; this is as against reactive depression, which arises from external influences on these same brain parts, e.g. adverse life events such as bereavements (the distinction is not at present clinically useful because the symptoms and current treatments of depression are largely independent of the aetiological relationship to outside events).

- '*Psychogenic pain*' becomes pain (itself a brain state) produced by changes in other parts of the brain mediating psychological functions, rather than by external noxious stimuli.

- '*Organic psychoses*' become psychotic disorders caused by gross pathology (tumour, endocrine disorders, reduced blood supply, etc.) affecting the brain. 'Functional', or 'non-organic', psychoses (e.g. schizophrenia) are caused by more subtle (and still putative) changes in the fine structure of the parts of the brain mediating psychological functions.

Brain–body dualism and Mrs Lazy

With brain–body dualism of this kind, then, there is no reason why the mind should not be fully understood, in time, by way of empirical investigations of the brain. Mrs Lazy's case seems to foreshadow this. Her case was unusual (it was written up for a newspaper), though such cases are far from rare. But those involved clearly felt that brain medicine, and by implication the medical (scientific) model, had shown its worth. As indeed it had. But now look at the final extract, indicating the eventual outcome.

EXERCISE 6   (10 minutes)

Read the whole article again, i.e. with the concluding paragraph added in:

> Anon (1996). Lazy wife has her head examined. *The Times*, 2 September (3)

Link with Reading 22.7

- Can all the implications of this case be safely drawn in terms of brain–body dualism?

- What is left out?

- Why could this be clinically, as well as philosophically, important?

As the report indicates, despite removing the tumour, Mrs Lazy did not regain her enthusiasm for housework. But what are we to make of this?

Clinically, the causal story offered by the surgeon, Mike Hanna, as reported, is entirely plausible. It is *possible* that the tumour was merely incidental to Mrs Lazy's change of personality; and antipsychiatry might want to press this point. But as noted earlier, tumours in this part of the brain (the frontal lobes) are known to produce changes in personality of just the kind shown by Mrs Lazy (the frontal lobe syndrome); and it is not unreasonable to believe that after 15 years, this large tumour (the largest Mike Hanna had ever seen), could indeed have affected Mrs Lazy's frontal lobes for good.

Another blow to antipsychiatry?

At first glance, then, cases like this seem to contradict antipsychiatry, at least of the extreme Szaszian kind that would make mental illness a myth. Szasz, as we saw earlier, would have to say that Mrs Lazy had a *brain* disease. And Boorse, Kendell, and others representing the equal and opposite extreme of the 'medical' model, would take Mrs Lazy's case as paradigmatic of the way psychiatry will develop as its scientific basis becomes more secure. This is Shorter's point, too (from the first reading in this chapter): brain science, *modern* brain science, will 'lay bare the mysteries of the mind'. It will reveal the causes of mental disorder, thus making possible medical treatments, not 'heroic' perhaps, but (we may imagine) precisely targeted physical manipulations by designer drugs, laser scalpels, nano-technological inserts, and the like.

There are, as Shorter would be the first to acknowledge, technological barriers to this brain-based future. Any form of 'talking therapy' would certainly have been 'aimless chat' as a treatment for Mrs Lazy's frontal lobe tumour. Cognitive therapy, on the other hand, is likely to remain a 'treatment of choice' for some time to come for a whole range of 'functional disorders'. However, granted the brain–body model of mental disorder, there should be no barrier of principle to physical treatments for all. Indeed, as noted earlier, on a brain–body model, 'talking therapies' themselves change how the brain functions.

The mind fights back

There is a clear signal, though, even in this brief report of an apparently obvious 'brain' case, that the mind side of the mind–body problem, cannot be so easily eliminated. This comes in the last paragraph of the second extract (linked with Exercise 5), in Mike Hanna's reference to depressive illness. A change in personality, he is reported as saying, is usually due to a 'depressive illness', but in perhaps less than one case in ten 'something may be going on in their brain'.

EXERCISE 7   (30 minutes)

Think about this comment before going on, in particular:

1 What 'model' of mental illness does it reflect?

2 Why does it signal that the mind cannot be so easily eliminated?

3 If the mind were eliminated, what would go with it, in Mrs Lazy's case and in general?

Mike Hanna's comment reflects the 'mental illness = mind = unreal' *versus* 'physical disease = body = real' antithesis noted in the last session (e.g. in relation to the Porter review of Shorter). If pressed, Mike Hanna would no doubt want to say that 'of course mental illness has a brain basis'. As we noted earlier, however, the cracks in ordinary usage give us a view through to our underlying concepts.

In this case, it is the mind that is showing through the crack. *Mental* illness, however strong our commitment to a medical-scientific model, carries with it the mind side of mind and body. It is this that Mike Hanna's contrast implies. Mental illness is 'on the cusp'. It really is *mind* and body.

Consciousness and responsibility

Once mind is allowed in through this crack, it brings with it everything that has been left out, of Mrs Lazy's story, and of the *brain–body* story in general. In the first place, it brings 'phenomenal consciousness'. Mrs Lazy's story reminds us that much that we take for granted about ourselves from ordinary introspection, is wrong. In mind-only accounts of persons, motivation (the 'will') is a central part of the model of an independent consciousness 'looking out', the 'Wizard of Oz' of our second reading ('A comet at heaven's gate'). Motivation, though, as Mrs Lazy's case and others like it show, is firmly located (at least in part) in the frontal lobes.

Mrs Lazy's case thus illustrates the way in which 'deficit states' may help us both to differentiate the components of consciousness, and to identify their brain basis. But, and this is another crucial 'but', when all that is said and done, are we any further to knowing what it is *like* to feel motivated or unmotivated, what it is like *from Mrs Lazy's perspective*, or for people in general? Surely not.

Even more significant clinically, though, is the fact that, with mind comes responsibility. This was the second characteristic of the mind, you will recall, which we explored in the two readings linked with Exercise 3 (*New Scientist* and *Sunday Times*) in the last session (there are other characteristics of the mind—see Session 3). These two readings illustrated the diametrically opposite ways we can take the implications of neuroscientific findings for responsibility (as either wholly irrelevant or as abolishing it). They also showed how reactions to a given case depend in part on our evaluation of the behaviour in question.

Responsibility and mental disorder

Just how we should resolve issues of responsibility, in Mrs Lazy's case or in general, is not clear. The problem of responsibility is, in a sense, the whole of the mind–body problem! At the same time, it is a very *practical* problem. As the *New Scientist* editorial 'Inadmissible evidence' (linked with Exercise 3) reminds us, it crops up all the time in forensic psychiatry, over issues of 'mad or bad'. But it is also at the heart of the ethical issues raised by involuntary psychiatric treatment.

Difficult as the problem may be, though, Mrs Lazy's case shows us how critically important it is not to foreclose on it, either to mind-only solutions or to brain-only solutions. Conversely, it also shows us how pathology can help us to identify and disentangle some of the components of the problem itself. One way to think about this is using the framework of ideas developed in the first part of this book and summarized in the diagram of the full-field model at the end of chapter 6.

EXERCISE 8   (60 minutes)

Go to the diagram at the end of chapter 6 (this is reproduced below as Figure 22.1) and think about Mrs Lazy's case in terms of the elements of the model summarized there. As we are thinking mainly about what is left out in the brain-only account of Mrs Lazy, think particularly about the left-field elements, i.e. values, the experience of illness, and agency. Also, think about these in relation to the clinical and scientific, as well as the conceptual, aspects of Mrs Lazy's case history.

This is a long exercise because there is a lot to it! As before, it is important to work through these points for yourself, and to write down your conclusions, before going on.

Given that mental disorder, and with it mental health practice, is on the cusp of the mind–body problem, we should not be surprised to find that the way in which we conceptualize mental disorder has a close connection with the way in which we conceptualize mind and body.

Mind, body and a 'full-field' model of mental disorder

Referring, then, to the full-field model, this is indeed what we find. Thus, the elements of what we called earlier the right-field of the model, reflecting the body, are evident enough in the story of Mrs Lazy as reported—facts, diseases (Mrs Lazy's tumour), and disease interpreted as disturbance of functioning of bodily parts and systems (Mike Hanna talks of the tumour pushing aside the tips of the frontal lobes where 'drive and motivation reside'). But what is left out of the story as reported (though showing through the crack of Mike Hanna's earlier reference to the contrast between depressive illness and something going on 'in the brain') are the three elements of the left-field. And all three of these elements are critically important in Mrs Lazy's case, i.e. values, the experience of illness, and illness interpreted as disturbance of agency or 'failure of action'. Taking these in turn:

1. *Values*. We noted, from the two readings linked with Exercise 3 above, the extent to which values drive ascriptions of responsibility. There is, perhaps, a deep *conceptual* connection here—Descartes' separation of mind and body can be identified with his (presumed) need to square the responsibility he recognized as a *moral being* (brought up by Jesuits) with his instincts as a *scientist*. And values, most now accept, are critical to the distinction between health and illness.

   But without getting drawn into these conceptual deep waters, there is a clear *clinical* requirement for not eliminating the value aspects of mind even from a 'brain-case' like Mrs Lazy. Once recognized, indeed, this runs right through the whole story. Evaluatively, it is presented as a *success* story. And no doubt Mrs Lazy was pleased to have had her tumour removed. This was, we all agree, a 'good thing'. But we are actually told nothing about *her* reaction. It is just assumed. The case report at no stage engages with *Mrs Lazy's* values, even though, initially, she rejected the idea that she was ill. We are not told of her response to being hijacked by her husband and 'the doctors'. How did she come to have a brain scan? Or the operation? And how did she take the outcome? Is she now, as she continues to feel unenthusiastic about housework, 'sick', 'disabled'; labelled and self-labelling in the 'sick role'? Or does she still see herself as having taken a perfectly reasonable decision to put her feet up?

   This is a brief case report. It may well be that in practice the clinical team were fully engaged in Mrs Lazy's perspective throughout. But this is certainly not reflected in the way Mrs Lazy's story is told. After the opening lines, Mrs Lazy (as a person) disappears. We see her brain, but we don't see her. This is exactly how many patients do feel—invisible as people—when they see their doctor.

2. *The experience of illness*. If values go with the 'mind', then it is clear that eliminating mind eliminates something that is critically important clinically. The same is true of other aspects of the patient's *experience*. There is a broad connection here, of course, with having a 'point of view'—you will recall from the last session that this is one of the features of mind that marks it out from matter. And the medical model, focusing on matter, is at risk of emphasizing objective scientific knowledge sometimes to the exclusion of the patient's subjective experience.

   Paying careful attention to each patient's experience, to their point of view as a unique individual, is important clinically. But it is also critical to straight thinking *scientifically*. Mike Hanna assumed that the tumour 'damaged' Mrs Lazy's frontal lobes. This indeed is very much how the story has been presented in this session. But all we can say (with reasonable certainty) is that the tumour *changed* the functioning of Mrs Lazy's frontal lobes. This is partly a matter of the value judgements involved in distinguishing health and pathology. We assume that Mrs Lazy's frontal lobes are now *under*active. But perhaps they were *over*active *before*. Perhaps she was pathologically conscientious about her housework, and the tumour has 'cured' her. There is a curious play on words (unintentional) in Mike Hanna's conclusion that the 'pressure may have changed her personality for good'. He meant *permanently*. Mrs Lazy may have said 'for the *better*'!

3. *Loss of agency (action-failure)*. All this is not to say that it was wrong to remove Mrs Lazy's tumour. It was, as Mike Hanna said, life-threatening. But just as it would have been wrong, clinically, to have left Mrs Lazy's values out of account, so it would have been wrong, scientifically, to assume that the effect of the tumour was to *impair* frontal lobe function.

This latter assumption arises from a conceptual confusion about the relationship between illness and disease noted in chapter 6. The medical model has it that illness (the patient's experience and behaviour) is defined by disease (underlying bodily changes). However, we saw in chapter 6 that a bodily change cannot (*logically* cannot) mark out a change in experience or behaviour as illness. The logical relationship, the relationship of meaning, between illness and disease is in fact the other way round—pathological changes in experience and behaviour mark out underlying bodily changes as disease. Mrs Lazy's case underlines this. For it shows that even an acknowledged *pathological* bodily change (a tumour) cannot, of itself, mark out a change in experience or behaviour as pathological.

Just what *does* mark out a change in experience or behaviour as pathological is of course the large question that we began to explore in Part I. The idea introduced there, that illness is to be understood in some way in terms of loss of agency, or failure of what Austin called 'ordinary doing', is important clinically. As we saw, this is especially so in giving us a range of conceptual tools appropriate to the complexity particularly of psychopathology (notably, delusion).

It is also important scientifically. This is proving increasingly the case in neuroscience. Again, as we saw in Part I, the results of recent work in brain imaging and artificial intelligence demand interpretation in terms of agency and action, the mode of operation of persons (and perhaps higher animals), rather than (directly) in terms of the functioning of their subparts and systems. And this in turn is tying the clinical and scientific firmly to the conceptual, much of what little we know about agency being derived (in part) from work in philosophy on the nature of action.

Minds, brains, and action-failure

The mind–brain problem, then, filtered through the concepts of illness and mental illness, comes down, in part but importantly, to a problem in the philosophy of action. This is not too surprising a result. Our notions of agency are equally mind based and brain (or body) based (see Fulford, 1989, chapter 7). They have to be, at least to the extent that the characteristic mode of operation of persons is action; and that persons, too, as we noted at the end of the last session, are equally mind based and brain based.

The philosophy of action itself reflects this. Like the agents with which it is concerned, it is a hybrid. In Austin's day it was part of *moral* philosophy. Now, with the rise of cross-disciplinary work between philosophy and neuroscience, it is seen as part of a philosophy of mind directly connected with the *brain sciences*! And it can be taken either way. The detailed work on agency

characteristic of modern action theory is critically important to neuroscience, including those areas concerned with abnormal aspects of consciousness, such as delusions. Work in other areas on agency, however, e.g. in the philosophy of law, is equally concerned with the 'free agency' of moral beings engaged in a world of persons.

Minds, brains, and persons

The bottom line of the last session, then, that mind and brain are equally essential to persons, is also the bottom line that we should take from the 'Case of Mrs Lazy'. It may be possible for some purposes to deal separately with mind and body, to adopt mind-only, or brain-only positions. Brain-only is the position of the more triumphalist among 'biological' psychiatrists, as we have seen. But what Mrs Lazy's case shows us is that it is *above all* in the case of pathology that we need both. Clinically, scientifically, and conceptually, there is no getting off the cusp of the mind–body problem. Uncomfortable as it is, this is where we must be; and for the best of all possible reasons, that we are concerned, inescapably, with *persons*.

Remember, this is not a 'solution' to the mind–body problem. It is a recognition merely that mind-only and brain-only solutions are no solutions, at least in mental health practice and research. A retreat to either extreme, excluding mind or brain, may be equally abusive. But just how we *contain* both, engaging fully in the scientific possibility of a completed neuroscience, while at the same time engaging fully in a moral world of free agents, is, as we put it at the start of this section, the mother of all philosophical problems. It is to philosophical attempts to tackle the mind–body problem that we turn next.

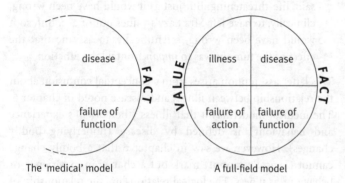

The 'medical' model   A full-field model

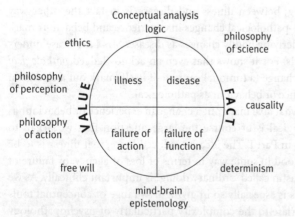

The full-field view in the philosophical context

Fig. 22.1 The full-field view in the philosophical context.

Reflection on the session and self-test questions

Write down your own reflections on the materials in this session drawing out any points that are particularly significant for you. Then write brief notes about the following:

1. Why did Mrs Lazy decide to give up housework?

2. Why did Mrs Lazy's family think that she was ill when she decided to give up housework? Why did her doctors agree with her family?

3. Does the concept of psychosomatic disorder as used in medicine depend on mind–body dualism?

4. What explanation of Mrs Lazy's decision was given by her doctors?

5. What did this leave out?

6. What is the wider message of Mrs Lazy's story for a neuroscience-led psychiatry?

Session 3 The mind–body problem: from ordinary use to philosophy

This session charts the development of the two paradigmatic philosophical perspectives on the relationship between mind and body, dualism and monism. We will be looking at readings from four major figures in the history of philosophy, namely Descartes, Berkeley, Hobbes, and Kant. Their ideas are crucial to understanding current debates in the philosophy of mind about the mind–body problem (to which we come in Session 4 and in chapter 23).

In J.L. Austin's neat aphorism, when a problem is solved in philosophy it gets 'kicked upstairs' (Womock, 1989, page 4). It becomes a new discipline—mathematics, natural science, and, more recently, psychology, logic, and linguistics, have all been 'kicked upstairs'.

The mind–body problem is still a long way from being kicked upstairs. The work of the last two sessions, therefore, has been no mere preliminary to the philosophical story. It has been concerned with identifying and making explicit the elements of the mind–body problem, (1) as they are with us *today* in ordinary usage (and, hence, in clinical practice and research); but also, (2) as they were tackled in the seventeenth century by *Descartes and his successors* (also his predecessors—see below); and (3) as they *continue to be tackled* in modern philosophy of mind.

The origins of the philosophy of mind

The problems with which the philosophy of mind is concerned have occupied philosophers since classical times. But the philosophy of mind emerged as a distinct subdiscipline in academic philosophy only in the late 1940s, with the work particularly of the Oxford philosopher Gilbert Ryle, and the Cambridge philosopher Ludwig Wittgenstein.

In Descartes' time, in the seventeenth century, the philosophy of mind was part of a debate on the nature of knowledge. This was a period when the primary concerns of general philosophy shifted from *metaphysics* (the inquiry into the fundamental basis of reality, or, alternatively, the exploration of what lies beyond our sense-experience), which had been central to Western philosophy since Plato and Aristotle, to *epistemology* (the inquiry into the limits, and possibility, of knowledge).

Like most movements in philosophy, this shift of interest was very much a product of the times. This was a period of radical challenges to traditional sources of authority—the Church, the State, moral tradition, were all being questioned. In the study of the natural world, the ideas of Newton had overthrown those of Aristotle. The Reformation had undermined the Pope's claim to be Holy Roman Emperor. And at about this time, too, the writings of the classical sceptical philosopher, Sextus Empiricus, were translated from Greek into Latin, and thus became available to all intellectuals in Europe. Sceptical ideas were suddenly the talk of the universities and academies. The very foundations on which

secure knowledge rested seemed in doubt. How then, could we *know* anything? What was our warrant?

We need to start, then, by seeing how the mind–body problem (and the two big theories in particular, dualism and monism) developed out of the larger debate concerning the nature of knowledge.

Rationalism versus empiricism

To a first approximation, we can say that in the seventeenth century two broadly opposed positions were taken on how we come to know things, *rationalism* and *empiricism*. Both reflected a model of the mind as a sort of vessel or container of knowledge.

Rationalists believed that this vessel had in-built tools (our rational capacities) for making sense of the world. Hence the foundations of knowledge lay in the exercise of our rational capacities, rather than in the sensations from which our experience of the world is derived. On this view, the rational subject comes into the world already equipped with the rational capacities to arrive at knowledge. We use these pre-existing rational capacities as tools to structure the raw data of our senses.

Empiricists saw things the other way around. They believed the vessel was empty until it has things put into it by our senses. Hence for empiricists, the foundations of knowledge are our experiences grounded on our senses, with the faculty of reason being a development from this. Thus the philosopher-physician, and arch-empiricist, John Locke, to whose work we return in chapter 28, believed the newborn child's mind was a *tabula rasa* (clean slate).

Both views are oversimplified models of how we gain knowledge. We, like other animals, are born with pre-existing capacities (as the rationalists believed); but (as the empiricists recognized) the full development of these capacities, and indeed the *way* they develop, is critically influenced by our experiences, particularly when we are young. Though it should also be said that the *philosophical* problem of knowledge (concerning our *warrant* for claiming that we really *know* anything), as distinct from the empirical problem of the developmental psychology of knowledge, is far from resolved.

(A valuable contemporary account of the developmental psychology of knowledge is Ed Hundert's *Philosophy, Psychiatry and Neuroscience: Three Approaches to the Mind* (1989). Ed Hundert is a philosopher-psychiatrist, currently Dean of the Harvard Medical School.)

René Descartes

An important early move in these epistemological debates, and the move that launched the mind–body problem in its present form, was made by the French philosopher, René Descartes.

Born in La Haye near Tours in France (now called La Haye-Descartes in his honour) in 1596, he was an extraordinary polymath. Besides founding the 'modern' period in philosophy, he

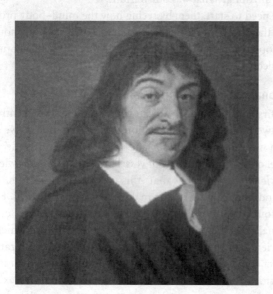

Fig. 22.2 René Descartes

invented the system of co-ordinate geometry that we still use today. Moreover, and contrary to his rationalist public image, he is now known to have been a keen experimentalist (see, for example, Clarke, 1982,; Garber, 1978, pp. 114–151).

Descartes did most of his definitive philosophical work between 1628 and 1649, living in Holland, after a period of seeing the world as a soldier. His key works on mind and body, published over this period, were the *Discourse on Method* (1637) and the *Meditations* (1641) (see Descartes, 1968) In 1649 (the year he published a *Treatise on the Passions*) he accepted an invitation to visit the Queen of Sweden to become her instructor in philosophy. He died the following year, apparently having succumbed to the rigorous climate. He never married but is believed to have had a daughter.

Descartes' project

Descartes' project, as we noted earlier, was epistemological. He wanted to find a secure foundation for knowledge. Much of the history of epistemology (from Greek philosophy onwards) has been a series of attempts to refute scepticism, the claim that we can *never* have *knowledge* of anything. This claim had been advanced in Descartes' time by the grandly named French humanist and essayist, Michel Equem de Montaigne (1533–92, usually just called Montaigne).

Montaigne had published a short but very influential essay *Apology for Raimond Sebond* in 1580. Using what was later to become known as the 'Oxford manoeuvre', of appearing to support philosophically what you are about to demolish,

Montaigne's *Apology* was in fact a demolition job on Sebond's (fifteenth century) attempt to show that the articles of the Christian faith could be established by reason. Montaigne drew on the sceptical arguments originally set out by the physician-philosopher Sextus Empiricus in the second century AD to argue for essentially sceptical conclusions about the possibility of knowledge in general, including that of religious faiths.

A virtuous scepticism

Montaigne's scepticism presented a deep challenge to an intelligentsia in the process of overthrowing the authorities of the Medieval world. As is the way with scepticism, though, it provoked fertile responses. You will recall from Part I, how the scepticism of Szasz and others in the 1960s and 1970s about mental illness, has brought us to a much deeper understanding of the subject. In the seventeenth century Montaigne's scepticism led both to empiricism in the form of Francis Bacon's 'inductive method' (see Part III, on The Philosophy of Science), and to Descartes' rationalism, in the form of his '*Method of Doubt*'.

There is no single extract from Descartes' work that can be taken as definitive of his method, but the next reading linked with Exercise 9 conveys much of the excitement of his approach.

EXERCISE 9	(30 minutes)

Read the two extracts from

Descartes (1996). Second meditation. In *Meditations* (ed. J. Cottingham). Cambridge: Cambridge University Press. (Extract, pp 16–18, 19.)

Link with Reading 22.8

Although this extract occurs early in the work (there are six meditations in all) it gives a flavour of the whole, with allusions to both the 'Cogito' (*cogito ego sum*—I think therefore I am) of the fourth meditation, and the 'malicious demon' thought experiment of the first meditation.

We return to both these below. But before you go on, think carefully about Descartes' arguments. Don't think of this reading as 'historical'. Take it seriously as tackling a contemporary problem.

As you read, make short notes on:

1. How Descartes sets up his thesis—he is concerned to show the fallibility of much that we ordinarily take to be true. He thus arrives at the conclusion that only a specific rational methodology can produce certain knowledge. How does he go about this?

2. What is the basic feature of this rational methodology? Are you convinced by it? How 'certain' is the knowledge that is thus produced?

Reading this piece we can see why Descartes' work ushered in what is now known as the 'modern' era in philosophy. Although not wholly original (even the 'cogito' was anticipated by St Augustine), the ideas that he brought together, and his vigorous independent style of argument, were truly revolutionary. There is nothing here of the obsession with spurious technicalities into which medieval scholastic philosophy, with its almost slavish reverence for Aristotelian principles (in which Descartes himself had been schooled by the Jesuits), had fallen. He embarks on an entirely novel course of subjecting every possible claim to critical inspection. This is his famous 'method of doubt'.

Descartes' method of doubt

In the 'Second Meditation', then, Descartes' begins by briefly reviewing the progress achieved in the First Meditation. (The reference to 'yesterday's meditation', by the way, is a literary device for adding veracity to the whole process. Many modern philosophers could learn from Descartes the value of contextualizing their work, of embedding it in a concrete situation to which their readers can relate. This is a real man struggling with real problems, however abstract!)

Descartes now goes on to assess to what degree any knowledge-claim is susceptible to doubt. This leads him to the (temporary) conclusion that *nothing at all* is certain. A glimmer of hope is provided by the thought that 'I myself may be perhaps the author of these thoughts' (p. 16). However, as the having of a thought cannot alter the radical doubts concerning the existence of the body of the thinker, all that is left is the mind, which, although it might be susceptible to deceit (the deceiver is introduced in the form of a 'malicious demon' in the 'First Meditation') seems to afford the license for speaking of 'I'.

But what is this 'I', Descartes asks? The problem, he acknowledges, is that the mind is constantly beset by imaginings, dreamings, and inventions, so that all here could be deceptive also . . . It is at this point that Descartes introduces his master-stroke. 'But what then am I?' he says, 'A thing that thinks. What is that? A thing that doubts, affirms, denies, is willing, is unwilling, and also . . . imagines and has sensory perceptions' (p. 19). The *contents* of this mind can still be deceptions—for if one relies on the mechanism of sensation to provide the objects that we take to be in the world, then deception is not only possible but all around us (things are never exactly as they seem, Descartes is saying). But the one feature of the mind which is beyond doubt or deception, argues Descartes, is the *act of judgement*. Thus, I cannot be deceived or in doubt that, when *making* a judgement, I am actually doing so (p. 21).

The 'cogito'

This is the pivot of Descartes' philosophy. He has set out to find certainty by this negative method of doubting everything that he can possibly doubt. Then he finds that the one thing he cannot doubt is that he is doubting. Even his 'malicious demon', capable of deceiving him on all else, cannot deceive him here. The British logical positionist (see Part III), A.J. Ayer, neatly summed up

Descartes' point thus: 'If one *doubts* whether there are acts of consciousness, it follows that there *are*, since doubting itself *is* such an act' (Ayer, [1973] 1976, p. 37, emphasis added). Hence, since doubting that one thinks is self-denying, I cannot doubt that I think; and if I think, Descartes concluded, there must be a thinker; it thus follows that 'I think therefore I am' or '*cogito ergo sum*'.

Much debate

The 'cogito' has become one of the most famous of all philosophical aphorisms, in popular culture no less than in philosophy. It continues to be hotly debated (for an excellent recent discussion, see Williams, 1978); and even at the time it aroused great interest, much of it hostile. The *Meditations* is possibly the first example of peer-group critical commentary in print, since the first edition appeared (in Latin) complete with several sets of anonymous 'Objections', alongside which were printed Descartes' replies—an early example of the format so successfully revived by the modern review journal, *Behavioural and Brain Sciences*, and on which *Philosophy, Psychiatry and Psychology* is based.

Descartes' philosophy has been criticized partly for the further consequences that he was to draw from the 'cogito': he claimed, for example, that it led to a proof of the existence of a perfect God, who, being perfect, guaranteed the veracity of 'clear and distinct' ideas as the basis of true knowledge. But the 'cogito' itself has also been extensively attacked. It has been said, for example, that it relies on an unjustified inference—the 'cogito', this criticism goes, shows only that *thinking* is, not that *I* think. This was a point made squarely by Immanuel Kant (see below). But the debates that Descartes sparked off have been highly productive. It is these debates, indeed, that have evolved into an important strand in the philosophy of mind.

Descartes sets the agenda

We can see this from the next reading linked with Exercise 10. This is a very short section from near the beginning of 'Discourse 4' in Descartes' *Discourse on Method* (this work was originally the introduction to a scientific work, *Dioptric, Meteors, and Geometry*, but quickly became established as a philosophical statement in its own right. It is Descartes' best known work).

EXERCISE 10	(20 minutes)

Read the two pages from

> Descartes (1968). Discourse 4. In *Discourse on Method and the Meditations* (trans. and with an introduction by F.E. Sutcliffe). London: Penguin Books. (Extract, pp. 53–54.)

Link with Reading 22.9

Descartes provides here a helpful summary of his philosophy. Take a few minutes to think carefully about what he says and try to spot as many topics in the philosophy of mind as you can.

Much of modern philosophy of mind, and most that is important to philosophy and mental health, is present, in microcosm, in this short extract.

First, there is the *mind–body problem*. This is what we will be concentrating on in the rest of this session. As we have seen, from the first two sessions in this chapter, the mind–body problem has a whole series of ramifications for clinical practice and research in mental health. But there are other items on the agenda. We will note these briefly here and return to some of them in more detail in later chapters.

1. *Personal identity*. Descartes writes 'I therefore concluded that I was a substance, of which the whole essence or nature consists in thinking...'. Well, *is* thinking the whole nature of what it is to be a person? Descartes meant by 'thinking' every aspect of conscious mental life. But even so, what about bodily continuity?

   This is the problem which in modern philosophy of mind, has become known as the problem of personal identity. There are in fact two subproblems here, both of which are critical in psychopathology:

   ◆ the problem of *re-identification*. This involves both how do I know that when you come back in the room you are the same person who went out and also that when I wake up I am the same person who went to sleep. This kind of problem is at the heart of delusional misidentifications, such as the Capgras syndrome (where the patient believes those around him, although apparently identical with his real friends and relatives, are imposters); it is also central to how we understand profound changes in personality, as in dementia (see, eg Hope, 1994).

   ◆ the problem of the *nature of persons*, or of 'personhood', i.e. what it is that is distinctive or characteristic of persons. This is central to a range of issues in psychopathology where aspects of mental life that we normally take to be essential to personhood appear to be absent. Again, dementia, when profound, may (though not necessarily justifiably) be seen to involve loss of personhood (Hope, 1994).

2. *Knowledge of other minds*. Descartes writes of the mind that '...it is easier to know than the body'. But is it? In a sense it is. We feel we have privileged access to our own thoughts. But what about unconscious thoughts? Am I always aware, say, of my dislike of a colleague? And as for other minds, how do I know that anyone else has a mind at all? Children with autism, it has been claimed, appear to lack just this knowledge.

   There are also two subproblems here, then: how (or to what extent) can I be said to know my own mind, and how can I have knowledge of other minds?

3. *The will*. As already noted, work on agency is an important strand in modern philosophy of mind. Descartes' approach is, on the surface, very cognitivist—it is all about thinking this, perceiving that, and so on. But remember that for Descartes 'thinking' broadly meant 'conscious mental activity'. And

notice that where he introduces the 'cogito' he writes that 'I *decided* thus to think...'. The emphasized word, decided, marks Descartes the agent. In the earlier reading (linked with Exercise 9), similarly, it was the *act* of judgement he could not deny. Once you start looking for them, you will find that the 'Second Meditation' (for example) is strewn with action verbs, so that the 'cogito' is not really an abstract proof but an embodied demonstration. We will see later that Immanuel Kant was to make much of this.

In all these areas, then, Descartes' 'cogito', while appearing to give him what he began by looking for (something indubitable on which to found knowledge), has set philosophical hares running which have yet to be caught. In fact, even as a foundation for knowledge, the 'cogito' fails. It fails because, as just noted, it shows, at most, that *thinking* is; and it shows even this, only for the *moment* of thinking (the *act* of the agent, note). Moreover, even granted this, there is nowhere to go with it. Descartes (in this last reading, linked with Exercise 10) tries to extract a principle of certain knowledge in his 'clear and distinct ideas'. But even he recognizes that he then has a problem with clearly identifying the 'clear'! In his system, as noted briefly above, he has to fall back on the idea of God.

So, Descartes has raised more doubts with his 'method of doubt' than he started with! This, though, is no criticism. It is often the case that an important idea is not important because it is true (in some absolute sense), still less because it is indubitable, but because it is *fruitful*. In the rest of this session we will be looking at some of the fruitful ideas on mind and body that emerged in the seventeenth and eighteenth centuries in the wake of Descartes' new agenda for philosophy.

The rest of this session

In the rest of this session, then, we will be surveying just a few of the mind–body 'solutions' that were advanced from Descartes' time through to the nineteenth century. This will introduce several of the other 'big names' in philosophy.

Dualism and monism

The philosophical influence of the mind–body problem, as set up by Descartes, is reflected in the extent to which it has continued to inspire debate over the centuries. As you might expect, the range of theories produced by so many ingenious minds can be somewhat bewildering. A good way to think about them, to get a sense of order, is in terms of one of the most widely used pairs of 'isms', dualism and monism.

◆ *Dualists* believe that there exist two distinct sorts of substance in the universe, matter and mind. Descartes was the original 'two-substance' dualist. Malebranche, Geulincx, and Leibniz (described below) were all dualists; the work of the Oxford analytic philosopher, P.F. Strawson, on personal identity, noted above, has dualist overtones.

◆ *Monists* hold that there is only one sort of substance in the universe, usually either *mind* (e.g. Berkeley's idealism, see below) or *matter*. The latter, or *materialist monism*, is by far the most influential mind—body theory in modern philosophy of mind (see chapter 23, in particular, on the current front-runner, *functionalism*); but there have been materialists throughout the history of philosophy (Thomas Hobbes, see below, was a contemporary of Descartes). A third kind of monism is *double-aspect theory*, according to which mind and matter are but two aspects of some more fundamental substance (see, e.g. Spinoza, below).

Malebranche's occasionalism

One of the principle philosophers who built on Descartes' dualism was the French philosopher-theologian Nicolas Malebranche (1638–1715). In 1674/5 he published *De La Recherche de la Vérité* in which he developed a theory of how mind and body are related, known as *occasionalism*. In effect, this continues the Cartesian project from where Descartes left off. Malebranche's occasionalism addresses the problem of the relation between mind and body.

Malebranche argued that causation is simply a convenient concept representing human attempts to account for the behaviour of objects. We have already seen (in Part III) that causation has proved extremely difficult to characterize. Most philosophers, nowadays, would go along with Malebranche, at least to the extent of arguing that there is no necessary connection between bodies that would afford a metaphysical account of causation. However, Malebranche went on to advance the radical view that in fact the human will has no power of causal interaction. What actually happens when the will is exercised in, say, moving one's arm, is that this exercise of will provides God with an *occasion to intervene* in the causal order of the universe, causing one's arm to move exactly as one wills it to move. It is God, not the will, which brings about what we take to be the effects of willing.

Malebranche's occasionalism, while stimulating fierce debate at the time (particularly among theologians), has not proved as enduring as Descartes' original ideas. If one accepts Malebranche's arguments, the mind—body problem is effectively solved, at least on the question of how Descartes' non-material substance (mind) could be related to a material substance (body). And the theory is certainly ingenious: to modern ears, it has something of the 'many worlds' account of quantum mechanics—this 'solves' the problem of the indeterminacy of quantum mechanics by arguing that each of the possible outcomes of a quantum mechanical process takes the form of a new universe (or world); so that each of the outcomes actually takes place, but each in its own universe.

As a 'solution', the 'many worlds' account of quantum mechanics works. But it is so extravagant that the cure seems worse than the disease! It is the cure being worse than the disease that has been the main objection to occasionalism. Moreover, while some physicists believe it may be possible to get experimental evidence to support the 'many worlds' theory, occasionalism, although advanced within a scientific world view (of causation etc.) is not open to test in the same way. Hence, few philosophers have been convinced by Malebranche's arguments, and the mind—body problem has continued to excite debate and stimulate ideas.

Geulincx's 'image of the two clocks'

Arnold Geulincx (1624–69), a Belgian philosopher and disciple of Descartes, addressed objections to Descartes' mind—body problem with his own version of occasionalism in his principle works *Ethica* (1675) and *Metaphysica* (1691).

Geulincx illustrated his response to the Cartesian mind—body problem with the image of two clocks that keep perfect time with each other (another philosophical thought experiment!). According to Geulincx, there are three possible explanations: (i) the clocks are in a relation of mutual influence; (ii) they are looked after by a minder who keeps them in perfect time; (iii) they each have a property of perfect timing, so that once set, they operate as if working in unity.

The two clocks (and their relation with one another) are a metaphor for the mind—body problem: (i) represents two-way interactionism, (ii) represents occasionalism, while (iii) represents harmonious parallel functioning.

Geulincx opted for (ii), necessitating, in his account, the introduction of Divine intervention as a means of keeping mind and body working together. Like Malebranche's occasionalism, Geulincx's ideas excited some debate at the time, but did not exercise an enduring influence on philosophy. However, his 'image of the two clocks' thought experiment prompted Leibniz's adoption of option (iii), which we will come to in a moment.

Spinoza's monism

Benedict Spinoza (1632–77) was a Dutch lens-grinder of Portuguese Jewish parents, who spent almost his entire life working in Holland. In 1656 the Jewish community expelled him for heresy (the Christians later banned his works on similar grounds). Spinoza, like Descartes, believed that explanation was basically deductive, and that therefore a purely rationalist account of the universe was possible.

Unlike Descartes, however, Spinoza, in his principle work the *Ethics* (1677), rejected substance dualism, arguing that there could, in principle, be only one substance, with various modes of being. This one substance was God. Individuals, claimed Spinoza, were simply finite modes of this one substance. Matter ('extension' in Spinoza's terminology) was simply *that which is extended*, whereas mind ('thought' in Spinoza's terminology) is simply *that which thinks*.

As the two were, in all respects, distinct and incommensurable as attributes of substance, Spinoza is really advancing an *attributive dualism*, while at the same time arguing that the two attributes functioned in harmony with each other. Extension and thought are not substances, therefore, and their relation is one of being attributes of the same infinite substance, which is God (for this reason Spinoza's philosophy has been described as 'pantheistic', as all things are in God—this is why both the Jews and the Christians rejected his ideas).

The fundamental subject matter of the philosophy of mind would therefore be, for Spinoza, the ideas that are thought, or, in his terminology, 'modes of thought'. However, Spinoza's commitment to determinism led him to reject free will, so in a sense the mind–body problem becomes merely academic. His views have been compared with some Eastern philosophies, and continue to be studied for their conceptual richness and complexity.

Leibniz's psychophysical parallelism

Gottfried Wilhelm Leibniz (1646–1716), a German philosopher and polymath who spent most of his life travelling as a diplomat and negotiator for German princes and nobility, nevertheless found time to make original contributions to philosophy, theology, mathematics, logic, epistemology, and the philosophy of mind. Perhaps not surprisingly, he never got around to writing a *magnum opus*, and his philosophical ideas are distributed over two books (*New Essays on the Human Understanding*, 1705; and *Theodicity*, 1710), and many short papers, originally produced as part of his voluminous correspondence with most of the intellectual giants of his time.

The Cartesian mind–body problem was of great interest to Leibniz. Like Spinoza, he took a strictly deterministic view of the universe, but nevertheless insisted that the will was free. Despite the fact that all is determined by God, Leibniz argues, we have a special responsibility to act in accordance with God's wishes. His inspiration comes in part from Geulincx's 'image of the two clocks' thought experiment, where he chooses option (iii), the harmonious parallel functioning. Leibniz's arguments for this solution, and the metaphysics involved, are, however, very strange indeed.

Rejecting Spinoza's claim that there was only one substance, Leibniz argued instead that there was an infinity of substances, or *monads*, in the universe (in his essay 'Monadology'). Each individual is a monad, and each monad is 'windowless', that is, sealed from the rest of the universe. But each monad contains an 'appetite' to express its own future, and in this way also reflects everything else in the universe, although every monad is causally independent of all others.

Unlike Descartes, Leibniz did not take consciousness to be an all-or-nothing affair, and monads are held to be soul-like atoms that constitute reality, and possess the capacity for perception and representation. Minds are a special subclass of monads that possess apperception or self-consciousness, and also possess 'petites perceptions' when not actively thinking. Minds appear to act upon the world (including the body), and vice-versa, because there is a pre-existing harmony between the two that relies on God—a psychophysical parallelism that gives the appearance that the two stand in a causal relation when in fact no causal relation exists at all.

Leibniz's philosophy has, quite rightly, been viewed as rather eccentric, and during the nineteenth century there was little interest in his work in the English-speaking world. However, in

1900 Bertrand Russell published *The Critical Exposition of the Philosophy of Leibniz*, in which he pointed out the original ideas on logic introduced by Leibniz in support of his metaphysics, thus prompting a degree of on-going debate about the value of Leibniz's contributions to logic. It must be said, however, that Leibniz's contribution to the mind–body problem has not attracted many supporters.

Berkeley's idealist monism

In contrast to Leibniz's extravagance of infinite substances, the Irish philosopher of English descent, Bishop George Berkeley, argued in 1710 that there was in fact no such thing as matter, and that the existence of material objects was founded upon our sensations. For material objects to exist, they must be perceived by a mind. All that can be said to exist, according to Berkeley, exists in the form of minds and their contents. This claim is one example of a thesis known as *idealism*.

Berkeley's idealism can be understood as an extreme metaphysical claim, or as a modest epistemological claim. It did not, however, find favour with his contemporaries, and has been controversial ever since.

Berkeley sets out his arguments in his great work 'Principles of human knowledge' ([1710] 1975). He begins by suggesting that the 'objects of human knowledge' are in fact ideas. He then argues that ideas rely for their existence on being perceived. What is unintelligible is that ideas should exist unperceived. 'Their *esse* is *percipi*'. But if this is the case, the 'objects' of knowledge, such as tables and trees, are but abstractions from their being perceived—the objects of sensation and the sensation itself are but one and the same thing 'the reader need only reflect and try to separate in his thoughts the being of a sensible thing from its being perceived'. The very notion of matter, argues Berkeley, involves a contradiction, as do all the other notions that together afford us knowledge of the world of material objects. The material objects we find in the world are products of our capacity for experience. The very notion of experience, Berkeley is in effect saying, is unintelligible outside of the mind. He concludes: 'the arguments foregoing plainly show it to be impossible that any colour or extension at all, or any other sensible quality whatsoever, should exist in an unthinking subject without the mind, or in truth, that there should be any such thing as an outward object'.

This view is exceedingly counterintuitive. It offends common sense. To Berkeley, however, it provided a convincing argument for the existence of God, who, he claimed, perceived everything all the time. His view was caricatured in a limerick by Ronald Knox, with a suitable reply from God:

> There was a young man who said, 'God
> Must think it exceedingly odd,
> If he finds that this tree
> Continues to be
> When there's no one about in the Quad.'

GOD'S REPLY:
Dear Sir:
Your astonishment's odd:
I am always about in the Quad.
And that's why the tree
Will continue to be,
Since observed by
Yours faithfully,
GOD.

Attributed to Ronald Knox, as reproduced
in Russell (1946, p. 623)

Although Berkeley's version of idealism has been accepted by very few thinkers, it is perhaps worthy of note that it foreshadowed the later doctrine known as *phenomenalism* (sometimes jokingly described as 'Berkeley without God'). Phenomenalism rejects any claim that there are inaccessible objects behind appearances, and reduces talk of perceived or perceivable things to talk of actual or possible experiences. Influential thinkers who propounded versions of phenomenalism included J.S. Mill, Ernst Mach, and A.J. Ayer (in his early work). Phenomenalist ideas have also surfaced in work on the conceptual foundations of quantum mechanics (see, e.g. the French theoretical physicist, d'Espagnat, 1983).

Thomas Hobbes: the first modern materialist?

Despite all these novel and sometimes eccentric contributions to the mind–body debate, there were, however, expressions of solid common-sense around in the seventeenth and eighteenth centuries.

The author of just such a view of the mind–body relation is the English political philosopher, Thomas Hobbes (1588–1679). The

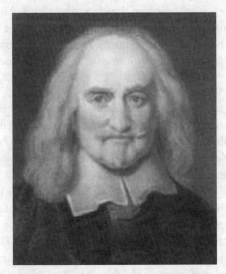

Fig. 22.3 Thomas Hobbes

son of a Wiltshire clergyman, Hobbes won a scholarship to Oxford and went on to become a disciple of the great English empiricist philosopher Francis Bacon. Hobbes was another great polymath, writing extensively on philosophy, ethics, religion, politics, mathematics, natural science, and the law. Most of his writing was done in his middle and later years, after the publication of Descartes' *Discourse* and *Meditations*. Indeed, he wrote a controversial set of objections to Descartes' *Meditations*, published, as we noted above, along with objections from other great Enlightenment thinkers, as an appendix to the first edition (in Latin).

In the next exercise, we will read the short extract from Hobbes' critique of Descortes. This comes from his 'Third Set of Objections' to Descartes' *Meditations*.

EXERCISE 11   (30 minutes)

Read the short extract from

Hobbes, T. (1984). 'Objections' to Descartes' *Meditations*. In *The Philosophical Writings of Descartes* (trans. J. Cottingham, R. Stoothoff, and D. Murdoch), Vol. 2. Cambridge: Cambridge University Press, pp. 122–123

Link with Reading 22.10

What are Hobbes objections to Descartes' cogito? What does he think it shows? What does he think it fails to show?

In the extract we have just read from Hobbes' 'Second Objection', he argues that Descartes (1) identifies the activity of thinking with the thing that thinks, and (2) then claims, on this basis that thinking entails the existence of a thinking thing, and, further, (3) that this thinking thing is a different substance from that which does not think. Hobbes contends that Descartes has gone further than logic will support with this argument, as all that follows from 'I think' or ' I am thinking' is that thinking is taking place, and it is I who thinks. But this does not entail that the thinker is a non-corporeal substance, any more than 'I walk' entails that the walker is a non-corporeal substance.

Hobbes argues that the reasonable conclusion to reach is, instead, that the thinker is corporeal, as we cannot conceive of an act without a subject, and the only subject presented to the senses is the corporeal subject (i.e. the only subject of propositions).

Further, Hobbes contends, unless we subject 'I think' to an iterative thought ('I think that I think that I think. . . .') we cannot make the subject the object of the thought. And yet, he writes, this is *not* how we know that we think—we know that we think because we are intimately engaged in the act of thinking, not by any iterative thought-process, which, in any case, leads simply to a vicious regress ('I think that I think that I think. . . .' *ad infinitum*). In fact, says Hobbes, the knowledge afforded by 'I think' is derived from knowledge of the act of thinking, and the knowledge we have of the author of the thought is derived from our senses, i.e. it is of a material thing. Thus mind and body are of the same substance, namely, matter.

In his 'Fourth Objection', Hobbes goes on to criticize Descartes for indulging in a game of word-play that amounts to shuffling around names connected with the verb 'is'. If that is all there is to Cartesian philosophy, says Hobbes, then the explanation for the mind–body problem consists in the motion of our bodily organs' (meaning the operation of the senses stimulating activity in the brain).

In his great work of political philosophy, *Leviathan*, Hobbes (1996) is even more explicit about his materialism: 'the Universe, that is to say, the whole mass of things that are, is corporeal, that is to say, body' (chapter 46, *Leviathan*, p. 689). Hobbes can therefore be seen as the forerunner of modern metaphysical materialism.

The null hypothesis

We have now looked at examples of each of the main ways of trying to solve the mind–body problem as it was set up by Descartes. We can summarize the Cartesian mind–body problem thus: mind and body, although clearly related in *some* way, also seem, in *other* ways, to be incompatible. Descartes, you will remember, regarded *extension* as the essence of matter; but the essence of mind, he argued, is thought, which is *extensionless*. The contemporary British Philosopher, Colin McGinn, gives a valuable account of how the problem can be understood in this way, including details of both the body-*like* and body-*unlike* features of mind, in chapter 2 of his introduction to the philosophy of mind, *The Character of Mind* (1982).

Now, if this is the *problem*, then we have only a limited range of possible solutions: either we explain how mind and body, despite appearing incompatible, can interact (i.e. dualism); or we reduce mind to brain (materialist monism) or brain to mind (idealist monism); or we hypothesize something more fundamental of which mind and matter (brain) are merely two aspects (double-aspect theory).

However, each of these 'solutions' has now been tried and found wanting. Of course, a solution along one or other lines may still be found (we will be looking at a modern form of materialism, *functionalism*, in detail in the next chapter). None the less, by analogy with experimental science, if none of the possible solutions appears to work, we might feel inclined to adopt the 'null hypothesis', i.e. to suppose that there is something wrong with the original problem, or at any rate with the way it has been set up.

Enter Immanuel Kant.

Kant's transcendental idealism

The Prussian philosopher Immanuel Kant (who we met first in Chapter 8) is justifiably among the most famous in the history of Western philosophy. Kant succeeded in reframing the entire philosophical problematic in 1781 with his *Critique of Pure Reason*.

Kant's project was in fact to unite the rationalist and empiricist views in the theory of knowledge, and to demonstrate the limitations of unaided reason, i.e. there comes a point at which reason must give way to faith (*Critique of Pure Reason*, 2nd edn, 'Preface'). Kant hoped to provide Newtonian science with a grounding in Christian faith. But in doing this, he put forward such a radical view of the human condition that it has continued to inspire analysis and criticism ever since.

We are going to read two short passages from the second edition of the *Critique of Pure Reason*, which fairly concisely summarize Kant's position on the relation between mind and body.

EXERCISE 12 (30 minutes)

Read two short extracts from:

Kant's Critique of Pure Reason, (Kant, 1 1929 [1781]) 'The paralogisms of pure reason' pp. 368–372 (B406–413) and 'Conclusion, in regard to the solution of the psychological paralogism', pp. 380–381 (B426–428)

Link with Reading 22.11

(Note that the original page numbering in this text is always referred to as 'A' (1st edn) and 'B' (2nd edn); a 'paralogism' is an error of reasoning of which the thinker is unaware.)

As you read, ask yourself what sort of claim Kant is making about the self or the subject of experience. It will help if you can identify what sort of argumentative strategy Kant is employing (clue: he is not using a conventional argument to a conclusion, but trying to demonstrate that such conventional arguments about the self actually presuppose certain conditions of possibility).

Kant's argument in the *Critique of Pure Reason* was stunningly original. The two passages we have just read give some of the flavour of this argument. Kant claims that the arguments we conventionally use are based on drawing conclusions about what is the case from what appears to be the case; whereas, he says, what we should be doing is identifying the logical preconditions for our being able to draw such conclusions at all (whether true or false).

Kant versus Descartes

In the passage we have just read, Kant offers a summary of his argument about the possibility of knowledge of the self, and the relation between mind and body. Kant's writing is notoriously obscure, and most people reading him for the first time tend to misunderstand his arguments. Here we will outline a brief summary.

One of Kant's more general arguments is that thinking alone does not give us knowledge of objects. Rather, knowledge comes about when we apply the unity of our consciousness—which is the character of thinking—to intuitions that are given to us through the senses. Knowledge, therefore, must consist of the determination of intuitions by thought. This includes knowledge of the self: I cannot gain knowledge of myself simply through thinking. In order to know myself, I must determine an intuition of myself through thought. In other words, I am conscious of myself as an *object* of consciousness. This seems to suggest that there are two selves: the determining, thinking self, and the determinable, intuited, objective self. Kant calls the former 'the determining subject' or 'the I that thinks', and calls the latter 'inner intuition'. The self that is known in self-consciousness is 'inner intuition'. The 'I think' is not an object to be known, but is the non-experienced structure that gives unity to experience.

Kant objects to the Cartesian 'cogito' on the grounds that Descartes does not recognize a distinction between the objective, intuited self, and the 'I think', and that Descartes therefore takes the 'I think', the mere *structure* of thought, to be the *object* of self consciousness. Kant sets out the relevant arguments on p. 389. They amount to four objections: Kant objects to Descartes' claims for the substantiality, simplicity, identity, and independence of the thinking self.

1. In the act of judgement, the 'I that thinks' must be understood as determining the unity of judgement. The 'I' is regarded always as the subject of thought, and never as a predicate or object of thought. However, the fact that the I as *subject* is a self-subsistent subject of thought, does not mean that the self as *object* is experienced as a self-subsistent subject of thought. I cannot deduce my existence as a self-subsistent being or substance, as Descartes claimed. (p. 369).

2. The 'I' that thinks is unitary, and is a logically simple subject. It is contained in the very concept of thought, and that the I is simple is an analytic proposition. But the self is not thereby a simple *substance*, as that concept ('substance') relates to things outside of thought, and such a proposition would therefore be synthetic. So again, Descartes is shown to be in error, as in the 'cogito' there are two kinds of conflation: (a) between abstract and concrete concepts ('I' and 'substance' respectively), and (b) between analytic and synthetic propositions, whereas the inclusion of 'substance' into the 'cogito' creates a synthetic proposition. Kant is, effectively, claiming that Descartes' argument is logically incoherent.

3. The previous two arguments entail that, when I claim I am conscious of myself, I am expressing an analytic proposition, which cannot indicate anything about the substance of my thinking being (i.e. personal identity, in the conventional sense; again, contra Descartes) (p. 369).

4. The claim that the self is distinct from the body is based on the presupposition that the self is a self-identical simple substance. But the characterization of the self in that way has been shown to be false by points 1–3.

The bottom line of these arguments is that the Cartesian claim is founded on a fallacy, in that it equivocates between the two senses of the self: one as an object of thought, as given through the senses, and therefore empirical; and the other as a logically reflexive subject, which is capable of grasping the precondition of unity as a possibility for the making of judgements (and therefore of self-consciousness) (p. 371).

In the second of the two passages (reading linked with Exercise 12), Kant makes explicit his central charge against Descartes: that in formulating the 'cogito', Descartes committed the error ('dialectical illusion') of confounding the psychology of thinking with the logic of thought (p. 380). Instead of arguing for the view that mind and body are separate, Kant says, we should instead be asking how what underlies the appearance of separateness comes together ('how a communion of the substances is possible'— p. 381). Kant leaves us with the thought that such knowledge lies outside both ordinary psychology, and human knowledge itself.

From Kant to modern philosophy of mind

Kant's philosophical corpus has provided the springboard for much of the agenda of academic philosophy ever since the end of the eighteenth century. Much philosophical work since Kant, in both the Analytic and Continental traditions, has been a development from his ideas or a reaction against them. The logical framework offered by Kant raised issues that dominated the philosophy of mind when it emerged as a distinct subdiscipline in the late 1940s. This is not to say the intervening 150 years can be totally ignored. Instead of taking a historical detour, however, we will point out the relevant events and ideas of this period as we explore the development of the philosophy of mind in Session 4.

Reflection on the session and self-test questions

Write down your own reflections on the materials in this session drawing out any points that are particularly significant for you. Then write brief notes about the following:

1. In the seventeenth century, what did rationalists believe and what did empiricists believe, about how we come to know things?

2. How was Descartes' philosophical project related to the contemporary debate about knowledge?

3. What method did Descartes adopt and to what did it lead?

4. How did his project launch the 'mind–body' debate in its modern form?

5. Name two early responses to Descartes' dualism. (We noted six.)

6. What was Kant's argumentative strategy in his *Critique of Pure Reason*.

7. What was the nub of his opposition to Descartes' cogito?

Session 4 A modern response to the Cartesian problem

In the previous session we looked at a number of early attempts to solve the mind–body problem. Although drawn mainly from the seventeenth and eighteenth centuries, these, as we saw, were tackling the problem as it is with us today. The readings from contemporary newspapers and science journals in Session 1 and the 'Case of Mrs Lazy' in Session 2 illustrated the features of the mind–body problem as essentially the same problem with which Descartes and his successors engaged.

In Chapter 23 we will look at some very recent approaches to the mind–body problem. We will find that just as the problem was the same in the seventeenth century as today, so the proposed solutions have essentially the same forms. The main difference is a particular emphasis on the need to relate minds to *brains*. This is important for mental health. The explosion of 'brain science' is both a resource for and a challenge to mental health practitioners, as experts on 'minds'. How we respond to that challenge will determine the very nature of mental health practice and research as ever more powerful ways of investigating the brain come on stream in the twenty-first century.

But we will conclude this historical introduction by looking at a mid twentieth century attempt to side-step some of the problems generated by a Cartesian approach.

A watershed in philosophy

We have seen that from the time Descartes published his ideas on mind and body, the most important feature of the specifically philosophical debate on these issues became the pervasive influence of the Cartesian 'cogito'. Almost every thinker who put pen to paper in the seventeenth and eighteenth centuries felt obliged to situate his thoughts in the context of the Cartesian project, even if in disagreement with Descartes' ideas.

In the nineteenth and early twentieth centuries although a time of enormous interest in the mind—all the big movements in psychology, including psychoanalysis and, indeed, psychiatry, have their origins in this period—there was relatively little concern with the mind–body problem as such. In the late 1940s, however, there was a decisive change in the way that philosophical enquiry into the mind was carried out, a change aimed at abolishing the Cartesian project.

Abolishing the Cartesian project

The book that most explicitly represented this change was by the Oxford philosopher, Gilbert Ryle (*The Concept of Mind*, 1949, Hutchinson). It established a perspective on the mind which became known as *logical behaviourism*. This was vehemently anti-Cartesian. It sought to relegate both epistemology and the mind–body problem to the second-rank of philosophical issues, putting in its place the analysis of the concepts of everyday language about the mind.

Ryle's book was quickly followed by a posthumous book by the Cambridge philosopher Ludwig Wittgenstein, which was to have more influence on philosophy in the English-speaking world than probably any other book this century. This was the *Philosophical Investigations* (1953), and it was again vehemently anti-Cartesian, although its epigrammatic structure made that moral less clear.

The ideas of these two philosophers, Ryle and Wittgenstein, stimulated a critical discussion that gave rise to much modern work in the philosophy of mind. It is, however, an open question whether they successfully shaped recent orthodoxy in the analytic philosophy of mind, which has tended to accept the problems Descartes gave rise to rather than, in the case of both Ryle and Wittgenstein, questioning the presuppositions of the accepted problem. We will be focusing on Ryle's work in this session and aspects of Wittgensteinian philosophy in later chapters.

The work of neither philosopher came out of the blue, of course. Ryle, in particular, was influenced by the current psychological theory, also called 'behaviourism', and a good way to understand logical (or philosophical) behaviourism, is by comparing and contrasting it with psychological behaviourism.

Psychological behaviourism

Psychological behaviourism is the view that publicly observable behaviour is the only proper subject matter for scientific psychology. This view was first advanced by the American psychologist J.B. Watson in the early 1900s (a definitive exposition of his views is given in his *Behaviourism*, 1930). An example of the ambitious claims of psychological behaviourism is the following quote from this book: 'Give me a dozen healthy infants, well-formed, and my own specified world to bring them up in, and I'll guarantee to take any one at random and train him to be any type of specialist I might—doctor, lawyer, artist, merchant, chef, and, yes, even beggar man and thief!' (ibid., p. 150).

The other major exponent of psychological behaviourism as a paradigm is another American, B.F. Skinner, whose book *The Behaviour of Organisms* (1938) was massively influential. Skinner was so ardent about behaviourism that he even published a book expounding the benefits of organizing society entirely according to behaviourist principles (Skinner, 1971); he had earlier produced a Utopian novel, *Walden Two* (Skinner, 1948) written along behaviourist lines.

Psychological behaviourism and philosophy

The proponents of behaviourism have at times made strong philosophical claims—Watson, for example, is famous for a remark that consciousness does not exist. But behaviourism as an approach in psychology is independent of philosophical theories of the mind. For example, psychological behaviourism rejects mind–body dualism as a *strategy* for developing a coherent approach to psychological research. But as a research strategy, this could be productive or unproductive irrespective of whether mind–body dualism is true or false as a philosophical theory of mind.

Perhaps the most useful way of understanding the relationship between psychological and logical behaviourism is to see logical behaviourism as an attempt to provide a philosophical legitimation of psychological behaviourism. For example, both Watson and Skinner believed that one of the features of science is the adoption of a publicly accessible source of data. In this

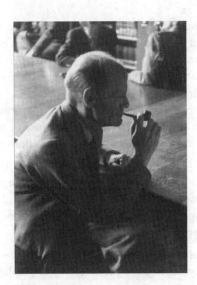

Fig. 22.4 Ryle

connection, logical behaviourism seems to offer a philosophically credible account of how the outward behaviour of humans could be sufficient to explain the 'impression' that we 'see' colours, 'feel' emotions, and so on. As we will see later, Ryle himself indicated the important influence of psychological behaviourism for philosophers of mind. On the other hand, however, Ryle's descriptions of behaviour make full use of mentally charged concepts. It does not attempt to reduce mind to behaviour described in a non-mental way. In other words Ryle's project is not reductionist in spirit in the way that much psychological behaviourism has been.

Ryle's model of the mind

To characterize Ryle's view of the mind in *The Concept of Mind* just as advocating a form of behaviourism would thus be to misrepresent a more sophisticated philosophical argument. Ryle did not merely aim to provide an answer to the mind–body problem as derived from Descartes. He aimed in part to provide a therapeutic dissolution of (rather than a theory-based solution to) the problem. In this his work can be seen as sharing the spirit of philosophical 'quietism' that marked the later Wittgenstein's work. Wittgenstein suggested that philosophy should 'leave everything as it is' and that it would not be possible to 'advance theses in philosophy' (*Philosophical Investigations* paragraphs 124 and 128). It is that desire both to explore and then relieve philosophical tensions that in part makes Wittgenstein's work so difficult. Ryle's work was less self-consciously 'quietist' and that explains both its strengths (accessibility, clarity) and its weaknesses (in the end it does advance an implausible philosophical thesis).

Ryle's central concern, then, was to lay the traditional conception of the mind–body problem (and, simultaneously, the problem of other minds) to rest by demonstrating that the problem itself was founded on a conceptual muddle arising *from the way language is used.*

Ryle's project was to identify and clarify the legitimate concepts that can be used in talk of the mind. This project, of conceptual clarification, adopts two assumptions that are relatively unproblematic. The first is that each individual with a mind already possesses a store of intuitive knowledge about what it is to have a mind. The second is that there is an identifiable 'logical geography' that characterizes the 'knowledge which we already possess'. These two assumptions are at the core of Ryle's methodology. Once the 'logical geography' of our concept of mind has been clearly set out, it will ensure that we avoid the errors of the past (Ryle, [1949] 1963, p. 9). All this is of course very much in the tradition of linguistic analysis, as we have already encountered it in J.L. Austin's work.

Category mistakes

So, what is the error, according to Ryle, which lies at the heart of mind–body dualism? It is what he calls a 'category mistake'—a confounding of 'one logical type or category (or range of types or categories)' with another. He describes this in the next reading.

EXERCISE 13   (15 minutes)

Read the three short extracts from

Ryle, G. ([1949] 1963). *The Concept of Mind*. London: Penguin. (Three Extracts, pp. 17–20).

Link with Reading 22.12

Think carefully about his example of a category mistake.

◆ Can you think of other examples?

◆ How does he apply this to the mind–body problem?

What the Cartesian, and others like him, have failed to notice, argues Ryle, is that our mental and physical concepts belong to different categories. This in itself indicates that the mental and physical belong to the same world—there are no grounds for the Cartesian claim that there is mind-stuff and body-stuff, each being radically different and distinct from the other. Cartesian introspection is a myth: there is mental activity but no mind within which it takes place, no Cartesian theatre in which to enjoy the show. These myths and misconceptions have arisen because we have been systematically misled by language into asking the wrong sorts of question about the mind.

We can summarize Ryle's own example of a category mistake thus: imagine a foreign visitor to Oxford or Cambridge who is taken on an extensive tour of colleges, libraries, and so on. After this the visitor asks: 'Where is the University?'. This question reveals that he has misconceived what sort of thing the University is. In fact, there is no one building or facility that can be called '*the* University'—the concept of the university combines all the diverse elements, which together form the functioning academic institution. So the foreign visitor already possesses an extensive knowledge of the university as a result of his guided tour. But he has been misled by our talk of such things as 'the University Library', into thinking that there is a university distinct from its parts. If we had spoken of 'Jones's library', it would be reasonable to suppose there was a separate 'Jones' after whom the library was named, or to whom it belonged. And it is this linguistic similarity between expressions such as these that misled the visitor into thinking that there was a distinct university separate from its parts. He mistakenly believes the university comes within the same category as a college or laboratory. He has made a category mistake.

The same sort of conceptual muddle, according to Ryle, lies behind our talk of 'mind' and 'body' as two separate things, when in fact they are conceptual elements in a single world. On this view, then, mind–body dualism (and, for that matter, materialism and idealism, and, indeed, the whole mind–body problem) is a conceptual muddle, which in turn is a consequence of a linguistic illusion produced by ordinary language (for example, Ryle calls the doctrine of mind–body dualism 'the dogma of the Ghost in the Machine').

Dispositions and occurrences

Up to this point, Ryle's argument amounts to a negative critique of mind–body dualism, and of the mind–body problem in general. But Ryle also made a positive contribution to the analysis of the concept of mind. At its most straightforward, it amounts to the claim that 'inner' mental states or processes can be analysed, ultimately, in terms of externally accessible dispositions to behave. In the following reading, we will explore Ryle's analysis of the concept of mental and physical activity in terms of dispositions.

EXERCISE 14   (30 minutes)

Read:

Ryle, G. ([1949] 1963). *The Concept of Mind*. London: Penguin, pp. 119–120

Link with Reading 22.13

As you read, make notes on the following questions:

1. How does Ryle characterize 'dispositions' and distinguish them in particular from laws?

2. In what way might the world 'satisfy' a dispositional statement?

3. What might a dispositional statement license us to do?

4. What arguments does Ryle give for dispositional statements not being identical to non-dispositional factual statements?

We can summarize the answers to the four questions in the exercise thus:

1. Dispositional statements are characterized by Ryle as statements describing a 'capacity, tendency, or propensity, or … liability' in a particular 'thing, beast or person' (p. 119). Dispositions are not laws, because they specify a particular individual, whereas a law must be applicable, in a limited way at least, across various instances of a phenomenon. To talk of a disposition is to say that something *would* or *might* happen in certain circumstances, and thus dispositions *resemble* laws in that they are partly 'variable' or 'open'.

2. The world 'satisfies' a dispositional statement if it makes it true. It does this if the 'actions, reactions and states of an object' display a tendency to conform to the description given in the dispositional statement.

3. Dispositional statements function as 'inference-tickets'. This means they license us to 'predict, retrodict, explain, and modify these actions, reactions, and states' (p. 119).

4. A dispositional statement is not an observation statement, nor a report of unobserved or unobservable mental states or processes. Dispositional statements are not factual in the way ordinary indicative statements are (p. 119). Thus, it may be the case that we are correct in stating 'John Doe knows French', even though there has never been a report of John Doe speaking or writing French. We know that John Doe knows French because he responds appropriately to spoken and written French (although, in this respect, his behaviour is no different from when he is responding to spoken and written English). However, the work of dispositional statements is closely connected with observation reports and narratives, because, if a dispositional statement is true, it will be satisfied by certain specific observation reports and narratives (e.g. 'John Doe is speaking French') (see pp. 119–120).

What this amounts to is that disposition statements cannot be identified with or reduced to any non-dispositional fact, or state of affairs, or pattern of occurrences (a dispositional statement may be true although there has never been an instance of its being satisfied). Yet dispositional statements can be satisfied by facts, or states of affairs, or pattern of occurrences, and as such their job is 'intimately connected' with narratives of incidents, because 'if true, they are satisfied by narrated incidents' (p. 120). None the less, it should be noted that an *occurrence* need not satisfy a dispositional statement: if Paul, a non-smoker, tries a cigarette, that occurrence does not mean that he has a disposition to smoke (the incident might confirm his loathing of, and revulsion at, cigarette smoking.). Occurrences and dispositions are different, yet it may be the case that there is a dependence between them (if Paul *does* have a disposition to smoke, then an occurrence of him smoking satisfies that disposition).

Rejecting Ryle

Important as Ryle's work was in reopening the debate about mind and body in the mid twentieth century, his positive contribution ultimately failed to carry conviction as a theory of mind.

One basic difficulty with his theory is that, despite his denials, it is behaviourist. The emphasis on behaviour seems to deny a basic phenomenological fact about the mind: that there is a subjective perspective to our mental lives. In a nutshell: there is nothing in Ryle's concept of dispositions to afford a distinction between actual pain behaviour and simulated pain behaviour. By extension, then, his theory fails also clinically. It leaves no room for anything that is characteristic of mind (e.g. subjectivity, a point of view, freedom, nor, even, phenomenal consciousness).

One way of thinking of this is that Ryle's account is not sufficiently radical in the way that it questions the framework of Cartesian dualism. With a distinction between the mind and body in place, it seems as though Ryle builds his conception of mind using materials from the body side of Descartes dualism rather than questioning that dualism. The account of behaviour looks to depend on the behaviour of a mindless body, the behaviour of a golem, perhaps.

The contemporary, Wittgenstein-inspired philosopher McDowell describes this sort of approach to a troubling dualism in this way:

> Ordinary modern philosophy addresses its derivative dualisms in a characteristic way. It takes its stand on one side of a gulf it aims to bridge, accepting without question the way its target dualism conceives the chosen side. Then it constructs something as close as possible to the conception of the other side that figured in the problems, out of materials that are unproblematically available where it has taken its stand. Of course there no longer seems to be a gulf, but the result is bound to look more or less revisionist. McDowell (1994, p. 94)

Ryle himself was clearly aware that the charge of behaviourism would be levelled against him. But despite that *The Concept of Mind* does not sufficiently address this concern.

Where does this leave the mind–body problem?

This chapter has examined the background to the mind–body problem both by looking at ordinary language use and by looking at the philosophical heritage. We have also looked at Ryle's work as an example of a philosopher in the analytic tradition attempting to provide an alternative view.

Ryle's discussion, however, does not succeed in providing a satisfactory account. What is more, the development of brain imagining techniques has brought the issue of the relation of mind and brain specifically onto the agenda of neuroscience (Andreasen, 2001). This will be the subject of Chapter 23, which starts with a reading based on recent brain imaging. While a future solution to the mind–body problem might indeed involve an element of dissolution as Ryle attempts, it will also need to address the attractions of modern materialism and the complexities raised by attempting to say that mental states are, or are determined by, brain states. That is what we will consider in the next chapter.

Reflection on the session and self-test questions

Write down your own reflections on the materials in this session drawing out any points that are particularly significant for you. Then write brief notes about the following:

1. How much interest was there in the mind–body problem in the nineteenth century?

2. Whose book is generally credited with re-igniting the debate within the analytic tradition?

3. How does logical behaviourism differ from psychological behaviourism? Give an exemplar of each.

4. What was the essence of Ryle's critique of Descartes?

5. How did Ryle characterize talk of mental states?

6. Why did Ryle not succeed in dissolving the mind–body problem?

Reading guide

Introductions to the philosophy of mind

There is a growing resource of accessible introductions to the philosophy of mind. Among them are: Braddon-Mitchell and Jackson (1996) *Philosophy of Mind and Cognition*; Burwood *et al.* (1999) *Philosophy of Mind*; Graham (1993) *Philosophy of Mind: an introduction*; McGinn (1982) *The Character of Mind*; and Rey (1997) *Contemporary Philosophy of Mind*.

A brief overview is given in chapters 4 and 5 of *Introduction to Philosophy* by William James Earle (1992).

Collections of essays on philosophy of mind

◆ Rosenthal (ed.) (1991) *The Nature of Mind* contains a comprehensive collection of journal papers and extracts from seminal texts ranging from Descartes up to about 1990.

◆ Less comprehensive but with better introductions to the topics is Lycan (ed.) (1990) *Mind and Cognition*.

◆ In William Lyons's (ed.) (1995) *Modern Philosophy of Mind*, the main texts consist of extracts from seminal works as well as journal papers, ranging from William James (1890) through to Colin McGinn (1989).

◆ A more historically focused collection is Robinson (1998) *The Mind*.

Cross-disciplinary and applied work

◆ Articles on many of the topics covered by this part of this book are included in George Graham and G. Lynn Stephens (1994) *Philosophical Psychopathology*.

• Colin Blakemore and Susan Greenfield's (ed.) (1987) *Mindwaves* includes a number of valuable articles on relevant topics especially in cognitive science.

• Kathleen Wilkes (1988) *Real People: philosophy without thought experiments* argues the case for philosophers basing their work more on the diversity of real mental phenomena represented by psychopathology and less on the traditional thought experiment.

The historical context of the recent resurgence of interest in psychiatry and abnormal psychology among philosophers (and vice-versa) is described briefly in Fulford's (1995) 'Introduction: just getting started' and in his 'Chapter 1: mind and madness: new directions in the philosophy of psychiatry' both in Phillips Griffiths (ed.) *Philosophy, Psychology and Psychiatry*.

Two recent books have made important contributions to the literature in this area by combining detailed case records with careful conceptual analysis: (1) Peter Halligan and John Marshall's (ed.) (1996) *Method in Madness: case studies in cognitive neuropsychiatry*, and (2) John Cutting's (1977) *Principles of Psychopathology*.

The history of philosophy of mind

A useful introduction to the general philosophical background of the ideas discussed in this session can be found in two volumes in the OUP Opus series *A History of Western Philosophy*. Volume 4, *The Rationalists* by John Cottingham (1988), and Volume 5, *The Empiricists* by R.S. Woolhouse (1988).

OUP also has a PastMasters series of introductory texts focusing on individual philosophers, the following being relevant to the topics of this session: *Descartes* by Tom Sorell (1984); *Berkeley* by J.O. Urmson (1982); *Hume* by A.J. Ayer (1980); and *Kant* by Roger Scruton (1980).

Two relatively short but rewarding texts on Descartes are: (1) John Cottingham (1986) *Descartes* and (2) Bernard Williams' (1978) *Descartes: the project of pure inquiry*.

An extremely useful text exploring the influence of scepticism on philosophy is Barry Stroud (1984) *The Significance of Philosophical Scepticism*, which offers a close examination of the sceptical techniques utilized by Descartes and other, more recent, philosophers.

References

Andreasen, N.C. (2001) *Brave New Brain: Conquering Mental Illness in the Era of the Genome*. Oxford: Oxford University Press.

Anon (1996) Lazy wife has her head examined. The Times. 2 September, page.

Anon (1997) Anorexia trigger found in the brain. *Sunday Times*, 13 April.

Ayer, A.J. (1973). *The Central Questions of Philosophy*. London: Weidenfeld and Nicholson. (Ayer, A.J. (1976). London: Pelican Books, p. 37.)

Ayer, A.J. (1980). *Hume*. PastMasters Series. Oxford: Oxford University Press.

Berkeley, G. ([1710] 1975). Principles of human knowledge. In *Philosophical Works*. London: Dent.

Blakemore, C. and Greenfield, S. (ed) (1987). *Mindwaves*. Oxford: Blackwell.

Braddon-Mitchell, D. and Jackson, F. (1996). *Philosophy of Mind and Cognition*. Oxford: Blackwell.

Burwood, S., Gilbert, P., and Lennon, K. (1999). *Philosophy of mind*. London: UCL.

Clarke, D. (1982). *Descartes' Philosophy of* Science. Manchester: Manchester University Press.

Cottingham, J. (1986). *Descartes*. Oxford: Basil Blackwell.

Cottingham, J. (1988). *The Rationalists*. Opus series: *A History of Western Philosophy*, Vol. 4. Oxford: Oxford University Press.

Cutting, J. (1977). *Principles of Psychopathology*. Oxford: Oxford University Press.

Dennett, D.C. (1993) *Consciousness Explained*. Illustrated by Paul Weiner. London: Penguin.

Descartes, R. (1637/1998). *Discourse on Method*. (Translated by Cress, D.A.). Indianapolis: Hackett.

Descartes, R. (1649/1988). *The passions of the soul*. (Translated by Voss, S.). Indianapolis: Hackett.

Descartes, R. (1968). *Discourse on Method and the Meditations* (transl., and with an introduction by F.E. Sutcliffe). London: Penguin Books.

Descartes, R. (1996). Second meditation. In *Meditations* (ed. J. Cottingham). Cambridge: Cambridge University Press.

Earle, W.J. (1992). *Introduction to Philosophy*. New York: McGraw-Hill Inc.

Editorial (1997a). A comet at heaven's gate. *New Scientist*, 5 April: 3.

Editorial (1997b). Inadmissible evidence. *New Scientist*, 22 March: 3.

d'Espagnat B. (1983). *In Search of Reality*. New York: Springer-Verlag.

Fulford, K.W.M. (1989). *Moral Theory and Medical Practice*. Cambridge: Cambridge University Press (paperback, 1995).

Fulford, K.W.M., (1995) Introduction: Just getting started. pps 1–3, Introduction to *Philosophy, Psychology, and Psychiatry*, ed. A. Phillips Griffiths. Cambridge: Cambridge University Press, for the Royal Institute of Philosophy.

Fulford, K.W.M. (2000). Disordered Minds, Diseased Brains and Real People. Chapter 4, in *Philosophy, Psyciatry and Psychopathy: Personal identity in mental disorder*. (ed. C. Heginbotham). Avebury series in Philosophy in association with The society for Applied Philosophy. Aldershot (England): Ashgate Publishing Ltd, pps 47–73.

Fulford, K.W.M., Morris, K.J., Sadler, J.Z., and Stanghellini, G. (2003). Past Improbable, Future Possible: the renaissance in philosophy and psychiatry. Chapter 1 (pps 1–41) in Fulford, K.W.M., Morris, K.J., Sadler, J.Z., and Stanghellini, G. (eds.) *Nature and Narrative: an Introduction to the New Philosophy of Psychiatry*. Oxford: Oxford University Press.

Garber, D. (1978). Science and certainty in Descartes. In *Descartes: critical and interpretive essays* (ed. M. Hooker). Baltimore, MD: Johns Hopkins University Press, pp. 114–151.

Graham, G. (1993, Second edition, 1998). *Philosophy of Mind: an introduction*. Oxford: Blackwell.

Graham, G. and Stephens, G.L. (1994). *Philosophical Psychopathology*. Cambridge, MA: MIT Press.

Halligan, P.W. and Marshall, J. (ed.) (1996). *Method in Madness: case studies in cognitive neuropsychiatry*. Hove, UK: Psychology Press.

Hobbes, T. (1984). 'Objections' to Descartes' *Meditations*. In *The Philosophical Writings of Descartes* (trans. J. Cottingham, R. Stoothoff, and D. Murdoch), Vol. 2. Cambridge: Cambridge University Press, pp. 122–126.

Hobbes, T. (1996). *Leviathan* (edited by Tuck, R.) Cambridge: Cambridge University Press.

Hope, T. (1994). Personal Identity and Psychiatric Illness, in *Philosophy, Psychology and Psychiatry*, ed. A. Phillips Griffiths, Cambridge: Cambridge University Press, for the Royal Institute of Philosophy Supplement 37: 131–143.

Hundert, E. (1989). *Philosophy, Psychiatry and Neuroscience: three approaches to the mind*. Oxford: Oxford University Press.

James, W. (1890). The stream of consciousness. *The Principles of Psychology* (2 vols). New York: Henry Holt.

Kant, I. ([1781] 1929). *Critique of Pure Reason* transl. N. Kemp Smith. Garden City, London: Macmillan.

Kenny, A.J.P. (1969). Mental health in Plato's republic. *Proceedings of the British Academy*, 5: 229–253.

Leibniz, G.W. (1705). *New Essays on the Human Understanding*. (paperback 1996) Cambridge: Cambridge University Press.

Leibniz, G.W. ([1710] 1988). *Theodicy*. Illinois: Open Court Publishing Company.

Locke, J. ([1690]1989). *An Essay concerning Human Understanding*. Ed P.H. Nidditch. Oxford: Clarendon Press.

Lycan, W. (ed.) (1990). *Mind and Cognition*. Oxford: Blackwell.

Lyons, W. (ed.) (1995). *Modern Philosophy of Mind*. London: Dent.

Malebranche, N. (1674–5) *De la recherche de la vérité*, in *Oeuvres*, vols 1–3, 6th edn, 1712; trans. T. Lennon and P.J. Olscamp as *The Search After Truth/Elucidations of the Search After Truth*, Columbus, OH: Ohio State University Press, 1980.

McDowell, J. (1994). *Mind and World*. Cambridge, MA: Harvard University Press.

McGinn, C. (1982). *The Character of Mind*. Oxford: Oxford University Press.

McGinn, C. (1989). 'Can we solve the mind-body problem?' *Mind*, 98, 349–366.

McGinn, C. (1993). Consciousness and cosmology: hyperdualism ventilated. In *Consciousness: Psychological and Philosophical Essays* (ed. M. Davies and G.W. Humphreys). Oxford: Blackwell.

Montaigne (2003 [1580]). *Apology for Raymond Sebond*. trans. R. Ariew and M. Grene. Hackett Publishing Co. Inc.

Nordenfelt, L. (1997a). The stoic conception of mental disorder: the case of Cicero. (with commentaries by Blackburn (1997), Leavy (1997), Mordini (1997), and Rhodes (1997), with a response from Nordenfelt (1997b, pp. 293–306) *Philosophy, Psychiatry & Psychology*, 4(4): 286–291.

Phillips Griffiths, A. (Ed) (1995). *Philosophy, Psychology and Psychiatry*. Cambridge: Cambridge University Press, for the Royal Institute of Philosophy.

Porter, R. (1997). Edward Shorter's *A History of Psychiatry*. Review in Evening Standard.

Quinton, A. (1985). Madness. In *Philosophy and Practice* (ed. A. Phillips Griffiths). Cambridge: Cambridge University Press, pp. 17–41.

Rey, G. (1997). *Contemporary Philosophy of Mind*. Oxford: Blackwell.

Robinson, D. (1998). *The Mind*. Oxford: Oxford University Press.

Rosenthal, D. (ed.) (1991). *The Nature of Mind*. Oxford: OUP.

Russell, B. (1900). *The Critical Exposition of the Philosophy of Leibniz*. London: Allen and Unwin.

Russell, B. (1946). *A History of Western Philosophy*. London: George Allen and Unwin.

Ryle, G. (1949). *The Concept of Mind*. London: Hutchinson. In paperback (1963). *The Concept of Mind*. London: Penguin.

Scruton, R. (1980). *Kant*. PastMasters Series. Oxford: Oxford University Press.

Skinner, B.F. (1938). *The Behaviour of Organisms*. New York: Appleton-Century-Crofts.

Skinner, B.F. ([1948] 2005). *Walden Two*. Indianapolis: Hackett.

Skinner, B.F. (1971). *Beyond Freedom and Dignity*. New York: Knopf.

Sorell, T. (1984). *Descartes*. PastMasters Series. Oxford: Oxford University Press.

Spinoza, B. ([1677] 2000) *Ethics*. Oxford: Oxford University Press.

Strawson, P.F. (1977) *Individuals: An Essay in Descriptive Metaphysics*. Oxford: Oxford University Press.]

Stroud, B. (1984). *The Significance of Philosophical Scepticism*. Oxford: Oxford University Press.

Urmson, J.O. (1982). *Berkeley*. PastMasters Series. Oxford: Oxford University Press.

Watson, J.B. (1930). *Behaviourism*. Rev. edn. New York: Harpers.

Wilkes, K. (1988). *Real People: philosophy without thought experiments*. Oxford: Oxford University Press.

Williams, B. (1978). *Descartes: The project of pure inquiry*. Brighton: Harnester Press.

Wittgenstein, L. (1953). *Philosophical Investigations*. Oxford: Basil Blackwell.

Woolhouse, R.S. (1988). *The Empiricists*. Opus series: *A History of Western Philosophy*, Vol. 5. Oxford: Oxford University Press.

CHAPTER 23

The mind–body problem and mental health, a philosophical update

Chapter contents

Introduction

The previous chapter provided an historical introduction to the mind–body problem. In this chapter we will return to the issue of the relation of mind and body and examine some of the rival contemporary approaches within the philosophy of mind. The aim of the chapter will be to shed light on the range of different ways that mind and body might be related and the kind of arguments, both based on a priori reasoning and on very general empirical evidence, that can be brought to bear on the issue. It will do this by examining a small sample of views and indicating the range of other choices that might be defended.

This chapter will also provide further introduction to the debates in later chapters. This is because the mind–body problem is one of the central issues in the philosophy of mind and views taken on this question will have ramifications into other debates. (By the same token, views here are influenced by views taken in those other debates.)

We will look at two influential views of the mind: functionalism, which is perhaps the most widely held view of philosophers who do *not* specialize in the philosophy of mind and the late Donald Davidson's 'Anomalous Monism'. We will also look at two general ideas about the relation of mind and body, which crop in different theories or models. The first is a codification of the view that mental states just are physical states. Mental states are identical to physical states: an *identity* thesis. The second is little more complex. Determining the physical properties of a person determines their mental properties but not vice versa. This is called *supervenience*. We will find that while there are a range of different models all face some difficulties. In other words, our intuitions about the relation of mind and body do not form a neat coherent set and accommodating some of them leaves others unsatisfied.

The plan of the chapter

This chapter will begin in *Session 1* by looking at some of the assumptions about the relation of mind and body found in neurology and neurologically informed psychiatry.

Session 2 will then review the advantages for holding a *functionalist* account of mind. This is the orthodox position (especially among philosophers who do not themselves specialize in the mind). It promises to underpin a science of the mind in which mental states are identified as second order physical states of the brain, picked out by their causal or functional roles. But it faces criticisms, the most important of which has to do with the role of rationality in the mind.

Session 3 will examine a more modest position: Donald Davidson's Anomalous Monism. This is modest in the sense that it holds out no promise of reducing mental properties to any other sorts of properties. (Functionalism, recall, identifies mental properties with functional properties, and these are just second order properties of the brain.) Nevertheless, Davidson argues that each individual mental state or event just is a physical state or event, differently described. That is why he calls his position a form of 'monism'.

However, Davidson's position comes under criticism partly because of his advocacy of a further claim about the relationship of mind and body: that the mind *supervenes* on the body. This is a constraint expressed by the claim that no two people who were physically identical could differ in their mental properties. There are arguments that the holding of both a token identity claim and supervenience is incompatible.

Session 4 examines two arguments against identity theories of mind and body. The first argues that if an identity theory were true it would have to be necessarily (rather than merely contingently) true. However, we have reason to believe that mental states might not have been physical and thus there can be no identity. The second argument focuses not on the nature of the relation but on what is related. It argues that even an identity claim as weak as a token-identity thesis (of which more below) is implausible.

Session 5 examines the arguments for the truth of supervenience: the claim that the physical properties of people or the world as a whole determine the mental properties. Even this modest claim turns out to be more problematic than it might at first appear.

Session 1 The mind–body problem in clinical neuropsychiatry

In the philosophy of mind, the relation of mind and body, the mental and the physical, is a contentious metaphysical issue. As we began to see in Chapter 22, some philosophers have argued that types of mental state are really types of physical state while others have argued that this cannot be so. In psychiatry, however, the connection between the mental and physical is not merely of academic interest. We begin with a reading that outlines the practical possibilities and current limitations in brain imaging techniques.

EXERCISE 1   (30 minutes)

Read the extract from:

> Posner, M.I. (1993). Seeing the mind. *Science*, 262: 673–674 (Extract p 673).

Link with Reading 23.1

In this exercise, we want you to start to think about the significance of the recent growth in the technology for *brain* imaging for making discoveries about the *mind*. Given the title of the reading, to what extent do the experimental techniques described reveal the nature of the mind? Is there an obvious *empirical* answer to this question? Think about the significance of the finding that local areas of brain activity often seem to be highly correlated with kinds of mental activity (such as speaking to oneself). Does this show that one is literally seeing the mind in a brain scan? If not, why not? Think also whether the relation between mind and brain could have been different. Could God have so designed the universe (so to speak) that there was a different relation?

Mental and physical correlations

Although there is some disagreement about the assumptions that underpin the interpretation of imaging techniques and expressing some scepticism about their validity, Posner presents a rosy picture. Take the following passage:

> It is a popularly held belief in psychology that the cognitive functions of the brain are widely distributed among different brain areas... Nevertheless, imaging studies reveal a startling degree of region-specific activity... When thought is analysed in terms of component mental operations, a beautiful localisation emerges. In word reading studies, words activate specific posterior visual areas that are not affected by consonant strings, and specific frontal and temporo-parietal areas are active when subjects are required to indicate the use of a noun... or its classification into a category. (p. 673)

On the assumption that such localization of brain activity correlated to specific mental activities is a genuine phenomenon of brain imagining what does this show about the relation of mind and brain?

It is interesting to note that that despite calling his short paper 'Seeing the mind', Posner does not go on to discuss at any length *how* the mind is seen. The implication, suggested in the passage above, is that brain activity can be correlated with mental activity (this is simply an empirical finding, according to Posner) and furthermore, imaging that brain activity just is imaging the mental activity. This second assumption deserves careful scrutiny. Is it clear that mental and physical correlations imply or justify in a weaker sense mental and physical identities?

Something like this latter assumption also underpins the very idea of cognitive neuropsychiatry. In the case studies described by Halligan and Marshall (1996), a clear, although implicit, connection between the mind and the body or brain is made simply through the juxtaposition of descriptions of patients' states of mind and behaviour and accounts of structural features of their brains. This implicit connection is a reflection of the key methodological assumption behind 'neuropsychiatry': structural accounts of the brain can shed light on psychiatric symptoms and vice versa.

But on the other hand, just what the nature of the connection is between neurology and psychiatry remains obscure. As the Introduction to *Method in Madness* notes

> We have no doubt that a neuropsychiatry is possible, despite the fact that many (or perhaps most) psychiatric conditions remain as yet 'functional'... [But] the disciplines of neurology and psychiatry seem to be investigating 'similar disorders viewed with different perspectives'. It will be a major challenge... to reconcile these perspectives... How much of a gap will always separate the two disciplines is debatable. Likewise, the extent to which the gap can be bridged by in vivo functional brain imaging is likely to remain highly controversial for some time to come. Halligan and Marshall (1996, p. 7)

Thus a discipline such as neuropsychiatry provides both the most concrete empirical evidence for the connection between mind and brain while at the same time demonstrating the still inconclusive nature of that evidence.

The element of cognitivism in the identity

It is also worth noting here that the connection speculated upon in the reading (Posner, 1993) is between *cognitive* psychology or psychiatry and neurophysiology. Posner says 'When thought is analysed in terms of component mental operations...' suggesting the same sort of cognitive analysis of thought processes.

So a first stage in the proposed connection will be the analysis of mental phenomena or states in cognitivist or information processing terms. This is a substantial assumption. Can the mental be described satisfactorily in these terms? An abstract form of cognitivism is a functionalist account of the mind. As we will see, however, in this chapter and Chapter 24, there are profound philosophical objections that functionalism would have to overcome for this assumption to prove correct.

One response to this marrying of bizarre psychological symptoms with underlying brain structures is to say—as we have already seen—that psychological and neurological descriptions are *different perspectives* on the *same phenomena*. There are not two sorts of phenomena—the mental and the physical—but one sort, which can be described in two different ways. This is not to say that the kinds of descriptions so far available can make this relation transparent. The connections between structural and functional descriptions of the brain and between those and functional or cognitivist descriptions of the mind cannot yet be filled out. But the underlying goal of a cognitive neuropsychiatry is precisely to articulate those connections. Furthermore, the kind of materialism expressed above may seem to be the best underpinning for such a project.

Such a materialist might seem to suggest that in, say, functional magnetic resonance imaging scans we see not only the working of the brain but also the working of the mind. It may seem that such a view is almost obligatory for any serious neurologically informed psychiatry because to doubt it would be to subscribe to some form of dualism of mind and matter. But as attention to the philosophical and metaphysical debate shows that is not a true opposition. Options in the mind–body debate do not comprise a binary opposition of a romantic dualism versus a serious minded scientific monism or materialism but comprise a range of different options that differ in the tightness of the connection of mental and physical properties. This chapter will steer a course through some of the recent debate in order to shed light on the range of available positions.

The next session will turn to functionalist accounts of mind. As well as being hinted at in the reading linked with Exercise 1 (Posner, 1993), these are also still the most popular accounts in the philosophy of mind.

Reflection on the session and self-test questions

Write down your own reflections on the materials in this session drawing out any points that are particularly significant for you. Then, thinking back over the chapter as a whole, write brief notes about the following:

1. How does empirical work contribute to our understanding of the relation of mind and brain?

2. What argument is given in the reading for the connection between mind and brain?

3. What suggestion is made about the connection between a cognitivist approach to the mind and the brain?

Session 2 Functionalist accounts of the mind

Introducing functionalism

This session introduces the current orthodoxy in the philosophy of mind: functionalism. It also considers some of the criticisms it faces. One of these criticisms is that functionalism cannot accommodate the essential connection between the mental and rationality. Such a connection will play an important role throughout this module while also introducing significant difficulties for the philosophy of psychiatry including, for example, an account for delusions.

The inspiration for functionalism is the computer. The basic idea is that mental states are software states, i.e. patterns of information-processing, whereas brain states are causal states of a physical substrate.

The attractiveness of this model is obvious. Unlike its main historical rival, behaviourism, it allows for a person's internal states to differ, although the outward behaviour may remain the same. Relatedly, it accounts for the fact that not all desires lead to action. Acting on one desire may be incompatible with satisfying another, perhaps stronger, desire. It also provides for internal states to drive or cause behaviour in some way. Unfortunately, though, as we will see, all these prima facie advantages have proved extremely difficult to pin down in a systematically consistent way.

Types and tokens

Functionalism can thus be seen as a way to avoid some of the objections to behaviourism. It also escapes an objection to crude forms of physicalism. Before summarizing its advantages over those positions it is worth revising the distinction between types and tokens. Talk of a *type* of mental state is a way of grouping together different individual or *token* mental states (at different times or in different people), which have a property in common.

Thus everyone who thinks that the prime minister is doing a good job has something in common. They all share the same *type* of belief. Everyone who has an ache in their left knee shares the same *type* of pain. But each person's pain is their own. One cannot, for example, give someone else one's pain in the knee (although one can cause them to have a pain of their own of the same sort). Each person has a different *token* state of the same general type. The same goes for beliefs.

A closely related distinction is between *qualitative* and *numerical* identity. Two ties can be qualitatively identical if they look exactly alike, are made of the same material and so on. But they cannot be numerically identical unless 'they' are the very same tie. Now it may seem that numerical identity is an idea of limited use as it seems to require both that there are two things (to stand in the *relation* of identity) and that really there is only one (as the relation is one of *identity*). But in fact there are often two different names or descriptions of the same thing whose coincidence comes as a discovery. In many cases, qualitative identity corresponds to sameness of type while numerical identity is sameness of token. (But this neat assimilation is complicated in the case of the putative identity of mental and physical *properties*: such as the claim that pain just is the firing of C-fibres. This is a claim about the numerical identity of properties: i.e. *types* of mental and physical state.)

With the distinction of type and token in place we can now summarize a key advantage that functionalism has over both behaviourism and physicalism.

Behaviourism as a type identity theory

Type identity versions of behaviourism identify types of mental state with types of behavioural disposition. Even Ryle's modest version of behaviourism described in Chapter 22 seems to require such a connection. However, as a mental state only results in action in the context of other mental states, a one to one correlation between mental states and dispositions to act is implausible. The desire for a drink of water may not lead to drinking if it is combined with the belief that the only available sources of water contain poison. But such a failure to drink does not imply that the desire for water did not exist after all, as a crude behaviourism would imply. Functionalism avoids this problem because it claims that mental states mediate between perceptions and actions as a network rather than individually. It also differs from behaviourism in that mental states are not merely disguised descriptions of behaviour but are internal states playing a genuinely causal role in the production of behaviour.

Type identity physicalism

Type identity physicalism identifies types of mental state with types of physical state. But this identification is implausibly *chauvinist* as it seems possible that creatures with very different physiology might possess the same mental states. Functionalism escapes this charge because it claims that what matters for the identity of a type of belief is a second order property rather than the first order properties of physical states. Nevertheless, it is still consistent with the more modest physicalist claim that each token (of a type of) mental state is a physical state.

Functionalism

Functionalism is the view that what make a mental state the state it is—whether a pain in the knee or a belief about frogs—are the causal relations holding between it, other mental states, perceptions, and behaviour. Thus each mental state is constituted by its functional relations to the rest of one's mental economy and the inputs and outputs to that economy.

What is the connection between functionalism and physicalism?

By concentrating on these causal or functional interrelations, functionalism *need not* take a view on what underpins these causal or functional relations. But in fact, some functionalists do commit themselves to materialism or physicalism. Ned Block (1980) makes a useful distinction between 'functional state identity theory' and 'functional specification' in his 'What is functionalism'. The former identifies pain, for example, with a functional state and inquires no further as to its underlying physical make up or ontology. Block ascribes this view to Putnam and Fodor. On this account pain just is the role or property. Such a view is consistent with a dualism of mental and physical substances. In other words, it provides no support for physicalism.

By contrast, functional specification uses functionalism to specify a role that is filled by some underlying and probably physical state with which mental states can then be identified. This is the view of Lewis and Armstrong. Pain, for example, is said by them to be the first order physical state or thing which has the second order role or property identified by functionalism. (This contrasts with saying simply that pain just is that second order role or property.) So construed, functionalism specifies a description that is satisfied by some physical state. Hence the philosopher David Lewis, for example, argues for an identity or for bridging laws between the mental and physical on the basis of functionalism. He claims, in other words, that, rather than conflicting with it, functionalism offers support for a kind of type-identity physicalism.

Lewis' argument goes like this:

1. Mental state M = occupant of causal role R (by definition of M)

2. Neural state N = occupant of causal role R (by physiological theory)

3. Therefore, mental state M = neural state N (by transitivity of identity)

Lewis claims that we can deduce identities rather than simply postulating them for ease or simplicity. (Unlike Saul Kripke—see later in this chapter—however, he does not go so far as to ascribe necessity to them.)

What justifies Lewis' extra claim that functionalism supports type–type physicalism? Consider the status of a putative identity of a type of mental state and a type of physical state in the face of possible discoveries about other creatures with very different physiologies. Lewis argues that such identities may be species specific. Thus some type of physical state will occupy a functional or causal role for a given population and will thus just be pain, say, for that population.

Mad pain

Interestingly, this suggests that if an instance of that type of physical state is realized in a person under abnormal circumstances and playing the 'wrong' causal or functional role, it will still be pain. Lewis calls this the possibility of 'mad pain' and imagines a person for whom characteristic pain behaviour was the solving of complex mathematical problems. By contrast, a behaviourist would have to say that such a person was not in pain.

Martian pain

And, in Lewis's picture Martian pain is also possible. This comprises a different type of physical state but one that plays the same causal role for Martians as our pain states do for us. Thus a variety of physicalism based on functional specification does not rule out the idea that creatures with very different physiologies might still share types of mental state with humans. It is not so chauvinistic.

It is not a fully physicalistic identity theory because what all pains have in common is not, however, any physical property. What makes Martian pain the same kind of state as our pain is not answered in physical terms. Hence Lewis's account is not in fact a victory for type-identity physicalism. In fact functionalism gives grounds for believing type-identity physicalism is false—we need not postulate sameness of physical state given that we can ascribe mentality on the basis of functional states. Given the possibility of the multiple realization of mental states, advocating type-identity physicalism is a needless epistemological risk. Thus functionalism looks at first sight an attractive account of the metaphysics of mind.

Can functionalism capture the experiential quality of mental states?

Two sorts of criticisms of functionalism

Functionalism has, however, faced a number of substantial criticisms. In 'Troubles with functionalism' Ned Block fires a broadside. His strategy has two main strands.

1. To argue that functionalism is fundamentally flawed as a model of mind as it privileges the quantitative aspects of mental states and processes (i.e. their measurable aspect) while ignoring or denying the qualitative aspects of mental states (e.g. belief-states, emotions).

2. To demonstrate that functionalism, in its various forms, is either too liberal (inclusive) or too chauvinistic (exclusive)—i.e. the functionalist project must include some systems without minds or exclude some with minds.

One criticism is that functionalism necessarily took no account of the *qualitative* aspects of some mental states. As well as mediating between certain sorts of causal inputs and behavioural outputs, pain, for example, has a characteristic feel. Similarly, it is often claimed that direct colour perception not only provides information about the ripeness of tomatoes but also involves a qualitative experience or *quale*. At first sight it seems that functionalism lacks the resources to articulate this aspect of our mental lives.

Block considers connecting the population of China together with two-way radios to mimic the functional organization of a human mind. They can then be connected to a robot body. In the thought experiment a single mind is staffed by a number of other minds and thus Block calls it a homunculi-headed system. But, he suggests, although this fits a functionalist criterion for a mind, it is not one.

> What makes the humunculi-headed system ... just described a prima facie counterexample to machine functionalism is that there is a prima facie doubt whether it has any mental states at all—especially whether it has what philosophers have variously called 'qualitative states', 'raw feels', or 'immediate phenomenal qualities'. (You ask: What is it that philosophers have called qualitative states? I answer, only half in jest: As Louis Armstrong said when asked what jazz is, 'If you got to ask, you aint never gonna get to know'). In Nagel's terms, there is a prima facie doubt whether there is anything which it is like to be the homunculi headed system. (p. 278)

In fact it is far from clear that this is a decisive objection. All turns on the kind of functional account of consciousness which may become available. (A defence of functionalism to this sort of objection is made in Van Gulick, 1994.)

A second objection to functionalism raised by Block is that it faced a fatal dilemma in specifying its inputs and outputs. The charge is that functionalism is guilty of either chauvinism or liberalism. It is chauvinistic if the inputs and outputs are so described that genuinely mental systems are wrongly ruled out. This is a danger if inputs and outputs are defined by analogy with the human case. This might be done in two different ways. One might define the outputs of a functional characterization of the mind as the movements of arms or legs. But this would imply that multiple amputees could not have minds. Or one might retreat to the outputs of the brain and describe the firings of the terminal neurones that normally cause bodily movement. But this would still be chauvinistic in that it would require that only those entities with human brains could have minds.

A radical alternative is not to describe the outputs to a functional system in physical terms at all. One might instead map out the system of functional interactions and then define the outputs in the most abstract and general terms: simply by numbering them, for example. But the danger now is one of liberalism. Such a formally described system could be instantiated by 'obviously' mindless systems such as economies. (One could equate output 1 with the inflation rate, and output 2 with the balance of trade, for example.)

Economic systems have inputs and outputs, e.g. influx and outflux of credits and debits. And economic systems also have a rich variety of internal states, e.g. having a rate of increase of GNP equal to double the Prime Rate. It does not seem impossible that a wealthy sheik could gain control of the economy of a small country, e.g. Bolivia, and manipulate its financial system to make it functionally equivalent to a person, e.g. himself. If this seems implausible, remember that the economic states, inputs, and outputs designated by the sheik to correspond to his mental state, inputs, and outputs, need not be 'natural' economic magnitudes...The mapping from psychological magnitudes to economic magnitudes could be as bizarre as the sheik requires. (p. 225)

This is a powerful dilemma. But it takes the form of a challenge to functionalism rather than a proof that a functionalist account of mind is impossible. The challenge of liberalism relies on the intuition that an abstract functional system equivalent to a human mind could be instantiated on a mindless system. A functionalist may reply that any such intuition relies on an oversimplified picture of what such a functional system will be like. A worked-out functional account of the mind will possess a complexity that precludes its instantiation by an economic system. If the objection is to prove decisive something more has to be added to it.

Syntax and semantics and Searle's Chinese room

One such addition stems from the fact that a functional system can be described in merely syntactic terms rather than semantic terms. (Syntax is the set of rules that govern the correct use and combinaton of symbols regardless of the meaning: the grammar, as it were. Semantics adds to those connections between words or sentences and parts of the world.) Thus describing the inputs and outputs to a functional system in purely formal terms does nothing to ensure that functional states possess intentionality or aboutness.

This is the heart of the philosopher John Searle's (1984) famous 'Chinese room' thought experiment. Searle likened artificial intelligence to a man in a closed room with a kind of Chinese phrase book but containing only questions and answers in Chinese. Phrases posted into the room could be paired with the same phrase in the book and a corresponding answer posted out. However, in the thought experiment, the man himself does not understand Chinese even though the box as a whole appears to. Searle suggests that the same applies to any artificial intelligence system brutally following a computer program. He called artificial intelligence simulated rather than real intelligence. (This thought experiment and Block's China thought experiment ask related questions. Searle asks: where is the intelligence, the meaning? Block asks: where are the qualia, the experiences, the point of view?)

Of course a functionalist may reply to this by saying that if mental states are functional states of the brain then they also *could* be described in merely syntactic terms but that does not show that they *cannot* also be described in semantic terms. Still, the challenge to functionalism is to show what grounds a semantic interpretation of its states.

Causal theories of reference

The standard contemporary answer is to add to a broadly functionalist account of the mind, a causal theory of reference. We will return to this idea in Chapter 24. But the basic idea is that internal functional states gain their semantic status by standing in causal relations to those things in the world that they are about. The causal theory of reference is problematic. But it provides a defence for this challenge to functionalism. The reason why economic systems lack intentionality is that they do not stand in the right additional causal relations to things in the world.

Block's dilemma and the reductionist hopes of functionalism

In fact, what makes functionalism vulnerable to Block's dilemma is that it attempts to characterize the mental in non-mental or reductionist terms. Reductionist forms of *behaviourism* attempt to define mental states in terms of behavioural dispositions. This presupposes that each state can be paired with a behavioural disposition. *Functionalism*, however, need not presuppose this because it recognizes that mental states only lead to action in the context of other mental states. One may be thirsty but this will not dispose one to drink fluid from a beaker if one also believes that it is poisoned. Thus mental states can only be defined in terms of perceptual inputs and behavioural outputs holistically. 'Ramsey sentences' provide a formal mechanism for defining the mental in non-mental terms but only as a whole.

The underlying motivation for this project is to shed light on the mental by defining it in terms of something supposedly less mysterious. For this reason, both inputs and outputs are described in non-mental terms. One does not describe an output as, for example, 'reaching one's hand out for the coffee cup' because the verb 'reaching' is purposive and implies possession of a mind. Instead this action has to be described in non-mental, non-intentional terms; perhaps as a movement of a five pouched manifold in an easterly direction at one metre per second. But the problem in realizing this reductionist project is that it may not be possible to define the mental in physical terms even at this holistic level. So far, however, we have only had Block's powerful intuition that that is so and not an argument that it must be the case.

Davidson's attack on reductionism

The American philosopher of language and mind Donald Davidson (1984) has put forward just such an argument. He claims that there is a principled reason why one cannot define the mental in non-mental terms. The mental is irreducible. His argument centres on the idea that rationality is a constitutive principle that necessarily governs the ascription of mental states. In making sense of each others' beliefs and actions we have to assume that we are largely rational. Thus, Davidson claims that the mental domain is governed by a constitutive principle of rationality while the physical is not. As a result, he claims, there can be no law-like relations between the two realms. But before moving on to Davidson's proposed solution to the mind–body

problem developed as a response to the claimed central role of rationality, it is worth noting a different response.

Can functionalism capture the rational character of mental states?

Non-reductionist functionalism?

Block claims, effectively, that functionalism cannot spell out inputs and outputs to a mental system both in non-mental terms and also in a way that avoids both chauvinism and liberalism. Thus one response might be to preserve something of functionalism by dropping the requirement of reductionism and allowing the inputs and outputs to be described in intentional or mind-involving terms. This would no longer shed light on the mental from the 'outside'. But it would at least provide an account of the metaphysics of mind. Such a position would stand to functionalism proper as non-reductive behaviourism of Gilbert Ryle stands to the behaviourism advocated by the psychologist B. F. Skinner (and some but not all of the writing of the philosopher W.V.O. Quine). It would, however, retain a key element of functionalism in construing mental states as internal functional states standing in nomic causal relations. As the following discussion shows, however, there is still something fundamentally wrong with this position.

McDowell's Davidsonian argument

The reading (linked with Exercise 2) is by the contemporary British philosopher John McDowell (1985). Examples of his work formed readings in Part 3. A running theme in those readings was the idea that the 'space of reasons' is different from the 'realm of law'. This had consequences for, among other things, the connection between observation and theory (Chapter 12) and the relation of the human and the natural sciences (Chapter 15). In this reading some of its consequences are explored in the context of the philosophy of mind.

EXERCISE 2 (30 minutes)

Read the extracts from:

McDowell, J. (1985). Functionalism and Anomalous Monism. In *Actions and Events* (ed. E. Lepore and B. McLaughlin). Oxford: Blackwell, pp. 387–398. Reprinted in McDowell, J. (1998) *Mind Value and Reality* Cambridge, M.A.: Harvard University Press, pp. 325–340 from which we have taken the extracts (Extracts pp. 328–331, 336–337)

Reading 23.2

This article is a criticism of a defence of functionalism by B. Loar in *Mind and Meaning*. But the key points can be understood independently of that book.

◆ What role does rationality play in McDowell's argument?

◆ What is the key difference between explanations in 'folk psychology' and natural science?

The key role of rationality

McDowell's (1985) attack on functionalism develops an argument from Donald Davidson (on whom more shortly) based on the role of rationality for the mind. Davidson focuses mainly on the reduction of the mental to the *physical*. McDowell is concerned with the reduction of the mental to the *functional*. But both agree that what prevents reduction is the constitutive role that rationality plays for the mind. McDowell argues in support of this by criticizing one particular functionalist account proposed by Brian Loar. He picks on Loar because Loar explicitly attempts to reduce at least some elements of rationality to a functionalist story. If Loar's project were successful then even though there is a close connection between meaning, mental content, and rationality this connection would not prevent a functionalist account. McDowell, however, argues that functionalism cannot after all account for the central role of rationality.

One of McDowell's arguments is quite straight forward. If functionalism is to capture the constitutive role that rationality plays for the mental it must capture the deductive links between an agent's beliefs. Loar claims that the deductive links between beliefs can be reduced to a formal structure or pattern. But as McDowell argues, one cannot in general reproduce these links without using an intentional language and describing the beliefs in terms of their contents. We know this because there is no general mechanical test for logical validity.

There is a mechanical test for validity of the simplest logical system: propositional logic. This is the logic that governs whole sentences and the logical connectives AND, OR, NOT, IF... THEN, etc. Valid arguments in propositional logic can be checked using truth tables in a way that can be mechanized. But there is no general mechanical method of determining whether arguments in predicate logic are valid. And there are arguments, based on Godel's theorem to show that this is not merely a matter of our ignorance. It is a necessary truth that there are no general mechanical tests for validity.

Furthermore, accounting for deductive logic is the easiest task for functionalism because it is the narrowest conception of rationality. But in claiming that mental states must necessarily stand in rational relations, Davidson includes the claim that the rationality of beliefs should also include induction and perception-based beliefs. There seems to be no prospect of providing a formal schema that abstracts away from the *content* of beliefs and prescribes when it is justified to form inductions or when one can form beliefs on the basis of direct perceptions. This is not to say that no such practical advice could be set down; however, it would turn on the *particular subject matter* of the inductions or perceptions.

Explanation by ideals and by subsumption under universals

McDowell (1985) argues that mental states stand in a different sort of structure to the nomological or law-like structure deployed by a causal functionalism. This is why the one structure cannot be mapped on to the other. McDowell goes on to provide a second argument against any such mapping, which has to do with the different kinds of explanation suitable for the different structures. It thus concerns the role of psychological explanations. McDowell argues that rationality also functions as a constitutive concept in explanation. Here the idea is that everyday folk psychological ways of making sense of each other are a species of *ideal* explanation. By contrast, explanation by subsumption under laws has a different 'logic'.

Explanation of speech and action works by fitting behaviour into a normative pattern of how rational subjects *ought* to act, given their beliefs and desires. One explains beliefs by citing what they ought to believe given other beliefs and perceptions. This use of 'ought' reflects the fact that psychological explanation turns on providing *good* reasons, reasons that one should have, which rationality ideally requires. Even mistaken beliefs are explained by providing a context of good reasons. This context is an a priori rational structure imposed on all folk psychological explanation.

This style of explanation by ideal contrasts with scientific or nomic explanation. The latter typically subsumes particular cases to be explained under a posteriori laws or generalizations as the covering law model attempts to formalize (Chapter 14). Unlike explanation by reference to ideal functioning, explanation by subsumption under generalizations is undermined by exceptions to the generalizations (unless they are merely statistical). But this is the way functionalism has to construe psychological explanation because of the law-like relations that functional states stand in. So functionalism cannot account for the ideal nature of psychological explanation.

Another way of making this claim is to point out that a functional specification of mental states is an empirical theory that charts their law-like structure. From this, however, it is impossible to milk a notion of having *good* reasons for beliefs or actions. Nor can it provide the resources for explaining how the relations that govern mental states mark the limits of intelligibility of other people. The relations between mental states that we employ in folk psychology do not comprise a merely contingent structure. If that were the case we could conceive of other relations holding. But in fact any widespread and significant deviation from the rational structure would be incomprehensible. (Quite how much divergence from rational belief formation and action is clearly an important matter for psychiatry.)

Functionalism is a form of Cartesianism!

McDowell (1985) provides an instructive diagnosis of what is wrong with a functionalist approach to the mind. He suggests, to begin with, that a broadly Cartesian account of mind results from thinking of reality as an objective realm while at the same time thinking of the mind as both real and subjective. Cartesianism attempts a quick ontological solution to this tension by construing the mind as real but immaterial. Functionalism is in no sense a dualist theory of mind but, like Cartesianism, it also tries to make the mental objective. It does this by suggesting that mental states are second order causal states of the body.

By contrast, recognizing that rationality plays a constitutive role makes the mental subjective for two reasons. First, it marks off mental states as both states *of* a subject and also *about* the world. And it makes the limits of intelligibility and mind forever open to further criticism and change. In short, McDowell's account of Davidson makes propositional attitudes as irreducible as qualia and as dependent on subject's points of view. (As mentioned above: functionalism has been criticized for being unable to account for the qualitative aspect of some mental state; however, most philosophers assumed that it was at least adequate to account for the intentional properties of mental states.) These dense comments will become clearer by examining Davidson's account of the mind: Anomalous Monism. Ironically it will turn out that McDowell's criticisms of functionalism also apply to Davidson's own account.

Reflection on the session and self-test questions

Write down your own reflections on the materials in this session drawing out any points that are particularly significant for you. Then write brief notes about the following:

1. What, in a nutshell, is a functionalist view of the mind. On what analogy is it based?

2. Does functionalism support or undermine a broadly physical or materialist view of mind? What is the relation of type and token versions of identity claims?

3. What is its relation to behaviourism?

4. What criticisms does it face? (We name two.)

Session 3 Davidson's Anomalous Monism

Functionalism is one account or model of how the mind might be related to the brain or body and thus serves as a potentially appropriate model for psychiatric research into the neurological underpinnings of mental illness. But, as we have seen, it faces considerable a priori criticism. The next reading (Davidson, 1980) introduces a different model: Donald Davidson's (1917–) more recent account of the metaphysics of mind.

Davidson was a recent American philosopher much influenced by W.V.O. Quine. His work can be divided very roughly into the philosophy of mind and the philosophy of language. He never wrote a book and his work comprises a series of articles in journals published since the 1960s many of which have been gathered into two collections *Essays on Actions and Events* and *Inquiries into Truth and Interpretation*. This reading comes from the collection that focuses on the philosophy of mind. (A clear introduction to Davidson's philosophy is in the Reading guide at the end of this chapter.)

What should be striking about Davidson's account is that it is a move to a more modest account. Whereas type identity physicalism or functionalism promise to explain mental properties as either physical properties or functional properties (and the latter are usually thought of as second order *physical* properties), Davidson assumes that mental properties cannot be reduced in this way. Types of mental state are not identical with any type of physical or functional state. But each *token* mental state is a (token) physical state.

Davidson thus presents, through a priori reasoning, an alternative to both a simple-minded assumption that mental properties are just physical properties seen from a different perspective and also to the more sophisticated view that mental properties are functional properties. Thus the issue for this session is whether Davidson's abstract conception of the relation of mind and body can provide a coherent model for clinical and research work in mental health.

EXERCISE 3 (30 minutes)

Read the extracts from:

Davidson, D. (1980). Mental events. In *Essays on Actions and Events*. Oxford: Oxford University Press, pp. 207–227 (Reprinted in N. Block (ed.), *Readings in Philosophy of Psychology*. Oxford: Oxford University Press, and in D. Rosenthal (ed.), (1991) *The Nature of Mind*. Oxford: Oxford University Press, pp. 247–256 from which we have taken the extracts (Extracts: pp. 247–248, 248–249, 250))

Link with Reading 23.3

◆ What are the three premisses or principles Davidson aims to reconcile?

◆ Would Davidson's account allow for neuropsychiatry?

The challenge

Davidson's account of mental states, Anomalous Monism, aims to reconcile three principles or assumptions:

1. that mental states stand in causal relations;

2. an underlying nomological account of causation;

3. the anomalism of mental; i.e. there are neither laws linking mental and physical or mental and mental properties.

At first sight, these assumptions appear to be in tension. The first premise is that mental states stand in causal relations. The second is that whenever there is causality, there are laws. But the third says that the mental realm is not governed by laws. Before summarizing Davidson's proposed reconciliation it is worth asking why he holds these principles. Given their at least apparent mutual tension, one response would be simply to reject one of the premises.

Davidson's three premises

Davidson's reasons for claiming that mental states stand in causal relations were first set out in his article 'Actions, reasons and causes' and are the subject of Chapter 26. Briefly his central argument is as follows. When we act for a reason, the reason *rationalizes* our action. It sheds light on why we acted by showing how the action is justified in light of our beliefs and desires. But it is also possible to hold a reason for acting, and act, but not act because of that reason but instead for some other reason. The question is, what is the difference between having a reason and acting (where 'and' is construed purely conjunctively) and acting because of the reason. As in both cases the reason would rationalize the action the difference between them must be something else. Davidson suggests that the only plausible candidate is that the reason why one acts is also the cause of the action.

The second ingredient of Anomalous Monism is a nomological account of causation. As we saw in Chapter 15 it is a widely held consequence of Hume's investigation that singular instances of causation require the existence of general laws. Davidson stresses that he is not assuming that saying that one thing causes another *means* that a general law-like relation exists. Nevertheless such a connection must exist.

The third ingredient is the claim that the mental is anomalous, i.e. it is not governed by laws that link mental properties. This involves a denial both of psychological laws (including those linking beliefs with other beliefs or with actions described in mental terms) and of psychophysical laws (linking types of mental states and types of underlying physical states—e.g. type-identity physicalism). One element of Davidson's motivation is his earlier work on testing and consequent criticisms of a Decision Theory approach (see his paper 'Psychology as philosophy' also in *Essays on Actions and Events*). But the justification for claiming that the mental is anomalous turns on the role of rationality in the ascription of mental states to which we will return in Chapter 25.

Davidson's token-identity theory

The solution that Davidson proposes to the problem of reconciling the three principles is to postulate a token-identity theory. Every mental event is identical to a physical event. Recall that in this context, the notion of identity is that of numerical rather than qualitative identity. (Two ties in a shop may be qualitatively identical while not being the very same tie. On the other hand I may wear the very same tie every Friday.) Here the claim is that each mental event just is the very same thing as a physical event. One way of thinking of this is to think of one sort of event having two different descriptions.

What makes it merely a token-identity theory is the claim that there is no alignment of types of mental event and physical event. If two people have the same type of mental state—perhaps they all share a deep respect for the Queen—then they will have two different tokens of that mental state type because one will be one person's respect and other will be the other's. In virtue of the token-identity theory these mental state tokens will be the very same things as physical state tokens. But because the mental is anomalous, there is no reason to believe that the physical state

tokens will have any physical properties in common. Types of mental state do not align with types of physical state.

Notice what a strong claim this is. It implies that there will be no physical laws linking types of psychological symptoms—for example, the phenomenon of thought insertion—with types of physical state, such as a type of brain lesion. Think of an analogy. It is like denying for a priori reasons that there might be a law-like relation between colours and wavelengths of light.

Anomalous Monism is *non-reductive* materialism

The reconciliation of the three premises for Anomalous Monism can now be quickly summarized. Mental states stand in causal relations. Therefore they are governed by general laws. There are no general laws that govern mental properties or mental types. But because each mental event is identical to a physical event it can be governed by a general law that connects its physical properties to other physical properties. Thus reasons can be causes even though the mental cannot be *reduced* to the physical. It cannot be reduced because mental properties cannot be

---

Box 23.1 **Davidson on events**

Davidson himself is careful to talk of a token-identity theory of mental and physical *events*. This concentration on events is partly the result of an investigation in the philosophy of language. It follows from the fact there is some difficulty in codifying deductions that involve adverbs. Adverbs form no part of first order predicate logic, the logic devised by Frege and which is best understood. From the statement that Jones buttered the toast carefully we can all infer that Jones buttered the toast. The difficulty is explaining why this is a valid inference. Davidson realized that this can be explained as a case of conjunction elimination in first order logic if these statements are interpreted as making claims about events. Thus: there was an event and the event was a buttering of toast and the event was by Jones and the event was careful. From this statement, the last conjunct can be eliminated in a deduction of the same form as if A and B are both true then A is true. Davidson concludes from this analysis that the world order comprises a succession of events. This is rather a startling claim. Davidson is drawing a conclusion about *ontology* or *what there is in the world* from an examination of which inferences can be codified in first order logic.

There is a second reason for talking of a token-identity theory of mental and physical events. This is that Davidson suggests that causation should be analysed as a dyadic relation between events. This account of causation differs, for example, from the Cambridge philosopher Hugh Mellor's claim that causation is a fact that relates facts. The relevance of causation to the token-identity theory will be made clear shortly, but we will speak more loosely and informally of a token-identity theory of *events* or *states* or *facts*.

equated with any physical properties. (In fact Davidson allows that mental and physical types could be aligned but this would be a matter of accident rather than law.) Thus Anomalous Monism might be called non-reductionist or non-reductive monism or materialism.

Supervenience

The role of supervenience in Davidson's philosophy

There is one other feature of Anomalous Monism that is merely hinted at in 'Mental events' but will be important shortly. This is the claim that the mental *supervenes* on the physical. During the last 30 years, Davidson has taken different views as to whether supervenience is an ingredient of Anomalous Monism or not. But it is defined in the following way: *determining or fixing the physical properties of a person (or possibly the person and their environment) determines or fixes their mental properties but the converse implication does not hold.*

One part of the reason to hold supervenience to be true is in response to the intuition that mental properties could be realized in more than one way. One of the things that makes this a plausible intuition is an analogy with computers. In their case, the same type of software state can be realized on *different* kinds of hardware and thus by different types of physical state. Thus determining the type of mental or software state does *not* determine the type of physical or hardware state. This explains the second half of the supervenience claim: that fixing the mental does *not* fix the physical. But why should one believe the first half? Why believe that determining the physical determines the mental? This will be the subject of Session 5 in this chapter. But a preliminary case can be made as follows.

Supervenience in ethics

Supervenience was first deployed in moral and aesthetic cases. There the analogue of the negative argument is the thought that moral values can be realized by different physical set-ups. The colour of the murderer's tie, for example, is of no consequence to the evil of the act. But on the other hand, imagine that all the physical properties that go to make up an act were reproduced: the movement of the hands, the trajectory of the knife, etc. Could the moral value of the act be different? Most of us would say no. Moral properties may not be reducible to physical properties but nevertheless they are not completely free floating. The same kind of intuition applies to the mental.

Here the analogous thought experiment is whether two people who were (qualitatively) identical with respect to their physical properties could differ in their mental states? By claiming that the mental is constrained by the physical through the relation of supervenience, Davidson attempts to demystify mental properties. As well as individual or token mental events being identical with physical events, mental properties are fixed by physical properties. As we will see shortly, there is a further reason for invoking supervenience. But the combination of token-identity thesis plus supervenience is not without its critics.

Mental properties and the charge of epiphenomenalism

Davidson aims, via Anomalous Monism, to reconcile the non-reducibility of the mental to the physical with a causal role for the mental. But one recent focus of criticism has been that he fails to make the mental causally relevant in the right sort of way. The problem might provisionally be put like this. Mental states rationalize and justify other beliefs or actions 'in virtue of' their mental properties. They are causally active 'in virtue of' their physical properties. But their mental *properties* are causally irrelevant. Suppose that the mental properties of an event are not essential to them being the event they are (in the way that the colour of a person's hair is not an essential property of them). Then an event would have just the same causal consequences whether or not it possessed its mental properties. They do not play a role in the causal order.

Davidson's twofold response

Davidson has made two complementary responses to this kind of criticism:

1. He emphasizes that causal relations are extensional. If one event causes another then they stand in a causal relation that holds of them no matter how they are described. This case contrasts with an intensional (with an 's') relation such as acting intentionally (with a 't'). Described one way an act may be intentional (turning a light on) while in another it may not (alerting a prowler). Because it is description-sensitive it is intensional. But causal relations are extensional. Thus one should not say that an event causes another 'in virtue of' its properties or description (as we did above for temporary clarity). It either causes it or not, however described. Thus mental events do not cause other events 'in virtue of' their physical properties at all.

2. He argues that providing the mental supervenes on the physical, if two events differ in mental properties (for example one has mental properties and the other does not) then they must differ in at least one physical property. Thus they will have different causal powers.

But are these adequate?

The relative strengths of the objection and Davidson's responses are by no means clear-cut (it is the main subject of the collection of essays edited by Heil and Mele in *Mental Causation*, 1993). But it is worth noting that the appeal to supervenience to ground causal efficacy may not be as convincing as it at first appears here. Think again of the intuition that moral properties supervene on physical properties. Thus if two events differ in moral properties then they must differ physically as well. A similar intuition might be thought to apply to aesthetic properties. If two pictures differ in their beauty then they must also differ in some physical property. (Although one might wonder whether a spectacularly good forgery was as good as a genuine Picasso. Financial worth certainly does *not* supervene on (non-relational) physical properties alone.) Granting for the sake of argument that these two other examples are cases of supervenience, does this imply that moral and aesthetic properties are causally relevant? Most people would think not. The supervenience relation is a metaphysical relation. It does not itself transmit causal relevance from physical properties to the properties that supervene on them.

If supervenience is not a satisfactory response to the claim that Davidson's account makes mental properties epiphenomenal, one possibility is to accept that mental properties are unlike physical properties and are not part of the causal order of the world. In this chapter we have simply assumed, so far, that the mental does play a causal role. This is a claim that Davidson makes explicit but which is also implicit in functionalism and type-identity forms of physicalism. We will return to arguments for and against causal accounts of the mind in Chapter 26.

Does supervenience cohere with Anomalous Monism anyway?

As well as the question of whether supervenience ensures the causal relevance of mental properties, Davidson's use of it has also come under separate criticism. One issue is whether it can be coherently combined with a merely token-identity theory. Another is whether supervenience is itself a coherent response to an underlying intuition about the relation of mind and body, or whether it 'inflates' into full-blown psychophysical laws. In the rest of this session we will begin to examine these in the context of Davidson's account.

Does supervenience imply psychophysical laws thus contradicting the claim of anomalousness?

A key tenet of Anomalous Monism is that there are no psychophysical laws. But, as Simon Evnine (1991, chapter 4) argues in his *Donald Davidson*, supervenience implies the existence of something like psychophysical laws. 'No mental change without physical change' implies 'same physical state implies same mental state'. Thus if supervenience holds, and if two people are in the same type of physical state, then they must be in the same type of mental state.

This, however, comprises 'half' of a psychophysical law in that it allows inferences to be drawn from the physical characteristics of a person to conclusions about their mental characteristics. This in turn seems to allow the ascription of mental states in ways that do not necessarily respect the central role of rationality in that ascription. One way of bringing out the worry here is to focus on the fact that it seems to be merely a contingent matter whether or not one could use a collection of these laws to ascribe wildly incompatible sets of beliefs to someone. This runs counter to the Davidson's view that it is an essential or necessary feature of mental states that they stand in rational relations.

(Consider the following thought. Suppose one person's neural state 123 is identical with the belief that it is raining and neural state 234 is identical with the belief that it is not. Now in general, according to Davidson, one cannot believe contradictory beliefs. This follows, he argues, from the claim that it would never be rational to ascribe such beliefs to another and such ascriptions are the only way of finding out about others' beliefs (see Chapter 25). But there seems no reason to hold that this necessary principle about the combination of mental states applies to physical states. Even if, as a matter of fact, neural states 123 and 234 were never combined in the person in the actual world, there seems to be no a priori reason why they could not be in some possible world. And now we can imagine that this might happen quite generally, contrary to Davidson's insistence about the overall rationality of the mental.)

William Child, however, proposes a response to this in *Causality Interpretation and the Mind* (1994, chapter 2, sections 1–3). The mental side of these half psychophysical laws still have to be arrived at in the normal way we ascribe mental states to one another. But these everyday methods of mutual interpretation respect the central role of rationality. Thus the link we establish between physical states and mental states always depends on first having interpreted the mental state using principles of rationality. Given that such interpretation depends on behaviour, it would always produce the same results for physically identical behaviour. Thus using the half psychophysical laws of supervenience is both subject to rational interpretation (to establish them) and will never deliver results that run counter to rational considerations.

Does supervenience inflate into psychophysical laws?

But there is another argument which Evnine (1991) aims against supervenience. This is that supervenience is an inadequate response to a particular metaphysical intuition. His argument is based upon progressive modifications to a thought experiment related to one we have already discussed. Imagine that there are two people with (perhaps only slightly) different *mental* properties. Supervenience guarantees that there must be at least one physical difference between these two. But would there be anything wrong with the story if we were told that this difference comprised merely the length of their eyelashes?

Evnine suggests that it would be inconsistent to insist that the mental supervenes on the physical but to be satisfied in this case that the physical difference accompanying mental difference might be something as irrelevant as eyelash length. But this objection would also apply if the physical difference concerned a part of the brain that has nothing to do with the mental properties concerned. One should only be satisfied by a difference in whatever parts of the brain are causally responsible for mental properties. In short, Evnine suggests that the metaphysical intuition that motivates the adoption of supervenience cannot be satisfied by anything short of full psychophysical laws, which in turn undermine Davidson's merely token-identity theory.

Given the kind of findings discussed in the first reading of this chapter (Posner, 1993), Evnine's argument is clearly relevant to any neurologically informed approach to psychiatry. What such an approach appears to show is that quite specific parts of the brain are involved in particular kinds of mental activity. Because of this, the claim that the mind supervenes on the brain appears to be a reasonable methodological assumption partly justified by subsequent empirical findings. But one might hold that, although parts of the brain were responsible for mental activity (either by causing it or by just being that very activity seen from a different perspective), there were no strict laws that linked mental types to underlying physical types. One motive for the latter doubt is the extent to which brains can differ in their physical properties. Evnine's argument appears to undercut such a modest middle ground. Supervenience inflates into either a type-identity theory or at least causal laws linking types of mental and physical state.

What is the moral of these objections?

Evnine's argument has a prima facie plausibility. On the assumption that one already believes in a token identity version of physicalism, supervenience adds a further constraint to the effect that the mental properties of (physical) events are themselves fixed by their physical properties. Without supervenience two physically identical persons could differ in mental properties. A token-identity theory by itself does not rule that out because they are numerically distinct persons (they are not the same person or they are at least temporally distinct stages of the same person) their mental states will not be numerically the same (the very same token of the same type of state) and thus there is no reason without supervenience to believe that they will be of the same type. But once supervenience is added it seems implausible to stop short of the claim that the mental properties of an event must supervene on a specific set of physical properties of that event (although so far unknown to us). Thus it inflates into a psychophysical law.

We will return to this claim a little later in the chapter. But one possible line of defence of supervenience is the thought that it is that constraint in combination with the token-identity thesis which is problematic. So one possibility is to keep supervenience and discard the token-identity thesis. We will look at arguments for that in Session 5.

As Evnine makes clear, supervenience need not be construed as an integral part of Anomalous Monism, which comprises at heart a token-identity theory and a denial of reductionism. It is an 'add-on' and thus one possible response to the arguments directed against it would be simply to dispense with it. (This is what Davidson has sometimes suggested despite also invoking it to explain the causal relevance of the mental.) Thus a different alternative is to abandon the supervenience claim while retaining the token identity claim. We will examine an argument against identity theses in the next session.

The many responses to dualism

What can already be seen from the discussion so far is how many different opposing positions there can be to Cartesian dualism and how much they can differ in their form of materialism. So to return to the issue raised in the discussion on clinical neuropsychiatry in the first session, it is not a straight-forward choice of hard line reduction of mind to brain or unscientific dualism. Philosophical reflection reveals both a number of different options and some critical arguments in addition to clinical findings, by which to judge them.

Consider Box 23.2 regarding some of the positions taken in the mind–body debate. So far we have encountered, in this and earlier modules, the first four positions.

In moving on to consider alternatives to Davidson's position it is worth bearing in mind what the other options are for explaining the relation of mind and body. If, for example, it turns out that even a token-identity theory makes too strong a connection between the mental and the physical then one will be forced to adopt a position lower down the order such as 5a or 5b, 6, or even 7.

Note also that the list in Box 23.2 contains only some of the available positions. Eliminativism, the view that psychological

Box 23.2 Some of the positions taken in the mind–body debate

1. *Type-identity physicalism.* Type of mental state/event are identified with types of physical state/event—so mental properties.

2. *Token-identity physicalism + type identity behaviourism.* Each individual mental event is a physical event + types of mental state are types of dispositions to behave.

3. *Token-identity physicalism + type identity functionalism.* Each individual mental event is a physical event + types of mental state are types of internal causal state individuated by their function (inputs and outputs).

4. *Token-identity physicalism + supervenience.* Each individual mental event is a physical event + fixing the physical state fixes the mental state but not vice versa. All world events are thus fixed by their physical properties only. A weak property dualism.

5a. *Supervenience without identity (weak supervenience).* The full mental history supervenes on the full physical history but no elements can be correlated/identified.

5b. *Token-identity physicalism without supervenience.* Each individual mental event is a physical event but fixing the physical history (of bodies? of whole worlds?) does not fix the mental history.

6. *Full property dualism (without supervenience).* Mental events are instantiations of mental properties which are as fundamental as physical properties—physical properties do not fix the history of worldly happenings.

7. *Substance dualism.*

mentalistic descriptions should be discarded in favour of physical or rather neurophysiological descriptions, is an obvious omission. (Perhaps it belongs at the very top as position 0.)

Reflection on the session and self-test questions

Write down your own reflections on the materials in this session drawing out any points that are particularly significant for you. Then write brief notes about the following:

1. What general philosophical claims does Davidson aim to reconcile?

2. How does his account of mind attempt this and what is it called?

3. What is supervenience? Is it compatible with Davidson's model of mind?

4. How many possible solutions are there to the mind–body problem?

Session 4 Arguments against mind–body identity theories

This session will examine two arguments against mind–body identity theories. The first is a general argument developed by Kripke from his work on the semantics of modal claims. In other words, it concerns the meaning of claims about necessity and possibility. Nevertheless it employs simple intuitions (which may or may not be correct!) about what is and what is not necessary and possible.

The second is an argument best set out by Child (1994) against Davidson's token-identity theory. It is, in effect, an application of one of the arguments from McDowell (1985) in the reading earlier in this chapter (in Session 2).

The development of some form of identity theory has been a key tool in contemporary materialist or physicalist accounts of the mind. Recall, the point of talking of an *identity* thesis is that this is a clear way of saying (with the first neuropsychiatric reading) that mental language and physical language are different ways of talking about *the very same things*, or events, or states. If it turns out that there are arguments against even such a weak construal of this approach as a token-identity then this is a significant blow to materialism.

In fact the two arguments considered here differ in their focus. Kripke argues against construing the *relation* between mental and physical states as one of strict identity. But, it will turn out, that this need not dramatically affect clinical findings. Child (1994), by contrast, attacks the very idea of aligning mental and physical states or events whatever the nature of the relation that is then supposed to hold between them. This does have profound consequences for what might be found clinically.

The background to Kripke's argument

Kripke's argument against mind–body identity

Saul Kripke is most famous for writing two books. One is an interpretation of Wittgenstein's later philosophy in which Kripke advocates a form of scepticism about meaning (see Chapter 25). The other, *Naming and Necessity*, is a prose interpretation of Kripke's own formal work on modal logic in which he explores the semantics (or rules governing the meaning) of names and descriptions. The two works are thus in some tension. The argument against mind–body identity theories is contained in the latter.

The background to Kripke's argument

In order to understand Kripke's argument against identity theories, one must first understand a little of the background that concerns the connection between names and necessity. The key claim that grounds the argument is that an identity statement that links natural kind terms—such as types of mental state and types of physical state—holds of necessity and the source of that necessity is genuinely metaphysical rather than the result of a linguistic convention.

In other words, statements of the form: 'necessarily X = Y' or 'necessarily X has feature Y' do not just report rules for the use of the symbols 'X' and 'Y'. Kripke rejects the idea that the source of the necessity in these lies in a connection forged in language and depends on the way the thing is described. This is called a *de dicto* account of necessity. In its place he favours a *de re* account, which is implicitly a form of essentialism. The origin of these claims about necessity in turn lies in his account of how names work especially within counter-factual conditional claims. (Remember, a counter-factual conditional claim is a claim about

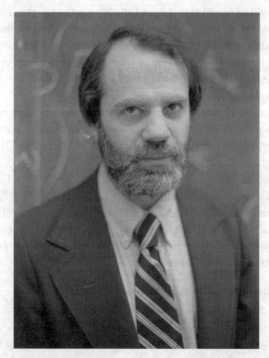

Fig 23.1 Saul Kripke

what would have been the case if some fact that is not or was not true had in fact been true. They were discussed in Chapter 15 on causation.)

Kripke's brief history of descriptive theories of names

Kripke gives the following potted history of the philosophy of names. (As an accurate intellectual history it leaves much to be desired but that is neither Kripke's nor our purpose here.) John Stuart Mill (whose inductive methods were discussed in Chapter 16) claimed that names have *denotation* but not *connotation* or *reference* but not *sense*. (This contrast will become clearer shortly.) But if so, the philosophers and logicians Frege and Russell asked at the turn of this century, *how* do we know what the name picks out? Or, to put the point less epistemologically, what is the connection between a name and a thing?

Frege and Russell instead proposed that what we generally take to be names stand for and mean some definite description such as the 'the leader of the Israelites'. (In fact there are important differences between Russell and Frege that Kripke ignores. Russell, for example, distinguished 'names' such as Napoleon for which this is true from 'logically proper names' like 'this', 'that', and 'I' but this need not concern us.)

But how should one pick out just one defining attribute? A natural modification of the idea is that names stand for a definite description is to employ instead a cluster of descriptions. The contemporary philosopher John Searle argued for such a position in the 1960s. Moses, for example, is that individual who possesses the majority of a cluster of descriptions for which his name stands: the leader of the Israelites, who was found in bulrushes, whose brother was Aaron, etc.

Theories of names of this sort aim to explain:

1. how a name can point to an individual person or thing including those who are no longer present or alive;

2. the content of identity statements such as that 'Hespherus is Phosporus' (the Greek names for what turns out to be the same planet: Venus). Such statements can be informative on this account because they connect two different sets of attributes.

Kripke's attack on descriptive theories of names

Kripke rejects outright the idea that names latch on to things via descriptions. His main argument is that that theory cannot account for how we can describe counter-factual possibilities. But there are a number of other criticisms worth note in passing:

1. We might not know any of the cluster descriptions associated with a name. Alternatively we might know of two people who share the few things we know. Perhaps all we know about Feynman is that he was a famous physicist. So were many others.

2. We might not be able to specify the attribute independently. If all we know about Einstein is that he devised 'Einstein's theory' and all we know of that is that it was Einstein's theory, we cannot latch on to Einstein.

3. Or properties may be satisfied by the wrong person. Columbus was not, after all, the first to discover America. But when we talk of 'Columbus' we do not mean the Vikings or whoever really first discovered it.

But the main objection Kripke raises to descriptive theories of names is that Moses *might not* have led the Israelites or done any of the cluster of things that we use to pick him out. Nevertheless if we talk about the counter-factual case in which Moses led a quiet life, we are still talking about *him* and contemplating possible circumstances for *him* (even if under those circumstances Aaron would have risen to the occasion and done those things actually done by Moses).

The moral

The conclusion Kripke draws is that definite descriptions or property clusters are a bad analysis of names because they behave differently in counter-factual circumstances. In another possible world the individual who satisfies the description 'the winner of the 1997 UK general election' might not have been Tony Blair. In such worlds Tony Blair might have narrowly lost the election, or might have taken no part in it having chosen to continue his earlier career in the law in which case various descriptions true of him in this world would not apply. In other circumstances he might not even have been called 'Tony Blair' if his parents had preferred the name 'Algenon'. But we could still talk about what Tony Blair would have done, had he been called 'Algenon' and been a successful lawyer. 'Tony Blair' always picks out the very same person in different possible worlds. But descriptions such as 'the winner of the 1997 UK general election' need not.

As Kripke puts it, names are rigid designators and definite descriptions or property clusters are non-rigid designators.

* *Rigid designators* (e.g. names): pick out the same individual in every possible world in which they pick out anything.

* *Non-rigid designators* (e.g. definite descriptions): pick out different individuals in different possible worlds.

Necessary identity statements

Given this definition then if two rigid designators pick out the same individual in one world, they will pick out that same individual in all worlds in which either applies. This follows from the definition of rigid designators that Kripke proposes. But it is supposed to answer a prior intuition we have. Thus if an identity statement such as 'Hespherus is Phosphorus' is true in any one possible world, there will be no possible world in which it is not true. There will be possible worlds in which neither name applies but none in which only one does. Thus if it holds it holds necessarily. By contrast 'Moses was the leader of Israelites' is not a necessary truth because it contains a non-rigid designator: 'the leader of the Israelites'.

Natural kind terms

One intuitive theory, similar to the cluster theory of names, defines natural kinds in terms of a cluster of properties. Gold, for example, might be a yellow, malleable metal. But, Kripke argues, we may *discover* that gold is not usually yellow. Or it might not have been usually yellow had other things been different. Or, similarly, we might find that some yellow-striped tiger-like things are really reptiles while others are not. In this case we should not conclude that some tigers are reptiles but that some of what we took to be tigers are not and are reptiles. Thus, Kripke argues that natural kind terms are not defined by clusters of properties but are also rigid designators (like names), which designate things or stuff with the same internal structure, whatever it is.

Natural kinds and identities

If natural kind terms are rigid designators then the same considerations which apply to identity statements linking names will also apply to identities between natural kinds. Thus if 'water is H_2O' is true in any possible world it will be necessarily true.

Some cautionary notes on possible worlds and other matters

1. Possible worlds are stipulated not observed. There is therefore no need to consider the epistemological question of how we could recognize individuals under other circumstances widely different from those in the actual world. Suppose we speculate on what would have happened if Tony Blair had become a plump sports commentator with no interest in politics who changed his name to 'Desmond'. One might think that this would raise a problem of how we might find him in this possible world. How would we recognize that that person was Tony Blair under different circumstances? But that is a mistake: we can simply specify that we are still talking about *him*!

2. Some *necessary* conditions govern stipulations about individuals in other possible worlds. Bill Clinton could not have been an armchair. (There might have been an armchair we called 'Clinton' for amusement.) Similarly, this! table (on which I am writing) could not have been made of ice. (A qualitatively identical one might have been ice but then it would have been this! table.)

3. Sometimes the reference of a name is fixed via a definite description, e.g. 'Hesperus is the evening star' but this description does not enter the meaning of the name—it doesn't have a meaning. Had Hesperus been hit by comet and pushed to a different orbit it would not have been an evening star but would still have been Hesperus (although presumably not called 'Hesperus' by the people in that possible world).

4. Recall the three distinctions between sorts of truth: necessary versus contingent, a priori versus a posteriori, analytic versus synthetic. These distinctions are, respectively, metaphysical, epistemological, and semantic. Since Hume there has been a school of thought that these distinctions classify truths into the same two sets. Any truth that is necessary will also be a priori and analytic. (Kant's claim that there are synthetic a priori truths is a notable exception.) There is an intuitive link between necessity and a priori and vice versa (if a truth is necessary, one does not need to look which world one is in) and analytic truths will be true in virtue of meaning in all possible worlds. Kripke claims instead that there are both a priori contingencies (the Paris bar is one metre) and a posteriori necessities (Hespherus is Phosphorus).

5. Kripke's positive account of naming depends on there being suitable causal relations between names and the objects named, mediated through the social use of the name. Causation provides the answer to the question the cluster theory was meant to answer. This is a notoriously problematic claim. How can the correct functioning of the causal claim be specified non-question beggingly? But it lies outside the scope of this book.

The argument against mind–body identity theories

We can now examine Kripke's argument about mind–body identity theories. Kripke argues that identity claims for natural kinds as well as for names express a posteriori necessities because natural kind terms are also rigid designators. Thus 'water = H_2O' is found by experiment but expresses a necessary linkage because both 'water' and 'H_2O' are rigid designators. But, he argues, this shows that the claim that pain is a certain type of neural state (e.g. state N) is not a true identity statement because we have independent reason to believe it is at best merely contingent. (Had it been true it would also have had to be necessarily true.)

EXERCISE 4	(30 minutes)

Read the extract from:

Kripke, S. (1980). *Naming and Necessity*. Reprinted in Rosenthal, D. (ed.) (1991). *The Nature of Mind*. Oxford: Oxford University Press, pp. 236–246. (Extract, pp. 242–243)

Link with Reading 23.4

◆ Try to identify the kernel of Kripke's argument.

◆ What is the role of the Cartesian intuition that one's mental states need not be physical states?

Kripke's argument against mind–body identity theories can be summarized like this:

i Assume that pain = neural state N.

ii If an identify holds between rigid designators then it is necessary.

iii Both 'pain' and 'neural state N' are rigid designators.

iv Therefore pain = neural state N is a necessary truth.

v But, by the Cartesisan intuition, pain = neural state N is (at best) contingent. (Note that all that is required is that the Cartesian claim is possible not that it is true.)

vi Therefore it is both necessary and not necessary. This is an absurdity so one premise must be rejected.

vii Therefore premiss (i)—the identity statement—is false.

Because this form of argument is *reductio ad absurdum* it is a matter of choice which premiss to reject. All that can be directly inferred is that at least one premiss must be false. But Kripke provides some argument that premisses (iii) and (v) are true and this leaves only (i) to be false.

Premiss (iii)

'Neural state N' names a natural kind (like electron) and thus picks out the same kind of state in every possible world. Thus it is a rigid designator. 'Pain' is also a rigid designator. Kripke says that if something is a pain it is essentially so. It would be absurd to suppose that a pain could have been some phenomenon other than it is. This contrasts with the case of 'the 42nd president of the USA', who might have been a different man.

The Cartesian intuition

This intuition is that either my pain state could have existed without some particular brain state or that my brain state could have existed without the pain—i.e. without consciousness. Either seems possible. How could this intuition be rejected for a principled reason? What would justify the counter claim that in no possible world could this pain have existed without its particular corresponding brain state?

Could the argument undermine the claim that water = H₂O?

Kripke's argument does, however, face an obvious counter objection to which he sets out a response. The objection is that there is a similar intuition to the Cartesian intuition available in the case of water and H₂O. We may claim to have a similar intuition here that would undermine the identity for water and H₂O, which, Kripke supposes, is a true identity. The argument would be of the same structure. If there is an identity between water and H₂O it must be a necessary identity. But it is at best contingent. Therefore there is no identity.

Kripke claims that one can defuse this second argument by explaining away the intuition on which it relies. He suggests that the intuition of contingency is the result of confusing the false thought that water might not have been H₂O with the true thought that a substance that brought about qualitatively identical experiences in us when we looked at, touched, and tasted it might not have been H₂O. But that substance would not have been water so there is no real Cartesian intuition here. Thus the identity is not undermined.

One might therefore think that the Cartesian intuition could also be explained away in a similar manner. But according to Kripke it cannot because if some state has the 'look and feel' of pain it simply is pain (whereas to look and feel like water is not necessarily to be water). If one has the experience as of pain, one has pain. Thus the intuition cannot be explained away and the identity of pain with any neural state cannot hold.

Responses to Kripke's argument

Two counter-arguments

Is Kripke's argument an elegant refutation of any identity theory of mind and body? If so, what is the connection—if any—between them? Kripke himself provides no positive account saying merely: 'I regard the mind–body problem as wide open and deeply confusing.'

McGinn's response to Kripke

One response to Kripke's argument is to argue that the Cartesian intuition on which it is based can in fact be explained away. In 'Anomalous Monism and Kripke's Cartesian intuitions' (1977), Colin McGinn argues that this is possible providing that one adopts a token rather than a type-identity theory of mind and body. He suggests that Kripke is right that if an identity theory is true then it is necessarily true. But this is consistent with a merely token identity. Thus, if a token mental state is identical with (i.e. it just is) a token physical state, it is so necessarily. Thus the Cartesian intuition that a particular pain might not have been a physical token is misleading because it is strictly false. But it can be explained away as the result of a confusion with the true claim that a state qualitatively (but *not* numerically) identical to a particular mental state might not have been this physical state nor a physical state like it with respect to its physical properties. Thus a token identity can explain away the Cartesian intuition in a similar way to Kripke's account of the case of water.

It is worth taking this again. If a merely token-identity theory is true, then mental state types gather together token states that are qualitatively the same as far as their mental properties go, but which are very different from a physical perspective. Thus the intuition that a particular mental state token could have had a physically different underpinning is strictly false but there is a true intuition with which it might be confused. That is that a mental token of the same mental type might have had a different physical basis.

Kripke, however, makes the point that there are two related broadly Cartesian intuitions. One is that one's mental states might not be physical. The other is that one's physical states might not be mental. McGinn can accommodate—by explaining away—the former, but not the latter.

Feldman's 'third-person response' to Kripke

Fred Feldman attempts to undermine Kripke's interpretation of the Cartesian claim that it is possible that a given mental state is not identical with any physical state in a different way (Feldman, 1980). He claims that it is possible that a token mental event might occur without any awareness of it by a subject. But this possibility depends on the idea that the qualitative, characteristically mental, aspect is not an essential property of the event. Thus construed a token-identity theory is a kind of contingent identity theory: all mental events are physical events but it is a contingent feature of these events that they are mental in the sense of having mental properties. A particular or token event that has mental properties in our world might have existed without having its mental properties in another possible world. A pain state or event would still be that very pain state or event but shorn of the contingent property of being felt by someone.

The idea that events have essential and non-essential properties fits with Kripke's general account of necessity as far described. It is a necessary property of Bill Clinton that he is a human. Bill Clinton could not have been a mouse (although there might have been a mouse called 'Bill Clinton'). But it is not a necessary property of him that he is or was the president, nor that he often wears a suit, nor even that he is his current height or weight. These latter properties could have been different. They are non-essential. Feldman claims that possession of mental properties is a non-essential element of the events which in our world have them. It is in this specific claim that he disagrees with Kripke.

Given this counter-intuitive account of mental events, Feldman can explain the other Cartesian intuition away and thus defuse Kripke's argument against identity theories. The intuition that the physical event could have occurred without the mental event is mistaken (as both are the very same event, if one happens, the 'other' *must* happen) but it is true that it could have occurred without its mental *properties* such as being felt. As Feldman advocates a token-identity theory he can employ McGinn's (1977) argument to defuse the other intuition that this pain, for example, might not have been a physical state.

What is the moral of Kripke's argument?

Kripke and Feldman trade opposing intuitions. Kripke claims that its painful feel is an essential property of every pain. Feldman denies this. One consideration in support of Feldman's position is this. Kripke's argument requires that both sides of identity statements are rigid designators. The physical description could well be. Types of neural state might be like types of atomic state in being natural kinds. One feature of them being natural kinds is that there is some independence between the underlying kinds and the way, relative to a given body of scientific knowledge, they are picked out. Particular experiential properties might turn out to be poor guides to the underlying kinds. (Kripke makes this point by saying that gold might turn out not always to be yellow and malleable.) But 'pain' does not seem to label a kind in the same way.

Two further considerations support this. First, there does not seem to be the same independence between the kind and how we pick it out. Kripke emphasizes this by saying that to feel like pain is to be pain. But if so this makes pain behave quite differently to other natural kinds. (To feel like gold is not to be gold.) Secondly, pain, unlike gold, does not seem to have a constant underlying *physical* structure. This stems from the thought that it could be

multiply realized. Why in that case should one think of it as a natural kind at all? What other underlying structure might it have?

On the other hand, to say that mental states possess mental properties only contingently presupposes the following sort of picture of mental states. They are free-standing internal states of the body, which also, contingently, possess the qualitative or intentional properties that they do. The question of whether this is a cogent conception of mental states is one to which we will return throughout this Part. It is a key element of an identity claim. But as will be made clearer in later chapters, the cost of this assumption is that it makes the answer to the question of how some mental states possess *intentionality* mysterious.

Note also that neither McGinn's argument nor that of Feldman can help with the intuition that a pain might have been non-physical. Token-identity physicalism is physicalist! So if physicalism amounts to the claim that the class of mental events is identical to a subclass of physical events, then Kripke's argument should apply to this class-wide identity claim.

What is the alternative to the *identity* of mind and brain?

If not identity then what? 'Composition' or 'realization'

It thus seems that if the modal intuitions on which Kripke bases his argument are correct then there cannot be an *identity* between mental states, events, or properties and physical states, events or properties. But if there cannot strictly be an identity theory, what sort of relation might there be between mind and body?

One possibility is to retreat to a less metaphysically loaded notion. Think of the relation between a car and its components. Suppose one were to claim that a car is simply identical to its components (perhaps in a working structural configuration). The reason for thinking this is that there is in some sense nothing more to the car than the components. Remove all the components from a driveway and one has ipso facto removed the car. But according to Leibnitz's Law, if two things are numerically identical (if they are really just the same thing) then they cannot differ in any properties. But the car I get back from a garage mechanic after a service may not have exactly the same properties (perhaps it now performs better) and it may not have the same components (because the brakes have been replaced). So if the 'first' car is identical to its components and the 'second' is to its components and these are not the same then the two cars are not the same.

As a result of such examples philosophers sometimes talk of the car being *composed* of its components while not being identical to it. Similarly, a ring may be composed of a certain amount of gold but is not identical to it. The ring can be destroyed in a furnace without destroying the gold for example. A building is also composed rather than identical to its bricks and concrete.

It seems, in other words, that Kripke's argument does not the count against *some* version of the claim that psychological and neurophysiological descriptions are different descriptions of the same thing. This might be true in the way that there could be descriptions of the historic buildings of England both in architectural and in stone-masonry terms. Retreating to constitution does not preclude some such relation of descriptions.

But there is some cost to the retreat to constitution. By contrast with the claim that water is H_2O (a strict identity claim) the claim that a ring is composed of its gold is less explanatory. The former identity explains the properties of water through the properties of H_2O. But while properties such as density and conductivity are transmitted from the gold to the ring, these do not fix others, such as its shape. And those properties are not transmitted from the ring to its substance—gold—in general. So if the mind is merely *constituted* by brain stuff, the brain stuff alone does not explain the nature of mind.

Child's non-modal argument against a token-identity theory

Kripke's argument turns on the following modal claim: since the identity between mind and body would be at best contingent, but since any identity statement linking such rigid designators must be necessary, there can be no such identity. As we have seen, one possible response to this is to retreat from the metaphysically loaded idea of identity and retreat to a weaker relation such as constitution. As this relation appears to work in the case of many objects and their parts, such a retreat appears to pose no threat to the direction of neuropsychiatric research. Child (1994, chapter 2 sections 4–6), however, takes a different tack in his *Causality, Interpretation and the Mind*. He argues against explicitly a token-identity theory not through consideration of the nature of the relation between the mental and physical but instead of what is linked by this relation. If Child is right, retreating to claims of constitution is irrelevant to the key problem that is *correlating* in whatever way mental and physical events or states.

> **EXERCISE 5**   (15 minutes)
>
> Look back at McDowell's (1985) argument against functionalism. Functionalism is a form of type-type identity theory. It relates types of mental state to types of functional state (states identified by their causal properties). Now think about Davidson's token identity physicalism. Could McDowell's arguments also apply to this weaker position? Think for yourself before going on.

Child (1994) presents an argument against the modest token-identity theory. Recall the reading linked with Exercise 2 (McDowell, 1985, reprinted in McDowell 1998, pp. 387–398). A central argument he raised against functionalism could be summarized roughly like this:

i Functionalism is a form of type-identity theory in which mental states are identified with functional states that are determined by codifiable functional relations, which resemble computer programs.

ii Mental states (intentional states at least) stand in a rational structure. Rationality plays a constitutive role for what mental states are.

iii But rationality cannot be codified.

iv Because functionalism is committed to the identity of mental and functional states it is committed to the codification of rationality.

v So functionalism is false.

vi And we might add: so is any identity theory that links mental states with states which are so codifiable such as physical states by physical theory.

Child applies the same kind of argument against even a token-identity theory. If a particular mental state (or event) is identical with a physical state (event) then the rational structure of mental states will have to be mirrored by an isomorphous structure of physical events (as each mental event will be a physical event and both will be governed by mental or physical relations). However, that impossibly presupposes the codifiability of rationality. Thus even token identity theories are false.

One way of putting this point is that it is just inconceivably unlikely that the structure of causal relations and rational relations will keep in step over time if they are not bound together by psychophysical laws.

The moral?

The moral of this argument is that the token-identity theory is an unstable middle ground between two more stable positions. One is a reductionist type identity theory that does offer some—albeit unsatisfactory—explanation of what keeps the mental and physical in step. The other position denies that any identification can be made between mental and physical states. Davidson's position has the initial attraction that it promises to reconcile antireductionism about mental properties with an account of how mental states can be causal in just the same way as physical events. However, it is not a stable middle ground because the identification of mental and physical elements requires a harmony that it no longer has the resources to explain.

If Child's (1994) argument is right—and it presupposes the central constitutive role for rationality in the mental domain for which we have so far encountered only limited argument—then no form of identity theory seems plausible. Child applies the argument to token- as well as type-identity theories. If that is the case, is anything left of a materialist account of the metaphysics of mind? One answer to that is supervenience, which is the subject of the next session. However, that claim is just that sameness of physical properties implies sameness of mental properties but not vice versa. Such a relation could obtain between two discrete realms of substances. An epiphenomenalist dualist of substance might hold that physical changes in the brain causal mental changes in one's thinking stuff such that sameness of physical state implies sameness of mental stuff. But this would be a dualist rather than a materialist position.

Reflection on the session and self-test questions

Write down your own reflections on the materials in this session drawing out any points that are particularly significant for you. Then write brief notes about the following:

1. What is Kripke's argument against the identity of mental and physical states? How is it based on his view of names and on possible worlds?

2. Is it necessary to believe that possible worlds are real?

3. What alternative view of the mind does he put forward instead?

4. Can the argument be refuted?

Session 5 Is there any reason to believe in supervenience?

If there are good reasons to doubt the soundness of an identity theory of mind and body, what is the relation between them? In addition to an identity (and more recently composition or realization), the other relation so far discussed has been that of supervenience. This session will consider the idea of supervenience in more detail.

EXERCISE 6 (10 minutes)

Supervenience was introduced above in the context of Davidson's Anomalous Monism as making the following claim: determining or fixing the physical properties of a person (or possibly the person and their environment) determines or fixes their mental properties but the converse implication does not hold.

♦ Could this claim be true in the absence of any sort of identity claim?

♦ What would supervene on what?

Haugeland's version of supervenience

It is easiest to think of supervenience in the context of an identity theory of some sort between the mental and the physical. But this is not necessary. All that is required for supervenience is something like this: the whole history of physical happenings determines or fixes the whole history of mental happenings without there being any further correlations. This latter thought amounts to this. There need be no event at the physical level that corresponds to a mental event. The two kinds of description of the world might not be commensurable. Again, the easiest way of expressing the supervenience relation does trade on something like an identity claim. One might say: there are two different descriptions—mental and physical—of the same events. But this initial description can then be modified by saying that there need not be identifiable elements—events—common to both descriptions.

The US philosopher of mind John Haugeland set out this view in an article called 'Weak supervenience' (1982). In it he attempts to articulate and motivate a weaker and less contentious version of physicalism than Davidson's token-identity thesis (a thesis that we have already seen reason to criticize). The paper does this by first attempting to undermine Davidson's argument for his position (which, to reiterate, is an argument based on the reconciliation of three assumptions). Then it presents an illustration of an case of supervenience without identity (the case of loop and arrow languages described below). Finally, it attempts to suggest that there will be a great difficulty in finding identities between the mental and the underlying physical given the considerations already put in place.

1. Haugeland's argument against Davidson turns on the charge that Davidson equivocates on the meaning of 'event' between the claim that mental events play a causal role and the claim that whenever events are related as cause and effect then there must be a strict law linking appropriate types. Haugeland argues that the first claim requires a robust construal of events as distinct disruptions, sudden changes or happenings. By contrast the second requires a mathematical construal of related gradual variations in properties. Haugeland's suggestion is that mental and physical 'events' are unlikely to be picked out in the same way. A distinct mental event might not correspond to any particular distinct physical event.

2. Haugeland provides an argument that supervenience need not require the identity of elements within the two sets of descriptions (or 'realms') by describing a single such case. A language of loops and a language of arrow vectors can both describe patterns in a two-dimensional world (you might think of pixels on a TV screen) but the loop language is a richer higher level language. But it supervenes on the arrow language because loops depend on pixels. However, the two languages do not share an ontology. There are no elements that feature as individual things in both descriptions. Supervenience is a relation of true descriptions (or truths) between complete histories rather than requiring an identity of a common grid of, say, mental and physical events or states.

3. Finally, Haugeland considers both the relation of waves on the motions of water molecules and chess playing behaviour on lines of programming code. In both cases he argues that the lower level description fixes or determines the higher level description while also arguing that there is no candidate at the lower level with which to identify 'robust' events of the higher level.

Haugeland, however, presents no positive argument for supervenience

Haugeland presents intuitive and illustrative support for the idea that one can have supervenience between two sets of properties without being able to correlate individual features, items, events, or states in both sets. It is an argument against the assumption that supervenience requires a token-identity thesis. So even if one gives up that claim about the identity of mind and body as too strong this does not preclude holding that the mental supervenes on the physical.

Haugeland's paper, however, does not provide a positive argument for mental supervenience. It simply removes a potential obstacle to holding that view. (The obstacle being the assumption that supervenience requires a token-identity theory, which is itself implausible.) If one were not already a supporter of supervenience then Haugeland's paper would not provide further argument in its favour. So why should one believe that mental facts are determined by physical facts? What independent justification is there for supervenience or, related by physicalism?

An argument for supervenience

Why should one believe in physicalism (the claim that the world contains just what a true complete physics would say it contains)? In response to an attack on physicalism initiated by the English metaphysicians and philosophers of mind Hugh Mellor and Tim Crane, there has been a flurry of discussion mainly conducted in the journal *Analysis*. We will consider a short statement and defence of physicalism and supervenience by David Papineau and a critical response by Tim Crane.

An argument for a token-identity thesis of sorts . . .

In an article called 'Why supervenience' (1990) David Papineau offers a defence of supervenience. In a sense the paper attempts to defend a combination that we have already rejected: a combination of a token-identity theory and supervenience. For the moment, however, that does not matter to the question of whether Papineau provides any positive support for supervenience.

Papineau provides the following argument first for a token-identity theory:

1. Mental occurrences have physical effects.
2. Physical effects also have physical causes.
3. Physical effects are not overdetermined—there are not two sufficient causes.
4. The physical and the mental cause are the same.

Note that Papineau takes a relaxed attitude to what the claim of sameness here amounts to. It does not matter whether it is a strict identity claim or a weaker claim such as that the mental is *realized* or *constituted* by the physical. These weaker relations still provide a way to avoid the overdetermination of physical effects by separate mental and physical causes. It is, however, a further question of whether the yet weaker claim that Haugeland puts

forward fits Papineau's argument, although that is better postponed until later.

This brief argument so far is based on an underlying claim about the *completeness of physics*: all physical events are determined entirely by prior physical events according to physical laws. This is a substantial assumption that will also merit further consideration. But first let us look at Papineau's further claim that supervenience can also be derived from this principle.

. . . and for supervenience

Papineau's argument for supervenience goes like this:

1. Consider a mental event or state, which is the cause of some physical effect.
2. Given the completeness of physics (CP), the physical effect must be determined by a physical cause in virtue of physical features.
3. Now consider the more complex case of a mental event or state that is the cause of a *mental* effect and that this has some further physical effect.
4. Therefore the original cause has a physical effect via an intermediate cause.
5. By CP the middle (mental) cause must cause its physical effect in virtue of its own physical features.
6. By CP these physical features must be caused by the physical features of the first cause.
7. Given that the final effect is caused by the intermediate cause (we say that the final event is caused via the intermediate cause rather than just saying it is caused via its physical features), the latter as a whole (not just its physical features) is determined by the physical features of the first. So there are no independent mental causal powers.
8. The mental is not complete in the same way so no similar result can show that physical effects are determined by mental features. Some mental effects are the result of non-mental causes.
9. Thus whenever a mental cause has an effect that effect is determined by physical features of the mental cause. By contrast, only some effects of physical causes are fixed by mental features of physical causes. Thus there are no mental differences without physical differences, whereas there are physical differences without mental differences.

This argument aims to show that whenever a mental event causes either a physical event or a mental event, its physical features would be sufficient to underpin that causal relation. Thus if two people were in different mental states there would have to be some physical difference between the two of them because being in different mental states would have different (physical) causal consequences and these differences in causal powers stem from physical differences.

In fact it should be clear that this argument does not require that mental and physical tokens are strictly identical or even merely *correlated*. The weaker claim that the mental *as a whole* is realized by the physical *as a whole* would suffice. No mention of identity is required to set out the underlying claim, which is that mental difference has to be accompanied by physical difference because otherwise there are events that are effects of non-physical causes. So on the assumption that the mental can play a causal role and that physics is complete, there can be an argument for supervenience, whether or not this is added to an identity claim. (And we have seen arguments that it should not be.)

A counter-argument

Crane's response

Tim Crane, however, responded to Papineau—in 'Why indeed: Papineau on supervenience' (1991a)—that the second assumption simply begs the question in favour of supervenience. His argument can be summarized as follows:

1. CP is just as contentious as supervenience. If one doubts the latter one will claim that some effects are determined by mental as well as physical causes. Such effects are *not* determined by physics alone and thus CP is not true.

2. 'Physics' cannot be defined in such a way that CP is both substantial and plausible. If it were simply (and *insubstantially*) defined as whatever would be included in an explanatorily complete science that need not rule out psychology as an essential part of a future complete science.

3. If, by contrast, physics is *substantially* defined by reference to the *micro*-sciences one could claim that by determining the micro-features of a situation one determines the macro-features. The motivation for this claim is the thought that at heart physics deals with the fundamental particles that make up matter and whose behaviour ultimately determines what happens in the universe. But if one simply assumes that micro-level phenomena determine what happens at the macroscopic level, and thus that the physical determines the non-physical this comes to assuming that there will be no macroscopic difference without microscopic difference. And this assumption is just supervenience again. One will in other words have simply assumed supervenience in the argument that was supposed to give it independent support.

Thus one needs an argument to establish the completeness of *physics* (hence *physicalism*) to establish supervenience in this way. What would one be? The alternative is that psychological factors may form part of a final theory of the world—the mental (mental properties) may be fundamental in a final description of the world.

A stalemate?

This dialogue between Papineau and Crane suggests a stalemate. If one can help oneself to the principle of the completeness of the physical then supervenience follows. But there seems little prospect of a truly independent argument for supervenience because that principle is too close to it. Now this need not matter.

All arguments start with premises or assumptions of one sort or another. So one response would simply be to say that supervenience is an assumption founded on the likely course of physical theory (this is what Papineau has subsequently said).

In fact Crane has gone on to argue that things are worse than that for supervenience. Whether or not he is successful, he highlights a very real question. In the absence of psychophysical laws, *how* is the physical supposed to determine the mental? Examining the issues raised by this last optional reading will help shed further light on the first of Papineau's assumption: the mental is causal.

In 'All God has to do' (1991b), Crane puts forward a dilemma for a defender of supervenience, which turns on a theological thought experiment. Having created the physical features properties and laws of the world, what more does God have to do to create the mental features? Does he have to create anything further? Specifically does he have to create further psychophysical laws?

> [D]oes God, in creating the physical facts, have to create laws linking those facts to the mental facts? If he does, then he has to do more than simply create the physical facts: he has to create laws in which mental properties figure. But if he doesn't, then the claim that he is creating genuine mental facts loses its bite: for if there are no mental laws, then arguable there are no genuine mental properties either. So the desired combination of physicalism and realism is unstable: the first horn of the dilemma threatens physicalism, while the second threatens realism.   (p. 237)

The first horn

Crane's dilemma has the following underpinning. Consider, for a start, the option that God *does* have to create psychophysical laws in order, in addition to having fixed the physical, to fix the psychological. If this is so, then in the act of so creating psychophysical laws, God effectively creates *in addition to the prior act of fixing the physical facts* the mental facts. This follows from the fact that such laws will characterize the mental facts by characterizing (at least partially) the mental properties that figure in them. If so, then the physical facts alone do not fix the mental facts and thus the mental floats free of the physical in contrast to the assumption of physicalist supervenience.

The second horn

But if, on the other hand, God does *not* have to fix anything other than the physical facts, then, at least according to Crane, that undermines the idea that there are any mental facts to be fixed. At this stage in this chapter, this is the horn which requires greater consideration. (The motivation for supervenience is in part the thought that there are no psychophysical laws but that the mental has, nevertheless, to be domesticated as part of the physical universe.)

Taking the first horn first. Crane argues that if God does have to add psychophysical laws to the physical facts then these laws will (partially) constitute the mental facts. So God will, in this second act of creation, create further mental facts.

The second horn presents more of a problem for the position that reflection on the readings of this chapter have tentatively supported: something like Haugeland's weak supervenience or Child's physicalism without identity thesis. Crane argues that if there are no psychophysical laws then there are no mental facts. Part of his argument here turns on rejecting Davidsonian arguments against psychophysical laws—which we have echoes of in McDowell's and Child's arguments against identity theories. But we will focus here on the claim that without psychophysical laws there would be no mental properties.

An analogy with aesthetic and ethical supervenience

Crane considers the analogies that defenders of mental supervenience draw on from the cases of aesthetics and ethics. (Recall that this is how mental supervenience was introduced above.) Crane makes two criticisms of the idea that supervenience in these two cases provide analogical support for psychophysical supervenience:

1. In those other cases the supervenience thesis is a necessary truth. Crane plausibly glosses this by saying that it is part of the *concept* of aesthetics that there is such a relation to the physical. Anyone who doubted aesthetic supervenience would have a different understanding of the aesthetic. By contrast, according to Crane, mental supervenience is a contingent matter. And if so, what underpins its contingent truth are the (psychophysical) laws of nature.

2. Mental properties are supposed to be part of the causal order. Thus, first, they need to instantiate laws and secondly this undermines the analogy with aesthetic and ethical properties, which are not directly part of the causal order.

Neither of these points are decisive but they do constrain appropriate responses. Further light will be shed on the nature of the mental throughout this book. But one preliminary response would be, on the one hand, to accept both these arguments. That is one would accept that the claim that the mental supervenes on the physical is a necessary truth. But on the other hand one could also deny that mental properties are causal at least in the way that physical properties are. The first claim can be made more plausible by considering the supervenience base of the mental to be physical properties that describe behaviour rather than simply brain states. It requires construing with the behaviourists that there is a necessary connection between mental states and behaviour. We will return to this issue in Chapter 27. The second requires an abandonment of one of the key assumptions of Davidson's Anomalous Monism. We will return to it in Chapter 26.

It is also worth considering the kind of picture Crane himself advocates. He suggests that mental properties are not reducible to physical properties but are related to them by laws. This is like saying that the gravitational facts about the universe are not reducible to the facts about electromagnetism but they are related by (in this case physical) laws. Such a position shares some features with type-type identity theories (higher up the earlier table) in that it accepts law-like relations between mental and physical properties or types. But unlike those positions, it does not accept that these law-like connections amount to ways of reducing mental properties to other properties (any more than electromagnetism can be reduced to gravity at least at the moment). So in another sense it is close to the bottom of the table in that mental properties are genuinely ontological distinct properties. There may not be mental substances but there are, according to Crane, distinct mental properties.

So what is the relation of mind and body?

The multiplicity of options

What the arguments in this chapter have shown is that there is very much more to the issue of thinking through what a sensible scientifically informed account of the relation of mind and brain might be. It is not, for example, a case of serious scientifically minded thinkers rejecting the absurdity of a substance dualist position and thus all agreeing on a common materialist position. There are many different forms that materialism can take.

But one of the general morals that the discussion in this chapter makes more plausible, if by no means obligatory, is that with respect to the general question of the relation of mind and brain, modesty is called for. The general trajectory of philosophical thinking in recent years has been away from the neat picture of type-type identity versions of physicalism. On such an approach, types of mental state simply are types of physical state. This promises a reduction of psychological properties to neurophysiological properties. But there is reason to believe that such an attractive picture is not true. As we have seen, it is much more likely that there are no such general connections between mental and physical descriptions.

A modest proposal

Now one response open to a philosophically informed neuropsychologist or psychiatrist is to accept such a general conclusion and make more restrictive claims about what brain imaging reveals. It does not reveal general connections between all forms of mentality and types of brain state. What it reveals are correlations applicable to humans (and their relatives) only. Thus it is still possible to discover fairly general connections between mental activity and brain activity, but these correlations are restricted to the human form of mind.

But the cost of this retreat is that it puts a key question beyond the reach of such studies. They will never show what it is that *all* forms mind have in common. They will not, that is, reveal what is fundamental to having a mind, or intentionality, or consciousness, or whatever. To restrict one's interpretation to human mindedness allows for empirical discoveries about the relevance of particular brain structures to our having minds but sheds more limited light on the general question.

A computational route to generality?

Now one way round that point is to follow Lewis and combine a more modest physicalism with functionalism. That has the advantage that a physical story can be told about the working of the human mind and brain and a more general account can be told of what it is for any species to have a mind in functional terms. We already saw in the first reading something like this approach in the thought that mental activities had first to be broken down into functional components, which were themselves to be identified with brain activity. This is how neuro-*computational* psychology works.

But as the second session argued, there are a priori arguments against functionalist accounts of mind. Mental states stand in a different sort of structure than the law-like structure described by functionalism.

Weaker physicalism?

What would be the consequences of the weaker philosophical positions for the interpretation of brain imaging techniques? Davidson's Anomalous Monism involves the denial that there can be any law-like connections between mental and physical types (and we saw that it could be extended to rule out functional types as well), but retains an identity claim at the more modest level of individual tokens. In fact, despite his general argument that there are no correlations between the mental and the physical as a matter of strict law, he has in recent years suggested that this is consistent with there being local correlations at the level of lore. This might seem, therefore, an attractive philosophical interpretation of the results of imaging experiments.

But Davidson's position does assert that mental states are identical with brain states and we have seen that there are arguments any such idea of identity, even merely token identity. These arguments suggest that when one looks at the brain one never sees the mind, because mental states are different sorts of state to freestanding brain states. A brain state can be the state it is independently of what happens outside the skull, but mental states are relational and world involving and thus cannot be found simply within the skull. And while brain states stand in nomic relations of cause and effect, mental states stand in rational relations.

This leaves a yet weaker claim. Although not identical with brain states, mental states supervene on them. Such a claim is probably a methodological assumption of anyone working in the neurosciences. (They may also believe some stronger claims about the relation as well.) Supervenience ensures that where there are mental differences between people (or in one person over time) then there must be some physical difference, but it

does not dictate just what kind of difference is involved. We also saw that this assumption is not unproblematic. It is far from clear that an independent argument can be given in its support. But it does provide a background against which more specific empirical findings can be viewed. Such findings might well unpack the kind of causal preconditions there are in localized areas of the brain for being able to think in certain ways. But, as we have seen, this does not imply that when we image the brain we image the mind. Things are more complicated than that.

One of the features of the rest of Part V is that it will shed light on how the mental is constrained by the physical. It will be a thread throughout the discussion of meanings in subsequent chapters.

Reflection on the session and self-test questions

Write down your own reflections on the materials in this session drawing out any points that are particularly significant for you. Then write brief notes about the following:

1. Supervenience was introduced in Session 4 in the context of an identity theory of mind and brain. Can it apply without even a token identity theory?

2. Is there an independent argument that the mind supervenes on physical states? If so, on what other claims might it be based?

3. What are the two horns of the dilemma that Crane argues faces arguments for supervenience?

Reading guide

◆ The mind–body problem is central to the philosophy of mind and covered in introductions such as: Braddon-Mitchell and Jackson (1996) *Philosophy of Mind and Cognition* (chapters 1–3), and Burwood *et al.* (1999) *Philosophy of Mind* (chapters 1 and 2).

◆ For a thorough, but difficult, introduction to the recent philosophical debate about the relation of mind and body together with an original contribution to that debate see: Macdonald (1989) *Mind-Body Identity Theories*.

◆ A very useful collection of modern readings is edited by Rosenthal (1991) *The Nature of Mind*.

Davidson's Anomalous Monism

◆ Davidson's philosophy is discussed in Evnine's (1991) excellent introduction *Donald Davidson*.

◆ A good collection of critical essays is edited by Lepore and McLaughlin (1985) *Actions and Events*.

Identity theories

◆ Kripke's argument about identity is discussed in Boyd's (1980) 'Materialism without reductionism' (in N. Block (ed.) *Readings in Philosophy of Psychology*).

◆ A more difficult discussion of Kripke occurs in Macdonald's (1989) *Mind-Body Identity Theories* (pp. 143–155).

◆ Debates about identity constitution realization and so forth form a difficult area of metaphysics. A good introduction to such issues is Loux (1998) *Metaphysics*.

Supervenience

◆ The locus classicus for discussion of supervenience is Kim's (1993) *Supervenience and Mind*.

◆ There are a number of essays on the connection between it and Davidson's Anomalous Monism in Heil and Mele (ed.) (1993) *Mental Causation*.

Applied work

◆ For an account of how neuroimaging and analysis of brain function impacts on the mind body problem see: Christen and Churchland (1992) *Neurophilosophy and Alzheimer's Disease*, and Northoff (1999) 'Psychomotor phenomena, functional brain organization, and the mind-body relationship: Do we need a 'philosophy of the brain'? (*Philosophy, Psychiatry, and Psychology*; with commentaries by Stein, Graham, and Spence, and a reply by Northoff).

◆ For a defence of the claim that how mind and body interact in depression should be treated as a medical rather than metaphysical mind–body problem see:

◆ Glannon (2002) 'Depression as a mind–body problem' (*Philosophy, Psychiatry, & Psychology*; with commentaries by Martin and Fuchs, and a response by Glannon). Among calls to leave the mind–body split behind, see Bracken and Thomas (2002), and Garnar and Hardcastle (2004).

References

Block, N. (1980). What is functionalism, and Troubles with Functionalism. In *Readings in Philosopohy of Psychology* (ed N. Block) London: Methuen, pp. 171–184, 268–306.

Block, N. (ed.) (1980). *Readings in Philosophy of Psychology*. London: Methuen.

Boyd, R. (1980). Materialism without reductionism. In *Readings in Philosophy of Psychology* (ed. N. Block). London: Methuen, pp. 67–106.

Bracken, P.J. and Thomas, P. (2002). Time to move beyond the mind–body split. *British Medical Journal*, 325: 1433–1434.

Braddon-Mitchell, D. and Jackson, F. (1996). *Philosophy of Mind and Cognition*. Oxford: Blackwell.

Burwood, S., Gilbert, P., and Lennon, K. (1999). *Philosophy of Mind*. London: UCL.

Child, B. (1994). *Interpretation, Causality and the Mind*. Oxford: Oxford University Press.

Christen, Y. and Churchland, P. (1992) *Neurophilosophy and Alzheimer's Disease*. Heidelberg: Springer-Verlag.

Crane, T. (1991a). Why indeed: Papineau on supervenience. *Analysis*, 51, 32–37.

Crane, T. (1991b). All God has to do. *Analysis*, 51, 235–244.

Davidson, D. (1980). *Essays on Actions and Events*. Oxford: Oxford University Press.

Davidson, D. (1984). *Inquiries into Truth and Interpretation*. Oxford: Oxford University Press.

Evnine, S. (1991). *Donald Davidson*. Oxford: Polity Press.

Feldman, F. (1980). Identity, necessity, and events. In *Readings in the Philosophy of Psychology* (ed. N. Block), Vol. 1. Cambridge, MA: Harvard University Press, pp. 148–155.

Fuchs, T. (2002). Mind, meaning, and the brain. (Commentary on Glannon, 2002a) *Philosophy, Psychiatry, & Psychology*, 9(3): 261–264.

Garnar, A. and Hardcastle, V.G. (2004). Neurobiological models: an unnecessary divide—neural models in psychiatry. In *The Philosophy of Psychiatry: a companion* (ed. J. Radden). New York: Oxford University Press, pp. 364–380.

Glannon, W. (2002a). Depression as a mind-body problem. (Commentaries by Martin, M.W. (2002, 255–260), Fuchs, T. (2002, 261–264), and response by Glannon, W. (2002, 265–270)) *Philosophy, Psychiatry, & Psychology*, 9(3): 243–254.

Glannon, W. (2002b). The psychology and physiology of depression. (Response to the Commentaries on Glannon, 2002a) *Philosophy, Psychiatry, & Psychology*, 9(3): 265–270.

Graham, G. (1999). Mind, brain, world. (Commentary on Northoff, 1999a) *Philosophy, Psychiatry, & Psychology*, 6(3): 223–226.

Halligan, P.W. and Marshall, J.C. (1996). *Method in Madness: case studies in cognitive neuropsychiatry*. Hove, UK: Psychology Press.

Haugeland, J. (1982). Weak supervenience. *American Philosophical Quarterly*, 19: 93–104.

Heil, J. and Mele, A. (ed.) (1993). *Mental Causation*. Oxford: Oxford University Press.

Kim, K. (1993). *Supervenience and Mind*. Cambridge: Cambridge University Press.

Kripke, S. (1980). *Naming and Necessity*. Oxford: Blackwell.

Lepore, E. and McLaughlin, B. (ed.) (1985). *Actions and Events*. Oxford: Blackwell.

Loar, B. (1981). *Mind and Meaning*. Cambridge: Cambridge University Press.

Loux, M.J. (1998). *Metaphysics*. London: Routledge.

Macdonald, C. (1989). *Mind-Body Identity Theories*. London: Routledge.

Martin, M.W. (2002). On the evolution of depression. (Commentary on Glannon, 2002a) *Philosophy, Psychiatry, & Psychology*, 9(3): 255–260.

McDowell, J. (1985). Functionalism and anomalous monism. In *Actions and Events* (eds E. Lepore and B. McLaughlin). Oxford: Blackwell, pp. 387–398. Reprinted in McDowell, J. (1998). *Mind Value and Reality*. Cambridge, MA: Harvard University Press, pp. 325–340.

McGinn, C. (1977). Anomalous monism and Kripke's Cartesian intuitions. *Analysis*, 37: 78–80.

Northoff, G. (1999a). Psychomotor phenomena, functional brain organization, and the mind-body relationship: Do we need a 'philosophy of the brain'? (Commentaries by Stein, D.J. (1999, 217–222), Graham, G. (1999, 223–226), Spence, S.A. (1999, 227–230), and reply by Northoff, G. (1999, 231–235) *Philosophy, Psychiatry, & Psychology*, 6(3): 199–216.

Northoff, G. (1999b). Neuropsychiatry, epistemology, and ontology of the brain: a response to the Commentaries on Northoff (1999a). *Philosophy, Psychiatry, & Psychology*, 6(3): 231–235.

Papineau, D. (1990). Why supervenience. *Analysis*, 50: 66–70.

Posner, M.I. (1993). Seeing the mind. *Science*, 262: 673–674.

Rosenthal, D.M. (ed.) (1991). *The Nature of Mind*. Oxford: Oxford University Press.

Searle, J. (1984). *Minds, Brains, and Science*. Cambridge, MA: Harvard University Press.

Spence, S.A. (1999). Does a philosophy of the brain tell us anything new about psychomotor disorders? (Commentary on Northoff, 1999a) *Philosophy, Psychiatry, & Psychology*, 6(3): 227–230.

Stein, D.J. (1999). Philosophy and cognitive neuropsychiatry. (Commentary on Northoff, 1999a) *Philosophy, Psychiatry, & Psychology*, 6(3): 217–222.

Van Gulick, R. (1994). Deficit studies and the function of phenomenal consciousness. In *Philosophical Psychopathology* (ed. G. Graham and G.L. Stephens). Cambridge, MA: MIT Press, pp. 25–50.

CHAPTER 24

Reasons and the content of mental states: 1. reductionist theories

Chapter contents

The central issue of locating meaning in nature

One of the underlying issues facing any science of the mind is to find a place in nature for the meaning, intentionality, or 'content' (as it is called) of mental states. This is certainly a challenge for psychiatry, which embraces at one extreme 'talking cures' from a psychoanalytic tradition and also both drug intervention and psychosurgery. The former deal with the meaningful and symbolic nature of mental states and symptoms. The latter pair both deal with causal effects that have no need for meanings. How can these different perspectives be reconciled? Both this chapter and the next will address the question of how meaningful or 'content-laden' mental states and utterances can be understood as part of the same nature, the same natural world, as causal interactions. (Chapter 26 will address a different but related issue: are reason explanations a species of causal explanation and how is this related to the idea of agency?)

The reason for dividing this topic between two chapters is this. In the *philosophy* of mind there have been two general approaches to accounting for the intentionality of mental states. These are reductionist and non-reductionist accounts. In brief, the former attempt to explain how meaning results from causal processes that can be described in non-intentional terms while the latter deny that any such reduction is possible. (We will return to this distinction shortly.)

These different approaches in the philosophy of mind fit different approaches in *psychiatric* theory and practice. Again very briefly, a reductionist approach to intentionality underpins many cognitivist accounts of both linguistic ability and disability while non-reductionist approaches fit better social or relational or 'discursive psychological' accounts in which the meaning of patients' utterances is constructed in the interaction of patient and clinician. Given these two fundamentally different approaches, the topic of intentionality will be divided between this and the next chapter. This chapter will examine reductionism in the philosophy of mind and cognitivism in psychiatry.

The plan of the chapter

This chapter explores the assumptions which lie behind cognitive approaches to understanding, meaning and thought and looks at philosophical theories which could be pressed into the service of cognitive psychology.

- *Session 1* examines a standard model drawn from cognitive psychology of both normal understanding of heard speech and related pathologies such as 'pure word deafness'. This model invokes but does not explain the working of a central 'semantic system'. It is this that explains our ability to understand the meaning of words.

- *Session 2* sets out in a preliminary way the general features of our 'intentionality', which are in need of clarification. 'Intentionality' includes our ability both to think thoughts and to make utterances *about* the world. By setting out its general characteristics we present a standard that any account of a central 'semantic system' should meet. These characteristics include the *normativity, rationality*, and *systematicity* of thought. In setting out the 'explananda', the session looks at Fodor's work, a philosopher whose theories most naturally dovetail with the assumptions of cognitive psychology. (In this chapter rationality will play a minor role. Its importance will be stressed in the contrasting view discussed in chapter 25.)

- *Session 3* contrasts, again in a preliminary way, two different very general strategies for explaining meaning or intentionality. *Reductionists* such as Fodor strive to explain the workings of a semantic system using concepts that do not presuppose the very properties of meaning or intentionality. (*Antireductionists* are examined in more detail in Chapter 25.) Fodor's version of an internal semantic system is then outlined. It deploys an infinite set of mental representations structured in a 'language of thought'. The account of mental representations outlined so far lacks a key feature, however. This is an account of what gives mental representations (processed in a semantic system) their meaning or *world-involving* nature.

- *Session 4* presents one solution: a causal theory of reference.

- *Session 5* presents a different solution: an evolutionary teleological theory. Both solutions are criticized, however, for failing to account for the normativity of thought and language. Finally, the lessons for a future cognitive neuropsychiatry are discussed.

Session 1   Aphasia, deficit studies, modularity, and meaning in cognitive psychiatry

The first reading (linked with Exercise 1—Ellis, 1996) is from a textbook on a cognitivist approach to psychology and psychiatry. Before looking at that, however, it will be worth thinking a little about what cognitive psychology is. Here is a passage from a different recent textbook:

> Cognitive psychology can be defined as the branch of psychology which attempts to provide scientific explanation of how the brain carries out complex mental functions such as vision, memory, language and thinking. Cognitive psychology arose at a time when computers were beginning to make a major impact on science and it was perhaps natural that cognitive psychologists should draw an analogy between computers and the human brain. The computer analogy was used frequently to draw up a model of the brain in which mental activity was characterized in terms of the flow of information between different stores.   Parkin (1996, p. 3)

Cognitive psychology, modules, and computers

This passage makes two interesting, and related, claims. One is that cognitive psychology has been very strongly influenced by developments in computer technology and computer science. The other is that it centres on the idea of information flow between different functional elements of the mind (or the brain?). This latter point presupposes that an analysis of mental capacities can assume a *modular* form. The mind comprises a series of functionally interrelated but also independent modules. As we will see this approach is revealed in the use of flow diagrams connecting modules (such as the 'auditory input lexicon') and showing how the output from one can feed into another.

This presupposition, and the kind of functional analyses it gives rise to, dovetails well with *deficit* studies. By studying mental disabilities, their consequences, and also what abilities are left intact, cognitive psychology can chart underlying functional systems that underpin these abilities. Such studies help to decompose 'normal' abilities into component elements through the examination of abnormal psychopathology.

It is worth noting, however, that there is a substantial assumption at work here. This is the assumption that the divisions that we might draw between abilities correspond to functional divisions between underlying independent (if interrelated) mental (or brain) systems. Now in part this assumption is tested by the future success or otherwise of cognitive psychology, but it is worth noting that there has also been some philosophical debate about whether the mind should be characterized as a system of modules or not. But while reading for that will be flagged at the end, it is not the subject of this chapter.

Talk of 'flow charts' of information flow between modules makes very clear why the computer has proved an influential metaphor. But as we will shortly see, it also encourages a further assumption about how this information flow works which has very important consequences for thinking about how the mind can deal with meanings or mental states with *world-involving* contents.

EXERCISE 1   (30 minutes)

Read the extract from:

Ellis, A. (1996). Recognising and understanding spoken words. In *Human Cognitive Neuropsychology: a textbook with readings*. Hove: Psychology Press, chapter 6. (Extract: pp. 143–146)

Link with Reading 24.1

- What is the relationship between pathologies of understanding and underlying modules?
- What account of normal successful understanding is given?

Recognizing *versus* understanding

Note first that the chapter title of this reading by Ellis (1996) is 'Recognising and understanding spoken words'. Given the modular

assumption of cognitive psychology, this might suggest that the chapter would concern two component abilities and thus two underlying functional systems responsible for, (1) recognizing, and (2) understanding words. Now it is worth thinking what sort of account might be given of the latter component. (It is the subject of the bulk of this and the next chapter and there will be time for further reflection.) But in fact, very little is explicitly said in the chapter about *understanding*. The module responsible for that lies at the innermost end of information flow lines (taking the heard word and speech to be at the outer ends) and is the 'semantic system'. Shortly we will return to what is said about its working but first think about the form of analysis offered for word *recognition*. Take this introductory passage:

> Imagine the case of recognizing a single word, clearly articulated and spoken in isolation. Unless that word is a homophone its sound pattern will be unique to it. To identify the word a listener will need to have stored in memory all the sound patterns of words he or she knows, and be able to compare the pattern just heard with these stored patterns to find the best match. What we are proposing is ... [a] word store or lexicon ... the auditory input lexicon.
> (p. 143)

The computer metaphor is at work in this passage in the assumptions it reveals about the underlying processing involved in word recognition. It says that a speaker (hearer) will need to have all the sound patterns of words he or she knows 'stored up in memory' and that these will then be compared with the pattern just heard to obtain the best match. But who has this memory and who does the comparing? One could imagine going about the laborious business of comparing sounds with, perhaps, a set of recordings of words spoken in a foreign language. But this is not what anyone actually does. Likewise, in order to recognize a word, one will have to remember what it sounds like but that is not to say that the sounds are 'stored' in memory.

This is not really a fair line of criticism. But what it reveals is a dangerous slippage between talk of a person's memory and the analogical talk of computer memory. Assumptions about computational processing underpin these strange locutions about comparing sounds with stored patterns.

Explanation of psychopathologies through the breakdown of functional connections

The chapter (Ellis, 1996) goes on to describe three different routes between hearing and repeating words. The most direct and shallow route with the least processing runs directly from a phonetic breakdown in the 'auditory analysis system' to the phoneme level of the output. This is the route used in the case of repeating nonsense words. The deepest route requires the recognition of words on the basis of phonemes by the auditory input lexicon, the understanding of the word in the semantic system, its activation of the speech output lexicon, and finally, activation of the phoneme level and speech. Psychopathological cases can then be explained through the selective breakdown of some but not all of these routes.

Given these different routes, a distinction between 'pure word blindness' and 'word meaning deafness' is then possible. The former involves 'impaired speech perception in the context of good speech production... and, importantly, intact perception of non-verbal environmental sounds' (p. 147). In such cases, subjects are unable to repeat words spoken to them. By contrast, word meaning deafness does not involve this last inability, although it does involve an inability to understand spoken words combined with an ability to understand written words.

1. The word must have undergone adequate acoustic analysis as evidenced by correct repetition.

2. The semantic representation of the word must be intact as evidenced by immediate comprehension of the word when presented in written form.

   Intact repetition of words and sentences implies an intact early stage of auditory analysis (the stage thought to be impaired with pure word deafness). Intact reading comprehension and spontaneous speech imply an intact semantic system and speech output lexicon... [W]ord-meaning deafness represents a complete or partial disconnection of the auditory input lexicon from the semantic system. (pp. 154–155)

Finally, there is the case of 'auditory phonological agnosia' in which subjects cannot repeat invented words but can repeat known real words. This can briefly be described as a breakdown of the direct connection between the auditory analysis system and the phoneme level of the output.

But is there an explanation of normal *understanding*?

These three types of psychopathological case help to support the particular functional hierarchy proposed. Both the component modules and their interconnections are derived from just such cases. In a sense, the comparison between normal and abnormal cases is an application of Mill's Method of Difference (see chapter 16). Thus the flow chart helps to shed light on what can go wrong with the recognition and understanding of words. But there is another sense in which it does not help shed much light on understanding because it does not break down what is going on in the central semantic system. It is one thing to explain a *failure* of understanding in the case of word meaning deafness by saying that there is a lack of information flow to the semantic system but quite another thing to say how that system underpins semantic understanding in other cases.

There are, however, some clues to the sort of account, which— if successful—would fit with a cognitive psychological approach. Think again about the sort of mention made of the semantic system in the reading (Ellis, 1996):

We propose that the first stage of auditory word recognition performed by an early auditory analysis system attempts to identify phonemes in the speech wave. The results of this analysis are transmitted to the auditory input lexicon where a match is sought against the stored characteristics of known words. If the match is a good one, the appropriate recognition unit in the auditory input lexicon will be activated. It, in turn, will then activate the representation of the meaning of the heard word in the semantic system...   (p. 144)

The key phrase here is: 'the representation of meaning of the heard word in the semantic system'. If there is to be a satisfactory account of how one can understand the meaning of a word on hearing it this comment would have to be unpacked. What is it to represent the meaning of a word? How could a module of the mind or brain represent meanings? Compare that issue with, for example, other modules that supposedly store acoustic properties of words. Is the *meaning* of a word a property akin to its acoustic properties? But it is also worth asking how an auditory analysis system could *represent* acoustic properties. We know how *people* might represent such properties. They might use a scientific vocabulary and notation and write down details using these. But how could a mindless *system* do this?

These are serious questions. But there is a clue to a possible approach to solving them that comes from the comment above that cognitive psychology was influenced by computers. These are machines that manipulate symbols in just such a way that information processing is possible. So perhaps answers to the question of how meaning or representation within a semantic system is possible can be answered by looking at the design of computers. That is the thought we will follow in the next session.

Reflection on the session and self-test questions

Write down your own reflections on the materials in this session drawing out any points that are particularly significant for you. Then write brief notes about the following:

1. What does the reading suggest about the challenge of explaining understanding in cognitive psychiatric terms?

Session 2 Preliminaries to a philosophical account of content

The first reading sets out what needs explanation

This session will begin to think about the general shape of the philosophy of thought, intentionality, or content. Chapter 23 looked at some accounts of the relation of mind and body or brain. But one feature of at least some mental states was largely absent from the discussion. This is that some mental states—e.g. thoughts—can be *about* things. One can think about one's cat Brix or one's next birthday (whether or not in fact one lives to see it). One can hope that one will have a nice party or that Brix will not eat too much cake. How is this possible?

The general characteristics of 'content'

In philosophy the word 'content' is used to refer to both mental content and linguistic meaning. What these both have in common is the possession of intentionality or 'aboutness'. Content-laden *mental* states—such as beliefs, intentions, and expectations—and *linguistic* entities—such as sentences and utterances—can be *about* distant or even non-existent states of affairs. In ascribing content to mental states or to groups of words, one ascribes this kind of general intentionality or 'aboutness'. In this broad philosophical sense, 'intentionality' refers to the capacity to be about something. This is a philosophical and non-standard use of the word. It should not be confused with the everyday sense of intentional, which means deliberate or with an intention. Intentions in that other sense are merely instances of mental states with the broader property of intentionality. The intention that one will read more philosophy possesses the broader property of intentionality because it concerns, and is about, one's intended future reading practice.

Brentano

There is a long philosophical tradition, attributed to Brentano's work at the turn of the century, which takes intentionality in this abstract general sense—the sense of 'aboutness'—to be the defining feature of the mental. Franz Brentano (1838–1917) was a philosopher and psychologist who repopularized the scholastic word 'intentionality' to characterize the world-relatedness of mental states. His most important work was his 1874 *Psychology from the Empirical Standpoint*.

Despite the close connections between the mind and intentionality, it is worth noting two qualifications of any such definition. First, it should not be taken to imply that the only forms of intentionality are forms of mental content. Sentences and utterances also possess intentionality. Secondly, there are mental states, such as sensations, which at least arguably lack intentionality. ('Arguably' because while it makes no sense to ask someone who has reported that they have a pain what it is about, one can ask where it is and this is something that the sensation itself tells them.) Nevertheless, accounting for the intentionality of mental states is an important philosophical task whether or not this takes the form of a reductionist explanation of intentionality. Brentano himself denied that intentional notions could be reduced to non-intentional terms.

'That-clauses'

A convenient way of spelling out the content of a mental states is the use of a 'that-clause'. The content of the belief that psychotherapy is cost-effective is, precisely, that *psychotherapy is cost-effective*. The content of the hope that the drug treatment will work is that *the drug treatment will work*. Using the content is clearly not the only way of *referring* to mental states. But contents as specified by 'that-clauses' are necessary individuating properties of content-laden mental states. Such specification also unpacks the intentionality that mental states possess. Both the object of the belief or the intentional object—psychotherapy—and what is attributed to it—its cost-effectiveness—are stated in the appropriate 'that-clause'.

As content can be stated using a that-clause it is often also called *propositional* content. Content-laden mental states are propositional attitudes because they can be individuated as attitudes or relations towards propositions. Smith's hope that the drug treatment will work is an attitude of hopefulness that Smith has towards the proposition *the drug treatment will work*. Smith is related via a relation of hope to that proposition. This form of analysis is clearly a move towards a philosophical rather than a pre-philosophical account of content. But it is a more or less natural development from and codification of the claim that content is what is stated by a 'that' clause.

Normativity

Spelling out intentionality in terms of propositional content highlights a further property or characteristic of intentional mental states or linguistic items. Propositional content is normative. This is clearest in the case of beliefs and assertions. A belief or assertion is either true or false in virtue of its content. It is true if its subject matter is as it takes it to be and false otherwise. It *prescribes* the condition that has to obtain for it to be true. However, other content-laden mental states are normative in that they prescribe what would satisfy them. Propositional attitudes specify a condition for the world to satisfy if the attitude is to be fulfilled. Linguistic meaning shares this normativity. Sentences and utterances also prescribe their truth conditions.

Fodor's account of mental states

Fodor's three criteria and the role of folk psychology

As we have seen, Fodor (1991) has his own list of essential properties of content-laden attitudes. He gives the following, different list in his *Psychosemantics* (1987, p. 10). These are:

1. Content-laden mental states are *semantically evaluable*. Fodor explains this by saying that they are the kinds of things that are true or false (beliefs), are fulfilled or frustrated (desires), turn out to be right or wrong (hunches), and so on. This is to emphasize the fact that they can be expressed by that-clauses and are normative. It is, in other words, an implicit part of what is ordinarily understood by content-laden mental states.

2. Fodor claims that propositional attitudes have *causal* powers. This is a more contentious claim. Indeed a later chapter will be given over exclusively to discussing it (Chapter 26). Whether or not mental states have causal properties will also be discussed as part of the discussion of reductionist theories in this chapter. But for now, it will be put to one side.

3. Mental states are governed by a common-sense belief desire psychology. Propositional attitude psychology is our everyday way of making sense of, explaining and predicting other people's behaviour. We explain the actions of others by attributing to them beliefs, desires, hopes, fears, and intentions. These can be used to make sense of or rationalize their actions. Because this method of action explanation is used in this everyday way it is often called folk psychology. It works by deploying a complex *system* of propositional attitudes to make sense of action and speech.

In his book *Mental Content* (1989), the philosopher of mind Colin McGinn (1950–) characterizes the connection between mental states and folk psychology in this way:

> First reference is made to a particular *person*; then some *attitude* is ascribed to that person; finally a *content* is specified for that attitude. Assertions of this form tell us who has what attitude towards which proposition. By making and receiving such assertions we come (it seems) to understand other people: what they do, why they want such and such, what made them hope for so and so, and so forth. Varying the three elements in the *person-attitude-content* structure gives us a seemingly powerful system for describing the minds of others (and our own), a system both antique and ubiquitous. Thinking of this system as a (tacit and unformalised) theory, we can say that folk psychology is a theory that centrally employs an explanatory ontology of persons and contentful attitudes; with these basic theoretical resources it sets about its explanatory and descriptive work.
>
> McGinn (1989, p. 120)

(Linguistic meaning dovetails with this system in the following way. Utterances provide the most important evidence for the ascription of propositional attitudes because people can *express* their mental states through language. The content of mental states can be put into words without remainder. There is

considerable philosophical dispute—based in part on a difference of pre-philosophical intuitions—about whether mental states also possess qualitative characteristics that are ineffable. Wittgenstein, for example, provides arguments against such a possibility. What matters in this context, however, is the *content* of beliefs and the claim that that is fully expressible is less controversial.)

Is folk psychology a *theory*?

On the assumption that folk psychology can be characterized as a *theory*, there has been much recent philosophical debate about whether it is a good theory. We will return to the question of its theoretical character in a later chapter. For now it is enough to note that folk psychology is a *systematic* interpretative stance, that it is used to explain behaviour and that it does this by ascribing content-laden mental states. (This is again a subject of Chapter 27 on how we can have access to others' mental states. Do we employ a interpretative theory or do we simulate what they are thinking by imaginatively putting ourselves into their position?)

Mental states possess a characteristic systematic structure

The systematicity of folk psychology just mentioned presupposes some relational structure between the content-laden mental states ascribed. It is worth mentioning two such connections here. One is that content is *rationally structured*. This is a claim forcefully stated by Frege. Mental states stand in logical and rational relations to one another. They are consistent, inconsistent, justificatory, disconfirmatory, and suchlike. As a result, the ascription of mental states in the explanation of speech and action through folk psychology is in part normative and prescriptive. The ascription turns in part on what people ought to think in the circumstances. The extent of this normativity is a philosophical matter, rather than merely a descriptive pre-philosophical one. For now, it suffices to say that the evidence for or against the ascription of an attitude to a person includes the rational connections between that attitude and the other attitudes already ascribed. Thus content-laden states are rationally structured.

There is a second and distinct respect in which content is structured, although this is clearly more of a philosophical claim, albeit one based on a powerful intuition. If one is able to understand the thought that a frog is green, one must also be able to understand thoughts to the effect that things other than frogs are green and that other frogs have colours other than green. Obviously, this is not to say that one must actually *hold* that this is the case. (One may have good reasons to hold that there is only one frog and one green thing left in the world.) But the ability to *understand* the first thought presupposes the ability to understand these other thoughts because understanding is a structured ability. The most influential statement of the claim that understanding a thought or, more generally entertaining a propositional attitude, is a structured ability that systematically presupposes connections to other thoughts or propositional attitudes is by the Oxford philosopher Gareth Evans (1946–80) in his difficult work *The Varieties of Reference* (1982, pp. 100–105). Consequently, it is often termed Evans's *Generality Constraint*. But the claim that content is systematic in this way is also emphasized by many others including Fodor (1987, pp. 147–153). (Linguistic meaning is also systematic. When one comes to understand a language—rather than simply knowing some phrases from a phrase book—one understands how to construct grammatically correct sentences from constituent words. It is criterial of this sort of understanding that if one can understand the sentence 'John loves Mary' then one will necessarily understand the sentence 'Mary loves John'. When one understands a language, one has a systematic ability to construct and understand novel sentences that employ known words in new structures. As we will see, Fodor uses the systematicity of our understanding of language to attempt to explain the systematicity of our mental states via the postulation of a 'language of thought'.)

The big question

These general characteristics of content-laden mental states present the challenge facing any philosophical explanation of content. How can there be states with just these properties?

Consider the sorts of properties that a chair has and compare this with those that a belief—perhaps a belief about a chair—has. The chair has mass, weight, length, and colour. It might also be to the left of the table or on top of the rug. The belief, by contrast, does not seem to have any of these properties. We would not normally say that a belief had a mass, length, or colour. And although the person having the belief may be to the left of the door or on top of the rug, we would not normally say that that was where the *belief* was. We don't normally say that beliefs are anywhere (except metaphorically perhaps at the back of my mind).

On the other hand, the belief is *about* the chair and it is held or entertained *by* a particular person. These are *relations* between the belief and parts of the world and the person holding it. Suppose the belief is that the chair is yellow. This looks like a relation between a person and the fact that *the chair is yellow*. Now some of the properties listed for the chair itself are also relational. The positional properties are clearly relational, linking the chair with the table and rug. Weight also turns on a gravitational field. It is arguable that even properties such as mass are really relations between different objects. But none of these relations mirror intentional relations. Note, for example, that the belief about the chair might be *false*. (Thus it would not be a relation to the yellowness of the chair: the chair is not yellow.) Or it might even be a belief about a non-existent chair. (The chair at the top of Mount Everest.) By contrast the relational properties of the chair have to link it to real things. So again the big question is: How can there be such things as beliefs with the properties they have?

Reflection on the session and self-test questions

Write down your own reflections on the materials in this session drawing out any points that are particularly significant for you. Then write brief notes about the following:

1. What mark of the mental did Brentano emphasize?

2. What are 'propositional attitudes'?

3. What aspects of mental states does Fodor stress?

4. What is the central question of the philosophy of content?

Session 3 **Naturalized or reductionist accounts of content**

What sort of account of content is needed?

The previous session attempted to give an everyday description of the features of content-laden mental states, or propositional attitudes. The next reading (linked with Exercise 3—Fodor, 1987) will begin to focus on one sort of philosophical approach to explaining how there can be states with these features. In effect, it provides one approach for augmenting cognitivist psychological theorizing about, for example, word recognition and understanding with an account of how the central 'semantic system' might work. It might thus shed light on how both linguistic understanding and the formation of mental contents (both of which are semantic) are possible.

What is the relation between the Representational Theory of Mind and functionalism?

This session will begin to examine a philosophical account of the meaning or content of mental states, which, like cognitive psychology, embraces the metaphor of the mind as computer. It is a form of cognitivism or representationalism that attempts to explain thought by postulating a system of internal mental representations within a structure of a language of thought. It is the contemporary American philosopher and psychologist Jerry Fodor's Representational Theory of Mind (RTM).

We have already examined one approach to the philosophy of mind based on an analogy with computers. That position was functionalism. (See Chapter 23.) It may be helpful to have an early hint at the difference between functionalism and the position that Fodor sets out, which is the subject of this session: the RTM. There are two key differences. (Do not worry if you do not understand these differences. They are the subject of this session.)

1. Functionalism is an answer to the question: What are mental states and how are they related to states of the body? Functionalism replies that mental states are second order states, individuated by their functional causal properties,

however those are realized. (We saw that some functionalists went on to argue that such states are physical, but that is a further argument.)

Fodor's RTM is an answer to the further question: How can mental states have meaning or content, how can they be *about* worldly states of affairs? A thorough functionalism would also have to answer this question but that is not how that position arose.

2. Functionalism individuates states by their functional properties. Mental states with different contents or meanings would have to be individuated by different functional properties. Thus the belief that coffee is good would have to have a different functional role to the belief that coffee is healthy. A functionalist would have to explain what this different property was without simply saying that one has the functional role of the belief that coffee is good while the other has the functional role that coffee is healthy, and go on to account for all other possible beliefs.

Fodor thinks that such an account will fail to cope with the infinity of potential belief types. He proposes instead to explain different mental contents through the idea of different internal mental representations, which are part of an inner innate *language* of thought. This move to talk of an inner language goes beyond the resources of functionalism proper. (Distinguishing carburettors from exhaust manifolds does not require talk of a *language* of motorcar components.)

The reading is taken from what is perhaps the clearest of Fodor's accounts of his views. Fodor has continued to develop and change his views and so this 1987 account from his short book *Psychosemantics* is not the most up to date, but it will help set out the general approach.

EXERCISE 3   (30 minutes)

Read the extract from:

Fodor, J.A. (1987). *Psychosemantics*. Cambridge, MA: MIT Press, chapter 4. (Extract: pp. 97–99)

Link with Reading 24.3

Think generally about the kind of explanation Fodor offers. What reason does Fodor give for the need for such a theory? What is the relation between explanatory priority of mental content and linguistic meaning?

Reductionist explanations of content

Fodor's account of mental content aims at a form of reductionism. Reductionist accounts aim to explain content by showing how it derives from processes that can be described without using, and thus presupposing, any intentional concepts. The aim is that the puzzling features of content can be reduced to processes which are not puzzling. Fodor characterizes this aim as

follows: 'What we want at a minimum is something of the form "R represents S" is true iff C where the vocabulary in which condition C is couched contains neither intentional nor semantic expressions.' (*Psychosemantics*, p. 32).

Reductionism aims at giving necessary and sufficient conditions (or failing that at least sufficient conditions) for content which can themselves be stated without using intentional concepts. If this could be achieved then it would provide a translation of the supposedly philosophically problematic intentional vocabulary into an unproblematic language and thus resolve the philosophical difficulties. Intentional states would be shown to comprise or derive from non-intentional states. But this raises the question: why think of talk of meaning, intentionality, or content as problematic?

Naturalism

A clue lies in the fact that reductionism here is sometimes called a 'naturalistic' account of content. Such a label reflects the belief that unless content can be explained in non-intentional terms then it cannot be an unmysterious part of the natural world. Fodor gives a clear expression of this methodological assumption in the following passage:

> I suppose that sooner or later the physicists will complete the catalogue they've been compiling of the ultimate and irreducible properties of things. When they do, the likes of *spin, charm* and *charge* will perhaps appear upon their list. But *aboutness* surely won't; intentionality simply doesn't go that deep. It's hard to see ... how one can be a Realist about intentionality without also being, to some extent or other, a Reductionist. If the semantic and intentional are real properties of things, it must be in virtue of their identity with ... properties that are *neither* intentional *nor* semantic. If aboutness is real, it must be really something else.   (p. 97)

Fodor's claim is thus that unless one can reduce or 'naturalize' the intentional, then the only other plausible view is to deny that it really exists. The motivation for this claim appears to be that, if it is not reducible to something else, nothing as strange and magical as meaning could itself form part of a respectable account of the world. Failing reduction, one would be forced to adopt an anti-realist reconstrual of content as a strictly fallacious way of speaking, a hangover from the pre-scientific age or as a sort of secondary quality existing only in the eye of the beholder. This is an assumption to which we will return in the next chapter but the connection with cognitive psychology should be clear.

Fodor and cognitive psychology share reductionist and naturalistic assumptions

Cognitive psychology also aims at a reductionist account of human mentality. This is implicit in its attempt to analyse human cognitive abilities in terms of information flow between different subpersonal systems. The very idea of talking of a semantic system as a subsystem of a whole person reveals the assumption that the semantic properties of mental states of whole people can be explained through lower level information processing. While Fodor makes explicit the motivation for a reductionist explanation of content-laden mental states, this motivation is shared at an implicit level by the assumptions made about cognitive psychological explanation. (This leads to the obvious question: if this motivation is questionable, what other kind of account of semantically evaluable states is possible. One such approach will be the subject of Chapter 25.)

Explanatory priority

A second preliminary observation of Fodor's approach is of the order of explanatory priority, which he assumes. Given that the aim is to provide a reductionist or 'naturalistic' account of intentionality, and given that both mental states but also linguistic items can possess intentionality, there are a number of different options for explanatory priority. What is to be explained in terms of what?

> **EXERCISE 4** (10 minutes)
>
> Stop! Before looking ahead think about the options available for a reductionist account of intentionality. What approaches might there be? Write down brief notes if you can on these points before going on.

Four explanatory options

There are four possible approaches to explanatory priority:

1. Assign explanatory priority to mental content and explain how linguistic meaning results from that.

2. Assign explanatory priority to linguistic meaning and explain how mental content results from that.

3. Explain mental content and linguistic meaning in the same way with equal priority.

4. Explain mental content and linguistic meaning in different ways with equal priority.

Option 1

The first option is to attempt to explain linguistic meaning by showing how it results from mental content. This is the strategy adopted by Fodor and the majority of reductionist theorists. Their hope is that conditions can be specified concerning the mental states of speakers, which are necessary and sufficient to establish linguistic meaning. The standard approach is to attempt to explain the meaning of sentences as an abstraction from the meaning of utterances made using them. The meaning of utterances is then supposed to be explained as deriving from the content of beliefs that the utterances were intended to convey. Given the content of these beliefs and intentions, the meaning of sentences can be derived and explained. A different and independent account would then have to be found of how mental states possess their content.

Examples of this strategy dominate contemporary philosophy of thought and language. This is partly the result of the influence of Grice's work in the 1950s (see for example Grice, 1969). Grice aimed to explain linguistic meaning as the result of speakers' beliefs and intentions. He attempted to articulate the conditions that have to be met for a speaker to intend to communicate a belief to an audience using a linguistic expression. The promise of the Gricean programme is that the meaning of conventional spoken words and sentences is explained as deriving from the content of the beliefs that the speaker intends to communicate and the audience realizes it is intended to share by means of established linguistic conventions. Thus linguistic meaning can be explained in terms of a speaker's beliefs and intentions. Attempts based upon Grice's work to reduce in this way the two problems of linguistic meaning and mental content to a single problem of mental content are called 'intentional based semantics'.

Once the two problems are reduced to one, reductionist accounts then attempt to provide a reductionist explanation of mental content in non-intentional terms. But it is worth noting that the question of the order of priority is independent of the question of whether to give a reductionist explanation or not. As we will see, however, the first order of priority fits most easily with reductionism.

Options 2 and 3

There are three other strategies concerning explanatory priority but only two of them are practical. The second is to reverse the above order and to explain mental content in terms of linguistic meaning. The third is to ascribe priority to neither side and to explain both in the same neutral way. While these are clearly different in principle, in practice it is difficult sharply to distinguish examples of them. Philosophers such as Wittgenstein and Davidson appear to subscribe to one or other of these two views but there are conflicting reasons for viewing their approaches as belonging to both the second and third strategy. (They are the subject of the next chapter but the reasons for ascribing to both the second and third position is this. Both Wittgenstein and Davidson provide an argument that the possession of a language is a precondition of any but the most rudimentary mental states. But they also explain linguistic meaning and mental content in the symmetric manner.)

For reasons that will become clearer, the second and third order of priority would be difficult to combine with a reductionist explanation of intentionality. Thus although they tie mental content and linguistic content together, they are not, as a matter of fact, the preliminary stage of a form of reductionism.

Option 4

There is also, in principle, a fourth possibility with respect to explanatory priority. One could assign no priority and offer two different and independent explanations of mental and linguistic content. Such a strategy has two clear practical disadvantages. First, it assumes from the start that the task is twice as difficult as the other three approaches. It assumes that two different accounts of content have to be given rather than that one will serve for both mind and language. Secondly, it faces the problem of explaining how the two distinct forms of content are related. Given that the content of a belief can be expressed by a sentence, some account of this congruence is required. It is unsurprising that examples of this strategy are difficult to find.

Fodor's representational theory of mind

The Representational Theory of Mind and the language of thought as a reductionist theory

So much then for the kinds of approach to a philosophical account of content. Let us return to Fodor's theory. In order to provide a reductionist explanation of how meaning or content can be part of the natural order, he deploys a causal theory of mental content, which he ties to the Language of Thought hypothesis.

The heart of the Representational Theory of Mind

Fodor suggests that the Representational Theory of Mind (RTM) is defined by two central claims. In *Psychosemantics* he says:

> At the heart of the theory is the postulation of a language of thought: an infinite set of 'mental representations' which function both as the immediate objects of propositional attitudes and as the domains of mental processes. More precisely, RTM [the Representationalist Theory of Mind] is the conjunction of two claims:
>
> *Claim 1* (the nature of propositional attitudes):
> For any organism O, and any attitude A toward the proposition P, there is a ('computational'/'functional') relation R and a mental representation MP such that
>
> MP means that P, and
>
> O has A iff O bears R to MP
>
> *Claim 2* (the nature of mental processes):
> Mental processes are causal sequences of tokenings of mental representations. (pp. 16–17)

What are mental representations?

On a first reading this may seem a rather daunting paragraph; however, it can be understood as a development of a functionalism in the philosophy of mind. Fodor claims that he can explain what it is to have a propositional attitude or content-laden mental state by invoking internal mental representations. As a first approximation, think of mental representations as internal second order states akin to functional states. There are some differences between Fodor's mental representations and functional states. This is signalled here by the phrase 'language of thought'. These differences, however, will become clearer shortly.

Mental representations are inner vehicles of content

Take the first of Fodor's claims. A person, O, has a propositional attitude or content laden mental state, A, if and only if they stand in a certain relation, R, to an internal mental representation MP. So Fodor *explains* what it is to have a mental state by hypothesizing

an internal state of the mind or brain, MP. The mental representation *encodes* the content of the propositional attitude. Thus it might somehow encode the content that *psychotherapy is cost-effective*. One way of construing encoding is to compare it with a written sentence or phrase. Take the sentence: 'Psychotherapy is cost-effective.' As a sentence it is composed of a number of words that are in turn made up of letters. The whole sentence is a squiggle on paper or a computer screen. But on the assumption that it is a sentence in English it says that *psychotherapy is cost-effective*. Those squiggles 'encode' that content. They are the vehicle of the content. Fodor thinks that in a similar way, mental content is carried by internal vehicles of content, which in this case are mental representations. These encode the contents of our mental states.

Relation R explains the differences between kinds of attitude

What of the relation R that mental representations are supposed to stand in? Fodor calls it a functional or computational relation. Here the idea is that the same content can be the object of different attitudes. One may believe, hope or fear that psychotherapy is cost-effective. In each case that content will have a different effect on one's mental economy. One acts differently on the basis of beliefs, hopes, and fears. Fodor suggests that these differences can be explained as the result of mental representations standing in different functional or computational relations.

So the role of mental representations is to explain how it is possible to have content-laden mental states. Part of the account employs functionalism in order to explain and distinguish the different 'psychological' attitudes described in folk psychology. So far, however, nothing has been said about how mental representations encode content. This is what Fodor's version of the causal theory of content is supposed to explain. As we will see, the basic idea of that is that mental representations encode contents by standing in suitable causal relations to those items in the external world which they are about. But before examining that theory, there is a further detail worth examining. This is how the structure of content is explained.

The role of the language of thought hypothesis

One of the pre-philosophical characteristics of content described earlier was its systematicity. If one is capable of thinking that John loves Mary then one must also be capable of thinking, or understanding the thought, that Mary loves John. One may not actually think this—as love may be unrequited—but one must be able to think it. Similarly, if one can understand the thought that coal is black, one must be able to understand the thought that something else is black. One must be able to understand the possibility of the more general application of the concept of black. What explanation can be given of these systematic abilities?

The systematicity of thought and language

The most explicit answer to these questions is provided by the language of thought hypothesis. According to this, mental representations are symbols in a language of thought with both a compositional syntax and semantics. The most direct motivation for this thesis is a swift response to the explanation of the systematicity of mental content. Such systematicity is also apparent in language. A language capable of representing the fact that John loves Mary (in English, by the sentence 'John loves Mary') is also capable of representing the fact that Mary loves John, by reversing the symbols for John and Mary in the representing sentence. So one obvious explanation for the systematicity of thought is to say that thinking comprises the manipulation of inner representational symbols in a language of thought. Thus as well as granting that the thought that John loves Mary is a structured thought, in accordance with Evans' Generality Constraint, the language of thought hypothesis claims that the internal bearer of this content is a structured or compositional symbol in an inner language.

Thus complex mental representations can be built up from more basic ones in a way that resembles the construction of complex from simple ideas in Locke's account of the mind.

The vehicles of content are structured

Fodor makes the distinction between the language of thought (LOT) hypothesis and other theories such as functionalism in the following passage:

> Practically everybody thinks that the *objects* of intentional states are in some way complex: for example, that what you believe when you believe that ... P & Q is ... something composite, whose elements are—as it might be—the proposition that P and the proposition that Q.
> But the (putative) complexity of the *intentional object* of a mental state does not, of course, entail the complexity of the mental state itself. It's here that LOT ventures beyond mere Intentional Realism ... LOT claims that *mental states*—and not just their propositional objects—*typically have constituent structure*. *Psychosemantics* (p. 136)

Such a claim ensures that those able to think the first thought are able to think the second thought because of the systematic relations between compositionally structured mental representations. So much then for the explanation of the systematicity of thought. But what of the rational structuring of thought? The systematicity of mental representations explains the fact that if one is able to think 'P and Q' one must also be able to think 'P' but not that one *ought* to think it. The language of thought hypothesis, however, also has an explanation of the rational or normative nature of our thinking.

The computer metaphor again

The computer provides an influential metaphor. Computers are machines that can be programmed to manipulate symbols so as to respect the semantic or rational relations of the contents that they encode. This manipulation, encoded in the lowest levels of computer programming languages, depends on causally relevant properties of the symbols, which, by design, correspond to their

syntax. Thus the harmony of the causal properties of symbols and the rational properties of contents is effected by the syntax of the symbols that encode those contents. This suggests that language of thought versions of representationalism can make use of a similar account to explain the rational structure of thought.

On this account, mental representations comprise symbols in a language of thought whose syntax governs their causal interactions such that the demands of rationality are respected. In other words, the mind is a computer whose computations involve the manipulation of internal symbols. Thinking comprises the causal manipulation of internal symbols according to a system of laws that matches the rational structure of the contents of thoughts encoded by the symbols.

Representational Theory of Mind and functionalism

The relation between Fodor's RTM, based on a language of thought differs from functionalism. Fodor thinks that the difference between hoping something and fearing it can be explained as a difference in the functional role of a mental representation. But he does not think that content of the attitude—what is hoped or feared—can be explained or determined by functionalism. That is instead explained as resulting from the combination of tokens in a language of thought.

Inner language or inner maps and models?

While the language of thought hypothesis is the most explicit representationalist attempt to explain the systematicity of thought, not all forms of representationalism are committed to it. An alternative explanation relies not on an inner linguistic structure but a structure based upon inner maps or models. Briefly, it has been argued that maps can also explain the systematicity and rational structure of thoughts. The same mapping conventions and symbols that enable a representation of Cambridge as to the east of Oxford could also represent Oxford as to the west of Cambridge. There is a systematicity in such mapping relations. An explanation of the rational structuring of thoughts based on maps is less clear than the language of thought explanation. But there is no reason in principle why a similar kind of story might not be developed. The harmony of the causal properties of map symbols and the rational properties of contents could be effected by a kind of spatial syntax of the mapping symbols, which, on this account, encode those contents. In what follows we will ignore the differences between language of thought and mental model theories of the mind.

There's still something missing!

Both the language of thought and the mental models hypotheses attempt to explain the structure of mental content through the structuring of internal states. But while these attempt to explain the 'syntactic' properties of thought (literally the syntax in the case of the language of thought and an 'internal' structure akin to syntax in the case of mental models), they do not explain the intentional or semantic properties of thought. That is, they do not explain how mental representations—thought of as second order states of the brain—can be *about* anything. The next two sessions will examine two different theoretical additions that attempt to explain how inner representations can be about the world. The first is a straight causal theory of reference. The second (in Session 5) is a teleological theory.

Session 4 Descriptive causal accounts of content

Semantics and the causal theory of reference

The representationalist picture of mind outlined so far postulates ontologically independent internal mental states standing in systematic causal relations one to another. They are 'ontologically independent' because their existence is not tied to any states of affairs in the outside world. (What is an ontologically *dependent* state? Think of the marriage of Posh and Becks. That state—their marriage—turns for its existence on the existence at some time of both parties. It is an essentially relational state.) But the very fact of their independence of the world raises a key problem: Why think of mental representations as representations *of* anything? Why think that they possess intentionality or semantic properties?

This question can be put in the context of the flow diagrams of the first reading in the chapter. At the heart of the modular and functional account of speech recognition and understanding was a 'semantic system'. On the assumption that such a system is thought of as a symbolic processor, operating on mental representations in the broad way Fodor describes, how does anything that goes on in there count as being about anything in the outer world? How could meanings be stored up in such a system as well as representations of words or the supposed *vehicles* of content? To answer these questions Fodor combines his account of RTM so far described with a causal theory of reference.

Fodor's RTM adds to the elements so far outlined a further claim. In addition to standing in causal relations to one another, mental representations also stand in causal relations to items in the external world. It is in virtue of their external causal relations that mental representations have intentional content.

Two roles for causal relations

In his book *The Representational Theory of Mind* the Australian philosopher K. Sterelny (1990) summarizes this idea as follows:

'Thoughts are inner representations; thinking is the processing of inner, mental representations. These representations have a double aspect ... [T]heir role within the mind depends on their individualist, perhaps their syntactic, properties ... [And] they are representations in virtue of relations with the world. Mental states represent in virtue of causal relations of some kind with what they represent.' (p. 39)

The basic idea is that mental representations gain their content by standing in suitable causal relations to items in the outside world. But simply adding additional external causal relations to the internal causal relations between mental representations does not explain how they come to possess intentionality.

Normativity and the disjunction problem

Representationalists do not generally attempt to tackle this problem directly. The problem that is generally acknowledged by representationalists is the problem of the *normativity* of beliefs. The assumption is something like this. If a representationalist theory of content cannot account for false beliefs, there is something fundamentally wrong with it. If the theory is not so falsified, then that may be some indication that it is indeed a theory of content. The problem of normativity is this. Beliefs can be both correct and incorrect. But a crude causal theory threatens to make false beliefs impossible if it simply identifies the content of a belief with what actually causes it. The theory will instead make all contents disjunctions of their causes. Thus the problem is often called the 'disjunction problem'.

To take an example. Suppose we want to be able to explain how is possible to have the false thought that there is a cow in front of one when in fact there is rather a plump horse. (Any theory that cannot allow such false thoughts is a bad account of fallible human thinking.) Suppose also that we adopt a representationalist assumption that such thoughts are in fact internal states of people (states of their brains perhaps). Then we need an account of how such and such a brain state *means* cow even though it is caused in this case by a plump horse. So a simple theory that says that a brain state means whatever causes it cannot account for this false thought.

There are two general approaches that are designed to meet this problem. Both work by adding an extra ingredient to the simple causal link. The first is to modify a pure descriptive theory. The second is to deploy the resources of biological teleological explanations. In the reading below Fodor briefly summarizes and criticizes one of each of these before putting forward his own descriptive causal theory. (Teleological theories will be the subject of the next session.)

Dretske's pure descriptive theory

In his influential 1981 book *Knowledge and the Flow of Information*, Fred Dretske (1932–) an engineer turned philosopher proposed a solution to the disjunction problem. He argued that a *learning process* establishes the correct causal connection between mental representations and what they are about. After an initial learning process, anything that causes a mental representation but that lies outside the correlation established during the learning time corresponds to an erroneous 'firing' of the mental representation rather than adding to the content it encodes.

But as Fodor argues, if a horse at night causes the mental representation that encodes 'cow'-thoughts to be tokened after the learning period, then presumably it would have caused it in the training period had it occurred then. Thus as one needs a counter-factual reading of the training period, this destroys the contrast between truth and error that this account was supposed to underpin.

Simple teleosemantics

Millikan's teleological reductionist account of mental content will be the subject of the next session. Fodor characterizes a slightly different form of that approach, which, for clarity, could be called a simple teleological solution. (See for example Papineau *Reality and Representation*, 1987, chapter 4.) Such a theory attempts to solve the disjunction problem by saying that the correlation that determines the content encoded by a mental representation is the causal connection that would occur under *optimal circumstances* where these are explicated through natural selection.

Fodor raises three objections to simple 'teleosemantics' (teleological semantics):

1. Why should what is optimal for belief fixing as far as natural selection is concerned be optimal for making them true? What about the selective advantage of fast but merely approximate thinking? And why should the conditions for optimality be the same for all beliefs? If not then the kind of circumstance in which mental representations are appropriately caused may have to be specified *after* settling their content.

2. Teleology merely replicates without solving the disjunction problem. Frogs could be described as responding to either flies or to little black things because in their environment the two coincide. Frogs of either type would survive equally well on earth. There is no material in actual historical natural selection to discriminate which is the *correct* intentional story.

3. This kind of account—which specifies conditions under which the causation corresponds to correct use—does not permit the *robustness* of meaning: that many things can cause me to think of cows quite correctly which are not cows (e.g. milk).

> **EXERCISE 5** (30 minutes)
>
> Read the extract from:
>
> Fodor, J.A. (1987). *Psychosemantics. Cambridge*, MA: MIT Press, pp. 106–108
>
> ---
>
> Link with Reading 24.4
>
> ---
>
> ◆ How satisfactory is Fodor's solution to the 'disjunction problem'?

Fodor's descriptive theory: asymmetric dependence

Fodor's preferred solution to the disjunction problem is to distinguish between causal connections that are constitutive of content and those that are not, in terms of asymmetric dependence. A type of mental representation has the content 'cow' if cows cause it to be tokened in the 'belief box' of a thinker and if those occasions on which it is caused by non-cows depend asymmetrically on the connection to cows. (Thus if the former connection had not existed—because the mental representation had a different content—then the latter would not have existed either.) Occasions when non-cows cause the 'cow' mental representation to be tokened can now be counted as errors.

Objections to Fodor's theory

Having now sketched out Fodor's positive theory we will turn, again rather briefly, to some standard objections. These can be divided between those that are more technical objections to the theory and for which some twiddling with the theory might be sufficient response and those that are fundamental objections and that aim to show that there is something inadequate about this whole approach to content, intentionality, or semantics.

Note first that a number of obvious objections to Fodor's theory can be avoided by making sure the dependence is specified in terms of *lawlike* connections between *properties* in the world. Thus a mental representation stands for cows if the property of cow-hood generally causes it. This allows, for example, for a mental representation to stand for unicorns even if it has never actually been tokened in the presence of a unicorn. It also helps avoid the following objection. If the mental representation that stands for horses has, as a matter of fact, only been produced by small horses—because these are the only horses so far experienced—does it really stand for small horses? Fodor replies that it does not providing it *would have been* caused by large horses had there been any.

Cats and robots

Lynne Rudder Baker raises an objection that introduces a disjunction back into the content encoded by mental representations based on an hypothetical example of cats and robot cats (Baker, 1991).

Sally has learnt the meaning of 'cat' from exposure to robot cats. (Thus her mental representations have been reliably caused by robot cats.) Suppose she now sees a normal biological cat. As it looks identical it will also cause a tokening of the 'cat' mental representation. What content does that representation encode then? Baker suggests the following options:

1. It correctly represents a cat and all the past tokens misrepresented robot cats as cats. But surely this gets the dependence relation the wrong way round?

2. It misrepresents this cat as a robot cat. But what of counterfactuals about what would have happened if she had seen this earlier?

3. It is disjunctive. Fodor opts for this. But this makes disjunction widespread. Most of us cannot distinguish horses and mules, for example. Also if it is disjunctive then Sally cannot later recognize her earlier application as an *error* when she finds out there are two sorts of thing. How do we get to asymmetric dependence from the earlier disjunction?

Causality and normativity

There are a number of similar arguments in the literature. Each tries to show that Fodor does not successfully solve the disjunction problem. But there is another more general problem highlighted by Godfrey-Smith (1989). He asks what resources a *purely causal* theory has for distinguishing between the independent causal relation that determines the content of a mental representation and those dependent causal relations that correspond to error?

Consider a mental representation that is caused by normal-looking horses, athletic cows, muddy zebras, and so forth. One obvious interpretation of this is that the representation encodes horse-thoughts and that the connections between it and some cows and zebras asymmetrically depends on the connection to horses. But there is another interpretation that is equally plausible given only the facts about causal connections. That is that the mental representation encodes a disjunctive content including normal looking horses, and some cows and zebras. There is, after all, a *reliable* causal connection between those animals and the representation. It is only *given* the content of the mental representation that one can determine which connections are fundamental and which are dependent, which would hold in nearby possible worlds and which would not. What this suggests is not just that there is a problem with Fodor's particular solution but that there is something generally wrong with attempts to reduce intentional notions to purely causal ones. Something is omitted by the causal account. It cannot determine which the *correct* application is.

Another way of looking at this last point is like this. Although Fodor may be correct to say that error depends on truth, the asymmetric dependence theory does not by itself explain how mental representations come to encode contents in the first place. If a mental representation has a certain meaning, then its application in errors will depend logically on a prior veridical use. But the causal story is itself insufficient to explain the antecedent. How is such encoding brought about? Asymmetric causal relations may be necessary but not sufficient for content.

To repeat, none of these objections would be accepted as decisive by Fodor. Think of his approach as a research programme in the Lakatosian sense (see Chapter 16). If so it is characterized by a central core of assumptions about how intentionality is to be explained and by less central hypotheses that spell this out. The technical objections threaten the latter outer hypotheses and thus might be countered by technical fixes of one sort or another. The more fundamental objections challenge the central core. But whether there are seen to be decisive will turn in part on what other options are available.

In general, however, the tide in reductionist philosophy of thought has turned against pure descriptive theories in favour of teleological evolutionary theories. We will now turn to one of these to see if it could explain how what might be processed in a 'semantic system' could possess intentionality.

Reflection on the session and self-test questions

Write down your own reflections on the materials in this session drawing out any points that are particularly significant for you. Then write brief notes about the following:

1. What needs to be added to the comparison with a computer for a reductionist account of intentionality?

2. What in broad outline is Fodor's solution and what further problem does he think it faces?

Session 5 Teleological causal accounts of content

One response to the charge that purely causal theories cannot account for the normativity of content is to think that a further ingredient has to be added. The most plausible explanation of what ensures that the causal connections between mental representations accord with their rational relations is the process of evolution. This is the motivation for a teleological causal theory. Although it adds an extra ingredient to account for the normativity of thought—the disjunction problem again—it is still part of a reductionist programme. It still seeks to explain in naturalistic terms derived from biological science how there can be meaning in the world, how there can be intentionality.

The most thorough version of a teleological account has been developed the American philosopher of thought and biology Ruth Garrett Millikan. The locus classicus is her book *Language, Thought and Other Biological Categories* (1984) and *White Queen Psychology* (1993) contains a number of more recent papers.

EXERCISE 6 (45 minutes)

Read the extract from:

Millikan, R. (1995). Biosemantics: explanation in biopsychology. In *Philosophy of Psychology* (ed. C. Macdonald and G. Macdonald). Oxford: Blackwell, pp. 253–276. (Extracts pp. 253, 255–258)

Link with Reading 24.5

This reading provides a concise introduction to Millikan's teleological explanation of content. Think what extra resources biological teleological explanations provide for 'naturalizing' content. What is the source of this conceptual extra?

Biological function

Teleological theories of content appear to have an important extra resource for explaining the normativity of content over and above those available to pure descriptive theories. They can employ the notion of a natural, proper, or biological function. There is some debate about how precisely to define such a function. Roughly speaking, however, it is that function that a particular trait of an organism exemplifies and explains the evolutionary success and survival value of that trait. Crucially, biological functions are distinct from dispositions. The biological function of a trait and its dispositions can diverge. Engineering limitations might cause the actual behavioural dispositions of a trait to diverge from the biological function it thus only partially exemplifies. The divergences might themselves be life threatening and play no positive part in explaining the value of the trait. The best explanation of the survival of that organism and those like it cites the *function* that helped propagation or predator evasion, for example, and not those aspects of its behavioural dispositions that diverged unhelpfully from it.

of and *for*

This point is sometimes put by saying that what matters is not what traits or dispositions are selected, but what *function* they are selected *for*. The distinction between 'selection of' and 'selection for' can be illustrated by the example of a child's toy (from Sober, 1984). A box allows objects of different shapes to be posted into it through differently shaped slots in the lid. The round slot thus allows the insertion of balls, for example. It may be that the actual balls allowed through or 'selected' in one case are all green. But they are *selected for* their round cross-section and not their green colour. Millikan stresses the fact that the biological function of a trait may be displayed in only a minority of actual cases. It is the function of sperm to fertilize an egg but the great majority of sperm fails in this regard (see Millikan, 1984, p. 34).

As biological functions can diverge from mere dispositions, teleological causal explanations of content have an extra resource to explain normativity. The distinction between correctness and incorrectness in the tokening of a mental representation can be defined by reference to its functioning in accord with its biological function. Its function may be to be caused only by cows, for example, and not by plump horses. Thus if it is caused by a plump horse that still does not make it *mean* plump horse. It means 'cow', although it can also be caused by horses when the lighting is poor. This, supposedly, solves the disjunction problem with respect to the content of mental representations.

A reduction of rationality?

It also seems that an appeal to biological function can also explain how mental representations stand in rational relations. Indeed, Millikan elsewhere goes further by suggesting that, given a teleological account, logic will become the first *natural* science (Millikan, 1984 p. 11). That is, teleology will underpin a psychologistic explanation of logic and rationality. What makes one thought logically follow from another or one number the correct result of a calculation depends, ultimately, on abstract rules that humans apply to experience and that have had survival value.

Teleology and cognitive psychology

Millikan's teleological theory differs from Fodor's in that it adds in an extra ingredient for explaining the semantics of mental states: their proper or biological function. But it still broadly shares Fodor's goal of explaining how the semantics or content of mental states arises from natural processes that can be described in non-intentional terms. As such, it could be combined with the sort of computational or representationalist account favoured by cognitive psychology. The 'semantic system' could be described using evolutionary terms in such a way as to answer the question raised earlier about why one should think that anything that goes on in it is really semantic or world-involving. The states processed by such a system are semantic because that is their biological function.

Objections to teleosemantics

Unsurprisingly, Millikan's account faces criticism. We will focus on a criticism that concerns the reductionist aspirations of Millikan's theory.

Fast thinking

There are, however, two fundamental objections to a teleological approach. One has already been raised by Fodor (see above). It is that a teleological approach presupposes that the requirements of survival and rationality must go hand in hand. It is far from clear that this is actually so or that it must be so. In some circumstances it seems much more likely that quick approximations will contribute more to survival than a slow derivation of the correct answer. But even if, by chance, rationality, and survival coincided in the evolutionary history of animals on earth, this would be a contingent matter and thus undermine the necessity of logic.

A general tension in teleosemantics

The second flaw stems from the real source of the teleological theory's apparent ability to account for normativity. As already suggested, this results from the fact that biological functions are not pure dispositions. The extra normative ingredient derives from this difference. Biological functions are defined by reference to what *explains* the selection of a trait. It is this idea of explanation that introduces the extra normative character of biological function. But two points are important here, which pull in different directions:

What matters in this explanation is what traits are selected *for* rather than just what the traits are that are actually selected. This follows from the fact that even traits that are favoured by evolutionary selection may have design flaws. Some behavioural dispositions that are the causal consequences of a successful trait might themselves have deleterious effects on survival.

But nothing should be counted part of the biological function of a trait which has not contributed to the causal explanation of survival of that trait. This follows from the fact that biological teleology is still really the result of normal non-teleological causal processes.

Peacocke on reduced content

This latter feature forms the basis of a criticism developed by Peacocke in *A Study of Concepts* (1992, pp. 129–132). Taking the case of a belief forming mechanism, he argues that the only consequences that can explain the success of such a mechanism are the consequences of beliefs formed that have a causal impact on organisms that have it. But the truth of the causally relevant consequences of a belief can fall short of the truth of a belief itself. Thus:

> In a nutshell, the problem of reduced content is this: how is the teleological theorist to block an incorrect assignment of content to beliefs, namely one that requires for its truth merely the truth of all the logical consequences of *p* that have a causal impact on the thinker, rather than the stronger condition of the truth of *p* itself? Peacocke (1992, p. 130)

Millikan's reply

Millikan's response is to stress again the first of the points above: what matters is not *what* mechanism is selected but what it is selected *for* (Millikan, 1995). She argues that the best explanation of the presence of any such belief forming mechanism will not ascribe to it a function of the limited form that Peacocke suggests. Its function is to represent *p* and not merely to select the consequences of *p* that have causal impact. But this response points, however, to a more fundamental problem. It turns on an argument from Wittgenstein mentioned in chapter 14 and discussed more fully in chapter 25 but the key point can be sketched out now.

Millikan and Wittgenstein

A teleological account of function is a form of *interpretational* theory because the characterization of the function that explains the survival of a trait is in effect an interpretation of the past behaviour. Past behaviour comprises signs to be interpreted. But

as will be made clearer in the next chapter, there is no limit on the different way a set of signs or one's own past behaviour can be interpreted. Like the interpretation of signs, such behaviour is *consistent* with an unlimited number of possible functions or rules. What ensures the determinacy of biological function—what selects just one of the rules—is an explanation of the presence of a trait couched in intentional terms that interprets what the trait is for. But finite past behaviour can be explained as exemplifying many different or 'bent' functions or rules, all of which would have been equally successful in the past. (The idea of a bent rule will be re-explained in the next chapter.)

Millikan dismisses these possible alternatives by stressing, this time, the second of the points above. The explanation of a trait turns on what caused it to survive in the past. Taking the case of the rules that govern a hoverfly's mating behaviour she argues:

> [The 'bent' rule] is not a rule the hoverfly has a biological purpose to follow. For it is not because their behaviour coincided with *that* rule that the hoverfly's ancestors managed to catch females, and hence to proliferate. In saying that, I don't have any particular theory of the nature of explanation up my sleeve. But surely, on any reasonable account, a complexity that can simply be dropped from the explanans without affecting the tightness of the relation of explanans to explanandum is not a *functioning* part of the explanation. Millikan (1993, p. 221)

The claim is that 'bent' rules introduce additional and unnecessary complexities that can be dispensed with without damaging the explanation of the success of a biological trait. But the claim that bent rules are overcomplex and can be rejected either presupposes a particular interpretation of past behaviour for comparison—in which case it is question-begging—or that judgements can be made about the simplicity of rules from an objective Platonist perspective. And that is an idea that Wittgenstein has demolished (we saw some of this in Chapter 14).

A dilemma for natural selective explanation

It is worth noting that in the case of the mental representations of observable states of affairs, the suggestion that their biological function can be specified objectively via the explanation of their survival is more attractive. But this is misleading because such explanation helps itself to natural kinds in the explanation of what it is that mental representations track. In the context of explaining content, such explanation faces a dilemma:

- *Either*: natural kinds are identified with the extension of mental representations, in which case they cannot be invoked to explain the content of mental representations.

- *Or*: they are identified with classification-independent groupings or patterns in the world. The idea here is that thought tracks groupings that already exist independently of human judgement. This resembles the Platonist theory that Wittgenstein criticizes in that it locates the standard of correctness for such judgements outside human practice. Thus it cannot account for the normativity of judgements about what does and does not belong to the classification. But a teleological theory faces a more specific difficulty. There is no reason to believe that the biological function of a representation will be to track such natural kinds as opposed to functional kinds. The categories that are useful for an organism may not align with natural kinds.

Natural and functional kinds

An example that has been used elsewhere helps emphasize this second point. Consider a mental representation that encodes the content poison. This seems to be a functional concept in that it denotes any substance that is toxic to the organism in question. But it is possible that in the circumstances in which it had survival value, all the causes of that representation belonged to the same natural kind, the same biological species. The problem now is what, according to a teleological theory, distinguishes representations that encode what are, pre-philosophically, functional kind contents from natural kind contents? It seems on reflection that even in the case of mental representations that concern detectable states of affairs, the teleological theory is no improvement on the pure descriptive causal theory. Neither can account for the normativity of content.

A deeper objection to reductionism

There is a further general Wittgensteinian objection to both descriptive and teleological causal theories of content. Both attempt to add something to internal mental states in order to explain their meaning or life. But what they add does not make the right sort of difference. The asymmetric dependence of the tokening of internal states on types of states of affairs does not explain why those states should be thought of as representational. Equally, the fact that internal states—which have the fortuitous causal consequences for movement—lead to natural selective advantage, does not explain why they are representational.

Chapter 23 noted that functionalism alone did not succeed in explaining the intentionality of mental states. Functionalism characterized them as merely a system of causal 'pushes and pulls in the head'. These 'horizontal' causal relationships could be sufficient to explain behaviour without the need to think of additional 'vertical' relationships of representation. Why think of the internal states so characterized by functionalism as about anything?

The teleological theory is supposed to provide an answer to precisely this question. The suggestion is that once an account has been given of 'vertical' causal relations between internal states and states in the world, the problem of naturalizing content will have been solved. But it does not. All it provides is a further specification of which internal causal states have causally advantageous consequences. It does not explain why the 'vertical' causal relations that it provides should, in addition to fulfilling this causal role, fulfil an intentional role.

The consequences for a cognitive psychological explanation of semantics

This chapter has examined philosophical explanations of mental content that have adopted one of two forms of reductionism. Neither has been successful at reducing intentional notions to non-intentional causal relations between internal mental representations and parts of the world. This, however, is the assumption behind cognitivist explanations of mental content. The idea is that the computer can be used as a metaphor for the mind in order to explain cognitive abilities in information-processing terms. But this idea faces a severe objection because computer-based information processing requires underlying states that can be processed. Real computers are so designed that their internal states possess causal properties that are designed to match syntactic or programming properties. But once one thinks of human mental states as explained by free-standing internal mental representations, this forces the question: Why think of these as having semantic properties? Simply postulating a 'semantic system' at the heart of mental processing does nothing to answer this question.

Both Fodor and Millikan attempt to resolve this issue by describing links between internal states and the external world, either through a purely causal connection or a teleological causal connection. Both of these attempts to explain intentional connections through causal connections, however, face grave difficulties. And this casts doubt on the very idea of explaining understanding through an internal 'semantic system'. But if this approach cannot work, what alternative is there?

The underlying motivation for reductionism identified earlier in this chapter was that without it, content could not form an unmagical part of the natural world. In the next chapter we will examine an alternative approach that takes the failure to reduce content as in no sense undermining a properly naturalistic sense of intentionality. But on the other hand, trying to explain semantic properties at a lower level using subpersonal systems has no prospect of success. Only whole people can have semantic states.

Reflection on the session and self-test questions

Write down your own reflections on the materials in this session drawing out any points that are particularly significant for you. Then write brief notes about the following:

1. What other broad approach to the reductionist explanation of intentionality is there aside from Fodor's causal approach?

2. What role does biological function have in such accounts? What is the importance of the distinction between selection of and selection for?

3. What problems does it face?

4. What consequences do these difficulties raise for cognitive psychiatric theories of meaning?

Reading guide

♦ Useful introductions to the philosophy of content or intentionality can be found in the general philosophy of mind textbook by Braddon-Mitchell and Jackson (1996) *Philosophy of Mind and Cognition* (chapters 10–11), as well as in textbooks on the philosophy of content specifically. See, for example, Luntley (1999) *Contemporary Philosophy of Thought*.

♦ For an introduction to the philosophy of language sympathetic to a reductionist, representationalist approach see Devitt and Sterelny (1999) *Language and Reality: an introduction to the philosophy of language*.

♦ Criticism of the very idea of a meaning-driven folk psychology in favour of eliminativism is found in P(atricia) Churchland's (1986) *Neurophilosophy*, and Stich's (1983) *From Folk Psychology to Cognitive Science* and Stich's (1992). What is a theory of mental representation? Mind 101: 243–261.

Representationalism

♦ Representationalism is set out in Sterelny's (1990) *The Representational Theory of Mind*.

♦ The language of thought is discussed in the appendix to Fodor's (1987) *Psychosemantics*.

♦ For a Wittgensteinian critique of representationalism see Thornton's (1998) *Wittgenstein on Language and Thought*.

♦ And for representationalist approaches in psychology see Thornton (2002).

♦ Ruth Millikan's work is set out fully in *Language Thought and other Biological Categories* (1984) and *White Queen Psychology* (1993). Concise introductions are G. Macdonald 'The biological turn' and Millikan 'Biosemantics: explanation in biopsychology', in C. Macdonald and G. Macdonald *Philosophy of Psychology*, pp. 238–276.

♦ For a more accessible introduction to a biological teleological approach to meaning ('teleosemantics') see Papineau (1987) *Reality and Representation*, and (1993) *Philosophical Naturalism*.

Clinical and interdisciplinary work

♦ Clinical work in a cognitive neuropsychological framework can be found in Caramazza (ed.) (1990) *Cognitive Neuropsychology and Neurolinguistics*.

♦ A philosophical attempt to set out the basis of a reconciliation of causal and information rich explanation for mental health practice is described in Bolton and Hill (1996) *Mind Meaning and Mental Disorder*.

♦ Interesting interdisciplinary work can be found in Carruthers and Boucher (1998) *Language and Thought: interdisciplinary*

themes, and in Bechtel and Graham (ed.) (1999) *A Companion to Cognitive Science*. Both of these contain discussions of modularity in cognitivist accounts of the mind.

References

Baker, L.R. (1991). Has content been naturalised? In *Meaning in Mind: Fodor and his critics* (ed. B. Loewer and G. Rey). Oxford: Blackwell, pp. 17–32.

Bechtel, W. and Graham, G. (ed.) (1999). *A Companion to Cognitive Science*. Oxford: Blackwell.

Bolton, D. and Hill, J. ([1996] 2nd edn 2004). *Mind Meaning and Mental Disorder*. Oxford: Oxford University Press.

Braddon-Mitchell, D. and Jackson, F. (1996). *Philosophy of Mind and Cognition*. Oxford: Blackwell.

Brentano, F. ([1874] 1995). *Psychology from an Empirical Standpoint*. (trans. Antos C. Rancurello, D.B. Terrell, and Linda L. McAlister). London: Routledge.

Caramazza, A. (ed.) (1990). *Cognitive Neuropsychology and Neurolinguistics*. Baltimore, MD: Johns Hopkins University.

Carruthers, P. and Boucher, J. (1998). *Language and Thought: interdisciplinary themes*. Cambridge: Cambridge University Press.

Churchland, P.S. (1989). *Neurophilosophy*. Cambridge. MA: MIT Press.

Devitt, M. and Sterelny, K. (1999). *Language and Reality: an introduction to the philosophy of language*. Oxford: Blackwell.

Dretske, F. (1981). *Knowledge and the Flow of Information*. Cambridge, Mass.: MIT Press.

Ellis, A. (1996). *Human Cognitive Neuropsychology: a textbook with readings*. Hove, UK: Psychology Press.

Evans, G. (1982). *The Varieties of Reference*. Oxford: Clarendon.

Fodor, J.A. (1987). *Psychosemantics*. Cambridge, MA: MIT Press.

Fodor, J.A. (1991). Propositional attitudes. In *The Nature of Mind* (ed. D. Rosenthal). Oxford: Oxford University Press, pp. 325–338.

Godfrey-Smith, (1989). Misinformation. *Canadian Journal of Philosophy*, 19: 533–550.

Grice, H.P. (1969). Utterer's meaning and intentions. *Philosophical Review*, 78: 147–177.

Luntley, M.O. (1999). *Contemporary Philosophy of Thought*. Oxford: Blackwell.

Macdonald, G. (1995). The biological turn. In *Philosophy of Psychology* (ed. C. Macdonald and G. Macdonald). Oxford: Blackwell, pp. 238–251.

McGinn, C. (1989). *Mental Content*. Oxford: Basil Blackwell.

Millikan, R. (1984). *Language Thought and other Biological Categories*. Cambridge, MA: MIT Press.

Millikan, R. (1993). *White Queen Psychology*. Cambridge. MA: MIT Press.

Millikan, R. (1995). Biosemantics: explanation in biopsychology. In *Philosophy of Psychology* (ed. C. Macdonald and G. Macdonald). Oxford: Blackwell, pp. 238–276.

Millikan, R.G. (1984). *Language, Thought and Other Biological Categories*. Cambridge, MA: MIT Press.

Millikan, R.G. (1993). *White Queen Psychology*. Cambridge, MA: MIT Press.

Papineau, D. (1987). *Reality and Representation*. Oxford: Blackwell.

Papineau, D. (1993). *Philosophical Naturalism*. Oxford: Blackwell.

Parkin, A.J. (1996). *Explorations in Cognitive Neuropsychology*. Oxford: Blackwell.

Peacocke, C. (1992). *A Study of Concepts*. Cambridge, Mass.: MIT Press

Sobere (1984). *The Nature of Selection*. Chicago: University of Chicago Press.

Sterelny, K. (1990). *The Representational Theory of Mind*. Oxford: Blackwell.

Stich, S. (1983). *From Folk Psychology to Cognitive Science*. Cambridge. MA: MIT Press.

Thornton, T. (1998). *Wittgenstein on Language and Thought*. EUP.

Thornton, T. (2002). Thought insertion, cognitivism and inner space. *Cognitive Neuropsychiatry*, 7: 237–249.

CHAPTER 25

Reasons and the content of mental states: 2. Antireductionism and discursive psychology

Chapter contents

While the previous chapter focused on cognitivist approaches to intentionality...

Chapter 24 examined the kind of approach to meaning and intentionality implicit in cognitive neuropsychology and cognitive neuropsychiatry. The underlying approach was characterizable using a term from the philosophy of thought and language as representationalism. Such an approach aims to shed light on how our mental states can have the meaning or content they do using a cognitivist model drawing heavily on an analogy with computing. A key idea is that the fact that people can have mental states such as beliefs can be explained at a lower subpersonal level in terms of information processing using inner mental representations: structural configurations in their brains. Because the intentionality—the world-involving nature—of the mental states of whole people is explained in terms of the causal processes acting on lower level parts of their brains, such an approach can be thought of as 'bottom up'.

...this chapter will explore an alternative non-reductionist perspective

This chapter will examine a contrasting view. In psychiatry this is sometimes called a 'discursive approach'. In one of the readings of the chapter (linked with Exercise 1) Steven Sabat and Rom Harré (1994) characterize this as the view that 'meanings are jointly constituted by the participants to a conversation'. The precise idea behind the phrase 'jointly constituted' will be subject to scrutiny, but whatever the details, if meanings are so constituted then they are not simply the result of causal processes going on in individual minds. Taking this talk of 'constitution' seriously implies that the kind of reductionist explanation of meaning, which is the aim of cognitivist approaches cannot succeed. Again, light will be shed on the general approach exemplified by discursive psychology by looking to some philosophical models that explore its underlying assumptions.

The philosophical alternative

In the philosophy of thought and language (also called the philosophy of content), an alternative to a cognitivist or representationalist theory of content has been developed by a number of different philosophers including Dennett, Davidson, Wittgenstein, McDowell, and the neo-Fregeans. These do not share a single, tightly defined, theory, but they do agree on a broad alternative strategy to representationalism, which could be called discursive. It might be characterized through four claims:

1. It is antireductionist, explaining intentionality not through internal brain states but as a way of acting in the world.

2. It grants an important role to the 'interpretation' of speech and action from an everyday third-person perspective.

3. As a result of points 1 and 2 it is called an 'externalist' approach.

4. There is a central connection between our intentionality and *rationality*.

These points will now be briefly summarized.

Antireductionism and the practical turn

The alternative to the philosophical project of naturalizing meaning or, more broadly, 'intentionality' through a reductionist account such as representationalism, is to provide a non-reductive account based on practice. Instead of construing thought as a system of internal representations, the alternative is to construe it as a systematic practical engagement with the world. Whereas representationalism or cognitivism aims to explain intentionality in meaning-free terms using causal relations between inner and outer states, the authors listed above share the view that intentionality cannot be broken down like that. It has instead to characterized in meaning-presupposing terms and pertaining to the behaviour of whole people not parts of their brains.

Meaning is necessarily available to a third person stance

In addition, Davidson, Dennett, and to some extent Wittgenstein and McDowell argue that an understanding of both thought and language requires understanding how behaviour is understandable from a mundane third person perspective. Light is shed on intentionality by examining the explanatory stance that we can take to other people to make sense of their speech and action. Thus Davidson (1984a) approaches intentionality by asking what the preconditions are for interpretation from scratch in 'Radical interpretation' while Dennett discusses the underpinnings of the 'Intentional Stance'.

An aside on the connection with epistemology in Chapter 27

Given this connection between intentionality and the third person perspective, there will be some connections between this chapter and Chapter 27 on autism and our knowledge of other minds. A key recent debate in the epistemological of mind has been between two opposing views of what our knowledge of other people's mental states is based. One approach, the 'theory-theory', is based on the idea that in everyday circumstances we apply a tacit *theory* of how minds in general work. The other approach, 'simulation theory', argues instead that we imaginatively reproduce what other people are thinking by seeing what we would think in those circumstances. On this latter view you do not need to have a *theory* of minds to know what other people are thinking just a *mind* yourself. In fact, although the authors that will be considered in this chapter emphasize the role of the third person perspective they do not all subscribe to a theory-theory. That is because the subject of this chapter is not epistemology but rather the ontology of minds. This point will become clearer in Chapter 27, however.

Externalism

One consequence of stressing the theoretical role of the third person stance in accounting for intentionality is externalism. Both internalists and externalists can agree that whether a belief is *true* or not depends on features of the external world (assuming that it is a belief about some feature of the external world). But external-ists, unlike internalists, argue that at least in the case of some beliefs, their very *content* depends on relations to the world. Thus, for example, they dispute Descartes' assumption in the *Meditations* that the content of one's thoughts could be just the same even if there were no external world. Descartes held that in the absence of the external world, many of one's beliefs would turn out to be false. Externalists hold that one could not even entertain many of the beliefs we do.

Rationality

Finally, an important element of thinking about the content of mental states in the antireductionist way discussed below is the central role of rationality. A key idea is that we adopt an interpretative or explanatory stance to other people, which differs from the stance appropriate to non-human objects such as chairs and tables (animals have an interesting intermediate status). In the case of humans (and some animals) we make *sense* of their behav-iour (and we might want to say *action* rather than *behaviour* to emphasize this point). But making sense of other people requires, as a constitute principle, that are able to find their behaviour broadly speaking *rational*. Thus rationality is of central importance in this chapter (by contrast with its modest role in Chapter 24). It is a precondition of being 'minded' that one is rational.

Plan of the chapter

- *Session 1* outlines in general terms the sort of alternative approach that will be discussed in this chapter.

- *Session 2* will examine three philosophical interpretations of the work of the later Wittgenstein. The aim will be both to sharpen the criticism of representationalist or cognitivist approaches discussed in Chapter 24 and to consider how best to understand Wittgenstein's alternative view of the mind and mental content.

- *Session 3* will examine the influential work of the American philosopher of mind Daniel Dennett.

- *Session 4* will examine the related but different view developed by Donald Davidson.

- *Session 5* will examine the key assumptions behind neo-Fregean approaches to thought.

- *Session 6* will return to the clinical reading from Session 1 on a Discursive Psychological approach to Alzheimer's disease and ask what general conclusions can be drawn.

Session 1　The discursive alternative

This short session will set the scene for the rest of the chapter. The extract linked with Exercise 1 below is just the first part of a paper, to which we will return in the final session (see reading linked with Exercise 8), by the psychologist Steven Sabat and the philosopher Rom Harré on Alzheimer's disease sufferers. However, this first part of the paper concerns the broader under-pinnings of their thinking about meaning.

EXERCISE 1 (15 minutes)

Read:

Sabat, S.R. and Harré, R. (1994). The Alzheimer's disease sufferer as a semiotic subject. *Philosophy, Psychiatry, & Psychology*, 1: 145–160. (Extract: pp 145–148)

Link with Reading 25.1

- What is the view of meaning to which the authors subscribe?

The view of meaning

There are a number of passages in which Sabat and Harré reveal their view of meaning and of the intentional nature of mental states in general. (Remember that in the context of the philosophy of thought and language, which is sometimes called the philosophy of content, the term 'intentionality' generally means the *aboutness* or *world-involving* nature of both mental states and linguistic utter-ances. This term was reintroduced to philosophy by Franz Brentano (1838–1917) a philosopher and psychologist. The gen-eral characteristics were discussed at some length in Chapter 24.)

The abstract to the paper comments that 'meanings are jointly constituted by the participants to a conversation'. However, also 'from a discursive point of view, psychological phenomena are not inner or hidden properties or processes of mind which discourse merely expresses. The discursive expression is, with some excep-tions, the psychological phenomenon itself' (p. 146). They recruit Leo Vygotsky (1896–1934), the Soviet psychologist, in support of the thesis that: ' "The mind" is no more than, but no less than, a privatised part of the "general conversation". Meanings are jointly constructed by competent actors in the course of projects that are realized within systems of public norms' (p. 146).

More precisely the paper reports that it uses the word 'mean-ing' in three different ways (p. 147):

1. for intention in acting,

2. for an interpretation of events and situations, and

3. for evaluations of events, situations, or actions.

Why are these three all regarded as senses of the same concept? Well in each case there is an idea of *significance* at work. Starting with the second point, the idea of interpreting events is simply that of seeing what the events are about or perhaps more broadly, just what the events are, such as, for example, a robbery, a wed-ding, a promise, etc. To construe the collection of sounds and movements involved as making up any of these actions is to fit them into a broader sense-giving context. (Because of what it is, a wedding ceremony has particular consequences that differ from those of a robbery.)

Once so construed, these actions and events can be evaluated in a variety of ways (point 3 above). These include the assessment of their desirability in the selfish idea of the wants and desires of an agent but also in the distinct sense of their rationality in the light of the agents other beliefs and desires. Although one may not approve of someone's voting intentions, one may be able to see how it is rational in the light of their other beliefs and about the world and their values. Finally (to take the first point), an agent can then act in response to or to bring about just such events, again because of the significance they have for him or her. What is more, an action is the action it is in part in virtue of the agents reasons for acting. (Administering a drug may ease a patient's pain and also hasten her death, but if the reason for administering the drug was the former and not the latter then the action is an action of easing pain rather than a killing.)

The contrast of emphasis with Chapter 24

Without going further into the paper, it is possible to see the sharp contrast in *emphasis* between this approach to meaning and the view discussed in Chapter 24. It is one thing to talk about the meaning of events, and to think of the actions of individuals in terms of events (bringing them about, preventing them, etc.) and quite another to talk of the meaning or content of psychological states in terms of second order structures within the brain, or computations over representations in an internal 'semantic system'.

But while there is a contrast in emphasis, is there really a clash in the underlying claims that these apparently different views take on meaning? Or might it be simply that they emphasize two different aspects of meaning that could, in fact, be reconciled in a future science of the mind? If meaning really is constituted jointly, how is this brought about? And what relation does this have to do with what goes on in the brain? Again to be clear about the underlying ideas it is useful to turn to contrasting philosophical models. These will help clarify the extent to which there might or might not be a reconciliation between the different perspectives on meaning and mental content.

A challenge to reductionists...

But to set the scene, think back to a challenge that was raised against reductionism in Chapter 24 and to which we will return towards the end of this chapter. The challenge is that thinking about meaning from the perspective of cognitivism arguably makes a mystery of the connection between states of mind and states of the world. As soon as one talks of internal mental representations meaning second order structures of the brain then it becomes mysterious how these have any bearing on the world. So if one wants to explain how it is possible for me to have thoughts about the cup in front of me, as soon as one postulates a state of my brain and suggests that it might be a representation of that cup, the question of how that configuration of neurones, for example, can have anything to do with the cup becomes pressing. Why isn't it *just* a configuration of neurones?

...and a reciprocal challenge to antireductionists

Nevertheless, there remains something problematic about the idea of intentionality to which the reductionists are, at least, sensitive. This was well captured by the quotation from Fodor in the previous chapter. As 'aboutness' is not likely to be one the explanatory

concepts used in a complete physics, then if it is a genuine feature of the world, it seems that it must really be or comprise something else. How else can something as mysterious as intentionality be part of the physical universe, on the assumption that we are not embracing an antiscientific dualism of mind and matter? This in turn raises a challenge to antireductionists. How can they make intentionality an unmysterious part of the world?

How can antireductionists fit meaning into nature?

As we saw in Chapter 24, one approach is to attempt a *reductionist* explanation of intentionality by devising causal and or evolutionary mechanisms to explain how internal states can take on or encode mental content. Such an approach has the advantage in that it aims to explain the problematic notions of content, meaning, and intentionality in supposedly better understood notions such as causation. But the alternative, which will be discussed in this chapter, takes a different tack. To anticipate, it aims to make these notions less mysterious by thinking instead about the everyday role of ascribing content-laden mental states to people. Thus both Dennett and Davidson suggest that the idea of content-laden mental states have to be understood as playing a role in the explanation and prediction of people's speech and action. They play a role within the overall interpretative strategy of either what Dennett calls the 'Intentional Stance' or what Davidson calls 'Radical Interpretation'. These will be the subject of Sessions 3 and 4 below.

Neither Dennett nor Davidson attempt to *reduce* the ideas of meaning, content, and intentionality to less problematic concepts. Neither the Intentional Stance nor Radical Interpretation can be characterized in merely causal terms, for example. They are instead approaches that can only be described as ways of finding patterns of meaning and significance in speech and action. Furthermore, as we will see, *rationality* plays an important central role in both accounts. So both approaches attempt to clarify connections between all these concepts but without showing how they might be reduced to the concepts of physical or even biological science.

Antireductionism and the discursive turn

How does this second general approach relate the comments in the reading above linked with Exercise 1 (Sabat and Harré, 1994, pp. 145–149) that meaning is constituted in interpersonal discourse? To a first approximation the answer is this. The philosophical view just sketched provides one way to unpack such a claim about how meaning is constituted. This is via the claim that it is a necessary feature of our speaking a meaningful language and having content-laden mental states, that our speech and action is interpretable by others in accordance with shared cannons of rationality. This latter claim is one way of insisting that meanings (construed broadly to include the meaning of action and the 'meanings' of our beliefs and desires) are public. They are necessarily the sorts of things that can be articulated from the everyday third person perspective we take when we explain people's actions.

In fact, stronger claims about the social constitution of meaning are sometimes made. One such claim is that the content of our minds and utterances are not just necessarily available to others but that they are actually constructed piecemeal in social negotiations. This sort of claim is a much more radical form of social constructionism. The weaker claim of the previous paragraph is consistent with the idea that when now I form the intention to end this sentence in an even number of words, that intention prescribes the range of satisfactory outcomes independently of any further social negotiation. It may be that it is necessarily the case that I could have been interpreted to have this intention (on the basis of what I say and do). But it is not necessary that I actually am so interpreted or that I speak to anyone about it to have the intention. Radical social constructionism by contrast insists that the connection between interpretation and mental states turns on what actually happens not on what could have happened. It will be touched on only rather briefly, however, because it is an implausible view.

Having now thought about the kind of alternative that might be available, the next session will turn to the later Wittgenstein's work via three different interpretations.

Reflection on the session and self-test questions

Write down your own reflections on the materials in this session drawing out any points that are particularly significant for you. Then write brief notes about the following:

1. What are the features of a discursive approach that relate specifically to meaning? What does it take meaning to be?

2. What prima facie advantages does this approach have over a cognitivist approach?

3. But is the approach really distinct from and incompatible with a cognitivist approach as described in Chapter 24?

Session 2   Wittgensteinian approaches to mental content

In order to clarify the idea of a social constructionist approach to meaning we will now turn to three interpretations of the work of the later Wittgenstein (1953) and his *Philosophical Investigations*. Wittgenstein's writing style is unusual: conversational German translated into conversational English with a minimum of technical terms. Nevertheless, it is not always easy to understand the general thread of his argument and thus there a number of rival interpretations.

One key idea, though, is that he stresses the public nature of meaning. But getting clear on what this entails is a matter for some work.

This session will outline some recent work on the later Wittgenstein's view of minds and meaning: by Saul Kripke, Crispin Wright, and John McDowell. The key positive idea is that understanding meaning should be thought of as a practical ability. This view is coupled with criticisms of the alternative discussed in Chapter 24: that having a meaning in mind is a matter of having an internal representation. To reach the positive account, however, it will be necessary to detour through that negative argument. The best place to begin is with Kripke's notorious sceptical interpretation of Wittgenstein's arguments.

Saul Kripke's interpretation of Wittgenstein

Kripke's sceptical interpretation of Wittgenstein

Saul Kripke, known primarily for work on modal logic and the semantics of names, wrote a short interpretation of a key part of Wittgenstein's *Philosophical Investigations* in the 1970s called *Wittgenstein on Rules and Private Language* (1982). This has proved highly influential, not because it has commanded agreement with its interpretation, but because it has stimulated philosophers to diagnose just how it can apparently justify a conclusion that is so obviously wrong. Like many sceptical arguments, the conclusion is clearly disastrous, but on first inspection, the argument in support of it appears to be sound. What is instructive for the philosophy of content is to determine which assumption leads to the sceptical conclusion. The moral that will be drawn here is that the possession of content-laden mental states depends at root on practical abilities rather than free-standing internal mental representations or symbols.

With that final destination in mind, we will concentrate first on the force of Kripke's argument about addition. We will return shortly to its application to meaning and content more generally.

Adding and quadding, plus and quus

Kripke's challenge is based on a simple thought experiment. How could you justify that replying '125' is the right answer to the question 'what is 57 + 68?'. Of course the first thing to do would be to ensure that there had been no mistake in carrying out the addition. One might best resolve this by setting out the addition using rows and columns, adding the units, correctly attending to the carry over and then adding the tens. But Kripke points out there is in principle a further 'meta-linguistic' error to be avoided that is giving the wrong interpretation to the sign '+'. He postulates a sceptic who proposes that in the past what you have meant by '+' was not the addition function but the 'quaddition' function which is defined thus:

$$x \text{ quus } y = x \text{ plus } y \text{ except where } x = 57 \text{ and } y = 68$$
$$\text{where } 57 \text{ quus } 68 = 5$$

The sceptic argues that as this has been the function you have been carrying out in the past, the correct response to the question: 'What is 57 + 68?' is '5'. The question becomes one of establishing what one meant in the past when one used that sign. How can one tell what function one has previously used that sign to represent? How does one know that in the past one meant addition by it rather than, in Kripke's example, the 'bent function' 'quaddition'?

EXERCISE 2 (10 minutes)

Think what answer you could give to Kripke's sceptic. What answer could you give show that you are right not to answer 5 to what is 57 + 68? What facts about your past performance or mental states show that you have meant addition rather than quaddition by '+' or 'plus'?

Adding and quadding, plus and quus again

Kripke's basic challenge stems from the fact that one's past behaviour is finite so one has only ever carried out a finite number of arithmetical operations. Thus the sceptical challenge is to say why writing '125' today is going on in the *same way* as one's past practice rather than, say, writing '5'. Sameness and difference depends on the rule or function that was previously applied. If previously one meant quaddition by '+' then writing '5' just is going on in the same way.

Kripke's two sceptical weapons

Kripke then deploys two sorts of consideration to undermine the efficacy of the most natural answers one might give to the sceptic. One device is the use of similar and ramifying (mis)interpretation of signs. The other is to stress the normativity implicit in the question. A satisfactory answer to the sceptic must show 'whether there is any fact that I meant plus not quus' (p. 11). But it must do this in such a way that it can 'show how I am *justified* in giving the answer 125' (p. 11). We will return to the role of this second element shortly.

The first tactic is evident in Kripke's responses to the following suggestions. In answer to the question, 'How does one now know which rule one was following in the past?', one might cite explicit instructions that one gave oneself. Perhaps one said (aloud): 'Now I'll *add* these numbers'. Obviously, this will not work because it simply repeats the problem. It only pins down one's past interpretation of the '+' sign if one can pin down the meaning of the spoken word 'add'. This problem applies equally whether the word is spoken aloud or silently to oneself.

The appeal to counting will not escape the problem of and quounting

One might hope instead to pin down the meaning of the sign '+' or the word 'add' by defining it—at some stage in the past—in more primitive counting terms. To add two numbers one counts on along the series of integers starting just after the first number and proceeding along by as many numbers as the second number. One might have repeated these instructions to oneself on some previous occasion. However, again this will not do because it will comprise a sequence of words that has correctly to be interpreted. Crucially as a way of distinguishing adding from quadding it depends what 'count' is taken to mean. If that really means *quount*—where to quount is the same as counting except where the numbers concerned are 57 and 68—the definition will serve to pick out quadding and not adding (Kripke, 1982, pp. 15–16).

It seems that any response to Kripkean scepticism that deploys any sort of sign or symbol that is spoken, written down or entertained in the mind will not work. Any sign could be misinterpreted to sustain a 'bent' rule.

Dispositionalism fails to address the normativity of the challenge

The other response, which Kripke considers and rejects, attempts to answer the sceptic by agreeing that meaning something by a sign cannot consist in having any occurrent mental phenomena but arguing that it is instead a dispositional state. There are a number of problems with this response but the central objection is this. Dispositions cannot meet the second requirement highlighted above. They cannot by themselves *justify* an answer as correct because one may be *disposed* to make an error.

The dispositionalist gives a *descriptive* account of this relation: if '+' meant addition, then I will answer '125'. But this is not the proper account of the relation, which is *normative*, not descriptive. The point is *not* that, if I meant addition by '+', I *will* answer '125' but rather that, if I intend to accord with my past meaning of '+' I *should* answer '125'. (pp. 160–161)

Kripke also makes a further—less decisive—objection to dispositional accounts. This is that one's dispositions are also finite. Thus given sufficiently large numbers to add, one is not disposed to give the correct answer because, for example, one cannot accurately remember the numbers or add them in the head. Thus one's actual dispositions do not fix the correct interpretation of the '+' sign.

Kripke's sceptical conclusion

Kripke goes on to draw the following substantial conclusion. Given that no fact can be called to mind to determine which function one previously meant by '+' or 'addition', there are no such facts. Furthermore, the same arguments could subsequently be deployed for one's present use of signs. Furthermore, nothing turns on the mathematical nature of the example chosen. The same argument applies to the use of any word and its meaning and to any speaker. As the meaning of any word must turn on what speakers mean by it, he concludes: 'There can be no such thing as meaning anything by any word. Each new application we make is a leap in the dark; any present intention could be interpreted so as to accord with anything we may choose to do. So there can be neither accord, nor conflict.' (p. 55).

Epistemology and ontology

The fact that he draws a metaphysical conclusion from merely epistemological considerations may seem startling. How can Kripke draw such a conclusion about the link between rules and applications from epistemological considerations? The answer is that an important assumption is built into the sceptical approach. If there were some fact that constituted the relation between a rule and its applications, it would be independently identifiable by the idealized subject that Kripke postulates. Kripke supposes, for the purpose of argument, that one may have all the possible information about one's past experiences, mental states, and inclinations. He then asks whether any of these would be sufficient to determine the rule that one were following. His conclusion, based on his interpretation of Wittgenstein's arguments, is that none would be. Given the idealizations involved, and the assumption that had any fact constituted the rule one were following one would have known it, then there is no such fact of the matter.

This sceptical interpretation of Wittgenstein is reinforced by Kripke's reading of Wittgenstein's *Philosophical Investigation* §201. Wittgenstein writes there:

> This was our paradox: no course of action could be determined by a rule, because every course of action can be made out to accord with the rule. The answer was: if everything can be made out to accord with the rule, then it can also be made out to conflict with it. And so there would be neither accord nor conflict here.   Wittgenstein (1953, §201)

Thus Kripke denies that, properly speaking, there are any facts about meaning. What a word means is never itself a matter of truth or falsity.

A positive account of meaning and social constructionism

Given that sceptical conclusion, what positive account does Kripke give of meaning? He suggests that while an individual cannot be thought of as following a rule in isolation, the individual can be treated as following a rule in the context of a community. As long as they do not conflict with the community's judgements then they can be so regarded. The key idea here is not that facts about meaning are genuinely ushered back onto the stage. Rather, individuals can be *dignified* as rule followers providing that they do not conflict with the wider community.

> It is essential to our concept of a rule that we maintain some such conditional as 'If Jones means addition by "+", then if he is asked for "68 + 57", he will reply "125"'… [T]he conditional as stated makes it appear that some mental state obtains in Jones that guarantees his performance of particular additions such as '68 + 57'—just what the sceptical argument denies. Wittgenstein's picture of the true situation concentrates on the contrapositive, and on justification conditions. If Jones does *not* come out with '125' when asked about '68 + 57', we cannot assert that he means addition by '+'.   Kripke (1982, pp. 94–95)

This view can be taken to support a social constructionist view of meaning. While the correct application of a word can be specified in advance, something akin to correct use emerges from communal practice.

Mental content

It should not take too much thought to realize how the sceptical argument might be generalized to apply not only to meaning something by a word but also to other intentional mental states. Meaning something by a word is a matter of intending to use it in a particular way. One can ask more generally by what token one knows the content or intentional object of past mental states. And again, it seems that the result will be the sceptical destruction of our everyday understanding of mental states. Anything that came to mind and that might be supposed to have fixed the content of what one was thinking could be interpreted in any number of ways. Thus there will be no facts of the matter about a person's content-laden states of mind.

What has gone wrong to lead to this drastic conclusion?

The main moral of Kripke for cognitive approaches to psychiatry

It is worth being clear what the purpose of looking at Kripke has been for this chapter. Aside from whatever intrinsic interest there is in Kripke's argument, one conclusion will remain intact despite the criticisms of Kripke described below. If one attempts to construe mental states as inner representations, then one will fall to Kripke's sceptical argument. That is a lasting consequence of the passages of Wittgenstein on which it is based. Kripke's own conclusion—that there is no such thing as meaning—can be resisted without this showing that nothing important has been learnt through his presentation of Wittgenstein's destructive arguments. Where Kripke goes wrong is in ignoring the conditional nature of the claim: *if* one construes mental states as inner representations…

We will now turn to two philosophers who have diagnosed what is wrong with Kripke's argument.

EXERCISE 3   (10 minutes)

Think about Kripke's sceptical argument. Especially keeping the analogy between following a rule or understanding a meaning on the one hand and having an intentional state on the other, can any argument be offered against it?

Defusing Kripke's argument: Wright and McDowell on Wittgenstein

Kripke himself distinguishes between two sorts of response to a sceptical argument. There are sceptical responses, which accept the force of the sceptical argument but suggest a way in which its consequences can be 'lived with'. Kripke suggests that Hume's response to his own argument about causation is such. On the other hand there are 'straight' responses. These diagnose a fault in the sceptical argument. We will now discuss two such responses that aim to diagnose a fundamental flaw in Kripke's argument.

Crispin Wright's interpretation of Wittgenstein

Wright's diagnosis of Kripke's argument

In 'On making up one's mind: Wittgenstein on intention' Crispin Wright (1987) points out that the assumption that guides the various responses to the sceptic that Kripke considers and rejects is that the relevant epistemology is *inferential*.

Except for the dispositional response, all the answers take the form of postulating internal signs from which the meaning that one attached to '+' or 'addition' is supposed to be *inferred*. Even dispositions are deployed as the source of an inference about meaning. The sceptical conclusion results from the fact that no such unique meaning can be determined by these resources.

The alternative to an inferential epistemology is instead a form of direct memory of a *sui generis* state. Now it may seem that such direct access to a state cannot be possible because of the peculiar properties of meaning. How can one have access to a state that normatively prescribes the correct use of a word? However,

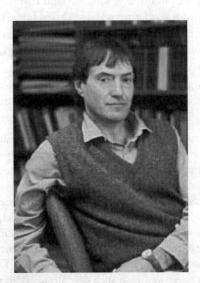

Fig 25.1 Crispin Wright

Wright points out that *intentions* have similar a property in that they *prescribe* the actions that satisfy them while we think of access to them as non-inferential.

> Had the sceptical argument been directed against intention in general, rather than at what it is tempting to regard as the special case of meaning, there is no doubt that the intuitive concept seems to contain the resources for a direct rebuttal. Since I can know of my present intentions non-inferentially, it is not question-begging to respond to the Sceptic's challenge to my knowledge of my past intentions to reply that I may simply remember them. (p. 395)

Thus Wright suggests that Kripke's sceptical argument can be defused by pointing out that it rests on the assumption that access is inferential and that this is an implausible assumption given our everyday notion of intentions more broadly. But he agrees with Kripke that there is a substantial philosophical question lurking here that stands in need of an answer. (In this he disagrees with John McDowell as we will see below.)

Wright's own version of Kripke's problem

The problem that Wright (1987) sees is this. The fact that intending serves as a good analogy for understanding rules or meanings cuts in two directions. The analogy can be used to block Kripke's sceptic but it invites a closely related question to that which motivates the rule-following considerations. How does an intention that can be arrived at in a flash normatively constrain those actions that would accord with it in the future? As we have emphasized, the normative connection between an intention and what accords with it seems as mysterious as that between understanding a rule and its correct applications. Wright, in other words, re-emphasizes the fundamental connection between the

problem of linguistic meaning and mental content. Wright deploys constructivism to explicate both.

In another paper Wright says:

> One of the most basic philosophical puzzles about intentional states is that they seem to straddle two conflicting paradigms: on the one hand they are avowable, so to that extent conform to the paradigm of sensation and other 'observable' phenomena of consciousness; on the other they answer constitutively to the ways in which the subject manifests them, and to that extent conform to the paradigm of psychological characteristics which, like irritability or modesty, are properly conceived as dispositional... It seems that neither an epistemology of observation—of pure introspection—nor one of inference can be harmonised with all aspects of the intentional. (p. 142)

Intention is only one example of a general phenomenon that also includes understanding, remembering, and deciding. In each case, the subject has a special non-inferential authority in ascribing these to herself which is, nevertheless, defeasible in the light of subsequent performance. Wright suggests that Wittgenstein's attack on reductionist explanations of such states shows that they cannot be modelled on a Cartesian picture of observation of private experiences. That is a significant result of even Kripke's summary of Wittgenstein's negative arguments. But if understanding, intending, and the like are to be modelled on abilities instead, as Wittgenstein seems to suggest but Kripke misses, how can the subject have special authority in ascribing these to herself in the light of the attack on reductionist explanation?

Wright's solution: constructivism

Wright's *constructivism* appears to provide a solution to this problem. The basic idea is to deny that there is any inner *epistemology* and to devise a constructivist account of intention instead:

> The authority which our self-ascriptions of meaning, intention, and decision assume is not based on any kind of cognitive advantage, expertise or achievement. Rather it is, as it were, a *concession*, unofficially granted to anyone whom one takes seriously as a rational subject. It is, so to speak, such a subject's right to declare what he intends, what he intended, and what satisfies his intentions; and his possession of this right consists in the conferral upon such declarations, other things being equal, of a *constitutive* rather than descriptive role. (p. 400)

All other things being equal, a speaker's sincere judgements constitute the content of the intention, understanding, or decision. They determine, rather than reflect, the content of the state concerned. This sort of approach fits well with the initial summary of a discursive psychological approach at the start of this chapter in which meanings are constructed in ongoing conversations rather than fixed in the head by mental representations. Meanings and mental states are constructed in ongoing conversations.

Wright's account of first person access is of independent interest whether or not it reflects Wittgenstein's concerns. But for now it is important to note that it assumes that there is a real problem to be overcome. It assumes that meanings are not the sort of thing that can be grasped without some further underlying story. To see how this assumption is not compelling, compare Wright's account of Kripke with that of McDowell.

John McDowell's interpretation of Wittgenstein

McDowell (1992) offers an initially similar diagnosis to Wright of the misleading assumption that underpins Kripke's argument. According to him, Kripke subscribes to a 'master thesis' about what can come before the mind: 'the thesis that whatever a person has in her mind, it is only by virtue of being interpreted in one of various possible ways that it can impose a sorting of extra-mental items into those that accord with it and those that do not' (p. 45).

Understanding meanings and mental states

This talk of 'sorting' is meant to capture the *normativity* implicit in understanding meaning. If one understands the meaning of a word one can sort the correct applications of it from the incorrect ones. One knows to which worldly items it applies. As McDowell (1992) emphasizes, this applies not only to understanding meaning but to intentionality in general. 'An intention, just as such, is something with which only certain future states of affairs would accord. Quite generally, a thought, just as such, is something with which only certain states of affairs would accord.' (pp. 45–46).

McDowell on Kripke's key assumption

Because Kripke assumes that the mind can only be populated by mental items that impose a normative constraint on worldly items once they have been interpreted, his sceptical deployment of a regress of interpretations is made possible. In other words, Kripke's assumption that the epistemology at play is based upon an inference follows from his view of what can come before the mind. Thus responses to the sceptic seem to have to attempt to justify knowledge of which rule guided past behaviour by inference from some free-standing mental item or state that could be interpreted in a number of different ways. Similarly access to one's current intentional states will require the interpretation of a mental item. 'The master thesis implies that whatever I have in my mind on this occasion, it cannot be something to whose very identity that normative link to the objective world is essential. It is at most something which *can* be interpreted in a way that introduces that normative link, although it can be interpreted differently.' (p. 46).

Scepticism defused

If the assumption that underlies the sceptical argument is that mental states require interpretation to connect them to actions or to the worldly items that satisfy them, then there is a way of escaping scepticism about meaning and intentionality. Instead of concluding from the fact that the normativity of meaning cannot be recovered from mental items that 'just stand there like a sign-post' that there are no facts about meaning, one can instead conclude that it cannot be *reduced* to non-normative phenomena. The alternative is, in other words, to claim that meaning something by a word is a *sui generis* state. The fact that Kripke rejects this alternative suggests that he subscribes to an assumption like Fodor's representationalist claim that if meaning is real it must really be something else.

The only argument that Kripke has against non-reductionism about content is an argument from 'queerness' similar to that of Fodor:

> Perhaps we may try to recoup, by arguing that meaning addition by 'plus' is a state even more *sui generis* than we have argued before. Perhaps it is simply a primitive state, not to be assimilated to sensations or headaches or any 'qualitative' states, nor to be assimilated to dispositions, but a state of a unique kind of its own ... Such a state would have to be a finite object, contained in our finite minds. It does not consist in my explicitly thinking of each case of the addition table, nor even of my encoding each separate case in the brain: we lack the capacity for that. Yet (§195) 'in a *queer* way' each such case already is 'in some sense present' ... What can that sense be? Can we conceive of a finite state which *could* not be interpreted in a quus-like way? How could that be?   Kripke (1982, pp. 51–52)

Kripke argues that any *sui generis* conception of meaning is too strange to form a natural part of the world. But in the passage just quoted he builds an important qualification into his description. A *sui generis* meaning would be a finite *object* contained in our finite minds. If this were the only model— meaning as a free-standing inner object—then Kripke would be right to reject a *sui generis* non-reducible conception of meaning. No object before the mind's eye could fix the normative consequences of meaning. But to assume that meaning must be conceived this way is already to be partially committed to the cognitivist or representationalist model. Effectively Kripke assumes that either a representationalist explanation of meaning is possible or, properly speaking, there is no such thing as meaning.

A hint towards a positive account

This diagnosis shows how scepticism can be avoided but it only gestures towards what a positive account of intentionality would be like. Wittgenstein provides one further clue in a passage the first half of which Kripke quotes. The passage continues:

> It can be seen that there is a misunderstanding here from the mere fact that in the course of our argument we give one interpretation after another; as if each one contented us at least for a moment, until we thought of yet another standing behind it. What this shews is that there is a way of grasping a rule which is *not* an *interpretation*, but which is exhibited in what we call 'obeying the rule' and 'going against it' in actual cases.
> Wittgenstein (1953, §201)

This passage begins to suggest a practical reorientation of the philosophy of content. Instead of thinking of mental states as free-standing internal states or mental representations, one should think of them as more like practical abilities. But how like an ability can a state like an expectation really be? How can such talk shed light on intentionality? Further light on this question will be shed in the rest of this chapter. But a clue can be found by noting what is at issue between McDowell and Wright.

An overview of Wright and McDowell

Wright thinks that Kripke (and perhaps Wittgenstein) raises an interesting question about how we can have access to normative and prescriptive mental states. How can there be such states given that we can have immediate if fallible access to them? Wright then sets about a philosophical building project in which the content of intentional states—and thus also linguistic meaning—is constructed from subsequent judgements.

McDowell, by contrast, blames the need for this philosophical construction on a restricted picture of the sort of mental items that can come before the mind. He says:

> The question 'How is it possible for meaning to reach ahead of any actual performance?' is just a specific form of the question 'How is it possible for the concept of accord to be in place in the way that the idea of meaning requires it to be?' The Wittgensteinian response is not that these are good questions, calling for constructive philosophy to answer them. The Wittgensteinian response is to draw attention to a defect in the way of thinking that makes it look as if there are problems here.   (p. 49)

There are two important conclusions to draw:

1. Wright and McDowell agree in broad outline on the diagnosis of what is question begging about Kripkean scepticism. There is no need to *infer* what one meant on previous occasions by one's words from evidence that can be characterized in non-intentional terms. The attempt to explain the intentionality of mental states by postulating free-standing internal items that need *interpretation* cannot succeed.

2. They disagree on what conclusion to draw. Wright then goes on to work within this conception to build a concept of meaning that does not require interpretation. One does not interpret one's past or present intentions but builds them from subsequent avowals. (Although it is arguable that this is itself akin to an 'inferentialist' conception.) McDowell, by contrast, rejects the assumption that both Kripke and Wright share about mental states or items. There is no need to take this restrictive and philosophically charged attitude to the nature of mental states.

But if McDowell is right, what light can be shed on the nature of mental states? What is the alternative to representationalism?

The clue that Wittgenstein gives instead is that meaning should be explained through practice. But to try to clarify what difference invoking practice makes to an account of intentionality that can serve as an alternative to representationalism, we will now

turn to examine two contemporary philosophers: Dennett and Davidson.

The connection between Wittgenstein and Davidson and Dennett

Both Dennett and Davidson share a fundamentally third personal account of intentionality. They both set about explaining the nature of intentional mental states by examining how such states are ascribed from a third person perspective. Dennett discusses the Intentional Stance while Davidson discusses Radical Interpretation. A key issue in assessing their views, however, will be closely related to that between McDowell and Wright.

Interpretation

McDowell and Wright disagree on the kinds of things that can be present to the mind, on whether mental states can be essentially connected to worldly states of affairs or whether they can only connect once they have been so interpreted. A key issue in the exegesis of Dennett and Davidson is the nature of the input for explanation and characterization via the Intentional Stance or Radical Interpretation. Is the input bare sounds and movements, which are then *interpreted* as being about something, as having meaning or being actions with purposes? Or is it that the input must always be thought of as intentionally characterized and ineliminably norm-laden? This question will be raised first with respect to Dennett's account and then investigated more thoroughly in the context of Wittgenstein-inspired criticism of Davidson. By answering it, fresh light will be shed on the kind of practical reorientation, which stands as an alternative to reductionist naturalism.

One important preliminary point: both Dennett and especially Davidson place a great deal of weight on the notion of interpretation. We have just seen, however, that there are good reasons for rejecting a picture of mental states as free-standing internal states that need interpreting. Wittgenstein summarizes this by saying that understanding is not a matter of interpretation. Thus it may seem that Wittgenstein has already refuted Davidson's whole approach. This is an important question. But for now it is worth noting two points:

1. The Intentional Stance and Radical Interpretation do not turn on the interpretation of *internal* mental items such as signs or symbols but are a matter of making sense of the behaviour of other people. Persons and their behaviour are the object of interpretation rather than bizarre denuded internal mental objects.

2. Even a Wittgensteinian account requires some explanation of how it is possible to have access to other minds and interpretation of behaviour seems at least a plausible start.

It is a matter of live debate whether the difference between the interpretation of inner mental objects and the behaviour of people is sufficient to defuse Wittgenstein's criticisms but we will put this issue aside initially.

Reflection on the session and self-test questions

Write down your own reflections on the materials in this session drawing out any points that are particularly significant for you. Then write brief notes about the following:

1. What is the relation between rules, meanings, and mental states?

2. How different are the interpretations of Wittgenstein put forward by Kripke, Wright, and McDowell?

3. Do they target the same thing?

4. What is Kripke's sceptical argument and can it be defused?

5. What positive lessons can be learnt? What is the connection to cognitivist approaches?

Session 3 Dennett and the Intentional Stance

Dennett's carving up of the philosophy of mind

Daniel Dennett, an empirically minded philosopher, has written on three main areas within the philosophy of mind (as well as other subjects). His account of consciousness is set out in *Consciousness Explained* (1991a). *Elbow Room* (1984) sets out his views on freedom of the will. *The Intentional Stance* (1987) gathers his papers on intentionality. These are the papers that are relevant here. More recently he has also written on Darwinian evolutionary theory.

The first reading in this session is the most definitive statement of Dennett's views on the problem of accounting for intentionality in the philosophy of thought and language. In it he sets out his version of an interpretation based, non-reductive, theory of the nature of mental content. As will become clearer it is rather a minimalist theory, although not quite so minimalist as it might at first appear.

EXERCISE 4 (30 minutes)

Read the extract from:

Dennett, D. (1987). True believers: the Intentional Strategy and why it works. In *The Intentional Stance*. Cambridge, MA: MIT Press, pp. 13–35. Reprinted in Rosenthal, D. M. (1991). *The Nature of Mind*. Oxford: Oxford University Press, pp. 339–349. (Extract: pp. 340–341)

Link with Reading 25.2

• What, according to Dennett, is it to be the possessor of content-laden mental states?

• To what extent is Dennett's account of mind and meaning realist?

Realism versus instrumentalism

Dennett suggests that there is a traditional distinction between realism and instrumentalism about mental states, which can be summarized as follows:

• *The realist strategy*: mental states are literally states in the head, whose existence is independent of our description. Mental states on this view are like micro-physical entities postulated by physical science. It is thus a completely objective matter what mental state someone has.

• *The instrumentalist strategy*: beliefs are 'merely' a product of our methods of interpreting each other. Such methods do not *describe* pre-existing entities and are interest relative. Hence the objectivity of ascriptions is doubly questionable.

Dennett suggests, by contrast, that his account is broadly realist without construing beliefs and other mental states as internal states. He claims that this follows providing he can show that the adoption of an interpretative stance based on ascribing mental states is an objective matter. (Of course it is one thing for him to *say* that he is realist. It is a matter of assessment whether he is successful in this splitting the difference between the two extremes.)

Two kinds of philosophy

Dennett (1987) also distinguishes between two sorts of philosophical clarification found in the philosophy of mind. One is a form of conceptual clarification while the other relies on the development of an underlying causal theory. The distinction does not require that causality plays no part in analysis. (Some concepts essentially involve causality as a part of their analysis. To be an autograph, for example, requires a particular kind of causal history. But for most, causality need not play a part in the *analysis* of mental concepts.) Thus there are two distinct kinds of approach to the philosophy of mind: the conceptual analysis of intentional concepts within folk psychology and the postulation of an underlying causal mechanism to explain folk psychology. Dennett's work on the intentional stance is a contribution to the first. He suggests that he has been influenced in this by Gilbert Ryle (whose work was discussed in Chapter 22).

It is worth noting that Dennett thinks that the second strategy is a perfectly reasonable enterprise but that no elements of the brain will correspond to the elements isolated in folk psychology. Intentional system theory is a normalization of folk psychology and subpersonal theory looks at lower level workings of the brain. *But there will be no identity between elements of these two accounts*.

A key distinction

In order to clarify the distinction between these two approaches to the philosophy of mind, and to flesh out the form of realism he intends to support, Dennett borrows a distinction from the philosopher of science and logical positivist Hans Reichenbach (1891–1953). This is between:

+ *abstracta*: calculation bound 'entities' or logical constructs such as centres of gravity; and

+ *illata*: posited theoretical entities such as electrons

The degree of Dennett's realism can now be described using this distinction. He holds that mental states are abstracta. They play a role in a calculus of human action in the way that centres of gravity play a role in mechanics. But they are not themselves internal states, which can play a causal role like illata. By contrast, representationalists like Fodor, are, in Dennett's phrase 'industrial strength realists' because they do posit internal states with causal powers.

Dennett's 'stance' approach to intentionality

If mental states are abstracta, something more has to said about the theoretical context in which they have their life. Dennett (1987) suggests that folk psychology, the network of lore that enables us to make sense of, explain and to some extent predict one another, should be clarified as a form of Intentional Stance. He clarifies this in turn, by contrast with two other stances.

Physical stance

One stance that one can take to predict and explain items or systems in the world is the physical stance. To predict the behaviour of a system determine its physical constitution, physical impingements, and physical laws. If *physicalism* is true (see Chapter 23), this stance should apply in principle to any system in the world. If all events are physical events, then the physical stance should have an unlimited field of application, again in principle. In practice, however, it is not always the best method of explaining or predicting. Suppose I wish to predict when my digital alarm clock will ring in the morning. One strategy would be to take it apart, investigate its circuits and chips, determine its voltages and currents and apply physical laws to make a prediction. In the case of an alarm clock this should work in principle because it is a physical mechanism whose behaviour is presumably fixed by (deterministic?) physical laws. In practice, however, the best way is to see what time the alarm has been set for and predict that that is the time at which it will ring. Hence the design stance.

Design stance

To predict the behaviour of a designed system ignore its physical details and predict that it will behave as it is designed to do. One adopts this stance for *pragmatic* reasons in the case of designed systems. Clearly, as not everything has been designed it has limited application. Even in the case of designed systems, it fails to apply when things break down and those breakages cannot be explained from this stance.

Intentional stance

Finally, in the case of some systems, even the design stance is 'practically inaccessible' and Dennett advocates instead the Intentional Stance. One adopts this in the case of rational systems. Determine what beliefs and desires it ought to have given its position in the world and determine what behaviour would further its ends and predict that it will behave like that. (Note that these are not so niche sensitive as the design stance.) Again the initial justification is pragmatic: one adopts it for practical ease.

The kind of explanation implicit in folk psychology as explained as the Intentional Stance is:

+ *justificatory*: explanations of behaviour provide rational justifications of it with respect to the beliefs and desires ascribed.

+ *idealized*: its explanations do not depend on subsumption under laws but by comparison with an ideal (cf. chapter 23 for a similar claim used as an objection to functionalism).

+ *abstract*: in that the states postulated need not be intervening distinguishable states of an internal causal system.

+ cashed out in terms of *evolutionary* biology. Dennett offers a biological explanation of why we are the sort of creatures for whom the Intentional Stance is predictive.

Dennett's bald key claim

Having set out this preliminary ground work, Dennett can then advance his central claim about the nature of mental states. In 'True believers' (1987) he sets out a bold central claim and then modifies it to take account of potential criticism. *To be a believer is to be explained by the Intentional Stance.* This view aims at the kind of relaxed view about entities which Pragmatists in the philosophy of science (such as James, Dewey, and Pierce) advocated. In Dennett's hands the view begins something like this: there is nothing more to the question as to the existence and nature of content-laden mental states, or intentionality in general, than the question of whether the Intentional Stance applies and what its nature is. As it is described simply as a useful way of predicting some 'systems' in accordance with an idealized rational structure, it seems that there is no specific philosophical worry left. Note also that such an account places meaning, construed in the broad sense of Sabat and Harré firmly in the public sphere. It is to be understood as internal to a public method of interpreting one another.

Despite the simplicity and appeal of this bald approach, Dennett is, however, forced some way away from such a fully pragmatist and minimalist account.

Dennett's bald claim modified

Further qualifications to the bald claim

The bald first statement of Dennett's view is of very wide scope and includes animals, chess playing computers, and plants, and even lightning. Keep in mind the attraction of such a bald claim. Like pragmatism about theoretical entities in the philosophy of science, it says that all there is to the question of the real existence of beliefs is that they appear in working theories of phenomena and there is no higher metaphysical standard. There is no further question about the realism of theoretical items beyond the fact that they appear in successful theories. But this advantage has to be diluted by responding to a number of objections that Dennett (1987) anticipates in 'True believers' (and elsewhere).

Objection 1

The crude definition is manifestly too wide because one can ascribe beliefs and desires to a lectern to predict its behaviour. Perhaps it desires to remain unnoticed and believes that by keeping still it will remain unnoticed. If the bald claim were correct then a lectern would have mental states as its staying still when not moved might be explained by ascribing to it the desire not to be noticed and the belief that by staying still it can best realize this.

Dennett's response

In response to this thought, Dennett narrows the claim as follows: To be a believer is to be predicted *with pragmatic advantage* by the Intentional Stance. We gain nothing by invoking the Intentional Stance in the lectern case that we did not have via the physical stance. The physical stance provides as quick a predictive hold.

Objection 2

Pragmatic advantage is, however, perspectival. It depends on what other explanatory resources are also available. Clever Martian neurologists and physicists might be able to predict our behaviour without deploying the Intentional Stance. So, *for them*, we have no mental states. So possession of beliefs is not an objective matter but depends upon the perspective of the interpreter.

(Note that for committed social constructionists this might be an acceptable view. They might well agree that whether I have mental states might always be a relative matter, depending on what you, for example, say about me.)

Dennett's response

Dennett, however, denies that there is no advantage even to the Martians of adopting the Intentional Stance. Without it, the Martians miss the *pattern* that is present in intentional action. Different ways of greeting share the fact that they are all greetings but lack any common physical basis. The same broad behaviour can be realized in different physical movements. This is the same point that was deployed as a criticism of type identity physicalism in chapter 23. (Compare this with what we can call 'financial transaction physicalism'. This is the claim that all monetary units are realized by physical states of some sort or other. But what physical properties do all the possible realizations of £500 have in common? Some are collections of coins, others notes, others handwritten cheques, others computer memory stores.) Thus even in the case of the Martian physicists, the Intentional Stance has pragmatic advantage. It is the only stance from which these patterns can be described. Thus there is no threat of perspectivalism and nothing wrong with Dennett's account of mental states.

Objection 3

Of course any such response raises an obvious counter response. One might argue that the Martians miss nothing by not adopting the Intentional Stance. Their predictions as to human sounds and movements, for example, are perfectly exact even though they cannot hear meanings in those sounds or see actions in those movements. In other words one might bite on the bullet and insist on an instrumental reading of the Intentional Stance such that the intentional pattern the Martians are supposed to miss is just an *artefact* of the theory and has no theory independent existence.

Adjudicating this disagreement largely depends on what sense can be given to the idea that there really are patterns in the affairs of humans which are not merely artefacts of our view of one another. One line of inquiry would be to press the claim that there is something wrong with the explanatory apparatus implicit in the Intentional Stance. This is the claim made by eliminativists that intentional vocabulary is misleading and the generalizations of folk psychology are largely false. (See Fodor's defence against such an attack in Chapter 24.) Dennett himself goes on to defend the reality of patterns in general and thus claims that the patterns of action are simply one case of that general phenomenon and we will now turn to a further paper of his. But it is also worth briefly flagging a related debate to which we will return in the next session on Davidson.

The next session will discuss Davidson's account of 'Radical Interpretation' and a Wittgenstein-inspired criticism of it. The criticism will turn on whether in interpretation, meaning or intentionality is read into bare sounds and movements, or whether in fact that conception of access to other minds is incoherent. If it is incoherent then the alternative view is that sounds and movements have always to be described in intentional terms. The same kind of worry and response can be made in Dennett's case. The worry is that if the Intentional Stance is construed as a way of reading meaning into bare sounds and movements that do not have any intrinsic meaning, it will face a similar Wittgensteinian objection. Thus one way of seeing Dennett's defence of real patterns in human behaviour is a way of heading off that criticism.

Thus while a first way of reading the Intentional Stance is as a way of interpreting more primitive hard behavioural data by reading into them an intentional pattern, in fact Dennett is driven to claim that the patterns are there anyway, whether we detect them of not. A similar transition seems to be present in Davidson's work. While the early Davidson (and some of his contemporary commentators) suggested that the input to Radical Interpretation comprised bare sounds and movements, the later Davidson suggests that this is not possible. Once the input is denuded of its meaning, there is no way to recover it. As we will see, this point is a reiteration of Davidson's general claim that intentional notions cannot be reduced to non-intentional notions. But we will return to this issue at the end of Session 4.

The Intentional Stance *describes* 'real patterns'

Although Dennett is classed as an instrumentalist in some textbooks and collections on the philosophy of mind, that places him too far from realism. Instrumentalism is, after all, usually characterized as the view that theoretical entities are postulated *merely* in order to save the observable phenomena and that theoretical statements are (literally construed) neither true nor false. But Dennett does not subscribe to such an antirealist view of mental states. He does not think that the pattern described from the Intentional Stance is merely in the eyes of the beholder. Dennett develops the idea of there being a real pattern in human action, which is *described* by the Intentional Stance in his paper 'Real patterns' (1991b).

Dennett starts by pointing out that we can use folk psychology to interpret the speech and actions of one another. But we can also use it successfully to predict action. Whence this power? Without some sort of pattern to events, nothing is predictable. So Dennett takes it upon himself in this paper to characterize further the kind of pattern that is on the one hand, there to be perceived from the Intentional Stance, but is on the other invisible from the Physical Stance.

Returning to the idea that mental states are abstracta (like centres of gravity, by contrast with illata like electrons), Dennett suggests that debate about whether abstract objects are real can take two separate paths:

1. metaphysically, do abstract objects in general exist?
2. scientifically, is a specific putative abstract object good in the sense of useful?

Dennett suggests, in a pragmatist tradition, that only the second is a useful and therefore good question. (It concerns usefulness after all.) Thus he suggests that the efficacy of the Intentional Stance can be attributed to the fact that the patterns it picks out are real, in the sense of being scientifically useful patterns. That is, the standard of reality to be appealed to. That is why Dennett invokes Fine's Natural Ontological Attitude, which insists on keeping such questions at the natural scientific level (see Chapter 13 for a discussion of Fine's 'NOA').

What is a pattern?

Using the analogy of a 'bar code' pattern of a series of black and white stripes partly degraded with black spots in the white bars and vice versa, Dennett (1991b) suggests that there is a real pattern 'if there is a description of the data that is more efficient than the bit map, whether or not anyone can concoct it' (p. 34). In the example at hand, it is more efficient to say that there is such and such a bar code of overall black and white stripes and then to pick out the exceptional spots than to describe each pixel individually. Thus there *really is* a pattern there to be perceived, despite the 'noise' obscuring the underlying 'signal'.

This talk of a real pattern obscures a further complication: perhaps there are several different ways of describing the fudged bar code, which differ in the way they pick out further patterns in the way apparently exceptional spots litter the wrong stripes. Dennett suggests that within this rivalry, decisions have to be made on pragmatic grounds of ease of use. This suggests a limit to the finality of questions of just *which* pattern is real. There may be no unique answer.

To give a particularly rich example of a pattern, Dennett discusses the 'Game of Life' developed by John Horton Conway,

John von Neumann Professor of Mathematics at Princeton University. The Game of Life is an example of a 'cellular automaton'. It is 'played' on a chessboard-like array of squares and is supposed to depict the life of cells on that array. Each cell is either briefly on or off. Each has eight neighbours. Three simple rules govern whether in the next 'turn' the cell is on or off. If two of its neighbours are on then it stays in its present state (whether off or on). If three are on then it turns on. For any other number it turns off.

Given these simple rules some initial shapes give rise to further stable patterns while others die away. Some patterns reproduce themselves slightly to one side and thus seem to move across the board. These are called 'gliders'. There are a number of other recognizable patterns. In principle, also, there are shapes that represent the functioning of a Turing machine or abstract computer.

This suggests different levels of description are available. One can describe the individual pixels of the Game of Life board. Or one can describe the patterns. Describing the pattern of development of patterns in the two-dimensional array of pixels using the vocabulary of stable shapes such as 'gliders' or more dramatically as describing an array of pixels as representing a Turing machine gives one much easier predictive power than relying on the piece-meal calculation of each generation of pixels. This provides an analogy for predictions of human behaviour using the Intentional Stance:

The scale of compression when one adopts the intentional stance toward the two-dimensional chess-playing computer galaxy is stupendous: it is the difference between figuring out in your head what white's most likely (best) move is versus calculating the state of a few trillion pixels through a few hundred thousand generations. But the scale of the savings is really no greater in the Life world than in our own. Predicting that someone will duck if you throw a brick at him is easy from the folk psychological stance; it is and will always be intractable if you have to trace the photons from brick to eyeball, the neurotransmitters from optic nerve to motor nerve and so forth (Dennett, 1991b, p. 42).

So is Dennett a realist then?

This leads back to the question of how realist or instrumentalist Dennett is. He himself provides a comparison with Fodor, Davidson, Rorty, and Churchland. Using the analogy of the hard lines of the bar code pattern for the 'determinacy' of ascriptions using the Intentional Stance he comments:

Fodor and others have claimed that an interior language of thought is the best explanation of the hard edges visible in 'propositional attitude psychology'. Churchland and I have offered an alternative explanation of these edges... The process that produces the data of folk psychology, we claim, is one in which the multidisciplinary complexities of the underlying processes are projected *through linguistic behaviour*, which creates an appearance of definiteness and precision, thanks to the discreteness of words.

So whereas Fodor's 'industrial strength realism' requires that the pattern detected by folk psychology is a reflection of a pattern in the head, Dennett thinks that there may be no under-lying pattern *there*. This means that no such pattern in the behaviour of neurological states can ever be detected by scanning techniques. Instead, the pattern of meaningful action, although caused by a variety of processes many of which are in the head, occurs at no deeper level than is observed in daily transactions.

The Intentional Stance and discursive psychology

So much then for Dennett's third person approach to meaning and intentionality. It provides one way of construing the claim in Sabat and Harré that meaning is constituted in conversations. But it is a weaker claim than those authors probably support. For Dennett, meaning is best understood as connected to its own special explanatory stance: the Intentional Stance. But this does not mean that meaning is merely read into otherwise intrinsically meaning-less sounds and movements. The pattern of meaning is there all along and is *described not constructed* by the Intentional Stance. Nevertheless it is a necessary feature of content-laden mental states that they are accessible to others because just what we mean by intentionality is that for which the Intentional Stance is the right strategy. To refine our understanding of this view, and the role of rationality in it, we will turn to another philosopher who shares many of the assumptions of Dennett: Donald Davidson.

Reflection on the session and self-test questions

Write down your own reflections on the materials in this session drawing out any points that are particularly significant for you. Then write brief notes about the following:

1. How does thinking about the Intentional Stance clarify the nature of meaning?

2. Are mental states real objects?

3. Are mental states, according to Dennett, merely aspects of a *theory* of human behaviour or are they independent of that?

4. Does the Intentional Stance construct or describe mental states?

Session 4 Davidson and Radical Interpretation

Davidson's overall philosophical profect

Donald Davidson's (1917–2003) philosophy can be roughly classi-fied as concerning the metaphysics of mind (early work on which is largely gathered in his *Essays on Actions and Events*, 1980) and the philosophy of thought and language (early work on which is largely gathered in his *Inquiries into Truth and Interpretation*,

1984). We have already met his contribution to the former: anomalous monism and the token identity theory, in Chapter 23. This chapter will focus instead on his account of content based around an account of 'Radical interpretation' (1984 pp. 125–141).

A full understanding of Davidson's account of intentionality would require a detour into the philosophy of language proper and Tarski's theory of truth. But that is not necessary for present purposes and the discussion here will focus on what another philosopher, and influential interpreter of Davidson, Richard Rorty has described as Davidson's 'philosophy of language of the field linguist'. We will say a little more about Davidson's relation to Tarski below. The reading sets out the key ingredients of Davidson's approach to the philosophy of content. It is quite dif-ficult on a first reading. Guides to Davidson's philosophy are listed in the Reading guide at the end of this chapter.

EXERCISE 5 (30 minutes)

Read the extracts from:

Davidson, D. (1984). Radical interpretation. In *Inquiries into Truth and Interpretation*. Oxford: Oxford University Press, pp 125–141. (Extracts: 125–126, 127–128, 136–137.)

Link with Reading 25.3

◆ What is the connection between ascriptions of beliefs and meanings?

◆ What is the evidence for Radical Interpretation?

◆ What is the role of rationality?

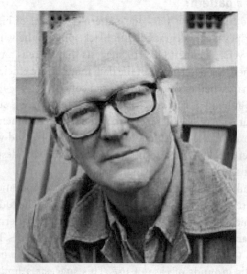

Fig 25.2 Donald Davidson

The nature of Radical Interpretation

Davidson's approach to content is based on the thought experiment of Radical Interpretation. In order to clarify what we understand when we understand our home language, Davidson considers the conditions of possibility of the Radical Interpretation of a foreign language. Radical interpretation is supposed to be interpretation from scratch. It is a philosophical abstraction from the kind of interpretation undertaken by a field linguist having first contact with an alien tribe. Such interpretation—it is assumed—cannot appeal to bilingual speakers or dictionaries. It precedes those resources. Furthermore, according to Davidson, it cannot make substantial use of the content of the mental states of speakers. Whatever the connection between mental content and linguistic meaning, Radical Interpretation must earn access to, and cannot simply assume, facts about both.

Instead, interpretation must rely only on the evidence of correlations between utterances and the circumstances which prompt them. As he says elsewhere: '[The radical interpreter] interprets sentences held true (which is not to be distinguished from attributing beliefs) according to the events and objects in the outside world that cause the sentence to be held true.' (Davidson, 'A coherence theory of truth and knowledge', p. 317).

Davidson and Quine

The idea of thinking about thought from the perspective of an anthropologist, which is central to Davidson's account of Radical Interpretation is a development from the American pragmatist philosopher W.V.O. Quine's (1908–2000) account of radical *translation* which Quine discussed in an influential book *Word and Object* (1960). There are, predictably, similarities between the accounts. But, without assuming knowledge of Quine, two key differences help shed light on Davidson's project. One is that Quine hoped that the thoughts ascribed by the imaginary anthropologist could be correlated by him or her to bodily stimuli construed as what things occur at the boundaries of the subject's body or proximal stimuli. The other is that Quine thought that the anthropologist need presuppose no mentality on the part of the subject and earn the right to ascribe mentality on the basis of mere descriptions of the subjects bodily reactions. Davidson rejects both of these behaviouristic and reductionistic assumptions (although he calls them 'details'!):

> The crucial point on which I am with Quine might be put: all the evidence for or against a theory of truth (interpretation, translation) comes in the form of facts about what events or situations in the world cause, or would cause, speakers to assent to, or dissent from, each sentence in the speaker's repertoire. We probably differ on some details. Quine describes the events or situations in terms of patterns of stimulation, while I prefer a description in terms more like those of the sentence being studied; Quine would give more weight to a grading of sentences in terms of observationality than I would; and where he likes assent and dissent because they suggest a behaviouristic test, I despair of behaviourism and accept frankly intensional attitudes toward sentences, such as holding true
>
> Davidson (1984, p. 230).

Davidson takes the evidence available to Radical Interpretation to be worldly facts and events in the environment of speakers together with the occasion of their utterances. The role that evidence plays is important and we will return to this issue having sketched in the underlying purpose of Radical Interpretation.

Davidson's methodology

Davidson's methodological claim for the philosophy of content is that one can clarify the nature of both linguistic meaning and mental content more generally by examining how it is determined in Radical Interpretation. 'What a fully informed interpreter could learn about what a speaker means is all there is to learn; the same goes for what the speaker believes.' ('A coherence theory' p. 315). Because it is intended to serve this philosophical purpose, Davidson concentrates on clear instances of Radical Interpretation—interpretation by field linguists—rather than the 'interpretation' that, he claims, takes place in daily life: 'All understanding of the speech of another involves Radical Interpretation. But it will help keep assumptions from going unnoticed to focus on cases where interpretation is most clearly called for: interpretation in one idiom of talk in another.' (*Inquiries*, pp. 125–126).

Nevertheless, Davidson also thinks that everyday understanding of language involves Radical Interpretation. That claim puts some strain on the initial characterization of Radical Interpretation as interpretation from scratch because it undermines the contrast that such a description presupposes. If everyday 'interpretation' is also really from scratch, what example could there be of interpretation which was not? But while Davidson makes this claim in part to defend his radical thesis that communal language plays no explanatory role in human understanding, it can also be seen as a reminder of the purpose of considering Radical Interpretation. That is to shed light on what is understood when we understand speech and action generally. (We will return to the question of whether everyday understanding can be called interpretation at all.)

Seen in this light, Davidson's account of Radical Interpretation serves as an example of reconstructive epistemology. It does not matter that our everyday understanding of other speakers does not proceed using the tools that Davidson describes. One might argue that everyday understanding works on the implicit and tacit assumption that others speak the same language as oneself. But Radical Interpretation does not aim at phenomenological accuracy. Similarly, it would not matter if real field linguists made use of interpretative heuristics less minimal than those Davidson describes. An example of that might be the assumption that any newly encountered human language has a good chance of being related to some previously encountered language. Such a principle would be useful if it turned out that all human languages sprang from a common source. As Radical Interpretation is really a piece of reconstructive epistemology, it concerns the ultimate *justification* of ascriptions of content whatever the actual process of reasoning that gives rise to them. It concerns the evidence that could be used to justify both the possible heuristic suggested above and also our everyday methods of understanding. Radical interpretation is supposed to explain what the assumption that other speakers speak the same language amounts to. (According to Davidson, one of its consequences is that such talk of shared languages is of no philosophical significance.) It is precisely because it plays a clarificatory—via a justificatory—role that Radical Interpretation is characterized in the austere terms that it is.

The connection between meaning and mental states

Davidson thinks that, ultimately, facts about mental content have to be determined in the same way as facts about linguistic meaning. The meanings of words and the contents of beliefs are interdependent. This presents a principled difficulty for Radical Interpretation:

> A speaker who holds a sentence to be true on an occasion does so in part because of what he means, or would mean, by an utterance of that sentence, and in part because of what he believes. If all we have to go on is the fact of honest utterance, we cannot infer the belief without knowing the meaning, and have no chance of inferring the meaning without the belief.   (*Inquiries* p. 142)

Thus the interpreter faces the task of unravelling two sets of unknowns—facts about meaning and facts about beliefs—with only one sort of evidence: linguistic actions which depend on both meaning and belief. How can the interpreter—to change the metaphor—break into this interdependent set of facts?

Davidson's twofold solution

Davidson's solution has two ingredients. First, he takes the evidential basis of Radical Interpretation to be the prompted assent of a speaker, which he characterizes as 'the causal relation between assenting to a sentence and the cause of such assent.' The reason for this is that it is possible to know that a speaker assents to a sentence without knowing what the sentence means and thus what belief is expressed by it (or vice versa). Characterizing a speaker as holding a particular sentence true is an intentional interpretation of what is going on—the speaker is described by relation to a propositional content—but it does not *presuppose* a semantic analysis of the sentence. That will be derived later.

The Principle of Charity

The second step is to restrain the degrees of freedom of possible beliefs in order to interpret linguistic meaning. The interpreter must impose his or her own standards of truth and coherence on ascriptions of beliefs and meanings. There must be a presumption that any utterance or belief held true really is true. Further, in a significant range of cases, the interpreter must assume that the object of an utterance, and the belief the utterance expresses, is the cause of the utterance and belief. (As Davidson remarks in a passage quoted above, the relevant cause is a worldly state of affairs rather than, as Quine (1960) suggests, proximal stimulation at the boundary of the body.) This complex of related assumptions governing the rationality imputed—generally briskly labelled the Principle of Charity—enables interpretation to get off the ground. If utterances are assumed by the interpreter to be generally true and to concern the worldly states of affairs that prompt them, then they can be correlated with those observed states of affairs. Their meaning can thus be determined. Given an overall interpretation, exceptional false beliefs can then be identified.

Holism

These a priori constraints on interpretation operate in a general manner but allow exceptions. Thus even the basic datum that a speaker holds a particular utterance true can be revised in the light of the subsequent interpretation of their other beliefs and meanings. The epistemology of interpretation is fallible and holistic. So the appeal to evidence should not be regarded as a foundational or reductive account of meaning.

(If language mastery is also holistic, such that one understands cluster of concepts, what happens if it breaks down in the case of Alzheimer's? We should expect great difficulty in understanding the speech of such sufferers. See Schwartz, M. (1990).)

The central role of rationality

But even though the constraints that Davidson points towards allow exceptions, they do suggest the following general constraint on possession of a mind. Only creatures whose behaviour and speech responses fit a general rational pattern towards others and towards the inanimate world can have minds. Minds are essentially generally rational. On the assumption that all the facts about the meanings of utterances and the contents of mental states (or about intentionality) are available to a third person radical interpreter, and on the assumption that Radical Interpretation is only possible by presupposing a largely rational pattern of behaviour, then possession of intentionality or mindedness in general presupposes an underlying rationality. The first assumption is justified by the claim that it is fundamentally our predicament if asked to justify our claims to know other people's minds, including those who taught us language. The second is justified by consideration of the constraints on the success of Radical Interpretation. Davidson's conclusion is that rationality plays a *constititive* role in what we understand by having a mind. We could not understand a creature as having a mind if their behaviour did not display such rationality. This claim is sometimes called the Constitutive Principle of Rationality.

An overview

Davidson's basic strategy can now be summarized as follows. On the assumption that Radical Interpretation has access to all the facts about content, content can be explicated by examining the conditions of possibility of Radical Interpretation. Thus Davidson assumes that content can be captured by a third person perspective and that it can be fully analysed through its connection to the action of agents in the world. In the weakest sense of the term, Davidson can be seen, in his philosophy of content at least, as promoting a form of philosophical behaviourism providing that this is not construed in its Quinean and reductive sense. Meaning is explicated through its role in human behaviour. (In fact, he adds to this picture of content a token identity theory in order to explain the *causal* role of content to which was discussed in Chapter 23.) This is why Rorty describes this basic approach as the 'philosophy of language of the field linguist'.

Box 25.1 Davidson's formal theory of meaning

A fuller understanding of Davidson would also require a detour into his more formal work. This box provides a brief optional sketch of how Davidson construes a theory of meaning. The Reading guide is listed at the end of the chapter.

Davidson suggests that the output of the process of Radical Interpretation can be regimented in a formal theory of meaning. He assumes that the theory can be extensional and employ merely the first order logic employed in Tarski's account of truth.

Although it plays a central role in his philosophy of language, Davidson fails to explain the purpose of the theory of meaning. What is it that such a theory explains? He makes two comments on the subject. One is that knowledge of such a theory would suffice for understanding (*Inquiries*, p. 125). The other is that it is a necessary condition for languages to be learnable that a constructive or compositional account of the language could be given (p. 3). But even taken together these do not explain how provision of a theory of meaning helps the philosophical enterprise of clarifying linguistic and mental content.

He is more explicit in his reasons why such a theory should be extensional. Theories of meaning of the form: s means m— where m refers to a meaning of a word or sentence—have proved to be of little use in showing how the meaning of parts of a sentence structurally determine the meaning of the whole. Things can be improved by modifying the theory's structure to be: s means that p, where p stands for a sentence. But this still leaves the problem that 'wrestling with the logic of the apparently non-extensional "means that" we will encounter problems as hard as, or perhaps identical with, the problems our theory is out to solve.' (p. 22). The solution is to realize that what matters for such a theory is not the nature of the connection between s and p but that the right s and p are connected:

> The theory will have done its work if it provides, for every sentence s in the language under study, a matching sentence (to replace 'p') that, in some way yet to be made clear, 'gives the meaning' of s. One obvious candidate for matching sentence is just s itself, if the object language is contained in the meta-language; otherwise a translation of s in the meta-language. As a final bold step, let us try treating the position occupied by 'p' extensionally: to implement this, sweep away the obscure means that, provide the sentence that replaces 'p' with a proper sentential connective, and supply the description that replaces 's' with its own predicate. The plausible result is

(T) s is T if and only if p. (p. 23)

Further reflection suggests that, if this is to serve as an interpretation, the appropriate predicate for T is truth. We want the sentence s to be true if and only if p.

The proposed theoretical schema has the further advantage (and motivation) that it dovetails with Tarski's account of truth. Tarski's account is pressed into service to show how the meanings of sentences are constructed from the meanings of words (which are themselves abstracted from the meanings of sentences). Davidson's use of Tarski inverts its normal explanatory priority. Tarski assumes that the notion of translation can be presupposed in the task of giving an extensional definition of truth in a language. By contrast, Davidson suggests that truth is a suitably primitive, transparent, and unitary notion to shed light on meaning. With this change of emphasis, Davidson can then borrow Tarski's technical machinery to articulate the structure of a given language.

Without going into its details it is worth noting one result of this strategy. Davidson replaces the intensional connective 'means that' with the extensional form s is true if and only if p. Clearly, however, the fact that the truth values of the left- and right-hand side of this conditional agree does not in itself ensure that the right-hand side provides an interpretation of the sentence mentioned on the left. In Tarski's use of the T schema, it can simply be assumed or stipulated that the right-hand side provides an interpretation by being the same sentence as, or a translation of, the sentence mentioned on the left. But Davidson has to earn the right to that claim. His suggestion is that instances of the T schema should not be thought of as interpretative in themselves (p. 61). Rather, it is the fact that each instance can be derived from an overall theory for the language, which also allows the derivation of many other instances of the T schema with the right matching of truth values, which is interpretative.

Given this regimentation, meaning is fundamentally holistic. As instances of the T schema are not interpretative in isolation, it makes no sense to ascribe meaning to elements of language in isolation from the rest. Only in the context of a language does a sentence (and therefore a word) have meaning. It is this, rather than the holistic epistemology of meaning ascription, which is the fundamental source of holism in Davidson.

Aside from the apparent benefits of escaping the intensionality of 'means that' and of the ability to make use of Tarski's formal machinery, Davidson's proposed structure for theories of meaning has another advantage. The formal machinery allows the derivation of a set of instances of the T schema. This seems to make it particularly apt for formalizing the output of Radical Interpretation because, as summarized above, that begins by assuming that uninterpreted utterances are held true. Thus it seems that this formal theory of meaning encapsulates the close relation between truth and meaning emphasized in Radical Interpretation.

It is worth noting here, however, that although Radical Interpretation and the formal theory of meaning sit fortuitously together, they are independent. Even if Radical Interpretation did not rely on the basic evidence of assertions but on imperatives instead, for example, its output might still be formalized using a theory of meaning based on Tarski. Reciprocally, Davidson's account of Radical Interpretation might be used to explicate meaning in general—its connection to action in the world, the connection between meaning and belief—without adopting the formal theory of meaning as a representation of language. The latter option what is pursued in this chapter.

Davidson on content-laden mental states

Having sketched out Davidson's account of the connection between determining meanings and determining beliefs via Radical Interpretation, we can now turn to a discussion of the clearest account that he gives of what ascribing mental states amounts to (Davidson, 1991).

Davidson's attack on 'inner objects' or mental representations

In 'What is present to the mind?' Davidson argues against the coherence of any picture of the mind which includes internal mental objects. The picture Davidson criticizes is this. To have a propositional attitude is to have an object, a propositional object, before, or present to, the mind. These objects have two roles: 'They *identify* a thought by fixing its content; and they *constitute* an essential aspect of the psychology of the thought by being grasped or otherwise known by the person with the thought.' (Davidson, 1991, p. 198).

Davidson argues that these two roles cannot be reconciled. The problem is that we take it for granted that we have authority over the content of our own mental states. But if their content is fixed by an object which is known to the thinker, then to know the content of one's own thoughts requires that one knows which object is before the mind: 'The trouble is that ignorance of even one property of an object can, under appropriate circumstances, count as not knowing which object it is.' (p. 198).

It is this difficulty that leads to the philosophical postulation of special objects, such as Fregean senses, which must be what they seem and seem what they are. But, as Davidson points out, there simply are no such objects. Thus: 'If the mind can think only by getting into the right relation to some object which it can for certain distinguish from all others, then thought is impossible. If a mind can know what it thinks only by flawlessly identifying the objects before it, then we must very often not know what we think.' (p. 201)

This argument clearly differs from Wittgenstein's or Kripke's argument against inner mental objects. Wittgenstein's argument turns not on problems with the identification of such inner objects but on the impossibility of them serving their supposed function in constituting thoughts. As Kripke makes clear, no object before the mind could have the normative connections that content-laden mental states have to their fulfilment conditions. But despite this difference in argument, the end result is the same. Thinking a thought is not a matter of having an internal object before the mind's eye. This convergence of critical views is more than just a matter of interest. The obvious question that follows from the negative result is: What then is it to have a content-laden mental state? Davidson provides a clear general account.

Davidson's response to the critical arguments is to accept the first role of objects and reject the second:

> It does not follow, from the facts that a thinker knows what he thinks and that what he thinks can be fixed by relating him to a certain object, that the thinker is acquainted with, or indeed knows anything at all about the object. It does not even follow that the thinker knows about any *object* at all. Someone who attributes a thought to another must ... relate that other to some object, and so the attributer must, of course, identify an appropriate object, either by pointing to it or describing it. But there is no reason why the attributer must stand in any special relation to the identifying object; all he has to do is refer to it in the way he refers to anything else. We specify the subjective state of the thinker by relating him to an object, but there is no reason to say that this object itself has a subjective status, that it is 'known' by the thinker, or is 'before the mind' of the thinker.   (p. 203)

The analogy with weights

He suggests that the ascription of propositional attitudes to people functions like the ascription of weights to objects. Objects stand in various relations of the form: weighing more than, weighing less than, weighing twice as much as. For simplicity, these relations and ratios can be represented by the use of a standard. This enables weights to be ascribed to objects directly using numbers. Thus one can say of an object that it weighs 5 kg. But this does not require the addition of *kilograms* into our ontology in addition to weighty objects. On this picture, numbers are in no sense *intrinsic* to the objects that have weight or *part* of them:

> What are basic are certain *relations* among objects: we conveniently keep track of these relations by assigning numbers to the objects ... In thinking and talking of the weights of physical objects we do not need to suppose there are such things as weights for objects to have. Similarly in thinking and talking about the beliefs of people we needn't suppose there are such entities as beliefs.   (p. 205)

The last sentence might be taken to imply some form of eliminativism. But it is clear from the context that that is not the position that Davidson supports. Instead he offers a picture that clarifies what should replace mental representations or internal objects in the metaphysics of thought. No objects come before the mind's eye. Nor are there internal states that encode propositional attitudes. But this implies neither eliminativism nor any crude behaviourism in which mental states can be identified one-to-one with dispositions to act. To be in a mental state with a certain content is for one's behaviour to be explicable from a third person perspective using a system of propositional attitudes. (This is a necessary condition. To rule out things that do not need to be so described but which could be—such as planets—Davidson would have to add some further condition. One such further condition might be that using the system of propositional attitudes must have pragmatic advantage over a merely physical description (cf. Dennett 1987, p. 23). However, the formal project of formally specifying necessary and sufficient conditions is not Davidson's purpose.)

Davidson and Wittgenstein

The general picture that Davidson suggests resembles a Wittgensteinian account in which behaviour is explained by reference to a system of content-laden states governed by normative and rational relations. It can also be coupled with Wittgenstein's claim that one learns new behaviour when one learns a language. One learns behavioural repertoires that essentially turn on one's linguistic abilities. And one also learns to describe oneself in the language of propositional attitudes. Thus there is no prospect of reducing content-laden mental states to behavioural dispositions that could be described without the resources of the language of propositional attitudes. But all that is essentially involved in having content-laden mental states is the possession of complex practical abilities and behaviour.

It is worth thinking back to the account of mental states discussed in Chapter 23 on the metaphysics of mind. There Davidson's account of anomalous monism was described as centring on the claim that mental states are identical with (i.e. they just are) physical events. Davidson claims that the account described above is also consistent with that identity theory. But given the criticisms of the identity claim, we can see this account of mental states as a possible alternative. Mental states are essentially relational states ascribed to people from a mundane third person perspective to make sense of their behaviour.

An objection to Davidson's account?

A phenomenological objection to talk of interpretation

We can now return to the objection mentioned earlier to the central notion of interpretation in Davidson, and which is also implicit in Dennett. This objection runs as follows: both Davidson and Dennett overintellectualize the 'process' of making sense of one another and thus get the phenomenology wrong. The experience of hearing meaning in someone's utterance does not feel like interpretation.

This is a criticism raised by Steven Mulhall (1990), a Wittgensteinian philosopher, on the basis of work both by Wittgenstein and Heidegger. Although it is an important criticism of approaches to meaning based on interpretation, and thus is a constraint on any form of 'discursive psychology', it will be argued below that it is not decisive.

EXERCISE 6	(15 minutes)

Read: the extract from Mulhall, S. (1990). *On Being in the World* London: Routledge. (Extract: pp. 99–106)

Link with Reading 25.4

Davidson deploys the idea of *interpretation* to shed light on the nature of meaning and understanding.

♦ To what extent do we interpret one another?

♦ How like Radical Interpretation is everyday understanding?

♦ Do the differences matter to Davidson's project?

The background to Mulhall's criticism is . . .

In *On Being in the World* (1990) Stephen Mulhall develops a phenomenological objection to Davidson on the basis of his (Mulhall's) reading of Wittgenstein.

The background to Mulhall's criticism is Wittgenstein's (1953) discussion of seeing aspects in part II section xi of the *Philosophical Investigations*. According to Mulhall, Wittgenstein's discussion of seeing aspects and aspect perception in the second half of the *Investigations* is of general importance. It attempts to characterize the immediacy with which we experience the significance of pictures, themes, words, actions, and the world more generally. The point of the discussion of cases of *changes* in aspect, such as Gestalt switches, is to illustrate the general nature of *continuous* aspect perception. The latter characterizes our normal immediate response to words and to the world. Forging a link with the Heideggerian notion of the ready-to-hand, Mulhall (1990) suggests that our experiences of the world are usually immediately charged with significance. They do not have to be interpreted.

. . . Wittgenstein's account of secondary sense

Wittgenstein describes this kind of immediate understanding of the meaning of a word in isolation as a form of understanding. But while this is not a metaphorical use of the word 'understanding' it is nevertheless a *secondary* use (Wittgenstein, 1953, p. 216). A secondary use is one which we find natural given the primary use, but which is discontinuous with, and could not be used to teach, the primary use. Nor is it metaphorical. An example is the use of 'fat' in the thought that Wednesday is fat. Clearly Wednesday cannot in any ordinary sense be compared with other fat or thin things. And it would be optimistic to attempt to teach the meaning of fat by giving Wednesday as an example. Nevertheless, many language users give spontaneous expression to the thought that Wednesday is a fat day.

Thus, although we may wish to say that a word or action can be immediately experienced as bearing a meaning in isolation, this does not contradict Wittgenstein's general connection of meaning with an extended practice or technique. The concept of meaning is used in its primary sense in the latter defining context and only in a secondary sense in the former. This distinction is important because Wittgenstein (1953) claims that, although as a matter of contingent fact it is not true of us, it would make sense to ascribe to someone understanding in the primary sense unaccompanied by the secondary aspect. He calls such a person 'aspect blind' (p. 213).

Mulhall (1990) argues that Davidson's use of Radical Interpretation to explicate meaning must be fundamentally mistaken because it presupposes that language users are all aspect blind:

[I]t is important to note that the metaphysics of the given—revealed as it is by Davidson's emphasis upon the concept of 'interpretation'—exemplifies to perfection the stance of the interlocutor in Section xi of the *Philosophical Investigations*. Incapable of finding a home for the notion of continuous aspect perception in his framework of thought, Davidson describes the everyday phenomenon of perceiving words and other human beings as if aspect-blindness were the normal human state. His emphasis on processes of theorizing as necessary in order to organize bare sounds and movements into words and actions... commits him implicitly to a general notion of visual perception as divided into what is really seen and what is interpreted, ie as divisible in precisely the way Wittgenstein rejects.   (p. 106)

A key idea here is that no account of understanding one another that turns on *interpretation* can be right because interpreting one another is an exceptional activity rather than the norm. Normally our understanding is instantaneous and requires no such activity. To think instead that understanding is always a matter of interpretation is to subscribe to what Mulhall labels an empiricist view in which one experiences bare sense data (whether visual or auditory) and then interprets it.

If Mulhall is right, this is a serious criticism. He is charging Davidson with commitment to the same sort of picture that was criticized in chapter 12 on the theory dependence of data. (Recall McDowell called just such a picture of the 'Myth of the Given' a general form of empiricism evident outside the philosophy of science.)

There is also a good Wittgensteinian criticism of any such picture. Recall the argument that Kripke (1982) used to show that if one tries to derive meanings from meaning-free states in the head that have to be subsequently interpreted, then scepticism about meaning is the result. A similar argument can be used on the idea that bare behaviour has to be interpreted as carrying meaning. If this were so, there would be no sense of interpreting correctly. Meanings really would just be in the eyes of the beholder (as Sabat and Harré, 1994, seem to suggest). But in fact there is good reason to think that this is an uncharitable interpretation of Davidson.

A defence of Davidson

Mulhall's argument is not a decisive criticism for three reasons:

1. It presupposes an uncharitable—if common—interpretation of Davidson that is not obligatory. While the early Davidson does indeed suggest that the evidence for Radical Interpretation should be described in neutral terms, the later Davidson explicitly criticizes the picture of any evidence for a belief 'whose character can be wholly specified without reference to what it is evidence for' (Davidson 'The myth of the subjective' p. 162). The division of perception into what is seen and what is interpreted is rejected as a (the third) dogma of empiricism.

2. Furthermore, those comments, which can be understood as expressions of Davidson's token identity theory, can be reconciled with Mulhall's criticism. The fact that meaningful utterances or actions—or even, according to Davidson, content-laden mental states—are identical with physical events or states does not imply that they are *experienced* as mere physical events and only subsequently interpreted.

3. The connection between the primary and secondary sense of meaning is far from clear. The fact that we experience the 'meaning' of words in isolation—in the secondary sense of 'meaning'—is a contingent feature of the phenomenology of meaning. Consequently, Davidson could simply reply that his account of Radical Interpretation is meant to capture only meaning proper, meaning in the primary sense. The phenomenology is a further matter. This fits with our interpretation of Radical Interpretation as merely *reconstructive* epistemology.

This third point may require a little more explanation. One of the problems of Mulhall's argument is that it is not clear what the presence or absence of the phenomenology amounts to. This is because it is difficult to describe what someone who is aspect-blind lacks without impinging on the primary sense of meaning. According to Wittgenstein, such a person cannot see aspects change, cannot see a cube 'as a cube', but nevertheless can recognize a cube (Wittgenstein *Philosophical Investigations*, pp. 213–214). Likewise she cannot experience a word as bearing a meaning in isolation but can nevertheless learn its technique of use because blindness to the secondary sense of meaning is not blindness to the first. But the moral of this separation is clear. Whatever the secondary experience consists in, as it is possible to understand and use a word without it, it is not a part of content proper. Thus it is not essential to the philosophy of content.

So even if an account of meaning or content emphasizes the role of interpretation, this need not be a fatal objection providing both that what is 'interpreted' is always conceived as meaningful—so meaning isn't merely read into it—and that talk of interpretation is not regarded as a phenomenologically accurate account of our experience. It can still be useful to talk of interpretation because it sheds light on the constraints that govern the way we make sense of each other including, for example, the central role of rationality at work here. This helps shed light on what could be meant by discursive psychology. But before returning to the first, clinical, reading, there is one other useful philosophical approach to consider.

Reflection on the session and self-test questions

Write down your own reflections on the materials in this session drawing out any points that are particularly significant for you. Then write brief notes about the following:

1. What thought experiment lies at the heart of Davidson's account of intentionality?

2. What does this presuppose about the accessibility of meaning? What key terms does Davidson deploy?

3. What effect does that have on Davidson's claims about mental states and meaning?

4. Does Davidson's account aim at phenomenological accuracy?

5. What is Davidson's attitude to inner mental representations?

Session 5 Singular thought and the division between mind and world

Another challenge to representationalism and cognitivism

This final philosophical session will examine a different kind of objection to representationalist theory of mind. This comes neither from Wittgensteinian argument about the normativity of thought (and thus that no world-independent inner state can sustain the normativity of thought), nor from advocacy of the mundane third person perspective on meaning taken by both Dennett and Davidson. Instead it is drawn largely from attention to a particular kind of thought that we all sometimes have: thoughts about objects identified merely by our direct perception of them. These are generally called 'singular thoughts'. (An example is the sort of thought you have about this page in front of you if you are thinking '*That* page is difficult!'.)

As the discussion in this session argues, the very possibility of such thoughts shows that the idea of the connection between mind and world underlying representationalism is mistaken.

Neo-Fregean theories of thought

The first reading in this session (linked with Exercise 7) is another from the work of the American-based English philosopher John McDowell. As well as being a commentator on the work of Wittgenstein, McDowell is also a key figure in an approach to the philosophy of content called *neo-Fregean* philosophy of thought and language. It is Fregean in that, as an approach to the philosophy of thought, its central concept is that of *sense*, which was introduced by Frege to stand in contrast to that of reference.

Sense and reference

The distinction between sense and reference was discussed as part of Kripke's theory of names in chapter 23. It was introduced by Frege as part of an account of what is understood by a speaker when they understand a name such as, in Greek, 'Hespherus', or the 'Evening Star' as it is translated. Because a speaker may know when to apply 'Hespherus' and also 'Phosphorus' (the 'Morning Star') but may not know that they stand for one and the same planet (Venus, in fact), Frege concluded that what is understood when a speaker understands a name is not simply what it refers to. (If it were so, then the Ancient Greeks would counterintuitively have understood the same thing by both 'Hespherus' and 'Phosphorus'.) Instead, he suggested, one knows its sense. As a way of fleshing out this term he suggested that the sense stands to a referent as the 'mode of presentation' construed as a viewpoint stands to what is so presented. And he gave, as an analogy, the idea of different views of the same object from different points or through different portholes.

In the example just given it is clear that the senses can be thought of as descriptive (the morning or evening star). The sense determines the object by containing a description.

McDowell following the work of the late Gareth Evans, has argued that in fact senses do not have to be construed as descriptions which specify worldly objects as we will shortly see.

Health warning

The next reading (linked with Exercise 7) is, perhaps, the most difficult piece of philosophy so far encountered in this chapter. There is much in the paper from which it is drawn that is not directly relevant to this chapter but the key message has important consequences for thinking about thought. It begins with some comments on Russell's theory of descriptions, which we will now summarize. Read these comments again after reading the article.

EXERCISE 7   (60 minutes)

Read the extract from section 8 of:

> McDowell, J. (1986). Singular thought and the extent of inner space. In *Subject, Thought and Context* (ed. P. Pettit and J. McDowell). Oxford: Oxford University Press, pp. 137–168. (Extract: pp. 158–161)

Link with Reading 25.5

◆ Try to work out what McDowell's objections are to a Cartesian picture of mind whether Descartes' or a modern materialist variant.

The Russellian background

A key background to the paper from which the extract is taken is discussed in the first four sections. Sir Bertrand Russell distinguished between what he called *logically proper names* and merely apparent names that have quite a different semantic structure. Logically proper names feature in *singular propositions*, which for simplicity we can think of as *singular thoughts*. A logically proper name is purely referential. It takes its meaning—what it contributes to a thought in which it features—simply by going proxy for the thing it named. As a result, if such a name fails to refer—for whatever reason—the singular thought it goes to make up would not be a proper thought at all. There would be something missing. It would be a kind of nonsense.

Russell argued that there are, however, very few logically proper names. Indeed he seems to have thought that only 'this', 'that' (when referring to sense data) and perhaps 'I' were such. A consequence of this (and probably its motivation) was that the sort of reference failure just envisaged was not possible (because one could not be so mistaken about the presence of sense data or oneself). So everything else that we would normally call a name, such as 'Moses', had to be construed differently. Russell deployed a logical analysis called the Theory of Descriptions to explain how such 'names' functioned.

The theory of descriptions

This logical 'theory' was first deployed by Russell to account for non-referring descriptive *phrases*. The most famous example of these is the sentence 'the present king of France is bald'. If an utterance of this sentence were successfully to have meaning it seems at first that it would have to be successful in referring to an individual—the king of France—and asserting of him that he is bald. But this first thought faces a problem. As there is no present king of France there would be something wrong with an utterance of the sentence now. It seems it would lack a clear meaning. To avoid this consequence, Russell analysed the sentence as making instead a conjunction of three claims:

1. There is one king of France.

2. There is no more than one King of France.

3. That thing is bald.

This conjunction of sentences (properly, utterances) is not meaningless. It is simply false because one of its conjuncts is false.

Russell suggested that apparent names such as 'Moses', which were not logically proper names, really stood for some such descriptive content as 'the leader of the Israelites'. Thus sentences about Moses could be analysed in the same way as those about the King of France.

Names, reference failure and two kinds of knowledge

McDowell (1986) points out that, although Russell realized the possibility of there being sentences or thoughts that were vulnerable to a radical form of failure—just in the case that the thing to which they refer does not exist—he deployed the Theory of Descriptions to make sure that this would never, as a matter of fact, happen. As the only sentences that contained genuine names referred to sense data, one would never be in error about them.

This distinction in the semantics of real and apparent names—in other words what they contribute to sentences containing them—was reinforced by an underlying epistemological distinction that Russell advocated. Russell suggested that thought made contact with everyday objects in two ways: either by specifying a description that the object satisfied or through direct contact or acquaintance. Hence the distinction between knowledge by description and knowledge by acquaintance. Russell supposed that one could only be directly acquainted with sense data and perhaps oneself. Thus the only logically proper names refer to these and all other 'names' are really disguised descriptions.

McDowell's extension of the idea of singular thoughts to everyday objects

McDowell (1986) suggests that the idea of object-dependent, or singular, thoughts can be taken from Russell and made more general. Instead of only being directly acquainted with sense data one can be directly acquainted with a range of everyday objects in direct perceptions and perceptual thoughts. The linguistic sign of such thoughts is a demonstrative expression of the form 'That cup is red!'.

> A typical visual experience of, say, a cat situates its object for the perceiver: in the first instance egocentrically, but, granting the perceiver a general capacity to locate himself, and the objects

he can locate egocentrically, in a non-egocentrically conceived world, we can see how the experience's placing of the cat equips the perceiver with knowledge of where in the world it is (even if the only answer he can give to the question where it is is 'There'). In view of the kind of object a cat is, there is nothing epistemologically problematic in suggesting that this locating perceptual knowledge of it suffices for knowledge of which object it is (again, even if the only answer the perceiver can give to the question is 'That one'). So those visual experiences of objects that situate their objects can be made out to fit the account I suggested of the notion of acquaintance: abandoning Russell's sense-datum epistemology, we can say that such objects are immediately present to the mind ...   (p. 140)

But as well as drawing the idea of direct acquaintance and singular thoughts from Russell, McDowell also draws on Fregean work on thought. (This is why he talks of singular *thoughts* rather than singular *propositions*.) Frege's outlook is characterized in the following way:

> Frege's doctrine that thoughts contain senses as constituents is a way of insisting on the theoretical role of thoughts (or contents) in characterizing a rationally organized psychological structure; and Russell's insight can perfectly well be formulated within this framework, by claiming that there are Fregean thought-constituents (singular senses) that are object-dependent, generating an object-dependence in the thoughts in which they figure.   (p. 233)

The first part of this quotation reiterates McDowell's methodological commitment to a Fregean or neo-Fregean philosophy of thought or content. This is centred round the notion of *sense* that McDowell here describes as playing a role in characterizing *a rationally organized psychological structure*. Recall the example of Hespherus and Phosphorus above. The same person could rationally take a different view to sentences that said the same thing about Hespherus and about Phosphorus because they may not realize that the sentences are about the same thing. This 'intuitive criterion of difference' marks out the thoughts expressed by the two sentences as being, or having, different contents. So in charting a person's rationally organized psychological structure one would want to individuate their thoughts with a finer grain than simply the level of the objects to which they refer. One needs also to take account of the senses, or the 'modes of presentation' of referents, which make up their thoughts.

What makes McDowell's remarks novel (albeit he is following the work of his late colleague Gareth Evans in making this point) is that a broadly Fregean focus on sense and not reference can be combined with the Russellian idea of singular thoughts (i.e. thoughts that are object-dependent) providing that one can think of some senses as fixing their referents more directly than by a description. (Recall that the Hespherus–Phosphorus example turns on associating different descriptions with the different names.) An example of a singular, or object-dependent, thought is what is expressed by the phrase 'this cup' in the sentence 'This cup is blue'. Think of this as how the cup is thought about when one thinks 'this cup ...'.

Russell's resistance to this is a sign of his Cartesianism

McDowell suggests, however, that this extension of singular thoughts to cover everyday objects would be rejected by Russell as nonsense for reasons that have to do with the Cartesian assumptions behind Russell's underlying view of the mind.

In a fully Cartesian picture, the inner life takes place in an autonomous realm, transparent to the introspective awareness of its subject; the access of subjectivity to the rest of the world becomes correspondingly problematic, in a way that has familiar manifestations in the mainstream of post-Cartesian epistemology. If we let there be quasi-Russellian singular propositions about, say, ordinary perceptible objects among the contents of inner space, we can no longer be regarding inner space as a locus of configurations which are self-standing, not beholden to external conditions; and there is now no question of a gulf, which it might be the task of philosophy to try to bridge, between the realm of subjectivity and the world of ordinary objects.

McDowell is here making two corresponding points:

1. In a Cartesian picture of the mind, there is no possibility of being in error about one's own thoughts in the way that is possible if there can be singular thoughts about everyday objects. Such thoughts might fail if there were no appropriate object to have thoughts about, because for example, of hallucination. The Cartesian picture can be more or less defined by the way in which it buys immunity to error here. It construes the mental or inner as a realm that is independent of the world of objects. (Of course it must *align* with the outer world if thoughts are to be *true*. But to *have* thoughts does not depend on standing in a relation to the world.) McDowell describes this picture as of a realm of configurations, which are self-standing, not beholden to external conditions.

2. But *if* one is prepared to accept the possibility that thoughts might fail in the way outlined, there is a corresponding gain. It is no longer the case that thought is cut off from the world. It is no longer the case that thoughts are construed as free-standing mental representations, which then have to be re-connected to the world through causal or evolutionary theories, for example.

Cartesian scepticism as the source of this picture

Section 5 of McDowell's (1986) paper attempts to diagnose how this conception of the inner came about, linking it to Descartes' sceptical project. The details of that historical project do not matter here but it is worth briefly noting one idea that has a bearing on epistemology. McDowell suggests that, on a Cartesian picture of the mind, our experience is taken to be notionally separable from the world that brings it about. Imagine two cases: one in which someone directly perceives a dagger before them and another in which they hallucinate that there is a dagger before them.

On a Cartesian picture, there is something in common to both cases: an experience as of a dagger, one might say. In the former

case this mental state is caused by a real dagger while in the latter it is not. This *highest common factor theory* contrasts with McDowell's preferred view: the *disjunctive theory* of experience. In this, experience is construed as either directly of a dagger or merely an appearance of such contact. The difference is that on the latter theory, in veridical experience, there is direct access between a subject and the world. The subject is not cut off from the world by a 'veil of ideas'. This is an important distinction for epistemology but not directly relevant to this Part except in the way it reinforces the general worry about the connection of mind and world.

McDowell's first (explicit) objection to the Cartesian picture

The final paragraph of section 5 brings out more clearly the connection between the highest common factor view of experience and the Cartesian view of the mind. It presents an underlying objection to a Cartesian account of experience. If one thinks of experience as self-standing and independent of the world (as it is in the highest common factor theory) then:

> This makes it quite unclear that the fully Cartesian picture is entitled to characterise its inner facts in content-involving terms—in terms of its seeming to one that things are thus and so—at all … there is a serious question about how it can be that experience, conceived from it own point of view, is not blank or blind, but purports to be revelatory of the world we live in.

So if one is in some sort of inner state that is common to both veridical experience and hallucination, what is it about that state which is about the world. If one can never have direct unmediated contact with the world of objects, how can one's inner states be about that world?

The same criticism applies to representationalism and cognitivism

Sections 6 and 8 of the paper apply these objection to a Cartesian picture of the mind to modern views. McDowell (1986) argues that modern pictures of the mind such as functionalism, representationalism, and cognitive science fall to the same underlying objection. While modern views are not dualist in the sense of embracing an immaterialist theory of mind, they nevertheless preserve the central idea that there is an inner realm (in this case literally spatially inner) that comprises self-standing items. As such they are open to the same charge of darkness.

A related objection cashed out in terms of sense

McDowell connects this objection to modern positions back to the central role of sense in neo-Fregean philosophy of thought and language. He points out that the idea of subjects having different thoughts with different senses standing for the same object in the world has to be explained in, say, representationalism by different internal happenings. It cannot be explained by what happens outside the subject because the same outside object may be involved in thoughts with different senses. But, McDowell

710 CHAPTER 25 2. ANTIREDUCTIONISM AND DISCURSIVE PSYCHOLOGY

argues, nothing that goes on inside in the way that representationalism construes it will help either because there is no reason to think of these self standing internal objects as carrying meaning, as being about the world. The inner realm in such accounts remains dark.

A summary so far

We can now stand back and think about the main point of this paper as far as this chapter and Part goes. McDowell attempts to undermine an underlying Cartesian assumption about the philosophy of mind that he thinks is present in the semantic theorizing of Russell and his more recent heirs (the latter are discussed more in later sections of the reading). This is the assumption that the mind is independent of the world. Once that assumption is in place, however, it makes thought's bearing on an outer world mysterious. Representationalists think that they can make some reply to this by devising causal mechanisms to explain how inner symbols become charged with meaning. But McDowell argues that such causal connections will still leave the inner world dark and meaningless.

It is this Cartesian assumption of world independence that stops Russell from drawing more general conclusions from his idea that some thoughts might indeed be object-dependent. But trapped within Cartesian thinking, Russell restricted such thoughts to those involving logically proper names whose scope was radically limited to pointing to sense data and thus not genuinely world-dependent thoughts after all. McDowell suggests that one should take seriously the idea that thoughts can be partly constituted through direct acquaintance with the world by construing such acquaintance as normal perception of objects (rather than of sense data). If so then the very idea of there being a gulf between an inner world of thoughts and an outer world of objects will be undermined. Singular thoughts are the thoughts that they are (such as the thought that that cup is red) partly in virtue of a perceptual ingredient that singles out the cup in front of me. They are essentially world-involving.

The second (implicit) criticism

This account of what is going on in McDowell's (1986) paper leaves one missing piece of the jigsaw. It concerns the difference between descriptive thoughts and singular thoughts. Now this distinction is found in Russell's logical work. But a rough and ready distinction can be brought out again making use of Frege's 'intuitive criterion of difference'. Two thoughts are distinct (i.e. they are, or have, different contents) just in the case that it could be rational for the same subject to take different views about their respective truth.

Now consider two assertions which I might now make using two different sentences,. Think whether these assertions express distinct thoughts or contents:

1. 'The cup in room S2.54 of the Warwick Philosophy department is red.'

2. '*That* cup is red.'

By Frege's intuitive criterion these do *not* express the same thought even if they say of the same object (the cup in my office) the same thing (that it is red). This is because it would be rational of me to accept the second but not the first if I did not realize that I was sitting in room S2.54 (although in fact I am).

The two thoughts expressed by these assertions are distinct in form. One is a *descriptive* thought that specifies the cup in question using a description: 'The cup in room S2.54 of the Warwick Philosophy department'. The other is a *singular* thought that specifies the cup in question directly from a perception (note that 'that!' is not a description). Singular thought theorists such as McDowell and Evans have argued that there is no way of specifying a descriptive content that would coincide with a singular thought such that it would never be rational to agree to one and reject the other. In other words they think that such disagreement would always be possible and thus that singular thoughts always have different content from descriptive contents.

Why singular thoughts cannot be accommodated within representationalism

With this additional piece of the jigsaw, we are, at last able to see why McDowell's view of the mind is incompatible with any broadly representationalist or cognitivist approach in which thoughts are identified with inner structures in the brain. If we, for the moment, disregard the criticism that self-standing configurations in the brain would not have content at all, and would remain dark, then it might be conceivable that descriptive thoughts could be modelled as blue prints realized by structures in the brain. That is, if we allow some content to internal symbols (how?!) they might underpin descriptive thoughts by coding descriptions that worldly objects could *satisfy*. Thus internal structures might come to be about worldly objects. (To repeat we still haven't said how even the descriptive elements get their content.) But as singular thoughts do not work like this, they cannot be fully linguistically coded in a description.

This suggests that there is a principled objection to the idea of explaining thoughts by invoking internal vehicles of content or mental representations. While such a programme might conceivably work for descriptive thoughts, it cannot work for singular thoughts because in their case there is nothing to be so coded. Worldly objects themselves partly constitute the content of singular thoughts and thus their content cannot be captured in internal symbols.

Two open questions

This argument is important because it forms one of the foci of much recent thinking about the philosophy of content in the UK. The neo-Fregean approach is obviously not without its critics. While exploring these would take us beyond the scope of this course, here are two lines of inquiry.

1. What is the role of real objects in constituting the content of thoughts? As we saw in Session 4, Davidson argues that while it is necessary for interpreters to relate subjects with objects in

propositional attitudes in order to make sense of their speech and action, it is not necessary for the subjects to have a 'psychological' or perhaps better a 'psychologistic' connection to them?

2. Can McDowell and the neo-Fregeans really reconcile the idea of acquaintance with the Fregean notion of sense? McDowell (1986) comments in the reading linked with Exercise 7 that this can be done providing one distinguishes between objects being constituents of thoughts (a Russellian idea) and objects figuring in thoughts (a neo-Fregean idea). But what is the distinction between these two. Why will senses not serve as just the sort of veil of ideas that the neo-Fregeans criticize in Cartesianism.

Summary of the 'philosophical' sessions on antireductionism

We can now return to examine the thrust of the more explicitly *philosophical* sessions in this chapter. Consider again the two challenges raised at the start of the chapter. One is the challenge to find a place in nature for meaning given that it is unlikely, to say the least, that 'aboutness' will feature in any final account of the world arrived at in physics. A reductionist response to this challenge is to attempt to explain how intentionality is itself the product of purely physical properties. Cognitivist neuropsychology shares just that aim. And like most reductionist philosophy, it starts with an assumption, motivated by an analogy with computers, that human information processing requires internal states or representations to carry that information. However, that raises the other challenge described again at the start of the chapter. The problem is that once one construes content-laden mental states as free-standing internal states standing in some causal relations, it becomes mysterious how they can also be about anything. (Trousers hanging in a wardrobe may be independent of the world but are not about it. How does adding in some causal relations bring 'light' to the inner world?) We saw one particular version of this challenge in the discussion of how inner states might share the normative properties of mental states.

The approach discussed in this chapter, broadly shared by both discursive psychology and by antireductionist philosophers of content aims to meet the first challenge without reducing intentional notions to non-intentional notions. It does this by reminding us how meaning plays a perfectly unmysterious role in the natural world even though that is not equated with the world as described by physical science. Intentional properties cannot be described by taking the physical stance but instead by taking the intentional stance, which answers to a different constitutive principle: rationality. So rather than looking for causal patterns within the head, antireductionists look to normative and rational patterns in human actions. It is this that is gestured at, with perhaps a little clumsiness in discursive psychology to which we will now turn again.

Reflection on the session and self-test questions

Write down your own reflections on the materials in this session drawing out any points that are particularly significant for you. Then write brief notes about the following:

1. How, according to Russell, can thoughts patch onto worldly objects? What theory does he advance for the analysis of descriptive thoughts?

2. What restrictions does Russell place on what can be known by acquaintance? How have they been relaxed by recent philosophers and why? What risk does this carry for the nature of thought?

3. What significance does Russell's account of thought have for the inner representation of thought and thus for cognitivist accounts of intentionality?

Session 6 Discursive psychology and Alzheimer's disease

This final session will return to the paper with which we began this chapter: Sabat and Harré's work on Alzheimer's disease sufferers as 'semiotic' subjects, but will also look at a more careful methodological textbook on discursive psychology written by Rom Harré and Grant Gillett, a neurosurgeon turned philosopher from New Zealand.

EXERCISE 8 (30 minutes)

Look back at Sabat and Harré (see the reading linked with Exercise 1, 'The Alzheimer's disease sufferer as a semiotic subject', 1994) at the start of this chapter and then this further extract: pp 150–152

Link with Reading 25.6

Think again about the range of claims made about meaning and mental states in the research paper.

- Are they consistent?
- What support do they receive from the discussion in the rest of this chapter?
- Could the empirical findings of the paper have been arrived at using different theoretical assumptions about meaning?
- What does the overview of discursive psychology in the chapter add?

What do discursive psychologists really say about meaning?

We are now in a much better position to assess the extent to which discursive psychology really does differ from the sort of cognitivist or representationalist models discussed in Chapter 24. The question is whether a discursive model is an alternative model that is inconsistent with that other approach or whether it is complementary, differing only in emphasis, focusing on the broader context rather than what goes on in the head.

Closer attention to the article reveals that it says a number of different things about the underpinning of meaning. So as was picked out in the first session Sabat and Harré say in the abstract that 'meanings are jointly constituted by the participants to a conversation' and 'from a discursive pint of view, psychological phenomena are not inner or hidden properties or processes of mind which discourse merely expresses'. These look at first as though they are saying the same sort of thing. But we can now see that strictly this is not the case.

If one adopts the view of Dennett, Davidson, Wittgensteinians, or neo-Fregeans, the second claim is necessarily true. This is the claim that psychological phenomena (or at least content-laden mental states, propositional attitudes) are necessarily the sort of things that can be described, explained or predicted from a mundane third person stance. In other words they are necessarily available to other members of the conversation (to put it metaphorically). However, that claim need not require that meanings are constituted in this activity of interpretation. One would need a further argument to establish that claim. Even talk of *joint* constitution threatens to undermine the idea that interpretation of others can be right or wrong. But being correct in their interpretation of Alzheimer's sufferers is surely something that Sabat and Harré aim at.

Some tensions in the characterization

On the other hand, despite such occasional radical claims about the social constitution of meaning, the authors also make use of a different sort of analogy. They say: 'It is our contention that a person suffering from Alzheimer's condition is like someone trying to cut wood with a blunt saw, or trying to play tennis with a racket with a warped frame. The basic intentions may be there, but the instrument for realising them is defective.' (p. 146).

But, as Tony Hope argued in a commentary on the paper, this does not sit well with the claim about the *social* constitution of meaning. To mean something by a word is a species of intention. One means or intends to use it in a particular way. So if this is intact, all that is left for other participants in the conversation to do is to *detect* it. And that is something for which Sabat's method of time compression seems particularly well suited. But in that case, the analyst is aiming simply to describe meanings that already exist, not partially to construct them.

So is discursive psychology consistent with cognitivism?

So far then it seems that discussion of the wider philosophical background has undermined the claims of discursive psychology. It either *is not or should not be* as radical as is sometimes claimed. So one possible response is to construe it as *consistent* with the approach described in Chapter 24. If the linguistic intentions of Alzheimer's sufferers are intact even if they are difficult to detect

and describe, perhaps the non-social facts that they consist in are those described in cognitivist terms.

But as both the criticisms of cognitivism discussed in Chapter 24 and the arguments described in this chapter suggest, that happy reconciliation cannot be true. While linguistic or other intentions need not await piecemeal construction by other participants in conversations, they are not the sorts of things that can consist in mental representations processed in a 'semantic system' in the head. They depend instead on normative patterns of speech and action in human transactions. They are essentially world-involving relational states that are necessarily describable from a third person perspective. They are not hidden internal states. *That* claim of discursive psychology has been supported by the consideration of this chapter.

A more careful statement of discursive psychology?

The brisk methodological remarks in the research paper are useful guides to some of the underlying beliefs of followers of discursive psychology. Presented without the caveats and restrictions of more formal methodological works, such hastier comments are often better guides to underlying thinking and assumptions. But in a more reflective philosophical text *The Discursive Mind*, Rom Harré (here with a different co-author: psychologist and philosopher Grant Gillet) presents a more cautious statement of the nature of discursive psychology, called here the 'second cognitive revolution'. At the centre of the more cautious view is the statement: 'In this sense, the psychological is not reducible to or replaceable by explanations in terms of physiology, physics, or any other point of view that does not reveal the structure of meanings existing in the lives of the human group to which the subject of an investigation belongs.' (p. 20).

This is a good statement of an antireductionist view of intentionality and also one that begins to gesture towards the reason why such reduction is impossible. It still leaves open the question more precisely *why* the structure of meanings cannot be mapped on to or reduced to the realm of law in the way that Fodor (and others from Chapter 24) promises. But we have begun to see in this chapter and in Chapter 24 some further reasons. Internal states cannot be *about* the external world because once such states are thought of as free-standing internal states they lose their normative connections to the world that cannot be reconstructed either by acts of interpretation or by merely causal resources. (Adding in teleology 'solves' the problem as long as it is construed as *presupposing* the same normative content that was supposed to be reduced. If not it is as powerless as a pure causal story.) And in this chapter we have begun to see an alternative account of the place of intentionality in nature: as revealed in one stance towards making sense of other people and ourselves.

But there are passages in the Harre & Gillett chapter that might seem to point beyond the general account developed in this chapter. Consider this:

Thus the experimenter or observer has to enter into a discourse with the people being studied and try to appreciate the shape of the subject's cognitive world. But at this point it no longer makes sense to talk of observers and subjects at all. They are only co-participants in the project of making sense of the world and our experience of it. (p. 21)

In the context of the research article this might sound like a statement of the ongoing social *construction* of meaning. But it does not *quite* say that. Being co-participants in a project of making sense of the world might not involve being co-creators of the realm of sense. It might involve jointly tracking or *detecting* the patterns that shape human behaviour. On the other hand, the more modest reading of the passage greatly reduces the motive for saying that 'it no longer makes sense to talk of observers and subjects at all'. There is no reason to reject this distinction (just try in a practical context of psychiatric inquiry dropping the distinction!) if keeping it does not imply that only the analyst is responsible for meanings and the 'subject' is an unwitting victim. And it does not. *Both* the observer and the subject may be tracking shared meanings in the social realm. This more modest claim does not require the idea that the meanings are made up as both parties go along.

Three principles of discursive psychology

In fact, one of the striking things about Harre & Gillett's work is just how difficult it is to pin down precisely what claims about the nature of psychological phenomena it wants to advance.

The three principles which characterize the discursive turn in psychology are summarized:

1. Many psychological phenomena are to be interpreted as properties or features of discourse, and that discourse might be public or private. As public, it is behaviour; as private, it is thought.

2. Individual and private uses of symbolic systems, which in this view constitute thinking, are derived from interpersonal discursive processes that are the main feature of the human environment.

3. The production of psychological phenomena, such as emotions, decisions, attitudes, personality displays, and so on, in discourse depends upon the skill of the actors, their relative moral standing in the community, and the story lines that unfold. (p. 27).

This summary involves a slippery use of the term 'discourse'. By construing psychological phenomena as 'properties or features of discourse' it appears to make a surprising and possibly socially constructionist claim. As we normally think of language as a public phenomenon, construing psychological phenomena as features of language makes them public also. But it then reconstrues 'discourse' in an equally surprising way—'as private, it is thought'—which undermines this. Unlike our normal understanding of language, discourse can simply *be* private thought.

The same slipperiness is present in the next paragraph (on p. 27), which says that: 'discursive phenomena, for example, acts of remembering, are not manifestations of hidden subjective, psychological phenomena. They are the psychological phenomena ... There is no necessary shadow world of mental

activity behind discourse in which one is working things out in private.' (p. 27).

This passage contains a claim that fits the general approach of this chapter. Mental phenomena do not take place in a hidden realm of mental representations. However, the passage also *suggests* a more radical claim that nothing stands behind the *expression in language* of say, remembering. (This is suggested by the phrase 'behind discourse'.) It *hints* at the view that there is no mental activity behind the linguistic act of announcing one's memory. But again it does not actually say this. What it does say is that 'acts of remembering ... are psychological phenomena'. And providing one takes an 'act of remembering' *not* to mean *saying* that one remembers but actually *remembering*, then there is nothing contentious in what is actually said.

A way to interpret the reading

But perhaps the best way to read practical accounts of discursive psychology (and, in fact, the others listed in the Reading guide at the end of this chapter) is as intermediate promissory statements located between empirical work, sharing the same emphasis on the social, the external, and the linguistic, and more explicitly philosophical work on the underpinnings of intentionality.

As such an intermediate statement it serves to summarize a general claim that has received support throughout the last two chapters. Content-laden mental states are not states of the brain. Utterances do not inherit their meaning by standing proxy for such inner states. The space of reasons (again to look to Sellars' and McDowell's phrase) is an essentially world-involving and potentially social space. It is best understood from a mundane perspective that charts the meaningful behaviour of whole people going about their lives.

Such an approach does however encourage the very careful attention to language used in context set out by, eg, Sabat in the case of Alzheimer's sufferers (Sabat 2001). Such careful empirical study does not need the further more radical claim that meaning is constructed, rather than relied upon, in dialogue.

Conclusions

We can step back from the details and take stock. Discursive psychology emphasizes the importance of a wider social context for making sense of the speech and actions of subjects. As the reading shows, this emphasis can be useful for empirical reasons. But on the face of it, one need not adopt all the claims sometimes made of discursive psychology to pursue such a programme. If linguistic intentions are in tact whether or not they can be realized, then perhaps they can be investigated using a cognitivist form of psychology.

Note also that even cognitivist approaches to mind and meaning could agree that social factors were *causally* important. It is surely plausible on any account that social factors in the form of education are developmentally important for being able to think thoughts about, say the balance of payments or electrons. This is a causal dependence.

But there is at least a strand of thinking within discursive psychology that makes the further claim that relations to things outside the head play a *constitutional* rather than merely a *causal* role. We have seen that if this is the claim that meanings are constituted through the interpretation of bare sounds then it is flawed. But if it is the claim that content-laden mental states are necessarily publicly accessible and world-involving then it receives support from a range of philosophical approaches to meaning. So the general result of the philosophical work surveyed over the last two chapters is that there is general a priori support for an approach to intentionality akin to a modest form of discursive psychology by contrast with the reductionist approaches of, say, cognitive neuropsychology. (This is not to say that every or even the majority of philosophers would agree with the arguments marshalled in these chapters.)

Reflection on the session and self-test questions

Write down your own reflections on the materials in this session drawing out any points that are particularly significant for you. Then write brief notes about the following:

1. What in general is the connection between the philosophical models of meaning provided by Wittgenstein, Dennett, Davidson, and McDowell and discursive approaches to psychology and psychiatry?

2. What support is given to social constructionism? Is social constructionism necessary to distinguish discursive psychology from cognitivism?

Reading guide

◆ The discursive approach to psychology is outlined in a number of places: Church (2004) 'Social constructionist models: making order out of disorder—on the social construction of madness' (in Radden (ed.) *The Philosophy of Psychiatry*); Edwards and Potter (1992) *Discursive Psychology*; Harré and Gillett (1994) *The Discursive Mind*; Sabat (2001) *The Experience of Alzheimer's Disease*; and Sabat and Harré (1994) 'The Alzheimer's disease sufferer as a semiotic subject'.

◆ It is further discussed in Gillett (1997a) 'A discursive account of multiple personality disorder', with a commentary by Braude and a response by Gillett.

◆ It is criticized from a distinct related perspective in Coulter (1999) 'Discourse and mind'.

◆ For an introduction to the philosophy of thought and language broadly consistent with discursive approach see Luntley (1999) *Contemporary Philosophy of Thought*, and Miller (1998) *Philosophy of Language*.

Wittgenstein on rules

◆ There is a very great deal written on the interpretation of Wittgenstein's (1953) *Philosophical Investigations*. A good place to start is McGinn's (1999) *Wittgenstein's Philosophical Investigations*, and Thornton's (1998) *Wittgenstein on Language and Thought*, which contains critical discussion of Kripke, Wright, and McDowell.

◆ For an interpretation of Wittgenstein that supports a radical social constructionism see Bloor's (1997) *Wittgenstein on Rules and Institutions*.

◆ See also Coulter (1979) *The Social Construction of Mind*.

◆ A good collection of essays on Wittgenstein's discussion of rules can be found in Miller and Wright (ed.) (2002) *Rule-Following and Meaning*.

Dennett and Davidson

◆ A useful beginning to Dennett's philosophy of mind is his *Kinds of Minds* (1996).

◆ Dennett's philosophy is discussed in Haugeland 'Pattern and being' and Rorty 'Holism, intrinsicality and the ambition of transcendence', both in Dahlbom (ed.) *Dennett and his Critics* (1993). A clear statement of Davidson's philosophy is Davidson's (1984b) 'Belief and the basis of meaning' in his *Inquiries into Truth and Interpretation*, pp. 141–154.

◆ Davidson's philosophy is introduced in Evnine (1991) *Donald Davidson*.

◆ There are useful critical essays in LePore and McLaughlin (ed.) (1985) *Actions and Events*.

◆ His formal theory of meaning is debated in Dummett (1993) 'What is a theory of meaning I and II' (in *The Seas of Language*), and McDowell (1999) 'In defence of modesty' (in *Meaning Knowledge and Reality*).

◆ The origins of neo-Fregean thinking are set out in the difficult Evans (1982) *The Varieties of Reference*.

The communicative or discourse failures of some victims of Alzheimer's are explored in Schwartz (1990). These sometimes include failures to grasp concepts holistically in webs of semantically related concepts, therein posing problems for the Davidsonian project of holistic interpretation.

References

Bloor, D. (1997). *Wittgenstein on Rules and Institutions*. London: Routledge.

Braude, S.E. (1997). A discursive account of multiple personality disorder. (Commentary on Gillett, 1997a) *Philosophy, Psychiatry, & Psychology*, 4(3): 223–226.

Church, J. (2004). Social constructionist models: making order out of disorder—on the social construction of madness. In *The Philosophy of Psychiatry* (ed. J. Radden). Oxford: Oxford University Press, p. 11.

Coulter, J. (1979). *The Social Construction of Mind*. London: Macmillan.

Coulter, J. (1999). Discourse and mind. *Human Studies*, 22: 163–81.

Davidson, D. (1980). *Essays on Actions and Events*. Oxford: Oxford University Press.

Davidson, D. (1984). *Inquiries into Truth and Interpretation*. Oxford: Oxford University Press.

Davidson, D. (1991). What is present to the mind? In *Consciousness* (ed. E. Villanueva). *Philosophical Issues*, Vol. 6: Ridgeview, pp. 197–213.

Dennett, D. (1984). *Elbow Room*. Cambridge, MA: MIT Press.

Dennett, D. (1987). True believers: the Intentional Strategy and why it works. In *The Intentional Stance*. Cambridge, MA: MIT Press, pp. 13–35.

Dennett, D. (1991a). *Consciousness Explained*. Boston: Little Brown.

Dennett, D. (1991b). Real patterns. *Journal of Philosophy*, 88: 27–51.

Dennett, D.C. (1996). *Kinds of Minds*. London: Weidenfeld & Nicolson.

Dummett, M. (1993). What is a theory of meaning I and II. In *The Seas of Language*. Oxford.

Edwards, D. and Potter, J. (1992). *Discursive Psychology*. London: Sage.

Evans, G. (1982). *The Varieties of Reference*. Oxford: Clarendon.

Evnine, S. (1991). *Donald Davidson*. Oxford: Polity.

Gillett, G. (1997a). A discursive account of multiple personality disorder. (Commentary by Braude, S.E. (1997, 223–226), and a response by Gillett, G. (1997, 227–230)) *Philosophy, Psychiatry, & Psychology*, 4(3): 213–222.

Gillett, G. (1997b). Response to the Commentary on Gillett (1997a). *Philosophy, Psychiatry, & Psychology*, 4(3): 227–230.

Harré, R. and Gillett, G. (1994). *The Discursive Mind*. London: Sage.

Haugeland, J. (1993). Pattern and being. In *Dennett and his Critics* (ed. B. Dahlbom). Oxford: Blackwell, pp. 53–69.

Kripke, S. (1982). *Wittgenstein on Rules and Private Language*. Oxford: Blackwell.

LePore, E. and McLaughlin, B. (ed.) (1985). *Actions and Events*. Oxford: Blackwell.

Luntley, M.O. (1999). *Contemporary Philosophy of Thought*. Oxford: Blackwell.

McDowell, J. (1986). Singular thought and the extent of inner space. In *Subject, Thought and Context* (eds P. Pettit and J. McDowell). Oxford: Oxford University Press, pp. 137–158.

McDowell, J. (1992). Meaning and intentionality in Wittgenstein's later philosophy. *Midwest Studies in Philosophy*, 17: 40–52.

McDowell, J. (1999). In defence of modesty. In *Meaning Knowledge and Reality*. Cambridge, MA: Harvard.

McGinn, M. (1999). *Wittgenstein's Philosophical Investigations*. Routledge.

McMillan, J. (1999). Cognitive psychology and hermeneutics: two irreconcilable approaches? *Philosophy, Psychiatry, & Psychology*, 6: 255–258.

Miller, A. (1998). *Philosophy of Language*. London: Routledge.

Miller, A. and Wright, C. (ed.) (2002). *Rule-following and Meaning*. Chesham: Acumen.

Mulhall, S. (1990). *On Being in the World*. London: Routledge.

Quine, W.V.O. (1960). *Word and Object*. Cambridge, MA: MIT Press.

Rosenthal, P.M. (1991). *The Nature of Mind*. Oxford: Oxford University Press.

Rorty, R. (1993). Holism, intrinsicality and the ambition of transcendence. In *Dennett and his Critics* (ed. B. Dahlbom). Oxford: Blackwell, pp. 184–202.

Sabat, S.R. (2001). *The Experience of Alzheimer's Disease*. Oxford: Blackwell.

Sabat, S.R. and Harré, R. (1994). The Alzheimer's disease sufferer as a semiotic subject. *Philosophy Psychiatry and Psychology*, 1: 145–160.

Schwartz, M. (ed) Modular deficits in Alzheimer's-type dementia. Cambridge MA: MIT Press.

Thornton, T. (1998). *Wittgenstein on Language and Thought*. Edinburgh: EUP.

Thornton, T. (2003). Psychopathology and two kinds of narrative accounts of the self. *Philosophy, Psychiatry, & Psychology*, 10: 361–367.

Wittgenstein, L. (1953). *Philosophical Investigations*. Oxford: Basil Blackwell.

Wright, C. (1987). On making up one's mind: Wittgenstein on intention. In *Logic, Philosophy of Science and Epistemology: Proceedings of the 11th international Wittgenstein symposium* (ed. P. Weingartner and G. Schurz). Vienna: Holder Pichler Tempsky, pp. 391–404.

Wright, C. (1991). Wittgenstein's later philosophy of mind. In *Meaning Scepticism* (ed. Puhl), pp. 126–147.

CHAPTER 26

Agency, causation, and freedom

Chapter contents

Introduction

One recurrent theme of this book is the relation between reasons and causes in psychiatry. Whereas many disciplines operate with one or other form of explanation and interpretation, psychiatry operates with both. Nowhere is the tension between the two as great as the issue of freedom versus causal determinism.

Giving, asking for, and acting on reasons appears to presuppose freedom. Summarizing Kant, McDowell (1994, p. 5) puts this connection like this: 'rational necessitation is not just compatible with freedom but constitutive of it. In a slogan, the space of reasons is the realm of freedom'.

But, as the first session of this chapter will outline, the success of recent brain imaging techniques looks to cast doubt on the possibility of such freedom. In other words, our increasing ability to explain neurological function in causal terms seems to put at risk the very possibility of freedom on which reasons depend.

This chapter will examine the connection between agency, causation, and freedom. The initial route into the area will by via consideration of some issues raised by research using brain imaging techniques into disorders of agency. The first reading (linked with Exercise 1—Spence, 1996a), which concerns the exact timing of mental and physical events, sheds light both on specific disorders of agency such as 'made actions' and thought insertion but may also shed light more generally on the very idea of the freedom of the will.

To put this in a broader context, there has been considerable and inconclusive philosophical debate about whether freedom—which is central to the idea of a responsible agent—really is compatible with our growing knowledge of the workings of the physical world at least since Hobbes' time. The basic issues of that debate are almost paradoxically easy to understand and yet give rise to no clear solutions. Assume for a moment that every event in the history of the world is the result of a prior cause. This is to assume the truth of 'determinism'. If so, then whenever I think that I have a free choice of action, since the action I do choose is an event in the history of the world, it is thus caused by prior events. One may want to say that it was always going to happen. And this seems to cast doubt on my freedom to choose.

Of course most scientists now believe that determinism is false at least at the level of the microscopic. (There is *no* causal explanation of why a particular radioactive particle decays at the moment it does. Radioactive decay is *indeterministic*.) However, this does not seem to make free will any the less problematic. Rather than being caused, our actions may be the result of indeterministic whimsy at the quantum level!

Agency: a more tractable issue?

Although we will return to the issue of freedom at the very end of the chapter, we will focus on a more tractable issue raised by the clinical research into made actions, thought insertion and such like. What is it to be the agent of an action, whether mental or physical? To approach this question we will set out some of the background to the debate on whether reasons are causes. Can the very same mental states, which are invoked to explain and justify speech and action, also play a *causal* role in generating that speech and action? Are mental states part of a mechanical mind, a system of causal pushes and pulls? Or are they instead part of a different kind of description, perhaps abstract elements in a broader calculus of action explanation? What connects this issue with that of freedom is that rather than running shy of causes, a number of philosophers have argued that the very idea of action requires that it is part of the causal order.

Agency and the mind-body problem

Different answers to the question of the relation between action and causation separate different positions taken up in the mind–body debate, which was discussed in Chapter 23. Functionalism, for example, holds that mental states are individuated by their causal roles or functions. Mental states are *caused* by perceptions and other mental states and *cause* actions and other mental states. Dennett's Intentional Stance, by contrast, holds that mental states are *abstracta* like centres of gravity, which are invoked for making predictions about behaviour but are not themselves causally active. (Dennett does think that there are causal accounts that are relevant to action, such as those provided by neurophysiology. But these do not talk of *mental* types.)

Agency, causes, and reasons

This chapter will approach the reasons–causes debate through the central issue of whether causality can be used in the analysis of agency as an answer to the question: What is the difference between action and mere movement? Roughly, a causal theory of action attempts to spell out this difference by saying that actions but not movements are caused by reasons. Thus what has to be added to a mere movement to make it an action is the fact that it was caused by beliefs and desires. So, for example, the mere movement of a hand in the direction of a coffee cup, is the *action* of *reaching for the cup* if it is caused by appropriate mental states. (These may be the desire to drink and the belief that by reaching for the cup one will be able to drink from it.) In fact, however, we will see that it has to be caused *in an appropriate way*. So psychopathological cases of 'made' actions—which result from reasons that the agent disowns—present interesting material for philosophical reflection.

A causal theory of action is an analytic project, aimed at shedding light on the notion of agency (of who or what are agents, of when a movement is an action and so on) by consideration of causality. But aside from that analytic project, the issue of whether mental states can have causal effects is also important for understanding the place of mind in nature as has just been suggested. One common guiding thought is that mental properties cannot be *real* properties, genuine parts of nature, if they cannot stand in such relations. So if this is disputed it will have important consequences for how we understand mental properties by comparison with other properties charted by the physical sciences and thus the status of psychology and psychiatry.

The plan of the chapter

◆ *Session 1* will examine agency and freedom from a neurological perspective.

◆ *Session 2* will examine non-causal philosophical accounts of agency from the 1960s.

◆ Session 3 will introduce Donald Davidson's influential causal theory.

◆ *Session 4* will consider in more detail just how a causal theory is supposed to work and consider whether it can shed light on irrational action.

◆ *Session 5* will examine recent criticism of a causal theory.

◆ Session 6 will return to the broader issue of the freedom presupposed by the notion of agency.

Session 1   Agency, freedom, and neuropsychiatry

The first reading attempts to draw conclusions for the nature both of agency and free will from both accounts of psychopathological symptoms and also neurological work. It is a challenging and very clear research paper by Sean Spence, a contemporary UK neurophysiologist specializing in brain imaging.

EXERCISE 1   (45 minutes)

Read the two extracts from:

Spence, S.A. (1996a). Free will in the light of neuropsychiatry. *Philosophy Psychiatry, & Psychology*, 3: pp. 75–90. (Extracts: pp. 78–81, 83–85)

Link with Reading 26.1

Take note of the brief clinical vignettes describing made action, thought insertion, and such like.

◆ What do these suggest about the nature of agency and freedom?

◆ How do these relate to the description of Libet's work on the timing of mental and neuronal events?

◆ What are the novel consequences of such brain imaging work for free will?

Neuropsychiatry and free will

The paper begins by outlining the philosophical problem of free will: that there is a conflict between our belief that we can freely choose how to act and our belief that what happens in the world, including our actions, is the result of antecedent causes. (Spence suggests that this way of putting the problem makes free will *merely* a belief. But talk of belief in the quotation could be replaced by 'putative fact'.)

Without further details, one can already begin to see the sort of problem that the paper might address, given its title. Given that research in neuropsychiatry will, no doubt, increasingly reveal the causal processes that 'underlie' mental activity, that research will increasingly focus attention on the already familiar philosophical paradox. (To say that physical processes 'underlie' mental processes is already to take up a stance in the mind–body problem. But it is at least widely accepted that possession of brain states is causally necessary to have mental states, at least for humans.)

The two strands of argument

In fact, Spence goes on to make two different kinds of more specific claim. One concerns what might be called the 'phenomenology' of agency. It is here that the case vignettes have their role. These imply that there is some continuity between non-pathological experiences of thoughts popping into one's mind and pathological experiences of made thoughts and made actions. The other concerns experiments based on work by Libet, on the relative timing of mental and physical phenomena. These suggest that conscious phenomena lag behind characteristic neurophysical precursors.

Experiences of altered volition

To take these two ideas in turn. There are perfectly normal cases of what Spence terms 'altered volition'. These are cases where, unlike a normal experience of deliberately saying or thinking something, one either blurts something out or a thought pops unbidden into one's mind. In these cases, the 'experience of voluntary action is diminished or lost'. Subjects 'do not experience as freely willed action the impulses which produced these acts' (p. 78).

Spence goes on to consider two kinds of pathological case: the alien hand syndrome and passivity phenomena. Having set out case examples of alien hand syndrome, he summarizes them thus:

> As may be seen from these accounts the alien hand is experienced as behaving in an autonomous and purposeful way. Its interference with normal activity is such as to provoke patients to developing strategies to restrain or 'distract' the hand. The patients acknowledge that the limb belongs to them but that its actions are not under their control. Yet they do not attribute its activity to outside forces (cf passivity)...The subject loses the *experience* of free will (with respect to the affected limb), and develops an accommodating abnormal experiential belief that the limb is autonomous.   (pp. 80–81)

Spence then turns to passivity phenomena: made thoughts, made actions, made affects, and made impulses, all of which are symptoms of schizophrenia but also found in other diseases. 'The subject experiences their thoughts, actions feelings and drives as having been influenced or replaced by those of external agencies' (p. 81). Spence suggests that these also are best understood as resulting from abnormal experiences of agency or will. Drawing on work by Frith, he suggests continuity between the idea that such subjects are abnormally 'monitoring' their own volitional processes (thoughts and actions) and that they might be *experiencing* their agency abnormally. In some cases subjects do not experience a sense of volition, despite acts occurring that appear purposeful. In others the act is experienced as volitional but resulting from an impulse that is not experienced as willed by its subject.

There are differences between these two sorts of pathological case and normal cases of a lack of experience of volition—central is the delusional elaboration of an outside locus of agency—but there is also continuity. Spence concludes that 'seemingly "purposeful" action and "insightful" thought may be...distinct from the sense of "will" or "ownership" which normally attends them' (p. 83).

Summing up the first strand

So this is one strand of the paper. Although we might think of exercises of free will in action and thought as always conscious, there are both normal and pathological instances where we have thoughts or we act apparently deliberately, but do not experience those acts or thoughts as consciously willed by us. This raises an interesting pair of questions: what is to *experience* thought or action as willed by oneself? and what is it for a thought or action to *be* willed by oneself? Light will be shed on these throughout the chapter. But first we will consider the second strand of Spence's work.

The second strand of Spence's argument

The connection between the two strands

In the second strand of the paper, Spence looks to the connection between the experience of freely willed action and neuronal events. In fact this separation into two strands is a little artificial. In the passage quoted above, Spence actually says: 'seemingly "purposeful" action and "insightful" thought may be *neurally* distinct from the sense of "will" or "ownership" which normally attends them'. But at that stage in the paper, it is not clear what justification there is for such a qualification (as opposed to saying simply that there is an experiential or conceptual distinctness).

Brain imaging results

The empirical work behind the second strand is Libet's work on the timing of mental and neuronal events. Subjects were asked to note when, according to a spatial clock they could see, they chose to make a decision to move part of their body. Meanwhile their EEG and EMG data were recorded. Libet noted that there was a characteristic electrical change 850 milliseconds prior to the actual movement but also 350 ms prior to the *subjective experience* of deciding to move. 'Thus Libet et al. conclude that volitional activity is initiated non-consciously' (p. 83).

This seems a radical conclusion. It suggests that what seemed like a free decision (that one will choose *now!* to move one's finger) is precipitated by a prior non-conscious neuronal event, 350 ms earlier. And this seems to imply that the conscious decision was not itself free. As Spence notes, there is no chance of preserving a role for conscious free choice as a *veto* for an action already initiated non-consciously because that conscious event would also have to be pre-empted by a suitable neuronal event. So

if there is free will, it happens at the level of non-conscious processing and not at a conscious level of act or thought initiation.

What if 350 ms were 35 seconds?

The time-lag described by Spence is very short and this can disguise the radical nature of his claims. One way to bring out the threat to free will is to imagine that the 350 ms were, say 3.5 seconds or even 35 seconds.

> **EXERCISE 2** (15 minutes)
>
> Before reading on, think what would be the consequences if the time-lag between the key measured brain event and the perceived experience of willing were much longer? Imagine yourself to be the experimental subject. What would happen if you were told when such an event had been detected? Could you change your mind?

Thirty-five seconds and freedom

If, unknown to a subject—you, say—Libet can predict 35 seconds before you make a decision that you will make it at a particular time, it does not seem that you are really free. You are a puppet of your neuronal events. To bring out the paradoxicality of this, now imagine that within this 35 second window, say 10 seconds before you are due to make your decision, Libet tells you exactly when you are going to make it. You cannot *now* stop making it in 10 seconds time, because that change of mind would require that there had already been another neuronal event 35 seconds before it (i.e. 10 seconds before the measured neuronal event). In fact if that new first event *had* already occurred, Libet would not have told you that you were going to make the decision as he originally predicted it. But if so, you would not now have changed your mind and so the new first event would not have occurred.

Such directly paradoxical possibilities are ruled out in the actual case by the small time interval actually found. There simply would not be time to react. But the fact we are saved from such counter-intuitive conclusions merely by the contingency of the time-scale should be small comfort.

Are the empirical findings secure?

We will return to the issues this paper raises for freedom of the will at the end of the chapter. But it is worth flagging two considerations. One is an empirical matter. Spence's conclusions could be resisted, and the subjective conscious experience of decision-initiation could be equated with the apparently earlier neuronal event if the there was an equal lag between looking at the clock and noting its time. If so, the apparent lag between the neuronal events that initiate action and the conscious experience could be explained away as the result of time taken subsequently to note the position of the clock.

A philosophical response

The other is a broader philosophical matter. Spence says that 'the reductionist, materialist perspective underlying the current research has been "pushed" to its logical conclusion. Consciousness is not the initiator of willed action' (p. 88). But in fact the diagrams of conscious experience lagging behind neuronal events looks more like an 'epiphenomenalist' position in which the mind is somehow the result of neuronal processes but separate from them. A materialist, reductionist will want to know just *what* the conscious processes are processes *of*. If a person changes mentally in the instant that he or she experiences a conscious decision (the result of a prior neuronal event), then surely there must be some *physical* change at the same time that explains that mental change. If not, it looks as though the mind really is separate from the brain. So a materialist would expect there to be further neuronal events, after the initial events found by Libet and coinciding with the change in conscious experience.

Let us suppose that there are such events and that they are caused by events 350 ms before them (the events identified by Libet). Does this undermine free will? It seems that it does not add anything further to the problem that already existed. If the brain is a deterministic machine then its states stand in potentially predictable causal relations. Add in the materialistic assumption that brain states somehow determine mental states and this alone gives the picture just outlined. For any mental state, there are simultaneous brain states that determine it, and these in turn are caused by prior brain states according to yet-to-be-discovered neurological laws.

What this suggests is that the problem of free will requires thinking about the relation between freedom and agency, on the one hand, and causal laws on the other (as in fact Spence says in his conclusion). So to shed light on that we will now turn to the nature of agency and its relation to causality. We will focus on the question of whether the reasons we have for acting in paradigmatic exercises of free will are also the causes of action. Are reasons causes? As will be illustrated, the current orthodoxy is that far from being in conflict, the very idea of agency is tied to that of causality. An action is caused by mental states.

Reflection on the session and self-test questions

Write down your own reflections on the materials in this session drawing out any points that are particularly significant for you. Then write brief notes about the following:

1. What do the case vignettes in Spence's paper suggest about the experience of free will? Is there a unified experience?

2. Does Libet's experiment really undermine free will? What interpretations could be offered, according to Spence?

3. What difference would imagining a greater time lag between prior brain event and conscious decision make?

4. Is Spence's interpretation of Libet a triumph of materialism, materialist analysis taken to the limit?

Session 2 Agency and volitions

Non-causal accounts in the 1950s

The first session outlined the apparent conflict between some recent experimental work on the timing of neural events and our everyday understanding of free will. This session will look at some influential arguments that aim to show that action explanation has nothing to do with causation. Historically this approach was promoted in the 1950s by a generation of philosophers of mind such as Gilbert Ryle (1900–76) and the American A.I. Melden (1910–91), working very much in the tradition of linguistic philosophy. They argue that understanding action is of a very different form than explaining events causally and thus stress the difference between the human and the natural sciences.

The current prevalence of causal approaches to the analysis of action was provoked by Donald Davidson's attack in 1969 on that previous non-causal orthodoxy. More recently, the current causal orthodoxy has itself come under fire again from non-causalists. So we will begin with the first generation of non-causalists. This will sharpen the conflict between the causal explanation of events that will increasingly be a feature of neurological science.

Cartesianism and causality

Ryle's work has already come under discussion in Chapter 22. Ryle was a key figure in the version of Anglo-American philosophy sometimes called Oxford or Ordinary Language Philosophy. We will examine a chapter from his attack on Cartesian philosophy of mind: *The Concept of Mind* (1963). In the course of this, Ryle attacks a causal construal of the role of reasons. Ryle's target here is what may seem the rather strange combination of Cartesian dualism and immaterialism. However, Ryle's arguments were also taken to count against materialist causal positions.

Ryle's critique of the Myth of Volitions

EXERCISE 3	(30 minutes)

Read the extract from:

> Ryle, G. (1963). *The Concept of Mind*. London: Penguin, pp. 61–80. (Extract: pp. 62–66)

Link with Reading 26.2

Isolate and assess Ryle's arguments against the Myth of Volitions. What account of action does he propose in its place? Think also whether Ryle's arguments would count against modern materialist causal theories of action such as functionalism.

The Myth of Volitions

The chapter of the *Concept of Mind* concerned with the will is a major plank of Ryle's argument in that book. In that chapter, Ryle aims to destroy a central element of the Cartesian picture of mind. The object of Ryle's fire is a philosophical theory of the will, construed as an 'executive' mental organ. It is this organ that mediates between thoughts or wishes that are 'unexecutive' and actions. The mental intermediaries that need to be added to a wish, for example, to generate action are *volitions*. These are special internal mental events and, Ryle suggests, are more specifically a special kind of mental action. (That they are really internal mental actions underpins one of Ryle's arguments against them.) It is the role of the faculty of will to generate these volitions. Hence Ryle's description of this theory as the 'Myth of Volitions'.

But it is worth focusing first on the problem for which the volitions were intended to be the solution. On a Cartesian world view, there are two possible explanations for changes in the motion of inanimate objects or for the movements of animate bodies. They can either be brought about by the motion of other matter. Or in the case of human beings they can result from 'thrusts of another kind' (p. 62). This other internal source for movement is the will. This general distinction corresponds to, and is meant to explain, the distinction between mere movements and actions. An action, on this theory, is a movement brought about in the right way: as a result of an inner mental episode.

A hint of a causal theory

Although this is not particularly emphasized by Ryle, he suggests that the relation between a volition and the movement (and thus the action) it produces is a *causal* relation.

> And so to say that a person pulled the trigger intentionally is to express at least a conjunctive proposition, asserting the occurrence of one act on the physical stage and another on the mental stage; and according to most versions of the myth, it is to express a *causal* proposition, asserting that the bodily act of pulling the trigger was the effect of the mental act of willing to pull the trigger.   (p. 62)

Contemporary causal theories of action continue with this last suggestion—despite Ryle's criticisms here—but outside the context of a specifically Cartesian conception of mind. One aim of a causal theory of mind is to explain the difference between deliberate actions and mere (involuntary) movements by specifying the defining difference in the causal aetiology of actions and mere movements. Thus one of the issues in assessing Ryle's attack on the myth of volitions is the extent to which it is successfully directed towards any causal theory of the mind or whether it turns on a Cartesian version of that kind of theory.

Four criticisms

Ryle offers four arguments against the Myth of Volitions. They are based on:

1. the lack of empirical evidence for volitions;

2. the impossibility of third person epistemology;

3. the inexplicable connection between volitions and actions;

4. a dilemma about their status as actions.

No evidence

Ryle offers a number of loosely related objections that are designed to undermine the general plausibility of the theory of volitions. He observes that contrary to what the theory would lead one to expect, no one ever offers descriptions of their own volitions. They never report undertaking slow or difficult ones, for example. Nor would they know what to say about them if pressed because the descriptions that apply to other actions seem to get no grip with volitions.

Ryle summarizes this objection in the following way. Volitions are never ordinarily reported; they lack non-academic names; there are no principles to determine their frequency, duration, or strength. Ryle concludes from these considerations that there is no empirical evidence for the existence of volitions or the will so construed. It must instead be the result of fallacious philosophical reasoning about what must be the case rather than everyday observations of what is the case.

No epistemology

Ryle's second objection is that if volitions really were internal mental acts, then it would never be possible to determine whether someone else's movements were caused in the right way to count as actions or not. The problem can be put this way. Imagine that you had no reason to believe whether the sounds and motions of those around you were deliberate actions or merely reflex movements. What evidence would be available to answer this question if the Myth were true? One could not look into another's mind to find out whether there were volitions causing their bodily movements. Even if they 'reported' that this were so it would not settle the matter. That would only help if one could determine whether the sounds made really were a sincere report that 'meant' what we would ordinarily take them to mean rather than being an exactly similar sounding but pattern of noises, which were not intended to convey any such thing. In other words, a report only helps if one already knows whether it is the result of a volition. But that is what is at issue. This objection is clearly a form of the Problem of Other Minds (see chapter 27).

No connection

The third objection is that the connection between volitions and actions is utterly mysterious. Ryle's objection here focuses specifically on a dualistic Cartesian picture that makes the interaction between the two sorts of substance particularly obscure. But it is worth noting as a more general challenge to monistic causal theories of mind. (Which is not to say that such theories cannot answer it.)

The mysteriousness of the connection between volitions and actions underpins the further epistemological claim that even in one's own case, one cannot know whether one's movements are actions. Even if introspection allows the detection of an inner volition preceding trigger pulling, that does not settle whether the volition really did cause the pulling. (We will see a related problem for causal theories later framed not in epistemological terms but as a problem in the analysis of action. If an action has by definition to be caused by an appropriate mental event, what is the precise nature of this relation? As we will see, there are some cases where mental states do seem to cause movement but cause them in the wrong way to count as deliberate actions.)

No answer

Fourthly, Ryle raises a dilemma for the Myth of Volitions. If volitions are mental happenings, are they themselves deliberate or not? If they are, then by the theory they should themselves be the result of antecedent volitions and this generates an infinite regress. If they are not themselves voluntary, then it seems absurd that the 'actions' they cause are voluntary. If a volition were inserted into one's mind by an outside agency and that volition were sufficient to cause an action, would the action be deliberate? Ryle suggests not.

Ryle's positive account

Having spelt out his critical attack on one philosophical explanation, Ryle goes on to offer some positive remarks about the distinction. He focuses mainly on the distinction between those actions that are *blameworthy* and those that are not. What might otherwise be a morally culpable action can be excused if it could not have been helped in the circumstances, if it was, in *that sense* involuntary. But one does not ask whether admirable actions are voluntary, are anyone's fault. Furthermore, Ryle suggests, the issue of voluntariness in this context is satisfied without appeal to inner mental items. One discovers instead the standing abilities and capacities and details in which they were exercised. Clearly, this sort of idea would have consequences for thinking about agency and freedom in the context of mental health.

Assessing Ryle's account

There are two things to consider when assessing Ryle's positive account. One is whether he gives a satisfactory account of the distinction on which he focuses. Does the appeal to the broader, generally social, context of the use of the distinction between the voluntary and involuntary suffice for an explanation of that distinction? We will return to this issue in the final reading of the chapter (linked with Exercise 7), by Sir Peter Strawson (1974).

The other issue is whether the distinction on which Ryle focuses captures the pre-philosophical puzzle with which we began. Ryle suggests that philosophers have stretched the use of 'voluntary' and it is only because of this that they feel the need to postulate volitions. Effectively, Ryle suggests that a Wittgensteinian move is called for. The philosophical problem that the myth of volitions is supposed to solve should instead be *dissolved*. Philosophical *therapy* is needed rather than philosophical theory. We will discuss this a little more below.

An issue may remain

But despite the claim that philosophical puzzlement stems from distorting the genuine and substantial question of whether an action is blameworthy, there does seem to be a different and genuinely puzzling issue, which remains even if that area is clarified.

What remains is the distinctions between actions and mere movements. This distinction is also mentioned in the reading (Ryle, 1963, pp. 71–72). It is the distinction between something that a person does and what is done to her. Ryle says: 'So sometimes the question "Voluntary or involuntary?" means 'Did the person do it, or was it done to him?'; sometimes it presupposes that he did it, but means 'Did he do it with or without heeding what he was doing?' or 'Did he do it inadvertently, mechanically, or instinctively, etc?' (p. 72).

So although Ryle offers good arguments against the Myth of Volitions, it is less clear whether he provides a resolution to the philosophical question: What is the difference between actions and mere movements? Note that this question is not the same as: How do we know whether something is a voluntary action rather than an involuntary movement? Rather, what does that distinction consist in?

It also worth reflecting here on the extent to which Ryle's argument against the Myth of Volitions, which he construes as involving a causal element, succeeds against causal theories which do not rely on an immaterial ghost in the machine. Think of reasons as material states of the brain, capable of causal pushes and pulls and think of actions as movements, which are caused by such reasons. Do Ryle's four arguments undermine this picture?

It is hard to give a precise answer to this question. But a modern causalist might argue in the following way. There is evidence for this new version of volitions: they are the reasons for our actions which we often report in daily life and we distinguish between those reasons on which we act and those which are idle fancies. We can tell when others have such states by asking them because the effects of reasons are detectable in the way that many hidden causes are detectable in the physical sciences: by their effects. The connection between reasons and causes is relatively straightforward. Whatever complex physical states mental states really are, they cause, in whatever normal account we have of causation, actions. Finally, there is no dilemma. Our actions are voluntary if we act for our reasons. Now although we may rationally scrutinize our reasons, many of our mental states are not themselves only the result of our own past actions. Looking around may be a deliberate action, but what I see is independent of me, and on the basis of what I see I will form beliefs that lead to actions. But this does not threaten the voluntary status of my subsequent actions.

In fact things are not as simple as these replies suggest. But to get a deeper understanding of the debate, a short summary of the work of another non-causalist, criticized by the causalist Davidson, will be helpful.

Melden's non-causal account of action

Melden's free action

In his book *Free Action* (1961), in particular chapter 13, the philosopher A.I. Melden sketches a Wittgensteinian picture of action that eschews causation.

One theme is an important metaphilosophical and methodological claim. Melden suggests that a major source of philosophical error is a natural tendency to 'suppose that the difficulty we may have in understanding what an intention or desire is, is the difficulty involved in the *discovery* of an elusive item in our experience' (p. 172, italics added). The idea is that, with this strategy in place, the solution to philosophical problems is taken to require *inferring* the existence of private mental items to explain the observed phenomena: public actions.

Action and meaning

Melden (1961) likens this approach to the nature of action to a similar move to explain meaning. There it involves the postulation of meanings or some other 'mental processes that ride piggy back, so to speak, on the words we utter' (p. 173). In that latter case, Wittgenstein's criticism (in his 1953 *Philosophical Investigations*) of mentalistic explanations of what needs to be added to sounds or symbols for them to possess, or for hearers to understand, their meaning has been increasingly influential. But Melden suggests that a similar moral applies also to the distinction between actions and mere movements. As in the case of special mental meanings so in the case of postulating internal volitions to explain actions: 'no such events could exhibit the requisite logical features of the concepts we employ' (p. 175).

Melden suggests instead (largely without further argument) that one should refrain from 'converting a question about meaning into an extremely questionable view about matters of psychological occurrence' (p. 175). Philosophers should instead 'examine carefully the manner in which terms like 'intention' and 'desire' operate in our familiar discourse about actions and agents' (p. 175). This approach should remind you of Austin's work, discussed in Part I.

The conceptual–connection argument

With these methodological preliminaries in place, Melden advances the following key claim. Because there are *logical* connections between mental items such as motives, desires, and intentions and actions, *causal* theories of action must be false. The logical connection or dependence is manifested in two ways. First, it is impossible to understand the former concepts independently of understanding the latter and vice versa. Secondly, *explanation* of action by appeal to such mental states differs significantly from the causal explanation of events in the physical sciences. Melden fills out the second a little later. He says:

> Where we are concerned with causal explanations, with events of which the happenings in question are effects in accordance with some law of causality, to that extent we are not concerned with human actions at all but, at best, with bodily movements or happenings; and where we are concerned with human action, there causal factors and causal laws in the sense in which, for example, these terms are employed in the biological sciences are wholly irrelevant to the understanding we seek. The reason is simple, namely, the radically different logical characteristics of these two bodies of discourse... (p. 184)

The underlying suggestion is this. The concepts of motive and action fit together with others in a structure that is different from and independent of the structure that relates cause, effect, and law. We have already encountered this idea in the distinction between the 'space of reasons' and the 'realm of law', which McDowell takes from the work of Sellars (see Part III). Melden argues that a causal theory of mind conflates two different conceptual structures. We will return to these arguments in the next session in order to assess both them and Davidson's counter arguments. But they are complemented by a further metaphilosophical methodological suggestion.

The primacy of persons

Melden suggests that the philosophy of action specifically, and of mind more generally, should begin with, or presuppose, the concept of a person: a practical being with a primitive ability to move his or her limbs and to act for reasons. Furthermore, persons or people typically act within a *social* framework of rules and customs. Again this starting point is proposed without much argument. But it is worth contrasting it with Descartes' starting point. Descartes assumes only first person access to the content of one's mental states and to sensations. The starting point is a purely mental point of consciousness. As we will see (in Chapter 27) there are strong arguments against the intelligibility of first person access independent of third person access or of the concept of an ego independently of that of an embodied person. Melden subscribes to these Wittgensteinian views and concludes that a satisfactory philosophy of mind should reject Descartes' abstraction and the explicitly epistemological concern that goes with it. Starting points in philosophy by definition resist justification. But one could argue meta-philosophically that Descartes' starting point has been tried throughout 300 years without great success and that this is reason enough to start somewhere else.

Given his starting point, Melden claims that the route to a clear understanding of action is clear. It turns on an analysis of the concepts used to justify or explain actions in everyday life. One should examine the broader space of reasons deployed in justification rather than events that take place at the very same time as actions. The latter focus is perfectly acceptable but only as an explanation of bodily movements, perhaps as pieces of physiological or neurophysiological inquiry.

Epistemology and interpretation

This leads to a further strand or argument. How is it possible to recognize an action as an action rather than as a mere movement? Melden likens this question to the question of how it is possible to see marks on paper or sounds as meaningful words. With that analogy in mind, Melden argues that it cannot be the case that one has to *interpret* movement as action. If that were so, he argues, there would be nothing left to justify an interpretation. Everything would hang in the air without conceivable support. This hint at an argument is a version of Wittgenstein's argument against using interpretation as the theoretical basis of meaning discussed in Chapters 24 and 25. In this case, however, one may ask what would be wrong with a theory that related inputs described in meaning-free terms with meaningful interpretations of them. Is it obvious that this is incoherent? May be this is not the best explanation of our ability? We will postpone discussion of this question because it is a matter of the *epistemology* of mind rather than the ontology of mind and the nature of action explanation. It will be the subject of Chapter 27.

This session has outlined two influential arguments that action explanation is not causal. If those arguments hold good, then the connection between the freedom that is a key aspect of the space of reasons—the metaphorical space that characterizes action explanation among other things—and causal determinism remains mysterious. But in fact philosophical accounts of action explanation have moved on and now causal theories hold greater influence. It is to these that we will now turn.

Reflection on the session and self-test questions

Write down your own reflections on the materials in this session drawing out any points that are particularly significant for you. Then write brief notes about the following:

1. What, according to Ryle, is the Myth of Volitions and what is its purpose?

2. What criticisms does Ryle offer of that myth and what positive account does he propose in its stead?

3. How does consideration of speech and meaning shed light on action according to Melden?

Session 3 Arguments for a causal theory of mind

The causal theory and reductionism

This session will outline the origins of recent causal theories of mind in Donald Davidson's seminal article 'Actions, reasons and causes' (1980 pp. 3–19). It is important first, however, to note a potential ambiguity in the use of the label 'causal theory of mind'. In some contexts it is used to refer to attempts to explain intentional concepts such as belief and meaning in non-intentional and usually causal terms. This is also called the project of 'naturalising' intentionality or providing a 'causal semantics' and was the subject of Chapter 24.

But even if one grants that that reductionist project is misguided, one can still subscribe to a causal theory of mind when this is construed in a different sense. One can argue that, although the intentional properties of mental states cannot be reduced to causal or other non-intentional properties, nevertheless the states or events that bare those properties still play a *causal* role in the

production of both action or other mental states, and are themselves caused by other mental states and perceptions.

Davidson's Anomalous Monism is perhaps the most influential example of such a theory. As we saw in Chapter 23, Davidson attempts to reconcile the view that mental concepts cannot be structured in natural laws with the view that the mental events to which they apply are still part of the causal fabric of the world. In what at first seems a counter-intuitive account, he attempts to have his cake and to eat it. We will see below that a key element of this causal theory of mind is that action explanation by citing reasons or propositional attitudes, is a species of causal explanation.

Although Chapter 23 introduced the metaphysical system by which Davidson hoped to reconcile the irreducibility of the mental with granting it a causal role, it did not discuss Davidson's argument for thinking that mental states are causes. That is the purpose of the next reading.

EXERCISE 4	(30 minutes)

Read the extract from:

Davidson, D. (1980). Actions, reasons and causes. In *Essays on Actions and Events*. Oxford: Oxford University Press, pp. 3–19. (Extract: pp 11–17)

Link with Reading 26.3

Summarize (on a piece of paper) Davidson's counter-arguments to previous arguments against granting reasons a causal role.

◆ What positive considerations does Davidson advance for saying that reasons actually are causes (as opposed simply to conceding that there are no good arguments against them being)?

◆ Can you think of a different response to Davidson's challenge?

Davidson's paper advances two general theses about action explanation via reasons:

1. For us to understand how a reason of any kind rationalizes an action it is necessary and sufficient that we see, at least in essential outline, how to construct a primary reason.

2. The primary reason for an action is its cause.

The first half of the paper (sections I–III) discusses the first while the second (section IV) focuses on the second: on the causal role of mental items.

The key idea that Davidson wants to defend is that an intentional action is one done for a reason. But to know that an action was intentional is not in itself sufficient to know the full reason for the action. To know that the action is intentional is to know that there is some reason, but not which one it is. Actions can be undertaken with different aims in view, different ends or effects of the same action. And even the same end can be desired, wished for or lusted for.

> By giving a reason for an action the action can be revealed as coherent, rational, connected with broader patterns of action: When we ask why someone acted as he did, we want to be provided with an interpretation. His behaviour seems strange, alien, outré, pointless, out of character, disconnected; or perhaps we cannot even recognise an action in it. When we learn his reason, we have an interpretation, a new description of what he did which fits into a familiar pattern.   (pp. 9–10)

Intentions and intensions

One reason why knowledge that an action was intentional is not in itself sufficient to imply the reason for which it was carried out is that intentional actions are also intensional with an 's'. (What follows turns on one particular way of individuating or counting actions; see shortly below.) The very same action can be described in many different ways. The action or event of turning on the light may also be an action or event of warning a prowler. The same event can be described in these different ways. But although the action is intentional under one description, it may not be under others. I may want to flick the switch and to turn the light on, but I may have no thoughts at all about warning any prowlers. I do not intend to warn the prowler although that is what I do by turning on the light. Davidson's thought here is that an action is intentional providing that there is some description under which fits into a reason explanation.

(That way of putting it clearly turns on an assumption about how to count actions. Davidson suggests that we count actions as events that may have different descriptions depending on their relational properties. Because the action of turning on the light has the broader consequence of alerting the prowler, it can also be called that. More narrowly, it can be called the action of flicking the switch. Narrower still it can be called the action of moving one's finger. That the switch is flicked depends on the causal structure of the world. It turns on the world doing us a favour. (In fact Davidson elsewhere suggests that we pick out a subclass of 'basic actions' that turn on no favours and do not extend beyond the skin.) But Davidson's approach to action-individuation is to group these all together as different relational ways of specifying the same action. In much the same way, the same individual can be somebody's brother, somebody's son, somebody's father. But an alternative approach is to say that these are all different actions because they all exemplify different properties. Thus turning the key and starting the car are different actions. In what follows, action individuation will play no role. For a discussion see the introduction to A.R. Mele *The Philosophy of Action*, 1997.)

Reasons as rationalizations

So far, Davidson's (1980) account of reason explanation sounds much like the broadly Wittgensteinian account suggested by both Ryle (1963) and Melden (1961). It presents action explanation as a method of fitting one action into a broader pattern. Reasons are

an appropriate spoonful of contextualizing information. They provide the resources for redescribing the action to be explained. Davidson formalizes the rationalizing property of reasons thus: 'C1. *R* is a primary reason why an agent performed the action *A* under the description *d* only if *R* consists of a pro attitude of the agent towards actions with a certain property, and a belief of the agent that *A*, under the description *d*, has that property.' (p. 5).

But he goes on to add to that picture an explicitly anti-Wittgensteinian element. He claims that reason explanation is also a form of causal explanation. The reason for an action is (part of) its cause. In order to ground this claim he needs to do two things. One is to overcome the (largely Wittgensteinian) arguments previously deployed to show that reasons cannot be causes. And he also needs to provide positive grounds for thinking that reasons actually are causes.

Against non-causalism

With respect to the first target, Davidson provides two key counter-arguments:

1. *Non-causalist claim.* The normative connection between mental states and behaviour is an obstacle to any causal account. Reasons and actions have to be described in a suitable way in order to display their rationalizing powers. This implies that there is an analytic or logical connection between reason and action whereas a causal link is contingent and empirical.

   Davidson's response. The analytic connection depends on how the facts are *described*. But the causal relation does not. The fact that an analytic connection can be made by a suitable choice of description cannot preclude a causal connection because any given causal relation can be so described. Suppose event A causes event B. Event A could be described as 'the cause of B' in the analytically true statement: the cause of B caused B. But this does not contradict the assumption that A caused B.

2. *Non-causalist claim.* The statement that someone acted in a particular way because of a particular reason does not imply that reasons of that type *generally* lead to actions of that type. But causation requires just such generality.

   Davidson's response. A Humean or nomological account of causation requires that some description of the two events is possible that connects them as a matter of law. But it does not require that the descriptions used to pick out cause and effect are suitable for inclusion in the law. It may be that the cause of an event that is reported on page 13 of the *Tribune* is itself reported on page 5 of *The Times*. But that does not imply that there is a linking law that uses the descriptions: 'events reported on page 13 of the *Tribune*' and 'events reported on page 5 of *The Times*'. Ignorance of the actual law does not, however, eliminate causal explanation.

Both of these counter-arguments are based on the following strong intuition or assumption. Unlike the intentionality of actions, their causality is extensional rather than intensional (again with an s). If one event causes another it does not matter how it is described. The underlying metaphysical facts about the causal structure of the world are indifferent to how we describe them. By contrast one may *not* have intentionally or deliberately killed one's father even if one deliberately struck an intruder over the head under circumstances where as a matter of fact in striking one killed and the intruder was one's father. Whether the action was intentional depends on how it is described. (Again, this account follows Davidson's way of individuating actions.)

Once the claim that causality is an extensional or description-independent relation is in place, Davidson has a general method for defusing the kind of argument that Melden deploys. Although the conceptual structure into which 'reason' and 'action' fits—the space of reasons—differs from the conceptual structure corresponding to the realm of law and including 'cause' 'effect' and 'law of nature' this does not imply that the two structures cannot apply to the very same items. They may structure them in different ways but, Davidson suggests, what is being structured is the same in the two cases.

As we have already seen (in Chapter 23), Davidson goes on to suggest that the (mental) events labelled by the mentalistic vocabulary of propositional attitudes just are the very same events that can also be picked out using the vocabulary of causes, effects, and strict or probabilistic laws. *Really*, there are only events and these can be picked both via their mental and also by their physical relations or properties. It is just that these two systems cannot be systematically related. But before accepting the need for his unifying metaphysics of events, we should ask a further question. What positive reason is there to think that reasons are causes?

Reasons as causes

Davidson provides two positive arguments. We will pick out one here and discuss the second below.

The first takes the form of a challenge to non-causal theories of mind based on the question: what is the difference between *a* reason for an action and *the* reason? The challenge Davidson puts forward is to explicate the difference between a case in which someone has a reason for an action *and* carries out that action—where the 'and' is read purely conjunctively—from cases where they act *because* of the reason, where the reason is 'active': '[A] person can have a reason for an action, and perform the action, and yet this reason not be the reason why he did it. Central to the relation between a reason and an action it explains is the idea that the agent performed the action *because* he had the reason.' (p. 9).

The philosophical issue here is to explain what this distinction amounts to. What constitutes the reason for an action as *the* reason?

This problem is not a matter of epistemology. It is not a question of how one *knows* which reason is *the* reason for an action. Davidson's implicit assumption is that epistemology is little guide to ontology here. How in practice one knows what the reason for

an action is, either in one's own case or for others, plays no part in the discussion. A philosophical account of the distinction need not postulate facts which help *guide* practical knowledge. (On the other hand, the account should not make knowledge here utterly mysterious or impossible.) Nor is the objection that one may always act for a number of reasons relevant. Providing that it is possible to act, and to have even one reason for that action which is *inactive*, then an account is owed as to what the difference between an active and an inactive reason is.

A reason versus *the* reason

Davidson argues that the rationalizing aspect of reasons is no help here. As we have seen, the rationalizing role of reasons is to make sense of action through contextualization. But if the rational power of reasons is understood in the way Davidson suggests and formalizes as condition C1 (above), it cannot constitute the difference between *a* reason and *the* reason. To be *a* reason is already to be a reason that is held by the person who acts and which rationalizes the action. Rationality has already been used in distinguishing between such reasons for action and mental states that have no bearing on the action whatsoever. It cannot also provide the extra ingredient sufficient for being the actual reason why someone acted.

Davidson suggests that one might augment the characterization of rational power so as simply to include the extra ingredient, whatever it is. But the cost of that assumption would be to make the rationalizing role of reasons mysterious. Davidson suggests that the rationalizing role should instead be construed in the transparent way already described and that something has to be added to the rationalizing role of reasons to answer the question.

Causation as the extra

Davidson's proposal is that the extra ingredient is causal efficacy. *The* reason for an action is the reason that causes it. Thus reasons have to meet a second non-rational condition: 'C2. A primary reason for an action is its cause.' (p. 12).

Thus the argument that Davidson puts forward is of the following form. Something needs to be added to the rationalizing force of reasons to distinguish between *a* reason for an action and *the* reason. The only candidate for this extra ingredient is causation. One way of putting this is that Davidson points out that there is a second necessary condition on reason explanation. But he gives no reason to believe that it is more than contingently true that this condition is satisfied by causation and little specific reason to believe that it is true of causation.

There is, however, implicit in some of his remarks in this paper a further argument why causality specifically has to be added to rationality to account for reason explanation. This has recently been made more explicit in a commentary by William Child (1994).

Child's version of the argument

In his book, *Causality Interpretation and the Mind*, Child (1994) develops and defends a causal theory of mind as that phrase is being used in this chapter: mental states play causal roles without any implication that mental properties can be analysed in causal terms.

Causes and explanation

Child reiterates the Davidsonian argument already described, but also goes on to make explicit another argument that is only hinted at by Davidson. This argument can be summarized baldly as follows:

1. an action explanation is an explanation of why something happened; but

2. no non-causal explanation can explain why something happened; so

3. action explanations must be causal.

Clearly this argument turns on the plausibility of its second premiss. There are two ways of testing this. One is to try to devise explanations that do not turn on citing causal explanations of why *non-mental* events occur. The other is to question whether the explanation of mental events and that of non-mental events must have the same underlying logical form.

With respect to the former, Child (1994) makes the following point:

> The idea that any explanation of the occurrence of an event must be causal is plausible case by case. For any putatively non-causal explanation of an event, we can always make the Davidsonian point: knowing this story allows us to fit the event into a pattern which potentially makes sense of it; but we are still left wanting to know why the event actually occurred, what made it happen when it did.
>
> (p. 92)

Thus Child proposes the following challenge to anyone who disputes the second premiss. Find a non-causal explanation of an event that is not merely an explanation of what constitutes it as the sort of event it is and really is an explanation of why it occurs. His claim is that all the non-causal explanations alluded to by the 1960s Wittgensteinians, for example, tell us something about the events in question but not why they happened.

Of course, this sort of argument has an essential modesty. Because Child cannot investigate every putative case of non-causal explanation, and because the only general rule he offers is the very one which is in dispute, he cannot provide a watertight justification of this principle. Nevertheless, his argument does provide strong intuitive support because of the *de facto* success of his challenge. For non-mental events, explanations of why they occur do seem to require the specification of causal information.

Child and Lewis

Child's argument is in accord with Lewis's account of natural scientific explanation, which was discussed in chapter 14. Lewis claims that all such explanation relies on the provision of part of the causal history of events. One of the criticisms made of Lewis's account there was that it was incomplete and did not cover all forms of explanation, such as mathematical or logical explanations which cite proofs. Child's argument is more limited because he restricts his concern to a subset of explanations: those concerned with why events occur, rather than anything else about them, and thus he escapes that sort of criticism.

But there is a second kind of response available. This is to concede Child's general claim with one important class of exceptions: the class of mental explanations. In other words, anyone who doubts that action explanation by reasons is a species of causal explanation might concede what Child claims *outside* that sphere but continue to dispute the relevance of those cases to the mental case. Even if explanations of why Atherton was bowled Leg Before Wicket, which explain why that event happened—by citing how the ball bounced on the dry earth, its speed, and the length of human reaction times—that need not show that *reason* explanations are causal. The explanation of why the bowler decided to try that kind of bowl by appeal to his plans, perceptions, and desires need not be causal.

To assess the force of this response requires further reflection on the nature of the claim that reasons are causes or that causality provides for a distinction between action and mere movement. As the next stage in this process of clarification, the following session considers the kind of causal theory of mind involved. Davidson argues that actions are caused by mental events while others argue that there is instead just a brute relation between an agent and there action.

Reflection on the session and self-test questions

Write down your own reflections on the materials in this session drawing out any points that are particularly significant for you. Then write brief notes about the following:

1. What are the two general ingredients that Davidson thinks are involved in action explanation (hint: not in this context belief and desire!).

2. What specific argument does he offer for the second element?

3. How does he defuse Wittgensteinian arguments against this?

Session 4 Event causation, agent causation, and irrationality

It is one thing to argue that reason explanation must be a species of causal explanation and another, further claim to explain how precisely this comes about: what reasons are or what is causally related. This session will look at two contrasting versions of a causal account. One is Davidson's account, already discussed in Chapter 23 in which causation links free-standing mental states and actions. The other is an account in which causation links a whole person to his or her actions.

Recap of Anomalous Monism

As we saw in Chapter 23, Davidson provides a novel reconciliation of three initially apparently irreconcilable claims:

1. that mental states stand in causal relations;

2. an underlying nomological account of causation;

3. the anomalism of mental states.

These appear to be in tension because the first and second together imply that there are laws that govern mental states while the third claims that there are no *mental laws*: no laws (or law statements to be precise) couched in mental terms. Davidson's solution is to claim that the very same states that are picked out using the mental vocabulary of reason explanation, can also be picked out in principle by their physical properties, which can be fitted into a structure of strict physical laws. The third claim remains true because there is no systematic way of relating mental properties to physical properties in such a way that the mental might be reduced to the physical. If there were bridge laws connecting mental and physical properties then given the existence of strict physical laws, there would also be strict mental laws. Thus to preserve the truth of the third claim—that there are no such laws—Davidson is forced to claim that there are no psychophysical laws.

Chapter 23 charted some of the objections that have been raised to Davidson's account of the metaphysics of mind. These include the objection that Anomalous Monism cannot provide an account of the causal efficacy of mental *properties* to which we will return shortly. But, on the initial assumption that these objections could be overcome, one strength of Davidson's account should now be clear. Davidson's general claim that reasons are causes relies on a straightforward construal of what causes are. Davidson simply means the same kind of causal relations that connect other non-mental events. Furthermore, he appeals to a familiar broadly Humean nomological account of causation. Thus the attraction of Davidson's account is the attraction of unification. The causal relations between mental states or between mental states and actions are of just the same kind as those described in the rest of the physical sciences. In saying that causation is an element of an account of agency, he means just the sort of causal relation that can connect events generally.

Agent-causation

Davidson's is not the only model of a causal theory of mind. Child (1994), discussed above argues for a causal theory but does not think it should link mental states to actions. Similarly, John Bishop Professor of Philosophy at Auckland defends a very different kind of causal theory of mind in this paper 'Agent-causation' (1983). On his account of agency, the causal relation connects not mental events or states to other states and actions, but, more primitively, it connects the agent herself to something else. (What is the other relatum? As he explains, the agent-causal relation cannot connect the agent to her action because the action is inclusively defined as the holding of the relation. He suggests that it connects her to her movement, narrowly described. The action is thus the whole fact of an agent standing in an agent-causal relation to a movement.)

There is a clear disadvantage of this approach as the contrast with Davidson should highlight. It does not provide the kind of unification to which Davidson's nomological event-causation account aspires. This follows from the fact that agent-causal relations—whatever they are—are not covered by standard nomological accounts of causation. Bishop defends the approach by arguing that the element of reduction implicit in Davidson's project fails because of an anomaly with which it cannot cope. Agent-causation is embraced as an alternative without any such reductionist intent. (Note that talk of reductionism here does not imply the reduction of mental-content to non-intentional concepts as it did in Chapter 24. It refers to the reduction of the concept of action to more primitive concepts such as rationalization plus causation.)

Causal deviance

The anomaly on which Bishop builds his argument is sketched out with admirably honesty by Davidson himself in a different essay:

> Let a single example serve. A climber might want to rid himself of the weight and danger of holding another man on a rope, and he might know that by loosening his hold on the rope he could rid himself of the weight and danger. This belief and want might so unnerve him to loosen his hold, and yet it might be the case that he never *chose* to loosen his hold, nor did he do it intentionally. It will not help, I think, to add that the belief and the want must combine to cause him to want to loosen his hold, for there will remain the *two* questions *how* the belief and the want caused the second want, and *how* wanting to loosen his hold caused him to loosen his hold.
>
> Davidson 'Freedom to Act' in *Essays on Actions and Events* (1980, p. 79)

Here is the problem. The first of the two arguments for a causal theory of mind isolated above took the form of a challenge. What has to be added to mere rationalizing force to distinguish *a* reason for action (which the agent may have) from *the* reason why she did the action? Davidson's suggestion is that causation is the relevant extra. But while causation may be a *necessary* extra ingredient for action, the example of the climber shows that it is not a *sufficient* addition—when added to the possession of reasons. In this example, and a host of others, the possession of reasons causally leads to some behaviour but leads to it in the wrong sort of way for it to count as intentional. The philosophical problem is that of spelling out what the right sort of way is which does not simply presuppose the concept of action.

To the normal range of cases that philosophers consider, we can add psychopathological cases such as made actions, made impulses, and so on. In such cases, subjects can 'act' and can have reasons for those actions which, if a causal theory is right, cause them. But there is still something pathological if the subject denies that they are the authors of their reasons.

In 'Agent-causation' (1983) John Bishop argues that the specification of causal deviance will always rely on a more primitive account of agent-causality. Thus in the climber example: 'He didn't let go intentionally, even though his intention to let go caused him to lose hold, because his nervousness prevented him from controlling his grip' is a reasonable off the cuff account of the deviance... [which] makes appeal to a notion of maintaining control which may well have agent-causal presuppositions.' (p. 68).

In general, diagnosis of which event-causal chains correspond to failures of intentional action will always rely on a prior and primitive theory of agent-causation.

Agent-causation and deviance

The substance of such an agent-causal account of agency turns on the nature of the primitive theory of agent-causality. Bishop (1983) spells this out as follows:

> [F]or M to Q intentionally, where this is a basic action, M must have the intention to Q, and M must exhibit behaviour which counts as Q-ing. But we require furthermore that, in behaving as he does M should himself be carrying out his intention to Q... Its satisfaction itself requires two further conditions be met, the *real capacity condition*, and the *non-pre-emption condition* ...
>
> There is a natural explication of such pre-emption... If, and only if, there are antecedent conditions causally sufficient for M to exhibit Q-ing behaviour which are *independent* of M's carrying out any proximate intention he may have to Q, then, if M *does* form such an intention, his opportunity to carry it out is pre-empted.   (pp. 75–76)

Bishop explicitly concedes that this sort of primitive theory is neither meant as a *reductive* explanation of intentional action nor deviant causation. Nevertheless, it is appropriate to ask what sort of elucidation Bishop's sketch of a theory succeeds in providing. The worry is this: it relies upon an unexplained notion of sufficient conditions for behaviour *independent* of intentional action. This casts doubt on the claim that agent-*causality* provides any unpacking of the notion of agency itself. While Davidson argues that light can be shed on what makes an action intentional by appeal to its causal origins, Bishop relies on a prior notion of intentional actions in order to diagnose whether behaviour caused by antecedent mental states is intentional or not.

But why agent-*causation*?

On the assumption that some form of causal theory of mind must be true and that causal theories must be of one form or another then Bishop's argument against Davidson's event-causality provides an argument for agent-causality instead. But this leaves another possibility. One might choose instead to reject the assumption that causality has anything to do with agency. As on Bishop's account causality only ever features as part of the primitive composite notion of agent-causality, why think of this as any form of causality rather than, say, agency? The primitive theory that he offers to form the backdrop for diagnosing what is wrong in the climber example could remain but reconstrued as a piece of conceptual analysis of what we all implicitly understand by agency. The next session will return to this possibility. For now we will consider a further difficulty of Davidson's causal theory. This turns on the distinction between mental content and the vehicle of mental content set out in Chapter 24.

Davidson on irrationality

The following extract (linked with Exercise 5) sets out a framework which Davidson (1982) suggests might help make sense of certain forms of irrationality: centrally weakness of will or 'akrasia'. It relies on the fact that Davidson's account allows a distinction between the rational and causal properties of mental states. One of the themes of this paper is that this distinction has consequences for the intelligibility of akrasia. A second is that any plausible account will also require the partitioning of the mind. For now, the first will provide a point of criticism of Davidson's account that shows a principled difficulty for causal theories of mind.

EXERCISE 5   (30 minutes)

Read the short extract from:

Davidson, D. (1982). Paradoxes of irrationality. In *Philosophical Essays on Freud* (ed. J. Hopkins and R. Wollheim). Cambridge: Cambridge University Press, pp. 289–305. (Extract: pp. 296–298)

Link with Reading 26.4

◆ What is the philosophical difficulty with understanding the very idea of irrational actions or beliefs?

◆ What is Davidson's key idea for accounting for them?

◆ What does this suggest about rational beliefs and actions?

Akrasia and paradox

As Davidson points out, the paradox of irrational actions or beliefs is that they are failures *within* what McDowell calls the space of reasons. If instead they were simply *non-rational* they would lie outside the sphere of rationality completely and would not be paradoxical. But irrational acting or thinking is subject to reason explanation and thus subject to the inbuilt rationality that that form of explanation carries. Irrational actions are, however, subject to merely *partial* reason explanations: reason explanations that fail to be fully rational. The philosophical difficulty is to account for this halfway house.

Davidson's solution is that irrationality is the result of reasons whose causal efficacy pathologically exceeds their rationalizing force. Taking the case of a man who goes out of his way to replace a branch he had moved in a park:

> The man who returns to the park to replace the branch has a reason: to remove a danger. But in doing this he ignores his principle of acting on what he thinks best, all things considered. And there is no denying that he has a motive for ignoring his principle, namely that he wants, perhaps very strongly, to return the branch to its original position... Irrationality entered when his desire to return made him ignore or override his principle.   (p. 297)

Whereas in normal cases, beliefs stand in both rational and causal relations to each other and to actions, in cases of irrationality some of the rational relations are distorted or overridden by merely causal relations. In the case of wishful thinking, for example, a reason—the wish to have a particular belief—which fails to offer rational support for that belief, serves as a reason, and is causally sufficient, for holding that belief. Irrational behaviour is sufficiently intelligible for interpretation via rational reasons still to be possible. The relevant causes of behaviour are still mental states—reasons—with semantic content, as displayed by their other rational connections. But the causal power of some of these reasons exceeds their rational power.

This looks at first a promising strategy for accounting more generally for content-laden psychopathological symptoms. The problem for philosophical elucidation is to account for the fact that symptoms can be meaningful, causal, and pathological. It seems at first plausible that these three constraints could be met by a suitable development of Davidson's ideas. Symptoms can be interpreted as meaningful by an analyst who charts a network of rational connections between them and the sufferer's mental economy. But not all the connections are rational or fully rational. In some cases the causal powers of mental states are out of proportion with their rational powers. It is this that leads to some outputs counting as symptoms rather than rational actions or utterances.

The mysterious harmony of causal and rational power

But a problem with this thought highlights a general problem with Davidson's reconciliation of reasons and causes. He provides no answer of why it is generally the case that the rational power and the causal power of reasons stand in proportion. There are simply no resources in his account to answer this question. As discussed in Chapter 23, Davidson fails to unite reasons and causes at the level of mental *properties*, which in turn casts doubt on the reconciliation achieved at the level of mental particulars.

This problem needs careful statement. As causal relations are extensional, it is not *in virtue of* its description as physical (or mental) that a mental event causes another event. Causal relations hold, of fail to hold, however the relata are described. Nevertheless, the properties that are invoked in the nomological account of the causal efficacy of mental events are exclusively physical. There are, according to Davidson, no strict laws linking mental properties. Thus mental *properties* play no part in causal explanations of action. But our standard model of the explanation of the occurrence of an event is that the properties that are cited—perhaps following the word 'because'—are causally relevant. It is in virtue of possessing those properties that the event happened. This is not true of Davidson's explanation of why reasons are causes. Thus he fails to unite reason explanation and causal explanation. The fact that events can play a role in both spaces is not sufficient to unite reasons and causes. While his account manages to display the rational structuring of reason and give an account of the causal role of reasons, it cannot explain how reason can itself play a role in causal explanation. He fails to reconcile or unite the rational and the causal.

Causal efficacy and mental *properties*

This is another way of bringing attention to the issue discussed in Chapter 23. Can a merely token identity of mental and physical events or states accommodate a suitable causal role for mental properties? (This is the central subject of the edited collection J. Heil and A. Mele *Mental Causation*, 1993.) Of course it is no problem for an account that eschews a causal role for the mental (to which we will turn in the next session). Nor is it a problem for causal theories of the mind, which are also reductionist about mental properties. If mental properties can be reduced to non-mental physical properties using bridge laws then they will play a causal role of just the same sort as physical properties. But it is a problem for any account that aims to be non-reductionist about mental content while advocating a causal interpretation of action explanation.

One way of making this point reflects back on a distinction made in Chapter 24. It is the distinction between (mental) content and the vehicles of that content. In Chapter 25 the McDowellian objection was raised that any attempt to reduce mental content through talk of the properties of free-standing internal states or events, which encoded mental content was open to the objection that it left the mind dark. If such states stand in a network of 'horizontal' causal relations, which fully explains their occurrence, why also attribute to them 'vertical' relations of meaning and reference? Why assume that these go hand in hand? A related objection can be raised in the current context. Davidson attributes both causal and rational properties to mental states construed as internal free-standing events. But why assume that these go hand in hand? And why think of the causal properties as having anything to do with the rational properties of the content that the events or states encode?

Given the objections raised against reductionist accounts of mental content in Chapters 24 and 25 and given the objections raised against Davidson's weaker token identity theory embedded in Anomalous Monism, it is time to reconsider what arguments there are for a causal theory of mind (in the modest sense of this chapter: the claim that reasons are causes). In Session 5 we will look at an article that rejects Davidson's claim that there is a need to invoke causation to explain action.

Reflection on the session and self-test questions

Write down your own reflections on the materials in this session drawing out any points that are particularly significant for you. Then write brief notes about the following:

1. Can the intuition that causation has something to do with agency be interpreted in ways other than Davidson's?

2. If so is it still clear that causation is playing a specific and characteristic role?

3. Can causation be used to explain irrationality?

Session 5 A non-causal account of agency?

In the light of the internal difficulties of causal theories, this session will re-examine the arguments that have been deployed in favour of the claim that reasons are causes.

Just as Davidson's paper 'Actions, reasons and causes' (1980 pp. 3–19) undermined an assumption that was held largely independently of particular compelling arguments that reasons could not be causes, more recent work, following Davidson, has almost universally held the converse. While Davidson himself did put forward genuine arguments for the claim, most philosophers of mind hold it instead as an article of faith, believing that Davidson's arguments are secure. The dominant approaches in philosophical accounts of mind such as functionalism or and Representationalism, described in Chapters 23 and 24, are examples of this. Thus arguments directed against Davidson in a recent paper by Julia Tanney are especially interesting because of the consequences they would have if successful.

EXERCISE 6   (30 minutes)

Read the extracts from:

Tanney, J. (1995). Why reasons may not be causes. *Mind and Language*, 10: 105–128. (Extracts pp. 108–110, 111–112, 113)

Link with Reading 26.5

Assess the strength of Tanney's counter arguments in the first half of the paper.

◆ What is the role that explanation plays in her choreography of Davidson in the middle section?

◆ What kind of account of mental explanation is suggested by her later remarks?

Tanney's arguments against Davidson's arguments for reasons being causes

This paper begins by recapping the general motives for Davidson's construal of reasons as causes as outlined earlier in this chapter. Something has to be added to the fact that a reason rationalizes an action or shows how it is reasonable to distinguish *a* reason for an action from *the* reason. And what has to be added is causation because only it promises to give an account of the 'mysterious connection' between reasons and actions. Tanney then goes on to question whether causation does provide a satisfactory addition and whether any addition is in fact needed.

First, taking the case of Oedipus unknowingly killing his father, there is no need to add causation into the account because it is not needed to distinguish between his reasons for killing the threatening old man and any more 'Oedipal' desires to kill his father. The latter are irrelevant to explaining his actions because

he does not believe the old man is his father. Thus it does not serve as part of a reason *he* has for killing the old man.

In the second case of overridden reasons, Tanney assumes that Oedipus does know that the old man is his father and that in addition to his Oedipal desires (to kill him) he also has moral qualms about killing his father. Nevertheless, these qualms are overridden by his own desire to survive when threatened and so he kills his father. Given this scenario, Oedipus's Oedipal desires do not form part of his reason for killing his father even though they are reasons he has. They are not his reason because they are *overridden* by his moral qualms. It is only because, in addition, he has a desire to survive and believes that he is threatened that he kills his father.

Davidson would explain this by saying that the Oedipal reason is not causally active in this case: that causation makes the difference between a reason and the reason. But as Tanney points out this assumption is unwarranted once an account of competing reasons is given that trades only on rational and motivational concepts. A difference in the space of reasons can make the difference (between *a* reason one has and *the* reason one acts) instead.

A distinct motive for introducing causal powers in addition to rational powers might stem from thinking about Buridan's Ass who has equal reasons for choosing either of a pair of exclusive choices. If we want to explain why one is chosen rather than the other, we may want to say that the reason for it was causally active while the other was not. But Tanney argues that the right response to such circumstances is to recognize that there simply is no reason for a choice of one over the other and the choice is thus not subject to reason explanation. It is rational to *pick* one or the other rather than becoming fixated on this one choice, but picking in this case is not a rational choice but like an arbitrary toss of a coin.

Nor, finally, does the case of weakness of will justify introducing causal powers. In such cases there may be a causal explanation of sorts (hormone imbalance, perhaps), but this is not part of a reason explanation, in the sense of a reason an agent has for an action. It may be necessary to complicate a purely rationalizing account by introducing competing subsets of beliefs, but this is not itself causal.

The role of weighted reasons

Tanney concludes that, once a more complex story of *weighted* reasons for actions is in place, there is no need to add a causal element to reason explanation. She then goes on, in Section 3, to suggest a deeper underlying motive for thinking that there must be some such causal addition. (She considers it only to reject it.) This is that there should be a determinate relation between reasons for action and action: that the former should be a sufficient condition for the latter. Tanney herself argues, on the basis of consideration of the Buridan's Ass case and that of weakness of will that this is too strong a requirement to place on rational explanation. Sometimes reasons are insufficient for action.

A further problem

Section 3 of the paper continues with a further criticism of Davidson's attempt to combine a causal theory of mind with the anomalousness of the mental. The first argument turns on the model of causation implicit in Davidson's account: Hempel's covering law account. Its basic idea is that whenever one event causes another there is a law-statement that taken with a suitable description of the occurrence of the first event implies that the second event occurs. Combining this with Anomalous Monism produces the following prima facie problem. As the laws that underpin the causality of the mental are physical, but the descriptions of events that feature in action explanation are mental, they will not 'fit together' to yield the right implications.

Now Davidson might respond to this objection in the following way. It does not matter that mental descriptions of events do not plug into the covering law account of causation. All that matters is that in principle there are pairs of suitable physical descriptions for the same events that do so fit. The cost of this response, however, is to sever the connection between this underlying metaphysical requirement and the reason explanations we give. As Tanney says of a slightly different point: 'But what any of this has to do with our original reason-attribution is left utterly mysterious since we haven't any idea how to identify the original event . . . as one that is apt both for the *appropriate* mental and physical predicates/properties to begin with.' (p. 119).

Where does this leave us?

So it seems both that Davidson's original arguments for a causal ingredient in reason explanation fail and that there would be something mysterious about the explanatory role of such an appeal even if further arguments could be found. Where does that leave us?

One possible line of response is to return to the sort of non-causal conception of mind with which the chapter started. Melden (1961) and Ryle (1963) argued that it was a mistake to think of mental states as the sorts of things that might stand in causal relations. Recall that Melden suggested that a major source of philosophical error was a natural tendency to 'suppose that the difficulty we may have in understanding what an intention or desire is, is the difficulty involved in the *discovery* of an elusive item in our experience' (p. 172, italics added).

But one virtue of Davidson's general account in the light of the first reading (linked with Exercise 1) by Spence (1996a) on neurophysiology was that it suggested a way of accommodating two different perspectives on action: the causal and the rational. It promised a picture of *how* freedom and determinism might be compatible by suggesting that these notions attached to different patterns of explanation of the very same events. In virtue of standing in a network of physical laws, mental events could be seen as physically determined. In virtue of standing in a rational pattern, they could be seen as expressions of autonomy. Furthermore, what makes mere movement into an action turns on its having the right kind of causal history: being caused (in the right way) by antecedent events. So one cost of giving up Davidson's causal theory of action and his token identity theory

of mental and physical events (i.e. there is just one set of events) is the loss of this response to the sort of worry raised by Spence (1996a). Recall, again, that this response was to suggest that Spence's challenge was just a specific instance of the more general problem of locating mind in nature and that Davidson provided that general account.

On the other hand, however, this kind of general picture of the dovetailing of the mental and the physical, with its core assumption about a causal theory of agency, might still seem to leave the general problem of reconciling freedom, which is a prerequisite of autonomous action, with the causal determinism highlighted by Spence. So in the last session we will return to Spence's paper and an influential paper by the Oxford philosopher Sir Peter Strawson.

Reflection on the session and self-test questions

Write down your own reflections on the materials in this session drawing out any points that are particularly significant for you. Then write brief notes about the following:

1. Does Davidson really establish a causal theory of mind?

2. Can his arguments be overturned?

3. If so what remains of his account?

Session 6   Freedom and determinacy

The position so far

Let us summarize the position so far. Spence (1996a) highlights a seeming conflict between our ideas of conscious freedom and neurological determinism. Rather than tackling that question head on, we turned to a debate in the philosophy of mind about the nature of action, as that is usually taken to require the relevant sense of autonomy and freedom. Here there has been debate between the position that formed the orthodoxy in the UK and the more recent Davidson-inspired orthodoxy. The first position holds that there is no connection between the characterization of a movement as an action and its causal antecedents. The second holds that, to the contrary, it is in virtue of being appropriately *caused* by mental states, that a movement is an action. The rare occasions that the rational and the causal properties of a state diverge comprise examples of weakness of will and thus Davidson's picture suggests an explanation of that phenomenon.

But, as we have seen, there are problems with Davidson's attempt to keep the rational and the causal properties of mental states or events in harmony. What explains the rarity of weakness of will? This suggests that there is something wrong with Davidson's way of explaining the nature of action.

Furthermore, even given Davidson's picture of the mind, there may remain the suspicion that Spence is right and that freedom and causal determinism are incompatible. This suspicion could be raised in the context of Anomalous Monism by saying that just because the rational and the causal properties of mental states are relatively autonomous, does not prevent causal determinism trumping the requirements of freedom at the rational level.

This final session will return to the question of freedom raised by Spence by examining an argument set out by the Oxford philosopher Sir Peter Strawson. This paper argues that, in so far as determinism is a coherent metaphysical doctrine, it cannot and should not threaten the idea of moral responsibility. Strawson argues for this without making any assumptions about the connection between mental and physical descriptions. In other words, if he is right, his conclusions apply independently of the correct view to take on whether reasons are causes.

EXERCISE 7

Read the extract from:

Strawson, P.F. (1974). Freedom and resentment. In *Freedom and Resentment, and Other Essays*. London: Methuen, pp. 1–25. (Extracts: pp 6–9, 10–11)

Link with Reading 26.6

- How does Strawson characterize the debate?
- What sort of response does he think should be given?
- Is he successful?

Strawson's twin aims

In this paper, Strawson attempts to carry out two related but separable tasks. One is to block the threat that determinism seems to pose to the idea of freedom and the various moral judgements that presuppose it. The other is to diagnose why it is that the choice between 'optimists' and 'pessimists' in that debate seems so stark. In this, Strawson aims at the therapeutic dissolution of a problem rather than providing a substantial justificatory philosophical theory to answer a genuine question. He wants to show why there is not a substantial problem concerning freedom, but without showing that we are in a strange sense *really* free.

Optimists and pessimists

Strawson characterizes the debate he wishes to assess as one between optimists and pessimists. Pessimists hold that if determinism is true then the concepts of moral obligation and responsibility lose their point. Optimists hold that this is not so. In fact Strawson further characterizes optimists as typically holding that moral concepts take their point from those moral practices that successfully regulate society. Both agree on the following further claim: that moral responsibility requires freedom. However, they disagree on what this freedom amounts to. Optimists think it is an absence of external compulsion and the presence of a coincidence of action

with the real wishes and intentions of agents. However, pessimists think that there is an extra sense to freedom that is incompatible with the truth of determinism, although, as Strawson points out, it is usually not possible to characterize this sense of freedom at all clearly. At this point an impasse is reached.

Strawson's therapeutic aim is then to provide the optimist with a further characterization of the grounding of moral concepts that will preclude the 'panicky metaphysics' of the pessimist. If something more can be said about the grounding of our moral concepts than merely their efficacy in regulating social practice, then perhaps there will be no need to invoke a queer sense of freedom to justify them.

Moral reactions

The first stage of Strawson's campaign (in section III of the paper) is to move away from more or less *intellectual* moral judgements to direct moral *reactions*. Here he notes that one's reactions to the actions of other depends greatly on their attitudes and intentions towards us. These affect whether one feels gratitude, resentment, and forgiveness, for example.

There are, however, occasions when one does not feel resentment, say, for an action that in other circumstances would prompt it. In one range of circumstances one takes the agent to be a morally responsible individual but the specific action to be one for which he or she was not responsible. Perhaps it was carried out under compulsion. In a second broad range of circumstances, one takes the agent not to be responsible: either because 'he was not himself' or because 'he's just a child' or suffering from schizophrenia. In this second range, of cases, instead of sharing a human relationship, one takes an objective attitude to the other: one treats them as someone to be managed, handled, or trained.

Strawson argues that we can also take this objective attitude to normal people, but not for long.

Moral reactions and determinism

With this context in place, Strawson goes on to ask what effect the truth of determinism should have upon our moral reactions or reactive attitudes. 'More specifically, would, or should, the acceptance of the truth of the thesis lead to the decay or the repudiation of all such attitudes? Would or should it mean the end of gratitude, resentment, and forgiveness?' (p. 10). This question amounts to whether the truth of determinism would or should justify the universal adoption of the objective attitude just described?

It does not seem to be self-contradictory to suppose that this might happen. So I suppose we must say that it is not absolutely inconceivable that it should happen. But I am strongly inclined to think that it is, for us as we are, practically inconceivable. The human commitment to participation in ordinary interpersonal relationships is, I think, too thorough going and deeply rooted for us to take seriously the thought that a general theoretical conviction might so change our world that, in it, there were no longer any such things as interpersonal relationships as we normally understand them; and being involved in interpersonal relationships as we normally understand them precisely is being exposed to the range of reactive attitudes and feelings that is in question (p. 11).

But there is a further implicit point that the paper goes on to draw out. When we normally adopt the objective attitude it is because we view the person who is to be controlled, rather than regarded as a moral agent, as incapacitated. It is not because we view them as 'determined' in the sense of the philosophical thesis of determinism. And in that sense, even if determinism were true it would not justify the objective attitude.

A niggling doubt?

Now there may remain a niggling doubt that Strawson has answered the wrong question: how we *would* react to the truth of determinism, not how we *should* react to its truth. But he claims to react in this way is to miss the point of his claims so far.

It might be said that all this leaves the real question unanswered, and that we cannot hope to answer it without knowing exactly what the thesis of determinism is. For the real question is not a question about what we actually do, or why we do it. It is not even a question about what we would *in fact* do if a certain theoretical conviction gained acceptance. It is a question about what it would be *rational* to do if determinism were true, a question about the rational justification of ordinary interpersonal attitudes in general. To this I shall reply, first, that such a question could seem real only to one who had utterly failed to grasp the purport of the preceding answer, the fact of our natural human commitment to ordinary interpersonal attitudes. This commitment is part of the general framework of human life, not something that comes up for review as particular cases can come up for review within this general framework. And I shall reply, second, that if we could imagine what we cannot have, namely, a choice in this matter, then we could rationally only in the light of an assessment of the gains and losses to human life, its enrichment or impoverishment; and the truth or falsity of a general thesis of determinism would not bear on the rationality of *this* choice (p. 13).

What optimists generally miss

The second half of Strawson's (1974) paper is argumentatively less dense. Broadly it goes on to argue that attention to the general framework of direct engaged reactions provides something that is often missing from an optimist's account of moral concepts. They instead base an account on a drier, less engaged account of human practice. Thus by adding in the basis of engaged reactions, Strawson hopes that he can give the pessimists that extra something, which they think must underpin moral judgements and which they construe as a genuine and deep sense of freedom.

This methodological claim, however, seems more a comment on the contingent way the philosophical debate has been conducted than on the underlying issues. Pessimists might agree that moral judgements run deep in our nature and are based on natural reactions and still call them into question if determinism is true. For that reason it is the argument halfway through the paper, and summarized above, which is the most crucial.

In summary

Strawson's paper is broadly in the same spirit as the work of Ryle (1963) and Meldon (1961) discussed at the start of this chapter and J.L. Austin from Part 1. It attempts, by more careful description of our (linguistic and other) practices to eschew the need for 'panicky metaphysics' (in this case, a sense of freedom which transcends the causal order). But does he really side-step the problems that Spence's (1996a) paper raises for freedom?

In the second half of his paper, Spence emphasizes the neural underpinnings of conscious free will, arguing that causal determinism is incompatible with there being any genuine sense of freedom of will. We are now in a position to give a response of sorts. We can argue that Spence's claim turns on a false opposition between the kind of freedom that we value and is a presupposition of moral responsibility, and the determinism that is a feature of the causal order. Despite first appearances, freedom in the former sense does not require the falsity of determinism. There is no connection between the discovery of the causal precursors to action and the justification of taking an objective attitude to subjects or agents.

This Strawsonian thought may or may not be combined with a causal theory of action, which would interact with the claims in the first half of Spence's paper. This was summarized earlier as the claim that, although we might think of exercises of free will in action and thought as always conscious, there are both normal and pathological instances where we have thoughts or we act apparently deliberately, but do not experience those acts or thoughts as consciously willed by us. A causal theory of action is an attempt to say what it is for action to be willed: it is for it to be caused (in the right way) by beliefs and desires. According to Davidson, these are in turn states of the body or brain. So one approach to Spence's clinical work is to fit it into just such a general philosophical account.

We have, however, seen that there are problems with arguments for a causal theory of mind in general and Davidson's version of monism in particular. So if instead the right moral is the adoption of a non-causal theory, Spence's results cannot be so accommodated. They would have instead to be taken to be attempting to join together two kinds of description—the mental and the causal—which are incommensurable. A non-causalist has yet to say just what it is for an action to be willed except in a negative way that it was not compelled or some such. Here further clinical work may well be very important. Nevertheless, to repeat the point just made, even the non-causalist account can help itself to Strawson's argument that there is not yet an intolerable threat to freedom raised by the results of brain imaging.

Reflection on the session and self-test questions

Write down your own reflections on the materials in this session drawing out any points that are particularly significant for you. Then write brief notes about the following:

1. What is the role of reactive attitudes in Strawson's account of the relation of freedom and determinacy?

2. How does the adoption, or not, of an objective attitude towards agents dovetail with the suspension of reactive attitudes like resentment?

3. What argument does he offer against the universal adoption of an objective outlook?

Reading guide

Useful collections concerning causal theories of action include:

◆ Alfred Mele (ed.) (1997) *The Philosophy of Action*.

◆ John Heil and Alfred Mele (ed.) (1993) *Mental Causation*.

◆ White's (1968) collection, *The Philosophy of Action*, includes Austin's (1956/7) *A Plea for Excuses* (see Part I) and Anscombe's (1959) *Intention*.

◆ Austin's (1966) *Three Ways of Spilling Ink*, Hampshire's (1959) *Thought and Action*, and Winch's (1972) *Ethics and Action*, are important classics.

◆ Jennifer Hornsby's (1980) *Actions* is more difficult but captures recent trends.

   (See also Reading guide to Chapter 6.)

Non-causal theories of action

The view of willing that inspired many non-causal theories of action can be found in: Wittgenstein (1953) *Philosophical Investigations*, §611–630.

   It is supported in:

◆ G.E.M. Anscombe (1959) 'Intention' (in *Proceedings of the Aristotelian Society*, and later reprinted in White's (ed.) (1968) *The Philosophy of Action*)

◆ Malcolm, N. (1968) The conceivability of mechanism *Philosophical Review*

◆ Melden, A.I. (1961) *Free Action*

◆ P. Winch's (1960) *The Idea of Social Science and its Relation to Philosophy* (2nd edn)

Causal theories of action

◆ Davidson's (1980) causal theory of action is set out in a number of essays collected in his *Essays on Actions and Events*.

◆ A useful introduction is Evnine's (1991) *Donald Davidson*.

◆ More specific work on Davidson's account can be found in Child's (1994) *Causality Interpretation and the Mind*, especially chapter 3, and in many of the essays in LePore and McLaughlin (1985) *Essays on Actions and Events*.

Freedom and determinism

The philosophical debate about freedom and determinism is set out in the following:

◆ Daniel C. Dennett (1984) *Elbow Room* and (2003) Freedom Evolves

◆ Ilham Dilman (1999) *Free Will: an historical and philosophical introduction*

◆ Robert Kane (ed.) (2001) *Free Will* (1996) The significance of free will

◆ Gary Watson (ed.) (2003) *Free Will*.

Applied work

◆ Spence's article: Spence (1996a) 'Free will in the light of neuropsychiatry' (*Philosophy, Psychiatry, & Psychology*, pp. 75–90); has commentaries by Frith (1996, pp. 91–94), Libet (1996, pp. 95–96), Stephens (1996, pp. 97–98), and reply by Spence (1996b, pp. 99–100).

◆ Spence's work is further developed in Spence (2001) 'Alien control: from phenomenology to cognitive neurobiology' (*Philosophy, Psychiatry, & Psychology*, pp. 163–172); with commentary by Pacherie (2001, pp. 173–176).

◆ Further applied work on free will includes: Waller (2004a) 'Neglected psychological elements of free will' (*Philosophy, Psychiatry, & Psychology*, pp. 111–118); with commentary by Lieberman (2004, pp. 119–124), and reply Waller (2004b, pp. 125–128).

◆ The Harvard psychologist Daniel Wegner sets out, in The Illusion of Conscious Will (2002), to deconstruct the idea that we consciously will our actions using experimental psychology.

◆ Stephens G.L. and Graham, G. (1996). Psychopathology, freedom and the experience of externality *Philosophical Topics* is an examination of just what our capacity to be alienated from our own states tells about us the importance of ownership of states for freedom & action.

References

Anscombe, G.E.M. (1959). Intention. *Proceedings of the Aristotelian Society* 57: 321–332. (Reprinted in White, A.R. (ed.) (1968). *The Philosophy of Action*. Oxford: Oxford University Press.)

Austin, J.L. (1956/7). A plea for excuses. *Proceedings of the Aristotelian Society*, 57: 1–30. (Reprinted in White, A.R. (ed.) (1968). *The Philosophy of Action*. Oxford: Oxford University Press, pp. 19–42.)

Austin, J.L. (1966). Three ways of spilling ink. *Philosophical Review*, 75: 427–440. (Reprinted in White, A.R. (ed.) (1968). *The Philosophy of Action*. Oxford: Oxford University Press.)

Bishop, J. (1983). Agent-causation. *Mind*, 92: 61–79.

Child, W. (1994). *Causality Interpretation and the Mind*. Oxford: Oxford University Press.

Davidson, D. (1980). *Essays on Actions and Events*. Oxford: Oxford University Press.

Davidson, D. (1982). Paradoxes of irrationality. In *Philosophical Essays on Freud* (ed. J. Hopkins and R. Wollheim). Cambridge: Cambridge University Press, pp. 289–305.

Dennett, D.C. (1984). *Elbow Room*. Cambridge, MA: MIT Press.

Dennett, D.C. (2003). *Freedom Evolves*. New York: Viking.

Dilman, I. (1999). *Free Will: an historical and philosophical introduction*. London: Routledge.

Evnine, S. (1991). *Donald Davidson*. Oxford: Polity.

Frith, C. (1996). Free will in the light of neuropsychiatry. (Commentary on Spence, 1996a) *Philosophy, Psychiatry, & Psychology*, 3(2): 91–94.

Hampshire, S. (1959). *Thought and Action*. London: Chatto and Windus. (Reprinted in White, A.R. (ed.) (1968). *The Philosophy of Action*. Oxford: Oxford University Press.)

Heil, J. and Mele, A. (ed.) (1993). *Mental Causation*. Oxford: Oxford University Press.

Hornsby, J. (1980). *Actions*. London: Routledge & Kegan Paul.

Kane, R. (1996). *The Significance of Free Will*. Oxford: OUP.

Kane, R. (ed.) (2001). *Free Will*. Oxford: Blackwell.

LePore, E. and McLaughlin, B. (1985). *Actions and Events*. Oxford: Blackwell.

Libet, B. (1996). Free will in the light of neuropsychiatry. (Commentary on Spence, 1996a) *Philosophy, Psychiatry, & Psychology*, 3(2): 95–96.

Lieberman, P.B. (2004). Action, belief, and empowerment. (Commentary on Waller, 2004a) *Philosophy, Psychiatry, & Psychology*, 11(2): 119–124.

Malcolm, N. (1968). The conceivability of mechanism. *Philosophical Review*, 77: 45–72.

McDowell, J. (1994). Mind and World. Cambridge, MA.: Harvard University Press.

Melden, A.I. (1961). *Free Action*. London: Routledge.

Mele, A.R. (1997). *The Philosophy of Action*. Oxford: Oxford University Press.

Pacherie, E. (2001). Agency lost and found: a commentary on Spence. (Commentary on Spence, 2001) *Philosophy, Psychiatry, & Psychology*, 8/2/3: 173–176.

Ryle, G. (1963). *The Concept of Mind*. London: Penguin.

Spence, S.A. (1996a). Free will in the light of neuropsychiatry. (Commentaries by Frith, C. (1996, pp. 91–94), Libet, B. (1996, pp. 95–96), and Stephens, G.L. (1996, pp. 97–98) and reply by Spence, S.A. (1996b, pp. 99–100)) *Philosophy, Psychiatry, & Psychology*, 3(2): 75–90.

Spence, S.A. (1996b). Response to the Commentaries (on Spence, 1996a). *Philosophy, Psychiatry, & Psychology*, 3(2): 99–100.

Spence, S. (2001). Alien control: from phenomenology to cognitive neurobiology. (with commentary by Pacherie, E. (2001, pp. 173–176)) *Philosophy, Psychiatry, & Psychology*, 8/2/3: 163–172.

Stephens, G.L. and Graham, G. (1996). Psychopathology, freedom and the experience of externality Philosophical Topics, 24: 159–182.

Strawson, P.F. (1974). Freedom and resentment. In *Freedom and Resentment, and Other Essays*. London: Methuen, pp. 1–25.

Tanney, J. (1995). Why reasons may not be causes. *Mind and Language*, 10: 105–128.

Waller, B.N. (2004a). Neglected psychological elements of free will. (Commentary by Lieberman, P.B. (2004, pp. 119–124) and reply Waller, B.N. (2004b, 125–128)) *Philosophy, Psychiatry, & Psychology*, 11(2): 111–118.

Waller, B.N. (2004b). Comparing psychoanalytic and cognitive-behavioral perspectives on control. (Response to Lieberman, 2004) *Philosophy, Psychiatry, & Psychology*, 11(2): 125–128.

Watson, G. (ed.) (2003). *Free Will*. Oxford: Oxford University Press.

White, A.R. (ed.) (1968). *The Philosophy of Action*. Oxford: Oxford University Press.

Winch, P. (1960). *The Idea of Social Science and its Relation to Philosophy*, (2nd edn). London: Routledge & Kegan Paul.

Winch, P. (1972). *Ethics and Action*. London: Routledge and Kegan Paul.

Wittgenstein, L. (1953). *Philosophical Investigations*. Oxford: Basil Blackwell.

CHAPTER 27

Knowledge of other minds

Chapter contents

So far the chapters in this part of the book have focused on the nature of the mind and mental states of central importance to psychiatry. The questions that they have addressed have included:

- What are mental states and how are they related to physical states including brain states?
- How are mental states *about* anything?
- In what sense is the aboutness or intentionality of the mind a *natural* property?
- What is the connection between thought and language?
- Can mental states cause actions?

Empirical versus metaphysical

These are all questions about the nature of mental phenomena, about their ontology. While they are not straightforwardly *empirical* questions we have looked at the bearing that empirical findings, such as the results of brain imaging or theories of mental function from cognitive psychiatry, have on them. However, they have all been questions of ontology, of the nature of what is. By contrast the subject matter of this chapter is the *epistemology* of mind of how we know about our and others' mental states.

Ontology versus epistemology

The focus of this chapter is how we can have *knowledge* of mental states rather than what mental states are. In fact, in the case of the philosophy of mind, the distinction between epistemology and ontology is not sharp. Getting clear on how we find out what we and other people think promises to shed light on the very nature of thought. However, the agenda will be set by following epistemological issues first.

The importance of the issue to mental health care

The question of how we know about the mental states of others is obviously important to an understanding of mental health care. Think, for example, of a clinical encounter between doctor and patient, or social worker and client. One of the key aims of the doctor or social worker is to find out about the state of mind of the patient or client. Now the Present State Examination is one attempt to increase the consistency (or inter-rater reliability) of such encounters. However, it does not raise the deep issue of how it is at all possible to know about someone else's mental states.

There is another source of interest in this question that results from clinical work. One of the central symptoms of autism is an impoverishment of a subject's ability to understand others. So if people who suffer autism have an impairment of an ability that non-sufferers enjoy, this promises to shed light on that ability. Just what is it that autistic people lack? What is the nature of their disability in this area?

Knowledge, access, and the role of justification

Given that we are concerned with epistemology: with how we know about other people's mental states there is a further preliminary point worth making. In general in philosophical discussion, epistemology is mainly concerned with *justification*. It addresses the *pedigree* of our beliefs (about the external world, the future, the past) by asking what justification can be given for them on the long-standing traditional assumption that justification (or something similar) is an element of knowledge. (The traditional thumbnail analysis is that knowledge is *justified true belief*.) This is reflected in a traditional question in the philosophy of mind: How can we *know* the contents of other minds, or know even whether other minds exist?

In this chapter we will be equally concerned with a question that appears to be prior to that of justification: How is it possible to form beliefs about the contents of other people's minds at all? How is any such access possible? In fact the question of access and the question of justification are closely related. As we do take ourselves to be justified in our beliefs about other minds, no account of access that leaves such judgements as having the status of mere guesswork will do. The very idea of talking about access to other minds implies some degree of reliability. Thus explaining how it is possible to form beliefs about mental states must dovetail with an explanation of why the method we generally deploy is justified.

Three main approaches

What gives the question of access to other minds its bite is the persuasive thought that we cannot literally see (into) the minds of others. Only I can directly access my mental states. Other people must *infer* them as I must infer both the existence and the contents of their mental states. On what basis and how can I draw inferences? To anticipate the rest of this chapter, there are currently two main rival responses to this question.

Theory-theory

One account replies that access to other minds is mediated by a *theory*. This takes as its input observable behaviour and, as its output, claims about unobservable mental states. Third-person access is thus akin to our access to the unobservable microstructure of the world provided by the theoretical physical sciences. In recent jargon this is called the 'theory-theory' approach.

Simulation theory

Its main rival is the 'simulation-theory' approach. This is based on a contrasting thought. Instead of deploying a *theoretical* knowledge of the workings of minds, we access other minds by *using* our own mental faculties. We put ourselves in the shoes of other people on the basis of an assessment of their situation, actions, and speech. Thus we simulate the mental states of others. Rather than *knowing* and applying general principles that govern the workings of minds, we simply *use* our own minds of whose working we might be ignorant.

These two sketches maximize the differences between theory-theory and simulation theory. As we will see later in the chapter, they may not be as different as all that. Very briefly: no theory theorist believes that the theory in question is a matter of *explicit* knowledge. The theory is, at most, *tacitly* known and codifies our abilities to ascribe mental states on the basis of behavioural evidence. It resembles the use of linguistic theory, which is supposed to codify our ability to use and understand grammatical sentences. Such linguistic theories—the stuff of Chomskian linguistics, for example—are not thought of as explicitly known by speakers but merely tacitly known. Likewise in this case the theory of others minds is tacit. But if so the ability it codifies may be an ability to simulate. At the same time, simulation theory requires that the results of the 'thought experiments' on which it depends are taken to be guides to how others think. It is open to question whether this can escape a theoretical inference that you are thinking the same thoughts as those I have just simulated.

What may serve as the clearest difference between these two approaches is the way rationality plays a constitutive role in the mind. But whether that role is best cashed out in either such theory is questionable.

Direct access?

There is also a lesser known third possibility. This is to deny that there is the fundamental epistemological barrier, that both of the preceding views presuppose, to the direct access to other's mental states. Spelling out this third option will require some care because there is something unarguable about the claim that we cannot directly observe other people's mental states. Nevertheless, this need not be seen as requiring the kind of explanatory account at which both the theory-theory and simulation theory aim.

But we will begin not with any of these contemporary views but with a piece of intellectual history.

The plan of the chapter

◆ *Session 1* examines the origin of the Problem of Other Minds in Descartes' account of the mind and the attempt to solve it using the Argument from Analogy.

◆ *Session 2* introduces the 'theory theory' approach.

◆ *Session 3* introduces the rival 'simulation theory' approach which emphasises the role of rationality.

◆ *Session 4* looks at the current state of the debate including the role of evidence from autism.

◆ *Session 5* examines a more direct approach to undermine the Problem of Other Minds.

Session 1 An historical starting point: Descartes and the argument from analogy

The origin of the Problem of Other Minds

In the Anglo-American tradition, the philosophy of mind, has until very recently, turned away from epistemological issues and concentrated instead on metaphysical and ontological questions about the nature of mental states. It has focused on the sorts of questions discussed in previous chapters. However, during the first half of the twentieth century, a central 'live' issue in the philosophy of mind was the Problem of Other Minds. How is it possible to account for our knowledge of the mental states of other people or even that they have them?

Like most philosophically sceptical questions, this question requires some initial stage setting for it to seem pressing. After all, it is obvious that in everyday life we routinely make judgements about other people's beliefs, moods, desires, and suchlike. Making arrangements to meet at a specific place and time requires just this sort of understanding. In law courts, evidence can be offered about the state of a person's mind with just as much claim to validity or objectivity as evidence about the state of their bank balance. Many human customs and practices would be impossible if it we were not able reliably to 'read' other people's minds. However, once one has been initiated into a characteristically philosophical way of thinking about the mind, this ability can come to seem mysterious or illusory.

Historically, the express route to the Problem of Other Minds was one or other form of Cartesian dualism. Descartes' arguments for a dualism of thinking non-extended stuff and extended non-thinking matter were touched on in Chapter 22. However, without thinking of the details of his argument—an argument whose validity is open to question—it is worth recalling generally its presuppositions.

EXERCISE 1	(30 minutes)

Read the short extract from the start of:

Descartes, R. ([1641] 1996). *Meditations on First Philosophy*. Cambridge: Cambridge University Press. (Extract: pp. 12–13.)

Link with Reading 27.1

◆ What is striking about the approach that Descartes adopts to doing philosophy?

◆ How might this affect his account of the mind?

The solitary starting point

Descartes' project is one that, he suggests, should be undertaken once in his life. He should examine his beliefs in order to establish some foundation for them. Thus he begins: '*I am here quite alone*, and at last will devote myself sincerely and without reservation to the general demolition of my opinions.' (p. 12, italics added)

What is striking about this starting point is its solitariness. In general we take the acquisition of knowledge to be a social endeavour. Scientists generally work in teams in large laboratories. The case conference is widely used in health care. Even individual scientific research is vetted and reproduced by others and the mark of its success turns on its wider publication in journals or at conferences. Descartes' project, by contrast, is one he undertakes alone. This is not to say that others might not also follow the same thought processes. However, they will also do it alone. As we will see, and as often happens in philosophy, his final account of the mind owes much to this apparently innocent choice of starting point.

Sources of scepticism

As should be familiar, Descartes then attempts to set aside any beliefs that can be the subject of doubt in order, he hopes, to arrive at a firm indubitable foundation on which to base his subsequent beliefs. Rather than attempting to run through his beliefs piecemeal and assess each individually, he thinks of three general sources of doubt about empirical beliefs. First, beliefs grounded in his senses are subject to perceptual illusions. Secondly, as at any moment he cannot reliably test that he is not dreaming, empirical beliefs based on the testimony of his senses or his memory may be false. Thirdly, he may be subject to delusion by an evil genie. 'I shall think that the sky, the air, the earth, colours, shapes, sounds and all external things are merely the delusions of dreams which he has devised to ensnare my judgement. I shall consider myself as not having hands, or eyes, or blood or senses…' (p. 15).

Thus all beliefs that turn on the reality of the external world are equally subject to doubt and are (temporally) rejected.

(One possible line of objection to Descartes' project is to object that there is no natural kind that comprises our knowledge of the external world. What Descartes presents as merely a short-cut is an essential presupposition. He seems to assume two things. First, that there is a logical gap between inner experience and the state of the outer world. It is this which enables him to say that we could not tell from inner experience alone that we were not deceived by an evil genie (or nowadays that we were not a brain in a vat). However, he also assumes that to counter scepticism, we must form justified beliefs about the outer world *from* our inner experience. He assumes, in other words, a form of foundationalism, which is far from mandatory. For this line of criticism see Williams (1996) *Unnatural Doubts*.)

The cogito

A sceptical loss of knowledge of the outer world is the dismal conclusion of the first meditation. In the second, Descartes continues in this sceptical vein but is stopped in his tracks by the following thought:

> But I have convinced myself that there is absolutely nothing in the world, no sky, no earth, no minds, no bodies. Does it follow that I too do not exist? No: if I convinced myself of something then I certainly existed. But there is a deceiver of supreme power and cunning who is deliberately and constantly deceiving me. In that case I too undoubtedly exist, if he is deceiving me; and let him deceive me as much as he can, he will never bring it about that I am nothing so long as I think that I am something. So after considering everything very thoroughly, I must conclude that this proposition, *I am, I exist*, is necessarily true whenever it is put forward by me or conceived in my mind.   (p. 17)

Thus the one thing that resists his sceptical attack is that he himself exists. It is another matter in what respect he exists: what he is. A similar procedure is followed to analyse this: 'I will then subtract anything capable of being weakened, even minimally, by the arrangements now introduced, so that what is left at the end may be exactly and only what is certain.'

As a result of this method, Descartes rejects definitions of himself as a rational animal or as embodied with a face, hands, and arms. All these substantial descriptions include elements whose existence cannot meet the strict epistemological pedigree imposed within the meditations. This leaves the minimal claim that he, Descartes, is a thing that thinks, that doubts, understands, affirms, and suchlike. It is worth briefly digressing here for a few paragraphs.

Digression on the validity of the argument

As has long been realized, if Descartes intends to ground a substantial negative conclusion that he Descartes is nothing more than a thinking thing, the argument suggested in the second meditation, is the wrong way to go about it. Using the resources available in this meditation, the best line of argument appears to be as follows:

1. One of the features or properties of myself is that its existence cannot be doubted by myself.

2. One of the features or properties of my body is that its existence can be doubted by myself.

3. If two apparently different things are really numerically identical (i.e. the very same thing) they must have all and only the same properties.

4. Therefore I am not my body.

This resembles a sound argument based on Leibnitz's law (the third premiss). I and my body differ in one property or feature and thus cannot be the very same thing. Suppose you were falsely accused of stealing a tie from a shop on an occasion when one but only one tie had been stolen and resembled the one carelessly tied around your own neck. One possible line of defence—if this were appropriate—would be to show that your tie and the one stolen differed in some feature. Perhaps the other (must have) had a 'St Michael' label and yours says 'Pierre Cardin'. If so, because they differ in this respect, they cannot really be one and the same and thus yours is not the stolen tie in question. (Perhaps you stole it from a different shop!)

In Descartes' case, however, this form of argument will not work. Consider (to use an oft-quoted example) that the Prime Minister were to awake suffering from amnesia. He might wonder who he was. Suppose he were to employ Descartes' method of doubt. Whimsically, or on the basis of some evidence found on the hospital ward, he might consider the possibility that he were, in fact, the Prime Minister. Now even if it were true that he were the Prime Minister, this fact would still be open to sceptical doubt. By contrast the fact of his own existence would not be open to him to doubt. By applying the same form of argument he could conclude that he were not the Prime Minister after all. As in this case true premisses would clearly lead to a false conclusion, the form of the argument in general cannot be valid.

The problem in Descartes' argument as formalized above is that the properties that plug into Leibnitz's law (whether in Descartes' case or the Prime Ministerial example) occur within what is called an 'intensional context' of a propositional attitude—in this case the Descartes *doubting that* such and such. In well behaved *extensional* contexts, substituting terms that refer to the same thing keeps the sentence true if it was true or false if it was false. Consider: 'The prime minister of the UK in 2005 was a man.' This is true. Thus so is: 'Tony Blair was a man.' These two sentences only differ in the substitution of 'Tony Blair' for 'The prime minister of the UK' which refer (in 2005) to the same man. But consider: 'Smith believes that the prime minister of the UK in 2005 was a man' and 'Smith believes that Tony Blair was a man'. It is perfectly possible that one is true and the other false.

Substituting co-referring terms within the content of mental states does not generally preserve the truth value of such reports. I may be a fan of the Roman orator Cicero and thus: I believe that *Cicero was a fine orator*. But it is not necessarily the case that: I believe that *Tully was a fine orator*, because I may not believe that Cicero was Tully (even though in fact 'Cicero' and 'Tully' are different names for the same person). Leibnitz's law does not apply to differences within intensional contexts.

End of digression

From the point of view of a sympathetic reading of Descartes, it is not clear that the fallacious argument set out above is what underpins his negative conclusion. In Meditation 6, he brings out the extent to which the assumption that God would not deceive him in his (Descartes') appraisal of what is and what is not possible. But what matters to this chapter is not so much Descartes' dualist conclusion, but the way his starting point shapes both his and others' assumptions about our epistemological predicament.

The origin of the Problem of Other Minds

Descartes builds a picture of the world outwards from a perspective even more alone than a philosopher sitting alone before the fire in his dressing gown. He is alone with his thoughts only, the existence of his body being a matter of inference that will (later) be underpinned by God. His account of the world starts from his own first-person perspective and builds outwards. A key presupposition is that this first perspective is not threatened or changed by scepticism about the outside world. In this assumption he differs from the externalists about content discussed in Chapter 25. They hold that the very ability to hold at least some thoughts requires that one stands in some actual relation to the 'outside' world. Descartes subscribes to an internalist assumption that although his beliefs will be false if there is no external world, they will remain the very same beliefs. Their existence is world-independent.

Now one problem, forcefully presented recently by the philosopher John McDowell, with this view of one's standing in the world is that it makes the ability of thoughts to concern worldly objects mysterious (see Reading guide). If mental states are free-standing elements in my mental wardrobe, why should they be any more *about* anything than my trousers? On Descartes' account, mental states are immaterial, but they retain a thing-like quality. If so how can they, as free-standing things be about anything?

However, even setting this fundamental problem aside leaves a long-standing further difficulty. How can one have knowledge of, or even access in some weaker sense to, other people's minds? If mental states are elements in a private theatre with only one spectator, how can others gain access to them? This is the Problem of Other Minds. The classic solution is the argument from analogy to which we will now turn.

An attempt to solve the Problem of Other Minds

> **EXERCISE 2** (10 minutes)
>
> Think about how one might know about other people's mental states if Descartes' account of the mind were true. How would access to your own mental states help? Try to take the problem seriously and consider what resources might be available to you. But also think how you do in fact experience other people's minds.

The argument from analogy

There are a number of plausible answers that might be given to the question: How can I know other people's mental states?

Perhaps the obvious answer is by *analogy* with my own. Of course another response is to assume in the face of Descartes' account of the mind as a private subjective realm that we do *not* know other people's minds. In other words, one might adopt a limited form of scepticism directed just at others' mental states while allowing knowledge of their outer behaviour. However, that is a radical and ultimately impractical line to take. (Try it!) Sir Bertrand Russell, for example, says:

> We are not content to think that we know only the space-time structure of our friends' minds, or their capacity for initiating causal chains that end in sensations of our own. A philosopher might pretend to think that he knew only this, but let him get cross with his wife and you will see that he does not regard her as a mere spatio-temporal edifice of which he knows the logical properties but not a glimmer of the intrinsic character. We are therefore justified in inferring that his skepticism is professional rather than sincere.
>
> Bertrand Russell 'Analogy' from *Human Knowledge: its scope and limits* ([1948] 1991, pp. 89–91)

Russell takes as the basic datum to be explained the fact that *we do know* the mental states, beliefs, moods, and desires of other people. We do not merely claim to know their physical properties, and their abilities to act (in the way that we know the dispositional properties of chemicals, for example). How is this possible, then? Russell sets out to articulate the principle on which such claims can be grounded given the basic Cartesian first-person perspective as a starting point.

His suggestion is that 'we must appeal to something that may be vaguely called "analogy". The behaviour of other people is in many ways analogous to our own, and we must suppose that it must have analogous causes.' Russell suggests that because he knows from his own case that his thirst is the normal cause of such an utterance, when he hears the sentence 'I'm thirsty' when he himself is not thirsty he can conclude that it is probable that someone else is. He assumes this the more readily given other behavioural factors such as seeing a hot drooping body. 'It is evident that my confidence in the "inference" is increased by increased complexity in the datum and also by increased certainty of the causal law derived from subjective observation.' (p. 90)

Russell sees this form of inference as akin to the reasoning from effects to causes in the physical sciences. While no such inference can be certain—because the same effect may be caused in different ways—it can, he suggests, be probable. The general principle is summarized as follows: 'If, whenever we can observe whether A and B are present or absent, we find that every case of B has an A as a causal antecedent, then it is probable that most B's have A's as causal antecedents, even in cases where observation does not enable us to know whether A is present or not.' (p. 91)

Against analogy

Although there is something initially attractive about the pairing of a Cartesian picture of mind with the argument from analogy, there are powerful arguments against this as a coherent position. Many are developments of remarks made by Wittgenstein about *criteria* to which we will turn shortly. But Wittgenstein himself also deployed two other considerations.

Wittgenstein's criticisms

A simple argument is that analogical reasoning provides poor justification. Unlike the establishment of correlations in physics, for example, there is in principle only *one* kind of correlation on which to base one's analogy: the connection between one's own mental states and behaviour. This goes no way towards undercutting the worry that only I have mental states in the first place: that there is a fundamental distinction between my experience and anyone else's.

Imagination

A different objection is raised in the following passage from the Wittgenstein's (1953) *Philosophical Investigations*:

> If one has to imagine someone else's pain on the model of one's own, this is none too easy a thing to do: for I have to imagine pain which I *do not feel* on the model of the pain which I *do feel*. That is, what I have to do is not simply make a transition in imagination from one place of pain to another. As, from pain in the hand to pain in the arm. For I am not to imagine that I feel pain in some region of his body (which would also be possible).   (§302)

The problem that Wittgenstein raises here is the difficulty of thinking of someone else's pain given only one's own experience of one's own pain. Given only this first-person starting point, what are the materials available to think of a pain that someone else experiences? It is not enough simply to imagine one's own pain in another body because this would be a case of feeling pain

on their leg, for instance. So how could one break out of a first-person grasp of pain as pain-as-I-feel it to imagine pain independently of my experience?

EXERCISE 3   (30 minutes)

Read the extract from:

Malcolm, N. (1958). Knowledge of other minds. *Journal of Philosophy*, 55. pp. 969–978. (Reprinted in Rosenthal, D (ed.) (1991). *The Nature of Mind*. Oxford: Oxford University Press, pp. 92–97 (whose page references are used below).) (Extract: pp. 92–93)

Link with Reading 27.2

- What is the force of Malcolm's criticism of the argument from analogy?
- What positive account of knowledge of other minds does Malcolm offer?

Norman Malcolm and third-person concepts

Norman Malcolm does not rely on the difficulty of *imagining* others' pain given the first-person starting point but on a related point based instead on one's *understanding* or conception of others' pain. (In passing he mentions but does not develop a more purely epistemological point that the argument from analogy is riskily based on inference from one case: one's own mental states.)

Malcolm's argument could be summarized like this. The argument from analogy helps itself to something to which it has no right. It is presented simply as an epistemological solution to an epistemological problem: How can I make judgements about Jones' mental states, his pains, for example? Russell (1991) specifies a principle, which, he argues, provides the necessary justification for such judgements. On the basis of my own experience of the causes of my pain-behaviour (my pains usually), I can infer from Jones' manifest pain-behaviour that 'Jones is in pain' is probably true. But, Malcolm argues, this presupposes that I already know what 'Jones is in pain' means. How?

One possible response is anticipated by Malcolm. The objector suggests that given that I understand what 'pain' means from my own case, I can infer what it means in the sentence 'he has pain' because it means just the same. But while the last claim is true, it is no help in this case until I understand what *sameness* here involves. As we have already seen, it does not involve my feeling pain in his body, for example.

Criteria...

Malcolm goes on to argue that 'Smith is in pain' can only be given meaning if the rules for its use are specified via third-person *criteria* for its correct application. But once such criteria are in place there is no need for an argument from analogy because the criteria will provide direct rules for judging when the state of affairs it describes obtains.

The use of the words 'criterion' and 'criteria' come from Wittgenstein. There has been much discussion of what these are supposed to mean and what philosophical work they can do. We will return to that debate later in this chapter (in Session 4). To begin with, though, criteria are rules for the employment of words, rules which thus determine their meaning. Malcolm's point is that only given such criteria does the phrase 'Smith is in pain' have a meaning but as these rules will specify the circumstances under which it can be applied they will undercut the need for analogical reasoning from one's own case. Instead of judging that Jones is in pain because he is behaving the way I behave when I am in pain, I make this judgement because I know it is licensed directly by Jones' behaviour. That such behaviour is sufficient, in normal circumstances, to warrant the judgement is something I know simply by knowing the meaning of the phrase 'Jones is in pain'.

...and symptoms

This last point is an important feature of criteria that Wittgenstein contrasts with what he calls symptoms. The connection between phenomena and their symptoms is a contingent matter, something to be investigated empirically. By contrast the connection between criteria and what they are criteria of is an a priori matter. Wittgenstein comments that criteria and symptoms can be swapped. What has previously been regarded as a contingent concomitant can come to be regarded instead as definitional. (A neurological indicator of a psychiatric disease may come to play an essential or definitional role, replacing behavioural signs.)

Are criteria defeasible?

Without pre-empting the later discussion of criteria, it is worth here noting one important feature of the connection between mental states and behaviour. Apparently qualitatively identical behaviour can sometimes be the expression of a mental state—such as pain—and can sometimes be a sham. It may, for example, be part of a play. So any account on which behaviour plays a criterial role will have to be one that also allows the relation between apparently identical behaviour and underlying mental states to come apart. For this reason, the first commentators described criteria as analytic but *defeasible* indicators.

Although it has epistemological consequences, what drives Malcolm's argument are considerations about meaning. The key idea is that Descartes' starting point—a necessarily isolated individual identifying his or her own sensations prior to identifying other people's—cannot yield a conception of other people's mental states. Thus, as an account of how we can know about other minds, it cannot be right because we do have a conception of other minds.

A slightly formal argument against a Cartesian account of other minds

In the UK in the 1960s arguments of this form were influential and gave rise to a form of logical behaviourism: roughly the view that there are logical analytic connections between descriptions of behaviour and descriptions of mental states. For a while it seemed that solutions to the Problem of Other Minds amounted to a choice between the scepticism that results from starting from a first-person perspective and then attempting to work outwards, or the behaviourism that resulted from starting from a third-person perspective. One can think of this choice as following from something like the following argument:

i   No one can perceive anyone else's sensations; (assumption).

ii All that can be perceived is behaviour (perhaps tautologically defined by what can be perceived); (assumption).

iii Knowledge of particular matters of fact is either directly perceived or inferred from direct perception; (assumption).

iv Others' sensations are not directly perceived; (from i).

v   Either they are not known or are inferred from behaviour; (from iv, iii, ii).

vi Inference is either deductive or inductive; (assumption).

vii Deductive inference involves logical truths; (assumption).

viii Inductive inference involves observed correlations; (assumption).

ix There are no observed correlations of others' sensations and behaviour; (from ii).

x   Either others' sensations are not known or there are logical truths relating sensations and behaviour, i.e. either scepticism or logical behaviourism (from ix, vi, v, vii).

But as we will see, there is another option: theory-theory.

Reflection on the session and self-test questions

Write down your own reflections on the materials in this session drawing out any points that are particularly significant for you. Then write brief notes about the following:

1. How does the central question of this chapter relate to the rest of Part V?

2. How does the Problem of Other Minds arise? How is it connected with a Cartesian picture of the mind?

3. How is the argument from analogy supposed to solve the problem? Is it successful?

Session 2 Introduction to the 'theory-theory' approach

Theory-theory as a response to logical behaviourism

This session introduces a very influential way of thinking about how we have knowledge of other minds now generally called the theory-theory approach. A clear way of understanding it is by contrasting it with the 1960s criteria-based accounts influenced by Wittgenstein discussed in the previous session. This is not to say that all theory theorists either then or now were explicitly reacting to logical behaviourism, but it is true of the first reading.

In brief, the theory-theory assumes that we access others' minds by employing a tacit theory, which postulates unobservable mental states in much the way that physical theory postulates unobserved particles to explain the behaviour of observable bodies.

In a paper discussed below (and the reading linked with Exercise 4) with 'Operationalism and ordinary language: a critique of Wittgenstein', Charles Chihara and Jerry Fodor attempt to undercut the dilemma that the Wittgensteinians attempted to impose: either scepticism about other minds or logical behaviourism. They press for a third option. Access to mental states is via an empirical theory. Their argument against the Wittgensteinian account is justified in part by an analogy between knowledge of others' mental states and knowledge of atomic particles.

The background: Chihara and Fodor on Wittgenstein and criteria

Chihara and Fodor (1991) summarize the Problem of Other Minds as traditionally turning on the assumption that there are no conceptual or logical connections between behavioural and mental predicates. Combined with the assumption that one can only have direct first-hand knowledge of one's own states, there will turn out to be insufficient justification for ascribing mental states to others. Hence a form of scepticism. The reason for this is that any justification would have to rely on an observed inductive correlation between mental states and behaviour and only *one* such correlation can be observed.

They go on to report that, in opposition to this, philosophers influenced by Wittgenstein denied the premiss and thus committed themselves to a form of logical behaviourism. Chihara and Fodor provide some general remarks about why this move fitted well into Wittgenstein's broader, operationalist approach to meaning. This, they suggest quite plausibly, is reinforced by and reinforces Wittgenstein's metaphilosophical claim that philosophical problems can be dissolved by attending to the way language is actually used, including cases where apparently similar grammatical forms mask very different uses. (Philosophical problems can result from assuming that there must be an underlying similarity.) Concentration on the use of words—such as 'pain' in 'Smith is in pain'—and on the way words are taught leads them to the role that criteria are supposed to play in a Wittgensteinian account of mind.

Wittgenstein's basic idea, they suggest, is that for mental concepts to be teachable, there must be criteria that can be invoked for their use and which are more basic than any inductive criteria. The reason for this dependence is that the correlations of, for example, symptoms with underlying conditions requires that one already understands the concepts of the kind of symptom and kind of underlying (mental state) condition in question. But one can only understand the latter in mental cases if one already understands criteria for it. They summarize the role of criteria thus: 'X is a criterion of Y in situations of type S if the very meaning or definition of "Y" justify the claim that one can recognise, see, detect, or determine the applicability of "Y" on the basis of X in *normal* situations of type S.' (p. 141)

The stress on normality is the result of the assumption that criteria are (on this reading of criteria) defeasible. That is, under the 'wrong' circumstances the criteria can be satisfied without the condition for which they are criteria being the case. Thus a ball going into the net may be the criterion of a goal but only in a game of football, when the ball is in play, when no player is off side and so forth. (We will return to a different interpretation of criteria later in the chapter.)

EXERCISE 4   (30 minutes)

Read the short extract from

Chihara, C.S. and Fodor, J.A. (1991). Operationalism and ordinary language: a critique of Wittgenstein. Reprinted in *The Nature of Mind* (ed. D. Rosenthal). Oxford: Oxford University Press, pp. 137–150. (Extract: pp. 145–146)

Link with Reading 27.3

This paper attempts both to explain a broadly Wittgensteinian, logical behaviourist account of knowledge of other minds and then to argue against it.

♦ What is the nature of the alternative that the authors set out in this passage?

♦ How plausible is the analogy on which it is based?

The theoretical alternative

In effect, Chihara and Fodor offer the following argument. The Problem of Other Minds originates from the assumption that the only justification for ascribing mental states to other people turns on observed inductive correlations and there are insufficient such correlations to achieve justification. The only alternative, according to logical behaviourism, is to say that the justification for the ascription of mental states to others turns on *criteria* for the application of mental concepts. It is a priori that in *normal* circumstances such and such behaviour is sufficient for ascribing so and so in the way of mental states. This flows from our understanding of the mental and behavioural concepts in question.

But, according to Chihara and Fodor, there is a third possible answer to the question of how we gain access to other people's mental states. This is neither by observed correlations nor by logical connections but instead through theoretical inference. The best explanation of the outward behaviour is the existence of inner states described by the theory of folk psychology. Thus third-person access is justified by the possession of an appropriate form of theory.

In fact this sort of approach has already been hinted at in two previous readings in previous chapters. By returning to those, a little more flesh can be put on the theory-theory.

EXERCISE 5 (60 minutes)

Re-read the extracts from Fodor and from Dennett from Chapters 24 and 25, i.e. extracts from:

Fodor, J.A. (1991). Propositional attitudes. In *The Nature of Mind* (ed. D. Rosenthal). Oxford: Oxford University Press, pp. 325–338

Dennett, D. (1987). True believers: the intentional strategy and why it works. In *The Intentional Stance*. Cambridge. MA: MIT Press, pp. 13–35

Now read the short extract from

Fodor, J.A. *Psychosemantics*. Cambridge, MA: MIT pp. 1–2

Link with Reading 27.4

◆ How might a theory of mind solve the Problem of Other Minds?

◆ What sort of theory is it?

Fodor on theory

In the paper 'Propositional attitudes' and further in his book *Psychosemantics*, Fodor presents a reductionist philosophical explanation of mental content. As we saw in Chapter 24, Fodor defends a particular philosophical theory of how the intentional properties of mental states (and thus derivatively, and in turn, of language) result from underlying causal connection between internal mental representations and worldly states of affairs. That is not the concern of this chapter. What is of concern is the way Fodor begins: with an account of the connection between mental states and the *theory* which he claims is implicit in folk psychology. Here he begins by arguing that our knowledge of the mental states of other people takes the form of an implicit theory that he calls 'folk psychology'.

(The argumentative strategy that Fodor continues in *Psychosemantics* as a whole is this. On the assumption that our knowledge of other people's minds can be codified in a theory, some explanation of why this theory works, of what features of the world it is true of, has to be given. Fodor argues that the explanation of this is that folk psychology is a theory that governs the internal mental representations described in Fodor's Representationalist Theory of Mind. This is how he attempts to ground a causal theory of the mind. We are here concerned with the first stage of that overall argument: the claim that our knowledge of other minds is codified in a theory of folk psychology.)

Folk psychology and folk explanation

Fodor argues that we can explain and predict the behaviour of others by postulating an underlying ontology of mental states.

(Fodor thinks that possession of a mental state can itself be explained by the possession of an internal mental representation. But that is a further stage.) The behaviour of these can be codified in the generalizations of folk psychology. One such generalization is that *if x is y's rival then x prefers y's discomfiture, all else being equal*. These fit together into a deductive structure to explain particular actions, broadly resembling the Deductive-Nomological model of explanation (see Chapter 14). Given knowledge of the particular circumstances of a person, we can apply generalizations to deduce their subsequent thoughts and actions. How is it possible to begin this process and have knowledge of particular matters? The answer is the same as how one knows of particular but unobservable matters in physical science: by a holistic fitting of the observed facts into a broader theory.

Fodor argues that in practice (and possibly in principle as well) there is no alternative to the deployment of this theory if one wants to explain and predict behaviour. How else could one predict that one would be met from an airport in 3 weeks' time, having made such an arrangement over the telephone? So folk psychology is *practically* compulsory. But as long as it is a more or less true theory of how we think and behave, it will underpin inferences from behaviour to their underlying mental causes. This is a matter not of observed correlations, nor of logical criteria, but of the best explanation of observable effects. It ties a variety of behavioural effects together in a plausible overall explanatory theory.

The analogy with a theory of meaning

It is worth noting that theories of this sort have been offered for other competencies. We have already briefly encountered one in Chapter 25. Davidson's formal theory of meaning is an attempt to codify the practical competence that speakers of a language have in the production and understanding of novel sentences. It has widely been assumed in recent analytic philosophy that such a theory goes some way to explain an ability by showing that it can be built up from component abilities: tacit knowledge of axioms of the theory, perhaps. What has not been explained is the precise explanatory burden such a theory is supposed to carry. Fodor is a rare exception in this regard. He is quite explicit that he thinks that corresponding to each of the elements described in a theory of grammar there will be mental elements, real mental entities. But other philosophers, including Davidson, have not wished to purchase clarity at this great cost. Given, however, that the theory-theory has been invoked explicitly in this chapter to explain third-person epistemology, one of its burdens will be to explain precisely how it is so explanatory. Before going on to examine a rival to the theory to ease just that assessment, we will briefly digress to revise Dennett's views on this issue.

Dennett on theory

Dennett agrees with Fodor in his emphasis on the importance of folk psychology as a predictive and explanatory strategy. To that extent it looks as though he shares a basic theory-theory approach. There are two important differences from Fodor and possibly theory-theory in general, however, in what he goes on to say. The first was touched on in Chapter 25. Dennett does not think that folk psychology as a theory stands in need of the further explanation that Fodor goes on to give. Dennett does not subscribe to Fodor's 'industrial strength realism' of *causally* active internal states. Folk psychological explanations are distinguished from those physical science explanations that cite the behaviour of unobservable *entities*. It thus does not require the further postulation of those entities to explain its success. Instead it resembles physical science explanations, which describe calculation bound entities or *abstracta*.

Explanation and rationality

This leads to a second difference from Fodor's account. Dennett stresses the claim that folk psychological explanations resemble explanation by comparison with an ideal rather than by subsumption under a generalization. Think of this as the difference between explanations by appeal to how people *ought ideally* to behave and those that chart the most *probable* ways in which people behave based perhaps on past statistical observations. Dennett's emphasis on the ideal results from the central role that *rationality* plays in the Intentional Stance. The idealizations involved are those of how people ought rationally to behave. In fact this is very pertinent to the subject matter of this chapter. It provides a reason for thinking that Dennett does not subscribe to a standard form of the theory-theory. But before that point can be explained, it will be useful to look first at its major competitor. (We will find a similar emphasis on the role of rationality in one of the founding papers of the rival to theory-theory.)

Reflection on the session and self-test questions

Write down your own reflections on the materials in this session drawing out any points that are particularly significant for you. Then write brief notes about the following:

1. How does theory-theory attempt to solve the Problem of Other Minds?

2. What is the connection between it and a functionalist account of mind?

Session 3 Simulation theory

Summary so far

The previous session presented the origins of theory-theory as a reaction to an argument that logical behaviourism was the only opposition to scepticism about other minds (conjoined with the claim that such scepticism was obviously false). The reaction stressed the broadly theoretical nature of folk psychology: those everyday generalizations and rationalizations that can be used to explain and predict behaviour. On the assumption that folk psychology can be classed as a theory, then the physics of the microscopic can provide an analogy of how we can know other people's mental states. We have a working theory of the underlying unobservable (mental) causes of observable (behavioural) effects. This underpins the inference from behaviour to mental states.

Theory-theory was also an attractive account of the epistemology of third-person access to mental states because it fitted into a broader programme of explaining complex abilities by breaking them up into component abilities in turn codified in a theory. If, for whatever reason, the existence of complex open-ended abilities requires the truth of a theory that articulates their structure, then why not assume that the use of that theory underpins more directly the relevant epistemology?

Simulation theory opposes these views at least with respect to reading other people's minds. Rather than relying on knowing a theory of mind, simulation theorists argue that we simply use the 'mental mechanisms' that theory theorists' theories were supposed to codify. The reading contains an extract from one of two seminal papers which, independently, arrived at broadly similar positions although for different reasons. The second is discussed below.

EXERCISE 6	(15 minutes)

Read the extract from the beginning of:

Heal, J. (1995). Replication and functionalism. In *Folk Psychology* (ed. M. Davies and T. Stone). Oxford: Blackwell, pp. 45–59. (Extract: pp. 45–47)

Link with Reading 27.5

◆ What is the role that rationality plays in Heal's argument against theory-theory?

◆ What is the alternative that Heal proposes?

◆ Does she avoid merely repeating the argument from analogy?

Heal's account of the motivation of theory-theory

Heal begins by summarizing what she sees to be the main motivation behind theory-theory. She does this by sketching out a broadly functionalist theory of mind. (It is worth asking whether all forms of theory-theory share the features that she identifies in functionalism. Think about the role of rationality in functionalism. This important issue will return shortly.) Functionalism provides a way of explaining the open-ended nature of our ability to ascribe mental states to other people. This ability is open-ended both because there is a vast number of different *kinds* of psychological state (beliefs, hopes, fears, desires, expectations, etc.) that can interact, but also because the *contents* of such states are not limited. I can believe that red is my favourite colour. And I can also believe that red is my favourite colour *and that* Paris is the capital of France. There is no limit on the number of different beliefs that can be achieved through conjunction alone. So how is it possible to be able to ascribe states of this complexity and open-ended multiplicity to other people?

A theory such as functionalism goes some way towards breaking this ability down into component parts standing in functional relations. A theory such as Fodor's Representationalist Theory of Mind, which deploys a language of thought, goes even further. It tries to explain how the content of complex beliefs is built up from component 'words' in a mental language. So here we have a connection between the subject matter of this chapter—the epistemology of mind—and that of Chapter 24. A theory of mental content explains how it is possible to entertain an unlimited open-ended number of different mental states. But if we already have tacit *knowledge* of such a theory, that would also explain our ability to handle complex *ascriptions* of mental states to others. Heal suggests that this is the motivation for what is now called a theory-theory approach (a label she does not herself use). But the motivation for ascribing tacit knowledge of such a massively complex theory (albeit one that reduces the complexity of the states it codifies) is undercut if there is a simpler explanation of our ability to 'read minds'.

Heal's alternative

The alternative that Heal suggests is 'replication' (or 'simulation' as the strategy has become known). Given that we have imaginative abilities to help us cope with a complex and unclear future by thinking through what it would be sensible to think and do in possible situations, we can use this to ascribe thoughts to others *without any further elaborate theorising about them.* (p. 47)

> I place myself in what I take to be his initial state by imagining the world as it would appear from his point of view and I then deliberate, reason and reflect to see what decision emerges... To get results from the method I require only that I have the ability to get myself into the same state as the person I wish to know about and that he and I are in fact relevantly similar. (p. 47)

What marks this strategy out is that one simply *uses* one's own 'mental machinery' in deliberating to find out what the other person thinks. One need not tacitly know a *theory* of how one's mind works.

Three objections

To defend this strategy, Heal has to show that it really is distinct from a theory-theory approach, that it does not presuppose theoretical knowledge. She suggests three potential criticisms and responses to them:

1. Replication, as Heal describes it, requires that one is able to put one's self in the same initial state as the other person, prior to running the simulation. But surely this will have to require an inference from behaviour to mental states and this simply smuggles a theory-theory back in.

   ♦ *Response*: Heal's response to this is, first, that there may be a more direct way of reading another's mental state than

theoretical inference. Secondly, the simulator can gauge the initial state by looking at how the world impacts on the other in order to simulate the initial state. As her first answer is not consistent with pure simulation theory but an example of the third general approach to the Problem of Other Minds we will postpone discussion of it until later.

2. Simulation will require putting oneself in a state of *make-believe belief*. Knowing what follows from some make-believe belief will surely itself be a piece of theoretical knowledge.

   ♦ *Response*: this is not so. We already use our imaginative abilities use our in practical reasoning about our own future experiences, thoughts, and actions. We do not employ theories to think what we should think under hypothetical circumstances, but simply reason directly. (This is called 'off line' reasoning by others.)

3. Working out what follows from an initial state will itself be a matter of deploying a theory of mind of applying principles of reasoning. Thinking is thus just first-person access to a theory of mind.

   ♦ *Response*: such principles are not causal generalizations but normative and rational principles about what ought to follow from what or what would make a particular belief true or desire satisfied. In part, this response stems from the way Heal characterizes her opponent as a functionalist rather than more broadly as a theory theorist. It turns, in other words, on assuming an opponent like Fodor rather than Dennett. This is brought out in section iii of her paper.

The role of rationality

In addition to the basic argument that replication is simpler and more plausible than ascribing tacit or implicit knowledge of a theory of mind that has yet to be articulated, Heal also deploys a positive argument in favour of replication over theory-theory. This turns on the role and nature of rationality in psychological explanation.

The basic idea is this: 'in giving a psychological explanation we render the thought or behaviour of the other intelligible, we exhibit them as having some point, some reasons to be cited in their defence. Another way of putting this truism is to say that we see them as exercises of cognitive competence or rationality.' (p. 52)

This claim resembles the distinction mentioned earlier in the chapter between explanation by subsumption and explanation by appeal to an ideal.

However, the presence of rationality makes a second difference. Heal suggests that the demands of rationality cannot be codified into any kind of theory that would serve the theory-theory. To be rational does not guarantee that any specific belief must be true. One can always ask the question: 'is this belief really true?' without that casting doubt on one's cognitive competence. Following Quine, we cannot pick out any belief as immune to future revision. But nor could rationality or competence be identified with making the correct application of particular rules of inference.

I can fail to follow simple and reliable inference rules and adopt some most unreliable ones, and recognise later that this was what I was doing, quite compatibly with continued trust in my then and present cognitive competence. The only constraint is that I should be able to make intelligible to myself why I failed to notice so-and-so or seemed to assume such-and-such.   (p. 53)

Either erroneous beliefs or erroneous inference rules can be made intelligible providing that one can give the right stage-setting. But what the right stage-setting is cannot itself be specified in advance or codified. Of course partial models of good thinking are encoded in, say, first order deductive logic, but failure to follow such models does not by itself imply a failure of overall cognitive competence.

If these thoughts are right and the demands of rationality cannot be codified, then the theory that any plausible theory theorist requires cannot be framed. This clearly counts against the theory-theory; however, it does not count against replication or simulation. In this alternative strategy, one assumption built into the replication is that others are like me in being rational. This is made no more problematic for the absence of a final account of what such rationality comprises.

Robert Gordon's account of simulation theory

Jane Heal was not the only philosopher to arrive at the idea of replication. Robert Gordon arrived at similar conclusions—although he coined the now more popular label 'simulation theory'—in R.M. Gordon (1995a) 'Folk psychology as simulation' (in Davies and Stone, ed. *Folk Psychology*).

Gordon's paper begins more straightforwardly and makes no explicit appeal to the connection between psychological explanation and rationality. (There is, however, an implicit connection through the role of practical reasoning.) However, he makes some interesting further claims towards the end.

While Heal appeals to the imaginative abilities we have to consider our own possible reactions to possible (distant) future events, Gordon starts with an appeal to our ability to predict our immediate future actions on the basis of our intentions to act. We can predict how we are about to act without the use of any theory, or general principles, which govern human action, except for the principle that we shall act as we intend, in general. As intentions are often the product of practical reasoning—reasons that justify or rationalize actions—simulated practical reasoning with hypothetical premises can serve as a predictive device of our own more distant future actions. The paper then suggests that this same ability can be put to use to predict the actions of others, 'As in the case of hypothetical self-prediction, the methodology essentially involves deciding *what to do*; but, extended to people of 'minds' different from one's own.' (p. 63)

So we can apply the very same non-theory-based ability to predict our own actions through the use of practical reasoning to predict the actions of others providing we can simulate their practical reasoning by 'putting ourselves in their shoes'. One projects oneself into another's situation *but without any attempt*

to project oneself into, as we say, the other's 'mind' (p. 63). Likewise it may not be possible for me ever to be in the situations of others whom I attempt to simulate—perhaps because the situations lie in the past—and so I do not have to decide what I myself would do or believe that I am in those circumstances. Instead I project myself into the other person's circumstances. Thus simulation does not involve implicit analogy with my own case. These final qualifications are important and we will return to them shortly. They are supposed to head off an objection that might have been niggling you so far in this session.

Simulation and concepts

So far we have focused on both Gordon's and Heal's epistemological arguments (although the latter's paper covers broader areas also). We have not touched on the question of what account of the *concepts* of various mental states can be given from the perspective of simulation theory. As well as accounting for our ability to ascribe mental states to others, can it also account for what it is that we conceive when we conceive of mental states (from a third-person point of view)?

This question can be brought into focus by drawing two different contrasts. Theory-theory provides not only an account of how we can know of others, mental states (answer: by implicit knowledge of such a theory of mind), but it also accounts for what beliefs are. They are just those (internal, causal) states described by the theory that have the inputs and outputs and general behaviour articulated in the theory. As simulation theory subscribes to no such theory, what account can it give?

Malcolm's Wittgensteinian attack on the argument from analogy discussed in Session 1 was based on the claim that the argument presupposed an account of the *concept* of a mental state characterized in third-person terms—such that Smith could be in pain—while precluding the materials to construct just such a concept. Malcolm concluded that unless one already had a more or less direct way of determining the third-person applicability of mental descriptions, arguing by analogy from one's own first-person case could not get started. Once one had those, there was no need for the argument from analogy. Can simulation theory escape a related charge and provide the resources for explaining the general concept of mental states such that they allow both first- and third-person ascription? (If the answer is no then it may be that the best account of the mind will involve elements of both simulation theory and theory-theory.) Gordon's paper provides one possible line of defence.

Gordon suggests that the concept of belief comes from the interaction of simulators. In order to distinguish a bona fide belief in *persona propria* from a statement of belief within the context of a simulation or pretence, some linguistic device is needed. One way of doing this would be to announce that one was about to run a simulation:

1 Let's do a Smith simulation. Ready? *Dewey won the election.*

The same task might be accomplished by saying:

2 *Smith believes that* Dewey won the election.

My suggestion is that (2) be read as saying the same thing as (1), though less explicitly… To attribute a belief to another person is to make an assertion, to state something as a fact, *within the context of practical simulation* (Gordon, 1995a, p. 68).

Empirical evidence

This is just the beginning of a suggestion about what concept of belief arises out of simulation rather than a worked out account. However, it leaves the following doubt unresolved. Is Gordon's account really sufficient to explain the concept of belief that we have, the concept of a state that can represent the world both truly and falsely and can serve as part of a reason for action? Gordon thinks that it is and suggests, furthermore, that there is some empirical evidence for this view.

1. The fact that children only learn to pass the false belief test at the age of 4 or 5, but are nevertheless able prior to that to make predictions based on true beliefs (or at least *shared* false beliefs) fits simulation theory better than theory-theory. According to the latter, to understand the very concept of beliefs is to understand a theoretical context. Thus Gordon argues that the *change* in children's ability can be explained as a development of a child's ability to simulate obstacles to other people believing what the child knows. By contrast a theory-theory has no account of this change. If a child can explain behaviour at all by ascribing mental states, the difference between true and false cases should be unimportant.

2. The fact that there is a correlation between a lack of understanding of others and a lack of imaginative play among autists fits a simulation account of third-person access. A lack of the latter would preclude the former.

We will return to whether empirical evidence supports simulation theory rather than theory-theory shortly. That debate is far from closed yet. However, Gordon's suggestion that empirical evidence also supports a simulation account of mental concepts appears less convincing. The problem is not so much that simulation theory could not underpin mental concepts but that no gesture has been given as to how it might. The false belief test, for example, suggests that children younger than 4 have not mastered the idea of beliefs as states whose contents can diverge from how the world is. But it is not clear that possessing the concept of beliefs or other mental states can be equated with an ability to simulate, or to form beliefs about the world in a pretend or off line mode. Perhaps simulation theory provides the materials for learning how to ascribe mental states to other people, but a full understanding of what such states are requires that children form a theoretical understanding of beliefs.

Is simulation theory just a version of the argument from analogy?

Putting matters like that, however, raises a further objection to simulation theory. Can it avoid the various objections raised against inferring from the first person to the third as an answer to the Problem of Other Minds? In fact Gordon (1995b) faces just this sort of objection in a different paper ('Simulation without introspection or inference from me to you' in Davies and Stone, ed., *Mental Simulation*).

There, Gordon claims that other philosophers who have developed simulation theory have subscribed to three principles all of which he rejects:

1. an analogical inference from oneself to others,

2. premissed on introspectively based ascriptions of mental states to oneself, and

3. requiring prior possession of the concepts of the mental states ascribed.

The first two views fit naturally together. As we saw earlier, the argument from analogy was deployed in conjunction with a broadly Cartesian model of first-person access. If one finds out about one's own mental states by a kind of inner perception of private mental items, it seems that the only hope of discovering the states of others is a form of analogical reasoning.

Gordon suggests that many other simulationists think along these lines. One first discovers what one would think in someone else's circumstances and one then reasons that they will think the same way. Gordon argues that this version of simulation theory will face some of the same objections that the argument from analogy faced. What justifies the inference from one's own case to others? How can one come to think of the mental states of others on the basis of one's own? He argues that either these objections will be impossible to overcome or if they can be overcome then the resultant theory will be a form of theory-theory. The inference from my own case to others, for example, will be a theoretical inference.

Gordon's proposed alternative works like this. Instead of imagining oneself in another person's position, seeing what state one is in and inferring that the other will be in the same type of state—an inference that requires one has a prior grasp on the concept of a type of mental state—one imagines that one is the other person in their position. One imagines, *in the first person*, the other person missing a flight or whatever. One does not transfer one's mental states to another, but transforms oneself into them, in imagination.

Similarly, Heal (1995) says of a related criticism that it 'misdescribes the direction of the gaze of the replicator. He is not looking at the subject to be understood but at the world around that subject. It is what the world makes the replicator think which is the basis for the beliefs which he attributes to the subject.' (p. 138) But she does also concede 'one simple assumption is needed: that they are like me in being thinkers' (p. 137).

So the question of whether Gordon's is really a coherent and plausible account of mental gymnastics is open to question. Can it escape the charge that there is still an analogical assumption present? Clearly, for example, there would be no question of confusing one's thoughts, arrived at by imagining the world surrounding the subject in question, with one's own. Their sorrow in the face of bereavement remains their sorrow even if one can imaginatively grasp its scope and object. Thus one line of objection to simulation theory is that it is not itself finally coherent. But in fact, that is not the most obvious difficulty which is instead to distinguish it from its main rival. It is to this question we will now turn.

Reflection on the session and self-test questions

Write down your own reflections on the materials in this session drawing out any points that are particularly significant for you. Then write brief notes about the following:

1. What is the main simulationist criticism of theory-theory?

2. How does simulation theory avoid this criticism itself?

3. Is simulation theory a version of the argument from analogy?

Session 4 The current state of the debate: evidence from autism

Summary

The previous two sessions have introduced both the theory-theory and simulation theory in the context of solving the Problem of Other Minds. The theory-theory likens our ability to 'read other minds' to a structure or body of knowledge we have of the mental workings of other people. Such a structure of knowledge underpins our ability to explain and predict their behaviour. It was introduced as an alternative to logical behaviourism: the view that there are logical connections between mental descriptions and behavioural descriptions, to which we will return in the final session.

Simulation theory is itself a reaction to theory-theory. It holds that our ability to read other people's minds turns on our non-theoretical ability to *use* our own minds in hypothetical practical reasoning. We saw that there was some risk that simulation theory is vulnerable to the argument from analogy, that it is really of a piece with a Cartesian theory of mind.

Evidence from autism

The discussion has, so far, been framed in largely philosophical terms. The arguments involved have concentrated on whether the various ideas are coherent, whether they would lead either to formal contradictions or informal absurdities. But the debate about theories of mind has also made much use of empirical findings. Some of the original research was done in the field of primatology. More recently, autism has been deployed as a rich source of empirical tests of philosophical theory. In this session we will examine some work on autism. One of the more apparent lessons

from this will be just how difficult it is to draw clear-cut conclusions once one steps away from pure philosophy and looks instead at the interplay between philosophy and an, as yet, unsettled empirical matter.

This session will consider a recent short summary of the debate and look towards the further applied work that has also been carried out. We will begin by examining how clear-cut the distinction between the two theories is.

EXERCISE 7 (30 minutes)

Read the extract from:

Stone, T. and Davies, M. (1996). The mental simulation debate: a progress report. In *Theories of Theories of Mind* (ed. P. Carruthers and P. Smith). Cambridge: Cambridge University Press, pp. 119–137. (Extract: pp. 131–134)

Link with Reading 27.6

◆ Is there really a clear distinction between theory-theory and simulation theory?

Stone and Davis set out a general overview of the opposition between theory-theory and simulation theory and then question—in the extract above—the state of play. What emerges is that, by contrast with the discussion in the previous session, there may be less of a clear distinction between the two explanations of our access to other minds than was at first thought.

Three forms of theory

What is particularly interesting is the discussion of just what sort of theory the theory-theory presupposes. The paper suggests that there are three dominant strategies varying from the most specific and tightly defined (and therefore least likely to be true) to the most relaxed view.

1. The first is to model the theory of folk psychology on a scientific theory: a tightly deductive theory that introduces entities in what are called Ramsey sentences. This view fits particularly with identifying psychological explanation construed as a form of regularizing explanation with a Deductive-Nomological model of scientific explanation. But as folk psychology differs from a scientific theory in various ways, this is also a (needlessly) implausible analogy.

2. More plausibly, one can compare folk psychology with the theory that is supposed to underpin our linguistic abilities and of which, according to much cognitive science, we have tacit knowledge. On the other hand the paper suggests, however, folk psychological explanation implies that we do have explicit knowledge of at least some of the principles in the theory. This marks a contrast with the linguistic case. In fact things are not so clear here as the paper here suggests, as Heal rightly emphasized, the principles contained in a theory-theory would have to include an unlimited number of detailed principles about

the behaviour of mental states according to their different contents. These would surely have to remain tacit and distinct from the principles used in everyday explanation.

3. Least contentiously, theory-theory can simply describe folk psychology as a body of knowledge akin to that of cookery, which explains our ability even if it cannot be deductively structured with the rigour demanded in the first case. Given this construal, to mark off a clear alternative simulation theory must deny that we negotiate the social world in virtue of some general principles about how people behave, and thus must assert that this differs from how we negotiate the physical world.

This summary of theory-theory encourages a twofold characterization of simulation theory (roughly how it has been described above). It involves an imaginative transference or transformation of perspective that requires the use of one's mental faculties rather than a theory of them. And it gives rise to forms of explanation that make sense of, or render intelligible, behaviour without subsuming it under statistical generalizations.

Three other dangers

There remain three dangers of the positions still blurring together which the paper picks out:

1. Much depends on the account of tacit knowledge of a theory if the ability to simulate others is not itself to count as such tacit knowledge.

2. In order to cut down on the complexity of their proposed theories, theory theories sometimes invoke an element of simulation within it. This is to enable an interpreter of another person's behaviour to understand the consequences of ascribing a belief with such and such content to them. Instead of having a massively complex theory of what each such content entails, an interpreter may simply simulate a belief of that content and see what it entails.

3. Most simulation theorists agree that some inductively based generalizations play some part in simulation.

Finally, Stone and Davies here are rare within the current debate on theory-theory and simulation in realizing that these positions do not exhaust all the possible contemporary positions. A third option is to abandon a 'regularising' conception of psychological explanation without thinking that this necessitates an imaginative identification with other people. One way of doing this is to subscribe to a form of *direct* access to which we will turn in the next and final session.

How is empirical evidence brought to bear?

The interdisciplinary debate about both the nature of autism, its explanation, and the light it sheds on the rest of the population is still wide open. We will shortly mention some representative recent papers. But the key issue to be clear on is *how* empirical evidence might shed light on such a debate and what the role of the philosophical theories is.

Take the case of autism and, especially, Wing's triad. This is a group of three symptoms that are centrally important in the diagnosis of autism. They comprise impairments of social competence; impairments of communication skills; and lack of pretend play. It is an empirical matter that these three distinct symptoms often occur together (in autism). This empirical finding might then be thought to shed light on how we have knowledge of other minds in something like the following way. Because it turns out that Wing's triad includes lack of pretend play, this suggests that the key deficit may be a lack of ability to simulate and it is this lack that explains the poor social competence. Thus, Wing's triad is evidence for simulation theory. (In fact a rival argument can be given that it supports theory-theory.)

The point is this. If it is legitimate to analyse a complex ability (such as the ability to read minds) as consisting in (and perhaps built from) simpler component abilities, then deficit studies should present evidence for or against particular analyses. The battle between simulation and theory theories is over which analysis is correct. Does both mind reading and pretend play turn on simulation or the possessing of theoretical 'metarepresentations' of others? Of course an alternative view is that there is something illicit or unnecessary about the attempt to analyse mind reading as dependent on lower but still mental skills. We will return to that option in the last session.

The complexity of the empirical findings

Two philosophers who have considered the role of empirical evidence and who take opposing views on it are Gregory Currie and Peter Carruthers. (See Currie 'Simulation-theory, theory-theory and the evidence from autism' and Carruthers 'Autism as mind-blindness' both in Carruthers and Smith, ed., *Theories of Theories of Mind*, 1996.)

Both Currie and Carruthers present some of the central or classic symptoms of autism and consider the relative merits of simulation theory and theory-theory in the light of them. As Currie comments at the very end of his paper: 'a fully satisfactory assessment of the simulation-versus-theory debate, even as confined to the present state of the evidence, would have to take into account the whole vast and bewildering range of autistic symptoms. Here I have focused on just a few of them.' (p. 256)

Thus, the extent to which he is able to marshall the evidence to present a case for one or other side may depend on careful selection only of 'Wing's triad' and some executive function deficits. The same consideration also applies to Carruthers.

This is the chief interest, in this context, of Boucher's paper also in Carruthers & Smith, (eds) 1996. It points out in some detail the clinical difficulties in pinning down just what is to be explained. Can autism really be tied to specific shared deficits, or are there a range of overlapping deficits but with no specific symptom or symptoms necessary and sufficient for such a diagnosis? The kind of explanation that both Currie and Carruthers aim at requires for its plausibility just such a clear clinical picture.

Wing's triad

Currie and Carruthers agree that both theories explain equally plausibly two of the deficits of Wing's triad: impairment in social relationships and in verbal and non-verbal communication. These features are named after Lorna Wing, a foremost autism researcher, who established the triad in the 1980s. However, both agree that there is at least a prima facie case that simulation theory can better explain the third: the absence of pretend play. It is reasonable to argue that pretend play just *is* the simulation of other roles: whether pirates or bears. Thus Carruthers, who attempts to defend a theory-theory, has to provide an account of this deficit using the explanatory prior idea that autists suffer from a deficit in their theory of mind. His idea is that autists do not engage in spontaneous pretence because they are deprived of the source of enjoyment in such play. This is, he claims, the manipulation of one's own mental states, which, he argues, requires consciousness of the pretence. Thus only those children able to form a second order belief (a belief about their beliefs) will be able to enjoy pretend play. The plausibility of this claim turns on the idea that this is what makes pretence pleasurable.

Problem solving

A further area of dispute is what better explains the findings that autists do worse at practical problem solving. Currie argues that while this is not at first an obvious consequence of deficits at simulation, a plausible connection can be found. Solving problems such as the Tower of Hanoi is generally a matter of simulated trial and error. One thinks through what the consequences would be of making a certain move, and what one ought to do as a result so as to eliminate bad strategies. Thus if autism is an inability to simulate, autists will also be bad at such practical problem solving.

Carruthers, however, suggests that an equally plausible explanation can be given that relates such cases to disruption of a theory of mind. Practical problem solving requires that one can both access and reflect on one's past thoughts and processes of reasoning. However, both of these abilities are mediated by a theory of mind module. Note that in saying this, Carruthers takes it that first-person access to one's past thoughts is a matter of theory, a view that Currie denies (and which is not part of the relaxed view of theory-theory discussed above). But whether or not this is so, it is at least consistent with theory-theory to say that the assessment of reasoning processes will require a working theory of mind.

So is there a difference between theory and simulation?

What the contemporary debate shows is that things are not as clear-cut as they may have at first seemed. In fact, this general debate is beginning to lose momentum as the participants, especially those in primate studies, begin to realize that the opposition between theory on the one hand and the ability to simulate on the other is not sharp. In the final session we will turn to a different tack that owes something to the Wittgensteinian account of the 1960s in its refusal to *theorize* at all. For now,

however, the following distinction in emphasis may be a helpful way of thinking about theory-theory and simulation theory. Simulation theory is better able to account for the role of rationality in mind.

Take Heal's argument for simulation theory. A key idea was that we can make sense of other people by thinking about what it would be rational to think in their position. We do this not by using a *theory* of rationality but just by using our rationality, our faculty of rationality, perhaps.

To use the language of a reading from Chapter 15 from McDowell, the structure of the 'space of reasons' is a rational structure. It concerns the support that beliefs give one another. Significant divergences from such a rational structure would not merely be unfortunate, they would be *unintelligible* as a structure of beliefs at all. But this idea that there are limits on what we could even understand finds no echo in the resources of natural laws, which would have to say merely that one sort of internal state tended to be followed by another. A sideways view of the rational structure could not explain how it marked the limits of intelligibility.

Of course this rational structure is a kind of ideal up to which we do not always live. Reason explanations have a different kind of logic to natural scientific nomological explanations. We *compare* with an ideal rather than *subsuming* under a universal law. We can make sense of virtually any mistaken beliefs they might have as long as we understand how they were thought to follow from their other beliefs. This elasticity in the structure of beliefs resists capture in a *theory* of other minds. It again brings out a difference between the structure of rationality that constitutes our thinking and a structure of laws. As an ideal we must also be alive to the thought that our conception of what follows from what, what gives reason for what, stands in need of correction and improvement. Again, this structure looks very different to the structure of a theory.

These considerations were deployed in Chapters 23 and 24 against the idea that mental states can be cashed out in functional terms. In other words, they were considered in the context of the *ontology* of mind. Do they also apply in the case of the *epistemology* of mind? Not entirely, but there is some sort of suggestive connection.

The reason they do not simply carry over is the difficulty of knowing what role a theory has and what constraints are put on the nature of that theory. No one thinks we explicitly use a theory to explain the everyday behaviour of others. It is at best tacit. And if a rational stance such as Dennett's Intentional Stance—which explicitly employs principles of rationality—counts as a theory, it is not clear that theory-theory cannot build rationality in. At the same time, however, it is against the spirit of theory-theory to acknowledge the central role of rationality given that its demands cannot be codified in a theory.

Having said that, both theory-theory and simulation theory assume that a philosophical account is needed in response to the Problem of Other Minds. In the final session we will turn to a different approach.

Reflection on the session and self-test questions

Write down your own reflections on the materials in this session drawing out any points that are particularly significant for you. Then write brief notes about the following:

1. How can the debate between simulation theory and theory theory be assessed?

2. What role does evidence for autism play?

3. Are the two positions really distinct?

Session 5 Rationality and direct access to mental states

This chapter began with the observation that the knowledge of other minds is central to mental health care. On the one hand, there are specific syndromes or conditions that involve a partial breakdown of our everyday ability to make judgements about others' minds. On the other hand, that general ability also underlies clinical practice. Only if one can form a picture of a client's state of mind is clinical intervention possible. We have examined the two dominant contemporary philosophical views and begun to see how empirical evidence from autism might impact on an assessment of their plausibility.

Is there a need for a substantial theory at this (mental) level?

The accounts of third-person access considered in the last two sessions have both assumed that there was a substantial problem to be addressed whose solution would require a philosophical theory. Both theory-theory and simulation theory are *substantial* theories in that they attempt to explain an ability that can seem mysterious: we are able to 'read other people's minds' despite the fact that minds are generally hidden. It is, in part, because of the assumption that mental states are not directly available to people other than their subjects that drives the need for an explanation of how we are able generally to know about mental states.

(Again, it is important to remember that this chapter has not investigated the question of how *first-person* 'access' to mental states is possible. But not that as some of the readings have suggested, some theory theorists argue that even this is a matter of theoretical *inference*.)

One of the advantages of such a construal both of the problem and of the general form of the solution is that it suggests that they may be an explanation of breakdowns of the ability to mind-read pitched at a mental level. If the full ability to understand and explain others' behaviour can be analysed as comprising more basic abilities, then there is the prospect of explaining failures of the full ability in terms of failures of these lower-level abilities, which still deserve mental descriptions. Contrast this case with a case where the breakdown has to be explained as a breakdown at an underlying physical level. (One very crude analogy is to think of the contrasts between software bugs and hardware faults in computing.)

However, there is a different kind of response that might be given to the original problem that will be briefly flagged in this final session. This is to construe the Problem of Other Minds as itself stemming from a dubious picture of the epistemological situation. Once this is rethought, there may be no problem remaining to be solved. (There may still be much neurological work to be carried out on how it is possible to hear meaning in others' speech or mental states in their behaviour. However, these explanations will be deployed using lower-level terms.)

In Heal's original paper, this possibility was suggested in her response to an anticipated criticism: that simulation required some other way of determining the initial conditions from which one runs one's simulated development. She suggested that it might be possible to read this initial state *without* the use of a theory that translated behavioural responses—thinly described as mere movements—into underlying mental states. She also cited McDowell in support of this view. The focus of discussion in this, final, session is therefore a paper by McDowell who puts forward just such a view in the context of re-evaluating Wittgenstein's use of the idea of criteria.

The standard view of criteria for other minds again

In 'Criteria, defeasibility, and knowledge' (1982) McDowell introduces a line of thinking about the Problem of Other Minds, of the relation between behaviour and mental states, and the role of Wittgenstein's notion of criteria here that generalizes to have important repercussions in epistemology more generally. Getting clear on the particular case of our epistemic standing with respect to other minds will clarify what happens when we open our eyes to the world in other cases, or so the hope goes. This connection makes McDowell's paper very important but it also helps to explain why it is more difficult than the others in this chapter.

McDowell begins by attempting to cast doubt on the coherence of the more widely held interpretation of criteria as a priori, conventional, but defeasible indicators or conditions of some (underlying) fact. The influential Wittgenstein exegete P.M.S. Hacker, writing in the *Oxford Companion to Philosophy*, defines a criterion thus:

A standard by which to judge something; a feature of a thing by which it can be judged to be thus and so. In the writings of the later Wittgenstein it is used as a quasi-technical term. Typically, something counts as a criterion for another thing if it is necessarily good evidence for it. Unlike inductive evidence, criterial support is determined by convention and is partly constitutive of the meaning of the expression for whose application it is a criterion. Unlike entailment, criterial support is characteristically defeasible. Wittgenstein argued that behavioural expressions of the 'inner', e.g. groaning or crying out in pain, are neither inductive evidence for the mental (Cartesianism), nor do they entail the instantiation of the relevant mental term (behaviourism), but are defeasible criteria for its application.

Key features of this definition are that the criteria of, for example, an 'inner' state such as pain are fixed by convention and are partly constitutive of what we mean by pain. Thus groaning and crying out are not mere symptoms but rather part of what we understand by pain. They are connected by definition not induction.

EXERCISE 8   (10 minutes)

On the standard view of criteria, the behavioural criteria for mental states provide some support, as a matter of meaning, for the ascription of mental states; however, they are also defeasible. Sometimes the criteria are satisfied when the subject is not in the relevant mental state. Before going on think whether this allows one ever to have knowledge of others' mental states? Think about the requirements one might make for someone in general to have knowledge (e.g. the analysis of knowledge as justified true belief). Can the criterial approach fit our normal beliefs about whether we have knowledge?

McDowell's objection to the standard view of criteria for other minds

McDowell's main objection is this. If a criterion can be satisfied while the underlying fact for which it is a criterion does not obtain, then knowing that the criterion is satisfied cannot legitimate (or legitimate 'criterially') the claim that one knows that the fact obtains. The problem is that if there is the slack between criteria and facts which the standard reading supposes then criteria cannot ever be *sufficient* for knowledge, whether or not there are conventions which supposedly declare this to be so.

McDowell attempts to bring out just what is wrong with this idea in the following thought experiment:

> Consider a pair of cases, in both of which someone competent in the use of some claim experiences the satisfaction of (undefeated) 'criteria' for it, but in only one of which the claim is true. According to the suggestion we are considering, the subject in the latter case knows that things are as the claim would represent them as being; the subject in the former case does not… However, the story is that the scope of experience is the same in each case: the fact itself is outside the reach of experience. And experience is the only mode of cognition—the only mode of acquisition of epistemic standing—that is operative; appeal to theory is excluded… How can a difference in respect of something conceived as cognitively inaccessible to both subjects… make it the case that one of them knows how things are in that inaccessible region while the other does not—rather than leaving them both, strictly speaking, ignorant on the matter?   (pp. 459–460)

(Appeal to *theory* is excluded because criteria are supposed to be conventional and a priori rather than a posteriori and contingent.)

The problem is the wedge between appearance and reality

The problem that McDowell picks out is that the standard view of criteria puts a wedge between experience and the knowledge that such experience is supposed to warrant or justify. Thus even in favourable circumstances where the fact that the criterion is a criterion for obtains, it seems that experiencing the criterion cannot make the right sort of difference to constitute knowledge as opposed to accidentally true belief.

> If experiencing the satisfaction of 'criteria' does legitimize ('criterially') a claim to know that things are thus and so, it cannot also be legitimate to admit that the position is one in which, for all one knows, things may be otherwise. But the difficulty is to see how the fact that 'criteria' are defeasible can be prevented from compelling that admission; in which case we can conclude, by contraposition, that experiencing the satisfaction of 'criteria' cannot legitimize a claim of knowledge. How can appeal to 'convention' somehow drive a wedge between accepting that everything that one has is compatible with things not being so, on the one hand, and admitting that one does not know that things are so, on the other?   McDowell (1982, p. 458; 1998, pp. 372–373)

(This objection resembles McDowell's claim that a conception of mental states as free-standing internal states makes their having a bearing on the world—possessing content—deeply mysterious. That argument was discussed in Chapter 25.)

The origin of the normal view of criteria

The main exegetical argument for the standard view of criteria is that Wittgenstein suggests that whether something is a criterion for something depends on the context or the particular circumstances. The standard view is that the background context can undermine a criterion (for some fact) that is satisfied. If so, then the criterion is defeated. However, McDowell suggests an alternative view in which the context determines whether some condition really is a criterion for a fact. What depends on context is not whether a satisfied criterion is defeated or not, but whether a condition really is a criterion in the first place. If it is, then it cannot be defeated by circumstances or context. Of course, what is at first taken for a criterion may turn out not to be.

McDowell supports this interpretative possibility by considering a passage in which Wittgenstein discusses criteria in a nonmental context.

> The fluctuation in grammar between criteria and symptoms makes it look as if there were nothing at all but symptoms. We say, for example: 'Experience teaches that there is rain when the barometer falls, but it also teaches that there is rain when we have certain sensations of wet and cold, or such-and-such visual impressions.' In defence of this one says that these sense-impressions can deceive us. But here one fails to reflect that the fact that the false appearance is precisely one of rain is founded on a definition.   Wittgenstein (1953, §354)

Wittgenstein here rejects the temptation to say that both the fall of a barometer and also sensations of wet and cold (or visual impressions) are mere *symptoms* of rain. Instead, and by contrast with the barometer fall, the connection between the sensations (or the visual impressions) and rain is definitional or criterial. They are used in an explanation of what 'rain' means. This thought can, however, be interpreted in two ways.

> Commentators often take this to imply that when our senses deceive us, criteria for rain are satisfied, although no rain is falling. But what the passage says is surely just this: for things, say, to look a certain way to us is, as a matter of 'definition' (or 'convention'…), for it to look to us as though it is raining; it would be a mistake to suppose that the 'sense-impressions' yield the judgement that it is raining merely symptomatically—that arriving at the judgement is mediated by an empirical theory. That is quite compatible with this thought… when our 'sense-impressions' deceive us, the fact is not that criteria for rain are satisfied but that they *appear* to be satisfied.
> McDowell (1982, p. 466; 1998, 381)

Similarly in the case of criteria for mental states, pretence can make it *seem* that the criteria for pain, for example, are satisfied when, in fact, they are not.

Appearances and the Problem of Other Minds

This idea is clarified in McDowell's response to a further argument for the standard view, which draws explicitly on assumptions about psychological descriptions central to this chapter. Quoting a case where Wittgenstein suggests that the criterion for someone else experiencing a mental image of redness is what they say and do, McDowell offers the following diagnosis of the usual interpretation. We ascribe mental states to other people on the basis of behavioural conditions that can be detected *independently* of (and antecedent to) their mental states. However, this does not follow from what Wittgenstein here says. The claim that one can tell what state someone is in by what they say and do does not imply that the latter is a 'condition that one might ascertain to be satisfied by someone independently of knowing that he has [e.g.] a red image' (p. 465). Nor is it the case that a specification of such a criterion gives a general recipe for generating other examples of criteria: namely anything which meets that specification. To repeat, criteria depend on *particular* circumstances.

McDowell suggests that the traditional view is of a piece with the Argument from Illusion, which is often used to ground a form of general scepticism. Instead of appearances in general, we here have bodily behaviour and instead of underlying reality in general, we have mental states, but the basic idea is the same. The latter is supposed to be epistemologically inaccessible in a way in which the former is not and the challenge is to try show how judgements about the former could ever warrant judgements about the latter. Rather than being a device deployed within this framework, McDowell suggests that criteria are a part of Wittgenstein's rejection of the sceptic's framework. We do not satisfy ourselves of the criteria for another's mental states as a route to finding out about their states. 'This flouts an idea that we are prone to find natural, that a basis for a judgement must be

something on which we have a firmer cognitive purchase than we do on the judgement itself; but although the idea can seem natural, it is an illusion to suppose that it is compulsory.' (p. 471)

Appearances and the Argument from Illusion

The third section of McDowell's paper draws some broader connection between this view of criteria and epistemology more generally. The Argument from Illusion is often taken to suggest the following picture of experience. As appearances can sometimes be deceptive, sometimes when it looks that such and such it is not in fact the case, although things seem just as they do when such and such is the case. Thus what is taken in in experience is the same in both cases: a mere appearance that is not the same as, and stops short of, the fact. He labels this the 'highest common factor' conception. It places a veil of ideas (in this case: appearance) between ourselves and the world. In its place, he suggests that the fact that experience is fallible only justifies the claim that experience is either of merely an appearance or it really is of the full fact: the disjunctive conception.

The main argument against the highest common factor conception is that it 'undermines the very idea of an appearance having as its content that things are thus and so in the world "beyond" appearances' (p. 474). Once one reifies appearances, then there being appearances of something becomes mysterious. Furthermore, our ability to have knowledge of the world is undercut because the facts we aim to know always remain 'blankly external' to our experiences.

What makes the highest common factor conception attractive in the first place is the following thought. Whether one is justified in a judgement cannot depend on something that could vary independently of how things are subjectively. This leads to the idea that one's 'epistemic entitlement ought to be something one could display for oneself… from within;… non-question-begging[ly] from a neutrally available starting point' (p. 475). McDowell argues that the first requirements can be met by the disjunctive conception while rejecting the second: 'When someone has a fact made manifest to him, the obtaining of the fact contributes to his epistemic standing on the question. But the obtaining of the fact is precisely not blankly external to his subjectivity, as it would be if the truth about that were exhausted by the highest common factor.' (p. 476)

This is because external facts can be taken in in veridical experience, so there is no need to attempt to fill out an account of justification, of reasons for belief, which make use of merely internal matters.

Finally, McDowell goes on to suggest that the Problem of Other Minds depends on reading the highest common factor conception of experience on to the gap between behaviour and minds. It turns both on thinking of persons as a product of the accessible behaviour of material bodies and inaccessible minds. Human bodies replace human beings (p. 469). This is in turn premised on the idea that human behaviour cannot be considered in itself expressive, any more than the behaviour of planets. However, once one abandons the highest common factor conception, other minds become accessible in their direct expression in behaviour. The behaviour does not merely license an *inference* to underlying mental states.

Summing up

We began the section with the origins of the Problem of Other Minds in Cartesian philosophy. But, although the Cartesian picture of the mind as a private inner realm observed only by a single person makes the Problem of Other Minds obvious, some such problem can seem mere common sense. We all want to say at some times in our lives that we are not understood by others, that they haven't grasped what things are like for us. Equally, we sometimes find it difficult to gauge other people's states of mind. It can be tempting to conclude informally, whether or not we know anything about Cartesian philosophy, that minds are private, hidden behind behaviour.

Such a thought, however, exaggerates the everyday Problem of Other Minds, allowing it to inflate into the philosophical Problem of Other Minds. It ignores much of our everyday experience of taking account of other people's mental states immediately, transparently. It ignores what McDowell calls the *expressive* character of behaviour. Even people who say when asked that minds are private, do not actually take that approach in practice. No one takes the Cartesian perspective seriously in living with others.

Whatever exactly the right account is of the source of our knowledge here, the one thing nearly all philosophers now agree on is that one should not begin an account of the mind from an individual first-person perspective. There is some difference in whether one should think of a third-person perspective, as in their different ways both Norman Malcolm and the theory theorists do, or as a shared first-person perspective as the simulation theorists and McDowell do. But the Cartesian perspective of a solitary, solipsistic ego is a hopeless non-starter.

But how does that leave the issue of the empirical findings from autism? Here much depends on what the role of a philosophical theory is. What is its explanatory force or role? If a theory-theory, what is the nature of our knowledge of it? If simulation theory, do we have unconsciously to simulate? Once this is settled there is then the further question of how deficit studies impact on normal cases. What is the sense in which complex abilities can be broken down into components? Is this a kind of logical analysis or does it actually reveal inner functional modules? Again, empirical work has a bearing on our understanding here, but no less than our getting clear on the concepts employed.

Reflection on the session and self-test questions

Write down your own reflections on the materials in this session drawing out any points that are particularly significant for you. Then write brief notes about the following:

1. What other options are there for solving the Problem of Other Minds?
2. What role can behaviour play? How is its description different from the description presupposed by theory-theory?

Reading guide

- A good place to start is the discussion of third-person access in Burwood, Gilbert, and Lennon (1999) *Philosophy of Mind*.
- A good historical approach is provided in Avramides (2000) *Other Minds*.

Theory-theory versus simulation theory

Theory-theory and simulation theory have recently been discussed as rival theories in a number of collections of papers:

- Davies and Stone's (ed.) (1995a) *Folk Psychology: a guide to the theory of mind debate*, and their (1995b) *Mental Simulation: evaluations and applications*.
- Carruthers and Smith (ed.) (1996) *Theories of Theories of Mind*.
- Hobson's (1991) *Against the 'Theory of Mind'*, and his (2002) *The Cradle of Thought*, provides important critiques.
- Stich, S. and Nichols, S. (2003) Folk psychology.

Direct access

- McDowell's account of direct experience of other people's minds is developed from a discussion of Wittgenstein. The most accessible source of this is in Wittgenstein (1972) *The Blue Book and Brown Books*.
- A traditional view of what Wittgensteinian meant by behavioural criteria for other minds is developed by the American philosopher Norman Malcolm in book length form in: Malcolm (1971) *Problems of Mind: Descartes to Wittgenstein*.
- And by the Oxford Wittgensteinian Peter Hacker (1972) in *Insight and Illusion*.
- For a number of essays arguing for a different view but in the same general area as McDowell, try Wright (ed.) (1986) *Realism Meaning and Truth*. This contains essays by Wright on Other Minds, on the use of theories to explain knowledge of a language and also epistemology more generally. It is quite difficult.
- For a different perspective try Glendinning (1998) *On Being with Others: Heidegger, Derrida, Wittgenstein*.

Empirical work

For work on the theory of mind and autism among other things see:

- Baron-Cohen (1995) *Mindblindness: an essay on autism and theory of mind*, and (1993) (ed.) *Understanding Other Minds: perspectives from autism*.
- Eilan *et al.* (ed.) (2005) *Joint Attention—Communication and Other Minds: issues in philosophy and psychology (consciousness & self-consciousness S.)*.

- Gordon and Barker (1995) Autism and the theory of mind debate (in Graham and Stevens (ed.) *Philosophical Psychopathology*).

References

Avramides, A. (2000). *Other Minds*. London: Routledge.

Baron-Cohen, S. (ed.) (1993). *Understanding Other Minds: perspectives from autism*. Oxford: Oxford University Press.

Baron-Cohen, S. (1995). *Mindblindness: an essay on autism and theory of mind*. Cambridge, MA: MIT Press.

Burwood, S., Gilbert, P., and Lennon, K. (1999). *Philosophy of Mind*. London: UCL.

Carruthers, P. (1996). Autism as mind-blindness. In *Theories of Theories of Mind* (ed. P. Carruthers and P. Smith). Cambridge: Cambridge University Press, 257–273.

Carruthers, P. and Smith, P.K. (ed.) (1996). *Theories of Theories of Mind*. Cambridge: Cambridge University Press.

Chihara, C.S. and Fodor, J.A. (1991). Operationalism and ordinary language: a critique of Wittgenstein. In *The Nature of Mind* (ed. D. Rosenthal). Oxford: Oxford University Press, 137–150.

Currie, G. (1996). Simulation-theory, theory-theory and the evidence from autism. In *Theories of Theories of Mind* (ed. P. Carruthers and P. Smith). Cambridge: Cambridge University Press, 242–256.

Davies, M. and Stone, T. (ed.) (1995a). *Folk Psychology: a guide to the theory of mind debate*. Oxford: Blackwell.

Davies, M. and Stone, T. (ed.) (1995b). *Mental Simulation: evaluations and applications*. Oxford: Blackwell.

Dennett, D. (1987). True believers: the intentional strategy and why it works. In *The Intentional Stance*. Cambridge. MA: MIT Press, pp. 13–35.

Descartes, R. (1996). *Meditations on First Philosophy*. Cambridge: Cambridge University Press.

Eilan, N., Hoerl, C., McCormack, T., and Roessler, J. (ed.) (2005). *Joint Attention—Communication and Other Minds: issues in philosophy and psychology* (*consciousness & self-consciousness S.*) Oxford: Oxford University Press.

Fodor, J.A. (1991). Propositional attitudes. In *The Nature of Mind* (ed. D. Rosenthal). Oxford: Oxford University Press, pp. 325–338.

Fodor, J.A. *Psychosemantics*. Cambridge, MA: MIT.

Gipps, R. (ed.) (2004). *Autism and Intersubjectivity* (Special issue). *Philosophy, Psychiatry, & Psychology*, 11(3).

Glendinning, S. (1998). *On Being With Others: Heidegger, Derrida, Wittgenstein*. London: Routledge.

Gordon, R.M. (1995a). Folk psychology as simulation. In *Folk Psychology* (ed. M. Davies and T. Stone). Oxford: Blackwell, pp. 60–73.

Gordon, R.M. (1995b). Simulation without introspection or inference from me to you. In *Mental Simulation* (ed. M. Davies and T. Stone). Oxford: Blackwell, pp 53–67

Gordon, R.M. and Barker, J.A. (1995). Autism and the theory of mind debate. In *Philosophical Psychopathology* (ed. G. Graham and G.L. Stephens). Harvard, MA: MIT Press, 163–181.

Hacker, P.M.S. (1972). *Insight and Illusion*. Oxford: Oxford University Press.

Hacker, P.M.S. (1995). Criteria. In *The Oxford Companion to Philosophy*, (ed. T. Honderich). Oxford: Oxford University Press.

Heal, J. (1995). Replication and functionalism. In *Folk Psychology* (ed. M. Davies and T. Stone). Oxford: Blackwell, pp. 45–59.

Hobson, R.P. (1991). Against the 'theory of mind'. *British Journal of Developmental Psychology*, 9: 33–51.

Hobson, R.P. (2002). *The Cradle of Thought*. London: MacMillan.

Malcolm, N. (1958). Knowledge of other minds. *Journal of Philosophy*, 55 pp. 969–978. (Reprinted in Rosenthal, D (ed.) (1991).
The Nature of Mind. Oxford: Oxford University Press, pp. 92–97.)

Malcolm. N. (1971). *Problems of Mind: Descartes to Wittgenstein*. London: Allen & Unwin.

McDowell, J. (1982). Criteria, defeasibility, and knowledge. *Proceedings of the British Academy*, 68 pp. 455–479 reprinted in Mc Dowell, J. (1998). Meaning knowledge and reality. Cambridge, MA: Harvard University Press, pp. 369–394.

Russell, B. (1948). Analogy (1948). In *Human Knowledge: its scope and limits* London: Allen & Unwin. London: Allen & Unwin. (Reprinted in Rosenthal, D (ed.) (1991). *The Nature of Mind*. Oxford: Oxford University Press, pp. 89–91.)

Stich, S. and Nichols, S. (2003). Folk psychology in The Blackwell Guide to the Philosophy of Mind (ed S. Stich and T. Warfield). Oxford: Blackwell, pp. 235–255.

Stone, T. and Davies, M. (1996). The mental simulation debate: a progress report. In *Theories of Theories of Mind* (ed. P. Carruthers and P. Smith). Cambridge: Cambridge University Press, 119–137.

Williams, M. (1996). *Unnatural Doubts*. Princeton. Princeton University Press.

Wittgenstein, L. (1953). *Philosophical Investigations*. Oxford: Basil Blackwell.

Wittgenstein, L. (1972). *The Blue Book and Brown Books*. Oxford: Blackwell.

Wright, C. (ed.) (1986). *Realism Meaning and Truth*. Oxford: Blackwell.

CHAPTER 28

Personal identity and schizophrenia

Chapter contents

What is this chapter about?

'One of the essential features of schizophrenia is the disturbances of the experiencing "I" ' (Bovet and Parnas, 1993, p. 589).

This chapter looks at another central concept drawn from the philosophy of mind, which can both inform and be informed by psychopathology. The concept of personal identity is central to the subject matter of psychiatry. However, it also exemplifies the relationship between empirical and conceptual work that has run throughout this book. While psychopathology can teach us a great deal about what is involved in the nature of persons and our identity through time—and thus what can threaten that—there is no simple experiment available to answer the question: What is a person? Instead empirical evidence and conceptual exploration go hand in hand.

In more detail, the chapter concerns what can be called the experiencing 'I' as well as the 'I' that is experienced. That is to say, it is about the self *identification* as well as the *identity* of one's person. It is also about the impact that mental illness, in general, and schizophrenia, in particular, may have on personal identity.

In this chapter as well as in the philosophical literature 'personal identity' or 'identity of a person' is taken to mean not a thing or property (like a driver's license or a sense of humor) that can be taken from you or altered in you, but what it takes for you as a person to persist from one time to another—for the *one and the same* person to exist at different times. What determines which future person, or which past person, is you?

Personal identity is a difficult topic. Yet it is or should be important to clinicians and mental health professionals. Suppose you have a patient in a clinic who is being hospitalized for onset of schizophrenia. Might this very person fail as the person he is to survive through the illness? Clearly you don't wish the illness to turn him into the psychologically fragmented remnant of a person. Or suppose a client presents herself to you with a diagnosis of dissociative (multiple) identity disorder. Could her body be the home of two, or three, or six different persons, each with its own temporal career? How could you find out if there are six persons in that body?

Plan of the Chapter

* *Session 1* introduces some of the basic issues about personal identity.

* *Session 2* sets out four different ways of denying that there is any such thing.

* *Session 3* introduces the idea that mental illness can impact on identity.

* *Session 4* looks at 4 positive theories of personal identity.

* *Session 5* concludes by looking again at how mental illness sheds light on identity.

Session 1 Personal identity: evidence and constitution

Context and bearings

One of the most famous case histories of schizophrenia is that of Daniel Schreber (1842–1911). Schreber was a judge in Leipzig who suffered from late-onset schizophrenia and was hospitalized in a sanatorium. He wrote an autobiographical account of his experiences called 'Memoirs of my nervous illness', which was discussed by Freud, Bleuler, and Jaspers, and is the subject of Sass's recent book *The Paradoxes of Delusion: Wittgenstein, Schreber and the Schizophrenic mind* (1995).

Screber's life was dominated by hallucinatory experiences and delusions. The director of the sanatorium wrote of Schreber's delusions as follows:

> He believed that he was dead and decomposing, that he was suffering from the plague; he asserted that his body was being handled in all kinds of revolting ways ... The patient was so much occupied with these pathological phenomena that he was inaccessible to any other impression and would sit perfectly rigid and motionless for hours.   Spitzer *et al.* (1981, p. 339)

Schreber sometimes acknowledged that his beliefs and attitudes were not normal. When not in the grips of an acute stage of his illness he wrote: 'I could even say with Jesus Christ: my kingdom is not of the world' (quote from Schreber's memoirs cited in Liddle, 2000, p. 571).

Schreber was profoundly muddled about and disturbed within himself. He had trouble identifying his own thoughts and deeds. He had difficulty distinguishing between what was part of him and what not. The 'I' whom he believed was dead and decomposing was, of course, alive. His body, which in fact moved of his own accord, he believed was moved or controlled by others. To compensate sometimes Schreber sat motionless.

Here is a remark from a second victim of schizophrenia:

> I get shaky in the knees and my chest is like a mountain in front of me, and my body actions are different. The arms and legs are apart and away from me, and they go on their own. That's when I feel I am the other person and copy their movements, or else stop and stand like a statue. I have to stop to find out whether my hand is in my pocket or not ... Sometimes the legs walk on by themselves or sometimes I let my arms roll to see where they will land.   Chapman (1966, p. 232)

Normally, we know when we perform our movements or actions. We tend immediately to recognize our deeds. In schizophrenia, by contrast, the ability to identify one's actions as one's own is severely disturbed. So, too, is recognition of mental activity as one's own. A young patient of the Canadian psychiatrist C.S. Mellor (1970) remarks: 'I cry, tears roll down my cheeks and I look happy, but inside I have a cold anger because they are using me in this way, and it is not me who is unhappy, but they are projecting unhappiness into my brain.'

What is the connection between being a person and being able to recognize one's actions, for example, as one's own? To get a preliminary idea about this consider the following pair of conceptual claims one sometimes comes across in philosophic discussions of personal identity, which suggest that the connection is *not* very close (they differ in the degree of separation proposed):

1. There is a distinction between the *identification* that we make of our selves or persons and our *identities* as persons. That I recognize my self or person in my thoughts or deeds is one thing. That I am who I am is another.

2. Those two facts (one about person identification and the other about identity) are not just distinguishable (or can be distinguished theoretically) but profoundly separable. Being me (my identity as a person) and conceiving me (my identification of my self) bear no relation one to the other.

The second point *surely* is mistaken or overstated even if the first, in some sense, is true. No relation? Victims of schizophrenia such as Schreber are disturbed in self identification. Perhaps it's not just self identification that is disordered in schizophrenia. Perhaps also the personal identity of a victim of schizophrenia is disintegrated—assuming that (contrary to the second point above) personal identity connects in some intimate manner with success or failure at identifying one's person.

Occasional failure to recognize my self in my thoughts and deeds may not affect my identity as a person. So, yes, that I self identify is one thing, my identity is another. However, persons are essentially self-identifying beings. Lynne Rudder Baker (1997), a philosopher at the University of Massachusetts at Amherst (USA), writes as follows: 'A being that cannot think of itself in a ... first-personal way is not a person' (p. 443). (See also Baker, 2000.) If so chronic or persistent failure to self identify is incompatible with being a person.

This raises a philosophical question about personal identity in schizophrenia, which can and also will be posed for other mental illnesses: Can personal identity withstand an illness such as schizophrenia in which self identification is profoundly muddled and disturbed? Can someone such as Schreber persist through the illness? Or is schizophrenia too much for a person, literally, disintegrating or dissolving him as the person he is? Some illnesses perhaps do have such a disintegrating impact. Advanced Alzheimer's dementia (as we will see) very well might. Does schizophrenia?

This not an easy question to answer. It is not even easy to understand. Let's begin by discussing the concept of personal identity.

The story of U

Suppose someone writes your biography. When would it—the biography and not the pre-biographical contextual material—begin? Presumably it would begin with your beginning. It would begin when you enter existence. When would it end? Presumably it would end when or if you exit from existence.

Call this biography (if you wish, imagine your own name here in the place of 'U'): *The Story of U*.

It is a presupposition of the Story of U—and more generally of the continued existence through time of any person—that *one and same person exists over time or at different moments in time*. The story of U begins with the entry into existence of U and ends with the exit from existence of this same person, the identical person, U.

Among statements in the story we might find some like the following:

(1) As a child, U was shy and socially withdrawn. However when U went to the university U's social personality changed. U became socially active and gregarious.

Such propositions are about U and say that U changed as U aged or matured. U's biography would also include statements such as:

(2) U had always been bright and curious. U had a gift for numbers. So no one was surprised, least of all U's parents, when U decided to become a university professor of mathematics. U now teaches topology at Warwick.

Such statements are about U, too, but unlike those in (1), those in (2) say that some features of U endured through adulthood. Some features did not change. U always was bright and curious.

Suppose U points to a photograph taken in childhood and says 'That's me winning the math prize in school.' 'I was surprised by the ease with which I could solve differential equations.' U's biographer may include this picture in U's biography. She may also include a picture, cherished by U's parents, of U as a young professional participating in an academic ceremony at Warwick in full regalia. Two pictures. One person. One U.

What does it mean for the same person to exist at different moments in time or throughout his or her span of existence? What is there—what 'persistence glue'—perhaps buried in a heap of biographical facts makes a person the same person at different moments in time? Philosophers call it *personal identity*. But what's that?

There are two conceptual possibilities. The first is that it is *nothing*. Personal identity is an illusion. Persons fail to persist over time; strictly speaking, there aren't persons. Peter Unger (1979) of New York University writes: 'I do not exist and neither do you' (p. 236). This possibility grossly violates common sense and Unger's enthusiastic embrace of the position may suggest to

---

EXERCISE 1   (10 minutes)

Think about the way the *Story of U* introduced above might be continued.

♦ What resources might we take from it to explain what the identity of U through time might consist in?

♦ What factors would we appeal to to determine whether we were still, at a later time, talking about the same person we had described earlier?

♦ What factors would U appeal to?

♦ What is the connection between how we know whether we are talking about the same person and the facts that underpin sameness?

some readers a form of mental illness. (Perhaps the Cotard delusion that consists, in part, in believing that one is dead or does not exist; see below.) However, Unger surely is not deluded. He is enunciating a philosophical thesis. Several very distinguished thinkers (to be noted below) have denied that, strictly speaking, they exist. These thinkers are paragons of sense and sensibility.

The second possibility is that personal identity is *something*. Persons persist over time; strictly speaking, there are persons. This of course is the common sense view and it also the view of most philosophers who have written on the subject of personal identity. However, the problem is articulating just what that something is, what personal identity consists in.

What then is the something that personal identity is?

Personal identity is not evidence

The answers to the questions in Exercise 1 are far from clear but we can make some preliminary points.

Personal identity is not a matter, for example, of having specific fingerprints. If someone 10 years from now has U's fingerprints, we may say that this person is U. However, having U's fingerprints is not the same as being U. It is *evidence* of U, but it is not the same as *being* U. It is possible to reproduce fingerprints or to transfer them from one person to another. We can imagine U saying 'Smith has my fingerprints but Smith is not me.' 'I alone am me.'

Other types of evidence for identity include physical and psychological similarities between past and present persons. If I met U in 1987 and then bump into someone in 2004 who looks and acts just like U, as I remember U, I have evidence that this present person is U. However, past U need not be like present U to be U. People do change. So, similarity is not *necessary* for identity. Neither does similarity *suffice* for identity. Identical twins may be utterly indistinguishable except for their locations, but they are not the same (identical) person. Just as the story of U is not the story of U's fingerprints, it is not the story of U's similarity over time or physical or psychological inalterability.

'We inquire,' writes Daniel Robinson (1998), past-president of the Division of Theoretical and Philosophical Psychology of the American Psychological Association, 'as to name and occupation, address, social security number, fingerprints, credit cards, and so on.' 'Following this investigation . . . we are prepared to assert that we know the actual identity of the person—the personal identity' (p. 353).

If Robinson is talking about *evidence* for identity, he is right. Such facts as those he cites are evidence of identity. Given the proper evidence we know who someone is. However, evidence for personal identity does not tell us what constitutes identity. What conditions make it up? What composes it? What is it?

If, by contrast, Robinson means to be talking about what *constitutes* personal identity, he is wrong. Personal identity is not a type of evidence. It is a *relation that no person can have to anything or anyone but himself or herself*. It is whatever it is that, in some sense, holds a person together over time and through alterations. Having fingerprints, say, of type T, fails to fit the bill, as more than one person can share T-type prints. Being similar to

someone fails to fit the bill. The same person can be similar to persons other than herself.

Thus we need to inquire a little deeper to find what might constitute identity. In the next session we will look at claims that, properly speaking, nothing does. This will help frame the discussion in the rest of the chapter. Responding to the challenge of 'identity antirealism' will give some clues for any plausible form of identity realism.

Reflection on the session and self-test questions

Write down your own reflections on the materials in this session drawing out any points that are particularly significant for you. Then write brief notes about the following:

1. What is the connection between psychopathology and personal identity?

2. What role does evidence of identity play in constituting personal identity?

Session 2 Four kinds of identity antirealism

Identity antirealism

In response to the question, 'What constitutes personal identity?', several very distinguished thinkers or philosophers have advanced versions of the view that, strictly, there is no such thing. 'Well, then,' they say, 'you can search for the composition of personal identity all you wish, but we're sorry to say that you will not find anything.' 'This is because when we refer to ourselves existing at different times—when we refer to our identity—we *refer to nothing*.' 'We don't persist.' 'Personal identity is an illusion, a myth. It's all nonsense.' 'Like witches, caloric fluid, phlogiston, and the gods of Roman religion, "personal identity" is the mistaken posit of a false theory of the metaphysics of personhood.'

Let's call this nihilistic view *personal identity antirealism* (hereafter 'PIAR' for short). It might also be called *identity fictionalism*, the idea being that personal identity is a fiction. It's a myth. The most common types of PIAR are of the following four sorts. They are:

PIAR-1

'The identity of my self or person' refers to nothing because if it did we should be able to find it in introspection. Introspection is the turning of the mind's eye inward. We can find nothing in introspection for the words 'I' or 'self' to refer to. What we find in introspection if we look carefully enough and without the naive prejudices of common sense are thoughts without thinkers, feelings, and emotions without selves or persons. We find collections or bundles of experiences but no 'experiencer'. We find no person, no 'I' or self with a temporal career.

The Scottish philosopher David Hume (1711–76), arguably the most influential English-speaking philosopher, held a version of

PIAR-1. We might call Hume's version *introspectionist antirealism*. Here in one of the most famous passages in the history of the philosophy of personal identity is Hume's report of his introspective search for self.

> For my part, when I enter most intimately into what I call myself, I always stumble on some particular perception or other, of heat or cold, light or shade, love or hatred, pain or pleasure. I never catch myself at any time without a perception, and never can observe any thing but the perception. When my perceptions are remov'd for any time, as by sound sleep; so long I am insensible of *myself*, and may truly be said not to exist. And were all my perceptions remov'd by death, and cou'd I neither think, nor feel, nor see, nor love, not hate after the dissolution of my body, I shou'd be entirely annihilate, nor do I conceive what is further requisite to make me a perfect nonentity. If any one upon serious and unprejudic'd reflexion, thinks he has a different notion of *himself*, I must confess I can reason no longer with him.... He may perhaps, perceive something simple and continu'd, which he calls *himself*, though I am certain there is no such principle in me.
>
> Hume, *A Treatise of Human Nature* (1967, Bk. I, pt. 4, ch. 6)

Only introspection can prove the existence of the self, Hume assumed. Nothing he found, he claims, was a *'continu'd'* him.

EXERCISE 2   (10 minutes)

As we saw in Chapter 3, the Canadian psychiatrist C.S. Mellor has studied schizophrenia in detail. A schizophrenic patient of his (Mellor, 1970, pp. 16–17) complained that her thoughts were 'sucked out of my mind by a... vacuum extractor, and there is nothing in my mind, it is empty.' Mellor's patient's disturbance is known as 'thought withdrawal'.

How different is Hume's account of his search for his self from Mellor's patient? Mellor's patient complained that her mind was devoid of thought. Suppose Hume complains that his mind is devoid of him. He cannot identify his self in his thoughts (or so he says). If you were to confront Hume as a psychiatric patient how would you construe his self-report? Can we make sense of his account of his search?

PIAR-2

Hume's claim is radical and initially surprising. How can there not be something that both underpins our personal identity—something that connects our thoughts etc.—and is also introspectible? But on the other hand, Hume's introspection surely stands for each of us as well. We would come to the same conclusion.

To assess Hume's scepticism about the idea of substantial self to unify ones thoughts or ideas we need to come up to date and think about the variety of forms of identity antirealism. We will, consider three other forms. The next, PIAR 2, is based on the following thought.

'My personal identity' refers to nothing because if it did we would use words like 'I' as referring expressions, but 'I' is not a referring expression. When I say something like 'I have a toothache', despite the fact that 'I' appears as the grammatical subject of a predicate ('have a toothache'), it is not serving a referring function at all. It may draw your attention to something (the toothache) but it does not report something about *me*. The word 'I' refers to nothing in a way rather like the way in which 'and' and 'furthermore' refer to nothing. It's a useful word but not a referring term.

One reason for advocating this initially surprising view is that first person avowals appear to have a particular kind of immunity to error. If I report that I am thinking such and such then it seems that I am normally immune to error as to *who* is thinking such and such. But if 'I' were a referring expression it would surely be possible to misapply it by referring to the wrong thing. That, after all, seems to be a feature of other referring expressions.

Ludwig Wittgenstein (1958) held a version of PIAR-2 and this position received an influential expression in a paper of Elizabeth Anscombe (1975) entitled 'The first person'. It may be called (appropriating a term from John Canfield's (1990, pp. 57–96) sympathetic discussion) *grammatical antirealism*.

PIAR-3

This is a more radical and general position. It holds that reality does not contain distinguishable things of ordinary day-to-day or familiar sorts (persons, cars, pieces of candy, rocks). The existence of such things (including persons) is an illusion.

Such a radical and general denial of ordinary things enjoys a surprisingly distinguished pedigree in the history of philosophy. The list of advocates includes Parmenides (a pre-Socratic Greek philosopher) and Buddha (the religious leader). Among contemporaries Peter Unger (1979a, 1979b) defends the denial. It may be called (as it is not restricted to persons) *anti-ordinary-things antirealism*. Reality may be one big individual (Very Big! a Blob perhaps), tiny subvisible particulars (microparticles perhaps), or something else entirely, but no particulars of ordinary or familiar sorts and thus no persons (including you and me) exist.

PIAR-4

'My identity' refers to nothing at all because if it did persons would be distinct from how they are conceived or represented and they are not. The furniture of the world includes planets and pebbles, fields and waves, sparrows and spices, theories and concepts. Planets, pebbles, and other real particulars are distinct from how they are conceived or represented. But persons are not distinct from how they are represented. Pebbles can sit on the beach but pebble *concepts* cannot. By contrast person concepts or person representations exist but persons, strictly speaking, do not exist. Person concepts or representations exist in human heads and culture but persons have no place in the real world at all.

A lot of interesting work has been done with PIAR-4 in the context of examining types of mental disorders. (The ambitious reader might want to read some of the following: Kathleen Wilkes (1988, 1991, 1999), Daniel Dennett (1991; Dennett and Humphrey, 1989), Owen Flanagan (1992, 1994; Hardcastle and Flanagan, 1999), and Thomas Metzinger (2000) for defences of the position. See Stephen Braude (1995) and George Graham (1999a,b, 2002) for critiques.) It may be called *representational antirealism*.

Daniel Dennett is a professor of philosophy at Tufts University in Massachusetts (USA). He is the author of many books and articles on the philosophy of mind and cognitive science. Here is how Dennett (in the context of discussing multiple personality disorder) with co-author Nicholas Humphrey conveys the tenor of representational antirealism.

Many people who find it convenient or compelling to talk about the 'self' would prefer not to be asked the emperor's-new-clothes question: just what exactly is the 'self'? . . . [But human beings] just find it useful to imagine the existence of this conscious inner 'I' when we try to account for behavior (and, in our own case, our private stream of consciousness). We might say that the self is rather like the 'center of narrative gravity' of a set of biographical events and tendencies; but, as with a center of physical gravity, there's really no such *thing* . . . Let's call this nonrealist picture of the self, the idea of a 'fictive-self'. [Brackets added.]

Dennett and Humphrey (1998, pp. 38–39)

> **EXERCISE 3** (10 minutes)
>
> What should be made of these four forms of PIAR? Should it persuade us that we ourselves are fictions or unreal? We don't persist. We *aren't*? What would be the consequences of this view? How might it be asserted, argued for and assessed.

Of course we cannot make a full and fair assessment of PIAR without looking at the arguments for various versions of this nihilistic doctrine, and we don't have room for that. However, there are at least two serious difficulties with PIAR that strongly suggest that the conclusion of a full and fair assessment of the position would be that PIAR is mistaken—seriously mistaken.

The first is that PIAR confronts those who endorse it with a kind of contradiction. Suppose you are reading something written by a philosopher who denies that persons persist. If you ask them whether they have written that personal identity is a myth, and they answer 'Yes, I wrote that', then this presupposes that (contrary to what they wrote) they believe persons persist—at least that *they* persist through the writing, the question, and the answer 'yes'.

Here is how Sir A.J. Ayer (1910–89), a distinguished British philosopher of the mid-twentieth century, expressed the contradiction: When it comes to the sentence 'I don't exist', he noted (and we are paraphrasing his remarks here), if one succeeds in making the statement, it must be false (Ayer, 1956, p. 50). 'I don't exist', say I. Peter Van Inwagen, a philosopher at the University of Notre Dame (2000) calls identity antirealism 'so much . . . arm-waving' (p. 176). One is tempted to agree with Van Inwagen. If a thesis cannot be stated without being false, it hardly seems to be a real thesis at all.

The second comment concerns Hume. Well, actually, it's more than a comment. It's a mini-exercise in introspection or in thinking about what it is like to undergo conscious experiences.

I-Thoughts

As noted Hume wrote that 'when I enter most intimately into what I call *myself* . . . I never catch *myself* at any time.' According to Hume the illusory idea of a self or person to whom, over time, experiences occur should be replaced with the idea of experiences occurring un-selfconsciously, impersonally.

Derek Parfit is Reader in Philosophy at the University of Oxford. Some comments of Parfit (1999; see also 1971, 1984) may be appropriated to explain the sorts of conscious activity that is consistent with a stream of consciousness of a card-carrying Humean identity antirealist: 'They would have no concept of themselves as the thinkers of . . . thoughts, or as agents of . . . acts.' 'And they would regard their experiences as occurring, rather than as being had.'

Parfit tries to convey the conscious tenor of how beings who did not regard themselves as persisting persons might identify thoughts in their stream of consciousness (but not as in episodes in *their* stream of consciousness). 'In place of the pronoun "I", these beings might have a special sense of "*this*" which referred to the sequence in which this use of "*this*" occurred. When one of us would say "I saw the Great Fire", one of them would say, "*This* included a seeing of the fire".'

In short, someone with a PIAR introspective consciousness would lack what are called 'I-thoughts'. Normally, of course, we think of ourselves as subjects of conscious states and attitudes. We entertain I-thoughts. We normally experience various thoughts, feelings, and actions as our own or (in the words of philosophers Roderick Chisholm (1976) and Syndey Shoemaker (1986)) as *adjectival* upon ourselves, our 'I's'. PIAR introspective consciousness operates with non-self, non-'I', or impersonal conscious awareness. Experiences occur but not as one's own. 'Instead of "I am angry", PIAR-ists would say "Anger has arisen here"' (Parfit, 1999).

Undergoing I-thoughts, strictly speaking, is incompatible with being a committed PIAR theorist in full control of one's antipersonal existence makeup. However, is it really possible let alone desirable to prune oneself of I-thoughts? Isn't there a second problem here comparable with the one mentioned above? If I admonish myself to experience no I-thoughts, and somehow succeed, aren't I responding to *my own* admonishment? If I fail to follow the admonition isn't this because, no, that's what I am. I am the sort of creature that can follow or fail to follow self directions. I am a person concerned to think in manner consistent with my beliefs, admonishments and commitments. I am, in Lynne Rudder Baker's terms, a being that can think of itself in a first-personal way. We will see later (in discussing John Locke and schizophrenia) that a capacity for I-thoughts may well play the central role in defining our persistence. The ways in which we think and speak of ourselves (the ways in which we identify ourselves as ourselves) may help to constitute who we are as persons existing across time.

Thus, although there have been a number of influential arguments against the reality of personhood, no such account can satisfactorily deal with the paradoxical consequences of such a denial. A guarded realism seems therefore a better approach to take. The next session will look at the consequences forms of mental illness for this discussion.

Reflection on the session and self-test questions

Write down your own reflections on the materials in this session drawing out any points that are particularly significant for you. Then write brief notes about the following:

1. What is puzzling about personal identity?

2. Why would any philosophers deny the existence of facts about personal identity?

3. Is such antirealism about personal identity itself coherent?

Session 3 Identity and mental illness

Gender identity disorder

In what follows we will assume that personal identity is a genuine feature of the world and thus that any form of PIAR should be rejected. This raises the question of whether personal identity can be lost. Suppose we wonder whether some mental illnesses or disorders eliminate or cause the disintegration of identity or persistence; others do not. Some, we fear, destroy personal persistence. Which ones? Is schizophrenia among them?

Let's consider two non-schizophrenia disorders first. Let's compare and contrast gender identity disorder with advanced stage Alzheimer's dementia. Alzheimer's is a progressive brain disease that in its advanced stage means victims have lost substantially all the memory of earlier lives and cannot, except occasionally and only in a fragmented way, respond appropriately to or recognize people to whom they have been close.

What is gender identity disorder? The *Desk Reference to the Diagnostic Criteria from DSM-IV* (APA, 1994) says that gender identity disorder consists, in part, in 'strong and persistent cross-gender identification' (p. 246). This may manifest itself in a preoccupation with eliminating and replacing primary and secondary sex characteristics (via e.g. requests for hormones or surgery). (See also Green 2000, pp. 211–217.)

'Charles' is the name of a hypothetical patient with transsexual gender identity disorder described in *DSM-III Case Book* (Spitzer *et al.*, 1981, pp. 63–64). Anatomically, Charles is a woman with normal female anatomy, but Charles feels her anatomy to be personally repulsive and emotionally incongruous. To Charles it is a source of chronic distress. She claims that she is a man. She wears a strap-on penis, upper garments that flatten her breasts, and seeks prescriptions for testosterone. She is the intimate other of a bisexual woman with two children, each of whom regards Charles as their stepfather.

As a young girl Charles was a tomboy. Let's call Charles as a tomboy 'Charlie'. Suppose that the story of this person is written. It refers to her as having been a tomboy named 'Charlie'. Once Charles begins trying to live as a member of the opposite sex, however, suppose that this hypothetical biography refers to Charlie as 'him'. The male pronoun is used because Charlie has replaced her gender identity with that of a man—'Charles'. 'Gender' is a potentially distinct category from 'sex'. 'Sex' is a term of anatomical reference. 'Gender' can be used as a socio-cultural term. It may identify people's preferences for how they wish to live and be perceived socially (as a man or as a woman). One and the same person can have different gender identities. But one and the same person cannot have different personal identities.

Alzheimer's disease

The DSM-IV reference manual also contains descriptions of Alzheimer's (APA, 1994, pp. 85–86). Symptoms include (among others): severe memory impairment, apraxia (victims may fall frequently or be unable to walk at all), and disturbance in executive functioning (they are incapable of sustaining plans or projects, their desires change rapidly). Does Alzheimer's bring an end to the existence of its victim as a person? Does it destroy the glue that binds a person over time? Can Alzheimer's cause the disintegration of personal identity?

When a person can acquire new memories, retain old ones, form and act on plans that are reasonably stable, and not inconsistent and self-defeating in the very short term, he or she readily is seen as a persisting person. If, however, in the grips of advanced Alzheimer's, someone's choices and desires, no matter the vigor of their expression, flatly contradict one another, reflect no coherent short-term plans, and so on, it is not so easy to see this particular being as a person. It is tempting to believe that a life lived in advanced dementia (with memory loss) is not the temporal career of a person. If we yield to this temptation, although gender identity disorder, we might say, is compatible with personal identity, advanced Alzheimer's, we will say, is not. The story of a person with such an illness ends when the advanced illness begins. A victim becomes a mere residue or remnant of a person.

EXERCISE 4 (10 minutes)

- With respect to personal identity, what are the differences between the two cases discussed so far in this session?

- Does either suggest reason to believe to a greater or lesser extent in the reality of personal identity?

More on the idea and importance of personal identity

One way of thinking about the differences between the two cases is that while gender identity disorder threatens the nature of the identity of a person, Alzheimer's, at least in its terminal form, threatens the possibility of any identity. Dementia looks to threaten the very idea of identity.

Perhaps the temptation to deny that a person can persist through advanced dementia will strike some readers as tendentious and contrived. So, before proceeding with this denial, we need to stop and say more about both the idea and the importance of personal identity.

Consider the following two pairs of statements:

- First person identity pair

    (fpi1) 'I will do that later'
    (fpi2) 'I did that earlier'

◆ Third person identity pair

    (tpi1) 'He will do that later'

    (tpi2) 'She did that earlier'

Now consider the following more specific examples of statements of each type:

    (FPI1) 'I will read the chapter tomorrow'

    (FPI2) 'I majored in philosophy thirty years ago'

    (TPI1) 'He will rob the bank tomorrow'

    (TPI2) 'She had an abortion two years ago'

Note that in each pair of statements the same person (me/you, the first person, in the first pair; he or she, other persons, in the second pair) is said to exist at different periods of time, roughly now, earlier, and later.

Note how deep our attachment is to the reality of the persistence of persons. We take it to be something substantial.

EXERCISE 5 (10 minutes)

Write down your own ideas about why personal persistence might matter to you as a person. Why, for example, is it important to you that you are the same person who has been reading this chapter for the last several minutes? If you are not the same person, what would that tell you about your powers of memory? That they could be grossly mistaken?

First, consider what it means to be a person. For one thing a person is a complex creature that can do many things. As a person I can act in various ways. I can hope, desire, and dream about many things. There are, also, things that can happen to me because I am a person. I can be joyous or forlorn. I can find myself in love, expectant, prideful or anxious.

Some of what happens in me, such as chemical activity in my kidneys, never enters my direct awareness, but much that happens to me and a great deal that I actively do deserves to be called 'conscious'. I will not climb trees because I am consciously and deathly afraid of falling. I will consciously attend to each key on the piano as I learn to play. I consciously desire, feel, intend, remember and act.

Now consider how much of our lives or existence as persons hinges on our persistence—requires personal identity across time. The possibility of intentional action requires that our actions as well as the intentions expressed in performing them are the actions and intentions of one and the same person. In voluntary behaviour our intentions help to cause our limbs to move. That is why we are able to say things like (FPI1) 'I will read the chapter tomorrow'. I can form the intention or decision today to read the chapter tomorrow. When I say as in (fpi1) 'I will do that later', I am presupposing that I expect later to act on a decision formed now. Second, the memory of my past presupposes the reality of personal identity across time. Events in which we were actively involved happen in the past and we may recollect them today. I say (FPI2) 'I majored in philosophy thirty years ago.' That memory, if true, is the result of a complex causal process involving activities in which I was engaged 30 years ago, the storage of information about that activity in the (my)

mind/brain, and its recall in the form of a memory report. If you remove the identity fact that I am the same person as the person who majored in philosophy 30 years ago, you eliminate my capacity for truly remembering the major as my major. You obliterate the 'my' of the major. I cannot remember something that I did unless I actually did it. I might *seem* to remember but I cannot really remember. Third, moral responsibility for good or bad deeds hinges on personal persistence. We persons stand morally accountable for things we've done or undone. We can be urged to act or to refrain from acting in certain ways under threat of punishment or prospect of praise. 'If you rob that bank tomorrow, and get caught, you will go to prison.' We assume that the same and only the same person as the criminal should go prison for the crime. Sending another person to prison for the robber's misdeed would be an injustice. Warning the potential robber that someone other than himself will go to prison likely would fall on deaf and unmoved ears.

What does it mean to be a person?

Some philosophers demand more from an analysis of the concept *person* than is offered above. George Graham and Terence Horgan (a philosopher at the University of Arizona in the USA) (1998) provide some terminology that can be deployed to characterize competing accounts of what it means to be a person. Accounts that depict concepts such as 'person' and other philosophically controversial concepts such as 'free will', 'mind', and so on, as making lot of detailed and substantive claims about the meaning of concepts, are *opulent* accounts, while accounts depicting concepts as requiring few semantic elements are *austere*. An austere account of the meaning of 'person' may appeal because accounts at the opulent end of the spectrum are likely to be excessively controversial or contestable. They have many elements and so have trouble avoiding debate. But how austere is desirable or feasible? We shouldn't and can't avoid any and all debate.

Consider a presupposition about personhood of Ronald Dworkin, who is a professor of both law and philosophy at both New York University and Oxford. In a chapter on 'Life past reason' in *Life's Dominion* (1993) Dworkin writes of anticipating the possibility of being a victim of advanced Alzheimer's dementia:

> I know that if I become demented, I will probably want to go on living, and that I may then still be capable of primitive experiential pleasures. Some dementia victims, it is true, lead frightful, painful lives, full of fear and paranoia. Some are brutally unpleasant and ungrateful to those who care for them. But even they continue to want to continue living. . . . (But others may) think a life ending like that is seriously marred. . . . They do not think like the childish pleasures of dementia would redeem its curse. . . . They would prefer not to live on.
>
> (pp. 230–231, parenthesis added).

Dworkin's hypothetical anticipation presupposes that he could become demented ('if I become demented'). If he is right in this supposition, the temptation to believe that dementia shatters personal persistence should be resisted. It doesn't. The question Dworkin then asks is whether he would want to persist as an advanced Alzheimer's victim. He says that he very well might.

Dworkin, no doubt, is operating with a fairly austere concept of person. He seems to be saying that to be a person—to be Dworkin with advanced dementia—it is enough to be a human organism that is capable of primitive experiential pleasures and of wanting to live. Not that such a creature would want to live but that it *could* want to live. That's enough.

Dworkin's reaction to the hypothetical prospect of advanced Alzheimer's confronts us with a dilemma: either we deny that a victim of advanced dementia (Alzheimer's) is a person, and hold that the concept of person is not *that* austere (as is presupposed in Dworkin's book), or we concede that a human organism that is capable of experiential pleasures and a desire to live is a person and endorse the notion that the persistence of a person can include dementia. How should we resolve this dilemma? And (speaking of schizophrenia again) what, if anything, does trying to escape from such a dilemma posed for persistence by Alzheimer's dementia reveal about the fate of personal identity in schizophrenia?

There is at least one theory of personal identity and of the conditions that obtain just when a person persists that promises a way out of this dilemma. It is owed to John Locke and insists on analysing the concept *person* so as, in effect, to enable us to decide whether a victim with advanced Alzheimer's could be *you*, a person. The decision is negative. Locke's is one theory of identity among those that will be mentioned below. We will look at this in the next session.

Reflection on the session and self-test questions

Write down your own reflections on the materials in this session drawing out any points that are particularly significant for you. Then write brief notes about the following:

1. With the preliminary work on personal identity of the previous session in mind, what impact do the psychopathologies discussed in this session have on personal identity or self-identification?

2. How can one resolve whether a condition such as severe dementia threatens the very identity of the sufferer?

Session 4 Theories of personal identity

Again: what constitutes personal identity? If the answer is something, what is this something?

There are four main possibilities each represented by a variety of different theories in the literature and variations on those theories. To keep things simple the theories are stated briefly.

1. *The physical approach.* The first is that our identity through time consists in the persistence of something physical. You are the past or future person that has your body, or that has the same brain as you do, or that is the same biological animal that you are. Whether you survive or persist has nothing to do with anything non-physical. We will call this the *physical approach.*

Defense of the physical approach may be found in Richard Taylor (1997), Peter van Inwagen (1990), and Eric Olson (1997, 1998). David Wiggins (1980) endorses a version of the physical approach (on one interpretation). So too did Aristotle (384–322 BC) (on one interpretation) and St Thomas Aquinas (1225–74) (on one interpretation). (We shall not explore the relevant interpretations here.) The physical approach may also be found in Bernard Williams (1970a,b).

2. *The spiritual approach.* The second is that our identity through time consists in the persistence of something non-physical. You are the past or future person that has your soul, or that has the same incorporeal ego as you do, or that is the same spirit that you are. Whether you survive or persist has nothing to do with something physical. We will call this the *spiritual approach.*

Advocates of the spiritual approach include Plato (427–347 BC), Descartes (1596–1650) (though see Baier, 1981), Locke, and Richard Swinburne (see Swinburne's contribution on dualism in Shoemaker and Swinburne, 1984).

3. *The capacity approach.* Both the physical and the spiritual approach agree that something (in the sense of some *object* either physical or spiritual) constitutes our persistence. Our identity through time primarily and necessarily follows from the survival of that something. A third view, in a sense, does not make a direct commitment to the type of object required—whether physical or spiritual. The primary glue for identity through time consists in the persistence of capacities that are distinctive and definitive of personhood. If such personal capacities are the capacities of something spiritual, this means that something spiritual must survive. However, if personal capacities are the capacities of something physical or need to be embodied in material of some sort (human bodies or brains), then something physical must survive. We will call this the *capacity approach.*

On this view, persons have personal capacities. These personal capacities mean that persons can perform certain activities that cannot be performed or performed as well or in the same manner by non-persons.

Not every advocate of the capacity approach agrees on the capacities that are supposed to be distinctive and definitive of personhood. So, the capacities must be identified and argued for. The most popular version of the capacity approach may be outlined as follows.

We persons are not just living animals or bodies. We are not even just beings that can feel and perceive. We are self conscious creatures that can identify ourselves as ourselves across time. We are aware of ourselves as our selves and we think of ourselves as having pasts and futures or lives of our own. We keep track of our selves as our selves over time. Our capacity to keep track of ourselves as ourselves over time is both distinctive and definitive of personhood. It is also—so this line of thought goes—the basis of personal persistence. Persons persist just so long as their *self tracking* capacity endures or persists. Facts about the persistence of persons are facts about the persistence of the self tracking capacity of persons.

Some advocates of the self tracking version of the capacity approach (such as John Locke) are immaterialists about persons and combine (3) with some version of (2) the spiritual approach. Other advocates insist on the embodiment of the capacity. They combine (3) with some version of (1) the physical approach. On this physicalist usage the capacity of persons to self track might be the capacity of the human brain. If so that which is tracking itself is the brain of a person (and then persons are identical with their brains). Additionally, the notion of self tracking has been analysed or described in different ways. Usually but not always self tracking is said to consist in autobiographical memory (sometimes also called 'experience memory'). Autobiographical memory occurs when I recollect some past action or event as involving me: as something that I did or witnessed and experienced. 'I majored in philosophy thirty years ago.'

Friends of the *self-tracking capacity approach* include philosophers such as H.P. Grice (1941), Anthony Quinton (1962), Sydney Shoemaker (1984, 1997), and Robert Nozick (1981) (on one interpretation).

4. *The closure approach.* A fourth view can be mentioned though it is difficult to pigeonhole and quite mysterious from a clinical or medical professional point of view. Our identity through time consists in something humanly unknowable and not analysable. Call this (for the sake of a label) the *identity basis.* The identity basis might be a microscopic object located somewhere in the brain. Or it might be a non-physical thing, a soul. Or it might be something else entirely. Either way, any way, there are no informative, tractable (knowable) persistence conditions for persons. Persons persist; identity antirealism is false. However, we just don't know how we persist. We just don't know what the identity basis is. With the emphasis on unanalysability this view is sometimes called the *simple view* (see Roderick Chisholm, 1976, pp. 108f; see also Chisholm, 1969) (although it is anything but simple). With the emphasis on unknowability it is sometimes labelled as an instance of 'cognitive closure' (human cognitive inaccessibility) (See Colin McGinn, 1999, and also see Dean Zimmerman, 1998.) The 'glue' of personal identity is unknowable by us. We will call this the *closure approach.*

Our intent in the rest of this chapter is not to discuss all these theories. They are listed so that the reader may be in a position to pursue theories that may intrigue or appeal to him or her. We will focus on the self-tracking capacity approach. This is because the self tracking approach has the most immediate or direct implications for how to understand the effect on identity of a number of different mental illnesses. We shall endorse (for the purposes of the chapter and as suggested earlier) the claim that persons are entities that can think of themselves in a first-personal (or 'I' thought) way. Such a claim perhaps is compatible with the spiritual approach, the physical approach, as well as the closure approach. However, it is

strikingly central to the self tracking capacity approach. So we will deploy the self tracking capacity approach.

Locke's identity

> ### EXERCISE 6 (15 minutes)
>
> Read the following extract from Locke's discussion of personal identity:
>
> Locke, J. (1989). *Essay Concerning Human Understanding* (ed. P. Nidditch). Oxford: Clarendon Press. Sections 17–26.
>
> ―――――――――――
> Link with Reading 28.1
> ―――――――――――
>
> ◆ How does he avoid Hume's challenge to the substantiality of personality set out earlier in this challenge?
>
> ◆ What insight does Locke suggest into the empirical cases discussed above?

There are two key passages in the reading linked with Exercise 6. Locke writes of personal identity as follows:

Self is that conscious thinking thing... which is sensible, or conscious of Pleasure and Pain, capable of Happiness or Misery, and so is concern'd for it *self*, as far as the consciousness extends.

(Essay II. XXVII.17)

Person, as I take it, is the name for this *self*. Where-ever a Man finds, what he calls *himself*, there I think another may say is the same *Person*.... This (person) extends it *self* beyond present Existence to what is past, only by consciousness, whereby it becomes concerned and accountable, owns and imputes to it *self* past Actions just upon the same ground, and for the same reason, that it does the present. (Essay II. XXVII.26)

Locke's claim that we can remember ourselves as ourselves in past times and that this is the defining condition of our being that past person is on to something about identity, though just what is open to debate. Efforts to clarify Locke's insight and to develop it into theory of personal identity have been undertaken by a number of philosophers. Some of these have been in response to some famous criticisms of Locke's claim offered in the eighteenth century by Thomas Reid and Joseph Butler (see the excerpts in Perry (1975) mentioned in the annotated list of recommended readings). Though our space is limited, let's make one such an effort at development here.

Identity in self-conscious Locke-step

Consider the experience that you are having at present. At the centre of it, say, is reading this chapter, but much else is happening as well. The experience may include such things as the following: the taste of the coffee that you are drinking as you read the chapter; the sight of words on the printed page; the touch or texture of the current page as you turn it; the sparkle of sunlight as it hits your desk, and so on. These components of taste, sunlight, and so on, in the experience are not disordered or jumbled, one hopes, but appear or occur as part of (what may be called) an experiential unity. You do

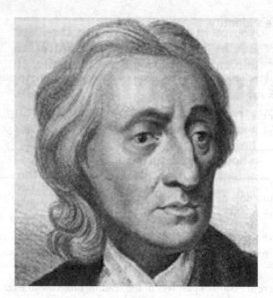

Fig 28.1 John Locke

not experience the words as dissociated from the page that you turn. You do not experience the sparkle of light as taking place at a different time than the taste of the coffee. Each is woven together in reading the chapter. Presumably also this experience of reading is presented to you as your experience. It's directly apparent either in the foreground or background of your conscious attention as *your* reading: as adjectival on you, as the taste to you of the coffee, the texture to you of the book page, the sunlight as it appears to you and so forth. If asked, for example, how the coffee tastes, you will reply, 'To me quite bitter.' The contrast would be between, for example, saying, 'To me quite bitter' and Hume- or Parfit-wise saying 'A bitter taste is occurring.' Of course we would not say such outlandish things (unless we were ill or in the depersonalized grips of PIAR). Our experiences appear to us as our own. As Locke notes: '... when we see, hear, smell, taste, feel, meditate, or will anything, we know that we do so.'

Here then is one interpretation of Locke's insight into the connection between (autobiographical) memory and identity. Just as my current experience of reading presents itself to me as mine, so the contents of my *past* experience in the form of autobiographical memories present themselves to me as belonging to my history. 'Yes, I did taste coffee yesterday and heard the ripple of rain on my window sill.' 'I am perfectly well aware that these experiences happened to me.' 'Today, however, sunlight has replaced the ripple of rain in the background as I read this book.' 'Yesterday I struggled to understand the paragraphs on PIAR.' 'Today I re-read those same paragraphs and believe that I understand them.'

Locke, if we are right, assigns to persons the power or capacity not just to appear to themselves *now* but to appear to themselves over time as themselves—as one and the same person as, for example, a past person. Indeed (and here is the connection between identity and memory) to be a persistent person, according to Locke, is to identify or experience one's self as persistent. Experiences that one has had (and may have in the future) are conceived as one's own.

Locke held that the capacity for self tracking or (as we may also call it) reflexively tensed self-consciousness ('I majored in philosophy thirty years ago', 'I will read the chapter tomorrow', etc.) is constitutive of us as persisting persons. That is, possessing the capacity is no mere evidence that we persist across time. It is what it means to persist.

James Cornman (1970, p. 178; cited in Canfield 1990, p. 33) once offered the following crisp critique of Hume's introspective antirealism. Cornman wrote: 'What Hume overlooked... is that self-awareness comes primarily, if not exclusively, when I am active; it is not some object that I find in introspection.... Someone is aware of himself when he is active, as in willing, just as surely as he is aware of any idea.'

Cornman's point is Lockian and it can be used to highlight something else that Locke says, which is (it may be recalled from the earlier quote from the *Essay*) that persons impute actions to themselves. Cornman is saying that it is by acting, by engaging in projects over time, forming intentions, making decisions, and acting on intentions and decisions, that our consciousness of ourselves is extended in temporal ways. When we act in the world we attribute to ourselves a past and anticipate a future. We think of ourselves as agents, as doers of deeds, instigators of movements. This consciousness of our selves makes possible (as Locke notes) praising and blaming people for deeds or misdeeds. If people were not capable of self awareness in action, the rationale for praise and blame would be lost. We would not be agents or doers.

On Locke's view an autobiographical-memory-less individual is not a person and cannot act as person or as a self-conscious agent in the world. Picturing such a complex and multitextured capacity for memory (for it supports, among other things, the capacity for deliberately acting in the world) as definitive of personal persistence is the basic Lockean admonition.

Reflection on the session and self-test questions

Write down your own reflections on the materials in this session drawing out any points that are particularly significant for you. Then write brief notes about the following:

1. What general approaches are there to answer the question: What does personal identity consist in?

2. What is the heart of Locke's account?

Session 5 Identity and mental illness again

Self tracking and Alzheimer's

What about mental illness? Locke's theory has negative implications for the fate of identity in advanced Alzheimer's.

To the Lockean, if a victim of advanced dementia is irreversibly deprived of relevant memories, the victim, conceived as a person, ceases to exist. What's left is a shell or remnant of a person, incapable of understanding themselves or that there is a world beyond them, let alone of keeping track of the course of their actions or projects. The dilemma extracted from Dworkin (1993) and mentioned earlier in the chapter thereupon is resolved in favour of a concept of person sufficiently opulent so as to reject the proposition that Dworkin or any person could persist through advanced Alzheimer's. To the Lockean, wanting to live but having utterly no sense of a past or future as one's own is insufficient for both being a person and personal persistence. Are there equally devastating implications for identity in schizophrenia?

We are very near to the point where we can explore the identity question of schizophrenia, but we are not quite there yet.

Two Locke variations

Two alternative versions of Locke's theory commit themselves to different ways in which the 'capacity to self track' and its connection with personal identity are understood. The two alternatives are these:

1. What makes a person one and the same person across time is that he or she remembers his or her past (especially his or her past deeds and experiences) and thinks of this past as his or her past.
2. One part of the body—namely, the neurobiologically living or functioning brain—is of crucial importance for realizing or embodying the autobiographical memory capacities of persons. The living or functioning brain controls and implements not merely individual acts of recall of the person, but the way in which people remember and the manner in which memory affects how a person acts, talks, and thinks. This physical basis of memory is what ultimately matters for personal identity. Only as the material basis functions to support self-tracking and persists, so, too, does the person.

Call the first version or theory *Pure Memory Theory* (hereafter 'PMT' for short). What matters for persistence is (autobiographical) memory period. PMT is compatible with the soul approach to personal identity. Locke himself, as noted, combined both the capacity and soul approaches. Call the second theory *Embodied Memory Theory* (EMT). What matters is matter: the functioning brainy substrate of the self-tracking capacity of persons.

According to PMT a person who is completely and utterly or irreversibly unable to remember the past does not continue to exist. One might as well say that they have been replaced by a non-person (if their body continues to exist and function) or a person remnant. If an individual lives without even a hint of autobiographical memory (not in the superficial way characteristic of temporary forgetfulness, but in a profound manner) this annihilates persistence.

According to EMT the functioning brain makes the defining contribution to the persistence—to personal identity across time.

The substratum must also be obliterated or irreversibly made memory-less if the person is to vanish from the face of existence. If the substratum can somehow function after a not irreversible loss of memory (perhaps the story behind the loss of memory is a dramatic type of motivationally repressed memory that somehow leaves the substratum intact and able, in time, to recover memories), the person persists.

EMT may be supplemented with the following idea. Although every major mental capacity (for autobiographical memory, deliberation, decision making, perceiving, reasoning, and so on) is implemented in some part or parts of the brain, diffusion reigns regarding the location of the neural basis that implements a capacity. It is now quite well established that, in the words of France's Joelle Proust (2000, p. 307), 'every mental function, even highly (encapsulated) ones, operates only on the background of other mental functions or cerebral systems' (parenthesis added). Proust's point is that the entanglement of the neural embodiment of a mental capacity, such as the capacity for autobiographical memory, with a variety of different cerebral systems (capacities for reasoning, perceiving, and so on), means that no mental capacity has a precisely circumscribed or isolated neural basis. Neural events in diffuse or distributed locales as well as other capacities are part of the ground or support system of autobiographical memory.

Neural entanglement is mirrored at a personal level of description. Consider, at the personal level of description, the psychological breadth of memory's entanglement in our lives. Suppose you intend to finish this chapter today. That project will involve: (1) a *desire* to read the chapter; (2) *belief* that you will read the chapter; (3) a *standing autobiographical memory* that you have not yet read the chapter; connected with (4) the background convictions and memories that you do know how to read, and so on. All such types of mental function (cognitive in the form of beliefs, motivational in the form of desires, etc.) are typically informed by—and wrapped up with—autobiographical memories of one sort or another (such as 3). Is it any wonder that the brain embodies memory's personal level entanglements?

Objections have been raised against Locke's autobiographical or self-tracking centred approach to personal identity. One of these is that the concept of autobiographical memory is too vague or obscure to bear the weight of a theory of personal identity. However, to reply, it must be noted that sometimes it is perfectly clear when memory deserves to be called 'autobiographical'. I remember going up the Eiffel Tower. This memory is of my past. It clearly is autobiographical. I do not autobiographically remember the First World War or the founding of Rome. I may claim to remember such events or (falsely) believe that I remember them. However, I was not present during them, so they cannot be (successfully) remembered as parts of my past.

We will not linger over misgivings with Locke's approach. The point of the chapter is not to defend a theory. It is to ponder the potential impact of mental illness on persistence. Schizophrenia is back on our doorstep. We should note, however, that EMT is to be preferred to PMT. PMT is vulnerable to an objection to which EMT is not vulnerable, arising from the possibility of false memories. Imagine that I memory-claim to have been prisoner of war in the First World War. Such a claim cannot prove that I existed during the war, although it may be fallible (albeit improbable) evidence for it. The memory claim needs to be checked, and so this leaves us needing to appeal to evidence other than apparent memories to determine whether I was a prisoner. My existence as a prisoner during the war is confirmed if it can be shown that certain effects of the war are somehow traceable or evident in my brain. Perhaps neural lesions associated with being a prisoner are observable in my substrate. Call these 'WWI Lesions'. WWI Lesions are the sorts of facts about the memory substrate and brain in general that EMT would say is relevant to my persistence as a person. As the lesions indicate that I was a prisoner, EMT would say that my past includes having been a prisoner of war.

What about PMT? PMT is a pure memory theory. No reference to an enduring substrate is part of the theory. Often, we need to determine which memories are real (true, veridical, successful) and which are merely apparent or alleged. If we have no means other than apparent memories for checking memory, we seem trapped in an unwelcome evidentiary circle—using one apparent memory to check another apparent memory. If I was a prisoner of war during the First World War, we cannot know this from my 'total claims to remember', because we don't know if my other memory claims are true.

So EMT is preferable to PMT. However, EMT is much more corporeal than Locke himself intended. Locke wished to detach the notion of personal identity from reference to the body. He is explicit about this, sharing with Descartes the assumption that what is constitutive of persons (memory or the backward reach of consciousness in Locke's case) is distinguishable from the material embodiment of persons. EMT takes the identity of a functioning material substrate to be constitutive of personal identity. EMT is in the self tracking capacity spirit of Locke, but certainly not in his letter. Like Locke, it honours the fact that persons appear to themselves over time as themselves. Unlike Locke, however, it pictures identity in terms, ultimately, of the persistence of the functioning substrate of this capacity.

Let us now return to schizophrenia and consider just what Locke's theory may tell us about the fate of personal identity in schizophrenia.

Identity in schizophrenia

Schizophrenia is a devastating mental illness. Christopher Frith (1998, p. 388), a neuropsychologist at the Institute of Neurology in London, calls it 'the most devastating' (parenthesis added). The most intimate thoughts, feelings, and actions of a schizophrenic are felt or experienced by the victim as imposed, known or shared by others. Hallucinatory voices may give a running commentary on a victim's behaviour. Speech may be incoherent.

There is a general clinical symptom associated with schizophrenia called *passivity experiences* or *delusions of passivity*. Some

(but alas not all) of the major difficulties that schizophrenics have with self identification are connected with this type of symptom. The patient experiences his own actions and thoughts as controlled not by himself but by some outside person or force. He believes that simple movements are made for him by another person or agent. He feels that thoughts are inserted into his stream of consciousness by another person. A patient of Mellor's (1970) remarks: 'I look out the window and I think the garden looks nice and the grass looks cool, but the thoughts of Eamon Andrews come into my mind. . . . He treats my mind like a screen and flashes his thought onto it.' Another complains: 'When I reach my hand for the comb it is my hand and arm which move, and my fingers pick up the pen, but I don't control them. . . . I sit there wanting them to move, and they are quite independent, what they do is nothing to do with me.'

Delusions of passivity are disturbances in the self tracking capacity of persons. Therein they are relevant to the persistence of persons and deeply relevant to a theory of identity like that of Locke, for whom the capacity to self track (both present and past in memory) is what it takes for a person to persist across time. Let's look specifically at a clinical phenomenon known as 'thought insertion', which is one of schizophrenia's typical passivity experiences. The remark about Eamon Andrews above is an instance of the phenomenon.

A person would normally couch a description of her thoughts in the language of self attribution. 'I am thinking of Paris'. 'I thought that you were going to buy my ticket.' However, in thought insertion a person fails to identify certain thoughts as her own and actually attributes them to another. A patient of Frith (1992, p. 66) remarks: 'Thoughts come into my head like 'Kill God'. It's just like my mind working, but it isn't.' Firth's patient continues: 'They come from this chap, Chris. They're his thoughts' (p. 66). Wing (1978, p. 105) reports: 'The symptom is not that (the patient) has been caused to have unusual thoughts . . . but that the thoughts *themselves* are not his.' (Parenthesis added.)

As a victim of thought insertion you might say something like: 'Thoughts of Paris are occurring in me. But they're not mine. They belong to Pierre.'

Louis Sass (1999, p. 319), a professor of clinical psychology at Rutgers University in New Jersey in the USA, writes that 'schizophrenics tend to lose their sense of integrated selfhood.' 'Even one's most intimate thoughts may appear to emanate from some external source.' Sass says that this is because victims of schizophrenia are severely disturbed in identifying themselves as themselves. This difficulty at self identification was noted at the beginning of the chapter. Does thought insertion help to disintegrate the personal identity of a victim of schizophrenia, assuming, with Locke, that self tracking is the essence of identity?

Imagine that someone is a victim of schizophrenia. Now a theorist of personal identity who believes, sceptically, that personal identity is destroyed or disintegrates in schizophrenia claims that this person does not persist across time. An argument for the sceptical conclusion may go something like the following.

The self experience of a victim of schizophrenia is a 'pandemonium phenomenon' (to appropriate an expression of Daniel Dennett, 1991). The thoughts and experiences (including actions) of the schizophrenic do not present themselves coherently and consistently to the victim as his own. A victim therein lacks appropriate autobiographical memories. He fails to experience or to remember himself as himself. 'All you have,' to appropriate some terms of Thomas Metzinger (2000, p. 301) written in an antirealist tone of voice, 'is a self-modeling system' which in schizophrenia is dissolved or disintegrated (p. 296). 'There is nobody... there' (p. 301). The person has ceased to exist and the human body is a person-less self-tracking-less fragment of a person.

That's crudely put, but the spirit is this. The thoughts and deeds of a victim of schizophrenia should not be described as the thoughts and deeds of *someone*—of a person. And the main reason for this? The profound breakdown in self-tracking associated with schizophrenia and as exhibited in thought insertion among numerous other symptoms.

Is *that* true? Does self tracking break down in schizophrenia? Is a schizophrenic without (to use Dennett's expression but not with its antirealist sense) a center of narrative gravity? This is a complex question and it can be asked not just of thought insertion but of many symptoms of schizophrenia (at least in advanced phases). Difficulty in self identification is exhibited, you may recall, in Schreber's bodily action delusions.

Does self-tracking break down in schizophrenia? Not necessarily. Again consider thought insertion. One half of the capacity for self identification or self tracking remains intact in thought insertion. One half of self tracking is more identity preservative than nothing. People suffering from inserted thoughts do recognize that 'inserted' thoughts occur in them. They appreciate that *they* are the subjects in whom thoughts occur or to whom certain conscious episodes are directly evident. Recall that Frith's patient says that thoughts with the content 'Kill God' occur in his head (1992, p. 66). It's just that Frith's patient believes that another person or agent is *doing* the thinking in his stream of consciousness. The patient's experience, as it were, gives him one-half the appropriate information about his conscious activity (namely that it occurs in him or is his in an 'in him' sense). It does not, however, give him a second half (namely, that he himself is *thinking* 'Kill God'). Such misattribution of mental activity to another reveals a dissociation or distinction within the conscious experience of a person between experiencing himself as the *subject* in whom thoughts occur and as the *agent* (person) who thinks. It is therein, to deploy words of John Campbell (1999, p. 611) of the philosophy department at the University of California at Berkeley, 'fundamentally a deficiency in the sense of agency.'

A victim of schizophrenia who suffers from thought insertion should therefore not be described as failing to self-track, but as tracking himself as subject without tracking himself as agent, namely, as 'having experiences with the right self as self-conscious subject but the wrong (i.e. misattributed) self as thinker.' (See G.L. Stephens and George Graham, 2000, as well as George

Graham, 2004, for related discussion.) Thought insertion does not obliterate self tracking. It truncates or distorts it.

General moral

We can distil a general moral from thought insertion that applies to any and all passivity experiences in schizophrenia. Whether such experiences mean that the self tracking capacity of a victim is obliterated depends upon whether *some* element of this capacity (such as in thought insertion the ability to experience one's self as subject in whom various conscious episodes occur) remains intact. Half a jar of identity glue is more binding than none. If some element of the capacity remains intact, arguably so does the victim of schizophrenia as a person.

Of course the mental life of schizophrenia does not consist just in experiences of thought insertion. Schizophrenia's devastation includes all sorts of other unfortunate symptoms and signs of illness. How then could each symptom be understood as consistent with a Lockean account of personal identity? This is not a question that we can answer here. The following exercise may help to convey the spirit of the challenge that the question poses and how best to respond to it.

EXERCISE 7 (15 minutes)

A schizophrenia exercise

Among the most disturbing clinical features of schizophrenia are the passivity experiences associated not with thought or feeling but with motivation, will, and action. These occur (among other places) in what are sometimes called cases of disjointed volition in schizophrenia. Disjointed volition is evident in grossly poorly organized or planned activities that appear to be prompted by impulse and may be attributed by the victim of schizophrenia to control by another person or outside force. Disjointed volition may also result in prolonged phases of inactivity. A victim of schizophrenia may lie in bed or sit motionless (as Schreber did) for hours.

One popular hypothesis for how best to understand disjointed volition is that it reflects an inability—given specific projects or intentions—to select appropriate behaviour and to inhibit inappropriate responses (see David, 2000, p. 577). Response selection and inhibition are (in part) memory skills requiring memory of past behaviour that has been successful or unsuccessful. If so, that is, if memory failure is involved in disjointed volition, disjointed volition represents a disturbance in the capacity of persons to self track. If as a victim of schizophrenia I cannot keep myself on task, perhaps this is because I have forgotten what I am intending to do or whether I should perform or repress a response.

Suppose, for the sake of hypothesis, that disjoined volition does represent a disturbance in the self-tracking capacity of persons. Mellor (1970) cites a case: a schizophrenic man (we will call him 'Frank') who experienced a sense of important opportunity while seated at a breakfast table in a boarding house. When another boarder offered the salt cellar to him, Frank suddenly blurted out that this meant that he should return home to greet the Pope who was visiting his family to thank him because his Lord and Savior was to be born again to one of the women in the house. Frank's consciousness was filled with I-thoughts (namely, he thought of his future and his house), although he was stimulated for action that was grossly inappropriate and unwise.

How might a Lockean argue that even if Frank went home to 'see the Pope' (certainly a bizarre act) he none the less acted as a persisting person with his capacity for autobiographical memory partially if not fully intact? Assume that Frank successfully returned to his home. Wouldn't this mean that he could differentiate between his home and another person's home? Frank might have thought to himself 'I intend to go to *my* home'. And he did. An important aspect of his autobiographical memory would seem to remain functional, would it not?

Prospects

Locke's *Essay* was first published in the late seventeenth century. So, it has been more than three centuries since his account of personal identity appeared in the literature. It will not be quick settling upon an appropriate theory of personal identity, although hopefully this will not take three hundred more years!

We human persons are not inanimate objects persisting through time, and we are not ephemeral events either, vanishing almost as soon as we appear. We are consciously persisting individuals with biographies. There are unfortunate individuals among us who for one reason or another suffer from mental illness and thus risk or undergo biographical upheaval in their temporal persistence as persons.

What more might be said about the uses of clinical data or of reference to such cases in constructing a theory of personal identity? It is not only schizophrenia, DID/multiple personality disorder, gender identity disorder, and Alzheimer's that need to be considered. The following is a partial list of additional disorders that may pose problems for personal identity if approached in terms of the capacity for self tracking.

1. *Depersonalization disorder.* Patients with depersonalization disorder often report that they do not feel like agents or persons. They experience a sense of disconnection or estrangement from their own body, feelings, thoughts, or behaviour. (APA, 1994, p. 231. See de Pauw, 2000, pp. 831–833.)

2. *Dissociative fugue.* Victims of dissociative fugue may try to assume a new social identity. The predominant disturbance is sudden, unexpected travel away from home or work, with the inability to recall one's past. (APA, 1994, p. 229. See Hacking, 2002.)

3. *Borderline personality disorder.* This is a heterogeneous syndrome marked by mood instability, impulsivity, persistently unstable sense of self, and chronically unstable interpersonal relationships. (APA, 1994, p. 280. See Carrasco and Lecic-Tosevki, 2000, pp. 934–937.)

Could I, this very person, survive the 'adventures' of such illnesses? Personal identity may be put under stress by features of the disorders mentioned above that concern disturbance or disorder in the identification or consciousness of self. A theory of personal identity like that of Locke needs to consider how various types of mental illness such as those (and others that could be mentioned) affect persistence.

More generally, placing Locke or the capacity approach to identity aside, an ideal partnership between philosophy and psychiatry should produce a conception of personal identity that honours both the properly understood or regimented meanings of concepts such as *person* and *identity* and relevant empirical or clinical facts. This is a tall order but it's one of the many projects towards which readers of this book now may be in a position to contribute either in theoretical research or analysis of clinical practice.

Reflection on the session and self-test questions

Write down your own reflections on the materials in this session drawing out any points that are particularly significant for you. Then write brief notes about the following:

1. With Locke's self-tracking account of personal identity in mind, what conditions threaten personal identity?

2. Are Alzheimer's disease and schizophrenia equally damaging to the existence of identity?

Reading guide

There has been so much work on personal identity in philosophy that the bibliographic citations (which are detailed in the Reference section below) in the text of the chapter are necessarily selective.

• Jonathan Glover's (1988) *I: The Philosophy and Psychology of Personal Identity*, provides a very readable and lively introduction to the main philosophical theories of personal identity.

• One of the best general introduction for students is: John Perry's (1978) *A Dialogue on Personal Identity and Immortality*. Perry focuses on the question of survival of bodily death, but canvasses arguments both for and against various approaches to personal identity.

- A very short but still informative inspection of the place of the idea of personal identity in psychiatry may be found in: Jennifer Radden's (1995) 'Personal identity: history and concepts' (in *Current Opinion in Psychiatry*, pp. 343–345). Radden (1996), who is a philosopher at the University of Massachusetts at Boston, probes relations between personal persistence and moral responsibility in *Divided Minds and Successive Selves: ethical issues in disorders of identity and personality*.

- Useful collections of papers and selections on personal identity (including classical and influential discussions) are John Perry's (ed.) (1975) *Personal Identity*, and Amelie Rorty's (ed.) (1976) *The Identities of Persons*. Heginbotham's (2000) edited collection combines philosophical and psychiatric sources. Harré's (1988) *Singular Self* develops an original discursive account.

Locke on personal identity

- More than one edition of Locke's *Essay* is available. A good one for a student reader is: John Locke's (1989) *Essay Concerning Human Understanding*.

- For discussions of Locke's views of persons and persistence, see Mackie's (1976) *Problems from Locke*, and Michael Ayers' (1991) *Locke, Volume II: Ontology*.

Schreber's memoir

- This in translation is available as Daniel Schreber's (2003) *Memoir of My Mental Illness*.

- The memoir is the subject of insightful commentary and discussion of schizophrenia in: Louis Sass (1993) *Paradoxes of Delusion: Wittgenstein, Schreber, and the schizophrenic mind*.

- Sass's account is criticized in Read (2001) 'On approaching schizophrenia through Wittgenstein' (*Philosophical psychology*).

Applied work on identity

There is a growing literature on personal identity, more than on any other aspect of psychopathology. Examples include:

- Thought insertion is the central question in Stephens and Graham (1994a). 'Self-consciousness, mental agency, and clinical psychopathology of thought-insertion' (*Philosophy, Psychiatry, & Psychology*, with a commentary by Wiggins (1994) and Chadwick (1994), and Stephens and Graham (1994b)).

- A broader Klinean perspective account of identity is the focus of Hinshelwood (1995). 'The social relocation of personal identity as shown by psychoanalytic observations of splitting, projection and introjection.' (*Philosophy, Psychiatry, & Psychology*, with commentaries by Braude, Gardner, and Lewis.

- A more philosophically minded approach to thought insertion is discussed in Coliva (2002a). 'Thought insertion and immunity to error through misidentification' (*Philosophy, Psychiatry, & Psychology*, with commentary by Campbell (2002), and response by Coliva (2002b)). Graham and Stephens (2000) *When Self-Consciousness Breaks* provides a careful philosophical account of the disturbances of consciousness experienced by people with schizophrenia. Laing's (1960) now classic *The Divided Self* is an ingenious analysis of the potential meaningfulness of these experiences.

- The moral implications of personal identity is discussed in Matthews (2003a). 'Establishing personal identity in cases of DID'. (*Philosophy, Psychiatry, & Psychology*, with commentaries by Braude (2003), Clark (2003), and Deeley (2003), and reply by Matthews (2003b)).

- Among the many potentially important topics not covered in this book is multiple personality disorder (MPD) or Dissociative Identity Disorder (DID). There has been much clinically informed philosophical work and philosophically informed clinical work on this rich vien in the philosophy of psychiatry.

- Of central importance is Kathy Wilkes' (1998). *Real People* which argues for the case for taking real empirical examples rather than thought experiments to underpin philosphical work.

Other book length contributions to the include:

- Ian Hacking's (1995). *Rewriting the Soul: Multiple Personality and the Sciences of Memory*.

- Radden's (1996b). *Divided Minds and Successive Selves: ethical issues in disorders of identity and personality* explores some of the ethical issues raised by MPD/DID.

- Stephen Braude (1995). *First person plural: multiple personality and the philosophy of mind* which charts the connections between dissociation and central philosophical issues in the philosophy of mind.

- A very different approach from the perspective of the Buddhist tradition of Theravada is Steven Collins (1982). *Selfless Persons: Imagery and Thought in Theravada Buddism*.

Papers in *Philosophy Psychology and Psychiatry* include:

- Braude, S. E. (1996). Multiple Personality and Moral Responsibility in *Philosophy, Psychiatry, & Psychology* 3: 37–54 (with commentaries by Clark, S. R. L. pp. 55–57 and Shuman, D. W. pp. 59–60).

♦ Clark, S. R. L. (1996). Minds, Memes, and Multiples *Philosophy, Psychiatry, & Psychology*, 3: 21–28 (with commentaries by Bavidge, M. pp. 29–30 and Sprigge, T. L. S. pp. 31–36).

♦ Gillett, G (1997). A Discursive Account of Multiple Personality Disorder *Philosophy, Psychiatry, & Psychology*, 4: 213–222 (with commentary by Braude, S. E. pp. 223–226).

♦ Matthews, S. (2003). Establishing Personal Identity in Cases of DID *Philosophy, Psychiatry, & Psychology*, 10: 143–151 (with commentaries by Braude, S. E. pp 153–156 Clark, S. R. L. pp. 157–159 Deeley, P. Q. pp. 161–167).

References

Anscombe, E. (1975). The first person. In *Mind and Language* (ed. S. Guttenplan). Oxford: Oxford University Press, pp. 45–65.

Anscombe, G.E.M. (1959). Intention. *Proceedings of the Aristotelian Society* 57: 321–332. (Reprinted in White, A.R. ed. (1968) *The philosophy of action*. Oxford: Oxford University Press.)

APA (1994). *Desk Reference to Diagnostic Criteria from DSM-IV*. Washington, DC: American Psychiatric Association.

Ayer, A.J. (1956). *The Problem of Knowledge*. London: Macmillan.

Ayers, M. (1991). *Locke, Volume II: Ontology*. London: Routledge.

Baier, A. (1981). Cartesian persons. *Philosophia*, 10: 169–188.

Baker, L.R. (1997). Persons in metaphysical perspective. In *The Philosophy of Roderick Chisholm* (ed. L. Hahn). Chicago, IL: Open Court, pp. 433–453.

Baker, L.R. (2000). *Persons and Bodies*. Cambridge: Cambridge University Press.

Bovet, P. and Parnas, J. (1993). Schizophrenic delusions: a phenomenological approach. *Schizophrenia Bulletin*, 19: 579–597.

Braude, S. (1995). *First person plural: multiple personality and the philosophy of mind*. Boston: Rowman & Littlefield Publishers.

Braude, S.E. (1995). The social relocation of personal identity. (Commentary on Hinshelwood, 1995) *Philosophy, Psychiatry, & Psychology*, 2(3): 205–208.

Braude, S.E. (2003). Counting persons and living with alters: Comments on Matthews. (Commentary on Matthews, 2003a) *Philosophy, Psychiatry, & Psychology*, 10(2): 153–156.

Campbell, J. (1999). Schizophrenia, the space of reasons, and thinking as a motor process. *The Monist*, 82(4): 609–625.

Campbell, J. (2002). The ownership of thoughts. (Commentary on Coliva, 2002a) *Philosophy, Psychiatry, & Psychology*, 9: 35–40.

Canfield, J. (1990). *The Looking Glass Self: an examination of self-awareness*. New York: Praeger.

Carrasco, J. and Lecic-Tosevski, D. (2000). Specific types of personality disorder. In *New Oxford Textbook of Psychiatry* (ed. M. Gelder, J. Lopez-Ibor, and N. Andraesen). Oxford: Oxford University Press, pp. 934–937.

Chadwick, R.F. (1994). Kant, thought insertion, and mental unity. *Philosophy, Psychiatry, & Psychology*, 1(2): 105–114.

Chapman, J. (1966). The early symptoms of schizophrenia. *British Journal of Psychiatry*, 112: 225–251.

Chisholm, R. (1969). The loose and popular and the strict and philosophical senses of identity. In *Perception and Personal Identity* (ed. N.S. Care and R.H. Grimm). Cleveland, OH: Case Western Reserve.

Chisholm, R. (1976). *Person and Object*. La Salle, IL: Open Court.

Clark, S.R.L. (2003). Constructing persons: the psycho-pathology of identity. (Commentary on Matthews, 2003a) *Philosophy, Psychiatry, & Psychology*, 10(2): 157–160.

Collins, S. (1982). *Selfless Persons: Imagery and Thought in Theravada Buddism*. Cambridge: CUP.

Coliva, A. (2002a). Thought insertion and immunity to error through misidentification. (Commentary by Campbell, J. (2002, pp. 35–40) and response by Coliva, A. (2002, pp. 41–46) *Philosophy, Psychiatry, & Psychology*, 9: 27–34.

Coliva, A. (2002b). On what there really is to our notion of ownership of a thought. (Response to Campbell, 2002) *Philosophy, Psychiatry, & Psychology*, 9: 41–46.

David, A. (2000). The clinical neuropsychology of schizophrenia. In *New Oxford Textbook of Psychiatry* (ed. M. Gelder, J. Lopez-Ibor, and N. Andraesen). Oxford: Oxford University Press, pp. 576–579.

De Pauw, K. (2000). Depersonalization disorder. In *New Oxford Textbook of Psychiatry* (ed. M. Gelder, J. Lopez-Ibor, and N. Andraesen). Oxford: Oxford University Press, pp. 831–833.

Deeley, P.Q. (2003). Social, cognitive, and neural constraints on subjectivity and agency: implications for dissociative identity disorder. (Commentary on Matthews, 2003a) *Philosophy, Psychiatry, & Psychology*, 10(2): 161–168.

Dennett, D. (1991). *Consciousness Explained*. Boston: Little, Brown.

Dennett, D. and Humphrey, N. (1998). Speaking for our selves. In *Brainchildren* (ed. D. Dennett). Cambridge, MA: MIT Press, pp. 31–58.

Duff, A. (1977). Psychopathy and moral understanding. *American Philosophical Quarterly* 14(3): 189–200.

Duff, R.A. (1990). *Intention, Agency and Criminal Liability*. Oxford: Blackwell.

Dworkin, R. (1993). Life past reason. In *Life's Dominion: an argument about abortion, euthanasia, and individual freedom*. New York: Knopf.

Flanagan, O. (1992). *Consciousness Reconsidered*. Cambridge, MA: MIT Press.

Flanagan, O. (1994). Multiple identity, character transformation, and self-reclamation. In *Philosophical Psychopathology* (ed. G. Graham and G.L. Stephens). Cambridge, MA: MIT Press, pp. 135–162.

Frith, C. (1992). *The Cognitive Neuropsychology of Schizophrenia*. Hillsdale, NJ: Lawrence Earlbaum.

Frith, C. (1998). Deficits and pathologies. In *A Companion to Cognitive Science* (ed. W. Bechtel and G. Graham). Oxford: Blackwell, pp. 380–390.

Gardner, S. (1995). The social relocation of personal identity. (Commentary on Hinshelwood, 1995) *Philosophy, Psychiatry, & Psychology*, 2(3): 209–214.

Glover, J. (1988). *I: The Philosophy and Psychology of Personal Identity*. London: The Penguin Group.

Graham, G. (1999a). Fuzzy faulty lines: selves in multiple personality disorder. *Philosophical Explorations*, 3: 159–174.

Graham, G. (1999b). Self-consciousness, psychopathology, and realism about the self. *Anthropology and Philosophy*, 24: 57–66.

Graham, G. (2002). Recent work in philosophical psychopathology. *American Philosophical Quarterly*, 39: 109–134.

Graham, G. (2004). Self-ascription: thought insertion. In *Oxford Companion to the Philosophy of Psychiatry* (ed. J. Radden). Oxford: Oxford University Press, pp. 89–105.

Graham, G. and Horgan, T. (1998). Southern fundamentalism and the end of philosophy. In *Rethinking Intuition: the psychology of intuition and its role in philosophical inquiry* (ed. M. DePaul and W. Ramsey). Lanham, MD: Rowman and Littlefield, pp. 271–292.

Green, R. (2000). Gender identity disorder in adults. In *New Oxford Textbook of Psychiatry* (ed. M. Gelder, J. Lopez-Ibor, and N. Andreasen). Oxford: Oxford University Press, pp. 913–917.

Grice, H.P. (1941). Personal identity. *Mind*, 50: 330–350.

Hacking, I. (1995). *Rewriting the Soul: Multiple Personality and the Sciences of Memory*. Princeton: Princeton University Press.

Hacking, I. (2002). *Mad Travelers: reflections on the reality of transient mental illness*. Cambridge, MA: Harvard University Press.

Hampshire, S. (1959). *Thought and Action*. London: Chatto and Windus.

Hardcastle, V. and Flanagan, O. (1999). Multiplex vs. multiple selves: distinguishing dissociative disorders. *The Monist*, 82: 645–657. (Special issue on cognitive theories of mental illness.)

Harré, R. (1988). *The Singular Self*. London: Sage.

Heginbotham, C. (ed.) (2000). *Philosophy, Psychiatry and Psychopathy: personal identity in mental disorder*. Avebury Series in Philosophy in association with The Society for Applied Philosophy. England: Ashgate Publishing Ltd.

Hinshelwood, R.D. (1995). The social relocation of personal identity as shown by psychoanalytic observations of splitting, projection and introjection. (Commentaries by Braude, S.E. (1995, pp. 205–208), Gardner, S. (1995, pp. 209–214), and Lewis, B. (1995, pp. 215–218) *Philosophy, Psychiatry, & Psychology*, 2(3): 185–204.

Hume, D. (1967). *A Treatise of Human Nature*, Book I, Part 4 (ed. L.A. Selby-Bigge). Oxford: Oxford University Press.

Laing, R.D. (1960). *The Divided Self*. London: Tavistock.

Lewis, B. (1995). The social relocation of personal identity. (Commentary on Hinshelwood, 1995) *Philosophy, Psychiatry, & Psychology*, 2(3): 215–218.

Liddle, P. (2000). Descriptive clinical features of schizophrenia in New Oxford Textbook of Psychiatry (ed M. Gelder, J. Lopoez-Ibor, and N. Andreasen), Oxford: OUP, pp. 571–576.

Locke, J. (1989). *Essay Concerning Human Understanding* (ed. P. Nidditch). Oxford: Clarendon Press.

Mackie, J. (1976). *Problems from Locke*. Oxford: Clarendon Press.

Matthews, S. (2003a). Establishing personal identity in cases of DID. *Philosophy, Psychiatry, & Psychology*, 10(2): 143–152. (Commentary by Braude, S.E. (2003, pp. 153–156), Clark, S.R.L. (2003, pp. 157–160), and Deeley, P.Q. (2003, pp. 161–168), and reply by Matthews, S. (2003, pp. 169–174).

Matthews, S. (2003b). Blaming agents and excusing persons: the case of DID. (Response to the Commentaries) *Philosophy, Psychiatry, & Psychology*, 10(2): 169–174.

McGinn, C. (1999). *The Mysterious Flame: conscious minds in a material world*. New York: Basic Books.

Mele, A.R. (2004). Action: volitional disorder and addiction. In *The Philosophy of Psychiatry: a companion* (ed. J. Radden). New York: Oxford University Press, pp. 78–88.

Mellor, C.S. (1970). First rank symptoms of schizophrenia. *British Journal of Psychiatry*, 117: 15–23.

Metzinger, T. (2000). The subjectivity of subjective experience: a representationalist analysis of the first-person perspective. In *Neural Correlates of Consciousness* (ed. T. Metzinger). Cambridge: MA: MIT Press, pp. 287–324.

Nozick, R. (1981). *Philosophical Explanations*. Cambridge, MA.: Harvard University Press.

Olson, E. (1997). *The Human Animal: personal identity without psychology*. Oxford: Oxford University Press.

Olson, E. (1998). There is no problem of the self. *Journal of Consciousness Studies*, 5: 645–657.

Parfit, D. (1971). Personal identity. *Philosophical Review*, 80: 3–27.

Parfit, D. (1984). *Reasons and Persons*. Oxford: Clarendon Press.

Parfit, D. (1999). Experiences, subjects, and conceptual schemes. *Philosophical Topics*, 26: 217–270.

Perry, J. (ed.) (1975). *Personal Identity*. Berkeley: University of California Press.

Perry, J. (1978). *A Dialogue on Personal Identity and Immortality*. Indianapolis: Hackett.

Proust, J. (2000). Awareness of agency: three levels of analysis. In *Neural Correlates of Consciousness* (ed. T. Metzinger). Cambridge, MA: MIT Press, pp. 307–324.

Quinton, A. (1962). The soul. *Journal of Philosophy*, 59: 393–403.

Radden, J. (1995). Personal identity: history and concepts. *Current Opinion in Psychiatry*, 8: 343–345.

Radden, J. (1996). *Divided Minds and Successive Selves: ethical issues in disorders of identity and personality*. Cambridge, MA: MIT Press.

Radden, J. (1996b). *Divided Minds and Successive Selves: ethical issues in disorders of identity and personality*. Cambridge, MA: MIT Press.

Read, R. (2001). On approaching schizophrenia through Wittgenstein. *Philosophical Psychology*, 14: 449–475.

Robinson, D. (1998). Cerebral plurality and the unity of self. In *The Mind* (ed. D. Robinson). Oxford: Oxford University Press, pp. 344–354.

Rorty, A. (ed.) (1976). *The Identities of Persons*. Berkeley, CA: University of California Press.

Sass, L. (1995). *The Paradoxes of Delusion: Wittgenstein, Schreber and the schizophrenic mind*. Ithaca, NY: Cornell University Press.

Sass, L. (1999). Schizophrenia, self-consciousness, and the modern mind. In *Models of the Self* (ed. S. Gallagher and J. Shear). Thoverton, UK: Imprint Academic.

Schreber, D. (2003). *Memoir of My Mental Illness*. New York: New York Review of Books.

Shoemaker, S. (1986). Introspection and the self. *Midwest Studies in Philosophy*, 10: 101–120.

Shoemaker, S. (1997). Self and substance. *Philosophical Perspectives*, 11: 283–304.

Shoemaker, S. and Swinburne, R. (1984). *Personal Identity*. Oxford: Blackwell.

Spence, S.A. (2002). Alien motor phenomena: a window on to agency. *Cognitive Neuropsychiatry*, 7(3): 211–220.

Spitzer, R., Skodol, A., Gibbon, M., and Williams J. (1981). *DSM-III Case Book*. Washington, DC: American Psychiatric Association.

Stephens, G.L. and Graham, G. (1994a). Self-consciousness, mental agency, and clinical psychopathology of thought-insertion. (Commentaries by Wiggins (1994) and Chadwick (1994), and Stephens and Graham (1994b) *Philosophy, Psychiatry, & Psychology*, 1: 1–10.

Stephens, G.L. and Graham, G. (1994b). Kant, thought insertion, and mental unity. (Commentary on Chadwick, 1994) *Philosophy, Psychiatry, & Psychology*, 1(2): 115–116.

Stephens, G.L. and Graham, G. (2000). *When Self-Consciousness Breaks: alien voices and inserted thoughts*. Cambridge, MA: MIT Press.

Taylor, R. (1997). Chisholm's idea of a person. In *The Philosophy of Roderick Chisholm* (ed. L. Hahn). Chicago: Open Court, pp. 45–51.

Unger, P. (1979a). There are no ordinary things. *Synthese*, 14: 117–154.

Unger, P. (1979b). I do not exist. In *Perception and Identity* (ed. G.F. MacDonald). Ithaca, NY: Cornell University Press, pp. 235–251.

Van Inwagen, P. (1990). *Material Beings*. Ithaca, NY: Cornell University Press.

Wiggins, D. (1980). *Sameness and Substance*. Cambridge, MA: Harvard University Press.

Wiggins, O.P. (1994). Commentary on Stephens and Graham, 1994a. *Philosophy, Psychiatry, & Psychology*, 1: 11–12.

Wilkes, K. (1988). *Real People: personal identity without thought experiments*. Oxford: Oxford University Press.

Wilkes, K. (1991). How many selves make me? In *Human Beings* (ed. D. Cockburn). Cambridge: Cambridge University Press.

Wilkes, K. (1999). Know thyself. In *Models of Self* (ed. S. Gallagher and J. Shear). Toverton, UK: Imprint Academic.

Williams, B. (1970a). Are persons bodies? *The Philosophy of the Body* (ed. S. Spicker). Chicago, IL: Quadrant Books, pp. 137–156.

Williams, B. (1970b). The self and the future. *Philosophical Review*, 79: 161–180.

Wing, J.K. (1978). *Reasoning about Madness*. Oxford: Oxford University Press.

Wittgenstein, L. (1958). *The Blue and the Brown Books*. New York: Harper.

Zimmerman, D. (1998). Criteria of identity and 'identity mystics'. *Erkenntnis*, 48: 281–301.

Conclusions to Part V

This part has looked to draw lessons drawn from psychiatry's own philosophy: the philosophy of mind. We have looked at some major debates from the philosophy of mind and philosophy of thought that impact at a fundamental level on our understanding of the subject matter of psychiatry.

One of the key tensions discussed in this part was a theme that has been repeated throughout the book: the relation between reasons and causes or, more precisely, the relation of the space of reasons and realm of natural law. It is this duality that makes the nature of mind and mind's place in nature so difficult to understand.

In the face of that intellectual challenge it is easy for views to become polarized. Some argue that it is of the very nature of mind that it stands distinct from the natural processes generally described by the sciences. There is something mysterious about the mind that resists incorporation into the rest of our picture of the world. Such a view is attributed to the 'New Mysterians': a group of philosophers who dismiss any such account of the mysteries of consciousness, etc. Although touched on in the Introduction to this part and Chapter 23, we have not concentrated on their work because it seems to be a premature retreat in the face of empirical evidence.

The opposing view, perhaps partly underpinned by recent advances in psychiatry, neuroimaging and so on, takes it as equally clear that the mind is simply another aspect of nature and one which will, in time, succumb to scientific explanation. This view often finds expression in forms of philosophical reductionism: the view that the mind is *nothing but* the brain, for example, or that mental processes are nothing but neurological processes.

Throughout the chapters that make up this part we have avoided both extremes of this forced choice. The opposition of science on the one hand and a proper sensitivity to the mysteries of the mind on the other is a false one.

We should not underestimate the genuine conceptual difficulties facing us. How can mental properties stand alongside physical properties? How can meanings be related to or underpinned by neurological mechanisms? Is freedom of the will compatible with a growing understanding of mechanisms? How can minds be manifested to others? How is personal identity constituted? These are all substantial problems that have been introduced but not resolved in this part. The one clear result is that there are no clear results!

However, at the same time, the interplay of empirical and conceptual work does suggest progress can be made. One can at least see how different aspects of the mind might be related according to different overall views. Thus Dennett's Intentional Stance sheds light on mental states and their meaning or intentionality but with the consequence, if true, that mental states do not play a causal role. Fodor's 'industrial strength realism' (in Dennett's phrase) allows that mental states might indeed be the causes of actions but, again if true, shows the need for a plausible account of neurological states can have meaning or intentionality.

However, just as *value* played a central role in Parts I, II, and IV and *judgement* played a central role in Part III so in this part a central role has been played by *rationality*. It is because connections between the rational properties of mental states and their meaning that, at one stage remove, the simple assimilation of mental to physical properties looks unconvincing (Chapters 22 and 23). Something would be lost in that translation. Similarly, the rational pattern of mental states makes a mechanistic account of meaning less likely (Chapters 24 and 25); makes the problem of free will particularly pressing (Chapter 26) and the codification of knowledge of other minds a theory of mind less plausible (Chapter 27) and the grasp of psychopathological symptoms such as thought insertion (Chapter 28).

To say that rationality makes a swift assimilation of the mind to the subject matter of the natural sciences implausible is not, however, to make either an antiscientific claim or to adopt some antediluvian form of dualism of mind and matter. It is to say that we should aim to respect the constitutive features of the mind even as we try to understand its place in a broader world view and to suggest that not every real feature of the world is best understood by explanation under natural laws. Psychiatry's genuine scientific advances have to go hand in hand with an understanding of the rational pattern that governs minds, a pattern that may well never be codified in a deductive scientific theory.

CHAPTER 29

Histories of the future

There are three kinds of clinical complexity, empirical, valuational, and conceptual. Medicine has traditionally been concerned mainly with complexity of the first kind, with the empirical challenges of the major pathologies, such as infections, cancer, and heart disease. Partly as a result of its growing success in meeting these challenges, however, late twentieth century medicine was marked by the emergence, first of valuational complexity, in the form of bioethics, and then, in the closing decade of the century, of conceptual complexity, in the form of a blossoming of new work in the cross-disciplinary field of philosophy of psychiatry.

The continuities and discontinuities between the new philosophy of psychiatry and the histories of its two parent disciplines in the twentieth century, back to Karl Jaspers and psychiatry's first philosophical phase, are set out in the opening chapter of the launch volume in this series, *Nature and Narrative*. The statistics, as described there, continue to impress: over thirty new academic groups around the world; new courses and training programmes; new book series (in the Netherlands, Germany, and France, as well as Britain and America); annual international conferences, in addition to many national and subject-based meetings; expansion of the journal, *Philosophy, Psychiatry, & Psychology*; the establishment of infrastructure support, in the International Network for Philosophy and Psychiatry and key sections in both the World Psychiatric Association and Association of European Psychiatrists; and, perhaps most significant of all, philosophy based developments in policy, training, clinical practice, and research in mental health.

Precisely why the philosophy of psychiatry should have blossomed at exactly this time is a matter for future historians to debate. After all, as we have indicated at several points in this book, historically there has been no shortage of cross-disciplinary contact. For much of the nineteenth century, as we noted in Part II, philosophy was not sharply distinct from psychology or indeed the psychiatry of the day. A key figure at the birth of biological psychiatry, in the early twentieth century, was Karl Jaspers, as much a philosopher as a psychiatrist, his twin disciplines being clearly reflected in the requirement for meaningful understanding as well as causal explanations in his foundational work on psychopathology, *Allgemeine Psychopathologie*. Meanings are also central to psychoanalysis, a dominant model in several parts of the world at different periods in the twentieth century, and the focus of much philosophical enquiry, both analytic (generally critical) and Continental (generally supportive). Again, outside of Britain and North America, phenomenology flourished through much of the twentieth century as a branch of philosophy crucial to psychiatry. Continental philosophy was important also to the antipsychiatry movement of the 1960s and 1970s, many aspects of which, as we saw in Part I, have been assimilated in modern user-centred and multidisciplinary models of service delivery. Szasz and Laing's critiques of psychiatry were analytic philosophical critiques in all but name, challenging as they did the dominant *conceptual* structures within which mental distress and disorder

were understood at the time. Among philosophers in the analytic tradition, there were occasional but repeated calls for engagement with psychiatry—J.L. Austin, Jonathan Glover, Anthony Quinton, Stephen Clark, and Kathleen Wilkes, for example, were all early in the field in this respect. And as we saw in Part III, the philosopher of science, Carl Hempel, made a crucial contribution to the development of modern symptom-based classifications of mental disorder.

Yet with hindsight it is perhaps not so surprising that the blossoming of new work in the philosophy of psychiatry should have started in the 1990s, heralded as this period was as the 'decade of the brain'. For one clear factor driving cross-disciplinary contact between philosophy and psychiatry has been the remarkable new technologies that began to emerge from the neurosciences at this time. As noted in Chapter 2, Nancy Andreasen is among leading figures in the neurosciences who have pointed to the ways in which functional neuroimaging, behavioural genetics, and brain prostheses (for Parkinsonism, for example, and depression), are pushing some of the deepest problems of philosophy to the top of the practical agenda of psychiatry: free will, personal identity, our knowledge of other minds, the structure of consciousness, the mind–body problem itself, are all now problems as much for the neurosciences and clinical psychiatry as for philosophy. And as we saw in Part V, this is an area of true partnership, an area in which psychopathology and the neurosciences have as much to teach philosophy as philosophy has to teach psychopathology and the neurosciences.

If the neurosciences have been one of the drivers of the new philosophy of psychiatry, however, equally important have been developments in our models of service delivery. The traditional doctor-led model is appropriate where the problems we face in health care are predominantly empirical in nature. As noted above, the major pathologies—infections, heart disease, cancer, and so forth—demand interventions that are guided primarily by the biological sciences. Even with such pathologies, of course, social and psychological factors may also be vitally important: public health measures, and high standards of nursing care, as much as antibiotics, are crucial to the control of infectious diseases, for example.

As we move, though, ever deeper into areas of health care in which valuational and conceptual, as well as empirical, problems become increasingly important practically, the dominant medical model must give way to more pluralistic approaches to service delivery. This is partly a matter of the need for a wider range of skills to meet the complex challenges of modern health care. Ethical and legal skills, for example, are increasingly crucial not only to setting policy and to dealing with 'hard cases', but in day-to-day clinical decision-making. It is also, though, and this is where philosophy comes in, a matter of matching services appropriately to the often very different needs and expectations of individual patients, informal carers and their communities.

Valuational complexity is important here. As we saw in Part IV, Values-Based Practice, derived from philosophical value theory, and drawing on substantive work on values from both empirical and phenomenological research, is currently one of two underpinning sources (the other being evidence-based practice) for training in the generic skills for user-centred and multidisciplinary models of mental health service delivery in the UK. Similarly with conceptual complexity: Tony Colombo's 'philosophical fieldwork', in Austin's phrase, combining linguistic-analytic with empirical social science methods, provides, as we described in Parts I and IV, a powerful policy and training framework for collaborative, rather than competitive, multidisciplinary and multiagency models of service delivery. Continental philosophy, too, as we saw in Part II, provides important exemplars of philosophy-into-practice: these include Pat Bracken's work, for example, with Amnesty International, drawing on Heideggerian phenomenology as the basis of new approaches to helping people who have survived severe trauma; and Rom Harré and Stephen Sabat's use of discursive methods to support communication with people with Alzheimer's disease.

It is important to emphasize how deeply scientific advances and developments in policy and practice in mental health, are intertwined in the new philosophy of psychiatry. Science, and not least medical science, has had an increasingly bad press recently. Bioethics, responding to public anxieties, has thus tended to assume a role, as in research ethics committees, of policing the boundaries of medical science. The new philosophy of psychiatry, by contrast, is a partner to medical science. It is a partner in research—phenomenology, for example, concerned with the structure of consciousness, is a partner to the neurosciences, concerned with brain functioning; and it is a partner also in the applications of the results of research to clinical practice, as in the complementary roles of values-based and evidence-based approaches to clinical decision-making outlined in Part IV.

In the twentieth century, the prominence of valuational and conceptual complexity in mental health was taken by many in medicine to be the mark of a defective, or at any rate primitive, science, the assumption being that with advances in medical science the valuational and conceptual complexities of mental health would recede. As we saw in Part I, such assumptions were the basis of deeply stigmatizing attitudes equally to those who use mental health services and to those who provide them. However, in the physical sciences, as we noted in Part III, conceptual complexity, at least, is a mark not of a deficient science, still less of a primitive science, but of an *advanced* science, a science at the cutting edge—theoretical physics, no less, being a case in point. And in the human sciences (including medicine), as we found in Part IV, advances in science and technology, far from reducing valuational complexity, actually *increase* it. This is because advances in science and technology open up new choices in medicine, and with choices go values—reproductive medicine, our example in Part IV, is an area in which, through the new choices opened up by advances in assisted reproduction, the full diversity of human values is already becoming a major factor in clinical decision-making.

Contrary, therefore, to twentieth century expectations, twenty-first century medicine, if it is to be both science-based and patient-centred, will have to embrace (just as mental health embraced in the twentieth century) valuational and conceptual complexity as well as empirical complexity. In mental health, notwithstanding the late twentieth century blossoming of cross-disciplinary work with philosophy, there is always the danger that we will lapse back into the relative simplicity of one or other traditional model. Biological, psychoanalytic, social, and cognitive-behavioural models are all currently competing for dominance; and the history of mental disorder, as we saw in Part II, is very much a history of repeated collapses into one or another single-message mythology. The new philosophy of psychiatry, just in being open and inclusive, offers no guarantee against ideology. But the inevitable growth of valuational and conceptual complexity, driven by scientific and technological advances, in all areas of twenty-first century medicine, means that in engaging with the new philosophy of psychiatry we are helping to write the histories of the future not only of mental health but of twenty-first century health care as a whole.

Key learning points

Part I Core concepts in philosophy and mental health

Chapter 2 Philosophical problems in mental health practice and research

Session 1 What is philosophy? What is psychiatry?

◆ Psychiatry is a medical discipline concerned primarily with disorders of the higher mental functions—mood, emotion, volition, belief, etc.—and associated disorders of behaviour.

◆ A clinical diagnostic formulation in psychiatry covers: differential diagnosis (based primarily on symptoms); aetiology; treatment; and prognosis.

◆ In so far as it is distinct from science, philosophy is concerned with conceptual problems, science is concerned with empirical problems.

◆ Among the more specific meanings of 'philosophy', those of particular relevance clinically include: the *Weltanschauung*, specific topic areas (jurisprudence, political philosophy, phenomenology, ethics, etc.), and conceptual analysis.

◆ The concepts of 'mental disorder', 'mental illness', etc., are at the interface between clinical problems, such as those presented by Mr AB in the session, and the deep problems of general philosophy.

Session 2 Fact, value, and the concept of mental disorder

◆ Mental disorders can be grouped together in the form of a conceptual 'map' representing what Gilbert Ryle called the 'logical geography' of the subject.

◆ Any proposed analysis of the meanings of our concepts of disorder must account for (either explaining or explaining away) the features of the 'map' as a whole.

◆ Among the main groups of mental disorders, we put organic conditions nearest to medical disorders (on the right of the map), non-organic (or functional) psychoses in the middle, and other groups around them.

◆ The four conceptually significant features of the map we identified were: wide diversity; variable conceptual distance from bodily disorder; variable illness status; variable degree of value-ladenness.

◆ There has been much debate both about the varieties of values and the overall logical relationship (or relationship of meaning) between fact and value. Putnam has argued that there is a distinction (an often useful distinction) between fact and value but that there is no fact/value dichotomy.

◆ Moving from right-field to left-field across the map, the three overall shifts towards value-ladenness are: from medicine to morals, from excusing conditions to conditions for which we are held responsible, from (apparently) value-free to (overtly) value-laden diagnostic criteria.

Session 3 Antipsychiatry and the debate about mental illness

◆ Szasz focused his arguments on the heart of what psychiatry is about, the very *concept* of mental illness: he argued that bodily illness is defined by factual norms (of anatomy and physiology) while mental illness (so called) is defined by ethical, legal, and social norms.

◆ His arguments, although now very wide ranging, have all been motivated by a concern that the medicalization of mental distress and disorder dehumanizes people.

◆ The three key structural features of Szasz's core argument can be summarized under problem, method, and conclusion, thus: (1) *problem*—Szasz assumed that mental illness is 'the problem' while bodily illness (by and large) is unproblematic, conceptually speaking; hence (2) his *method* was to argue by comparing and contrasting mental illness with bodily illness, and then, as he finds mental illness to be different from bodily illness (in particular, in being more value-laden), (3) he *concluded* that mental illness is a myth.

◆ Among the strengths of Szasz' arguments, he has (1) prompted widespread reflection and debate about the conceptual foundations of psychiatry, in particular its more value-laden nature compared with bodily illness, and (2) contributed to the development of a stronger 'user voice' in service development.

◆ Among the weaknesses of Szasz' arguments are: (1) his characterization of bodily illness as being defined by value-free anatomical and physiological norms is (at the least) widely contested; and (2) his rejection of *any* role for medicine in relation to mental health issues would, if taken literally, cut off an important resource (among many others) for those with mental health problems.

◆ There are many alternatives to the medical model (we noted psychological, labelling, social, hidden meanings, unconscious mental processes and 'political').

◆ These different models are all important in reflecting particular parts of the conceptual map of mental disorder but (taken separately) they fail to account for the features of the map as a whole.

◆ Although some have claimed 'antipsychiatry' to be 'dead', many of its themes in the 1960s and 1970s have now been integrated into policy and practice in different areas of mental health.

Session 4 The medical model (and beyond)

◆ Kendell developed his arguments about the meaning of mental illness as a direct rejoinder to Szasz's early work on the 'myth of mental illness'.

◆ He took the core of his ideas from the work of Scadding (a chest physician) and others in bodily medicine.

◆ Kendell differed from Szasz in concluding that mental illness is essentially similar to bodily illness because (adopting Scadding's arguments from bodily medicine) (many) mental illnesses are, like bodily illnesses, associated with 'biological disadvantage' as measured by the evolutionary norms of reduced fertility and increased mortality.

- Kendell adopted an essentially similar form of argument to Szasz: he assumed that mental illness is *the* problem and bodily illness (relatively speaking) unproblematic; and, hence, argued by comparing (candidate) mental illnesses with (the assumed paradigm of) bodily illness.

- The critical difference between Szasz and Kendell is not over the meaning of mental illness but over that of *bodily* illness. Szasz defined bodily illness by reference to norms of anatomy and physiology; Kendell defined bodily illness by reference to evolutionary norms (as above). Hence, the debate turns out (in a sense we will be exploring further in Chapter 4) to be, after all, a debate not about mental illness but about bodily illness!

Chapter 3 Experiences good and bad: an introduction to psychopathology, classification and diagnosis for philosophers

Session 1 Diagnosis in medicine and psychiatry

- The four key purposes of diagnosis in medicine are: descriptive (of symptoms, signs etc.), aetiological (assigning causes), therapeutic (indicating what treatments and other interventions may be helpful), and prognostic (likely course and outcome).

- Diagnostic categories in psychiatry are defined primarily in terms of symptoms and signs rather than in terms of causal disease processes (hence they are like, e.g. 'migraine' rather than, e.g. 'pneumococcal pneumonia').

- A positive interpretation of the differences between diagnostic categories in psychiatry and in bodily medicine is that the sciences underpinning psychiatry are more *difficult* (empirically as well as conceptually).

- A negative interpretation is that the sciences underpinning psychiatry have been slower to develop and that psychiatry thus remains relatively *deficient*, scientifically speaking, compared with areas of bodily medicine such as cardiology and gastroenterology.

Session 2 Descriptive psychopathology

- The main groups of psychological symptoms widely recognized in psychiatry are: disorders of mood (anxiety and affect, i.e. happy/sad), thought (stream of thought, connections between thoughts, possession of thoughts, and content, i.e. delusions and related phenomena), perception (hallucinations and related phenomena in all five sense modalities), and cognitive functions (orientation, attention, memory and general IQ).

- There is a growing and increasingly rich body of user-narrative literature on experiences of mental distress and disorder. This is the most important of the wide range of resources available from both philosophy and mental health practice for interdisciplinary work on different areas of psychopathology.

- The term insight is used in connection with psychopathology in a number of different senses.

- Traditionally, loss of insight has marked psychotic from non-psychotic disorders: a psychotic disorder is characterized by symptoms (paradigmatically delusion) in which the person concerned understands 'what is wrong' not as something *psychologically wrong with* themselves but as something (generally negative but in hypomania often partly positive) that they *have done* or that is *being done or is happening to them.*

- A recurring worry that one has done 'something wrong' could be (among other symptoms) a delusion (a psychotic symptom) or an obsession (a non-psychotic symptom). The person with the delusion really believes that they have done something wrong (this would be a delusion of guilt), whereas the person with the obsession experiences their worry as irrational and hence as something for which they might seek medical help.

- Psychiatry is concerned with a wide range of bodily signs and symptoms. Diagnosis in all areas of medicine should always be 'holistic', i.e. focusing, as appropriate, equally on bodily, psychological, and social contributions to disorder.

Session 3 Categories of mental disorder

- The main categories of adult mental disorder are: organic (e.g. dementia, etc.); alcohol- and drug-related disorders; psychotic disorders other than affective and organic; affective disorders (depression, hypomania, etc.); anxiety and related disorders (the latter including obsessive-compulsive, associative and somatoform); and disorders of vegetative functions (e.g. anorexia nervosa, disorders of sexual function and of sleep).

- Just as personality is relatively stable long term, so a personality *disorder* is a long-term maladaptive pattern of experience and/or behaviour.

- A stress-induced disorder differs from the main categories of adult mental disorder much as, in bodily medicine, 'wounds' or 'trauma' differ from illnesses: i.e. a stress-induced disorder is one in which the person's symptoms are clearly a response to major stressful experiences.

- Disorders of childhood and adolescence include: learning difficulties and specific developmental delays; pervasive disorders; emotional disorders of childhood; behavioural disorders (e.g. conduct disorder); and disorders of physiological functions (e.g. enuresis).

- The main stages in developing a diagnosis in psychiatry are: (1) clarification of symptoms; (2) exclusion of drug/alcohol-related disorders, personality and stress-induced disorders; and (3) differential diagnosis mainly according to symptoms (including those symptoms that point to the possibility of underlying major bodily pathology).

- Psychiatric assessment should always include the possibility that a person's experiences and behaviour, even if distressing, may be neither pathological nor, even, wholly negative.

Chapter 4 **Philosophical methods in mental health practice and research**

Session 1 **Better definitions: philosophy as 'an unusually stubborn effort to think clearly'**

◆ Dictionary definitions of everyday objects such as 'chairs' are broadly consistent but differ in many details.

◆ Two particular difficulties with defining everyday objects such as 'chairs' arise from the necessity of trading, (1) specificity *versus* range of use, and (2) breadth *versus* depth of understanding. Two further difficulties arise from, (3) the hierarchy of embedded terms, and (4) the increasingly abstract terms that arise as one moves up the hierarchy.

◆ Difficulties of these kinds are generic to all definitions including those of mental health terms.

◆ Among many different ways of 'first defining your terms' we noted seven major categories of definition: ostentive, conventional, persuasive, declarative, contextual, essential and semantic.

◆ All these categories of definition are important in different ways in health care: for example, all but formal semantic definitions, are to be found in major psychiatric classifications of mental disorder.

◆ 'First define your terms' should be understood as 'be alert to difficulties of meaning' rather than as a 'clearing up' of all problems of meaning before starting on the 'serious' business of empirical research.

◆ Definitions are meaningful only to the extent that we already understand the meanings of the terms (further up the hierarchy) in which they are cast. But definitions are none the less useful within given contexts and for particular purposes.

Session 2 **Use and definition: J.L. Austin and the Linguistic Analytic (Oxford) move in philosophy**

◆ The facility with which we *use* a term does not run parallel with the extent to which we are able to give a clear explicit *definition* of it. For example, we can use the concept of 'time' without being able to define it; conversely, we can define 'depressive affect' but it remains difficult to use (depression is in practice difficult to distinguish from anxiety).

◆ The fact that the use of the concept of 'illness' in psychological medicine is more problematic than in bodily medicine, far from being a sign that psychological medicine is relatively primitive scientifically, is a sign that it is more complex conceptually (there are corresponding conceptual difficulties about 'time' in theoretical physics but not in mechanical engineering).

◆ Austin called focusing on the use of concepts as a guide to their meanings, 'philosophical fieldwork'.

◆ Focusing on the use of concepts allows us to develop a more complete picture of the 'logical geography' (see Chapter 2); but it is not a panacea—it is, as Austin emphasized, only one particular way of getting started with some kinds of philosophical problem!

◆ Much of the literature on concepts of disorder has focused on the relatively unproblematic (in use) 'bodily disorder'. However, we are more likely to gain insight into the meaning of 'illness' through the more problematic (in use) 'mental illness' (recall Austin's comment that it is when there are difficulties in the use of a concept that we break through the 'blinding veil of ease and obviousness').

◆ Ordinary usage in 'Austin's philosophical fieldwork' means any non-reflective use of a term (in both lay and professional/technical contexts) as distinct from reflective attempts to provide explicit definitions (whether by philosophers or others).

Session 3 **Illness and disease: definition and ordinary usage**

◆ The terms 'illness' and 'disease' are often used as synonyms in everyday usage. However, they are also used to mark the distinction between people's individual *experiences* of illness and professionals' generalized *knowledge* of disease.

◆ In Boorse's theory, 'disease' (defined by reduced fertility and/or increased mortality) is a value-free concept covering the scientific theory at the core of medicine, while 'illness' is a value-laden concept covering people's experiences of illness when a disease process becomes serious enough to cause incapacity.

◆ In developing the distinction between illness and disease, Boorse is able to contain in a single model both value-laden individual experiences and (supposedly) value-free medical-scientific theory. He thus bridges between the polarities of the traditional psychiatry versus antipsychiatry debate in regard to the concept of mental illness.

◆ Boorse *defines* 'disease' stipulatively in value-free terms; however, he none the less *uses* the concept with evaluative connotations (the value-free term 'deviation' becomes the 'value-laden deficiency'; the value-free 'environmental causes' becomes the value-laden 'hostile environment').

◆ If use is a better guide to meaning than definition (as Austin's 'philosophical fieldwork' approach suggests), Boorse's value-laden use of 'disease', despite his value-free definition of the term, suggests that the meaning of 'disease' (the linguistic *work* that the term does for us in both professional and lay contexts) depends (in part but essentially) on an evaluative element in the meaning of the term.

Session 4 **Anglo-American and Continental philosophy**

◆ In so far as they are distinct, Anglo-American philosophy is analytic (including formal logic—see chapter 5) while Continental philosophy is more text-based.

- The three major 'schools' of Continental philosophy are:

  1. *phenomenology*, concerned with the structure of subjective experience (as illustrated in the work of Merleau-Ponty on disorders of speech, perception, etc.—and phenomenology, through Karl Jaspers, is also the basis of descriptive psychopathology);

  2. *existentialism*, concerned with putting 'existence' (including our powers of self-initiation of action) ahead of 'essence' (hence it sustains an empowering ethic of choice, as illustrated in the critique of Freud by Jean-Paul Sartre); and

  3. *hermeneutics*, a set of techniques for analysing the meaning of discourse, as illustrated by Paul Ricoeur's hermeneutic reconstruction of psychoanalysis.

- An important factor in the convergence of Continental and Anglo-American philosophy towards the end of the twentieth century has been the recognition among analytic philosophers of the importance of focusing, as Continental philosophy has always done, on real people. This is why *both* traditions are so crucial to the new interdisciplinary field of philosophy and mental health.

- Philosophical-analytic and empirical-scientific methods are essentially complementary.

Chapter 5 Arguments good and bad: an introduction to philosophical logic for practitioners

Session 1 An introduction to deductive reasoning and formal logic

- The aim of deductive argument is to preserve truth. True premisses should never lead to a false conclusion.

- A valid argument is one where if the premises are true then the conclusion must also be true. A sound argument is a valid argument with, in addition, true premises. The conclusion of a sound argument must be true.

- One way to assess a deductive argument is to see whether it shares the same structure or form as a known valid argument.

- Syllogism is one family of forms of deductive argument whose codification dates back to the Greeks; however, more recently propositional and predicate logics have been formulated.

- Propositional logic is the logic of simple logical connectives such as 'and', 'or', 'not'. These can be represented using truth tables, which can be used as a mechanical test for the validity of an argument in propositional logic.

Session 2 An introduction to the philosophy of logic: What underpins deductive logic?

- The strength of deductive argument is that the conclusions do not 'add anything' to the premises. The corollary is that such argument is, strictly, uninformative: it does not tell us anything not contained in the premises.

- But that does not undermine its usefulness in testing knowledge claims. The purpose of logical argument is to avoid reaching false conclusions from true premises.

- Although forms of valid argument are well known, there remains some philosophical dispute about how exactly logical inference is underpinned.

- An influential approach connects logical inference to the meanings of terms used as codified in truth tables; however, using truth tables to justify inferences is typically circular.

Session 3 Implication and entailment

- Formal logic has a clear structure that enables clear-cut assessment of whether arguments are valid or not. One cost of this, however, is that there are some seemingly paradoxical aspects of logical inferences associated with implication and the connective 'if . . . then'.

- A central paradox of formal logic is the 'paradox of material implication': for any statement A, if A is false then, if A then B is true for any statement B. In other words, *any* statement can be derived from a *false* statement.

- How to resolve this paradox remains an area of active discussion. Attempts to tighten the relationship between the meaning of statements in an implication (A and B, in the above) through strict implication and 'relevance logic' still face similar difficulties.

Chapter 6 Philosophical outputs in mental health practice and research

Session 1 'I wonder if this headache is mine?'

- In conceptually difficult areas (such as mental health) testing what we take to be self-evident is an important part of improving practice (although not in the face of an immediate practical emergency!)

- As a young man, Bertrand Russell represented the overoptimistic approach to the practical returns from philosophy (broadly along the lines of providing necessary foundations).

- Kurt Göedel showed that even mathematics cannot be put on totally secure foundations in logic (his 'undecidability' theorems).

- Ludwig Wittgenstein is among philosophers who have been too pessimistic about the practical value of philosophy, his work suggesting that philosophical problems are an artefact of philosophy itself.

- A balance between overoptimistic and overpessimistic views of the practical pay-off from philosophy, is that it gives us a *more complete understanding* of the meanings of the complex higher-level concepts in terms of which we organize and make sense of the world around us and of other people (noting that 'more complete' does *not* mean 'complete'!).

Session 2 Adding value to fact

◆ People have shared values over some things but often very different values over others: the degree of agreement falls on a spectrum.

◆ R.M. Hare suggested that a value *term* (e.g. 'good' in 'this is a good strawberry') expresses a value *judgement* (e.g. I commend this strawberry) the criteria for which are *descriptions* of the object of the evaluation (e.g. the descriptive criterion 'this strawberry is sweet').

◆ Hare showed that value terms may come to look like purely descriptive terms where the descriptive criteria for the value judgements they express are very widely shared. A non-medical example is 'good apple'; a medical example is 'disease'.

◆ *Illness*, *disease*, *dys*function, and other terms of *dis*order, as evaluative expressions, appear purely descriptive (hence purely 'scientific') to the extent that they are used of aspects of experience (e.g. bodily pain) over which people's values are very largely shared.

◆ Correspondingly, mental illness, and related concepts of mental disorder, are more value-laden than their bodily counterparts, not because they are less 'scientific' but because they cover aspects of human experience and behaviour (emotion, desire, volition, etc.) over which human values are highly diverse.

◆ This conceptual insight adds values to facts: it puts people's values on an equal footing with the scientifically derived facts emphasized by the traditional medical model of disorder.

Session 3 Adding illness to disease

◆ Adding values to facts in our understanding of the conceptual structure of medicine is important but not sufficient because the medical concepts express a *particular kind* of negative value judgement (illness is different from, e.g. foolishness).

◆ Moral descriptivism, the theory that in some circumstances, evaluations may be reduced to descriptions, would provide for a value-free way of defining the medical concepts while still allowing them to express evaluative meaning.

◆ In a non-descriptivist account of the relationship between illness and disease, disease processes *cause* experiences of illness, but (negatively evaluated) experiences of illness *define* which underlying causal processes are (negatively evaluated and hence) diseases.

◆ Asymptomatic diseases, according to this non-descriptivist account, are defined secondarily, i.e. as changes in bodily structure or functioning that tend to *cause* experiences of illness. (Recall that as A.J. Ayer said, causal connections in general are 'connections of tendency'.)

◆ A non-descriptivist account of the relationship between descriptive and evaluative meaning adds patients' experiences of illness to the professionals' knowledge of disease as emphasized in the traditional medical-scientific model.

Session 4 Adding action to function

◆ Among the features that mark out an experience as being one of illness are: (1) negative evaluation; (2) intensity and duration; (3) that it is not a 'done or happens to' type of experience; and (4) that, at the same time, it is not a 'done by' type of experience, i.e. something that the person concerned experiences as something that they are doing.

◆ The experience of illness (as incapacity) can be understood as a failure of what Austin called 'ordinary doing', i.e. a failure of the things that we are normally able to do without thinking about them.

◆ An analysis of the experience of illness as a failure of a particular kind of agency might be thought (1) to be little different from the medical model analysis of disease in terms of failure of function, and (2) to be appropriate only for illnesses involving disturbance of movement.

◆ An analysis of the experience of illness in terms of a particular kind of disturbance of agency is related to the analysis of disease in terms of disturbance of functioning in the same way that the actions of whole agents are related to the functioning of the parts and systems of which they are made up.

◆ An analysis of the experience of illness in terms of a particular kind of loss of agency can be generalized from illness experiences involving movement (and lack of movement) to other kinds of illness experience (including the rich variety of psychopathologies) by drawing on the fact that different illness experiences involve different parts (sensations, perceptions, memory, appetites, etc.) of what Austin called the 'machinery of action'.

◆ An analysis of the experience of illness as a particular kind of disturbance of agency completes a 'full-field' model of the conceptual structure of medicine by adding to the scientific resources of the traditional medical model, concerned with failures of functioning of bodily parts and systems, the resources of philosophical analysis concerned with failures of action as reflecting the agency of whole organism.

Part II A philosophical history of psychopathology

Chapter 7 A brief history of mental disorder

Session 1 Introduction and overview

◆ Mental disorders have been recognized across most cultures and historical periods back at least to classical times (with Plato).

◆ Interpretations of mental disorder over this period have swung to and fro between medical-scientific and moral-spiritual models.

Session 2 The main historical periods

- Examples of moral conceptions of madness in classical Greek and Roman thought include, respectively, Plato ('harmony of the soul') and the Stoics. Corresponding medical conceptions include, respectively, Hippocrates and Galen ('harmony of the humours').

- In the early Mediaeval period, moral conceptions of madness were dominant in the Christian West and medical conceptions in Islamic cultures.

- The Renaissance and Reformation were the period of the 'witch trials' in Europe.

- The Enlightenment saw a reassertion of medical conceptions of madness and the early asylums.

- This was followed by rapid expansion of the asylum movement over the mid-eighteenth to mid-nineteenth centuries, coinciding with the Industrial Revolution.

- Karl Jaspers' work in the philosophy of psychiatry was a response to psychiatry's first biological phase (at the turn of the twentieth century).

- Current developments in the philosophy of psychiatry are (in part) a response to psychiatry's second biological phase (at the turn of the twenty-first century).

Chapter 8 Karl Jaspers and General Psychopathology

Session 1 The clinical context of Jaspers' thought

- Experiences and behaviours associated with mental distress and disorder come in a wide variety of different kinds.

- Jaspers sought to categorize and order these experiences drawing on four key distinctions, namely between: (1) meaningful and causal connection; (2) understanding and explanation; (3) objective and subjective phenomena; and (4) form and content.

Session 2 Karl Jaspers the man

- Karl Jaspers (1883–1969) worked for much of his life in the University of Heidelberg.

- As a young man at the time of psychiatry's first biological phase, Jaspers wrote a textbook, *Allgemeine Psychopathologie* (or *General Psychopathology*). First published in 1913, this was to have a formative influence on modern descriptive psychopathology.

- Jaspers was a philosopher as well as psychiatrist and for much of his life, he was better known as a philosopher.

Session 3 Causal and meaningful connections

- A particular influence on Jaspers' work was the 'Methodenstreit', a debate about method in the social sciences that ran through much of the nineteenth century.

- Responding to the challenges of the new 'biological psychiatry', Jaspers wrote two key papers, (1) on causal and meaningful connections (arguing that both are needed in psychopathology), and (2) on phenomenology (arguing that this is a method of enquiry uniquely adapted to exploring subjectivity and, hence, psychopathology). The themes of these two papers run through *Allgemeine Psychopathologie*.

Session 4 Phenomenology

- The second of Jaspers' two key papers written in response to the challenge of biological psychiatry, his paper on phenomenology, introduces the distinctions between (1) objective and subjective symptoms, and (2) form and content.

- The distinction between form and content in modern descriptive psychopathology is derived from Jaspers' work.

- This distinction is subject to a number of different philosophical interpretations—particularly in Kant and in Husserl—and the philosophical influences on Jaspers himself have correspondingly been much debated.

Chapter 9 Phenomenology and psychopathology

Session 1 Jaspers' phenomenological approach to psychopathology

- Objective symptoms are those that are either manifest physically or grasped (understood) through rational thought without the need for empathy; subjective symptoms are accessed only through the exercise of empathy.

- Empathy is spontaneous understanding of 'what it's like' from the other's point of view (as opposed to understanding through rational reflection).

- Phenomenology is part of subjective psychology; it is concerned with both 'static' (i.e. cross-sectional) and 'genetic' (i.e. longitudinal) understanding of mental symptoms.

- The aim of phenomenology for Jaspers is to make as vivid as possible the diversity of mental life (this was in reaction to the tendency of objective science to reduce phenomena to the smallest number of kinds).

- Phenomenology (as Jaspers uses the term) is limited to the description and understanding of mental states (as opposed to explanations of the kind provided, for example, by neurophysiology).

Session 2 The background to Husserl's phenomenology

- Husserl's early work was in the philosophy of arithmetic and the 'problem of psychologism'.

- Psychologism is the view that logical and/or mathematical truths ultimately have a psychological basis.

- Husserl argued that logic is normative while psychology is not and hence that psychologism is mistaken.

- There none the less remains debate about the extent to which Husserl's work is psychologistic in character.

Session 3 Husserl's conception of phenomenology

◆ Husserl's phenomenology seeks to define the essential features of experience (in contrast to psychology, which studies particular instances of experience). Husserl thus conceives of phenomenology as an a priori discipline such as logic or arithmetic.

◆ Husserl argued that phenomenology precedes abstract thinking by analysing the 'essential types' of mental acts from which the wide variety of *particular* acts are derived. Again, he had in mind a parallel with the way in which the abstractions of geometry related to particular objects in the world.

◆ Husserl called his method, his way of using phenomenology 'ideational abstraction': this involves reflecting on one's mental states (e.g. *reflecting* on 'seeing a chair' as opposed to simply *seeing* a chair).

◆ For Husserl, the 'knowing subject' is the object of phenomenology.

◆ In Husserl's later work he introduced the idea of 'bracketing'. This is nowadays often used to mean setting aside our pre-suppositions in an attempt to get to the pure essences of things.

◆ Husserlian 'bracketing' is a more subtle concept that involves treating our pre-suppositions as an object of phenomenological study in their own right.

◆ Phenomenology (following Brentano) identifies 'intentionality' as the key and characteristic feature of mental states. Mental states are intentional in the sense that they are always *about* or *of* something.

Session 4 Assessment of Husserl's influence on Jaspers

◆ Debate continues about the extent of Husserl's influence on Jaspers.

◆ There are a number of important differences as well as similarities between their phenomenologies.

◆ An important difference of particular relevance to psychopathology is that Jaspers' phenomenological method is partly empirical, whereas Husserl regarded phenomenology as entirely a priori.

Session 5 Conclusions: the contemporary reference of the phenomenological tradition in psychiatry

◆ Besides Jaspers, the German philosopher, Martin Heidegger, had an important influence on psychotherapy through the work particularly of Ludwig Binswanger and Medard Boss.

◆ A key concept in Heidegger's phenomenology is 'dasein', literally 'being there'.

◆ Heidegger employed the concept of 'dasein' in an attempt to bridge the Cartesian separation of subject from the world, by focusing attention on our normally seamless engagement with everyday things through embedded practices.

◆ A rich diversity of other phenomenological traditions developed through the twentieth century particularly in Continental Europe, Japan, and South America.

Chapter 10 Psychopathology and the 'Methodenstreit'

Session 1 Understanding, explanation, and the 'Methodenstreit'

◆ At the heart of Jaspers' psychopathology is a distinction between understanding the meaning of an experience and explaining it in causal terms.

◆ While our uses of 'explain' and 'understand' overlap in everyday language, there are also differences between causal explanations (invoking laws as in the natural sciences) and making sense of social phenomena (by intuitive understanding as in disciplines such as history).

◆ Both sides of this distinction continue to raise many conceptual difficulties. What counts as 'understandable', in particular, has increasingly been recognized to be more complex than Jaspers had realized and continues to resist simple analysis.

◆ Philosophers such as Mill have argued that there is no fundamental difference between understanding and explanation.

Session 2 Understanding and explanation in Jaspers' psychopathology

◆ Jaspers takes from Wilhelm Dilthey (1833–1911) the idea that empathy is important to understanding.

◆ However, Jaspers was also influenced by Heinrich Rickert (1863–1936) and by the sociologist Max Weber (1864–1920), neither of whom believed that empathy is important to understanding.

◆ Weber believed that understanding involved evaluation rather than empathy.

◆ These and other conflicting influences in Jaspers' thinking are reflected in inconsistencies in his treatments of empathy and understanding.

◆ Jaspers also employs Weber's concept of an ideal type: a normative model incorporating current values and beliefs as opposed to the causal models of natural science.

◆ The evaluative model of ideal types derived from Weber feeds into Jaspers' account of 'meaningful' as distinct from causal explanation.

◆ A further unresolved tension in Jaspers' work is between the view that meanings are in *principle* irreducible to causes or only irreducible in *practice* (i.e. because of the limitations of the neuroscience of the day).

◆ The unresolved tensions in Jaspers' work continue to be reflected in modern philosophy: in the philosophy of science, for example, on the role of values in the natural sciences (see Part III); and in the philosophy of mind on the relationship between meanings and causes (see Part V).

Session 3 Conclusions: Jaspers, the *Methodenstreit*, and psychiatry today

- A first tension in Jaspers' thought is broadly that between a Dilthean (empathy-based) approach to understanding and a Rickert–Weber (evaluation-based) approach.

- A second tension is between different (empathy-based and evaluation-based) types of understanding.

- A third tension is around whether the difficulty of reducing meanings to causes is a difficulty of principle or only a contingent difficulty, a difficulty of practice.

- A fourth tension is between Jaspers' 'values out' account of understanding and what in the terminology of Part I, we may now call the 'values in' account of Weber and Rickert.

Part III Philosophy of science and mental health

Chapter 11 Psychoanalysis: an introduction to the philosophy of science

Session 1 Science: What is it and what's the problem?

- The conceptual difficulties about the scientific status of psychoanalysis (and psychiatry) suggest, following Austin (in Part I), (1) that these are relatively difficult (not deficient) sciences, and (2) that exploring these difficulties in psychoanalysis (and psychiatry) may shed light on the nature of science as a whole.

- 'Science' is a higher-level concept (in the terms of Part I). Hence when people try to 'define' it, they come up with different definitions reflecting different parts of its 'logical geography' (Ryle's term, Part I).

- The four stages of the traditional model of science are,
  - *Stage 1*: Data collection
  - *Stage 2*: Theory building, by
    - *Substage (A)* defining patterns, and/or
    - *Substage (B)* identifying underlying causes.
  - *Stage 3*: Theory testing (involves further data applied either at Substage A or Substage B),
  - *Stage 4*: Advancement of knowledge (negatively if the theory fails, positively if it succeeds).

Session 2 Psychiatry as science

- A traditional model of 'science' is strongly reflected in psychiatry's core textbooks in the second half of the twentieth century, in such words and phrases as 'observation', 'fact', 'hypothesis', 'explanatory', and 'prediction'.

- In these same textbooks, science (concerned with generalizable knowledge) in medicine and psychiatry is often contrasted with 'art' and the humanities generally (concerned with individuals).

- Science was seen as, (1) a barrier against bias and prejudice, and (2) the basis for focusing on medical rather than other kinds of mental problems.

- Contrary to expectations, while neuroscience has indeed made dramatic advances since these textbooks were written, the humanities, far from becoming less important in psychiatry, have flourished.

- This suggests a future for psychiatric science in which, as in other complex sciences, empirical and conceptual methods will go increasingly hand-in-hand.

- Negative reactions to the greater conceptual complexity of psychiatry have included, denial (ignoring it), proscription (placing it outside psychiatry's professional remit), and displacement (pushing it on to a related discipline, such as psychoanalysis).

Session 3 Scientific psychiatry and the case of psychoanalysis

- Psychoanalysis is unscientific, so its critics have claimed, at each of the four stages of the traditional model: its data are subjective (Stage 1); its theoretical terms have different meanings for different 'schools' (Stage 2); it is not experimental (Stage 3); and it shows few signs of a progressive consensus (Stage 4).

- Although rejecting his early neurological model (in the unpublished 'Project'), Freud remained committed to a traditional model of psychoanalytic science.

- Dora was an 18-year-old woman brought to Freud by her father (between 1896 and 1900) because she was troubled by obsessive thoughts about a friend of the family, Herr K.

- Freud's initial 'data collection' in his account of Dora differs from Stage 1 of the traditional model in being, (1) theory dependent, and (2) goal directed.

- In psychopathology, the pattern recognition required by Stage 2A of the traditional model, is complicated, among other ways, (1) by difficulties of separating the parts (of a mental state) from the whole, and (2) by value-norms (defining pathology, e.g. by epistemic values).

- The explanatory theories of Stage 2B of the traditional model are (in general) in the natural sciences, causal theories; but in the human sciences (including psychiatry) the explanations we give of why people do things are also in terms of reasons.

Session 4 Theory testing and the progress of knowledge

- The equivalent of 'testing' a theory, broadly construed, in Freud's report of his work with Dora, is the interpretation: the therapist interprets the patient's experiences and behaviours in terms of a hypothetical (partially repressed, hence hidden) mental 'cause' and gauges the success or otherwise of the theory according to how the patient reacts.

♦ The dominant account of how science tests its theories at the time of Dora was verificationism, essentially that scientific theories are confirmed (verified) by evidence. Sir Karl Popper argued that a theory could never be confirmed because there could always be disconfirming evidence waiting to be discovered.

♦ Thomas Kuhn was an American historian of science who showed that sciences do not progress continuously but through a series of paradigm shifts between which there may be relatively long periods of 'normal science' governed by the paradigm of the day.

♦ A paradigm (as it has come to be interpreted) has four components: (1) a set of symbolic generalizations (e.g. the definition of the Watt); (2) a set of metaphysical beliefs (e.g. the atomic structure of matter); (3) a set of values (e.g. epistemic values); and (4) a set of exemplars for problem-solving (e.g. the 'double helix' discovery).

♦ Kuhn's work (and subsequent work by Rom Harré and others), shows the extent to which, contrary to Popper's falsificationist criterion, scientists are in practice resistant to disconfirming evidence during periods of 'normal science' governed by a given paradigm.

♦ This, (1) brings psychoanalysis closer to sciences such as physics than Popper believed, and (2) illustrates the general point that the difficulties of developing a science of the mind point to difficulties in science as a whole, but (3) this neither proves nor disproves that psychoanalysis is a genuinely scientific theory of the mind.

Session 5 Psychoanalysis without science

♦ A sustained hermeneutic reconstruction of psychoanalysis was developed by the French philosopher, Paul Ricoeur.

♦ Ricoeur's hermeneutic account of psychoanalysis is part of a wider hermeneutic reconstruction of science (as in the work of Jurgen Habermas).

♦ Hermeneutic reconstructions of science emphasize the interpretative nature of science within a local discourse as distinct from the universal explanations of the traditional model.

♦ The American philosopher Adolf Grunbaum has argued (contra both Popper and Ricoeur) that psychoanalysis is a science but a *failed* science.

♦ 'Folk psychology' is our everyday understanding of people's psychology (our own and others): it includes attributing reasons for actions.

♦ Sebastian Gardner (building particularly on the work of James Hopkins and Richard Wollheim) has drawn on analytic work in the philosophy of mind to argue that psychoanalysis is properly understood as an extension of folk psychology.

Chapter 12 Psychopathology and the theory dependence of data

Session 1 The theory dependence of everyday observations and psychopathology

♦ Even a straightforward observational exercise reveals that observations have to be selected from a potential infinity according to one's needs and purposes. The practical context of an observation sets standards of, for example, the right level of precision. Thus even in a case as simple as this, observation is not merely a matter of 'drinking in' the data.

♦ The PSE is a thorough going attempt to place observation at the heart of clinical practice and to codify its role so as to maximize reliability. It can thus be seen as a sophisticated version of the traditional model of science from Chapter 11.

♦ One prima facie difference between observation in psychiatry and in other sciences is the active engagement of both parties to the observation: it is not a passive process.

Session 2 An Empiricist model of scientific theory

♦ Logical Empiricism was a sophisticated attempt closely associated with members of the Vienna Circle to articulate a broadly traditional model of science developed from the 1920s, which made space for, as a form of empiricism, a central role for observation.

♦ Observations might be used to confirm or according to 'Falsification' to refute scientific theory.

♦ Logical Empiricism attempted to underpin the objectivity of science both by stressing the role of public observation statements and by arguing that the language of observation should be separable from and prior to the language of theory. This is a two language model of theory and observation. A semantic distinction between the languages is used to defend the epistemological claim of the independence of observation.

♦ The aim of separating observation and theory has also played an influential role in psychopathology. However, while the Logical Empiricists aimed to separate observation and all theory, in psychopathology the aim is usually the more modest separation of observation and aetiological theory.

Session 3 Arguments for the theory dependence of observation statements

♦ There are a number of related claims that are made under the label of the theory dependence of observation.

♦ Duhem powerfully suggests that scientific observation statements are typically theory-laden. However, he does not preclude falling back to neutral observations in the case of disagreement.

♦ Paul Churchland shows that consideration of how we would translate alien languages emphasizes the role of theories held by speakers rather than their inner sensations in the case of perceptual reports. Nevertheless, there remains at least the possibility that such theories might concern observational properties of the world.

- Hesse, however, provides a powerful challenge to any such split. She suggests, partly on the basis of historical example, that while a distinction can be drawn at any particular time between theoretical and observational properties, the distinction drawn depends on the theories held. Thus it cannot serve as a neutral arbiter in the case of theoretical disagreement.

- This suggests that, to the extent to which there can be observations underpinning scientific claims, they are not unconceptualized raw data. So whatever the division between observation and aetiological theory in psychopathology, psychiatric observations cannot be a matter of raw data.

Session 4 Arguments for the theory dependence of the content of the process or experience of observations

- It is well known that expectations can change what people report they see or hear; however, this does not necessarily imply a fundamental connection between concepts and experiences.

- The duck–rabbit figure, introduced by Gestalt psychologists and discussed by Wittgenstein, suggests a more fundamental connection between what we can experience and our concepts. 'Seeing as' is conceptually structured. Possession of the concepts of 'duck' and 'rabbit' affect the experience of observers of the duck–rabbit figure.

- The dawning of an aspect, however, involves an immediate phenomenological effect, which appears to be a contingent feature of human experience over an above the idea that experience is conceptually structured. But attention to this phenomenon enables a better understanding of Hanson's and Churchland's disagreement about Kepler and Tycho observing the sunrise.

- There is a more general Kantian idea that suggests experience is never a matter of receiving brute raw data but is always, instead, conceptually structured. The argument, in a nutshell is that that is the only way experience can have a rational effect on our beliefs. This provides a way of connecting experience and observation statements: both are conceptually structured.

Session 5 The consequences for observation in psychiatry and physics

- Recent theoretical work in physics (as in the EPR paradox) suggests that the nature and role of observation is itself a contentious scientific issue.

- The analogy with work on observation in physics suggests that there is a middle ground between denying that observation is a complex matter and denying it any role at all. Efforts such as the PSE's to underpin the reliability of observation against a theoretical background are part of this work.

Chapter 13 Natural classifications, realism, and psychiatric science

Session 1 Hempel and two new agendas for psychiatric classifications

- The 'big issue' in the Research Agenda for DSM-V, as reflected in the Editor's introduction, is *validity*, i.e. the development of an 'aetiologically based, scientifically sound' classification.

- *Conceptual issues*, although prominent in the Research Agenda for DSM-V, are not named as such, it being assumed that a valid classification can be developed on the basis of empirical research alone.

- The feature of the Logical Empiricist account of what it is to be scientific by which modern psychiatric classifications have been most deeply influenced, is the separation of observational statements (i.e. descriptions of symptoms being the basis of modern classifications) from statements of theory (i.e. aetiological theories being the basis of earlier classifications).

- The influence of Logical Empiricism on modern psychiatric classifications was mediated by the American philosopher, Carl Hempel, the British psychiatrist, Aubrey Lewis, and the WHO official, Norman Sartorius.

- The first classification to reflect the influence of Logical Empiricism, by switching from a theoretical (aetiological) to a descriptive (symptom) basis, was the ICD-8.

- Subsequent classifications have added, (1) operationalized inclusion and exclusion criteria and a dimensional (axial) structure (especially DSM-III), and (2) an explicit evidence-based process for changing criteria and categories (especially DSM-IV).

- The 'big issue' on the agenda of psychiatric classification in the run-up to ICD-9 (and right through to DSM-IV) was *reliability* (inter-rater and test–retest agreement).

- Three limitations of operationalism in psychiatry (pointed out by Hempel) are:

  1. '*mere observation*'—that clinical observation rather than an operational procedure is the basis of clinical assessment;

  2. '*partial criteria of application*'—that different operational definitions are needed across different ranges of severity and for use in different contexts;

  3. '*antecedently understood terms*'—that for an operational (or any other) definition to be meaningful, the terms in which it is cast must already be understood.

  Limitation 1 applies particularly to psychiatry; Limitations 2 and 3 are generic.

- The major respect in which psychiatric classifications have developed differently from Hempel's expectations as a Logical Empiricist philosopher, is that they have become more *descriptive* (symptom-based) rather than more theoretical (aetiology-based).

Other respects include: (1) the greater emphasis on reliability; (2) the greater reliance on operationalism; and (3) the persistence of qualitative (rather than quantitative) criteria.

Session 2 Values, natural classifications, and the Absolute Conception

♦ Hempel (writing in 1959) argued that value terms were evident in psychiatric classifications of the day; that this risked reducing their scientific status (particularly though not only through reduced reliability); and hence that value terms would become less prominent in future psychiatric classifications as psychiatric science advanced.

♦ Szasz argued (like Hempel) that the prominence of values in psychiatric diagnostic concepts showed them to be 'unscientific'; but (unlike Hempel) he took values to show psychiatry to be unscientific primarily because (he believed) they undermined the *validity* (hence the 'reality') of its diagnostic concepts rather than (as Hempel argued) their reliability.

♦ Crispin Wright has argued that humour is not objective because it lacks 'cognitive command'.

♦ Bernard Williams' Absolute Conception is the conception of the world as it really is 'anyway', i.e. as distinct from how we may see it. It is a conception that we reach through progress in science.

♦ Williams employed the distinction between primary and secondary qualities to define 'progress' in science. He argued that progress in science consists in progressively stripping away the secondary qualities that we are aware of from this or that particular perspective (or 'local' conceptions, as determined by our sense organs, psychology, etc), in favour of the primary qualities that are there 'anyway' independent of any such local conception of what the world is like.

♦ J.L. Mackie, and others, have taken Williams' Absolute Conception to show that values (like secondary qualities) have no place in science.

♦ John McDowell's three arguments (noted here) against Williams' Absolute Conception are:

1. that secondary qualities may, contrary to the assumption guiding the Absolute Conception, be *both* subjective (in McDowell's sense of being conceptually connected with our experiences) *and* part of the fabric of the world;

2. that there is a tension within the idea of the Absolute Conception itself, namely, that we cannot even know what it is that the Absolute Conception is designed to explain without adopting the local perspective (essential to knowing what a secondary quality is) that is precluded by the Absolute Conception; and

3. that invoking the progress of science to resolve a dilemma generated by the Absolute Conception merely leaves us with a new dilemma in essentially the same form, generated by the progress of science itself.

♦ The implication of John McDowell's arguments is that Williams' Absolute Conception fails to provide, as Mackie and others have suggested, a 'knock-down' argument against values having a proper place in science. (Others, e.g. Dancy, have provided free-standing arguments to the same conclusion.)

Session 3 Scientific realism in physics

♦ Van Fraassen developed an account of science that aimed to replace Logical Empiricism with what has come to be called 'constructive empiricism': this combines three elements:

1. *semantic realism*—the theoretical statements of science really do (literally) make claims about the world;

2. *ontological realism*—the theoretical statements of science are true or false to the extent that they correspond with how the world really is;

3. *epistemological antirealism*—we can never have sufficient evidence to know, finally, which of science's theoretical statements actually are true or false.

♦ Constructive empiricism suggests that scientific theories should be judged by criteria of 'empirical adequacy', i.e. we should accept theoretical statements to the extent that, in Duhem's phrase, they 'save the phenomena'.

♦ Boyd and McMullen are among those who have sought to retain a traditional realist stance based on the idea that science shows us what is really there by way 'inferences to the best explanation'.

♦ Cartwright is a realist about causal entities.

♦ Hacking is a realist about what we can manipulate.

♦ Fine attacks the traditional realist/antirealist opposition arguing that we should adopt the attitude of practising scientists and accept local criteria for theory choice as they are developed within each discipline (his Natural Ontological Attitude or NOA).

♦ Recent debates about realism in science have been focused particularly on physics. They, (1) show that there are no simple unambiguous criteria of validity even in physics, and (2) suggest a number of fruitful aspects of validity for further exploration (e.g. Hacking's 'manipulability') in psychiatric science.

♦ Fine's work suggests that whatever we can learn from other sciences, local considerations will always be relevant to developing criteria of validity in psychiatric (as in any other) science.

Session 4 The Third New Agenda—an Agenda modelled on the philosophy of physics

♦ The Agenda (developed here) for an *Extended Family of Classifications* carried over from the Agenda for ICD-9 the 'big issue' of *reliability* as a small but important step towards the 'big issue' on the Agenda for DSM-V, *validity*.

♦ Conceptual issues are recognized to be important in psychiatric classification in the Agenda for ICD-9 *and* named as such. Conceptual issues are even more evident in the Agenda for DSM-V but are *not* (generally) named as such.

- The big issue on our Agenda for an Extended Family of Classifications is *good process* aimed at basing our classifications more securely, not on received authority, but on observation.

- Making explicit the importance of conceptual as well as empirical issues, and focusing on 'good process' based on the principles of observational science, in the development of an Extended Family of Classifications leads to:

  (1) rejection of a deficit model of psychiatric science in favour of a strengths model;

  (2) an opening up of psychiatric science to conceptual alongside empirical research methods; and

  (3) a more equal relationship between patients and other users of services, as 'experts by experience', and professionals as 'experts by training', as the basis of a genuinely *scientific* classification.

Chapter 14 Diagnosis, explanation, and tacit knowledge

Session 1 The Deductive-Nomological model of explanation

- One way to understand what diagnosis adds to a description of a patient's signs and symptoms is to think of it as an explanation of them and hence an inference from them.

- At least some forms of diagnosis are also explicitly causal. Others might be 'merely' a matter of pattern recognition when there is no clear aetiological theory developed.

- Hempel provides a logical model of explanation that likens it to a sound logical argument for what it explains. His model suggests the possibility of a formal model of diagnosis.

- Hempel's model is formal in that it gives clear necessary and sufficient conditions for an explanation, including the idea that general laws play an essential role. Hence the label 'covering law' model of explanation.

- These conditions make explanation and prediction symmetric.

- However, Hempel's model faces a number of counter-examples, many of which turn on the implicit idea that explanation is causal. This really seems to be an aspect of our everyday understanding of explanation brought out in the counter-instances to Hempel's model that causes cannot be explained in terms of their effects.

Session 2 A causal model of explanation

- Building on the counter-examples to Hempel's models outlined in the previous session, Lewis suggests that explanation of why events happen is always a matter of providing causal information.

- However, given that different aspects of the causal history can be given depending on the context of interest, there is no one explanation. Good explanation is a matter of judgement in selecting relevant causal information.

- Despite the differences, Lewis suggests that something like Hempel's models might be one way of providing that information.

- Van Fraassen goes further in suggesting that explanation always presupposes a particular context. For that reason he concludes that science itself which is not context independent does not contain explanations.

- If context does play an essential role in explanation, this suggests that it will not be possible to draw up a formal, context-free, model. Explanation will depend on good judgement.

Session 3 Clinical skills and tacit knowledge

- Collins' empirical work suggests that there is an element of tacit knowledge at the heart of a central aspect of scientific process: replication. Further, he describes this in the context of hard physical or engineering science.

- Collins suggests that one reason that tacit knowledge is present is that replication involves doing things that are relevantly similar although not the very same (because that would be impossible); however, it is impossible to specify all the relevant factors.

- Kuhn outlines the role of tacit knowledge in an intellectual, rather than practical, context. Puzzling solving in scientific education involves tacitly learning how to extrapolate from examples.

- Collins and Kuhn's arguments are mainly empirical and thus mainly suggest that tacit knowledge is, as a matter of fact, important in science. Wittgenstein, whom Collins invokes, provides a principled reason for there to be an ineliminable aspect of tacit knowledge, or judgement, in applying concepts or following rules. Explicit knowledge rests essentially on implicit practical skills. Thus all science, including scientific psychiatry, rests on tacit knowledge or judgement.

Session 4 Tacit knowledge, diagnosis, and a possible link to phenomenology?

- Kraus argues that psychiatric diagnosis is more a matter of a 'top-down' recognition of a patient's whole state than a 'bottom-up' recognition of individual symptoms. If true, this suggests that the expertise involved cannot be codified as involving more basic elements.

- Phenomenology has in general emphasized the importance of holism. This complements the approach taken in this chapter that emphasizes the role of implicit knowledge or judgement in general.

Chapter 15 Causes, laws, and reasons in psychiatric aetiology

Session 1 An introduction to philosophical accounts of causation

- As Chapter 14 began to outline, causation plays an important part in diagnostic reasoning and manipulating cause–effect relations is central to treatment and management but the concept of causation is itself surprisingly complex.

- The modern philosophy of causation begins with Hume's sceptical and unsuccessful search for the source of our idea of a necessary connection between events: a kind of causal glue. This reflects Hume's general philosophical method that ideas can be traced back to corresponding impressions. However, in this case, there does not seem to be any such impression either by looking to 'outer' events such as billiard ball collisions or 'inner' events.

- Failing to find an impression, Hume gives different definitions of causation—although he implies they are the same—based either on the idea of regularity or constant conjunction or on a 'counterfactual conditional': had the cause not occurred then neither would the effect, all other things being equal. The definitions are:

  1. an object, followed by another, and where all the objects similar to the first are followed by objects similar to the second. (p. 76)

  2. or in other words where, if the first object had not been, the second never had existed. (p. 76)

  3. an object followed by another, and whose appearance always conveys the thought to that other. (p. 77)

- More recently Mackie has offered a definition of causation based on the logical ideas of necessity and sufficiency: causation is an INUS condition. However, although it uses the word 'necessary' it is also consistent with Hume's failure to find the source of that idea in the context of causation and based instead on Hume's regularity approach to causation.

- Humean regularity theories owe an account, however, of which regularities correspond to laws of nature and can underpin causal connections, and which are mere accidents. One proposed solution depends on balancing the simplicity and universality of scientific theories. Another connects it to the justification of induction.

Session 2 A probabilistict view of causation?

- Hume's two definitions of causation provide the clue for two different modern approaches: regularity theories based on laws (described in Session 1), and Lewis' account based on counterfactual conditionals. A counter-factual conditional is a conditional whose antecedent runs counter to the facts.

- For Lewis' account to be a real alternative to a regularity theory, he needs to able to analyse counter-factual conditionals in a way that does not presuppose laws of nature.

- However, it is not clear that his analysis in terms of possible worlds really is more basic than the terms he is trying to explain.

- The connection between causation and raising the probability of effects suggests a different approach. It fits with the use of statistical tests for causal relations in medicine.

- However, Cartwright argues that it is not possible to *define* causation this way because cause only raises the chances of its

effects if there are no other causal factors present. Specifying that condition makes use of, and thus does not define, causation.

- Even if it is possible to define causation in a way that does not presuppose regularities or, more precisely, natural laws, there is still a plausible argument for a connection between them. The kind of events that stand in need of causal explanation can only be specified against a background of law.

Session 3 The realm of law and the space of reasons

- McDowell suggests that a consequence of the success of the rise of the natural sciences in modern times has been the assumption that nature is fully captured using their characteristic tools including explanation by subsumption under natural laws. This leaves phenomena which are normally interpreted as belonging to the 'space of reasons' looking less real. This in turn has led to a variety of approaches to reconcile them, including the attempted reduction of the 'space of reasons' to the 'realm of law'.

- McDowell himself advocates accepting a distinction between the 'realm of law' and 'space of reasons' but expanding our conception of what is part of nature to include the latter.

- Winch outlines a number of Wittgenstein-inspired differences between the natural and human science, which turn on the role of rules in making sense of social science phenomena.

- Bolton and Hill argue that the gulf between reasons and laws can be bridged with the assumption that meanings or reasons are encoded in the brain; however, this leaves the challenge of explaining how.

- Brown and Harris suggest a more practical rapprochement: devising a causal model of depression that includes meaningful elements.

- It remains an open question whether there can be a more principled reconciliation of these central and apparently distinct aspects of psychiatry.

Chapter 16 Knowledge, research, and evidence-based medicine

Session 1 Evidence-based medicine, Hume, and the problem of induction

- The basic aim of evidence-based medicine is to articulate the best ways of learning from past experience to guide future practice. It is thus part of a long-standing debate that evidence from the past can be brought to bear on the future. The modern philosophical discussion begins with Hume's problem of induction.

- Hume's Fork is the distinction between 'matters of fact' and 'relations of ideas'. The former, unlike the latter, requires experience. The latter, unlike the former, are necessary truths.

- Hume questions the status of some matters of fact: not matters of direct experience or perception but rather reasoning about, e.g. future events from past events.

- The problem of induction arises from the fact that there seems to be no non-circular justification of its use as a form of inference. A deductive justification of induction seems impossible. However, an inductive justification of induction seems to be circular.

Session 2 Philosophy of science responses to the problem of induction

- The philosophy of science has responded to Hume's problem of induction by attempting to articulate a model of scientific rationality for theory appraisal. The problem is not itself undermined but practical methods for side-stepping it are outlined.

- Falsificationism is an influential approach. It side-steps the problem of induction by suggesting that science should aim at the refutation of false theories, using deduction, rather than the confirmation of true theories, using induction.

- However, even falsification is more complex than it might at first seem. Theories can only be refuted in conjunction with other assumptions and observation statements themselves are fallible. Thus a realistic falsificationist methodology cannot offer clear-cut prescriptions.

- Kuhn argues that science proceeds through periods of occasional revolution interspersed by cumulative phases of problem solving. While there is no rational measure of progress across revolutions, there are agreed standards between such disruptions.

- Sociological study of science suggests that there is no context-independent account of scientific rationality and argues that it has to be studied in its historical setting. This need not be taken to undermine scientific rationality so much as to suggest that there is no simple model of it.

Session 3 Epistemological responses to the problem of induction

- Epistemological responses to the problem of induction have generally attempted to diagnose why there is not really a problem.

- One proposal is to deny an intuitive idea that to know something requires that one also knows that one knows it. By denying that, Hume's scepticism is, in part at least, defused. Thus Mellor argues that knowledge by induction is possible providing that there are causal connections from past to future, whether or not we also know that additional general fact.

- McDowell agrees with Mellor's 'externalist' approach to knowledge but stresses the idea that knowledge still requires reasons. However, he suggests that having good reason need not involve

being able, single-handedly, to offer an argument from first principles for every piece of knowledge. Knowledge can rub off on other people.

- Wittgenstein suggests that our knowledge is founded on a motley of inherited claims and background certainties.

Session 4 Evidence-based medicine and clinical trials

- The chapter has shown that the context of evidence plays an important part in assessing theory.

- The evidence-based medicine hierarchy of different forms of evidence can be given some support by looking at Mill's Method of Difference. These provide an a priori model of rationality. But Mill's Methods cannot be applied in practice without approximations that undermine their a priori status.

- The evidence-based medicine hierarchy itself contains an implicit empirical claim. It is thus subject to the same kind of evidence-based scientific assessment as any other claim. And this suggests the need for boots-strapping and hence judgement in assessing its status.

Part IV Values, ethics, and mental health

Chapter 17 Tools of the trade: an introduction to psychiatric ethics

Session 1 Ethical and conceptual issues in psychiatry: aims and objectives

- Just as in Chapter 2 conceptual issues were found to be not always self-evident, so, here, in Chapter 17, a first point to note is that ethical issues are not always self-evident.

- Also as in Chapter 2, philosophy (as distinct from other disciplines basic to ethics, such as the social sciences and religion) can help to give us a more complete picture particularly of the conceptual difficulties underpinning ethical problems in mental health.

- Four intermediate objectives for training in mental health ethics are: raising awareness, changing attitudes, increasing knowledge, and improving thinking skills. Of these, increasing the knowledge base of ethical reasoning is particularly important for strengthening the user voice because it puts the facts about what users of services really value at the centre of decision-making.

- Hare distinguished Level 1, spontaneous 'reflex' ethical reasoning appropriate for day-to-day practice, from Level 2, the more measured reflective reasoning that we are able to undertake in training and research by way of preparation for practice. Conceptual analysis is part of Level 2 reasoning.

Session 2 Conceptual difficulties and mental health ethics

◆ Bioethics, like biomedicine, has tended to neglect mental health issues, and in part for the same reason, namely that both have neglected the *conceptual* issues that are at the heart of the particular difficulty of mental health.

◆ Most authors define two conditions for consent: information and voluntariness (with freedom from coercion sometimes split out as a third condition). Both conditions are made more complicated in mental health by the effects of many different kinds of psychopathology.

◆ Delusion, historically and cross-culturally, has been the mark of the particular kind of irrationality that has been taken to undermine a person's responsibility for his or her actions: it is thus, equally, an *invalidating* condition for consent and an *excusing* condition in law.

◆ In addition to issues of consent, confidentiality, as an ethical problem, is complicated conceptually in mental health by the fact that the 'locus' of disorder may be distributed (e.g. within a family) rather than confined within a particular individual.

◆ In practice, the value of confidentiality (in mental health and in other areas) has to be balanced against the value of sharing information as the basis of multidisciplinary and multiagency teamwork.

Session 3 Conceptual difficulties and mental health law

◆ The philosophical fieldwork with which we started this session was our own response to a series of case vignettes involving (possible) involuntary treatment.

◆ The overall result was that (consistently with everyday practice) it was people particularly with psychotic symptoms who were most likely to be picked out as warranting involuntary treatment.

◆ This result is consistent across many different groups, including user groups; it is also a stable pattern historically and cross-culturally.

◆ The result is not sufficiently explained by mental health law, which, as standardly drawn, requires only two conditions for compulsion, (1) mental disorder, and (2) risk. These two conditions are thus considerably over-*inclusive* (allowing for too many people to be subject to compulsion).

◆ Strengthening the standard mental health law criteria, of mental disorder and risk, by adding a bioethical criterion of 'immediately life threatening' as a measure of seriousness, fails to explain the result, because, this time, it would be too *exclusive*, i.e. it would exclude those who (in the vignettes as in practice) would be subject to compulsion.

◆ The Butler criteria were, essentially, the presence of psychotic symptoms used as a measure of 'seriousness' appropriate to the particular issues of loss of responsibility raised by mental

disorder. Proposed by a Government Committee in the UK in the 1970s, they fit the results from our philosophical fieldwork, the case vignette questionnaire, perfectly. However, this begs the key question practically, namely, of what lies behind the cases where people's responses are split.

◆ Among the many possible reasons for the neglect of mental health issues by bioethics, the specifically *conceptual* reason is that bioethics has (implicitly) adopted the same medical-scientific, 'left-field', model as biomedicine: hence it has assumed (wrongly, we have argued) that the 'tools' for ethical reasoning developed in bodily medicine can be applied essentially unchanged in mental health.

Chapter 18 From bioethics to values-based practice

Session 1 Bioethics and health care

◆ Among a number of historical factors, modern bioethics developed as a response to advances in the sciences and technology underpinning medicine: this prompted the need for the shift from 'medical beneficence' to 'patient autonomy' which is at the heart of modern bioethics.

◆ Although an important development, the growth of ethical rules and legal regulation as the principal 'tool' for connecting bioethics with practice, has had three downsides: (1) code inflation; (2) practitioner deflation; and (in some cases) (3) problem conflation (in particular, disadvantaging users of services).

◆ Code inflation reflects a failure to recognize that conceptual difficulties cannot be fully resolved by explicit rules (this is an aspect of the difference between definition and use explored in Part I).

◆ Practitioner deflation arises from a failure to acknowledge the importance of tacit knowledge and skills derived from experience as a key contribution to health-care decision-making (we covered implicit knowledge in Part III).

◆ Problem conflation shows the need for other tools in the ethical 'toolkit' in addition to rules and regulation.

◆ Three methods of ethical reasoning have been found to be particularly helpful in practice: principles (top-down reasoning), casuistry (or case-based bottom-up reasoning), and perspectives (focusing on the different perspectives of those involved in a particular situation).

◆ Each of these has strengths and weaknesses but used together they offer complementary ways of reasoning about ethical issues in health care.

Session 2 Bioethics and mental health

◆ The 'four principles', introduced by Beauchamp and Childress, are autonomy, beneficence, non-maleficence, and justice.

- Beauchamp and Childress are unusual (in the bioethics literature) in focusing on the particular conceptual difficulties of consent in mental health. They analyse involuntary treatment as being justified where the competencies for autonomous decision-making are impaired by psychopathology: the principle of autonomy is thus outweighed (mainly) by the principle of beneficence (doing good).

- However, Beauchamp and Childress' analysis of the relevant psychopathology, which is in essentially cognitive terms, although fitting their own case example (of dementia), fails to fit the functional cases picked out in the responses to our case vignettes in Chapter 17.

- Casuistry (case-based) reasoning 'works', i.e. people come to agreed ethical conclusions, because and to the extent that their implicit values are shared.

- This makes casuistry a possibly dangerous tool in mental health ethics because mental health, as we saw in Part I, is an area in which people's values are particularly diverse. Hence if used unreflectingly, casuistry could be used to impose the values of the majority on minorities.

- The emphasis on individual differences of values in perspectives reasoning is helpful in mental health ethics. But some of the most difficult problems (including involuntary treatment) arise where (as with 'loss of insight') the perspectives of the person concerned differs radically from the perspectives of everyone else.

- All three methods, principles, casuistry, and perspectives, thus have strengths and weaknesses for mental health ethics, but, neither separately nor together, do they offer a panacea.

Session 3 Philosophical ethical theory

- Deontology is rights-based ethics, involving rights and responsibilities. It is the basis of legal and regulatory ethics.

- Consequentialism focuses on outcomes. Utilitarianism (the 'greatest good of the greatest number') is a form of consequentialism that is the basis of health economic models aimed at fair distribution of resources (e.g. QALYs).

- Analytic ethics focuses not on substantive ethical conclusions (about what is right, fair, etc.) but on the meanings and implications (the 'logic') of value terms.

- Analytic ethics is important generally in mental health because of the extra conceptual difficulties with which mental health is associated.

- The extra 'tools' that analytic ethics delivers are a set of ideas about working with differences of values (called Values-Based Practice—see next Session), such differences representing a particular aspect of the greater conceptual difficulty of mental health ethics.

- Substantive ethical theory seeks to provide 'answers', i.e. substantive outcome values, such as autonomy, by which decisions should be guided. Analytic ethical theory focuses rather on good process. The key shift required to work equally effectively with both types of ethical theory, substantive and analytic, is thus a shift from 'right outcomes' to 'good process'.

Session 4 Values-based practice

- Values-Based Practice is the theory and skills base for effective health-care decision-making where different, and hence potentially conflicting, values are in play.

- Where substantive ethics start from particular values (such as autonomy), Values-Based Practice starts (like a democracy) from respect from different values and relies (again, like a democracy) on good process for effective decision-making.

- Good process in Values-Based Practice includes three principles linking it closely with Evidence-Based Practice: the 'two feet' principle (all decisions rest on values as well as facts); the 'squeaky wheel' principle (we notice values, or facts, only when they cause difficulty); and the 'science driven' principle (that the increasingly complex values involved in health care are a result of scientific progress opening up ever-wider choices).

- Good process in Values-Based Practice depends on a model of service delivery that is user-centred (starting from the values of individual service users, families, etc.) and multidisciplinary/agency (different disciplines/agencies providing different value perspectives as the basis of balanced decision-making where values conflict).

- Four particular clinical skills are required to support good process in Values-Based Practice: (1) raised awareness of values (and of differences of values); (2) knowledge of values (including 'evidence-based' research knowledge); (3) reasoning about values (using ethical reasoning to explore differences of values rather than to get the 'right' answer); and (4) communication skills (both for exploring values and for resolving differences).

- Bioethics, as an extension of medical law, has tended to see itself as a 'guardian' of patients' rights against the exercise of medical power. Combining Values-Based with Evidence-Based approaches to health-care decision-making seeks to restore partnership is decison-making between users and providers of services.

Chapter 19 It's the law! Rationality and consent as a case study in values and mental health law

Session 1 The legal basis of consent

- The law on consent in health care is derived from the need to balance patient autonomy (the right to self-determination) with medical beneficence (the duty to act in the patient's 'best interest'). The roots of these two principles lie in the moral and cultural traditions of medicine back to the Hippocratic 'Oath'.

◆ The legal embodiment of these two principles is often in the form of 'rights'.

◆ Legal consent may be: (1) express; (2) implied; or, in English law at least, (3) by 'estoppel' (a form of 'reasonable person' test).

◆ Current legal doctrine requires that for consent to be valid: (1) the person concerned has the *capacity* to consent; (2) they have sufficient *information* on which to base their consent; and (3) they made their decision *voluntarily*.

◆ A 'status' test is one that determines whether a person's consent is valid according to their status: e.g. a child below a certain age (and/or maturity) may not have the status to give (or withhold) valid consent; more contentiously, in many administrations a person with a mental disorder may not have the status to give (or withhold) valid consent for their mental disorder.

Session 2 Capacity, information, and causes of action

◆ The four key elements of decision-making capacity defined in *ReC* are: (1) understanding and retaining the relevant information; (2) believing it; (3) weighing the information; and (4) arriving at a clear choice.

◆ Although intended as an objective test of capacity, i.e. one that is independent of the 'rights or wrongs' of the actual decision the patient makes, values come into this test, *inter alia*, implicitly in the concept of rationality underlying the element of 'understanding', and explicitly in the element of 'weighing'.

◆ Causes of action for unlawful treatment without consent include, in criminal law an action for battery, and in civil law an action either for trespass (civil battery) or negligence.

◆ Battery involves three elements: (1) touching; (2) damage; and (3) reasonable forseeability of damage.

◆ The elements of negligence are: (1) duty of care; (2) breach of the relevant standard of care; and (3) causation.

◆ The Bolam test is an example of a 'prudent doctor' standard of care: a doctor will not be liable for negligence if he or she acted '. . . in accordance with a practice accepted as proper by a responsible body of medical practitioners' skilled in that particular area.

◆ A prudent patient test asks only what a 'prudent' or 'reasonable' patient would want to know in the circumstances.

◆ The courts in recent rulings have been clear that, while retaining a prudent doctor test, medical opinion in a given case has to be in the court's view, reasonable, responsible, and respectable.

Session 3 Consent, voluntariness, and best interests

◆ Cases of enforced Caesarean section focus on issues such as capacity and rationality as vehicles for the exercise of (implicit) judicial values.

◆ So long as judicial values remain implicit, they may be problematic where the values, respectively, of the courts, of doctors and of patients, are all likely to be different (cf. Part I).

◆ Generic incapacity legislation seeks to reconcile different tests of capacity developed in different contexts for different purposes, within a single test.

◆ The legal concept of 'best interests', although rightly requiring decision-makers to consider a range of relevant information about the actual (or likely) values of the person(s) concerned, makes explicit the deep issues of value lying behind legal judgments.

Chapter 20 Values in psychiatric diagnosis

Session 1 The central place of values in psychiatric diagnosis: the case of Simon

◆ A values-based model of medical diagnosis adds values rather than subtracting facts.

◆ The PSE defines a delusional perception as a delusion that is 'based on sensory experiences' and involves 'suddenly becoming convinced that a particular set of events has a special meaning'.

◆ In the ICD-10 diagnostic manual, a delusional perception is among the symptom-criteria that (with other criteria such as a particular duration) are sufficient for a diagnosis of schizophrenia (or related psychotic disorder, depending on other co-present symptoms).

◆ DSM adds to the (otherwise essentially similar) criteria for schizophrenia in ICD, a Criterion B of 'social/occupational dysfunction'.

◆ The DSM-IV explicitly claims to be strongly evidence based. It *is* strongly evidence based. But, like the ICD it uses many terms with clear evaluative connotations. Further, with the introduction of criteria of social/occupational *dys*function into the diagnosis of psychotic disorders, the DSM-IV in effect puts values at the heart of psychiatric diagnosis. The DSM-IV is thus both evidence based and values based.

Session 2 Generalization: the pervasiveness and importance of values in psychiatric diagnosis

◆ Values are all pervasive in DSM: in its definition of disorder; in the value-laden terms used in many criteria; and centrally in the explicitly evaluative judgements involved in applying criteria of social/occupational dysfunction (such as Criterion B) for psychotic disorders.

◆ DSM's criterion of 'clinical significance' does not provide an escape route for the medical model from values because the criterion is not defined (other than as being 'an inherently difficult clinical judgement'—which might well itself involve one or more *value* judgements).

- Positing underlying (actual or hypothetical) bodily causes does not provide an escape route from values for the medical model because, as we saw in Part I, it is the (negatively evaluated) experience of illness that marks out an underlying bodily cause of that experience as a *pathological* cause, not vice versa. (*All* experiences, normal and pathological, being caused.)

- Moral descriptivism is the claim in philosophical value theory that at least in some circumstances values can be redefined in terms of facts.

- There is no escape route from values for the fact-only medical model in moral descriptivism. This is because, in addition to the general arguments against moral descriptivism outlined in Part I, the moral descriptivist redefinition of values in terms of facts depends on people's values being *shared*, whereas psychiatry, and hence psychiatric diagnosis, is concerned with areas in which people's values are highly *diverse*.

- A moral descriptivist 'escape route' for the medical model, like other attempts to mask the importance of values in psychiatric diagnosis, risks abusive consequences arising either from over-use or underuse of psychiatric diagnostic concepts.

- The alternative is not to seek an escape route at all, but to adopt a *non*-descriptivist logical framework in which fact and value, description and evaluation, are understood to have equal and complementary roles in psychiatric diagnosis.

Session 3 Bioethics and values in psychiatric diagnosis

- Reich identifies (explicitly or implicitly) a number of important positive points about psychiatric diagnosis: (1) that it is ethically laden; (2) that it is indeed ethically central; (3) that misdiagnosis can take several distinct forms; (4) that non-purposeful misdiagnoses are even more significant ethically than purposeful misdiagnosis; (5) that there are many empirical difficulties also; (6) that the misuse of psychiatric diagnosis in the former USSR has lessons for us all; (7) that psychiatric diagnosis may have a number of positive and helpful implications; and (8) that the problems of psychiatric diagnosis have their origins in our common human nature. (*Note*: each of these really *is* a key learning point!)

- Reich presents each of these points not as positive but as negative points about psychiatry: it is ethically laden, hence unscientific, etc.

Chapter 21 From bioethics to values-based practice in psychiatric diagnosis

Session 1 Philosophy, values, and psychiatric diagnosis

- In her review of philosophical issues in psychiatric classification and diagnosis, Radden focuses particularly on the philosophy of science.

- Like Szasz and Kendell, on opposite sides in the debate about mental illness (in Part I), Reich assumes in relation to psychiatric diagnosis, (1) that mental illness is *the* problem, and (2) that physical illness, relatively speaking, is *not* a problem.

- As with medical diagnosis (see Chapter 20, Session 1), a values-based understanding of psychiatric classification and diagnosis, adds values rather than substracting facts.

Session 2 From fact-only to fact+value model of psychiatric diagnosis

- Behind Reich's essentially negative take on psychiatric diagnosis lies his (implicit) adoption of the fact-only medical model.

- If the problems of psychiatric diagnosis arise (at least equally) from its evaluative as from its descriptive aspects, an approach guided by the fact-only (or fact-centred) medical model may be blind to these problems.

- Reich, along with many others in 'Western' bioethics, assumes that Soviet psychiatric science was peculiarly deficient: this is why, the assumption goes, abuses of psychiatric diagnosis became widespread in the former USSR.

- Closer inspection, however, suggests that Soviet psychiatric science was not essentially different from the corresponding psychiatric sciences of the day in Britain and North America.

- Guided by a fact-only medical model, Reich implies that the 'cure' for misuses of psychiatric diagnosis lie in strengthening its scientific basis in particular *by excluding values* from it.

- An alternative approach to reducing the misuses of psychiatric diagnosis is to *focus on its evaluative aspects* and to take seriously the implications for diagnosis of the particular diversity of human values in the areas with which psychiatry is concerned.

Session 3 Reversing Reich

- All of Reich's points in his list of the (ironically named) 'beauties' of psychiatric diagnosis, could, in principle, though sometimes to a lesser degree, be made as points about diagnosis in bodily medicine.

- In the terms of a 'diagnostic formulation' (Chapter 2), (1) Reich's 'diagnosis' of the abuses of psychiatric diagnosis is that it offers a way out for people trying to evade problems, (2) his 'aetiological theory' is thus that such abuses arise from the frailty of human nature, and (3) his 'treatment' is to stiffen up standards with (a) ethical and legal rules and regulation, and (b) tighter scientific standards.

- Stiffening up scientific standards in itself can only make abuses less likely. However, focusing on the scientific side of diagnosis *at the expense of* its evaluative side, could lead to neglect of an important source of the difficulties of psychiatric diagnosis (i.e. differences of values) and hence increase the risks of abuses.

♦ While a framework of law and ethics is always important, such a framework (in reflecting shared values) could increase the risks of abuses if applied unreflectingly across areas (such as mental health) where values are inherently diverse.

Session 4 Practical applications: values-based practice and psychiatric diagnosis

♦ Values-based psychiatric diagnosis involves: (1) identifying and understanding the values of the person (or family) concerned; (2) being able to draw on different value perspectives (as represented by the multidisciplinary or multiagency service models) to come to a balanced judgement where values conflict; and (3) an 'open society' of mental health stakeholders in which a dynamic of mutual checks and balances is maintained.

♦ In research, values-based practice involves drawing on a wide range of methods—philosophical, empirical and mixed—to explore the values actually operative in different situations.

♦ Values-based (as well as evidence-based) approaches to diagnosis are relevant in all areas of psychiatric research, including the neurosciences.

♦ Adopting a values-based as well as evidence-based approach to classification would not alter the *descriptive* elements in the criteria in existing classifications (though there might be other reasons for altering them). Rather, a values-based approach would, (1) make the existing *evaluative* elements in these criteria more fully explicit, and (2) indicate key features of the 'good process' required to work with both evaluative and descriptive elements equally effectively.

Part V Philosophy of mind and mental health

Chapter 22 Mind, brain, and mental illness: an introduction to the philosophy of mind

Session 1 The mind–body problem in ordinary usage

♦ Among other adverse effects on mental health, the difficulty of the mind–body problem has: (1) been the basis of (some) antipsychiatry attacks, particularly by way of the contrast between 'real' bodily diseases and mental illnesses that are ' all in the mind'; (2) deepened divides between different models adopted by different 'schools' of psychiatry (e.g. psychoanalytic versus biological); and (3) encouraged slides towards eliminativist positions (mind-only or brain-only), that are both, (a) equally conceptually untenable, and (b) practically dangerous (leading to unbalanced and abusive practice).

♦ People have drawn equal and opposite implications from putative neuroscientific discoveries of the brain basis of particular behaviours; some reject, while others embrace, the idea that such discoveries show that people are not responsible for the behaviour in question.

♦ It is a feature of the logical geography of our ordinary usage that the concept of a 'person' involves both brain-talk and mind-talk. Strawson argued that persons are (logically) primitive, i.e. that brain-talk and mind-talk are both dependent on the concept of a person.

Session 2 The mind–body problem: the case of Mrs Lazy

♦ 'Mrs Lazy' decided to give up housework because she was fed up with it.

♦ Her family thought she was ill because this was so out of character; her doctors agreed because diseases affecting the brain (especially the frontal lobes) can cause changes of personality.

♦ Causal stories of this kind, although called in medicine 'psychosomatic', depend on brain–body dualism not mind–body dualism.

♦ When a tumour in Mrs Lazy's frontal lobes was found, this was consistent with the medical–causal explanation of the change in her personality.

♦ But this account of her decision, in neglecting Mrs Lazy's values, experience, and agency, left out the person, the real Mrs Lazy.

♦ The wider significance of Mrs Lazy's story is this: it is *above all* where we can give a causal explanation of someone's behaviour, important *not* to neglect the values and other aspects of their experience that are essential to who they are as unique individuals.

♦ In other words, Mrs Lazy's story shows the increased danger that arises when we are able to explain the brain basis of some aspect of a person's experience or behaviour, of neglecting the values and experiences of that person, and thus failing to relate to them as real people.

Session 3 The mind–body problem: from ordinary usage to philosophy

♦ In the seventeenth century, rationalists and empiricists both conceived of the mind as a vessel for knowledge: rationalists believed the vessel had in-built tools ('rational capacities') for making sense of the world; empiricists believed the vessel started off empty and that knowledge was based on experiences gained through the senses.

♦ Descartes' philosophical project was a response to scepticism (especially Montaigne's scepticism) about the very possibility of (secure) knowledge.

♦ His 'method of doubt' led him to his *cogito*, 'I think, therefore I am'.

♦ The supposed indubitable nature of the (mental) *cogito* seemed to suggest that mind must be different in kind (a different *substance*) from matter (including brains). It is this 'Cartesian dualism' and the many responses to it that have generated together the mind–body problem in its modern form.

- Among the best known early responses to Descartes' dualism are:
  1. Malebranche's *Occasionalism* (an extension of dualism to include God's interventions),
  2. Geulincx's '*two clocks*' (that mind and brain tick together),
  3. Spinoza's *Monism* (that mind and matter are two aspects of the same substance),
  4. Leibniz's *Psychophysical Parallelism* (a version of the 'two clocks' in which mind and brain function harmoniously in parallel),
  5. Berkeley's *Idealist Monism* (that the essence of things is to be perceived—thus resolving dualism in favour of the mind), and
  6. Hobbes' *materialism* (that 'I think' depends on knowledge of the author of thought—thus resolving dualism in favour of matter).

- In his *Critique of Pure Reason*, Kant sought the logical preconditions that make all conventional arguments (from premises to conclusions) possible.

- The nub of Kant's argument against Descartes is that the apparent force of the 'cogito' depends on an equivocation between two senses (a logical and an empirical sense) of the self.

Session 4 A modern response to the Cartesian problem

- Psychology was a growth industry in the nineteenth century but there was relatively little interest in the philosophical mind–body debate.

- The re-igniting of the debate is generally attributed to Gilbert Ryle's book *The Concept of Mind*.

- Ryle's position is generally (and Wittgenstein's by some) considered to be a form of *logical behaviourism*, i.e. the claim that meanings are nothing more than publicly observable behaviours, as distinct from *psychological behaviourism*, i.e. the claim that psychology should be concerned with nothing more than publicly observable behaviours (as in the work of J.B. Watson and B.F. Skinner).

- Ryle argued that mind–body dualism arises from a *category mistake* equivalent to the visitor to a university, who, having seen all the parts of the institution (the university library, etc.), still insists on being shown '*the* university'. He has made the mistake of thinking that the 'the university' is a thing of the same kind (category) as 'the university library'.

- Ryle characterized mental states as '*dispositional statements*', i.e. statements of the dispositions (the propensities, capacities, etc.) of things to show certain behaviours or to react in certain ways.

- More recent commentators have argued that Ryle's position, his denials notwithstanding, is behaviourist. It thus exploits one side of the mind–body dualism (the body side) rather resolving the problem of how they might be related.

Chapter 23 The mind–body problem and mental health, a philosophical update

Session 1 The mind–body problem in clinical neuropsychiatry

- Work in psychiatry, especially in neuroimaging, suggests close and specific connections between the mind and the brain; however, it does not, of itself, suggest a perspicuous account of how the mind and brain are related.

- That the connection is thought to be close is suggested by the fact that Posner provides no argument to connect seeing the brain with the mind: he merely assumes it.

- Mind and brain may be connected according to a particular analysis of mental states such as a cognitivist analysis that analyses mental states as information states.

Session 2 Functionalist accounts of the mind

- Functionalism compares the relationship of mental states and brain states with computer software and hardware. Mental states are functional states: defined by their inputs (perceptions and other mental states) and outputs (behaviour and other mental states).

- It is compatible with physicalism (the view that everything is ultimately physical); however, it need not be taken to imply physicalism.

- A type identity theory connects mental states and physical states as types. A type or generality of mental states is identified with a type or generality of mental states. A token identity claim merely claims that each individual mental state is a physical state. This distinction is akin to that between numerical and qualitative identity.

- Functionalism escapes an objection to behaviourism by loosening the connection between mental states and behaviour. But it maintains a relation between mental states and behaviour as a whole.

- One influential criticism of functionalism is that merely describing the relational properties of mental states omits their intrinsic qualities or qualia. This point is emphasized in arguments about the functional equivalence of systems with inverted or missing qualia.

- A second objection is that the rational character of mental states cannot be captured in functional relations. Davidson stressed the rational and normative basis of mental states and hence their irreducibility to physical patterns. McDowell stressed the different patterns of explanation that comprise comparison with an ideal (in the mental case) and subsumption under a law (in the physical).

Session 3 Davidson's Anomalous Monism

◆ Davidson aims to reconcile three plausible but apparently incompatible claims: (1) a nomological account of causation; (2) the claim that mental states have causal powers; and (3) the denial that there are psychological or psychophysical laws.

◆ He claims that each mental state is a physical state while denying that types of mental state can be reduced to or mapped on to types of mental state. Thus he calls his account: Anomalous Monism. It is monistic in that there is only one kind of stuff but it is anomalous because there are no laws linking physical and mental types. It is thus a form of token identity thesis.

◆ Supervenience is the thesis that determining or fixing the physical properties of a person (or possibly the person and their environment) determines or fixes their mental properties but the converse implication does not hold. It was first applied in the case of ethics.

◆ Davidson adds supervenience to his basic claim that mental states are token-identical to physical states in part to head off the charge that his is a form of epiphenomenalism: mental states are caused by physical states but have no causal powers themselves.

◆ However, there is some tension in the combination of a token identity thesis and supervenience.

◆ Consideration of functionalist and Davidsonian theories already suggest that there are a number of possible responses to the mind–body problem.

Session 4 Arguments against mind–body identity theories

◆ Kripke argues that some names are 'rigid designators', which pick out their referents essentially. Identity claims expressed using rigid designators express de re necessities: they are necessarily true, or true in all possible worlds, even if they can only be known through experience or a posteriori.

◆ Although Kripke explains these claims by talking of possible worlds it is not necessary to think that these are real. Nevertheless, strict rules have to be followed in describing them.

◆ Kripke argues that if identity statements expressed using rigid designators hold necessarily but if the putative identity of mind and brain is at best contingently true, as Descartes plausibly suggests, then there is no identity between mind and brain.

◆ Kripke does not himself suggest what relation this leaves.

◆ Assessing Kripke's argument depends on assessing the essential properties of mental states: centrally whether there is more to mental states than their felt qualities.

◆ There are ways of linking mental and physical states that are weaker than identity such as 'constitution' but even these are threatened by the difference between the rational pattern into which mental states fit and the law-like relations that are assumed to characterize physical states.

Session 5 Is there any reason to believe in supervenience?

◆ The claim that the mental supervenes on the physical can be made without there being any way of correlating mental and physical elements. The totality of mental events may supervene on the totality of physical events without the events correlating even at the level of tokens.

◆ Papineau suggests that the thesis that physics could be a complete account of the world implies the truth of the supervenience of mental events on physical events. His argument is based on the claim that physics can be complete.

◆ But, according to Crane, the claim that physics is complete is just as contentious and cannot justify supervenience.

◆ Crane argues that a dilemma can be outlined by asking, metaphorically, what God would have to do to fix the mental facts having fixed the physical facts. If he has to create further laws these will create further mental facts and thus the physical facts alone do not determine the mental. If he does not then, according to Crane, this undermines the idea that there are any mental facts. While not decisive, this argument makes supervenience less well founded than might first appear, and hence the mind-body problem remains open.

Chapter 24 Reasons and the content of mental states: 1. Reductionist theories

Session 1 Aphasia, deficit studies, modularity, and meaning in cognitive psychiatry

◆ While the modular approach to the mind helpfully explains the relations of mental abilities or deficits it raises the question of how mental states possess intentionality in the first place.

◆ Talk of representations of words and representations of their meaning merely disguises the problem of how representation of meaning is possible.

Session 2 Preliminaries to a philosophical account of content

◆ Since Brentano, intentionality or 'aboutness' has been a central focus of the philosophy of mind.

◆ At least some mental states can be thought of as propositional attitudes. A subject has an attitude towards a proposition. The attitude might be hope, fear, believe, etc. The proposition might be something like: that it is raining, that an election is coming, that the sun will rise, etc.

◆ Fodor suggests that mental states are semantically evaluable— that is, like other meaningful items they can be, for example, true or false—they have causal powers and are governed by common sense psychology.

- The central question of the philosophy of content is how intentionality so described is possible.

Session 3 Naturalized or reductionist accounts of content

- The attempt to reduce intentional concepts to more basic concepts raises a number of preliminary questions. Central is the question of whether linguistic meaning or mental content is more basic. Either could be explained in terms of the other.

- Reductionist approaches generally assume that mental content is more basic and that linguistic meaning can then be explained through the intentions of speakers: intention-based semantics.

- Fodor's representational theory of mind is an attempt, based on the idea that the mind is a kind of computer, to describe mental operations as operations of internal mental representations.

- But unlike functionalism, Fodor does not think that the fine-grained content of mental states can be explained in functional terms even though the difference between different sorts of attitude can be.

- Propositional attitudes are encoded in different functional attitudes towards different propositions, themselves encoded in mental representations.

Session 4 Descriptive causal accounts of content

- Reductionism about mental content needs to add a further ingredient to the computer metaphor. It needs to explain how internal mental representations—neural states, probably—have intentionality. Fodor advocates a causal theory: mental representations have the meaning or content they do because they are the effects of features of the world. They are about what causes them.

- However, a causal theory faces the disjunction problem: explaining how *false* beliefs are possible.

- Fodor's theory faces a number of different objections, however. The difficulties suggests the kind of problem any reductionist theory of meaning must face and thus the challenge for a thorough cognitivist psychiatry.

Session 5 Teleological causal accounts of content

- A more recent reductionist approach to meaning invokes evolutionary theory to account for the meaning of mental representations. It is sometimes called teleosemantics.

- Like the evolutionary theory approach to mental disorder it deploys the idea of biological or proper function. The proper function of a mental representation gives its meaning. The function is what a biological trait is selected for, now what is actually selected.

- Again, however, this approach faces difficulties crucially in specifying the biological function of mental representations in ways that mirror content without begging the question of what they mean.

- These objections suggest that the attempt to break the notion of meaning or intentionality down to something more basic may be mistaken. Instead it may be that it is an irreducible notion tied to the idea of personhood. If so it may be a mistake to think that meaning is encoded in mental representations.

Chapter 25 Reasons and the content of mental states: 2. Antireductionism and discursive psychology

Session 1 The discursive alternative

- Discursive psychology presents an alternative view of meaning and mental states to that provided more cognitivist psychiatric models of mind and brain.

- Discursive psychology links meaning and mental states to conversations or discourse: outer and public rather than inner and private phenomena. It thus avoids the challenge to cognitivist accounts of explaining how inner states can be about external states of affairs.

- As in the case of the latter, discussed in Chapter 24, there are philosophical models of meaning that help shed light on the issue.

- A question for assessment is, however, whether the discursive view of meaning merely places a different emphasis on social and public aspects of meaning or whether it is strictly incompatible with the cognitivist approach discussed in Chapter 24. One way to distinguish the claims is to construe discursive psychology as committed to a form of social constructionism: meaning is constructed in conversations. That is a radical view of meaning.

Session 2 Wittgensteinian approaches to mental content

- A social constructionist version of discursive psychology often looks to Wittgenstein for support.

- Wittgenstein's work has been interpreted as supporting a number of different, conflicting claims. However, all agree that because understanding a word means understanding how to use it correctly, there is an important connection between rules and meanings. Both are normative. There is also a connection to mental states because they prescribe what they are about.

- Kripke argues that Wittgenstein's discussion contains a sceptical attack on the very idea of meaning. He bases this claim on an argument about how we know what mathematical rules we have followed in the past. It seems that there is no evidence we can appeal to which will uniquely determine a mathematical function. Also, similar considerations would apply to our knowledge of the rules governing the use of other everyday words.

- Wright suggests that Kripke's sceptical argument can be partially defused by an analogy with intentions. If asked how we know what we previously intended we would not hesitate to say we simply remembered the intention directly rather than via an inference.

- However, Wright suggests that intentions are philosophically baffling because they lie between dispositional states and direct avowals. As a result he suggests that they are constructed rather than reported by the utterances of speakers.

- Contrary to both Kripke and Wright, McDowell argues that Wittgenstein's target is not our everyday understanding of meaning. It is a particular explanation of meaning that postulates internal mental states that need interpretation. Without giving way to that, the sceptical argument can be defused using Wright's suggestion. However, it provides no support for social constructionism.

- The critical aspect corresponds to the challenge faced by cognitivist approaches described in Chapter 24: How can internal or neural states possess intentionality?

- The positive aspect suggests that meaning is publicly available; however, this idea can be expanded by looking to other recent philosophers.

Session 3 Dennett and the Intentional Stance

- Dennett aims to make sense of intentional mental states by articulating the explanatory stance that deploys them. The Intentional Stance is contrasted with two others: the physical stance and the design stance.

- On this view, mental states are abstract rather than concrete entities. They are real as are centres of gravity but they are not concrete entities and do not have causal powers.

- The bald initial claim that mental states are nothing but what are deployed in the Intentional Stance has to be modified to suggest that they have separate existence in the patterns of human behaviour that are there whether or not anyone deploys the Intentional Stance.

- Dennett claims that such patterns really exist independently of our describing them.

- Thus he does not support radical social construction of meaning and mental states.

Session 4 Davidson and Radical Interpretation

- Davidson's account of linguistic meaning and mental content is based on the idea of Radical Interpretation: interpretation by an anthropologist from scratch. This is derived from Quine's radical translation.

- Davidson assumes that the full facts about meaning are available to this public perspective. This is akin to discursive psychology.

- His theoretical approach emphasizes both the interdependence of meaning and mental content and the central role of rationality for both. The ideas of the Principle of Charity and the Constitutive Principle of Rationality mark the role of rationality in both detecting minds and meanings and in their very nature.

- Davidson's account may look to falsify everyday phenomenology. Normally our understanding of other people's speech proceeds without any conscious interpretation. However, it need not be construed as actually postulating the active interpretation of otherwise meaningless data. Rather it is a rational reconstruction to reveal what could justify ascriptions of mental states and meanings whether or not we normally appeal to it.

- Davidson argues that inner mental representations are unnecessary to explain mental states and meanings.

Session 5 Singular thought and the division between mind and world

- According to Russell, thoughts can latch on to objects through descriptions or through direct acquaintance. The Theory of Descriptions is designed to explain the meaning of sentences such as 'the present King of France is bald' where there is no object corresponding to the apparent subject of the sentence: no King of France.

- Thoughts that depend on direct acquaintance depend for their very existence on a contextual connection to real objects.

- While, for Cartesian reasons, Russell restricted such thoughts to sense data and I-thoughts, more recent philosophers have argued that they also apply to everyday singular thoughts based, e.g. on the perception of objects. The argument for this is that it is the only way to make sense of the speech and action of subjects. If so, however, it is possible to be in error about the kind of thought one is thinking if no such object actually exists. And this seems to run counter to Cartesian assumptions about the mind.

- If singular thoughts exist and depend for their existence not on inner representations—perhaps corresponding to Russell's Theory of Descriptions—but on contextual relations to real objects then they cannot be represented by any internal mental representation. They would thus comprise an objection to cognitivist accounts of the mind according to which thoughts can be encoded in mental representations.

Session 6 Discursive psychology and Alzheimer's disease

- The philosophical discussion of the chapter allows a distinction between two versions of a discursive approach to the mind.

- In one, meanings are constructed in conversations; however, this faces philosophical objections drawn from an interpretation of Wittgenstein.

- A more plausible alternative, however, is one in which meanings are necessarily publicly available, available to conversations, but not constructed in those conversations. There are a family of philosophical approaches to meaning that differ in detail but share this common approach.

Chapter 26 Agency, causation, and freedom

Session 1 Agency, freedom, and neuropsychiatry

- Although we might think of exercises of free will in action and thought as always conscious, there are both normal and pathological instances where we have thoughts or we act apparently deliberately, but do not experience those acts or thoughts as consciously willed by us.

- Libet's experimental work appears to imply that there is no such thing as a conscious exercise of free will because the timing of the conscious will seems to follow a prior brain event. This is a striking consequence and invites reflection on the general relation between freedom and causal determinism.

- Spence suggests that it may be possible to retain a notion of freedom but separate it from a conscious experience. Equally we might decide that there is no genuine freedom.

- Imaging a longer time lag between brain event and conscious experience reinforces the paradoxical nature of the case because it would seem to provide time to change one's mind, but that would in turn require another, again earlier, brain event.

- There is reason to doubt Spence's claim that he has taken a materialist analysis to the limit. Where in the materialist order of things is the conscious experience of making a decision, whether or not this is already determined by non-conscious brain events? Again, this calls for further reflection on the model of the relation of mind and brain.

Session 2 Agency and volitions

- Ryle criticizes an intuitive explanation of actions based on mental causes. According to the Myth of Volitions, actions unlike movements are brought about by volitions.

- Ryle lists four criticisms of which the most important is that it starts a vicious regress because volitions would themselves have to be deliberate mental acts and thus require prior volitions and so on.

- Ryle's positive account of the difference between actions and mere movements depends on broader social and environmental factors that might overturn the ascription of voluntariness. This might not seem to be a response to the central question of what is the difference between voluntary action and what is not so much as an attempt to turn that problem aside.

- Melden usefully compares action with meaningful speech and suggests that neither requires additional mental elements either to animate linguistic signs or to make movements into actions.

Session 3 Arguments for a causal theory of mind

- Davidson suggests that action-explanation involves a rationalizing element: a reason for the action. But, in addition, he suggests that something else needs to be added to the account to distinguish a reason for an action from the reason why the act is actually committed. He suggests that the only plausible extra ingredient is causation: the reason for an action not only justifies but also causes it.

- Although there are arguments based on the logical connection between descriptions of reasons and actions, which suggest that the connection cannot be also contingent and causal, Davidson argues that these do not undermine the causal connection of the events so described. He distinguishes between how events are described and the events themselves.

- Davidson's arguments for the causal connection of reason and action fits Lewis' arguments for a causal model of explanation more generally.

Session 4 Event causation, agent causation, and irrationality

- Even given a causal model of action-explanation, the basic idea can be 'unpacked' in more than one way. While Davidson's claim that actions are caused by mental states, there are other accounts in which actions are caused by the agents themselves (i.e. the subjects who act).

- The idea of 'agent causation', however, is different from a standard Humean analysis of causation and is difficult further to explain. This threatens the idea that it is really a form of causation rather than an unanalysed notion of agency that causation was supposed to help explain.

- Davidson's separation of the causal and rational powers of mental states suggests a model for weakness of will and other partial breakdowns of reason. The causal powers of some reasons can outweigh their rational powers.

- This account of irrationality raises the general question of what normally keeps the two powers in step in Davidson's account. This suggests that Davidson's account may not be stable.

Session 5 A non-causal account of agency?

- Although Davidson's arguments against non-causal theories of action seem plausible, his argument for a causal connection is less strong. Davidson's main argument for a causal analysis of action turned on distinguishing a reason for an action from the reason.

- But according to Tanney, the same work can be done by talking of the competing motivational powers of conflicting reasons rather than separating out their rational and causal powers.

- If we reject Davidson's in other ways attractive account of mind and body this might leave something more like Ryle and Melden's picture. But if so, what response can be given to

Spence's arguments from Session 1 about the compatibility or otherwise of causal determinism and freedom of the will?

Session 6 Freedom and determinacy

- Strawson argues that the debate between freedom and determinism is hampered by a lack of clarity about the thesis of determinism; however, he suggests that appeal to moral reactions helps clarify the issue. He uses such attitudes to investigate what taking determinism seriously would be like.

- As a matter of fact we sometimes suspend natural reactive attitudes such as resentment with those we do not think are responsible for actions that impinge on us. This may be because the action was carried out under external compulsion or because the subject is not generally responsible. In such cases we adopt an objective attitude.

- Strawson suggests that putting such reactions into abeyance in general by adopting an 'objective attitude' is not an option for us. Thus we could not give up the notion of freedom in the face of a thesis of determinism. Whether this really resolves the issue of whether freedom actually is immune to determinism remains open to question.

- Strawson's approach is akin to that of Ryle and Melden. Rather than giving a substantial answer to the question of what the difference between voluntary action and mere movement consist in they all instead attempt to remind us of how the everyday distinctions are made: both in ordinary life and clinical practice.

Chapter 27 Knowledge of other minds

Session 1 An historical starting point: Cartesian theatres and the argument from analogy

- The questions addressed so far in Part V have largely concerned the ontology of mind. This chapter concerns epistemology.

- Descartes' approach to the nature of mind makes the Problem of Other Minds particularly vivid. By characterizing mental states as states in a kind of private theatre Descartes casts doubt on our access to other people's mental states.

- One influential solution appeals to an argument from analogy. The idea is that one can infer that other people are in a particular mental state because of a connection in one's own case between the nature of one's mental states and one's behaviour. By analogy with that connection one can infer the nature of another person's mental state from their outward behaviour.

- But as the Wittgensteinian philosopher Norman Malcolm argued, the argument from analogy can only work if one already knows what it means to say that someone else is, for example, in pain. And it is unclear that even that is possible given Descartes' starting point.

Session 2 Introduction to the 'theory-theory' approach

- A more recent solution likens knowledge of other minds to knowledge of unobservable entities in the physical sciences. Knowledge of other minds is thus described as theoretical knowledge, based on a theory of mental function that we are all supposed to possess.

- Thus theory-theory uses a broadly functionalist approach to the ontology of mind to solve the epistemological problem of knowledge of other minds.

Session 3 Simulation theory

- Simulation theory is an alternative to theory-theory motivated in part by the complexity of the theory that the latter presupposes. Simulationists argue that the theory presupposed by theory-theory would, for example, have to have some way to represent every belief another person might have.

- Rather than having a theory of mind, 'simulationists' suggest that one needs merely to be in possession of mind. One can use this imaginatively to put oneself in the position of others, discover what one would think oneself under such circumstances and ascribe that thought to others.

- While defenders of simulation theory stress that it is not a version of the argument from analogy because it encourages instead a gaze towards the world rather than others' mental states, this remains a matter of debate.

Session 4 The current state of the debate: evidence from autism

- Although solutions to the problems of other minds such as theory-theory and simulation theory are philosophical models, evidence can be brought from psychopathology to assess their rival claims.

- Autism has played a central role in this case. Empirical evidence from the study of autism can be brought to bear by looking, for example, at the relative ease with which they explain Wing's triad of disabilities

- One complication, however, in assessing the choice between theory-theory and simulation theory is the danger of the two positions collapsing into one. If the theory described in the former position is known merely implicitly then it is not clear that it really is incompatible with simulation theory. The difference may be one of emphasis.

- In the case of simulation theory and theory-theory the opposing views become blurred if knowledge of the theory in question in the latter case is construed as implicit knowledge and if the ability to simulate in the former case can be described through a regimented theory.

Session 5 Rationality and direct access to mental states

- While the responding to the Problem of Other Minds has suggested theoretically promising work on autism, there is reason to doubt that it is really or empirically a pressing problem.

- A third option—in addition to theory-theory and simulation theory—suggests that mental states can be expressed in behaviour.

- Unlike other approaches, this approach does not take the description of behaviour to be independent of a description of underlying mental states. It is not, in other words, reductionist.

On this approach, one can take in in experience the fact that someone else is, for example, in pain. This approach may reconcile our everyday untroubled talk of other minds with a philosophical model.

Chapter 28 Personal identity and schizophrenia

Session 1 Personal identity: evidence and constitution

- While they are distinct, there is a plausible connection between personal identity and the ability to identify oneself and one's actions.

- Self-identification and, arguably self-identity, can be fragmented in psychopathology.

- While evidence such as fingerprints can help identity people, such evidence does not *constitute* personal identity.

Session 2 Four kinds of identity antirealism

- There are a number of philosophical positions that hold that there is no such thing as personal identity.

- David Hume argues for a form of antirealism about personal identity on the basis of introspection. He only ever experienced particular thoughts and never a uniting subject of them.

- However, denying personal identity seems to be paradoxical and self-undermining.

Session 3 Identity and mental illness

- Psychopathology presents conditions that threaten the nature of the personal identity or self-identification who suffers them.

However, there are also conditions, such as Alzheimer's that may threaten the very possibility of the continued existence of a person.

- To settle whether severe dementia really does threaten the existence of a person depends on deciding what personal identity involves.

Session 4 Theories of personal identity

- There are a number of ways of answering the question: What does personal identity consist in? Approaches include: physical, spiritual, capacity, and what we called 'closure'.

- Locke's influential account places the burden on autobiographical memory. Possession of such memory is a necessary condition of identity through time. To be a person is to have self-awareness in action.

Session 5 Identity and mental illness again

- Alzheimer's disease threatens a subject's ability to think of themselves as the same through time and thus threatens the very idea of their continued identity as a person.

- Things are not so clear-cut in the case of schizophrenia. While thought disorder suggests some difficulty with self tracking it is possible to distinguish between identifying oneself as a subject and identifying oneself as an agent. If so schizophrenia may threaten only one aspect of personal identity, on a Lockean account.

- The impact of other conditions on personal identity depends on one's analysis of identity, which remains very much a matter of philosophical debate informed by clinical findings.

References

Abbany, Z. (2001). Caught in a trap. *New Scientist*, 169 (2283): 46–49.

Adshead, G. (1996). Psychopathy, other-regarding moral beliefs, and responsibility. (Commentary on Fields, 1996). *Philosophy, Psychiatry, & Psychology*, 3(4): 279–282.

Adshead, G. (1997). Pathological autobiographies. (Commentary on Harré, 1997). *Philosophy, Psychiatry, & Psychology*, 4(2): 111–114.

Adshead, G. (1999). Psychopaths and other-regarding beliefs. (Commentary on Benn, 1999). *Philosophy, Psychiatry, & Psychology*, 6(1): 41–44.

Adshead, G. (2000). Commentary on Case 7.1, 'Alan Masterson—clear and present danger'. In *In Two Minds: A casebook of psychiatric ethics* (ed. D. Dickenson and K.W.M. Fulford). Oxford: Oxford University Press, pp. 233–236.

Adshead, G. (2001). Commentary on 'Impossible things before breakfast': (Commentary on Burman (2001) and Richmond (2001)). *Philosophy, Psychiatry, & Psychology*, 8/1: 33–38.

Adshead, G. (2002). Through a glass, darkly: Commentary on Ward. (Commentary on Ward, 2002). *Philosophy, Psychiatry, & Psychology*, 9(1): 15–18.

Adshead, G. (2003). Measuring moral identities: psychopaths and responsibility. (Commentary on Ciocchetti, 2003). *Philosophy, Psychiatry, & Psychology*, 10(2): 185–188.

Agich, G.J. (1983). Disease and Value: A rejection of the Value-neutrality Thesis. *Theoretical Medicine*, 4, 27–41.

Agich, G.J. (1993). *Autonomy and Long-term Care*. Oxford: Oxford University Press.

Agich, G.J. (1994). Key Concepts: autonomy. *Philosophy, Psychiatry, & Psychology*, 1(4): 267–270.

Alarcón, R.D., Bell, C.C., Kirmayer, L.J., Lin, K-M., Üstün, B., and Wisner, K.L. (2002). Beyond the funhouse mirrors: research agenda on culture and psychiatric diagnosis. In *A Research Agenda for DSM-V* (ed. D.J. Kupfer, M.B. First, and D.E. Regier). Washington, DC: American Psychiatric Association, pp. 219–282.

Alderson, P. (1990). *Choosing for Children: parents' consent to surgery*. Oxford: Oxford University Press.

Alderson, P. (1994). *Children's Consent to Surgery*. Buckingham: Open University Press.

Allen, B. (1995). *Truth in Philosophy*. London: Harvard University Press.

Allott, P., Loganathan, L., and Fulford, K.W.M. (2002). Discovering hope for recovery. In *Innovation in Community Mental Health: international perspectives*. Special Issue. *Canadian Journal of Community Mental Health*, 21(2): 13–33.

Amador, X.F. and David, A.S. (1998). *Insight and Psychosis*. Oxford: Oxford University Press.

American Group for the Advancement of Psychiatry (1990). *A Casebook for Psychiatric Ethics*. New York: Brunner and Mazel.

American Psychiatric Association (1952). *Diagnostic and Statistical Manual of Mental Disorders* (1st edn, DSM-I). Washington, DC: American Psychiatric Association.

American Psychiatric Association (1968). *Diagnostic and Statistical Manual of Mental Disorders* (2nd edn, DSM-II). Washington, DC: American Psychiatric Association.

American Psychiatric Association (1980). *Diagnostic and Statistical Manual of Mental Disorders* (3rd edn, DSM-III). Washington, DC: American Psychiatric Association.

American Psychiatric Association (1987). *Diagnostic and Statistical Manual of Mental Disorders*, (3rd edn, revised DSM-III-R). Washington DC: American Psychiatric Association.

American Psychiatric Association (1994). *Desk Reference to Diagnostic Criteria from DSM-IV*. Washington, DC: American Psychiatric Association.

American Psychiatric Association (1994). *Diagnostic and Statistical Manual Of Mental Disorders* (4th edn, DSM–IV). Washington, DC: American Psychiatric Association.

American Psychiatric Association (2000) *Diagnostic and Statistical Manual of Mental Disorders*, 4th edn, text revised (DSM-IV-TR). Washington, DC: American Psychiatric Association.

Anastasi, A. (1968). *Psychological Testing*, 3rd ed. New York: Macmillan.

Andreasen, N.C. (2001). *Brave New Brain: Conquering Mental Illness in the Era of the Genome*. Oxford: Oxford University Press.

Anon (1996). Lazy wife has her head examined. *The Times*. 2 September.

Anon (1997). Editorial: The crisis in psychiatry. *Lancet*, 5 April.

Anon (1997) Anorexia trigger found in the brain. *Sunday Times*, 13 April.

Anscombe, G.E.M. (1975). The first person. In *Mind and Language* (ed. S. Guttenplan). Oxford: Oxford University Press, pp. 45–65.

Anscombe, G.E.M. (1959). Intention. *Proceedings of the Aristotelian Society* 57: 321–332. (Reprinted in White, A.R. (ed.) (1968). *The Philosophy of Action*. Oxford: Oxford University Press.)

Anzia, D.J. and La Puma, J. (1991). An annotated bibliography of psychiatric medical ethics. *Academic Psychiatry*, 15: 1–7.

Arens, K. (1996). Wilhelm Griesinger: psychiatry between philosophy and praxis. (Commentary by Aaron Mishara, 1996) *Philosophy, Psychiatry, & Psychology*, 3: 147–164.

Aristotle (2000). *Nicomachean Ethics* (ed Crisp, R.) Cambridge: Cambridge University Press.

Atkinson, A.P. (2001). Pathological beliefs, damaged brains: a review of Max Coltheart and Martin Davies, Ed., Pathologies of Belief. *Philosophy, Psychiatry, & Psychology*, 8/2(3): 225–230.

Audi, R. (ed.) (1999). *The Cambridge Dictionary of Philosophy*. Cambridge: Cambridge University Press.

Austin, J.L. (1956–7). A plea for excuses. *Proceedings of the Aristotelian Society* 57:1–30. (Reprinted in White, A.R., ed. (1968) *The Philosophy of Action*. Oxford: Oxford University Press.)

Austin, J.L. (1966). Three ways of spilling ink. *Philosophical Review*, 75: 427–440. (Reprinted in White, A.R. (ed.) (1968). *The Philosophy of Action*. Oxford: Oxford University Press.)

Austin, J.L. (1968). A plea for excuses. In *The Philosophy of Action* (ed. A.R. White). Oxford: Oxford University Press, pp. 19–42.

Avramides, A. (2000). *Other Minds*. London: Routledge.

Ayer, A.J. (1936). *Language, Truth and Logic*. London: Victor Gollancz.

Ayer, A.J. (1956). *The Problem of Knowledge*. London: Macmillan.

Ayer, A.J. (1973). *The Central Questions of Philosophy*. London: Weidenfeld and Nicholson. (Ayer, A.J. (1976). London: Pelican Books.)

Ayer, A.J. (1980). *Hume*. PastMasters Series. Oxford: Oxford University Press.

Ayers, M. (1991). *Locke, Volume II: Ontology*. London: Routledge.

Baggini, J. and Fosl, P.S. (2003). *The Philosopher's Toolkit: a compendium of philosophical concepts and methods*. Oxford: Blackwell Publishing.

Baier, A. (1981). Cartesian persons. *Philosophia*, 10: 169–188.

Baker, G. (2003). Wittgenstein's method and psychoanalysis. In *Nature and Narrative: an introduction to the new philosophy of psychiatry* (ed. K.W.M. Fulford, K.J. Morris, J.Z. Sadler, and G. Stanghellini). Oxford: Oxford University Press, Chapter 3.

Baker, L.R. (1991). Has content been naturalised? In *Meaning in Mind: Fodor and his critics* (ed. B. Loewer and G. Rey). Oxford: Blackwell.

Baker, L.R. (1997). Persons in metaphysical perspective. In *The Philosophy of Roderick Chisholm* (ed. L. Hahn). Chicago, IL: Open Court, pp. 433–453.

Baker, L.R. (2000). *Persons and Bodies*. Cambridge: Cambridge University Press.

Banzato, C.E.M., and Pereira, M.E.C. (2005). Eyes and ears wide open: values in the clinical setting. *World Psychiatry*, 4(2): 90.

Barnes, B. (1974). *Scientific Knowledge and Sociological Theory*. London: Routledge.

Baron, M.W., Petit, P., and Slote, M. (1997). *Three Methods of Ethics*. Oxford: Blackwell.

Baron-Cohen, S. (ed.) (1993). *Understanding Other Minds: perspectives from autism*. Oxford: Oxford University Press.

Baron-Cohen, S. (1995). *Mindblindness: an essay on autism and theory of mind*. Cambridge, MA: MIT Press.

Barondess, J.A. (1979). Disease and illness – a crucial distinction. *The American Journal of Medicine* 66: 375–376.

Bayley, J. (1999). *Iris and Her Friends: a memoir of memory and desire*. New York: W.W.Norton.

Bayne, T. and Pacherie, E. (2004). Bottom-up or top-down? Campbell's rationalist account of monothematic delusions. *Philosophy, Psychiatry, & Psychology*, 11(1): 1–12.

Bayne, T. and Pacherie, E. (2004). Experience, belief, and the interpretive Fold. *Philosophy, Psychiatry, & Psychology*, 11(1): 81–86.

Beauchamp T. (1999). The philosophical basis of psychiatric ethics. In *Psychiatric Ethics* (ed. S. Bloch, P. Chodoff, and S.A. Green), (3rd edn). Oxford: Oxford University Press, Chapter 3.

Beauchamp, T.L. and Childress, J.F. (1989; 4th edn 1994). *Principles of Biomedical Ethics*. Oxford: Oxford University Press.

Bebbington, PE. (1997). Psychiatry: science, meaning and purpose. *British Journal of Psychiatry* 130: 222–228

Bebbington, P.E. and Broome, M.R. (2004). Exploiting the Interface between Philosophy and Psychiatry. *International Review of Psychiatry*, 16, 3:179–183.

Bechtel, W. (1988). *Philosophy of Science: an overview for cognitive science*. Hillsdale, NJ: Lawrence Erlbaum.

Bechtel, W. and Graham, G. (ed.) (1999). *A Companion to Cognitive Science*. Oxford: Blackwell.

Beck, A.T., Ward, C., Mendelson, M., Mock, J., and Erbaugh, J. (1961). An inventory for measuring depression. *Archives of General Psychiatry*, 4: 561–571.

Beer, M.D. (1996). The dichotomies: psychosis/neurosis and functional/organic: a historical perspective. *History of Psychiatry*, vii, 231–255.

Beer, M.D. (2000). The Nature, Causes, and Types of Ecstasy. (Commentary on Wolff, 2000). *Philosophy, Psychiatry, & Psychology*, 7(4): 311–316.

Belnap, N. (1961–62). Tonk, Plonk and Plink. *Analysis*, 22: 130–134.

Bendelow, G. (2004). Commentary: Sociology and concepts of mental illness. (Commentary on Fulford and Colombo, 2004a) *Philosophy, Psychiatry, & Psychology*, 11(2): 145–146.

Benn, P. (1999). Commentary on Matthews (1999). Moral vision. *Philosophy, Psychiatry, & Psychology*, 6(4): 317–320.

Benn, P. (1999). Freedom, resentment, and the psychopath. *Philosophy, Psychiatry, & Psychology*, 6(1): 29–40.

Benn, P. (1999). Response to the Commentaries. *Philosophy, Psychiatry, & Psychology*, 6(1): 57–58.

Benn, P. (2003). The responsibility of the psychopathic offender: a comment on Ciocchetti. (Commentary on Ciocchetti, 2003). *Philosophy, Psychiatry, & Psychology*, 10(2): 189–192.

Bentall, R.P. (1992). A proposal to classify happiness as a psychiatric disorder. *Journal of Medical Ethics*, 18: 94–98.

Bentall, R.P. (2003). *Madness Explained*. London: Penguin.

Berghmans, R. (1998). Suicide, euthanasia, and the psychiatrist (Commentary on Burgess and Hawton, 1998). *Philosophy, Psychiatry, & Psychology*, 5(2): 131–136.

Bergo, B. (2004). Psychoanalytic models: Freud's debt to philosophy and his Copernican revolution. In T*he Philosophy of Psychiatry: a companion* (ed. J. Radden). New York: Oxford University Press, pp. 338–350.

Bergson, H. (1927) *Essai sur les données immédiates de la conscience*. Paris: Presses Universitaire de France.

Berkeley, G. ([1710] 1975). Principles of human knowledge. In *Philosophical Works*. London: Dent.

Bermudez, J.L. (2001). Normativity and rationality in delusional psychiatric disorders. *Mind & Language*, 16(5): 457–493.

Bernet, R., Kern, I., and Marbach, E. (1993). *An Introduction to Husserlian Phenomenology*. Evanston: Northwestern University Press.

Berrios, G.E. (1992). Phenomenology, Psychopathology and Jaspers: a Conceptual History. *History of Psychiatry*, 3:303–28.

Berrios, G.E. (1993). Phenomenology and psychopathology: Was there ever a relationship? *Comprehensive Psychiatry* 34: 213–220.

Berrios, G.E. (1996). *The History of Mental Symptoms. Descriptive psychopathology since the nineteenth century*. Cambridge: Cambridge University Press.

Berrios, G.E. and Freeman, H. (ed.). (1991) *150 Years of British Psychiatry: 1841–1991*. London: Gaskell.

Berrios, G.E. and Porter, R. (ed.) (1995). *History of Clinical Psychiatry: the origin and history of psychiatric disorders*. London: Athlone Press.

Bettelheim, B. (1982). *Freud and Man's Soul*. London: Penguin Books.

Bhugra, D. (1996). *Psychiatry and Religion*. London and New York: Routledge.

Bin, K. (1992) *Essais de psychopathologie phénoménologique*. Paris: Presse Universitaire de France.

Bin, K. (2001). Cogito and I: a bio-logical approach. *Philosophy, Psychiatry, & Psychology*, 8(4): 331–336.

Bindman, J., Maingay, S., and Szmukler, G. (2003). The Human Rights Act and mental health legislation. *British Journal of Psychiatry*, 182: 91–94.

Binns, P. (1994). Affect, agency, engagement: conceptions of the person in philosophy, neuropsychiatry, and psychotherapy', with a response by Peter Caws (1994). *Philosophy, Psychiatry, & Psychology*, 1(1): 13–23.

Binswanger, L. (1975). *Being in the World*. (trans. J. Needleman). London: Souvenir Press.

Bird, A. (1998) *The Philosophy of Science*. London: Routledge.

Bird, A. (2001). *Thomas Kuhn*. Chesham: Acumen.

Birley, J. (2000). 'Psychiatric ethics: an international open society'. Chapter 11, in *In Two Minds: a casebook of psychiatric ethics* (ed. D. Dickenson and K.W.M. Fulford). Oxford: Oxford University Press, pp. 327–335.

Birley, J.L.T. (1993) Invited response to Bentall, R. (1993). *British Journal of Psychiatry*, 162: 540–541.

Bishop, J.L.T. (1983). Agent-causation. *Mind*, 92. 61–79

Biswanger, L. (1963). *Being-in-the-World*. New York: Basic Books.

Blackburn, S. (1994) *The Oxford Dictionary of Philosophy*. Oxford: Oxford University Press.

Blackburn, S. (2001) *Think: a compelling introduction to philosophy*. Oxford: Oxford Paperbacks.

Blakemore, C. and Greenfield, S. (ed) (1987). *Mindwaves*. Oxford: Blackwell.

Blankenburg, W. (1971) *Der Verlust der Natuerlichen Selbstverstaendlichkeit. Ein Beitrag zur Psychopathologie Symptomarmer Schizophrenien*. Stuttgart: Enke.

Blankenburg, W. (2001). First steps toward a psychopathology of common sense. *Philosophy, Psychiatry, & Psychology*, 8(4): 303–316.

Bleuler, E. (1911). *Dementia Praecox; or the group of schizophrenias*. New York: International Universities Press. (Translated and printed by IUP in 1950.)

Bloch, S. and Chodoff, P. (1981 second edition 1991). *Psychiatric ethics* (first edition). Oxford: Oxford University Press.

Bloch, S. and Porgiter, R. (1999). Codes of ethics in psychiatry. In *Psychiatric Ethics* (ed. S. Bloch, P. Chodoff, and S.A. Green). Oxford: Oxford University Press, Chapter 6.

Bloch, S. and Reddaway, P. (1977). *Russia's Political Hospitals: The abuse of psychiatry in the Soviet Union*. London: Victor Gollancz.

Bloch, S., Chodoff, P., and Green, S. A., (1999) *Psychiatric ethics* (third edition). Oxford: Oxford University Press.

Block, N. (ed.) (1980). What is functionalism. In *Readings in Philosophy of Psychology*. Cambridge, MA: Harvard University Press. p 171–184.

Bloor, D. (1976). *Knowledge and Social Imagery*. London: Routledge. Reprinted (1991). *Knowledge and Social Imagery*. Chicago: Chicago University Press.

Bloor, D. (1997). *Wittgenstein, Rules and Institutions*. London: Routledge.

Bluglass, R. and Boden, P. (1990). *Principles and Practice of Forensic Psychiatry*. Edinburgh: Churchill Livingstone.

Bolton, D. (1997). Encoding of meaning: deconstructing the meaning/causality distinction. (With commentaries by Segal, 1997, with a response by Bolton, 1997, and by Wiggins and Schwartz, 1997, with a further response by Bolton, 1997). *Philosophy, Psychiatry, & Psychology*, 4(4): 255–268.

Bolton, D. (1997). Response to the Commentary by Segal (1997). *Philosophy, Psychiatry, & Psychology*, 4(4): 273–276.

Bolton, D. (1997). Response to the Commentary by Wiggins and Schwartz (1997). *Philosophy, Psychiatry, & Psychology*, 4(4): 283–284.

Bolton, D. (2000). Continuing commentary alternatives to disorder. *Philosophy, Psychiatry, & Psychology*, 7(2): 141–154.

Bolton, D. (2004). Shifts in the philosophical foundations of psychiatry since Jaspers: implications for psychopathology and psychotherapy. *International Review of Psychiatry*, 16(3): 184–189.

Bolton, D. and Hill, J. (1997). Commentary on 'Reasons and causes'. *Philosophy, Psychiatry, & Psychology*, 4(4): 319–322.

Bolton, D. and Hill, J. ([1996] 2005). *Mind, Meaning and Mental Disorder*. 2nd Edition Oxford: Oxford University Press.

Boorse, C. (1975). On the distinction between disease and illness. *Philosophy and Public Affairs*, 5: 49–68.

Boorse, C. (1976) Wright on functions. *Philosophy Review*, 85, 70–86

Boorse, C. (1976). What a theory of mental health should be. *Journal of Theory and Social Behaviour*, 6: 61–84.

Boorse, C. (1977) Health as a theoretical concept. *Philosophy of Science*, 44, 542–573.

Boorse, C. (1997) A Rebuttal on Health. Ch 1 in Humber J.M. and Almeder, R.F. eds *What is Disease?* Totowa, New Jersey: Humana Press, pps 1–134.

Boss, M. (1963) *Psychoanalysis and Daseinalaysis*. (Transl by Lefebre, L. New York: Basic Books.

Boss, M. (1963). *Daseinanalysis*. New York: Basic Books.

Boss, M. (1984) Existential Foundations of Medicine and Psychology (transl by Conway, S. and Cleaves, A). New York: Jason Aronson.

Bovet, P. and Parnas, J. (1993). Schizophrenic delusions: a phenomenological approach. *Schizophrenia Bulletin*, 19: 579–597.

Bowie, M. (1991). *Lacan*. London: Fontana.

Boyd, R. (1980). Materialism without reductionism. In *Readings in Philosophy of Psychology* (ed. N. Block). London: Methuen.

Boyd, R. (1999). On the current status of scientific realism. In *The Philosophy of Science* (ed. R. Boyd, P. Gaspar, and J.D. Trout). Cambridge, MA: MIT Press, pp. 195–222.

Boyd, R., Gasper, P. and Trout, J.D. (ed.) (1991). *The Philosophy of Science*. Cambridge, MA: MIT Press.

Boyne, R. (1990) *Foucault and Derrida: the other side of reason*. London: Unwin Hyman.

Bracken, P. (1999). Phenomenology and psychiatry. *Current Opinion in Psychiatry*, 12: 593–596.

Bracken, P. (2001). Post modernity and post traumatic stress disorder. *Social Science and Medicine*, 53: 733–743.

Bracken, P. (2001). The radical possibilities of home treatment: postpsychiatry in action. In *Acute Mental Health Care in the Community: intensive home treatment* (ed. N. Brimblecombe). London: Whurr Publishers.

Bracken, P. (2002) *Trauma: Culture, Meaning and Philosophy*. London: Whurr Publishers.

Bracken, P. (2002). Commentary on 'Listening to Foucault'. (Commentary on Lilleleht, 2002). *Philosophy, Psychiatry, & Psychology*, 9(2): 187–188.

Bracken, P. and Petty, C. (ed.) (1998). *Rethinking the Trauma of War*. London: Free Association Books.

Bracken, P. and Thomas, P. (2001). Postpsychiatry: a new direction for mental health. *British Medical Journal*, 322: 724–727.

Bracken, P. and Thomas, P. (2002). Time to move beyond the mind-body split. *British Medical Journal*, 325: 1433–1434.

Bracken, P. and Thomas, P. (2005) *Postpsychiatry*. Oxford: Oxford University Press.

Bracken, P., Giller, J., and Summerfield, D. (1997). Rethinking mental health: work with survivors of wartime violence and refugees. *Journal of Refugee Studies*, 10: 431–442

Bracken, P.J. (1995). Beyond Liberation: Michael Foucault and the Notion of a Critical Psychiatry. *Philosophy, Psychiatry, & Psychology*, 2(1): 1–14.

Bracken, P.J. (1998) Hidden Agendas: Deconstructing Post Traumatic Stress Disorder. Chapter 2 in Bracken, P.J. and Petty, C. (eds) *Rethinking the Trauma of War*. London and New York: Free Association Books, pps 38–59.

Bracken, P.J. (1999). Phenomenology and psychiatry. *Current Opinion in Psychiatry*, 12: 593–596.

Bracken, P.J. (1999). The importance of Heidegger for psychiatry. (Commentary on Svenaeus, 1999). *Philosophy, Psychiatry, & Psychology*, 6(2): 83–86.

Braddon-Mitchell, D. and Jackson, F. (1996). *Philosophy of Mind and Cognition*. Oxford: Blackwell.

Brandom, R. (1998). Knowledge and the social articulation of the space of reasons. *Philosophical and Phenomenological Research* 55: 895–908.

Braude, S.E. (1995) *First person plural: multiple personality and the philosophy of mind* Boston: Rowman & Littlefield Publishers

Braude, S.E. (1995). The social relocation of personal identity. (Commentary on Hinshelwood, 1995) *Philosophy, Psychiatry, & Psychology*, 2(3): 205–208.

Braude, S.E. (1996). Multiple personality and moral responsibility. Commentary by Clark, S.R.L. pp. 106–117 and Shuman, D.W. pp. 59–60. *Philosophy, Psychiatry, & Psychology*, 3(1): 137–54.

Braude, S.E. (1997). A discursive account of multiple personality disorder. (Commentary on Gillett, 1997a) *Philosophy, Psychiatry, & Psychology*, 4(3): 223–226.

Braude, S.E. (1998). False memory syndrome. (Commentary on Hamilton, 1998) *Philosophy, Psychiatry, & Psychology*, 5(4): 299–304.

Braude, S.E. (2003). Counting persons and living with alters: Comments on Matthews. (Commentary on Matthews, 2003) *Philosophy, Psychiatry, & Psychology*, 10(2): 153–156.

Brazier, M. (1992). *Medicine, Patients and the Law*. London: Penguin.

Brazier, M. (1995). Who should be committable? (Commentary on Lavin, 1995). *Philosophy, Psychiatry, & Psychology*, 2(1): 49–50.

Brendel, D.H. (2003). A pragmatic consideration of depression and melancholia. (Commentary on Radden, 2003). *Philosophy, Psychiatry, & Psychology*, 10(1): 53–56.

Brentano, F. ([1874] 1995). *Psychology from an Empirical Standpoint* (trans. Antos C. Rancurello, D.B. Terrell, and Linda L. McAlister). London: Routledge.

Brett, C. (2002). Psychotic and mystical states of being: connections and distinctions. (Commentary on Brettford, 2002a). *Philosophy, Psychiatry, & Psychology*, 9(4): 321–342.

Brett, C. (2002). Spiritual experience and psychopathology: dichotomy or interaction? (Commentary on Marzanski and Bratton, 2002). *Philosophy, Psychiatry, & Psychology*, 9(4): 373–380.

Brett, C. (2002). Response to the commentaries. The application of nondual epistemology to anomalous experience in psychosis. *Philosophy, Psychiatry, & Psychology*, 9(4): 353–358.

Breuer, J. and Freud, S. *Studies in Hysteria*. In Freud (1955). London: The Hogarth Press.

Brewer, W.F. and Lambert, B. (2001). The theory-ladenness of observation and the theory-ladenness of the rest of the scientific process. *Philosophy of Science*, 68.

Bridgman, P.W. (1927). *The Logic of Modern Physics*. New York: Macmillan.

British Medical Association (2002). *Medical Ethics Today: its Practice and Philosophy*. London: British Medical Association.

Brock, D.W. (1998). Time frame of preferences, dispositions, and advance directives.(Commentary on Savulescu and Dickenson, 1998). *Philosophy, Psychiatry, & Psychology*, 5(3): 251–254.

Brockmeier, J. (1997). Autobiography, narrative, and the Freudian concept of life history. (with commentaries by Holmes, 1997, pp. 201–204, and Robinson, 1997, pp. 205–208, and response Brockmeier, 1997, pp. 209–212). *Philosophy, Psychiatry, & Psychology*, 4(3): 175–200.

Brockmeier, J. (1997). Response to the Commentaries. *Philosophy, Psychiatry, & Psychology*, 4(3): 209–212.

Broekman, J. (2000). Unordered lives. (Commentary on Robinson, 2000). *Philosophy, Psychiatry, & Psychology*, 7(3): 223–228.

Broome, M.R. (2004). The rationality of psychosis and understanding the deluded. (Commentary for Special Issue on Delusion). *Philosophy, Psychiatry, & Psychology*, 11(1): 35–42.

Brown, G.W. and Harris, T. (1978). *Social Origins of Depression*. London: Tavistock.

Brown, G.W., Birley, J.L.T., and Wing. J.K. (1972). The influence of family life on the course of schizophrenia. *Journal of Health and Social Behaviour*, 9: 203–214.

Brown, H. (1977). *Perception Theory and Commitment*. Chicago, IL: University of Chicago Press.

Brown, S., Collinson, D., and Wilkinson, R. (ed.). (1996). *Dictionary of Twentieth Century Philosophers*. London: Routledge.

Burgess, S. (1998). Time frame of preferences, dispositions, and advance directives. (Commentary on Savulescu and Dickenson, 1998). *Philosophy, Psychiatry, & Psychology*, 5(3): 255–258.

Burgess, S. and Hawton, K. (1998). Suicide, euthanasia, and the psychiatrist. *Philosophy, Psychiatry, & Psychology*, 5(2): 113–126.

Burgess, S. and Hawton, K. (1998). Response to the Commentaries. *Philosophy, Psychiatry, & Psychology*, 5(2): 151–152.

Burman, E. (2001). Reframing current controversies around memory: feminist contributions. *Philosophy, Psychiatry, & Psychology*, 8(1): 21–32.

Burman, E. (2001). Remembering feminisms: a response to the commentary. *Philosophy, Psychiatry, & Psychology*, 8(1): 39–40.

Burnside, J.W. (1998). Suicide, euthanasia, and the psychiatrist (Commentary on Burgess and Hawton, 1998). *Philosophy, Psychiatry, & Psychology*, 5(2): 141–144.

Burton, N. (forthcoming) *Psychiatry*. Oxford: Blackwell.

Burwood, S., Gilbert, P., and Lennon, K. (1999). *Philosophy of mind* London: University College London.

Butler, Rt. Hon., the Lord. (1975). Chairman, *Report of the Committee on Mentally Abnormal Offenders*, Cmnd. 6244. London: HMSO.

Bynam, W.F. (1983). Psychiatry in its historical context. In *Handbook of Psychiatry*, Vl. 5 (ed. M. Shepherd and O.L. Zangwill). Cambridge: Cambridge University Press.

Calnan, M. (1987). *Health and Illness: the lay perspective*. London: Routledge.

Campbell, A.B. and Higgs, R. (1982). *In That Case: Medical Ethics in Everyday Practice*. London: Darton, Longman and Todd.

Campbell, A.V. (1994). Dependency: the foundational value in medical ethics. In *Medicine and Moral Reasoning* (ed. K.W.M. Fulford, G.R. Gillett, and J.M. Soskice). Cambridge: Cambridge University Press, p. 184.

Campbell, E.J., Scadding, J.G., and Roberts, R.S. (1979). The concept of disease. *British Medical Journal*, 2: 757–762.

Campbell, J. (1999). Schizophrenia, the space of reasons and thinking as a motor process. *The Monist*, 82: 609–625.

Campbell, J. (2001). Rationality, meaning, and the analysis of delusion. *Philosophy, Psychiatry, & Psychology*, 8(2–3): 89–100.

Campbell, J. (2002). The ownership of thoughts. (Commentary on Coliva, 2002) *Philosophy, Psychiatry, & Psychology*, 9: 35–40.

Campbell, P.G. (1996). What we want from crisis services. In *Speaking Our Minds: an anthology* (ed. J. Read and J. Reynolds). Basingstoke: Macmillan for The Open University, pp. 180–183.

Campbell, P.G. (2002). What we want from crisis services. In *Healthcare Ethics and Human Values* (ed. K.W.M. Fulford, D. Dickenson, and T.H. Murray). Oxford: Blackwell Science.

Campbell, P.G. (2000). Diagnosing agency. *Philosophy, Psychiatry, & Psychology*, 7(2): 107–120.

Campbell, P.G. (2000). Naturalizing agency: a response to the Commentary. *Philosophy, Psychiatry, & Psychology*, 7(2): 123–124.

Campbell, R. (ed.) (1992). *Mental Lives: case studies in cognition*. Oxford: Blackwell.

Canfield, J. (1990). *The Looking Glass Self: an examination of self-awareness*. New York: Praeger.

Caplan, A.L., Engelhardt, H.J., and McCartney, J.J. (ed.) (1981). *Concepts of Health and Disease*. Reading, MA: Addison-Wesley Publishing Co.

Caramazza, A. (ed.) (1990). *Cognitive Neuropsychology and Neurolinguistics*. Baltimore, MD: Johns Hopkins University.

Carrasco, J. and Lecic-Tosevski, D. (2000). Specific types of personality disorder. In *New Oxford Textbook of Psychiatry* (ed. M. Gelder, J. Lopez-Ibor, and N. Andraesen). Oxford: Oxford University Press, pp. 934–937.

Carruthers, P. (1996). Autism as mind-blindness. In *Theories of Theories of Mind* (ed. P. Carruthers and P. Smith). Cambridge: Cambridge University Press, 257–273.

Carruthers, P. and Boucher, J. (1998). *Language and Thought: interdisciplinary themes*. Cambridge: Cambridge University Press.

Carruthers, P. and Smith, P.K. (ed.) (1996). *Theories of Theories of Mind*. Cambridge: Cambridge University Press.

Cartwright, N. (1983). *How the Laws of Physics Lie*. Oxford: Oxford University Press.

Cartwright, N. (1999). The reality of causes in a world of instrumental laws. In *The Philosophy of Science* (ed. R. Boyd, P. Gasker, and J.D. Trout). Cambridge, MA: MIT Press, pp. 379–386.

Cartwright, N. (2000). *The Dappled World : a study of the boundaries of science*. Cambridge: Cambridge University Press.

Casenave, G. (2003). Death, disability, and dialogue. (Commentary on Clegg, J. and Lansdall-Welfare, R., 2003) *Philosophy, Psychiatry, & Psychology*, 10(1): 87–90.

Caws, P. (1979) *Sartre*. London: Routledge.

Caws, P., (1994) Commentary on Binns, P. (1994) ''Affect, Agency, and Engagement'', *Philosophy, Psychiatry, & Psychology*, 1(1), 25–26.

Chadwick, R.F. (1994). *Ethics and the Professions*. Aldershot: Avebury.

Chadwick, R.F. (1994). Kant, thought insertion, and mental unity. *Philosophy, Psychiatry, & Psychology*, 1(2): 105–114.

Chadwick, R.F. (1995). Commentary: Karl Jaspers and Edmund Husserl—III (Walker, 1995). *Philosophy, Psychiatry, & Psychology*, 2: 83–84.

Chadwick, R.F. (1998). Commentary on 'Is Mr Spock mentally competent?'. (Commentary on Charland, 1998) *Philosophy, Psychiatry, & Psychology*, 5(1): 83–86.

Chalmers, A. (1999). *What is this thing called science?* Buckingham: Open University Press.

Chapman, J. (1966). The early symptoms of schizophrenia. *British Journal of Psychiatry*, 112: 225–251.

Charland, L.C. (1998). Is Mr Spock mentally competent? Competence to consent and emotion. *Philosophy, Psychiatry, & Psychology*, 5(1): 67–82.

Charland, L.C. (1998). Response to the Commentaries. *Philosophy, Psychiatry, & Psychology*, 5(1): 93–96.

Charland, L.C. (2004). Character: moral treatment and the personality disorders. In *The Philosophy of Psychiatry: a companion* (ed. J. Radden). New York: Oxford University Press, pp. 64–77.

Charland, L.C. (2002). Commentary on Tuke's healing discipline. (Commentary on Lilleleht, 2002). *Philosophy, Psychiatry, & Psychology*, 9(2): 183–186.

Charney, D.S., Barlow, D.H., Botteron, K., Cohen, J.D., Goldman, D., Gur, R.E., Lin, K-M, López, J.F., Meador-Woodruff, J.H., Moldin, S.O., Nestler, E.J., Watson, S.J., and Zalcman, S.J. (2002). Neuroscience Research Agenda to Guide Development of a Pathophysiologically Based Classification System. In *A Research Agenda for DSM-V* (ed. D.J. Kupfer, M.B. First, and D.E. Regier). Washington, DC: American Psychiatric Association, pp. 31–84.

Chihara, C.S. and Fodor, J.A. (1991). Operationalism and ordinary language: a critique of Wittgenstein. In *The Nature of Mind* (ed. D. Rosenthal). Oxford: Oxford University Press. 137–150.

Child, W. (1994). *Causality, Interpretation and the Mind*. Oxford: Oxford University Press.

Chisholm, R. (1969). The loose and popular and the strict and philosophical senses of identity. In *Perception and Personal Identity* (ed. N.S. Care and R.H. Grimm). Cleveland, OH: Case Western Reserve.

Chisholm, R. (1976). *Person and Object*. La Salle, IL: Open Court.

Chodoff, P. (1999). Misuse and abuse of psychiatry: an overview. In *Psychiatric ethics*, (3rd edn). (ed. S. Bloch, P. Chodoff, and S.A. Green). Oxford: Oxford University Press, Chapter 4.

Christen, Y. and Churchland, P. (1992) *Neurophilosophy and Alzheimer's Disease*. Heidelberg: Springer-Verlag.

Christodoulou, G.N. (1977). The syndrome of Capgras. *British Journal of Psychiatry*, 130: 556–64.

Church, J. (2004). Social constructionist models: making order out of disorder—on the social construction of madness. In *The Philosophy of Psychiatry: a companion* (ed. J. Radden). New York: Oxford University Press, pp. 393–408.

Churchland, P. (1979). *Scientific Realism and the Plasticity of Mind*. Cambridge: Cambridge University Press.

Churchland, P.S. (1989). *Neurophilosophy*. Cambridge, MA: MIT Press.

Ciocchetti, C. (2003). The responsibility of the psychopathic offender. *Philosophy, Psychiatry, & Psychology*, 10(2): 175–184.

Ciocchetti, C. (2003). Some thoughts on diverse psychopathic offenders and legal responsibility. (Response to commentaries). *Philosophy, Psychiatry, & Psychology*, 10(2): 195–198.

Cioffi, F. (1988). Exegetical myth-making in Grunbaum's Indictment of Popper and Exoneration of Freud. In Clark and Wright (1988). Oxford: Blackwell, pp. 61–87.

Clare, A. (1979). The disease concept in psychiatry. In *Essentials of Postgraduate Psychiatry* (ed. P. Hill, R. Murray, and A. Thorley). New York: Academic Press, Grune & Stratton.

Clark, P. and Wright, C. (ed.) (1988). *Mind, Psychoanalysis and Science*. Oxford: Blackwell.

Clark, S.R.L. (1996). Multiple personality and moral responsibility. (Commentary on Braude, 1996). *Philosophy, Psychiatry, & Psychology*, 3(1): 55–58.

Clark, S.R.L. (2003). Constructing persons: the psychopathology of identity. (Commentary on Matthews, 2003) *Philosophy, Psychiatry, & Psychology*, 10(2): 157–160.

Clarke, D. (1982). *Descartes' Philosophy of* Science. Manchester: Manchester University Press.

Clegg, J. and Lansdall-Welfare, R. (2003). Death, disability, and dogma. *Philosophy, Psychiatry, & Psychology*, 10/1: 67–80.

Clegg, J. and Lansdall-Welfare, R. (2003). Commentary on 'Living with contested knowledge and partial authority'. *Philosophy, Psychiatry, & Psychology*, 10(1): 99–102.

Coate, M. (1964). *Beyond All Reason*. London: Constable.

Code, L. (1996). Loopholes, gaps, and what is held fast. (Commentary on Potter, 1996). *Philosophy, Psychiatry, & Psychology*, 3(4): 255–260.

Coetzee, J.M. (2003) Commentary "Fictional Beings". *Philosophy, Psychiatry, & Psychology*, 10(2): 133–134.

Coetzee, P.H. and Roux, A.P.J. (eds) (2002) *Philosophy from Africa*. 2nd edition. Cape Town: Oxford University Press.

Coliva, A. (2002). Thought insertion and immunity to error through misidentification. (Commentary by Campbell, J. (2002, pp. 35–40) and response by Coliva, A. (2002, pp. 41–46) *Philosophy, Psychiatry, & Psychology*, 9: 27–34.

Coliva, A. (2002). On what there really is to our notion of ownership of a thought. (Response to Campbell, 2002) *Philosophy, Psychiatry, & Psychology*, 9: 41–46.

Collins, H. (1985). *Changing Order*. London: Sage.

Collins, S. (1982) *Selfless Persons: Imagery and Thought in Theravada Buddhism* Cambridge: Cambridge University Press.

Colman, S. (2003). What's in the box then, Mum?—Death, Disability and Dogma. (Commentary on Clegg, J. and Lansdall-Welfare, R., 2003) *Philosophy, Psychiatry, & Psychology*, 10(1): 81–86.

Colombo, A. (1997). *Understanding Mentally Disordered Offenders: a multi-agency perspective*. Aldershot, UK: Ashgate.

Colombo, A., Bendelow, G., Fulford, K.W.M., and Williams, S. (2003). Evaluating the influence of implicit models of mental disorder on processes of shared decision making within community-based multi-disciplinary teams. *Social Science & Medicine*, 56: 1557–1570.

Colombo, A., Bendelow, G., Fulford, K.W.M., and Williams, S. (2003). Model behaviour. *Openmind*, 125: 10–12.

Coltheart, M. and Davies, M. (eds). (2000). *Pathologies of Belief*. Oxford: Blackwell.

Cooper, J. (1999) Chapter 2 in *Promoting Mental Health Internationally*, (eds.) Eisenberg, L., Goldberg, D., De Girolamo, G., and Cooper, J. London: Hayuards Heath Gaskell.

Cooper, J. (2003) Editorial: Prospects for Chapter V of ICD-11 and DSM-V. *British Journal of Psychiatry*, vol 183:379–381.

Cooper, J.E., Kendell, R.E., Gurland, B.J., Sharpe, L., Copeland, J.R.M., and Simon, R. (1972). *Psychiatric Diagnosis in New York and London*. Maudsley Monograph No. 20. London: Oxford University Press.

Cordess, C. (ed.) (2001). *Confidentiality and Mental Health*. London: Jessica Kingsley Publishers.

Cornwell, J. (ed.) (2004). *Explanations* Oxford: Oxford University Press.

Corvi, R. (1997). *An Introduction to the Thought of Karl Popper*. London: Routledge.

Cottingham, J. (1986). *Descartes*. Oxford: Blackwell.

Cottingham, J. (1988). *The Rationalists*. Opus series: *A History of Western Philosophy*, Vol. 4. Oxford: Oxford University Press.

Coulter, J. (1979). *The Social Construction of Mind*. London: Macmillan.

Coulter, J. (1999). Discourse and mind. *Human Studies*, 22: 163–81.

Cox, J., Campbell, A. V., and Fulford, K.W.M. (eds) (forthcoming) *Medicine of the Person: Faith, Science and Values in Healthcare Provision*. London: Jessica Kingsley.

Crammer, J.L. (1994). English asylums and English doctors: Where Scull is wrong. *History of Psychiatry*, 5: 103–115.

Crane, T. (1991). Why indeed: Papineau on supervenience. *Analysis*, 51: 32–37.

Crane, T. (1991). All God has to do. *Analysis*, 51. 235–44

Crary, A. and Read, R. (eds) (2000) *The New Wittgenstein*. London: Routledge.

Crisp, R. (1994). How should we measure need? (Commentary on Marshall, 1994) *Philosophy, Psychiatry, & Psychology*, 1(1): 37–38.

Crisp, R. (1994). Quality of life and health care. In *Medicine and Moral Reasoning* (ed. K.W.M. Fulford, G.R. Gillett, and J.M. Soskice). Cambridge: Cambridge University Press.

Culver, C.M. and Gert, B. (2004). Competence. In *The Philosophy of Psychiatry: a companion* (ed. J. Radden). New York: Oxford University Press, pp. 258–270.

Currie, G. (1996). Simulation-theory, theory-theory and the evidence from autism. In *Theories of Theories of Mind* (ed. P. Carruthers and P. Smith). Cambridge: Cambridge University Press, 242–256.

Currie, G. and Jureidini, J. (2001). Delusion, Rationality, Empathy: A Commentary on Davies *et al.* (2001). *Philosophy, Psychiatry, & Psychology*, 8(2–3): 159–162.

Cutting, J. (1997). *Principles of Psychopathology: two worlds-two minds-two hemispheres*. Oxford: Oxford University Press.

Cutting, J. (1999). *Psychopathology and Modern Philosophy*. The Forest Publishing Company.

Cutting, J. (2001). On Kimura's Ecrits de psychopathologie phénomenologique. (Commentary on Bin, 2001). *Philosophy, Psychiatry, & Psychology*, 8(4): 337–338.

D'Amico (1995). Is disease a natural kind? *Journal of Medicine and Philosophy*, 20: 551–569.

Dancy, J. (1985). *An Introduction to Contemporary Epistemology*. Oxford: Blackwell.

Dancy, J. (1993). *Moral Reasons*. Oxford: Blackwell.

David, A.S. (1990). Insight and psychosis. *British Journal of Psychiatry*, 156: 798–808.

David, A.S. (1994). Insight, delusion, and belief. (Commentary on Gillett, 1994) *Philosophy, Psychiatry, & Psychology*, 1(4): 237–240.

David, A.S. (1999). On the impossibility of defining delusions. (Commentary on Jones, 1999) *Philosophy, Psychiatry, & Psychology*, 6(1): 17–20.

David, A. (2000). The clinical neuropsychology of schizophrenia. In *New Oxford Textbook of Psychiatry* (ed. M. Gelder, J. Lopez-Ibor, and N. Andraesen). Oxford: Oxford University Press, pp. 576–579.

Davidovskii, I.V. (1962) *Problems of Causality in Medicine*. Moscow: The State Medical Publisher.

Davidovskii, I.V. and Snezhnevsky, A.V. (1972) *Schizophrenia*. Moscow: News of the Academy of Medical Science.

Davidson, D. (1980). *Essays on Actions and Events*. Oxford: Oxford University Press.

Davidson, D. (1982). Paradoxes of irrationality. In *Philosophical Essays on Freud* (ed. J. Hopkins and R. Wollheim). Cambridge: Cambridge University Press, pp. 289–305.

Davidson, D. (1984). *Inquiries into Truth and Interpretation*. Oxford: Oxford University Press.

Davidson, D. (1991). What is present to the mind? In *Consciousness* (ed. E. Villanueva). *Philosophical Issues*, 6: 197–213.

Davidson, D. (1995). Laws and cause. *Dialectica*, 49: 263–279.

Davidson, L. (1994). Insight, delusion, and belief. (Commentary on Gillett, 1994) *Philosophy, Psychiatry, & Psychology*, 1(4): 243–244.

Davies, M. (1996). Textbook on Medical Law. London: Blackwell.

Davies, M. (forthcoming) *The Mind*. Oxford: Oxford University Press.

Davies, M. and Coltheart, M. (2000). Introduction: pathologies of belief. In *Pathologies of Belief* (ed. M. Coltheart and M. Davies). Oxford: Blackwell, Chapter 1.

Davies, M. and Stone, T. (ed.) (1995). *Folk Psychology: a guide to the theory of mind debate*. Oxford: Blackwell.

Davies, M. and Stone, T. (ed.) (1995). *Mental Simulation: evaluations and applications*. Oxford: Blackwell.

Davies, M., Coltheart, M., Langdon, R., and Breen, N. (2001). Monothematic delusions: towards a two-factor account. *Philosophy, Psychiatry, & Psychology*, 8(2–3): 133–158.

Davies, P.C.W. and Brown, J.R. (1986). *The Ghost in the Atom*. Cambridge: Cambridge University Press.

Davis, R. (1997). *The Gift of Dyslexia*. London: Souvenir.

de Boer, T. (1978). *The Development of Husserl's Thought* (trans. by Theodore Plantinga). The Hague: Martinus Nijhoff.

De Pauw, K. (2000). Depersonalization disorder. In *New Oxford Textbook of Psychiatry* (ed. M. Gelder, J. Lopez-Ibor, and N. Andraesen). Oxford: Oxford University Press, pp. 831–833.

Deeley, P.Q. (1999). Ecological understandings of mental and physical illness. *Philosophy, Psychiatry, & Psychology*, 6(2): 109–124.

Deeley, P.Q. (1999). Response to the Commentaries. *Philosophy, Psychiatry, & Psychology*, 6(2): 135–144.

Deeley, P.Q. (2003) Social, cognitive, and neural constraints on subjectivity and agency: implications for dissociative identity disorder. (Commentary on Matthews, 2003a) *Philosophy, Psychiatry, & Psychology*, 10(2): 161–168.

Dennett, D. (1984). *Elbow Room*. Cambridge, MA: MIT Press.

Dennett, D. (1987). True believers: the *Intentional Strategy* and why it works. In *The Intentional Stance*. Cambridge, MA: MIT Press, pp. 13–35.

Dennett, D. (1991). *Consciousness Explained*. Boston: Little, Brown.

Dennett, D. (1991). Real patterns. *Journal of Philosophy*, 88: 27–51.

Dennett, D. (1996). *Kinds of Minds*. London: Weidenfeld & Nicolson.

Dennett, D. (2003). *Freedom Evolves* New York: Viking.

Dennett, D. and Humphrey, N. (1998). Speaking for our selves. In *Brainchildren* (ed. D. Dennett). Cambridge, MA: MIT Press, pp. 31–58.

Department of Health (1999). *National Service Framework for Mental Health: Modern Standards and Service Models*. London: Department of Health.

Department of Health (2000). *The NHS Plan, A plan for investment, A plan for reform*. London: The stationery office.

Department of Health (2002). *Draft Mental Health Bill*. Cm5538-I. London: The stationery office.

Department of Health (2002). *Improvement, Expansion and Reform: the next 3 years. Priorities and Planning Framework, 2003–06*. London: Department of Health.

Department of Health (2003). *Inspiring Hope: recognising the importance of spirituality in a whole person approach to mental health*. National Institute for Mental Health in England.

Department of Health (2004) *NIMHE Guiding Statement on Recovery*. London: Department of Health.

Department of Health (2004). *Mental Health Care Group Workforce Team: national mental health workforce strategy*. London: National Institute for Mental Health in England.

Department of Health (2004). *The Ten Essential Shared Capabilities: a framework for the whole of the mental health workforce*. London: The Sainsbury Centre for Mental Health, the NHSU (National Health Service University), and the NIMHE (National Institute for Mental Health in England).

Department of Health (2004). *Interim Report of the National Steering Group: guidance on new ways of working for psychiatrists in a multi-disciplinary and multi-agency context*. London: The Royal College of Psychiatrists, National Institute of Mental Health in England, and the Modernisation Agency—Changing Workforce Programme.

Department of Health (2003). *Meeting the Spiritual and Religious Needs of Patients and Staff: Guidance for Staff*. London: The stationery office.

Department of Health and Welsh Office (1993) *Code of Practice: Mental Health Act* 1983. London: HMSO.

Depraz, N. (2003). Putting the *époché* into practice: schizophrenic experience as illustrating the phenomenological exploration of consciousness. In *Nature and Narrative: an introduction to the new philosophy of psychiatry* (ed. K.W.M. Fulford, K.J. Morris, J.Z. Sadler, and G. Stanghellini). Oxford: Oxford University Press, Chapter 12.

Descartes, R. ([1637]1998) *Discourse on Method*. (Translated by Cress, D.A.) Indianapolis: Hackett.

Descartes, R. ([1649]1988) *The passions of the soul*. (Translated by Voss, S.) Indianapolis: Hackett.

Descartes, R. ([1641]1996). *Meditations on First Philosophy*. Cambridge: Cambridge University Press.

d'Espagnat, B. (1976). *Conceptual Foundations of Quantum Mechanics*, (2nd edn). Reading, MA: W.A. Benjamin Inc.

d'Espagnat B. (1983). *In Search of Reality*. New York: Springer-Verlag.

Devitt, M. and Sterelny, K. (1999). *Language and Reality: an introduction to the philosophy of language*. Oxford: Blackwell.

Diamond, J. (1993). Born to be gay? *The Sunday Times*, 15 July.

Dickenson, D. (1994) Children's Informed Consent to Treatment: Is the Law an Ass? (1994) Guest Editorial, *Journal of Medical Ethics*, 20(4): 205–206.

Dickenson, D. (1997) *Property, Women, and Politics: Subjects or Objects?* Cambridge: Polity Press.

Dickenson, D. (1997). Rationality and its discontents. In *Property, Women and Politics: subjects or objects?* Cambridge: Polity Press, pp. 148–152.

Dickenson, D. and Fulford, K.W.M. (2000). *In Two Minds: a casebook of psychiatric ethics*. Oxford: Oxford University Press.

Dickenson, D. and Johnson, M. (ed.). (1993). *Death, Dying and Bereavement*. London: Sage Publications in association with The Open University.

Dickenson, D. and Jones, D. (1995). True wishes: the philosophy and developmental psychology of children's informed consent. *Philosophy, Psychiatry, & Psychology*, 2(4): 287–303.

Dilling, H. (2000) Classification. Chapter 1.11 in Geder, M.G. *et al*, 2000 *New Oxford Textbook of Psychiatry*. Oxford: Oxford University Press.

Dilman, I. (1999). *Free Will: an historical and philosophical introduction*. London: Routledge.

Dilthey, W. (1976). *Selected Writings* (ed. and trans. H.P. Rickman). Cambridge: Cambridge University Press.

Dilthey, W. (1977). Ideas concerning a descriptive and analytic psychology. In *Descriptive Psychology and Historical Understanding* (trans. R.M. Zaner and K.L. Heiges). The Hague: Martinus Nijhoff, pp. 21–120.

Dingwall, R. (1976). *Aspects of Illness*. London: Martin Robertson.

Discussion, Various Contributors (1961). In *Field Studies in the Mental Disorders* (ed. J. Zubin). New York: Grune and Stratton, pp. 23–50.

Dodd, J. (2000) *An identity theory of truth*. London: MacMillan.

Dominion, J. (1994). Commentary on normal grief: Good or bad? Health or disease? (Commentary on Kopelman, 1994). *Philosophy, Psychiatry, & Psychology*, 1(4): 221–222.

Dorland's American Illustrated Medical Dictionary, (25th edn). (1974). Philadelphia, PA: Saunders.

Dray, W. (1957). *Laws and Explanation in History* Oxford: Oxford University Press.

Dray, W. (1964). *Philosophy of History*. Englewood Cliffs, N.J.: Prentice Hall.

Dreijmanis, J. (1989). *Karl Jaspers on Max Weber*. New York: Paragon House.

Dresser, R. (1998). Time frame of preferences, dispositions, and advance directives. (Commentary on Savulescu and Dickenson, 1998). *Philosophy, Psychiatry, & Psychology*, 5(3): 247–250.

Dretske, F. (1981). *Knowledge and the Flow of Information*. Cambridge, MA: MIT Press.

Dretske, F. (1991). *Explaining Behavior: reasons in a world of causes*. Cambridge, MA: MIT Press.

Dreyfus, H.L. (1991). *Being-in-the-World: A commentary on Heidegger's Being and Time*. Division 1. Cambridge, MA: MIT Press.

Drury, J. (1994). Cognitive science and hermeneutic explanation: symbiotic or incompatible frameworks. *Philosophy, Psychiatry, & Psychology*, 1(1): 41–50.

Duff, A. (1977). Psychopathy and moral understanding. *American Philosophical Quarterly* 14(3): 189–200.

Duff, R.A. (1986). *Trials and Punishments*. Cambridge: Cambridge University Press.

Duff, R.A. (1990). *Intention, Agency and Criminal Liability*. Oxford: Blackwell.

Duff, R.A. (1996). Psychopathy, other-regarding moral beliefs, and responsibility. (Commentary on Fields, 1996). *Philosophy, Psychiatry, & Psychology*, 3(4): 283–286.

Duhem, P. (1962). *The Aim and Structure of Physical Theory*. New York: Atheneum.

Duhem, P. (1985). *To Save the Phenomena: an essay on the idea of physical theory from Plato to Galileo*. Chicago: University of Chicago Press.

Dummett, M. (1981). *The Interpretation of Frege's Philosophy*. London: Duckworth.

Dummett, M. (1993). *Origins of Analytical Philosophy*. London: Duckworth.

Dummett, M. (1993). What is a theory of meaning I and II? In *The Seas of Language*. Oxford: Oxford University Press.

Dworkin, R. (1993). Life past reason. In *Life's Dominion: an argument about abortion, euthanasia, and individual freedom*. New York: Knopf, pp. 218–229.

Dyer, A. (1999). Psychiatry as a profession. In *Psychiatric Ethics* (ed. S. Bloch, P. Chodoff, and S.A. Green), (3rd edn). Oxford: Oxford University Press, Chapter 5.

Eacott, M.J. (1998). False memory syndrome. (Commentary on Hamilton, 1998) *Philosophy, Psychiatry, & Psychology*, 5(4): 305–308.

Earle, W.J. (1992). *Introduction to Philosophy*. New York: McGraw–Hill.

Eastman, N.L.G. and Peay, J. (1999). (Eds) *Law Without Enforcement: integrating mental health and justice*. Oxford and Portland, OR: Hart Publishing.

Eastman, N.L.G. (1998). Time frame of preferences, dispositions, and advance directives. (Commentary on Savulescu and Dickenson, 1998). *Philosophy, Psychiatry, & Psychology*, 5(3): 259–262.

Eastman, N.L.G. and Hope, R.A. (1988). Ethics of enforced medical treatment: the balance model. *Journal of Applied Philosophy*, 5: 49–59.

Edie, J.M. (ed) (1964). *The Primacy of Perception*. (trans. various)

Editorial (1997). A comet at heaven's gate. *New Scientist*, 5 April.

Editorial (1997). Inadmissible evidence. *New Scientist*, 22 March.

Edwards, D. and Potter, J. (1992). *Discursive Psychology*. London: Sage.

Edwards, P. and Pap, A. (ed.). (1973). *A Modern Introduction to Philosophy*, 3rd edn. New York: The Free Press/London: Collier Macmillan Publishers.

Edwards, R.B. (Ed) (1982) *Psychiatry and ethics: insanity, rational autonomy, and mental health care*. New York: Prometheus Books.

Eekelaar, J. (1995). True wishes. (Commentary on Dickenson and Jones, 1995). *Philosophy, Psychiatry, & Psychology*, 2(4): 305–308.

Ehrlich, E., Ehrlich, L., and Pepper, G.B. (ed.) (1986). *Karl Jaspers: basic philosophical writings*. Athens, OH: Ohio University Press.

Eigen, M. (2001). *Ecstasy*. Middletown, CT: Wesleyan University Press.

Eilan, N. (2001). Meaning, truth, and the self: A Commentary on Campbell (2001) and Parnas and Sass (2001). *Philosophy, Psychiatry, & Psychology*, 8(2–3): 121–132.

Eilan, N., Hoerl, C., McCormack, T., and Roessler, J. (ed.) (2005). *Joint Attention—Communication and Other Minds: issues in philosophy and psychology*. Oxford: Oxford University Press.

Ellenberger, H. (1970). *The Discovery of the Unconscious*. New York: Basic Books. (London: Fontana, 1994.)

Elliott, C. (1994). Puppetmasters and personality disorders: Wittgenstein, mechanism, and moral responsibility. *Philosophy, Psychiatry, & Psychology*, 1(2): 91–100.

Elliott, C. (1996). Key Concepts: Criminal Responsibility. *Philosophy, Psychiatry, & Psychology*, 3(4): 305–308.

Elliott, C. (1998). Commentary on 'Is Mr Spock mentally competent?'. (Commentary on Charland, 1998) *Philosophy, Psychiatry, & Psychology*, 5(1): 87–88.

Elliott, C. (1999). *A Philosophical Disease: bioethics, culture and identity*. London: Routledge.

Ellis, A. (1996). *Human Cognitive Neuropsychology: a textbook with readings*. Hove, UK: Psychology Press.

Engelhardt, H.T. Jr. (1975) The concepts of health and disease. In Engelhardt, H.T., Jr. and Spicker, S.F. eds. *Evaluation and explanation in the biological sciences*. Dordrecht, Holland: D. Reidel.

Erwin, E. (1996) *A Final Accounting: Philosophical and Empirical Issues in Freudian Psychology*. Cambridge, Mass, USA: MIT Press.

Erwin, E. (ed) (2002) *The Freud Encyclopedia*. New York: Routledge.

Evans, G. (1980). Things without the mind. In *Philosophical subjects: essays presented to P.F. Strawson* (ed. Z. van Straaten). Oxford: Clarendon Press.

Evans, G. (1982). *The Varieties of Reference*. Oxford: Clarenden

Evnine, S. (1991). *Donald Davidson*. Oxford: Polity Press.

Ey, H. (1954) *Etudes Psychiatriques*. Paris: Desclee de Brouwer.

Eysenck, H.J. (1968). Classification and the problems of diagnosis. In *Handbook of Abnormal Psychology*. London: Pitman Medical, Chapter 1.

Eysenck, H.J. (1985). *Decline and Fall of the Freudian Empire*. London: Penguin.

Eysenck, H.J. and Wilson, G.D. (ed.) (1973). *The Experimental Study of Freudian Theories*. London: Methuen.

Fabrega Jr. H. (1999). Elegant case history analysis or original contribution? (Commentary on Deeley, 1999) *Philosophy, Psychiatry, & Psychology*, 6(2): 125–128.

Fabrega, H. (1972). The study of disease in relation to culture. *Behavioural Science*, 17: 183–203.

Fairbairn, G.J. (1998). Suicide, language, and clinical practice. *Philosophy, Psychiatry, & Psychology*, 5(2): 157–170.

Fairbairn, G.J. (1998). Response to the Commentaries. *Philosophy, Psychiatry, & Psychology*, 5(2): 179–180.

Falzer, P. and Davidson, L. (2002). Language, logic, and recovery: a commentary on Van Staden. (Commentary on Van Staden, 2002) *Philosophy, Psychiatry, & Psychology*, 9(2): 131–136.

Falzer, P. and Davidson, L. (2002). Language, logic, and recovery: a commentary on Van Staden. (Commentary on Van Staden, 2002). *Philosophy, Psychiatry, & Psychology*, 9(2): 131–136.

Fann, K.T. (1969) (ed) *Symposium on J. L. Austin*. London: Routledge and Kegan Paul.

Farias, V. (1989). *Heidegger and Nazism*. Philadelphia: Temple University Press.

Farmer, A., McGuffin P., and Williams, J. (2002). *Measuring Psychopathology*. Oxford: Oxford University Press.

Feinberg, J. (1986). *Harm to Self: the moral limits of the criminal law*. Oxford: Oxford University Press.

Feldman, F. (1980). Identity, necessity, and events. In *Readings in the Philosophy of Psychology* (ed. N. Block), Vol. 1. Cambridge, MA: Harvard University Press. pp 148–55

Fields, L. (1996). Psychopathy, other-regarding moral beliefs, and responsibility. *Philosophy, Psychiatry, & Psychology*, 3(4): 261–278.

Fields, L. (1996). Response to the Commentaries. *Philosophy, Psychiatry, & Psychology*, 3(4): 291–292.

Fields, L. (1996). Sanity and irresponsibility. (Commentary on Wilson, 1996). *Philosophy, Psychiatry, & Psychology*, 3(4): 303–304.

Fine, A. (1984) 'And not anti-realism either'. *Nous* 19, 51–65 reprinted in (1988, pp. 359–368). *Scientific Knowledge: basic issues in the philosophy of science* (ed J.A. Kournay). Belmont, CA: Wadsworth Publishing Company.

Fine, A. (1999). The natural ontological attitude. In *The Philosophy of Science* (ed. R. Boyd, P. Gasker, and J.D. Trout). Cambridge, MA: MIT Press, pp. 261–277.

Fingarette, H. (1972). Insanity and responsibility. *Inquiry*, 15: 6–29.

First, M.B. (2005) Keeping an eye on clinical utility. *World Psychiatry*, 4(2): 87.

First, M.B., Bell, C.C., Cuthbert, B., Krystal, J.H., Malison, R., and Offord, D.R. (2002). Personality disorders and relational disorders: a research agenda for addressing crucial gaps in DSM. In *A Research Agenda for DSM-V* (ed. D.J. Kupfer, M.B. First, and D.E. Regier). Washington, DC: American Psychiatric Association, pp. 123–200.

Fisher, S. and Greenberg, R. (1977). *The Scientific Credibility of Freud's Theories and Therapy*. New York: Columbia University Press.

Fitzpatrick, R., Hinton, J., Newman, S., Scrambler, G., and Thompson, J. (1984). *The Experience of Illness*. London: Tavistock Publications.

Flanagan, O. (1992). *Consciousness Reconsidered*. Cambridge, MA: MIT Press.

Flanagan, O. (1994). Multiple identity, character transformation, and self-reclamation. In *Philosophical Psychopathology* (ed. G. Graham and G.L. Stephens). Cambridge, MA: MIT Press, pp. 135–162.

Flew, A. (1973). *Crime or Disease?* New York: Barnes and Noble.

Fodor, J.A. (1984). Observation reconsidered. *Philosophy of Science*, 51: 23–43.

Fodor, J.A. (1987). *Psychosemantics*. Cambridge, MA: MIT Press.

Fodor, J.A. (1991). Propositional attitudes. In *The Nature of Mind* (ed. D. Rosenthal). Oxford: Oxford University Press, pp. 325–338.

Foot, P. (ed.) (1967). Moral beliefs. In *Theories of Ethics*. Oxford: Oxford University Press, pp. 83–92.

Foucault, M. (1965). *Madness and Civilization* (trans. R. Savage). New York: Mentor Books.

Foucault, M. (1989). *Madness and Civilisation*. London: Routledge.

Fourcher, L.A. (1998). Relativism and the social-constructivist paradigm. (Commentary on Gillett, 1998). *Philosophy, Psychiatry, & Psychology*, 5(1): 49–54.

Freedman, A.M. and Halpern, A.L. (1999) The Psychiatrist's Dilemma: a Conflict of Roles in Executions. *Australian and New Zealand Journal of Psychiatry*, 33, 629–635.

Frege, G. (1892). *On Sense and Reference* (Reprinted in Geach, P. and Black, M. Translations from the writings of Gottlob Frege Oxford: Blackwell, 1960).

Frege, G. (1980). *Foundations of Arithmetic* (trans. J.L. Austin). Oxford: Blackwell.

Freud, S. ([1894] 1962). *The Neuro-Psychoses of Defence* (Freud, 1955), Vol. III.

Freud, S. (1900) *The Interpretation of Dreams* (Freud, 1955), Vol. IV.

Freud, S. (1955) *Standard Edition of the Complete Psychological Works of Sigmund Freud*. London: Hogarth Press.

Freud, S. (1963). *Analytic Therapy* (Freud, 1955), Vol. XVI; also in Pelican Freud Library, Vol. 1(1973), London: Penguin.

Freud, S. (1966). *Project for a Scientific Psychology* (Freud, 1955), Vol I.

Freud, S. (1973). 'Introductory Lectures on *Psychoanalysis*. Pelican Freud Library, Vol. 1. London: Penguin.

Freud, S. (1977). 'Dora' case study. In *Case Histories I*. The Pelican Freud Library, Vol. 8. London: Penguin, pp. 41, 45–49.

Frith, C. (1992). *The Cognitive Neuropsychology of Schizophrenia*. Hillsdale, NJ: Lawrence Earlbaum.

Frith, C. (1996). Free will in the light of neuropsychiatry. (Commentary on Spence, 1996) *Philosophy, Psychiatry, & Psychology*, 3(2): 91–94.

Frith, C. (1998). Deficits and pathologies. In *A Companion to Cognitive Science* (ed. W. Bechtel and G. Graham). Oxford: Blackwell, pp. 380–390.

Fuchs, T. (2001). The Tacit dimension. (Commentary on Blankenburg, 2001). *Philosophy, Psychiatry, & Psychology*, 8(4): 323–326.

Fuchs, T. (2002). Mind, meaning, and the brain. (Commentary on Glannon, 2002) *Philosophy, Psychiatry, & Psychology*, 9(3): 261–264.

Fulford, K.W.M. (1988) Diagnosis, Classification and Phenomenology of Mental Illness. Ch. 1 in Rose, N. (ed) *Essential Psychiatry*. Oxford: Blackwell Scientific Publications.

Fulford, K.W.M. (1989, reprinted 1999). *Moral Theory and Medical Practice*. Cambridge: Cambridge University Press.

Fulford, K.W.M. (1990) Philosophy and Medicine: The Oxford Connection. *British Journal of Psychiatry*, 157, pp. 111–115.

Fulford, K.W.M. (1991). Evaluative delusions: their significance for philosophy and psychiatry. *British Journal of Psychiatry*, 159 (Suppl. 14): 108–112.

Fulford, K.W.M. (1992). Thought insertion and insight: disease and illness paradigms of psychotic disorder. In *Phenomenology, Language and Schizophrenia* (eds M. Spitzer, F. Vehlen, M.A. Schwartz, and C. Mund). New York: Springer-Verlag, p. 358.

Fulford, K.W.M. (1993). Bioethical blind spots: four flaws in the field of view of traditional bioethics. *Healthcare Analysis*, 1: 155–162.

Fulford, K.W.M. (1993). Invited response to Bentall R. A proposal to classify happiness disease as a psychiatric disorder (*Journal of Medical Ethics*, 1992; 18: 94–98). *British Journal of Psychiatry*, 162: 541–542.

Fulford, K.W.M. (1993). Praxis makes perfect: illness as a bridge between biological concepts of disease and social conceptions of health. *Theoretical Medicine*, 14: 321–324.

Fulford, K.W.M. (1993). Value, action, mental illness and the law. In *Action and Value in Criminal Law* (ed. S. Shute, J. Gardner, and J. Horder). Oxford: Oxford University Press, pp. 279–310.

Fulford, K.W.M. (1994 [1988]) Diagnosis, classification and phenomenology of mental illness. Chapter 1 In *Essential Psychiatry*, 2nd Edition, (ed. N.D.B. Rose), Oxford: Blackwell Scientific Publications.

Fulford, K.W.M. (1995). Psychiatry, compulsory treatment and the value-based model of mental health. In *Introductory Applied Ethics* (ed. B. Almond). Oxford: Blackwell.

Fulford, K.W.M. (1995). The concept of disease and the meaning of patient-centred care. Chapter 1, In *Essential Practice in*

Patient-Centred Care (ed. K.W.M. Fulford, S. Ersser, and T. Hope). Oxford: Blackwell Science.

Fulford, K.W.M., (1995) Introduction: Just getting started. pps 1–3, Introduction to *Philosophy, Psychology, and Psychiatry*, ed. A. Phillips Griffiths. Cambridge: Cambridge University Press, for the Royal Institute of Philosophy.

Fulford, K.W.M. (1995) Mind and Madness: New Directions in the Philosophy of Psychiatry. Chapter 1 in *Philosophy, Psychology and Psychiatry*, Phillips Griffiths, A ed., Cambridge: Cambridge University Press, for the Royal Institute of Philosophy.

Fulford, K.W.M. (1996). Value, illness and action: delusions in the new philosophical psychopathology. In *Philosophical Psychopathology* (ed. G. Graham and G Lynn Stephens). Cambridge, MA: MIT Press.

Fulford, K.W.M. (1998) Mental illness, Concept of. 5000 word entry for R. Chadwick (ed), *Encylopedia of Applied Ethics*. Vol 3, pps 213–233. San Diego: Academic Press

Fulford, K.W.M. (1998). Commentary: Aristotle's function argument and the concept of mental illness. *Philosophy, Psychiatry, & Psychology*, 5(3): 215–220.

Fulford, K.W.M. (1998). Dissent and dissensus: the limits of consensus formation in psychiatry. In *Consensus Formation in Health Care Ethics* (ed. H.A.M.J. ten Have and H.-M. Saas). Philosophy and Medicine Series. Dordrecht: Kluwer, pp. 175–192.

Fulford, K.W.M. (1998). Replacing the Mental Health Act 1983? How to change the game without losing the baby with the bath water or shooting ourselves in the foot. *Psychiatric Bulletin*, 22: 666–668.

Fulford, K.W.M., and Sadler, J.Z. (eds.) (1998) Special Issue on Euthanasia. *Philosophy, Psychiatry, & Psychology*, 5(2).

Fulford, K. W. M. (1999) *From Culturally Sensitive to Culturally Competent: A Seminar in Philosophy and Practice Skills*. Ch 3 in Bhui, K. and Olajide, D. eds. *Mental Health Service Provision for a Multi-cultural Society*. pp 21–42. London: W.B. Saunders Company Ltd.

Fulford, K.W.M. (2000) Teleology without Tears: Naturalism, Neo-Naturalism and Evaluationism in the Analysis of Function Statements in Biology (and a Bet on the Twenty-first Century). *Philosophy, Psychiatry, & Psychology* 7(1): 77–94.

Fulford, K.W.M. (2000). Disordered minds, diseased brains and real people. Chapter 4, in *Philosophy, Psychiatry and Psychopathy: personal identity in mental disorder* (ed. C. Heginbotham). Avebury Series in Philosophy in association with The Society for Applied Philosophy. Aldershot: Ashgate Publishing Ltd, pp. 47–73.

Fulford, K.W.M. (2001) Philosophy into practice: the case for ordinary language philosophy. Part 2. In *Health, Science and Ordinary Language* (ed. L. Nordenfelt). Amsterdam: Rodopi, pp. 171–208.

Fulford, K.W.M. (2001). The paradoxes of confidentiality. a philosophical introduction. In *Confidentiality and Mental Health* (ed. C. Cordess). London: Jessica Kingsley Publishers, pp. 7–23.

Fulford, K.W.M. (2002). Report to the Chair of the DSM-VI Task Force from the Editors of *Philosophy, Psychiatry, & Psychology* on 'Contentious and noncontentious evaluative language in psychiatric diagnosis' (Dateline 2010). In *Descriptions & Prescriptions: Values, Mental Disorders, and the DSMs* (ed. J.Z. Sadler). Baltimore, MD: The Johns Hopkins University Press, Chapter 21.

Fulford, K.W.M. (2002). Values in psychiatric diagnosis: Executive Summary of a Report to the Chair of the ICD-12/DSM-VI Coordination Task Force (Dateline 2010). *Psychopathology*, 35: 132–138.

Fulford, K.W.M. (2003). *Mental Illness: definition, use and meaning*. Long entry for Post, S. G. (ed.). *Encyclopedia of Bioethics*, (3rd edn). New York: Macmillan.

Fulford, K.W.M. (2004) Values-Based Medicine: Thomas Szasz's Legacy to Twenty-First Century Psychiatry. Ch 2 in Schaler, J.A (ed) *Szasz Under Fire: The Psychiatric Abolitionist Faces His Critics*, pps 57–92. Chicago and La Salle, Illinois: Open Court Publishers.

Fulford, K.W.M. (2004). Insight and delusion: from Jaspers to Kraepelin and back again via Austin. In *Insight and Psychosis*, (2nd edn) (ed. X.F. Amador and A.S. David). New York: Oxford University Press.

Fulford, K.W.M. (2004). Ten principles of values-based medicine. Chapter 14, In *The Philosophy of Psychiatry: a companion* (ed. J. Radden). New York: Oxford University Press.

Fulford, K.W.M. (2005) Values in Psychiatric Diagnosis: Developments in Policy, Training and Research. *Psychopathology* 38(4): 171–176.

Fulford, K.W.M. And Benington, J. (2005). VBM[2]: a collaborative values-based model of health care decision making combining medical and management perspectives. Chapter 5, In *Medical and Management Perspectives in Child and Adolescent Psychiatry* (ed. G. Williams). Oxford: Oxford University Press.

Fulford, K.W.M. and Bloch, S. (2000). Psychiatric ethics: codes, concepts, and clinical practice skills. In *New Oxford Textbook of Psychiatry* (ed. M. Gelder, J.J. Lopez-Ibor, and N. Andreasen). Oxford: Oxford University Press, pp. 27–32.

Fulford, K.W.M. and Colombo, A. (2004). Six models of mental disorder: a study combining linguistic–analytic and empirical methods. *Philosophy, Psychiatry, & Psychology*, 11(2): 129–144.

Fulford, K.W.M. and Colombo. A. (2004). Professional judgment, critical realism, real people, and, yes, two wrongs can make a right! *Philosophy, Psychiatry, & Psychology*, 11(2): 165–174.

Fulford, K.W.M. and Hope, R.A. (1994). Psychiatric ethics: a bioethical ugly duckling? Chapter 58, In *Principles of Health Care Ethics* (ed. R. Gillon and A. Lloyd). Chichester: John Wiley. pp. 681–695.

Fulford, K.W.M. and Hope, T. (1996). Control and practical experience. In *Informed Consent in Psychiatry: European perspectives on ethics, law and clinical practice* (ed. H.-G. Koch, S. Reiter-Theil, and H. Helmchen). Baden-Baden: Nomos Verlagsgesellschaft, pp. 349–377.

Fulford, K.W.M. and Howse, K. (1993). Ethics of research with psychiatric patients: principles, problems and the primary responsibilities of researchers. *Journal of Medical Ethics*, 19: 85–91.

Fulford, K.W.M. and Radden, J. (ed.) (2002). Bioethics: Special Issue on psychiatric ethics. *Bioethics*, 16: 5.

Fulford, K.W.M. and Williams, R. (2003). Values-based child and adolescent mental health services? *Current Opinion in Psychiatry*, 16: 369–376.

Fulford, K.W.M., Broome, M., Stanghellini, G., and Thornton, T. (2005) Looking With Both Eyes Open: Fact *and* Value in Psychiatric Diagnosis? *World Psychiatry*, 4(2): 78–86.

Fulford, K.W.M., Dickenson, D. and Murray, T.H. (ed.) (2002). *Healthcare Ethics and Human Values: an introductory text with readings and case studies*. Malden, USA and Oxford, UK: Blackwell.

Fulford, K.W.M., Dickenson, D., and Murray, T.H. (2002). Many voices: human values in healthcare ethics. pps 1–19, In *Healthcare Ethics and Human Values: an introductory text with readings and case studies* (ed. K.W.M. Fulford, D. Dickenson, and T.H. Murray). Malden, MA: Blackwell Publishers, pp. 1–19.

Fulford, K.W.M., Morris, K.J., Sadler, J.Z. and Stanghellini, G. (eds.) (2003) *Nature and Narrative: an Introduction to The New Philosophy of Psychiatry*. Oxford: Oxford University Press.

Fulford, K.W.M., Morris, K.J., Sadler, J.Z., and Stanghellini, G. (2003a) *Past Improbable, Future Possible: the renaissance in philosophy and psychiatry*. Chapter 1 (pps 1–41), in Fulford, K.W.M., Morris, K.J., Sadler, J.Z., and Stanghellini, G. (eds.) *Nature and Narrative: an Introduction to the New Philosophy of Psychiatry*. Oxford: Oxford University Press.

Fulford, K.W.M., Smirnoff, A.Y.U., and Snow, E. (1993). Concepts of disease and the abuse of psychiatry in the USSR. *British Journal of Psychiatry*, 162: 801–810.

Fulford, K.W.M., Stanghellini, G. and Broome, M. (2004) What can philosophy do for psychiatry? Special Article for *World Psychiatry* (WPA), Oct 2004, pps 130–135.

Fulford, K.W.M., Williamson, T. and Woodbridge, K. (2002). Values-added practice (a values-awareness workshop). *Mental Health Today*, October: 25–27.

Fulwiler, C. and Folstein, M.F. (1995). Commentary: Chris Walkers (1995). Interpretation of Karl Jaspers phenomenology. *Philosophy, Psychiatry, & Psychology*, 2(4): 345–347.

Gallagher, S. (1996). Body schema and intentionality. In *The Body and The Self* (ed. N. Eilen). Cambridge, MA: MIT Press.

Gallagher, S. (2000). Self reference and schizophrenia: a cognitive model of immunity to error through misidentification. In *Exploring the Self*. (ed. D. Zahavi). Amsterdam: John Benjamins Publishing Company.

Gallagher, S. (2003). Self-narrative in schizophrenia. In *The Self in Neuroscience and Psychiatry* (ed. T. Kircher and A. David). Cambridge: Cambridge University Press, pp. 336–357.

Gallagher, S. and Cole, J. (1995). Body schema and body image in a deafferented subject. *Journal of Mind and Behaviour*, 16: 365–390.

Gane, M. (2002). Normativity and pathology. (Commentary on Margree, 2002). *Philosophy, Psychiatry, & Psychology*, 9(4): 313–316.

Garber, D. (1978). Science and certainty in Descartes. In *Descartes: critical and interpretive essays* (ed. M. Hooker). Baltimore, MD: Johns Hopkins University Press, pp. 114–151.

Gardner, S. (1993). *Irrationality and the Philosophy of Psychoanalysis*. Cambridge: Cambridge University Press.

Gardner, S. (1995). Psychoanalysis, science, and consciousness. (With commentaries by Hinshelwood, 1995, pp. 115–118, and Snelling, 1995, pp. 119–222) *Philosophy, Psychiatry, & Psychology*, 2(2): 93–114.

Gardner, S. (1995). The social relocation of personal identity. (Commentary on Hinshelwood, 1995) *Philosophy, Psychiatry, & Psychology*, 2(3): 209–214.

Garety, P.A. and Freeman, D. (1999). Cognitive approaches to delusions: a critical review of theories and evidence, *British Journal of Clinical Psychology*, 38: 113–154.

Garner, A. and Hardcastle, V.G. (2004). Neurobiological models: an unnecessary divide—neural models in psychiatry. In *The Philosophy of Psychiatry: a companion* (ed. J. Radden). New York: Oxford University Press, pp. 364–380.

Gbadegesin, S. (1991) *African Philosophy: Traditional Yoruba Philosophy and Contemporary African Realities*. New York and London: Peter Lang.

Geddes, J.R. and Carney, S.M. (2001). Recent advances in evidence-based psychiatry. *Canadian Journal of Psychiatry*, 46(5): 403–406.

Geddes, J.R. and Harrison, P.J. (1997). Evidence-based psychiatry: closing the gap between research and practice. *British Journal of Psychiatry*, 171: 220–225.

Gelder, M.G., Gath, D., and Mayou, R. (1994). The *Concise Oxford Textbook of Psychiatry*. Oxford: Oxford University Press.

Gelder, M.G., Mayou, R., and Cowen, P. (2001). *Shorter Oxford Textbook of Psychiatry*, (4th edn). Oxford: Oxford University Press.

Gelder, M.G., Gath, G., and Mayou, R.A.M. (1983). Signs and symptoms of mental disorder. In *The Oxford Textbook of Psychiatry* (1st edn). Oxford: Oxford University Press.

Gelder, M.G., Lopez-Ibor, J.J., and Andreasen, N. (ed.). (2000). *New Oxford Textbook of Psychiatry*. Oxford: Oxford University Press.

General Register Office (1968) *A Glossary of Mental Disorders. Studies on Medical and Population Subjects.* 22, London: HMSO.

Gennery, B. (2005) Academic clinical research in the new regulatory environment. *Clinical Medicine: Journal of the Royal College of Physicians of London.* 5:39–41.

Georgaca, E. (2004). Factualization and plausibility in delusional discourse. *Philosophy, Psychiatry, & Psychology*, 11(1): 13–24.

Georgaca, E. (2004). Talk and the nature of delusions: defending sociocultural perspectives on mental illness. *Philosophy, Psychiatry, & Psychology*, 11(1): 87–94.

Gerrans, P. (2002). A one-stage explanation of the Cotard delusion. *Philosophy, Psychiatry, & Psychology*, 9(1): 47–54.

Gerrans, P. (2002). Multiples paths to delusion. *Philosophy, Psychiatry, & Psychology*, 9(1): 65–72.

Gerrans, P. (2004). Cognitive architecture and the limits of interpretationism. (Commentary for Special Issue on delusion) *Philosophy, Psychiatry, & Psychology*, 11(1): 43–48.

Gert, B. and Culver, C.M. (2004). Defining mental disorder. In *The Philosophy of Psychiatry: a companion* (ed. J. Radden). New York: Oxford University Press, pp. 415–425.

Ghaemi, S.N. (1999). Depression: insight, illusion, and psychopharmacological Calvinism. (Commentary on Martin, 1999) *Philosophy, Psychiatry, & Psychology*, 6(4): 287–294.

Ghaemi, S.N. (1999). An empirical approach to understanding delusions. (Commentary on Jones, 1999) *Philosophy, Psychiatry, & Psychology*, 6(1): 21–24.

Ghaemi, S.N. (2004). The perils of belief: delusions reexamined. (Commentary for Special Issue on delusion) *Philosophy, Psychiatry, & Psychology*, 11(1): 49–54.

Gibbs, P.J. (2000). Thought insertion and the inseparability thesis. *Philosophy, Psychiatry, & Psychology*, 7(3): 195–202.

Gibbs, P.J. (2000). The limits of subjectivity: a response to the Commentary. *Philosophy, Psychiatry, & Psychology*, 7(3): 207–208.

Gillet, G.R. (1990). Neuroscience and meaning in psychiatry, *Journal of Medicine and Philosophy*, 15: 21–39.

Gillett, C. and Loewer, B. (2001). *Physicalism and Its Discontents*. Cambridge: Cambridge University Press.

Gillett, E. (1998). Relativism and the social-constructivist paradigm. *Philosophy, Psychiatry, & Psychology*, 5(1): 37–48.

Gillett, E. (1998). Response to the Commentaries. *Philosophy, Psychiatry, & Psychology*, 5(1): 61–66.

Gillett, G. (1989). *Reasonable Care*. Bristol: The Bristol Press.

Gillett, G. (1994). Insight, delusion, and belief. *Philosophy, Psychiatry, & Psychology*, 1(4): 227–236.

Gillett, G. (1994). Puppetmasters and personality disorders. (Commentary on Elliott, 1994). *Philosophy, Psychiatry, & Psychology*, 1(2): 101–104.

Gillett, G. (1997). A discursive account of multiple personality disorder. (Commentary by Braude, S.E. (1997, 223–226),

and a response by Gillett, G. (1997, 227–230)) *Philosophy, Psychiatry, & Psychology*, 4(3): 213–222.

Gillett, G. (1997). Response to the Commentary on Gillett (1997). *Philosophy, Psychiatry, & Psychology*, 4(3): 227–230.

Gillett, G. (1999). *The Mind and its Discontents*. Oxford: Oxford University Press.

Gillett, G. (1999). Benn-ding the rules of resentment. (Commentary on Benn, 1999). *Philosophy, Psychiatry, & Psychology*, 6(1): 49–52.

Gillett, G. (2002). The self as relatum in life and language. (Commentary on Van Staden, 2002) *Philosophy, Psychiatry, & Psychology*, 9(2): 123–126.

Gillett, G. (2003). Form and content: the role of discourse in mental disorder. In *Nature and Narrative: an introduction to the new philosophy of psychiatry* (ed. K.W.M. Fulford, K.J. Morris, J.Z. Sadler, and G. Stanghellini). Oxford: Oxford University Press, Chapter 9.

Gilligan, C. (1993) *In a Different Voice: Psychological Theory and Women's Development* (second edition). Cambridge, MA: Harvard University Press.

Gillon, R. (1986). *Philosophical Medical Ethics*. Chichester: John Wiley and sons.

Gillon, R. (1994) Preface: Medical Ethics and the Four Principles, pages xxi–xxxi, in in Gillon, R. and Lloyd, A., (eds) *Principles of Health Care Ethics*, Chichester Wiley.

Gillon, R. (1996). Ethical theory, ethnography and differences between doctors and nurses in approaches to patient care. *Journal of Medical Ethics*, 22: 292–299.

Gillon, R. and Lloyd, A. (ed.) (1994). *Principles of Health Care Ethics*. Chichester: Wiley.

Gipps, R.G.T. (2003). Illnesses and likenesses. (Commentary on Pickering, 2003). *Philosophy, Psychiatry, & Psychology*, 10(3): 255–260.

Gipps, R.G.T. (ed.) (2004). Autism and Intersubjectivity (Special issue). *Philosophy, Psychiatry, & Psychology*, 11(3).

Gipps, R.G.T. and Fulford, K.W.M. (2004). Understanding the clinical concept of delusion: from an estranged to an engaged epistemology. *International Review of Psychiatry*, 16(3): 225–235.

Glannon, W. (2002). Depression as a mind-body problem. (Commentaries by Martin, M.W. (2002, 255–260), Fuchs, T. (2002, 261–264), and response by Glannon, W. (2002, 265–270)) *Philosophy, Psychiatry, & Psychology*, 9(3): 243–254.

Glannon, W. (2002). The psychology and physiology of depression. (Response to the Commentaries on Glannon, 2002) *Philosophy, Psychiatry, & Psychology*, 9(3): 265–270.

Glas, G. (2003). Anxiety—animal reactions and the embodiment of meaning. In *Nature and Narrative: an introduction to the new philosophy of psychiatry* (ed. K.W.M. Fulford, K.J. Morris, J.Z. Sadler, and G. Stanghellini). Oxford: Oxford University Press, pp. 231–249.

Glas, G. (2003). Idem, ipse, and loss of the self (Commentary on Wells, 2003, Kennett and Matthews, 2003, Phillips, 2003 and Wooding, 2003). *Philosophy, Psychiatry, & Psychology*, 10(4): 347–352.

Glendinning, S. (1998). *On Being With Others: Heidegger, Derrida, Wittgenstein*. London: Routledge.

Glendinning, S. (forthcoming) *Derrida*. Oxford: Oxford University Press.

Glover, J. (1970) *Responsibility*. London: Routledge.

Glover, J. (1977). *Causing Death and Saving Lives*. England: Penguin (2nd edn 1992).

Glover, J. (1988) *I: The Philosophy and Psychology of Personal Identity*. London: Penguin.

Godfrey-Smith, (1989). Misinformation. *Canadian Journal of Philosophy*, 19: 533–550.

Goodman, N. (1983). *Fact Fiction and Forecast*. Harvard, MA: Harvard University Press.

Goodwin, G. (2002). Hypomania: what's in a name? *British Journal of Psychiatry*, 181: 94–95.

Gordon, R.M. (1995). Folk psychology as simulation. In *Folk Psychology* (ed. M. Davies and T. Stone). Oxford: Blackwell. pp 60–73.

Gordon, R.M. (1995). Simulation without introspection or inference from me to you. In *Mental Simulation* (ed. M. Davies and T. Stone). Oxford: Blackwell. pp 53–67.

Gordon, R.M. and Barker, J.A. (1995). Autism and the theory of mind debate. In *Philosophical Psychopathology* (ed. G. Graham and G.L. Stephens). Harvard, MA: MIT Press. pp. 163–181.

Graham, G. (1993, Second edition, 1998). *Philosophy of Mind: an introduction*. Oxford: Blackwell.

Graham, G. (1999). Mind, brain, world. (Commentary on Northoff, 1999) *Philosophy, Psychiatry, & Psychology*, 6(3): 223–226.

Graham, G. (1999). Fuzzy faulty lines: selves in multiple personality disorder. *Philosophical Explorations*, 3: 159–174.

Graham, G. (1999). Self-consciousness, psychopathology, and realism about the self. *Anthropology and Philosophy*, 24: 57–66.

Graham, G. (2002). Recent work in philosophical psychopathology. *American Philosophical Quarterly*, 39: 109–134.

Graham, G. (2004). Thinking inserted thoughts. In *Oxford Companion to the Philosophy of Psychiatry* (ed. J. Radden). Oxford: Oxford University Press.

Graham, G. and Horgan, T. (1998). Southern fundamentalism and the end of philosophy. In *Rethinking Intuition: the psychology of intuition and its role in philosophical inquiry* (ed. M. DePaul and W. Ramsey). Lanham, MD: Rowman and Littlefield, pp. 271–292.

Graham, G. and Stephens, G. Lynn. (1994). *Philosophical Psychopathology*. Cambridge, MA: MIT Press.

Green, R. (2000). Gender identity disorder in adults. In *New Oxford Textbook of Psychiatry* (ed. M. Gelder, J. Lopez-Ibor, and N. Andreasen). Oxford: Oxford University Press, pp. 913–917.

Greenberg, W.M. (1994). Commentary on Sabat and Harré (1994), The Alzheimer's disease sufferer as semiotic subject. *Philosophy, Psychiatry, & Psychology*, 1(3): 163–164.

Greenhalgh, T. and Hurwitz, B. (1998) *Narrative Based Medicine: Dialogue and Discourse in Clinical Practice*. London: BMJ Books.

Grice, H.P. (1941). Personal identity. *Mind*, 50: 330–350.

Grice, H.P. (1969). Utterer's meaning and intentions. *Philosophical Review*, 78. 147–177.

Griesinger, W. ([1867] 1882). *Mental Pathology and Therapeutics* (trans. C.L. Robertson and J. Rutherford) New York: William Wood and Co.

Griffin, J. (1990). *Well-being: its meaning, measurement and moral importance*. Oxford: Clarendon Press.

Griffiths, A.P. (ed.). (1985). *Philosophy and Practice*. Cambridge: Cambridge University Press.

Griffiths, A.P. (ed) (1989) *Key Themes in Philosophy*. Cambridge: Cambridge University Press, for the Royal Institute of Philosophy.

Griffiths, A.P. (ed) (1995) *Philosophy, Psychology, and Psychiatry*. Cambridge: Cambridge University Press, for the Royal Institute of Philosophy.

Grisso, T. and Appelbaum, P.S. (1998). *Assessing Competence to Consent to Treatment: a guide for clinicians and other health professionals*. New York: Oxford University Press.

Grosskurth, P. (1991). *The Secret Ring*. London: Jonathan Cape.

Group for the Advancement of Psychiatry (1990). *A Casebook for Psychiatric Ethics*. New York: Brunner and Mazel.

Grunbaum, A. (1984). *The Foundations of Psychoanalysis*. Berkeley, CA: University of California Press.

Grunbaum, A. (1988). Precis of *The Foundations of Psychoanalysis*. In *Mind, Psychoanalysis and Science* (ed. P. Clark and C. Wright). Oxford: Blackwell.

Grunbaum, A. (1993). *Validation in the Clinical Theory of Psychoanalysis*. Madison, CT: International Universities Press.

Gunn, J. and Taylor, P.J. (1993). *Forensic Psychiatry: clinical, legal and ethical issues*. Oxford: Butterworth-Heinemann.

Gunther, Y.H. (2003). *Essays on Nonconceptual Content*. Cambridge MA: MIT Press.

Gupta, M. and Kay, L.R. (2002). The impact of phenomenology on North American psychiatric assessment. *Philosophy, Psychiatry, & Psychology*, 9(1): 73–86.

Gupta, M. and Kay. L.R. (2002). Phenomenological methods in psychiatry: a necessary first step. (Response to the commentaries). *Philosophy, Psychiatry, & Psychology*, 9(1): 93–96.

Guttenplan, S. (1997). *The Languages of Logic: an introduction to formal logic*. Oxford: Blackwell.

Guttenplan, S., Hornsby, J., and Janaway, C. (2003). *Reading Philosophy: selected texts with a method for beginners*. Blackwell.

Haack, S. (1976). The justification of deduction. *Mind*, 83: 112–19.

Haack, S. (1978). *Philosophy of Logics*. Cambridge: Cambridge University Press.

Hacker, P.M.S. (1972). *Insight and Illusion*. Oxford: Oxford University Press.

Hacker, P.M.S. (1987). *Appearance and Reality*. Oxford: Blackwell.

Hacker, P.M.S. (2004). The conceptual framework for the investigation of emotions. *International Review of Psychiatry*, 16(3): 199–208.

Hacker, P.M.S. (1995) in Honderich, T. (ed) *Oxford Companion to Philosophy*. Oxford: Oxford University Press.

Hacking, I. (1982) Experimentation and Scientific Realism. *Philosophical Topics*, 13: 154–172.

Hacking, I. (1983) *Representing and Intervening*. Cambridge: Cambridge University Press.

Hacking, I. (1990) *The Taming of Chance*. Cambridge: Cambridge University Press.

Hacking, I. (1995) *Rewriting the Soul: Multiple Personality and the Sciences of Memory* Princeton: Princeton University Press

Hacking, I. (1998) *Mad Travelers: Reflections on the Reality of Transient Mental Illnesses*. Charlottesville and London: University Press of Virginia.

Hacking, I. (1999). Experimentation and Scientific realism. In *The Philosophy of Science* (ed. R. Boyd, P. Gaspar, and J.D. Trout). Cambridge, MA: MIT Press, pp. 247–260.

Hales, S.D. and Welshon, R. (1999). Nietzsche, perspectivism, and mental health. (Commentary on Lehrer, 1999) *Philosophy, Psychiatry, & Psychology*, 6(3): 173–178.

Halligan, P.W. and Marshall, J.C. (ed.) (1996). *Method in Madness: case studies in cognitive neuropsychiatry*. Oxford: Psychology Press.

Hamilton, A. (1998). False memory syndrome and the authority of personal memory-claims: a philosophical perspective. *Philosophy, Psychiatry, & Psychology*, 5(4): 283–298.

Hamilton, A. (1998). Response to the Commentaries. *Philosophy, Psychiatry, & Psychology*, 5(4): 311–316.

Hammond, M., Howarth, J. and Keat, R. (eds) (1991) *Understanding Phenomenology*. Oxford, UK and Cambridge, MA: Blackwell.

Hampshire, S. (1959). *Thought and Action*. London: Chatto and Windus.

Hanfling, O. (ed) (1981). *Essential Readings in Logical Positivism*. Oxford: Blackwell.

Hansen, J. (2003). Listening to people or listening to prozac? Another consideration of causal classifications. (Commentary on Radden, 2003). *Philosophy, Psychiatry, & Psychology*, 10(1): 57–62.

Hanson, N.R. (1958) *Patterns of Discovery* Cambridge: Cambridge University Press.

Hardcastle, V. and Flanagan, O. (1999). Multiplex vs. multiple selves: distinguishing dissociative disorders. *The Monist*, 82: 645–657. (Special issue on cognitive theories of mental illness.)

Hardcastle, V.G. (2003). Emotions and Narrative Selves. (Commentary on articles in the Special Issue on agency, narrative, and self) *Philosophy, Psychiatry, & Psychology*, 10(4): 353–356.

Hare, R.M. (1952). *The Language of Morals*. Oxford: Oxford University Press.

Hare, R.M. (1963). Descriptivism. *Proceedings of the British Academy*, 49: 115–134. (Reprinted in Hare, R.M., 1972, London: Macmillan.)

Hare, R.M. (1963) *Freedom and Reason*. Oxford: Oxford University Press.

Hare, R.M. (1964). Pain and evil. *Aristotelian Society Supplement*, XXXVIII. (Reprinted as in Hare, R.M., 1972.)

Hare, R.M. (1972). *Essays on the Moral Concepts*. London: The Macmillan.

Hare, R.M. (1981). *Moral Thinking: its levels, methods and point*. Oxford: Oxford University Press.

Hare, R.M. (1993). Medical ethics, can the moral philosopher help? In *Essays on Bioethics*. Oxford: Clarendon Press, pp. 1–14.

Hare, R.M. (1993). The philosophical basis of psychiatric ethics. In *Essays on Bioethics*. Oxford: Clarendon Press, pp. 15–30.

Hare, R.M. (1997) *Sorting out Ethics*. Oxford: Oxford University Press.

Harold, J. and Elliott, C. (1999). Travelers, mercenaries, and psychopaths. (Commentary on Benn, 1999). *Philosophy, Psychiatry, & Psychology*, 6(1): 45–48.

Harper, D.J. (2004). Delusions and discourse: moving beyond the constraints of the modernist paradigm. (Commentary for Special Issue on delusion). *Philosophy, Psychiatry, & Psychology*, 11: 55–64.

Harré, R. (1988). *The Singular Self*. London: Sage.

Harré, R. (1993). *Laws of Nature*. London: Duckworth.

Harré, R. (1997). Pathological autobiographies. *Philosophy, Psychiatry, & Psychology*, 4(2): 99–110.

Harré, R. (1997). Response to the Commentaries. *Philosophy, Psychiatry, & Psychology*, 4(2): 119–120.

Harré, R. (1998). Suicide, language, and clinical practice. (Commentary on Fairbairn, 1998). *Philosophy, Psychiatry, & Psychology*, 5(2): 171–174.

Harré, R. (1999). Bringing relations to life. (Commentary on Deeley, 1999). *Philosophy, Psychiatry, & Psychology*, 6(2): 129–132.

Harré, R. and Gillett, G. (1994). *The Discursive Mind*. London: Sage.

Harré, R. and Lamb, D. (ed.). (1987). *Dictionary of Philosophy and Psychology*. Oxford: Blackwell.

Hart, H.L.A. (1968) *Punishment and responsibility: essays in the philosophy of law*. Oxford: Oxford University Press.

Haugeland, J. (1982). Weak supervenience. *American Philosophical Quarterly*, 19: 93–104.

Haugeland, J. (1993). Pattern and being. In *Dennett and his Critics* (ed. B. Dahlbom). Oxford: Blackwell.

Hawton, K., Salkovskis, P.M., Kirk, J. and Clark, D.M. (1989) *Cognitive Behaviour Therapy for Psychiatric Problems: a Practical Guide*, Oxford, England: Oxford University Press.

Heal, J. (1995). Replication and functionalism. In *Folk Psychology* (ed. M. Davies and T. Stone). Oxford: Blackwell, pp. 45–59.

Healy, D. (1990). *The Suspended Revolution: psychiatry and psychotherapy re-examined*. London: Faber and Faber.

Heaton, J. and Groves, J. (1994). *Wittgenstein for Beginners*. Cambridge, UK: Icon Books.

Heginbotham, C. (1998). Suicide, euthanasia, and the psychiatrist (Commentary on Burgess and Hawton, 1998a). *Philosophy, Psychiatry, & Psychology*, 5(2): 137–140.

Heginbotham, C. (ed.) (2000). *Philosophy, Psychiatry and Psychopathy: personal identity in mental disorder*. Avebury Series in Philosophy in association with The Society for Applied Philosophy. Avebury: Ashgate Publishing Ltd.

Heginbotham, C. (2004) 'Psychiatric Dasein'. *Philosophy, Psychiatry, & Psychology*, 11(2), 147–150.

Heidegger, M. ([1927] 1962). *Being and Time* (transl. J. Macquarrie and E. Robinson). Oxford: Blackwell.

Heidegger, M. (1985). *History of the Concept of Time: Prolegomena* (trans. by T. Kisiel). Bloomington, IN: Indiana University Press.

Heidegger, M. (1987). *Zollikoner Seminare: Protokolle—Gespräche—Briefe* (ed. M. Boss). Frankfurt am Main: Klostermann.

Heidegger, M. (1988). On adequate understanding of daseinsanalysis: excerpts from Martin Heidegger's zollikon teaching (trans. by Michael Eldred). *Humanistic Psychologist*, 16: 75–98.

Heil, J. and Mele, A. (ed.) (1993). *Mental Causation*. Oxford: Oxford University Press.

Heinimaa, M. (2003). Incomprehensibility. In *Nature and Narrative: an introduction to the new philosophy of psychiatry* (ed. K.W.M. Fulford, K.J. Morris, J.Z.S. Sadler, and G. Stanghellini). Oxford: Oxford University Press, Chapter 14.

Heinze, M. (1995). Commentary on 'Moralist or therapist?' (Matthews, 1995). *Philosophy, Psychiatry, & Psychology*, 2(1): 31–32.

Helman, C.G. (1981). Disease versus illness in general practice. *Journal of the Royal College of Practitioners*, 230(3): 548–552.

Helman, C.G. (2000). *Culture, Health and Illness: an introduction for health professionals* (4th edn). Oxford: Butterworth-Heinemann.

Hempel, C.G. (1961). Introduction to problems of taxonomy. In *Field Studies in the Mental Disorders*. New York: Grune and Stratton, pp. 3–22. (Reprinted in Sadler, J.Z., Wiggins, O.P., and Schwartz, M.A. (1994).)

Hempel, C.G. ([1942] 1965). The Function of general laws in history. In *Aspects of Scientific Explanation and Other Essays in the Philosophy of Science*. London: Collier-MacMillan, pp. 231–243.

Hempel, C.G. (1965). *Aspects of Scientific explanation*. London: Free Press.

Hempel, C.G. (1966). *Philosophy of natural science*. London: Prentice-Hall.

Hempel, C.G. ([1962] 1993). Explanation in science and in history. In *Explanation* (ed. R. David-Hillel). Oxford: Oxford University Press.

Hempel, C.G. (1994). Fundamentals of taxonomy. In *Philosophical Perspectives on Psychiatric Diagnostic Classification* (ed. J.S. Sadler, O.P. Wiggins, and M.A. Schwartz). Baltimore, MD: Johns Hopkins University Press.

Hempel, C.G. (1999). Laws and their role in scientific explanation. In *Philosophy of Science* (ed. R. Boyd, P. Gasker, and J.D. Trout). Cambridge, MA: MIT Press, pp. 299–315.

Hert, M. De, Thys, E., Magiels, G., and Wyckaert, S. (2004). *Anything or Nothing: self-guide for people with bipolar disorder*. Antwerp: Janssen-Cilag/Organon.

Hesse, M. (1980). *Revolutions and Reconstructions in the Philosophy of Science*. Brighton: Harvester.

Hill, D. (1968) Depression: disease, reaction or posture? *American Journal of Psychiatry* 125: 445–57.

Hinshelwood, R.D. (1995). Psychoanalysis, science, and commonsense. (Commentary on Gardner, 1995) *Philosophy, Psychiatry, & Psychology*, 2(2): 115–118.

Hinshelwood, R.D. (1995). The social relocation of personal identity as shown by psychoanalytic observations of splitting, projection and introjection. (Commentaries by Braude, S.E. (1995, pp. 205–208), Gardner, S. (1995, pp. 209–214), and Lewis, B. (1995, pp. 215–218) *Philosophy, Psychiatry, & Psychology*, 2(3): 185–204.

Hinshelwood, R.D. (1997). Primitive mental processes: psychoanalysis and the ethics of integration. (With commentaries by Mace (1997), Sturdee (1997), and Thornton (1997), and a detailed response (Hinshelwood, 1997) *Philosophy, Psychiatry, & Psychology* 4(2): 121–144.

Hinshelwood, R.D. (1997) Response to the Commentaries. *Philosophy, Psychiatry, & Psychology*, 4(2): 159–166.

Hinshelwood, R.D. (1997). *Therapy or Coercion? Does Psychoanalysis Differ from Brainwashing?* London: H. Karnac (Books) Ltd.

Hinshelwood, R.D. (2001). A Kleinian contribution to the external world. (Commentary on Richmond, 2001). *Philosophy, Psychiatry, & Psychology*, 8(1): 17–20.

HMSO (1995). *Report of the Clinical Standards Advisory Group on Schizophrenia*, Volume 1, London: HSMO.

Hobbes, T. (1984). 'Objections' to Descartes' *Meditations*. In *The Philosophical Writings of Descartes* (trans. J. Cottingham, R. Stoothoff, and D. Murdoch), Vol. 2. Cambridge: Cambridge University Press, pp. 122–126.

Hobbes, T. ([1651]1996) *Leviathan* (edited by Tuck, R.) Cambridge: Cambridge University Press.

Hobbs, A. (1998). Commentary: Aristotle's function argument and the concept of mental illness. *Philosophy, Psychiatry, & Psychology*, 5(3): 209–214.

Hobson, R.P., Patrick, M.P.H., and Valentine, J.D. (1998). Objectivity in psychoanalytic judgements. *British Journal of Psychiatry*, 173: 172–177.

Hobson, R.P. (1991). Against the 'theory of mind'. *British Journal of Developmental Psychology*, 9: 33–51.

Hobson, R.P. (2002). *The Cradle of Thought*. London: Macmillan

Hodges, H.A. (1952). *The Philosophy of Wilhelm Dilthey*. London: Routledge and Kegan Paul.

Hoenig, J. (1965). Karl Jaspers and psychopathology. *Philosophy and Phenomenological Research*, 26: 216–229.

Hoerl, C. (2001a). Introduction: understanding, explaining, and intersubjectivity in schizophrenia. *Philosophy, Psychiatry, & Psychology*, 8(2–3): 83–88.

Hoerl, C. (2001b). On thought insertion. *Philosophy, Psychiatry, & Psychology*, 8(2–3): 189–200.

Hoff, P. (2005). Die psychopathologische Perspektive. In *Ethische Aspekte der Forschung in Psychiatrie und Psychotherapie* (ed. M. Bormuth and U. Wiesing). Cologne: Deutscher Aerzte–Verlag, pp. 71–79.

Hohwy, J. (2004). Top-down and bottom-up in delusion formation. (Commentary for Special Issue on delusion). *Philosophy, Psychiatry, & Psychology*, 11: 65–70.

Hollis, M. (1985, reprinted 1992) *Invitation to Philosophy*. Oxford: Blackwell.

Holmes, J. (1997). Commentary on 'Autobiography, narrative, and the Freudian concept of life history'. (Commentary on Brockmeier, 1997) *Philosophy, Psychiatry, & Psychology*, 4(3): 201–204.

Holmes, J. and Lindlay, R. (1989). *The Values of Psychotherapy*. Oxford: Oxford University Press.

Honderich, T. (ed). (1995). *The Oxford Companion to Philosophy*. Oxford: Oxford University Press.

Hook, S. (1959). *Psychoanalysis, Scientific Method, and Philosophy*. New York: New York University Press.

Hooker, B. and Little, M.O. (ed.). (2000). *Moral Particularism*. Oxford: Clarendon Press.

Hope, R.A. (1990). Ethical philosophy as applied to psychiatry. *Current Opinion in Psychiatry*, 3: 673–676.

Hope, T. (1994). Commentary on Sabat and Harré (1994), The Alzheimer's disease sufferer as semiotic subject. *Philosophy, Psychiatry, & Psychology*, 1(3): 161–162.

Hope, T., (1994) Personal Identity and Psychiatric Illness, in *Philosophy, Psychology and Psychiatry*, ed. A.P. Griffiths (1995), Cambridge: Cambridge University Press.

Hope, T. (2004). *Medical Ethics: a very short introduction*. Oxford: Oxford University Press.

Hope, T. and Fulford, K.W.M. (1994). Medical education: patients, principles and practice skills. In *Principles of Health Care Ethics* (ed. R. Gillon). Chichester: Wiley, Chapter 59.

Hope, T., Fulford, K. W. M. and Yates, A. (1996). *The Oxford Practice Skills Course: Ethics, Law and Communication Skills in Health Care Education*. Oxford: Oxford University Press.

Hopkins, J. (1988) Epistemology and Depth Psychology: Critical Notes on The Foundations of Psychoanalysis, Part One, Section 2, p33, in P. Clark and C. Wright (eds) *Mind, Psychoanalysis and Science*. Oxford: Blackwell.

Hornsby, J. (1980). *Actions*. London: Routledge and Kegan Paul.

Horwich, P. (1990). *Truth*. Oxford: Blackwell.

Howson, C. (2000). *Hume's Problem: induction and the justification of belief*. Oxford: Clarendon Press.

Hudson Jones, A. (1999). Narrative in medical ethics. *British Journal of Medicine*.

Hughes, J.C., Louw, S.J., Sabat, S.R. (eds) (2006) *Dementia: Mind, Meaning, and the Person*. Oxford: Oxford University Press.

Human Rights Watch/Geneva Initiative on Psychiatry (2002). *Dangerous Minds: political psychiatry in China today and its origins in the Mao era*. New York: Human Rights Watch.

Hume, D. ([1739–40] 1967). *A Treatise of Human Nature*, (ed. L.A. Selby-Bigge). Oxford: Oxford University Press.

Hume, D. ([1748] 1975). *Enquiries Concerning Human Understanding and Concerning the Principles of Morals*. Oxford: Oxford University Press.

Hundert, E.M. (1989). *Philosophy, Psychiatry and Neuroscience: three approaches to the mind*. Oxford: Oxford University Press.

Hunink, M.G.M. and Glasziou, P.P. (2001) *Decision making in health and medicine: Integrating evidence and values*. Cambridge: Cambridge University Press.

Hunter, R. and McAlpine, I. (1963). *Three Hundred Years of Psychiatry: 1535–1860*. London: Oxford University Press.

Husserl, E. (1927). Phenomenology. Edmund Husserl's Article for the *Encyclopaedia Britannica* (revised translation by Richard E. Palmer). In *Husserl: Shorter Works*. Indiana: University of Notre Dame Press (1981), pp. 21–35. (Reprinted from (1971) *Journal of the British Society for Phenomenology*, 2: 77–90.

Husserl, E. ([1931] 1960). *Cartesian Meditations* (transl. D. Cairns). The Hague: Nijhoff.

Husserl, E. (1970). Investigation IV. In *Logical Investigations* (trans. by J.N. Findlay), 2 vols. London: Routledge and Kegan Paul.

Husserl, E. (1970). *Philosophie der Arithmetik* (ed. L. Eley). The Hague: Martinus Nijhoff.

Husserl, E. ([1900–1] 1970). *Logical Investigations* (transl. J.N. Findlay). London: Routledge.

Husserl, E. (1975). *Introduction to the Logical Investigations* (trans. P.J. Bossert and C.H. Peters) (ed. E. Fink). The Hague: Martinus Nijhoff.

Husserl, E. (1977). The task and the significance of the *Logical Investigations* (trans. by J.N.Findlay). In *Readings on Edmund Husserl's 'Logical Investigations'* (ed. J.N. Mohanty). The Hague: Martinus Nijhoff, pp. 197–215.

Husserl, E. (1981). Philosophy as a rigorous science. In *Husserl: Shorter Works* (trans. by Quentin Lauer). Indiana: University of Notre Dame Press, pp. 166–197. (Also in Husserl, E. (1965) *Phenomenology and the Crisis of Philosophy*. New York: Harper & Row, pp. 71–147.)

Husserl, E. ([1931] 1982). *Ideas Pertaining to a Pure Phenomenology and to a Phenomenological Philosophy, First Book* (transl. in English by F. Kersten). Dordrecht: Kluwer.

Hyman, J. (1992). The causal theory of perception. *The Philosophical Quarterly*, 42(168): 277–296.

Hyman, S.E. and Fenton, W.D. (2003). What are the right targets for psychopharmacology? *Science*, 299: 350–351.

Jackson, M.C. (1997). Benign schizotypy? The case of spiritual experience. In *Schizotypy: relations to illness and health* (ed. G.S. Claridge). Oxford: Oxford University Press.

Jackson, M.C. and Fulford, K.W.M. (1997). Spiritual experience and psychopathology. *Philosophy, Psychiatry, & Psychology*, 4(1): 41–66.

Jackson, M.C. and Fulford K.W.M. (1997). Response to the Commentaries. *Philosophy, Psychiatry, & Psychology*, 4(1): 87–90.

Jackson, M.C. and Fulford, K.W.M. (2002). Psychosis good and bad: values-based practice and the distinction between pathological and nonpathological forms of psychotic experience. *Philosophy, Psychiatry, & Psychology*, 9(4): 387–394.

Jackson, M.C. and Fulford, K.W.M. (2002). Spiritual Experience and Psychopathology. Chapter 20 pps 141–149 in Fulford, K.W.M., Dickenson, D. and Murray, T.H. (eds) *Healthcare Ethics and Human Values: An Introductory Text with Readings and Case Studies*. Maiden, MC, and Oxford, UK: Blackwell.

Jacoby, R. and Oppenheimer, C. (1996). *Psychiatry in the Elderly*. Oxford: Oxford University Press.

James, W. (1890). The stream of consciousness. *The Principles of Psychology* (2 vols). New York: Henry Holt.

James, W. (1902). *The varieties of religious experience*. New York: Longmans.

Jamison, K.R. (1996). *Touched With Fire: manic depressive illness and the artistic temperament*. California: Touchstone Books.

Jamison, K.R. (1996). *An Unquiet Mind: a memoir of moods and madness*. New York: Free Press.

Jaspers, K. ([1911] 1963). Zur Analyse der Trugwahrnehmungen' (The Analysis of False Perceptions). In *Gesammelte Schriften zur Psychopathologie*. Berlin: Springer-Verlag, pp. 191–251.

Jaspers, K. ([1913] 1963/1997). *Allgemeine Psychopathologie* (4th edn). Berlin: Springer-Verlag; *General Psychopathology* (trans. J. Hoenig and M. W. Hamilton). Chicago: University of Chicago Press. New edition with a Foreword by Paul R. McHugh (1997) Baltimore: The Johns Hopkins University Press.

Jaspers, K. ([1912] 1968). The phenomenological approach in psychopathology (trans. of 'Die phänomenologische Forschungsrichtung in der Psychopathologie); reprinted in *Gesammelte Schriften zur Pschopathologie* (*Collected Writings in Psychopathology*), pp. 314–328; anonymously translated in *British Journal of Psychiatry*, 1968; 114: 1313–1323.

Jaspers, K. ([1913] 1974). Causal and 'meaningful' connections between life history and psychosis (Kausale und verständliche Zusammenhänge zwischen Schicksal und Psychose bei der Dementia praecox). Translated with an introduction and postscript by J. Hoenig. In *Themes and Variations in European Psychiatry* (ed. S.R. Hirsch and M. Shepherd). Bristol: Wright, pp. 80–93.

Jaspers, K.([1919] 2005). *Psychologie der Weltanschauungen* (*The Psychology of World Views*) Berlin: Springer-verlag.

Jaspers, K. ([1920] 1951). *Max Weber*. Reprinted in *Rechenschaft und Ausblick*. Munich: Piper.

Jaspers, K. ([1932] 1969). *Philosophie*. Translated as *Philosophy* (trans. by E.B. Ashton). Chicago, IL: University of Chicago Press.

Jaspers, K. (1936). *Nietzsche: Einführung in das Verständnis seines Philosophierens* (*Nietzsche: An Introduction to the Understanding of His Philosophical Activity*) (trans. C.F. Wallruff and F.J. Schmitz). Baltimore, MD: Johns Hopkins University Press.

Jaspers, K. (1957). Philosophical autobiography. In *The Philosophy of Karl Jaspers* (ed. P. Schilpp). LaSalle, IL: Open Court.

Jaspers, K. (1962). *Kant: Leben, Werk, Wirkung*. Munich: Piper. (Trans. as *Kant*, Vol. II of *The Great Philosophers*, trans. by R. Mannheim. New York: Harcourt, Brace and World.).

Jellineck, E.M. (1960). *The Disease Concept of Alcoholism*. New Haven, CT: College and University Press.

Jensen, U.J. (1987). *Practice & Progress: a theory for the modern health-care system*. Oxford: Blackwell Scientific Publications.

Jones, E. (1938). The theory of symbolism. In *Papers on Psychoanalysis*. London: Ballière Tindall.

Jones, E. (1999). The phenomenology of abnormal belief: a philosophical and psychiatric inquiry. *Philosophy, Psychiatry, & Psychology*, 6(1): 1–16.

Jones, E. (1999). Response to the Commentaries. *Philosophy, Psychiatry, & Psychology*, 6(1): 27–28.

Jonsen, A.R. and Toulmin, S. (1988). *The Abuse of Casuistry: a history of moral reasoning*. University of California Press.

Joseph, D. and Orek, J. (1999). The ethical aspects of confidentiality in psychiatry. In *Psychiatric Ethics* (ed. S. Bloch, P. Chodoff, and S.A. Green), (3rd edn). Oxford, Oxford University Press, Chapter 7.

Kane, R. (1996) *The significance of free will*. Oxford: Oxford University Press.

Kane, R. (ed.) (2001). *Free Will*. Oxford: Blackwell.

Kant, I. ([1781] 1929). *Critique of Pure Reason* (trans. N. Kemp Smith). London: Macmillan.

Kaplan, B. (ed.) (1964). *The Inner World of Mental Illness: a series of first-person accounts of what it was like*. New York: Harper & Row.

Käsler, D. (1988). *Max Weber: an introduction to his life and work* (trans. by Philippa Hurd). Cambridge: Polity Press.

Kelleher, M.J. (1998). Suicide, euthanasia, and the psychiatrist (Commentary on Burgess and Hawton, 1998). *Philosophy, Psychiatry, & Psychology*, 5(2): 145–150.

Kendall, T. (1995). Commentary on 'Beyond liberation'. (Bracken, 1995). *Philosophy, Psychiatry, & Psychology*, 2: 15–18.

Kendell, R.E. (1975) The concept of disease and its implications for psychiatry. *British Journal of Psychiatry*, 127: 305–315

Kendell, R.E. (1975). *The Role of Diagnosis in Psychiatry*. Oxford: Blackwell Scientific Publications.

Kendell, R.E. and Jablensky, A. (2003). Distinguishing between the validity and utility of psychiatric diagnoses. *American Journal of Psychiatry*, 160: 4–12.

Kennedy, I. (1981). *The Unmasking of Medicine*. London: George Allen and Unwin.

Kennedy, I. (1996[1988]). *Treat Me Right: essays in medical law and ethics*. Oxford: Clarendon Press.

Kennedy, I. and Grubb, A. (1998). *Principles of Medical Law*. Oxford: Oxford University Press.

Kennedy, I. and Grubb, A. (2000). *Medical Law: text with materials*, (3rd edn). London: Butterworths.

Kennett, J. and Matthews, S. (2003). The unity and disunity of agency. *Philosophy, Psychiatry, & Psychology*, 10(4): 305–312.

Kenny, A.J.P. (1969). Mental health in Plato's Republic. *Proceedings of the Aristotelian Society*, 229–241.

Kesey, K. (1963) *One Flew over the Cuckoo's Nest*. New York: Penguin.

Kierkegaard, S. (1981). *The Concept of Anxiety*. Princeton: Princeton University Press.

Kierkegaard, S. (1983). *The Sickness Unto Death*. Princeton: Princeton University Press.

Kiloh, L. and Garside, R. (1963). The independence of neurotic depression and endogenous depression. *British Journal of Psychiatry*, 109: 451–463.

Kim, K. (1993). *Supervenience and Mind*. Cambridge: Cambridge University Press.

King, C. (2005) Coloring our eyes. *World Psychiatry*, 4(2): 95.

Kirkham, R.L. (1995). *Theories of Truth: a critical introduction*. London: MIT Press.

Kitamura, T. (2005) Looking with both the eyes and heart open: the meaning of life in psychiatric diagnosis. *World Psychiatry*, 4(2): 93.

Klee, R. (2004). Why some delusions are necessarily inexplicable beliefs. *Philosophy, Psychiatry, & Psychology*, 11(1): 25–34.

Klee, R. (2004). Delusional content and the public nature of meaning. *Philosophy, Psychiatry, & Psychology*, 11(1): 95–100.

Kleinman, A. (1996). How is culture important for DSM-IV? In *Culture and Psychiatric Diagnosis: a DSM-IV perspective* (ed. J.E. Mezzich, A. Kleinman, H. Fabrega, and D.L. Parron). Washington: American Psychiatric Press Inc., Chapter 2.

Kline, P. (1972). *Fact and Fantasy in Freudian Theory*. London: Methuen.

Komesaroff, P.A. and Wiltshire, J. (1998). Commentary: A phenomenology of dyslexia. *Philosophy, Psychiatry, & Psychology*, 5(1): 21–24.

Kopelman, L. (1994). Normal Grief: Good or Bad? Health or Disease (with commentaries by Dominion, 1994, and Wise, 1994, and a response by Kopelman, 1994 *Philosophy, Psychiatry, & Psychology*, 1(4): 209–220.

Kopelman, L. (1994). Rejoinder (to Commentaries on Kopelman, 1994). *Philosophy, Psychiatry, & Psychology*, 1(4): 225–226.

Kopelman, L.M. (1989). Moral problems in psychiatry. In *Medical Ethics* (ed. R. Veatch). London: Jones and Bartlett.

Kopelman, L.M. (ed.) (1992) Philosophical Issues Concerning Psychiatric Diagnosis. *The Journal of Medicine and Philosophy*, 17 (2).

Kopelman, L.M. (1994) Normal Grief: Good or Bad? Health or Disease? *Philosophy, Psychiatry, and Psychology*, 1, 209–220

Kopelman, L.M. (1994). Case method and casuistry: the problem of bias. *Theoretical Medicine*, 15: 7–9.

Kopelman, L.M. (1994). Normal grief: good or bad? Health or disease? (Commentaries by Dominian, J. and Wise, T.N. pp. 221–224; response by Kopelman, pp. 226–227) *Philosophy, Psychiatry, & Psychology*, 1(4): 209–220.

Kovel, J. (1995). Commentary on 'Beyond liberation' (Bracken, 1995). and 'Moral therapist?' (Matthews, 1995). *Philosophy, Psychiatry, & Psychology*, 2(1): 33–34.

Köhnke, K.C. (1991). *The Rise of Neo-Kantianism* (trans. by R.J.Hollingdale). Cambridge: Cambridge University Press.

Kraepelin, E. (1902) *Clinical Psychiatry: a text-book for students and physicians*. New York: Macmillan. Translation by A. Ross of the 6th edition of Emil Kraepelin's *Lehrbuch der Psychiatrie*.

Kramer, H. and Sprenger, J. (1996). *Malleus Maleficarum*. London: Bracken Books.

Kramer, M. (1969) Cross-National Study of Diagnosis of the Mental Disorders: origin of the problem. *American Journal of Psychiatry*, 125 (suppl.): 1–11.

Kramer, M., Sartorius, N. Jablensky, A., Gulbinat, W. (1979) The ICD-9 Classification of Mental Disorders: A Review of its Development and Contents. *Acta Psychiatrica Scandinavica*, 59: 241–262.

Kraus, A. (1994). Phenomenological and criteriological diagnosis. In *Philosophical Perspectives on Psychiatric Diagnostic Classification* (ed. J.S. Sadler, O.P. Wiggins, and M.A. Schwartz). Baltimore, MD: Johns Hopkins University Press, pp. 148–162.

Kraus, A. (2003). How can the phenomenological-anthropological approach contribute to diagnosis and classification in psychiatry? In *Nature and Narrative: an introduction to the new philosophy of psychiatry* (ed. K.W.M. Fulford, K.J. Morris, J.Z. Sadler, and G. Stanghellini). Oxford: Oxford University Press, pp. 199–216.

Kreitman, N., Sainsbury, P., Morrissey, J., Towers, J., and Scrivener, J. (1961). The reliability of psychiatric assessment: an analysis. *Journal of Mental Science*, 107: 887–908.

Kripke, S. (1980). *Naming and Necessity*. Oxford: Blackwell.

Kripke, S. (1982). *Wittgenstein on Rules and Private Language*. Oxford: Blackwell.

Kroll, J. (1995). Essay review: the histriography of the history of psychiatry. *Philosophy, Psychiatry, & Psychology*, 2(3): 267–276.

Kruger, C. (2003). Self-injury: symbolic sacrifice/self-assertion renders clinicians helpless. (Commentary on Potter, 2003). *Philosophy, Psychiatry, & Psychology*, 10/1: 17–22.

Kuhn, T.S. (1962, 2nd edn/1970 revised and enlarged). *The Structure of Scientific Revolutions*. Chicago: Chicago University Press.

Kuhn, T.S. (1970). Logic of discovery or psychology of research? In *Criticism and the Growth of Knowledge* (ed. I. Lakatos and A. Musgrave). Cambridge: Cambridge University Press, pp. 1–23.

Kuninski, M. (1979). The methodological status of the cultural sciences according to Heinrich Rickert and Max Weber (trans. by T. Kadenacy). *Reports on Philosophy*, 3: 71–85.

Kupfer, D.J., First, M., and Regier, D. (ed.). (2002). *A Research Agenda for DSM-V*. Washington, DC: American Psychiatric Association.

Kupfer, D.J., First, M.B., and Regier, D.E. (2002). Introduction. In *A Research Agenda for DSM-V* (ed. D.J. Kupfer, M.B. First, and D.E. Regier). Washington, DC: American Psychiatric Association, pp. xv–xvii.

Kushner, T.K. and Thomasma, D.C. (2001). *Ward ethics: dilemmas for medical students and doctors in training*. Cambridge: Cambridge University Press.

Kutchins, H. and Kirk, S.A. (1997). *Making Us Crazy: DSM—the psychiatric bible and the creation of mental disorder*. London: Constable.

Lacan, J. ([1966] 1977). *Ecrits: A selection* (trans. Alan Sheridan). London: Tavistock Publications.

Lacan, J. (1977). *The Four Fundamental Concepts of Psychoanalysis* (ed. Jacques-Alain Miller, trans. Alan Sheridan). London: Hogarth Press.

Ladyman, J. (2002). *Understanding Philosophy of Science*. London: Routledge.

Laing, R.D. (1960). *The Divided Self*. London: Tavistock.

Lakatos, I. (1970). Falsification and the methodology of scientific research programmes. In *Criticism and the Growth of Knowledge* (ed. I. Lakatos and A. Musgrave). Cambridge: Cambridge University Press, pp. 91–195.

Langer, M. (1989) *Merleau-Ponty's Phenomenology of Perception: a guide and commentary*. Basingstoke: Macmillan.

Langford, C.H. (1942). *The Notion of Analysis in Moores Philosophy*. In Schilpp, P.A. (ed) (1968) *The Philosophy of G.E. Moore* (third edition), La Salle, IL: Open pp. 321–342.

Lansky, M.R. (1999). Perspectives on perspectivism. (Commentary on Lehrer, 1999) *Philosophy, Psychiatry, & Psychology*, 6(3): 179–180.

Lanteri-Laura, G. (1998) *Essai sur les paradigms de la psychiatrie modeme*. Paris: Editions du temps.

Laor and Agassi, (1990). Ethics of diagnostic systems. In *Diagnosis: philosophical and medical perspectives*. Episteme Book Series, Vol. 15. Dordrecht: Kluwer.

Laplanche, J. and Pontalis, J.-B. (1973). *The Language of Psychoanalysis*. London: The Hogarth Press.

Larvor, B. (1998). *Lakatos: an introduction* London: Routledge.

Latour, B. (1987). *Science in Action: how to follow scientists and engineers through society* Cambridge, MA: Harvard University Press.

Latour, B. and Woolgar, S. (1992). *Laboratory Life: construction of scientific facts*. Princeton: Princeton University Press.

Laudan, L. (1977). *Progress and its Problems*. Berkeley, CA: University of California.

Lavin, M. (1995). Who should be committable? *Philosophy, Psychiatry, & Psychology*, 2(1): 35–48.

Law, S. (2004) *The Philosophy Files*. London: Orion Children's.

Leavy, S.A. (1997). Commentary: The stoic conception of mental disorder. *Philosophy, Psychiatry, & Psychology*, 4(4): 295–296.

Leff, J.P. and Vaughn, C.E. (ed.). (1985). *Expressed Emotion in Families: its significance for mental illness*. New York: Guildford Press.

Leff, J.P. and Isaacs, A.D. (1978, third edition, 1990). *Psychiatric examination in clinical practice*. Oxford: Blackwell Scientific Publications.

Lehman. A.F., Alexopoulos, G.S., Goldman, H., Jeste, D., and Üstün, B. (2002). Mental disorders and disability: time to reevaluate the relationship? In *A Research Agenda for DSM-V* (ed. D.J. Kupfer, M.B. First, and D.E. Regier). Washington, DC: American Psychiatric Association, pp. 201–218.

Lehrer, R. (1999). Perspectivism and psychodynamic psychotherapy. (With commentaries by Pearson, 1999, pp. 167–172; Hales and Welshon, 1999, pp. 173–178; Lansky, 1999, pp. 179–180; Lieberman, 1999, pp. 181–186; and Mace, 1999, pp. 187–190) *Philosophy, Psychiatry, & Psychology*, 6(3): 155–166.

Lehrer, R. (1999). Response to the Commentaries. *Philosophy, Psychiatry, & Psychology*, 6(3): 191–198.

Leibniz, G.W. (1705). *New Essays on the Human Understanding*.

Leibniz, G.W. ([1710] 1988) *Theodicity*. Illinois: Open Court Publishing Company.

Lemmon, E.J. (1965). *Beginning Logic*. London: Van Nostrand Reinhold.

Leplin, J. (ed.) (1984). *Scientific Realism*. Berkeley, CA: University of California.

Lepore, E. and McLaughlin, B. (1985). *Actions and Events*. Oxford: Blackwell.

LeVay, S. (1993) *The Sexual Brain*. Cambridge: MIT Press

Levy, D. (1996). *Freud Among the Philosophers*. New Haven, CT: Yale University Press.

Levy, N. and Bayne, T. (2004). Doing without deliberation: automatism, automaticity, and moral accountability. *International Review of Psychiatry*, 16(3): 209–215.

Lewis, A.J. (1934). On the psychopathology of insight. *British Journal of Medicine and Psychology*, 14: 332–348.

Lewis, A.J. (1953). Health as a social concept. *British Journal of Sociology*, 4: 109–24.

Lewis, B. (1995). The social relocation of personal identity. (Commentary on Hinshelwood, 1995) *Philosophy, Psychiatry, & Psychology*, 2(3): 215–218.

Lewis, C.I. and Langford, C.H. (1932). *Symbolic Logic*. New York: The Century Co.

Lewis, D. (1973). Causation. *Journal of Philosophy*, 70: 556–567 (Reprinted in *Causation* (ed. E. Sosa and M. Tooley). Oxford: Oxford University Press, 1993, pp. 193–204.)

Lewis, D. (1986). Causal explanation. In *Philosophical Papers*, Vol. II. Oxford: Oxford University Press. (Reprinted in Ruben, D.-H. (ed.) (1993). *Explanation*. Oxford: Oxford University Press, pp. 182–206.)

Libet, B. (1996). Free will in the light of neuropsychiatry. (Commentary on Spence, 1996) *Philosophy, Psychiatry, & Psychology*, 3(2): 95–96.

Liddle, P. (2000). Descriptive Clinical features of Schizophrenia in *New Oxford Text Book of Psychiatry* (Gelder, M.G. 2000), pp. 571–576. Oxford: Oxford University Press.

Lieberman, P.B. (1999). Perspectivism, realism, and psychotherapy. (Commentary on Lehrer, 1999) *Philosophy, Psychiatry, & Psychology*, 6(3): 181–186.

Lieberman, P.B. (2004). Action, belief, and empowerment. (Commentary on Waller, 2004) *Philosophy, Psychiatry, & Psychology*, 11(2): 119–124.

Lilleleht, E. (2002). Progress and power: exploring the disciplinary connections between moral treatment and psychiatric rehabilitation. *Philosophy, Psychiatry, & Psychology*, 9(2): 167–182.

Lilleleht, E. (2002). Listening, acting, and the quest for alternatives: a response to Charland and Bracken. *Philosophy, Psychiatry, & Psychology*, 9(2): 189–192.

Lindahl, B.I.B. and Johansson, L.A. (1994). Multiple cause-of-death data as a tool for detecting artificial trends in the underlying cause statistics: a methodological study. *Scandinavian Journal of Social Medicine*, 22(2): 145–158.

Lindahl, B.I.B. and Nordenfelt, L. (ed.) (1984). *Health, Disease, and Causal Explanations in Medicine*, Vol. 16. In *Philosophy and Medicine Book Series* (series ed. H.T. Engelhardt and S.F. Spicker). Dordrecht-Holland: D. Reidel Publishing Company.

Lipton, P. (1991). *Inference to the Best Explanation*. London: Routledge.

Lishman, A.W. (1978). (1997 paperback). *Organic psychiatry*. Oxford: Blackwell Scientific Publications.

Littlewood, R. (1997) Spiritual experience and psychopathology. (Commentary on Jackson and Fulford, 1997). *Philosophy, Psychiatry, & Psychology*, 4/1: 67–74.

Littlewood, R. (1999). Ecological understandings and cultural context. (Commentary on Deeley, 1999). *Philosophy, Psychiatry, & Psychology*, 6(2): 133–134.

Livesley, W.J., (1996) Commentary on "Epistemic Value Commitments". *Philosophy, Psychiatry, & Psychology*, 3(3), 223–226.

Loar, B. (1981) *Mind and Meaning*. Cambridge

Locke, J. ([1690] 1989). *Essay Concerning Human Understanding* (ed. P. Nidditch). Oxford: Clarendon Press.

Locker, D. (1981). The construction of illness. In *Symptoms and Illness*. London: Tavistock Publications, pp. 93–101.

Loewenstein, K. (1965). *Max Weber's Political Ideas in the Perspective of Our Time*. Amherst, MA: University of Massachusetts Press.

Loizzo, J. (1994). Insight, delusion, and belief. (Commentary on Gillett, 1994). *Philosophy, Psychiatry, & Psychology*, 1(4): 241–242.

Loizzo, J. (2000). Guarding patient agency. (Commentary on Campbell, 2000). *Philosophy, Psychiatry, & Psychology*, 7(2): 121–122.

Lord Chancellor's Department (1997). *Who Decides? Making Decisions on Behalf of Mentally Incapacitated Adults*, CM 3803, London: The Stationery Office Ltd.

Losee, J. (1980). *A Historical Introduction to the Philosophy of Science*, (2nd edn). Oxford: Oxford University Press.

Loughlin, M. (2003). Contingency, arbitrariness, and failure. (Commentary on Pickering, 2003). *Philosophy, Psychiatry, & Psychology*, 10(3): 261–264.

Louhiala, P. and Stenman, S. (ed.). (2000). *Philosophy Meets Medicine*. Helsinki: Helsinki University Press.

Loux, M.J. (1998). *Metaphysics*. London: Routledge.

Lowe, E.J. (1998). False memory syndrome. (Commentary on Hamilton, 1998). *Philosophy, Psychiatry, & Psychology*, 5(4): 309–310.

Lu, F.G., Lukoff, D., and Turner, R.P. (1997). Commentary on 'Spiritual experience and psychopathology'. (Commentary on Jackson and Fulford, 1997). *Philosophy, Psychiatry, & Psychology*, 4(1): 75–78.

Lucas, F.R. (1993). *Responsibility*. Oxford: Clarendon Press.

Luntley, M.O. (1996) Commentary on "Epistemic Value Commitments". *Philosophy, Psychiatry, & Psychology*, 3(3), 227–230.

Luntley, M.O. (2002). Knowing how to manage: expertise and embedded knowledge. *Reason in Practice*, 2(3): 3–14.

Luntley, M.O. (1999). *Contemporary Philosophy of Thought*. Oxford: Blackwell.

Lycan, W. (ed.) (1990). *Mind and Cognition*. Oxford: Blackwell.

Lyons, W. (ed.) (1995). *Modern Philosophy of Mind*. London: Dent.

Macdonald, C. (1989). *Mind-Body Identity Theories*. London: Routledge.

Macdonald, G. (1995). The biological turn. In *Philosophy of Psychology* (ed. C. Macdonald and G. Macdonald). Oxford: Blackwell, pp. 238–252.

Mace, C. (1997). Primitive mental processes: psychoanalysis and the ethics of integration. (Commentary on Hinshelwood, 1997) *Philosophy, Psychiatry, & Psychology*, 4(2): 145–150.

Mace, C. (1999). On putting psychoanalysis into a Nietzschean perspective. (Commentary on Lehrer, 1999) *Philosophy, Psychiatry, & Psychology*, 6(3): 187–190.

MacIntyre, A. (1982). *After Virtue*. London: Duckworth.

Mackie, J.L. (1976). *Problems from Locke*. Oxford: Clarendon Press.

Mackie, J.L. (1977) *Ethics: inventing right and wrong*. New York: Viking.

Mackie, J.L. (1993). Causes and conditions. In *Causation* (ed. E. Sosa and M. Tooley). Oxford: Oxford University Press, pp. 33–50.

Macklin (1973). The medical model in psychoanalysis and psychotherapy. *Comprehensive Psychiatry*, 14: 49–69.

MacQuarrie, J. (1973) *Existentialism*. London: Penguin Books.

Maehle, A-H. and Geyer-Kordesch, J. (ed.) (2002). Historical and philosophical perspectives on biomedical ethics. *Historical and Philosophical Perspectives on Biomedical Ethics: from Paternalism to Autonomy?* Aldershot, Ashgate Publishing Limited.

Magee, B. (1987). *The Great Philosophers: an introduction to Western philosophy*. London: BBC Books.

Makkreel, R.A. (1969). Wilhelm Dilthey and the neo-Kantians: the distinction of the Geisteswissenschaften and the Kulturwissenschaften. *Journal of the History of Philosophy*, 7: 423–440.

Makkreel, R.A. (1975). *Dilthey: philosopher of the human studies*. Princeton: Princeton University Press.

Malcolm, N. (1958). Knowledge of other minds. *Journal of Philosophy*, 55. (Reprinted in Rosenthal, D (ed.) (1991). *The Nature of Mind*. Oxford: Oxford University Press, pp. 92–97.)

Malcolm, N. (1968) The conceivability of mechanism *Philosophical Review* 77: 45–72.

Malcolm. N. (1971). *Problems of Mind: Descartes to Wittgenstein*. London: Allen & Unwin.

Malebranche, N. (1674–5) *De la recherche de la vérité*, in *Oeuvres*, vols 1–3, 6th edn, 1712; trans. T. Lennon and P.J. Olscamp as *The Search After Truth/Elucidations of the Search After Truth*, Columbus, OH: Ohio State University Press, 1980.

Malter, R. (1981). Main currents in the German interpretation of the *Critique of Pure Reason* since the beginnings of neo-Kantianism. *Journal of the History of Ideas*, 42: 531–551.

Margree, V. (2002). Normal and abnormal: Georges Canguilhem and the question of mental pathology. *Philosophy, Psychiatry, & Psychology*, 9(4): 299–312.

Margree, V. (2002). Canguilhem and social pathology: a response to the Commentary. *Philosophy, Psychiatry, & Psychology*, 9(4): 317–320.

Marina, J.A. (1999). The problem of values in psychiatry. In *Archivos de Psiquiatria: Introduccion al Proyecto: Hechos y Valores en Psiquiatria. Suplemento 3*. (Facts and Values in Psychiatry: an introduction) (ed. J. Ortega y Gasset, G.R. Lafora, and J.M. Sacristan). Madrid: Editorial Triacastela, 3: 55–68.

Marshall, M. (1994). How should we measure need? Concept and practice in the development of a standardized assessment schedule. *Philosophy, Psychiatry, & Psychology*, 1(1): 27–36.

Martin, M.W. (1999). Depression: illness, insight, and identity. *Philosophy, Psychiatry, & Psychology*, 6(4): 271–286.

Martin, M.W. (1999). Response to the Commentary. *Philosophy, Psychiatry, & Psychology*, 6(4): 295–298.

Martin, M.W. (2002). On the evolution of depression. (Commentary on Glannon, 2002) *Philosophy, Psychiatry, & Psychology*, 9(3): 255–260.

Martins, F., Costa, A. and Porto, K. (2000) Delusion according to the theory of speech acts. *Psicologia: Reflexao e Critica* 13: 189–198.

Marx, M.J. and Johnson, J.L. (1991). *The Illness Experience: Dimensions of Suffering*. Newbury Park, London: Sage Publications.

Marzanski, M. and Bratton, M. (2002). Commentary: Minding your language: a response to Caroline Brett and Stephen Sykes. *Philosophy, Psychiatry, & Psychology*, 9(4): 383–386.

Marzanski, M. and Bratton, M. (2002). Psychopathological symptoms and religious experience: a critique of Jackson and Fulford. *Philosophy, Psychiatry, & Psychology*, 9(4): 359–372.

Marzanski, M. and Bratton, M. (2002) Commentary on 'Mystical states or mystical life? Buddhist, Christian, and Hindu perspectives. *Philosophy, Psychiatry, & Psychology*, 9(4): 349–352.

Mason, J.K. and McCall Smith, R.A. (1999). *Law and Medical Ethics*. London: Butterworths.

Mason, P. (1996). Agoraphobia: letting go. In *Speaking Our Minds: an anthology* (ed. J. Read and J. Reynolds). London: Macmillan Press Ltd, for the Open University, pp. 3–8.

Matthews, E. (1995). Moralist or therapist? Foucault and the critique of psychiatry. *Philosophy, Psychiatry, & Psychology*, 2(1): 19–30.

Matthews, E. (1996) *Twentieth Century French Philosophy*. Oxford: Oxford University Press.

Matthews, E. (1998). Choosing death: philosophical observations on suicide and euthanasia. *Philosophy, Psychiatry, & Psychology*, 5(2): 107–112.

Matthews, E. (1999) Mental and Physical Illness: An Unsustainable Separation? In Eastman, N. and Peay, J. (eds) *Law without Enforcement: Integrating mental health and justice*, Oxford and Portland, OR: Hart Publishing.

Matthews, E. (1999). Moral vision and the idea of mental illness. *Philosophy, Psychiatry, & Psychology*, 6(4): 299–310.

Matthews, E. (1999). Disordered minds: a response to the commentaries. *Philosophy, Psychiatry, & Psychology*, 6(4): 321–322.

Matthews, E. (2003). How can a mind be sick? In *Nature and Narrative: an introduction to the new philosophy of psychiatry* (ed. K.W.M. Fulford, K.J. Morris, J.Z.S. Sadler, and G. Stanghellini). Oxford: Oxford University Press, Chapter 4.

Matthews, E.H. (2004) Merleau-Ponty's body-subject and psychiatry. *International Review of Psychiatry*, 16, 3:190–198.

Matthews, S. (2003). Establishing personal identity in cases of DID. *Philosophy, Psychiatry, & Psychology*, 10(2): 143–152. (Commentary by Braude, S.E. (2003, pp. 153–156), Clark, S.R.L. (2003, pp. 157–160), and Deeley, P.Q. (2003, pp. 161–168), and reply by Matthews, S. (2003, pp. 169–174).

Matthews, S. (2003). Blaming agents and excusing persons: the case of DID. (Response to the Commentaries) *Philosophy, Psychiatry, & Psychology*, 10(2): 169–174.

May, W. (1982). The virtues in a professional setting. In *After Virtue*. London: Duckworth.

May, W.F. (1994). The virtues in a professional setting. In *Medicine and Moral Reasoning* (ed. K.W.M. Fulford, G.R. Gillett, and J.M. Soskice). Cambridge: Cambridge University Press, Chapter 6.

McCormick, S. (1995). True wishes. (Commentary on Dickenson and Jones, 1995). *Philosophy, Psychiatry, & Psychology*, 2(4): 309–310.

McDowell, J. (1982). Criteria, defeasibility, and knowledge. *Proceedings of the British Academy*, 68.

McDowell, J. (1985). Functionalism and anomalous monism. In *Actions and Events* (eds E. Lepore and B. McLaughlin). Oxford: Blackwell, pp. 387–398.

McDowell, J. (1986). Singular thought and the extent of inner space. In *Subject Thought and Context* (ed. J. McDowell and P. Pettit). Oxford: Oxford University Press, pp. 137–168.

McDowell, J. (1992). Meaning and intentionality in Wittgenstein's later philosophy. *Midwest Studies in Philosophy*, 17: 40–52.

McDowell, J. (1994). *Mind and World*. Cambridge, MA: Harvard University Press.

McDowell, J. (1998). *Mind, Value, and Reality*. Cambridge, MA: Harvard University Press.

McDowell, J. (1998). *Meaning Knowledge and Reality*. Cambridge, MA: Harvard University Press.

McGhee, M. (2002). Commentary on 'Mysticism and psychosis: descriptions and distinctions.' (Commentary on Brett, 2002). *Philosophy, Psychiatry, & Psychology*, 9(4): 343–348.

McGhee, M. (2002). Mysticism and psychosis: descriptions and distinctions. (Commentary on Brett 2002a). *Philosophy, Psychiatry, & Psychology*, 9(4): 343–348.

McGinn, C. (1977). Anomalous monism and Kripke's Cartesian intuitions. *Analysis*, 37: 78–80

McGinn, C. (1982). *The Character of Mind*. Oxford: Oxford University Press.

McGinn, C. (1989), 'Can we solve the mind-body problem?' *Mind*, 98: 349–366.

McGinn, C. (1989). *Mental Content*. Oxford: Blackwell.

McGinn, C. (1993). Consciousness and cosmology: hyperdualism ventilated. In *Consciousness: Psychological and Philosophical Essays* (ed. M. Davies and G.W. Humphreys). Oxford: Blackwell.

McGinn, C. (1999). *The Mysterious Flame: conscious minds in a material world*. New York: Basic Books.

McGinn, M. (1989). *Sense and Certainty*. Oxford: Blackwell.

McGinn, M. (1997). *Wittgenstein and the Philosophical Investigations*. London: Routledge.

McGinn, M. (1999). *Wittgenstein's Philosophical Investigations*. London: Routledge.

McHale, J., Fox, M., and Murphy, J. (1999). *Health Care Law: text and materials*. London: Sweet and Maxwell.

McHugh, P. R. and Slavney, P. R. (1983) *The Perspectives of Psychiatry*. Baltimore, USA: The Johns Hopkins University Press.

McMillan, J. (1999). Cognitive psychology and hermeneutics: two irreconcilable approaches? (Commentary on Widdershoven, 1999) *Philosophy, Psychiatry, & Psychology*, 6(4): 255–258.

McMillan, J. (1999). Commentary: Cognitive psychology and hermeneutics: two irreconcilable approaches? *Philosophy, Psychiatry, & Psychology*, 6(4): 255–258.

McMillan, J. (2002). Jaspers and defining phenomenology. (Commentary on Gupta and Kay, 2001). *Philosophy, Psychiatry, & Psychology*, 9(1): 91–92.

McMillan, J. (2003). Dangerousness, mental disorder, and responsibility. *Journal of Medical Ethics*, 29: 232–235.

McMullin, E. (1987). Explanatory success and the truth of theory. In *Scientific Inquiry in Philosophical Perspective* (ed. N. Rescher). New York: University Press of America, pp. 51–73.

Meares, R. (2003). Towards a psyche for psychiatry. In *Nature and Narrative: an introduction to the new philosophy of psychiatry* (ed. K.W.M. Fulford, K.J. Morris, J.Z.S. Sadler, and G. Stanghellini). Oxford: Oxford University Press, Chapter 2.

Mechanic, D. (1981). The social dimension. In *Psychiatric Ethics*, (1st edn) (ed. S. Bloch and P. Chodoff). Oxford: Oxford University Press, pp. 46–59.

Megone, C. (1998). Aristotle's function argument and the concept of mental illness. *Philosophy, Psychiatry, and Psychology*, 5(3): 187–202.

Megone, C. (1998). Aristotle's function argument and the concept of mental illness. (Commentaries by Szasz (1998), Hobbs (1998) and Fulford (1998) and a response (Megone, 1998). *Philosophy, Psychiatry, & Psychology*, 5(3): 187–202.

Megone, C. (1998). Response to the Commentaries. *Philosophy, Psychiatry, & Psychology*, 5(3): 221–224.

Megone, C. (2000). Mental illness, human function, and values. *Philosophy, Psychiatry, and Psychology*, 7(1): 45–66.

Melden, A.I. (1961). *Free Action*. London: Routledge.

Mele, A.R. (1997). *The Philosophy of Action*. Oxford: Oxford University Press.

Mele, A.R. (2004). Action: volitional disorder and addiction. In *The Philosophy of Psychiatry: a companion* (ed. J. Radden). New York: Oxford University Press, pp. 78–88.

Mellor, C.S. (1970). First rank symptoms of schizophrenia. *British Journal of Psychiatry*, 117: 15–23.

Mellor, D.H. (1991). *Matters of Metaphysics*. Cambridge: Cambridge University Press.

Mellor, D.H. (1991). The warrant of induction. In *Matters of Metaphysics*. London: Routledge.

Melville Woody, J. and Phillips, J. (1995) Freud's project for a scientific psychology after 100 years: the unconscious mind in the era of cognitive science. *Philosophy, Psychiatry, & Psychology*, 2(2): 123–134.

Mental Health Act Commission (2003). *Placed Amongst Strangers. Tenth Biennial Report 2001–2003. Twenty years of the Mental Health Act 1983 and the future for psychiatric compulsion.*' London: The Stationery Office.

Mental Health Foundation (1999). *The Courage to Bare our Souls*. London: Mental Health Foundation.

Mental Health Foundation (2002). *The Somerset Spirituality Project*. London: Mental Health Foundation.

Menzies, P. (1996). Probabilistic causation and the pre-emption problem. *Mind*, 105: 85–117.

Menzies, P. (1999). Intrinsic versus extrinsic conceptions of causation. In *Causation and Laws of Nature* (ed. H. Sankey). Kluwer Academic Publishers, pp. 313–329.

Merleau-Ponty, M. ([1945] 1962, 1996). *The Phenomenology of Perception* (transl. Colin Smith). London: Routledge.

Merleau-Ponty, M. (1963) *The Structure of Behaviour*. A. L. Fisher (trans.) Boston, MA: Beacon Press.

Merleau-Ponty, M. (1964) *Le Visible et l'invisible* (Paris: Gallimard), edited byt Claude Lefort, English trans. *The Visible and the Invisible*, trans. Alphonso Lingis, (Evanston, IL: Northwestern University Press, 1968).

Merleau-Ponty, M. in McCleary, R. C. (trans) *Signs*. (1964 Evanston, Ill: Northwestern University Press; original French edition 1960). *The Structure of Behaviour*. A. L. Fisher (trans.) Boston, MA: Beacon Press, 1963 and London: Methuen, 1965.

Metzinger, T. (2000). The subjectivity of subjective experience: a representationalist analysis of the first-person perspective. In *Neural Correlates of Consciousness* (ed. T. Metzinger). Cambridge: MA: MIT Press, pp. 287–324.

Mezzich, J. E. (2002) Comprehensive diagnosis: a conceptual basis for future diagnostic systems. *Psychopathology*, 35(2–3):162–5.

Mezzich, J.E. (2005) Values and comprehensive diagnosis. *World Psychiatry*, 4(2): 91.

Mezzich, J.E. Kleinman, A, Fabrega, H. and Parron, D.L. (eds) (1996) *Culture and Psychiatric Diagnosis: A DSM-IV Perspective*. Washington: American Psychiatric Press Inc.

Mezzich, J.E., Berganza, C.E., Von Cranach, M., Jorge, M.R., Kastrup, M.C., Murthy, R.S., Okasha, A., Pull, C., Sartorius, N., Skodol, A., and Zaudig, M. (2003) IGDA. 8: Idiographic (personalised) diagnostic formulation. In *Essentials of the World Psychiatric Association's International Guidelines for Diagnostic Assessment (IGD). The British Journal of Psychiatry*, 182(Suppl. 45): 55–57.

Mezzich, J.E., Kleinman, A, Fabrega, H., and Parron, D.L. (ed.) (1996). *Culture and Psychiatric Diagnosis: a DSM-IV perspective*. Washington, DC: American Psychiatric Press Inc.

Michels, R. and Kelly, K. (1999). In *Psychiatric Ethics* (ed. S. Bloch, P. Chodoff, and S.A. Green), (3rd edn). Oxford, Oxford University Press, Chapter 24.

Mill, J.S. (1879). *A System of Logic*. London: Longman.

Mill, J.S. (1974). *Collected Works of John Stuart Mill*, Vol. VIII: *A System of Logic, Ratiocinative and Inductive* (ed. J.M. Robson). London: Routledge and Kegan Paul, Books IV–VI and Appendices.

Miller, A. (1998). *Philosophy of Language*. London: Routledge.

Miller, A. and Wright, C. (ed.) (2002). *Rule-following and Meaning*. Chesham: Acumen.

Milligan, S. and Clare, A. (1993). *Depression and How to Survive It*. London: Arrow.

Millikan, R.G. (1984). *Language, Thought and Other Biological Categories*. Cambridge, MA: MIT Press.

Millikan, R.G. (1993). *White Queen Psychology*. Cambridge, MA: MIT Press.

Millikan, R.G. (1995). Biosemantics: explanation in biopsychology. In *Philosophy of Psychology* (ed. C. Macdonald and G. Macdonald). Oxford: Blackwell, pp. 238–276.

Minkowski, E. (1927) *La Schizophrenie. Psychopathologie des Schizoides et des Schizophrenes*. Payot: Paris.

Minkowski, E. (1968) *Le Temps Vecu*. Paris: Presse Universitaire de France.

Minkowski, E. and Targowla, R. (2001). A contribution to the study of autism: the interrogative attitude. *Philosophy, Psychiatry, & Psychology*, 8(4): 271–278.

Minsky, L. (1933). The mental symptoms associated with 58 cases of cerebral tumour. *Journal of Neurology and Psychopathology*, 13: 330–343.

Mishara, A. (1996). William Griesinger. (Commentary on Arens, 1996). *Philosophy, Psychiatry, and Psychology*, 3(3): 165–168.

Mishara, A.L. (2001). On Wolfgang Blankenburg, common sense, and schizophrenia. (Commentary on Blankenburg, 2001). *Philosophy, Psychiatry, & Psychology*, 8(4): 317–322.

Mitchell, J. (1998). Neurosis and the historic quest for security: a social-role analysis. *Philosophy, Psychiatry, & Psychology*, 5(4): 317–328.

Mitchell, J. (1998). Response to the Commentary. *Philosophy, Psychiatry, & Psychology*, 5(4): 333–336.

Mitchell, J. (2001). Anorexia: social world and the internal woman. (Commentary on Richmond, 2001). *Philosophy, Psychiatry, & Psychology*, 8(1): 13–16.

Mohl, P. (1995). Freud's Project for a scientific psychology after 100 years. (Commentary on Woody and Phillips, 1995) *Philosophy, Psychiatry, & Psychology*, 2(2): 135–136.

Montaigne ([1580] 2003). *Apology for Raymond Sebond*. Trans. R. Ariew and M Grene. Hackett Publishing Co. Inc.

Montgomery, J. (1996). Patients first: the role of rights. In *Essential Practice in Patient-centred Care* (ed. K.W.M. Fulford, S. Ersser, and T. Hope). Oxford: Blackwell Science, Chapter 9.

Montgomery J. (1997). *Health Care Law*. Oxford: Oxford University Press.

Montgomery, J. (1998). Suicide, euthanasia, and the psychiatrist: a legal footnote. *Philosophy, Psychiatry, & Psychology*, 5(2): 153–156.

Moore, A. (1997). Psychological courage. (Commentary on Putnam, 1997). *Philosophy, Psychiatry, & Psychology*, 4(1): 13–14.

Moore, A., Hope, T., and Fulford, K.W.M. (1994). Mild mania and well-being. *Philosophy, Psychiatry, & Psychology*, 1(3): 165–178.

Moore, G.E. (1980[1903]). *Principia Ethica*. Cambridge: Cambridge University Press.

Moore, M.S. (1984). *Law and Psychiatry: rethinking the relationship*. Cambridge: Cambridge University Press.

Mordini, E. (1997). Commentary on 'The stoic conception of mental disorder'. *Philosophy, Psychiatry, & Psychology*, 4(4): 297–302.

Morgan, J. (1994). Commentary on 'How should we measure need?' *Philosophy, Psychiatry, and Psychology*, 1(1): 39–40.

Morley, J. (2002). Phenomenological and biological psychiatry: complementary or mutual? (Commentary on Gupta and Kay, 2001). *Philosophy, Psychiatry, & Psychology*, 9(1): 87–90.

Morris, K.J. (2003). Commentary on 'Did you hurt yourself?' (Commentary on Potter, 2003). *Philosophy, Psychiatry, & Psychology*, 10(1): 23–24.

Morris, K.J. (2003) The phenomenology of body dysmorphic disorder: a Sartrean analysis. Chapter 11 in Fulford, K. W. M., Morris, K.J., Sadler, J.Z., and Stanghellini, G. (eds.) *Nature and Narrative: An Introduction to the New Philosophy of Psychiatry*. Oxford: Oxford University Press, pp. 270–274.

Mulhall, S. (1990). *On Being in the World*. London: Routledge.

Mulhall, S. (1996). *The Routledge Philosophy Guidebook to Heidegger and 'Being and Time'*. London: Routledge.

Mullen, P.E. (2002). Moral principles don't signify. (Commentary on Ward, 2002). *Philosophy, Psychiatry, & Psychology*, 9(1): 19–22.

Mullen, R. (2003). Definition is limited and values inescapable. (Commentary on Pickering, 2003). *Philosophy, Psychiatry, & Psychology*, 10(3): 265–266.

Mundt, C.H. (2003). Editorial: Common language and local diversities of psychopathological concepts—alternatives or complements? P*sychopathology*, 36(3): 111–113.

Mundt, C.H. and Spitzer, M. (2001). Psychopathology today. In: *Contemporary Psychiatry*, Vol. 1 *Foundations of Psychiatry* (ed. F. Henn, N. Sartorius, H. Helmchen, and H. Lauter). Berlin: Springer-Verlag, pp. 1–28.

Murphy, D. and Woolfolk, R.L. (2000). The harmful dysfunction analysis of mental disorder. *Philosophy, Psychiatry, & Psychology*, 7(4): 241–252.

Murphy, D., and Woolfolk, R.L. (2000). Conceptual analysis versus scientific understanding: an assessment of Wakefield's folk psychiatry. *Philosophy, Psychiatry, & Psychology*, 7(4): 271–294.

Murray, T.H. (1994). Medical ethics, moral philosophy and moral tradition. In *Medicine and Moral Reasoning* (ed. K.W.M. Fulford, G. Gillett, and J.M. Soskice). Cambridge: Cambridge University Press, pp. 91–105.

Murray, T.H. (1995). Commentary on true wishes. (Commentary on Dickenson and Jones, 1995). *Philosophy, Psychiatry, & Psychology*, 2(4): 311–312.

Musalek, M. (2003) Meanings and causes of delusions. Chapter 10 in Fulford, K. W. M., Morris, K. J., Sadler, J. Z., and Stanghellini, G. (eds.) *Nature and Narrative: An Introduction to the New Philosophy of Psychiatry*. Oxford: Oxford University Press.

Muse, K.R. (1991). Edmund Husserls impact on Max Weber. In *Max Weber: critical assessments*, Vol. 2 (ed. P. Hamilton). London: Routledge, pp. 254–263.

Nagel, T. (1986). *The View from Nowhere*. Oxford: Oxford University Press.

Nagel, T. (1987). *What does it all mean? A very short introduction to philosophy*. Oxford: Oxford University Press.

National Institute for Mental Health England, The Sainsbury Centre for Mental Health and the NHSU (2004). *The Ten Essential Shared Capabilities for Mental Health Practice*. London: Sainsbury Centre for Mental Health.

Naudin, J. and Azorin, J.-M. (1997). Commentary on Wiggins and Schwartz, 1997, Edmund Husserls influence on Karl Jaspers's phenomenology. *Philosophy, Psychiatry, & Psychology*, 4: 37–40.

Naudin, J. and Azorin, J.-M. (2001). Schizophrenia and the void. (Commentary on Minkowski and Targowla, 2001). *Philosophy, Psychiatry, & Psychology*, 8(4): 291–294.

Neurath, O. (1932). Protokollsaetze. *Erkenntnis*, 3: 204–214.

Nissim-Sabat, M. (1999). Phenomenology and mental disorders: Heidegger or Husserl? (Commentary on Svenaeus, 1999). *Philosophy, Psychiatry, & Psychology*, 6(2): 101–104.

Nissim-Sabat, M. (2001). Psychiatry, psychoanalysis, and race. *Philosophy, Psychiatry, & Psychology*, 8(1): 45–60.

Nordenfelt, L. (1987). *On the Nature of Health: an action-theoretic account of health*. Dordrecht: D. Reidel Publishing Co.

Nordenfelt, L. (1994). Mild mania and theory of health. (Commentary on Moore *et al.*, 1994) *Philosophy, Psychiatry, & Psychology*, 1(3): 179–184.

Nordenfelt, L. (1997) *Talking about Health: A Philosophical Dialogue*. Amsterdam: Rodopi.

Nordenfelt, L. (1997). The stoic conception of mental disorder: the case of Cicero. *Philosophy, Psychiatry, & Psychology*, 4(4): 285–292.

Nordenfelt, L. (1997). Response to the commentaries. *Philosophy, Psychiatry, & Psychology*, 4(4): 305–306.

Nordenfelt, L. (2001) *Health, Science, and Ordinary Language*. Amsterdam: Rodopi.

Norrie, A. (1997). Pathological autobiographies. (Commentary on Harré, 1997). *Philosophy, Psychiatry, & Psychology* 4(2): 115–118.

Northoff, G. (1999). Psychomotor phenomena, functional brain organization, and the mind-body relationship: Do we need a 'philosophy of the brain'? *Philosophy, Psychiatry, & Psychology*, 6(3): 199–215.

Northoff, G. (1999). Neuropsychiatry, epistemology, and ontology of the brain: a response to the Commentaries on Northoff (1999). *Philosophy, Psychiatry, & Psychology*, 6(3): 231–235.

Nozick, R. (1981). *Philosophical Explanations*. Cambridge, MA.: Harvard University Press.

Oakes, G. (1988). *Weber and Rickert: concept formation in the cultural sciences*. Cambridge, MA: MIT Press.

O'Brien, B. (1976). *Operators and Things: the inner life of a schizophrenic*. London: Sphere Books Ltd.

O'Hear, A. (1985) *What Philosophy Is*. Harmondsworth, England: Penguin Books.

Okasha, A. (2000). Ethics of psychiatric practice: consent, compulsion and confidentiality. *Current Opinion in Psychiatry*, 13: 693–698.

Okasha, A. and Maj, M. (ed.). (2001). *Images in Psychiatry: an Arab perspective*. World Psychiatric Association. Egypt: Scientific Book House.

Olson, E. (1997). *The Human Animal: personal identity without psychology*. Oxford: Oxford University Press.

Olson, E. (1998). There is no problem of the self. *Journal of Consciousness Studies*, 5: 645–657.

Ormiston, G. and Schrift, A. (eds.) (1989) *Transforming the Hermeneutic Context*. New York: State University of New York Press.

Ormiston, G. and Schrift, A. (eds.) (1990) *The Hermeneutic Tradition*. New York: State University of New York Press.

Osborn, D. (1999). Research and ethics: leaving exclusion behind. *Current Opinion in Psychiatry*, 12(5): 601–604.

Ott, H. (1993). *Martin Heidegger: a political life* (trans. by A. Blunden). London: Fontana Press.

Pacherie, E. (2001). Agency lost and found: a commentary on Spence. (Commentary on Spence, 2001) *Philosophy, Psychiatry, & Psychology*, 8(2–3): 173–176.

Pachoud, B. (2001). Reading Minkowski with Husserl. (Commentary on Minkowski and Targowla, 2001). *Philosophy, Psychiatry, & Psychology*, 8(4): 299–302.

Papineau, D. (1986). Laws and accidents. In *Fact, Science and Morality* (ed. G. MacDonald and C. Wright). Oxford: Blackwell, pp. 190–191.

Papineau, D. (1987). *For Science in the Social Sciences*. Basingstoke: Palgrave.

Papineau, D. (1987). *Reality and Representation* Oxford: Blackwell.

Papineau, D. (1990). Why supervenience. *Analysis*, 50: 66–70.

Papineau, D. (1993). *Philosophical Naturalism*. Oxford: Blackwell.

Parfit, D. (1971). Personal identity. *Philosophical Review*, 80: 3–27.

Parfit, D. (1984). *Reasons and Persons*. Oxford: Clarendon Press.

Parfit, D. (1999). Experiences, subjects, and conceptual schemes. *Philosophical Topics*, 26: 217–270.

Parker, M. (1995). True wishes. (Commentary on Dickenson and Jones, 1995). *Philosophy, Psychiatry, & Psychology*, 2(4): 313–314.

Parker, M. (1999). *Ethics and Community in the Health Care Professions*. London: Routledge.

Parker, M. and Dickenson, D. (2000). *The Cambridge Workbook in Medical Ethics*. Cambridge: Cambridge University Press.

Parkin, A.J. (1996). *Explorations in Cognitive Neuropsychology*. Oxford: Blackwell.

Parnas, J. and Sass, L.A. (2001). Self, solipsism, and schizophrenic delusions. *Philosophy, Psychiatry, & Psychology*, 8/2/3, 101–120.

Parnas, J. and Zahavi, D. (2000). The link: philosophy–psychopathology–phenomenology. In *Exploring The Self* (ed. D. Zahavi). Amsterdam: Benjamins, pp. 1–16.

Parnas, J., Sass, L. and Stanghellini, G. and Fuchs, T. (forthcoming) *The Vulnerable Self: the clinical phenomenology of the schizophrenic and affective spectrum disorders*. Oxford: Oxford University Press.

Parry-Jones, W. (1972). *The Trade in Lunacy*. London: Routledge and Kegan Paul.

Parsons, T. (1951). *The Social System*. Glencoe, IL: Free Press.

Peacocke. (1992). *A Study in Concepts*. Cambridge, MA: MIT Press.

Pears, D. (1990). *Hume's System*. Oxford: Oxford University Press.

Pearson, G. (1975). *The Deviant Imagination*. London: Macmillan.

Pearson, K.A. (1999). Perspectivism and relativism beyond the postmodern condition. (Commentary on Lehrer, 1999) *Philosophy, Psychiatry, & Psychology*, 6(3): 167–172.

Peay, J. (2003) *Decisions and Dilemmas: Working with Mental Health Law*. Portland, OR: Hart Publishing.

Peele, R. and Chodoff, P. (1999). 'The ethics of involuntary treatment'. In *Psychiatric Ethics* (ed. S. Bloch, P. Chodoff, and S.A. Green), (3rd edn). Oxford: Oxford University Press, Chapter 20.

Perkins, R. (2001). What constitutes success? The relative priority of service users' and clinicians' views of mental health services. *British Journal of Psychiatry*, 179: 9–10.

Perkins, R. and Moodley, P. (1993). The arrogance of insight. *Psychiatric Bulletin*, 17: 233–234.

Perkins, R., and Repper, J. (1998). *Dilemmas in Community Mental Health Practice: Choice or Control*. Aberdeen: Radcliffe Medical Press.

Perring, C. (2004). Development: disorders of childhood and youth. In *The Philosophy of Psychiatry: A Companion* (ed. J. Radden, J.). New York: Oxford University Press, pp. 147–162.

Perry, J. (1978). *A Dialogue on Personal Identity and Immortality*. Indianapolis: Hackett.

Perry, J. (ed.) (1975). *Personal Identity*. Berkeley: University of California Press.

Persaud, A. (1999). *Respect for Privacy, Dignity and Religious and Cultural Beliefs*. Wiltshire: Wiltshire Health Authority.

Petitot, J., Varela, F., Pachoud, B., and Roy, J.-M. (ed.) (2000). *Naturalizing Phenomenology: issues in contemporary phenomenology and cognitive science*. Cambridge: Cambridge University Press.

Phillips, J. (1996). Key concepts: hermeneutics. *Philosophy, Psychiatry, & Psychology*, 3(1): 61–70.

Phillips, J. (1998). Commentary on 'Relativism and the social-constructivist paradigm'. *Philosophy, Psychiatry, & Psychology*, 5(1): 55–60.

Phillips, J. (1999). The hermeneutical critique of cognitive psychology. (Commentary on Widdershoven, 1999) *Philosophy, Psychiatry, & Psychology*, 6(4): 259–264.

Phillips, J. (2001). Kimura Bin on schizophrenia. (Commentary on Bin, 2001). *Philosophy, Psychiatry, & Psychology*, 8(4): 343–346.

Phillips, J. (2002). Arguing from neuroscience in psychiatry. (Commentary on Gerrans, 2002). *Philosophy, Psychiatry, & Psychology*, 9: 61–64.

Phillips, J. (2003). Psychopathology and the narrative self. *Philosophy, Psychiatry, & Psychology*, 10(4): 313–328.

Phillips, J. (2004). Understanding/explanation. In *The Philosophy of Psychiatry: a companion* (ed. J. Radden). New York: Oxford University Press, pp. 180–190.

Phillips, J. and Morley, J. (ed.). (2003). *Imagination and Its Pathologies*. Cambridge, MA: MIT Press.

Philpott, M.J. (1998). A phenomenology of dyslexia: the lived-body, ambiguity, and the breakdown of expression. *Philosophy, Psychiatry, & Psychology*, 5(1): 1–20.

Philpott, M.J. (1998). Response to the Commentaries. *Philosophy, Psychiatry, & Psychology*, 5(1): 33–36.

Philpott, M.J. (1999). The how and why of phenomenology. (Commentary on Svenaeus, 1999). *Philosophy, Psychiatry, & Psychology*, 6(2): 87–94.

Pickering, N. (2003). The likeness argument and the reality of mental illness. *Philosophy, Psychiatry, & Psychology*, 10(3): 243–254.

Pickering, N. (2003). The likeness argument: reminders, roles, and reasons for use. (A response to the commentaries). *Philosophy, Psychiatry, & Psychology*, 10(3): 273–276.

Pickering, N. (2006) *The Metaphor of Mental Illness*. Oxford: Oxford University Press.

Pigden, C.R. (1993). Naturalism. In *A Companion to Ethics* (ed. P. Singer). Oxford: Blackwell.

Pine, D.S., Alegria, M., Cook, E.H. Jr, Costello, E.J., Dahl, R.E., Koretz, D., Merikangas, K.R., Reiss, A.L., and Vitiello, B. (2002). Advances in developmental science and DSM-V. In

A Research Agenda for DSM-V (ed. D.J. Kupfer, M.B. First, and D.E. Regier). Washington, DC: American Psychiatric Association, pp. 85–122.

Plato. (2003) *The Republic*. Harmondsworth, England: Penguin Books Limited.

Pocock, S.J. (1983). *Clinical Trials: a practical approach*. Chichester: Wiley.

Polanyi, M. ([1958] 1974). *Personal Knowledge: towards a post-critical philosophy*. Chicago, IL: University of Chicago Press.

Polt, R. (1999). *Heidegger: an introduction*. London: University of London Press.

Popper, K. ([1934] expanded text, 1959). *The Logic of Scientific Discovery*. London: Hutcheson.

Popper, K. (1962). *The Open Society and Its Enemies*, Vol. 1. Princeton: Princeton University Press.

Popper, K. (1963). *Conjectures and Refutations*. London: Routledge.

Popper, K. (1972). Conjectural knowledge: my solution to the problem of induction in *Objective Knowledge*. Oxford: Oxford University Press. pps 1–31.

Porter, R. (1987). From fools to outsiders. In *A Social History of Madness*. London: Weidenfeld and Nicolson.

Porter, R. (1997) A review of Edward Shorter's *A History of Psychiatry*. *Evening Standard*.

Porter, R. and Shepherd, M. (1985). *The Anatomy of Madness*, (2 vols). London: Tavistock.

Posner, M.I. (1993). Seeing the mind. *Science*, 262: 673–674.

Potter, N.N. (1996). Loopholes, gaps, and what is held fast: democratic epistemology and claims to recovered memories. *Philosophy, Psychiatry, & Psychology*, 3(4): 237–254.

Potter, N.N. (2001). Feminism. *Philosophy, Psychiatry, & Psychology*, 8(1): 61–72.

Potter, N.N. (2003). Commodity/body/sign: borderline personality disorder and the signification of self-injurious behavior. *Philosophy, Psychiatry, & Psychology*, 10(1): 1–16.

Potter, N.N. (2003). Moral tourists and world travelers: some epistemological issues in understanding patients' worlds. *Philosophy, Psychiatry, & Psychology*, 10(3): 209–224. Commentaries by Cassell (2003), Jaeger (2003), Spitz (2003), and with a response by Potter (2003).

Potter, N.N. (2003). In the spirit of giving uptake. Response to the commentaries. *Philosophy, Psychiatry, & Psychology*, 10/1: 33–36.

Potter, N.N. (2004). Gender. In *The Philosophy of Psychiatry: a companion* (ed. J. Radden). New York: Oxford University Press, pp. 237–243.

Pringuey, D. and Kohl, F.S. (ed.) 2002 *Phenomenology of human identity and schizophrenia*. Collection Pheno sous la direction de Georges Charbonneau. France: Association Le Cercle Herméneutique, Société d'Anthropologie Phénologique et d'Herméneutique Générale.

Prior, A. (1960). The runabout inference-ticket. *Analysis* 21: 38–39. (Reprinted in Strawson (ed.), (1967) *Philosophical Logic*. Oxford: Oxford University Press.)

Proust, J. (ed.) (1999). Special Issue of *The Monist*.

Proust, J. (2000). Awareness of agency: three levels of analysis. In *Neural Correlates of Consciousness* (ed. T. Metzinger). Cambridge, MA: MIT Press, pp. 307–324.

Putnam, D. (1997). Psychological courage. *Philosophy, Psychiatry, & Psychology*, 4(1): 1–12.

Putnam, H. (1995). *Renewing Philosophy*. Cambridge, MA: Harvard University Press.

Putnam, H. (1996). In *Words and Life* (ed. J. Conant), (3rd edn). Cambridge, MA: Harvard University Press.

Putnam, H. (2002). *The Collapse of the Fact/Value Dichotomy and other Essays*. Cambridge, MA: Harvard University Press.

Quine, W.V.O. (1960). *Word and Object*. Cambridge, MA: London MIT Press.

Quine, W.V.O. (1975) On Empirically Equivalent Systems of the World. *Erkenntnis*, 9: pp 313–328.

Quinton, A. (1962). The soul. *Journal of Philosophy*, 59: 393–403.

Quinton, A. (1985). Madness. Chapter 2, in *Philosophy and Practice* (ed. A. Phillips Griffiths). Cambridge: Cambridge University Press, pp. 17–41.

Rachels, J. (2003) *The Elements of Moral Philosophy*, 4th Edition. Boston: McGraw-Hill.

Rachels, J. (2005) *Problems from Philosophy*. Boston: McGraw Hill.

Radden, J. (1994). Recent criticism of psychiatric nosology: a review. *Philosophy, Psychiatry, & Psychology*, 1(3): 193–200.

Radden, J. (1995). Personal identity: history and concepts. *Current Opinion in Psychiatry*, 8: 343–345.

Radden, J. (1996). *Divided Minds and Successive Selves: ethical issues in disorders of identity and personality*. Cambridge, MA: MIT Press.

Radden, J. (1996). Psychopathy, other-regarding moral beliefs, and responsibility. (Commentary on Fields, 1996). *Philosophy, Psychiatry, & Psychology*, 3(4): 287–290.

Radden, J. (2003). Learning from disunity. (Commentary on Wells, 2003, Kennett and Matthews, 2003, Phillips, 2003, and Wooding, 2003). *Philosophy, Psychiatry, & Psychology*, 10(4): 357–360.

Radden, J. (2003). Is this Dame Melancholy? Equating today's depression and past melancholia. *Philosophy, Psychiatry, & Psychology*, 10(1): 37–52.

Radden, J. (2003). The pragmatics of psychiatry, and the psychiatry of cross-cultural suffering. (Response to the commentaries on Radden, 2003). *Philosophy, Psychiatry, & Psychology*, 10(1): 63–66.

Radden, J. (2004) (Ed) *The Philosophy of Psychiatry: A Companion*. New York: Oxford University Press.

Ramsey, F. (1927). Facts and propositions. *Proceedings of the Aristotelian Society*, 7 (Suppl.): 153–170.

Raphael, D. D., (1994) (Second Edition) *Moral Philosophy*. Oxford, Oxford University Press.

Read, R. (2001). On approaching schizophrenia through Wittgenstein. *Philosophical Psychology*, 14: 449–475

Read, R. (2003). Literature as philosophy of psychopathology: William Faulkner as Wittgensteinian. *Philosophy, Psychiatry, & Psychology*, 10(2): 115–124.

Read, R. (2003) On Delusions of Sense: A Response to Coetzee and Sass. *Philosophy, Psychiatry, & Psychology*, 10(2): 135–142.

Reber, A. (1995). *Implicit Learning and Tacit Knowledge: an essay on the cognitive unconscious*. New York: Oxford University Press.

Reich, W. (1999). Psychiatric diagnosis as an ethical problem. *Psychiatric Ethics* (3rd edn), (ed. S. Bloch, P. Chodoff, and S. Green). Oxford: Oxford University Press, pp. 193–224.

Reichenbach, H. (1951). *The Rise of Scientific Philosophy*. Berkeley, CA: University of California Press.

Reinders, H. (2003). The ambiguities of 'meaning'. (Commentary on Clegg and Lansdall-Welfare, 2003). *Philosophy, Psychiatry, & Psychology*, 10(1): 91–98.

Reset, J.L. and Gracia, D. (ed.) (1992). *The Ethics of Diagnosis*. Philosophy and Medicine Book Series, Vol. 40 (series ed. T. Engelhardt and S. Spicker). Dordrecht: Kluwer.

Rey, G. (1997). *Contemporary Philosophy of Mind*. Oxford: Blackwell.

Reznek, L. (1987). *The Nature of Disease*. London: Routledge.

Reznek, L. (1991) *The Philosophical Defence of Psychiatry*, London: Routledge.

Reznek, L. (1995). Dis-ease about kinds: reply to D'Amico. *Journal of Medicine and Philosophy*, 20: 571–584.

Reznek, L. (1997) *Evil or Ill?*. London: Routledge.

Rhoden, N, (1986). The Judge in the delivery room: the emergence of court ordered caesareans, *California Law Review*, 74: 1951.

Rhodes, R. (1997). Commentary on 'The stoic conception of mental disorder'. *Philosophy, Psychiatry, & Psychology*, 4(4): 303–304.

Richmond, S. (2001). Psychoanalysis and feminism: anorexia, the social world, and the internal world. *Philosophy, Psychiatry, & Psychology*, 8(1): 1–12.

Richmond, S. (2001). A Response to Mitchell (2001), Hinshelwood (2001), and Adshead (2001). *Philosophy, Psychiatry, & Psychology*, 8(1): 41–44.

Rickert, H. (1962). *Science and History: a critique of positivist epistemology* (trans. G. Reisman). New Jersey: D. Van Nostrand.

Rickert, H. (1986). *The Limits of Concept Formation in the Natural Sciences: a logical introduction to the historical sciences* (trans. Guy Oakes). Cambridge: Cambridge University Press.

Rickman, H.P. (1987). The philosophical basis of psychiatry: Jaspers and Dilthey. In *Philosophy of the Social Sciences*, 17: 173–196.

Ricoeur, P. (1970). *Freud and Philosophy* (trans. D. Savage). London: Yale University Press.

Rippon, G. (1998). A phenomenology of dyslexia. (Commentary on Philpott, 1998). *Philosophy, Psychiatry, & Psychology*, 5(1): 25–28.

Rizzi, D.A. (1994). Causal reasoning and the diagnostic process. *Theoretical Medicine*, 15: 315–333.

Robbins, E. and Guze, S.B. (1970) Establishment of diagnostic validity in psychiatric illness: its application to schizophrenia. *American Journal of Psychiatry*, 126: 983–987.

Robertson, D. (1996). Ethical theory, ethnography and differences between doctors and nurses in approaches to patient care. *Journal of Medical Ethics*, 22: 292–299.

Robertson, S. (2004) Philosophy and History of Psychiatry, chapter 27, pps 551–568. in C. Fear (ed) *Essential Revision notes in Psychiatry for the MRCPsych* Knutsford, England: Pastest Ltd.

Robinson, D. (1996). *Wild Beasts and Idle Humours: the insanity defense from antiquity to the present*. Cambridge, MA: Harvard University Press.

Robinson, D. (1998). *The Mind*. Oxford: Oxford University Press.

Robinson, D. (1998). Cerebral plurality and the unity of self. In *The Mind* (ed. D. Robinson). Oxford: Oxford University Press, pp. 344–354.

Robinson, D.N. (1997). Commentary on 'Autobiography, narrative, and the Freudian concept of life history.' (Commentary on Brockmeier, 1997) *Philosophy, Psychiatry, & Psychology*, 4(3): 205–208.

Robinson, D.N. (2000). Madness, badness, and fitness: law and psychiatry (again). *Philosophy, Psychiatry, & Psychology*, 7(3): 209–222.

Robinson, D.N. (2000). Stories as tales and as histories: A response to the commentary. (Commentary on Robinson, 2000). *Philosophy, Psychiatry, & Psychology*, 7(3): 229–230.

Robinson, D.N. (2003). Psychiatry and law. In *Nature and Narrative: An Introduction to the New Philosophy of Psychiatry* (eds K.W.M. Fulford, K.J. Morris, J.Z. Sadler, and G. Stanghellini). Oxford: Oxford University Press.

Roessler, J. (2001). Understanding delusions of alien control. *Philosophy, Psychiatry, & Psychology*, 8(2–3): 177–188.

Rogers, A., Pilgrim, D., and Lacey, R. (1993). Getting the treatment. In *Experiencing Psychiatry: Users' Views of Services*. London: Macmillan, in association with Mind Publications.

Rogers, A., Pilgrim., D., and Lacey, R. (1993). *Experiencing Psychiatry: users' views of services*. London: Macmillan.

Rorty, A. (ed.) (1976). *The Identities of Persons*. Berkeley, CA: University of California Press.

Rorty, R. (1993). Holism, intrinsicality and the ambition of transcendence. In *Dennett and his Critics* (ed. B. Dahlbom). Oxford: Blackwell.

Rorty, R. (1998). *Truth and Progress*. Cambridge: Cambridge University Press.

Rosenhan, D. (1973). On being sane in insane places. *Science*, 179: 250–258.

Rosenthal, D.M. (ed.) (1991). *The Nature of Mind*. Oxford: Oxford University Press.

Rossi, P. (2003) Magic, science, and equality of human wits. In *Nature and Narrative: an introduction to the new philosophy of psychiatry* (ed. K.W.M. Fulford, K.J. Morris, J.Z.S. Sadler, and G. Stanghellini). Oxford: Oxford University Press, Chapter 17.

Roth, M. and Kroll, G. (1986). *The Reality of Mental Illness*. Cambridge: Cambridge University Press.

Roth, M. (2000). Ecstasy and abnormal happiness: the two main syndromes defined by Mayer-Gross. (Commentary by Wolff, 2000). *Philosophy, Psychiatry, & Psychology*, 7(4): 317–322.

Rounsaville, B.J., Alarcón, R.D., Andrews, G., Jackson, J.S., Kendell, R.E., and Kendler, K. (2002). Basic nomenclature issues for DSM-V. In *A Research Agenda for DSM-V* (ed. D.J. Kupfer, M.B. First, and D.E. Regier). Washington, DC: American Psychiatric Association, pp. 1–30.

Royal Australian and New Zealand College of Psychiatrists (1998) *Code of Ethics* (2nd edn). Melbourne: Royal Australian and New Zealand College of Psychiatrists.

Royal College of Psychiatrists (2000) *CR85. Good Practice Guidance on Confidentiality*. London: Royal College of Psychiatrists.

Ruben, D. (ed.) (1993). *Explanation*. Oxford Readings in Philosophy. Oxford: Oxford University Press.

Russell, B. (1912). The value of philosophy. In *The Problems of Philosophy*. London: Williams and Northgate, pp. 237–250.

Russell, B. (1946). *A History of Western Philosophy*. London: George Allen and Unwin.

Russell, B. ([1900] 1958). *The Critical Exposition of the Philosophy of Leibniz*. London: George Allen and Unwin.

Russell, B. (1962). *An Inquiry into Meaning and Truth*. London: Penguin Books.

Russell, B. Analogy (1948). In *Human Knowledge: its scope and limits*. (Reprinted in Rosenthal, D (ed.) (1991). pp. 89–91.) London: Geore Allen and Unwin.

Rust, J. and Golombok, S. (1989) *Modern psychometrics*. London: Routledge.

Ryan, A. (1970). *The Philosophy of the Social Sciences*. London: Macmillan Press.

Rycroft, C. (1972). *A Critical Dictionary of Psychoanalysis*. London: Penguin.

Ryle, G. ([1949] 1963). *The Concept of Mind*. London: Penguin.

Sabat, S.R. (2001) *The Experience of Alzheimer's Disease: Life Through a Tangled Veil*. Oxford: Blackwell.

Sabat, S.R. and Harré, R. (1994). The Alzheimer's disease sufferer as a semiotic subject. *Philosophy, Psychiatry, & Psychology*, 1(3): 145–160.

Sackett, D.L., Straus, S.E., Scott Richardson, W., Rosenberg, W., and Haynes, R.B. (2000). *Evidence-Based Medicine: how to practice and teach EBM*, (2nd edn). London: Churchill Livingstone.

Sadler, J.Z., Wiggins O.P., and Schwartz, M.A. (ed.) (1994). *Philosophical Perspectives on Psychiatric Diagnostic Classification*. Baltimore, MD: The Johns Hopkins University Press.

Sadler, J.Z. (1996). Epistemic value commitments in the debate over categorical vs. dimensional personality diagnosis. 3(3): 203–222.

Sadler, J.Z. (1998). Suicide, language, and clinical practice. (Commentary on Fairbairn, 1998). *Philosophy, Psychiatry, & Psychology*, 5(2): 175–178.

Sadler, J.Z. (ed.) (2002). *Descriptions & Prescriptions: values, mental disorders, and the DSMs*. Baltimore, MD: Johns Hopkins University Press.

Sadler, J.Z. (2004) *Values and Psychiatric Diagnosis*. Oxford: Oxford University Press.

Sadler, J.Z. (2004). Diagnosis/antidiagnosis. In *The Philosophy of Psychiatry: a companion* (ed. J. Radden). New York: Oxford University Press, pp. 163–179.

Sadler, J.Z. (2005) Bug-eyed and breathless: emerging crises involving values. *World Psychiatry*, 4(2): 87.

Sadler, J.Z. and Agich, G.J. (1995). Dysfunction as a value-free concept: a Reply to Sadler and Agich. *Philosophy, Psychiatry, & Psychology*, 2: 233–246.

Sadler, J.Z. and Fulford, K.W.M. (2000). Editors' Introduction. *Philosophy, Psychiatry, & Psychology*, 7(1): 1–2.

Sadler, J.Z. and Fulford, K.W.M. (2000). *Aristotle, Function and Mental Disorder* (with contributions by Szasz, 2000, Wakefield, 2000, Megone, 2000, Thornton, 2000, and Fulford, 2000) . *Philosophy, Psychiatry, & Psychology*, 7(1).

Sadler, J.Z. and Fulford, K.W.M. (2003). Agency, narrative, and self: a philosophical case conference. *Philosophy, Psychiatry, & Psychology*, 10(4): 295–296.

Sadler, J.Z. and Fulford, K.W.M. (2004). Should Patients and Their Families Contribute to the DSM-V Process? *Psychiatric Services*, Vol 55(2): 133–138.

Sadler, J.Z., and Agich, G.J. (1995). Diseases, functions, values and psychiatric classification. *Philosophy, Psychiatry, & Psychology*, 2(3): 219–232.

Sadler, J.Z., Wiggins, O.P., & Schwartz, M.A. (eds) (1994) *Philosophical Perspectives on Psychiatric Diagnostic Classification*. Baltimore: Johns Hopkins University Press.

Sainsbury, R.M. (1988). *Paradoxes*. Cambridge: Cambridge University Press.

Salmon, W. (1989). *Four Decades of Scientific Explanation*. Minneapolis: University of Minnesota Press.

Sargent, C. (2003). Gender, body, meaning: anthropological perspectives on self-injury and borderline personality disorder. (Commentary on Potter, 2003). *Philosophy, Psychiatry, & Psychology*, 10(1): 25–28.

Sartorius, N. (1976). Modifications and New Approaches to Taxonomy in Long-Term Care: Advantages and Limitations of the ICD. *Medical Care*, 14: 109–115, Supplement 5.

Sartorius, N. (1991). The classification of mental disorders in the Tenth Revision of the International Classification of Diseases. *European Psychiatry*, 6: 315–322.

Sartorius, N. (1992) Preface to World Health Organization (1992) *The ICD-10 Classification of Mental and Behavioural Disorders: Clinical Descriptions and Diagnostic Guidelines*. Geneva: World Health Organization.

Sartorius, N. (1995). *Understanding the ICD-10 Classification of Mental Disorders. A Pocket Reference*. London: Science Press Limited, (Also published in Polish, Russian and Ukrainian).

Sartorius, N. (2004). Personal Communication (at the World Psychiatric Association conference in Florence, November 10–13, on Treatments in Psychiatry: an Update.)

Sartorius, N. (2005). Recognizing that values matter. *World Psychiatry*, 4(2): 90.

Sartre, J-P. (1956). *Being and Nothingness* (transl. H.E. Barries). New York: The Citadel Press.

Sartre, J-P. (1967). Consciousness of self and knowledge of self. In *Readings in Phenomenological Psychology* (ed. N. Lawrence and D. O'Connor) (1967) Englewood cliffs, NJ: Prentice-Hall.

Sass, L.A. (1994). *Madness and Modernism: insanity in the light of modern art, literature, and thought*. Cambridge, MA: Harvard University Press.

Sass, L.A. (1995). *The Paradoxes of Delusion: Wittgenstein, Schreber and the schizophrenic mind*. Ithaca, NY: Cornell University Press.

Sass, L.A. (1999). Schizophrenia, self-consciousness, and the modern mind. In *Models of the Self* (ed. S. Gallagher and J. Shear). Thoverton, UK: Imprint Academic.

Sass, L.A. (2001). Commentary: Pathogenesis, common sense, and the cultural framework (Commentary on Stanghellini, 2001). *Philosophy, Psychiatry, & Psychology*, 8(2–3): 219–224.

Sass, L.A. (2001). Self and world in schizophrenia: three classic approaches. *Philosophy, Psychiatry, & Psychology*, 8(4): 251–270.

Sass, L.A. (2003). Incomprehensibility and understanding: on the interpretation of severe mental illness. (Commentary on Read, 2003). *Philosophy, Psychiatry, & Psychology*, 10(2): 125–132.

Sass, L.A. (2004). Some reflections on the (analytic) philosophical approach to delusion. (Commentary for Special Issue on Delusion). *Philosophy, Psychiatry, & Psychology*, 11(1:) 71–80.

Sass, L.A. and Parnas, J. (2001). Phenomenology of self-disturbances in schizophrenia: some research findings and directions. *Philosophy, Psychiatry, & Psychology*, 8(4): 347–356.

Savulescu J. (2001) Taking the Plunge, *New Scientist*, 3: 50–51.

Savulescu, J. and Dickenson, D. (1998). The time frame of preferences, dispositions, and the validity of advance directives for the mentally ill. *Philosophy, Psychiatry, & Psychology*, 5(3): 225–246.

Savulescu, J., and Dickenson, D. (1998). Response to the Commentaries. *Philosophy, Psychiatry, & Psychology*, 5(3): 263–266.

Sayce, L. (1998). Transcending mental health law. *Psychiatric Bulletin*, 22: 666–670.

Schaffer, J. (2000). Trumping preemption, *Journal of Philosophy*, 9: 165–181.

Schaffner, K.F. (ed.) (1986). *Logic of Discovery and Diagnosis in Medicine*. Pittsburgh Series in Philosophy & History of Science. Berkley, CA: University of California Press.

Schaffner, K.F. (1993). *Discovery and Explanation in Biology and Medicine. Science & Its Conceptual Foundations*. Chicago: University of Chicago Press.

Schaler, J.A. (ed.) (2004). *Szasz Under Fire: the psychiatric abolitionist faces his critics*. Chicago, IL: Open Court Publishers.

Scheff, T. (1974). The labelling theory of mental illness. *American Sociological Review*, 39, 444–452.

Schiller, L. and Bennett, A. (1996). *The Quiet Room: a journey out of the torment of madness*. New York: Warner Books.

Schlick, M. (1981). Meaning and verification. In *Essential Readings in Logical Positivism* (ed. O. Hanfling). Oxford: Blackwell.

Schlipp, P.A. (1981). *The Philosophy of Karl Jaspers*. LaSalle, IL: Open Court.

Schmidt, G. (1987). A review of the German Literature on delusion Between 1914 and 1939. In *The Clinical Roots of the Schizophrenia Concept* (ed. J. Cutting and M. Shepherd). Cambridge: Cambridge University Press, pp. 101–134.

Schmidt, J. (1985). *Maurice Merleau-Ponty: between phenomenology and structuralism*. New York: St Martin's Press.

Schmitt, F.F. (1995). *Truth: a primer*. Oxford: Westview.

Schmitt, W. (1986). Karl Jaspers' influence on psychiatry. *Journal of the British Society for Phenomenology*, 17: 36–51.

Schnädelbach, H. (1984). *Philosophy in Germany 1831–1933* (trans. by E. Matthews). Cambridge: Cambridge University Press.

Schneider, K. (1959). *Clinical Psychopathology* (trans. M.W. Hamilton). New York: Grune & Stratton.

Schreber, D.P. (2000). *Memoir of My Mental Illness*. New York: New York Review Books.

Schwartz, M. (ed) (1990) *Modular deficits in Alzheimer-type dementia* Cambridge MA: MIT Press.

Schwartz, M.A. and Wiggins, O.P. (1998). Neurosis and the historic quest for security. (Commentary on Mitchell, 1998). *Philosophy, Psychiatry, & Psychology*, 5(4): 329–332.

Schwartz, M.A. and Wiggins, O.P. (2004). *Phenomenological and Hermeneutic Models: understanding and interpretation in psychiatry*. Ch. 24 in Radden, J. (ed) The Philosophy of psychiatry: A Companion, pp. 351–363. New York: Oxford University Press.

Schwartz, S.H. (2004). Basic human values: their content and structure across countries. In *Valores e trabalho* [Values and work] (ed. A. Tamayo, A. and J. Porto). Brazil: Universidade de Brasilia.

Scriven, M. (1959). Truisms as the grounds for historical explanation. In *Theories of History* (ed. P. Gardiner). New York, pp. 443–468.

Scruton, R. (1980). *Kant*. PastMasters Series. Oxford: Oxford University Press.

Scull, A. (1995). Psychiatrists and the historical facts. Part two: re-writing the history of asylumdom, *History of Psychiatry*, 6: 387–394.

Searle, J. (1967). How to derive 'ought' from 'is'. In *Theories of Ethics* (ed. P. Foot). Oxford: Oxford University Press.

Searle, J. (1969). *Speech Acts: an essay in the philosophy of language*. Cambridge: Cambridge University Press.

Searle, J. (1984). *Minds, Brains, and Science*. Cambridge, MA: Harvard University Press.

Sechehaye, M. (1994). *Autobiography of a Schizophrenic Girl: the true story of 'Renee'*. New York: Penguin.

Sedgwick, P. (1973). 'Illness – Mental and Otherwise', *The Hastings Center Studies* I (3), 19 – 40 (New York: Institute of Society, Ethics and Life Sciences, Hastings-on-Hudson).

Seedhouse, D. (1994). The trouble with well-being: a response to mild mania and well-being. *Philosophy, Psychiatry, & Psychology*, 1(3): 185–192.

Segal, G.M.A. (1997). Commentary on 'Encoding of meaning'. *Philosophy, Psychiatry, & Psychology*, 4(4): 269–272.

Segal, G.M.A. (1997). Encoding of meaning. (Commentary on Bolton, 1997) *Philosophy, Psychiatry, & Psychology*, 4(4): 269–272.

Sen A. (1987). *On Ethics and Economics*. Oxford: Blackwell.

Sensky, T., Hughes, T., and Hirsch, S. (1991). Compulsory psychiatric treatment in the community, Part 1. A controlled a study of compulsory community treatment with extended leave under the Mental Health Act: and special characteristics of patients treated and impact of treatment. *British Journal of Psychiatry*, 158: 792.

Sheehan, T. (1988). Heidegger and the Nazis. *New York Review of Books*, June 16.

Shepherd, M. (1990). *Karl Jaspers: general psychopathology, conceptual issues in psychological medicine*. London: Tavistock.

Shoemaker, S. (1968). Self-reference and self-awareness. *Journal of Philosophy*, 65(19): 555–567.

Shoemaker, S. (1986). Introspection and the self. *Midwest Studies in Philosophy*, 10: 101–120.

Shoemaker, S. (1997). Self and substance. *Philosophical Perspectives*, 11: 283–304.

Shoemaker, S. and Swinburne, R. (1984). *Personal Identity*. Oxford: Blackwell

Shorter, E. (1997). *A History of Psychiatry: from the era of the asylum to the age of prozac*. New York: John Wiley and Sons.

Shuman, D.W. (1996). Multiple personality and moral responsibility. (Commentary on Braude, 1996). *Philosophy, Psychiatry, & Psychology*, 3(1): 59–60.

Shuman, D.W. (2003). A Comment on Christopher Ciocchetti: The responsibility of the psychopathic offender. (Commentary on Ciocchetti, 2003). *Philosophy, Psychiatry, & Psychology*, 10(2): 193–194.

Simpson, R.L. (1988). *Essentials of Symbolic Logic*. London: Routledge.

Sims, A. (1988). *Symptoms in the Mind: an introduction to descriptive psychopathology*. London: Baillière Tindall.

Sims, A. (1997). Commentary on 'Spiritual experience and psychopathology'. (Commentary on Jackson and Fulford, 1997). *Philosophy, Psychiatry, & Psychology*, 4(1): 79–82.

Sims, A., Mundt, C. Berner, P. and Barocka, A. (2000). Descriptive phenomenology. In *New Oxford Textbook of Psychiatry*, (Gelder et al, 2000).

Skinner, B.F. (1938). *The Behaviour of Organisms*. New York: Appleton-Century-Crofts.

Skinner, B.F. ([1948] 2005) *Walden Two*. Indianapolis: Hackett.

Skinner, B.F. (1971). *Beyond Freedom and Dignity*. New York: Knopf.

Slater, E. (1972). The psychiatrists in search of a science; I Early thinkers at the Maudsley. *British Journal of Psychiatry*, 121: 591–598.

Slater, E. (1973). The psychiatrists in search of a science; II Developments in the logic and the sociology of science. *British Journal of Psychiatry*, 122: 625–636.

Slater, E. (1975). The psychiatrists in search of a science; III The depth psychologies. *British Journal of Psychiatry*, 126: 205–224.

Slater, E. and Roth, M. (1969). *Mayer-Gross, Slater and Roth: clinical psychiatry* (3rd edn). London: Ballière Tindall and Cassell.

Slovenko, R. (1999). Responsibility of the psychopath. (Commentary on Benn, 1999). *Philosophy, Psychiatry, & Psychology*, 6(1): 53–56.

Snelling, D. (1995). Psychoanalysis, science, and commonsense. (Commentary on Gardner, 1995) *Philosophy, Psychiatry, & Psychology*, 2(2): 119–122.

Sober (1984). *The Nature of Selection*. Chicago: University of Chicago Press.

Somerset Spirituality Project Group (2002). It would have been good to talk. *Mental Health Today*, October 2002.

Sorell, T. (1984). *Descartes*. PastMasters Series. Oxford: Oxford University Press.

Sosa, E. and Tooley, M. (ed.) (1993). *Causation*. Oxford: Oxford University Press.

Spence, S.A. (1996). Free will in the light of neuropsychiatry. (Commentaries by Frith, C. (1996, pp. 91–94), Libet, B. (1996, pp. 95–96), and Stephens, G.L. (1996, pp. 97–98) and reply by Spence, S.A. (1996, pp. 99–100)) *Philosophy, Psychiatry, & Psychology*, 3(2): 75–90.

Spence, S.A. (1996). Response to the Commentaries (on Spence, 1996). *Philosophy, Psychiatry, & Psychology*, 3(2): 99–100.

Spence, S.A. (1999). Does a philosophy of the brain tell us anything new about psychomotor disorders? (Commentary on Northoff, 1999a) *Philosophy, Psychiatry, & Psychology*, 6(3): 227–230.

Spence, S.A. (2001). Alien control: from phenomenology to cognitive neurobiology. *Philosophy, Psychiatry, & Psychology*, 8(2–3): 163–172.

Spence, S.A. (2002). Alien motor phenomena: a window on to agency. *Cognitive Neuropsychiatry*, 7(3): 211–220.

Spinoza, B. ([1677] 2000) *Ethics*. Oxford: Oxford University Press.

Spitz, D. (1999). Commentary on 'How to cut the psychiatric pie: the dilemma of character. (Matthews, 1999). *Philosophy, Psychiatry, & Psychology*, 6(4): 311–316.

Spitzer, M. (1990). On defining delusions. *Comprehensive Psychiatry*, 31(5): 377–397.

Spitzer, M. (1994). The basis of psychiatric diagnosis. In *Philosophical Perspectives on Psychiatric Diagnostic Classification* (ed. J.Z. Sadler, O.P. Wiggins, and M.A. Schwartz). London: Johns Hopkins University Press.

Spitzer, M., Uehlein, F., Schwartz, M.A., and Mundt, C. (ed.) (1993). *Phenomenology Language and Schizophrenia*. New York: Springer-Verlag.

Spitzer, R.L., Skodol, A., Gibbon, M., and Williams J. (1981). *DSM-III Case Book*. Washington, DC: American Psychiatric Association.

Spitzer, R.L. (2005) Recipe for disaster: professional and patient equally sharing responsibility for developing psychiatric diagnosis. *World Psychiatry*, 4(2): 89.

St Augustine. ([397] 2002) *Confessions*, New York: Dover.

Stainton Rogers, W. (1992). *Explaining Illness*. Milton Keynes: Open University Press.

Stanghellini, G. (2000). At issue: vulnerability to schizophrenia and lack of common sense. *Schizophrenia Bulletin*, 26(4): 775–787.

Stanghellini, G. (2001). Psychopathology of common sense. *Philosophy, Psychiatry, & Psychology*, 8(2–3): 201–218.

Stanghellini, G. (2001). A dialectical conception of autism. (Commentary on Minkowski and Targowla, 2001). *Philosophy, Psychiatry, & Psychology*, 8(4): 295–298.

Stanghellini, G. (2004). *Deanimated bodies and Disembodied Spirits. Essays on the psychopathology of common sense*. Oxford: Oxford University Press.

Stein, D.J. (1999). Philosophy and cognitive neuropsychiatry. (Commentary on Northoff, 1999) *Philosophy, Psychiatry, & Psychology*, 6(3): 217–222.

Stengel, E. (1959). Classification of mental disorders. *Bulletin of the World Health Organization*, 21: 601–663.

Stephens. G.L. (1999). Defining Delusion. (Commentary on Jones, 1999) *Philosophy, Psychiatry, & Psychology*, 6(1): 25–26.

Stephens, G.L. (2000). Thought insertion and subjectivity. (Commentary on Gibbs, 2000) *Philosophy, Psychiatry, & Psychology*, 7(3): 203–206.

Stephens, G.L. and Graham, G. (1994). Self-consciousness, mental agency, and clinical psychopathology of thought-insertion. (Commentaries by Wiggins (1994) and Chadwick (1994), and Stephens and Graham (1994) *Philosophy, Psychiatry, & Psychology*, 1(1): 1–10.

Stephens, G.L. and Graham, G. (1994). Kant, thought insertion, and mental unity. (Commentary on Chadwick, 1994) *Philosophy, Psychiatry, & Psychology*, 1(2): 115–116.

Stephens, G.L. and Graham, G. (1996) Psychopathology, Freedom and the experience of externality. *Philosophical Topics* 24: 159–182.

Stephens, G.L. and Graham, G. (2000). *When Self-Consciousness Breaks: alien voices and inserted thoughts*. Cambridge, MA: MIT Press.

Stephens, G.L. and Graham, G. (2004). Reconceiving delusion. *International Review of Psychiatry*, 16(3): 236–241.

Sterelny, K. (1990). *The Representational Theory of Mind*. Oxford: Blackwell.

Stern, K (1993). Court-ordered Caesarian sections: in whose interests? *Modern Law Review* 56: 238–243.

Stevenson, J. (1961). Roundabout the runabout inference ticket. *Analysis* 21: 124–128.

Stich, S. (1983). *From Folk Psychology to Cognitive Science*. Cambridge, MA: MIT Press.

Stich, S. and Nichols, S. (2003) Folk psychology in *The Blackwell Guide to the Philosophy of Mind* (ed S. Stich and T. Warfield) Oxford: Blackwell pp 235–255.

Stocker, M. (1997). Aristotelian *Akrasia* and psychoanalytic regression. (Commentary by P.G. Sturdee, pp. 243–246) *Philosophy, Psychiatry, & Psychology*, 4(3): 231–242.

Stone, A. (1984). *Law, Psychiatry, and Morality*. Washington, DC: American Psychiatric Press.

Stone, T. and Davies, M. (1996). The mental simulation debate: a progress report. In *Theories of Theories of Mind* (ed. P. Carruthers and P. Smith). Cambridge: Cambridge University Press. 119–137.

Storr, A. (1989). *Freud*. Oxford: Oxford University Press.

Storr, A. (1997). Commentary on 'Spiritual experience and psychopathology'. (Commentary on Jackson and Fulford, 1997a). *Philosophy, Psychiatry, & Psychology*, 4(1): 83–86.

Stranson, P.F. (ed) (1967) *Philosophic Logic,* Oxford: Oxford University Press.

Straus, E.W. (1958). Aesthesiology and hallucinations. In *Existence: a new dimension in psychiatry and psychology* (ed. R. May, E. Angel, and H.F. Ellenberger). New York: Basic Books, pp. 139–169.

Strawson, G. (1989). *The Secret Connexion: causation, realism and David Hume.* Oxford: Oxford University Press.

Strawson, P.F. (1974). Freedom and resentment. In *Freedom and Resentment, and Other Essays.* London: Methuen, pp. 1–25.

Strawson, P.F. (1977). *Individuals: An Essay in Descriptive Metaphysics.* Oxford: Oxford University Press.

Strenger, C. (1991). *Between Hermeneutics and Science: An Essay on the Epistemology of Psychoanalysis.* Madison, CT: International Universities Press

Stroud, B. (1977). *Hume.* London: Routledge and Kegan Paul.

Stroud, B. (1984). *The Significance of Philosophical Scepticism* Oxford: Oxford University Press.

Sturdee, P.G. (1997). Primitive mental processes: psychoanalysis and the ethics of integration. (Commentary on Hinshelwood, 1997). *Philosophy, Psychiatry, & Psychology,* 4(2): 151–154.

Sturdee, P.G. (1997). Aristotelian akrasia and psychoanalytic regression. (Commentary on Stocker, 1997). *Philosophy, Psychiatry, & Psychology,* 4(3): 243–246.

Sturdee, P.G. (1999). There has to be a pattern. (Commentary on Svenaeus, 1999). *Philosophy, Psychiatry, & Psychology,* 6(2): 95–100.

Styron, W. (1991). *Darkness Visible*: *a memoir of madness.* London: Jonathan Cape.

Sullivan, M.D. (1995). Key concepts: pain. *Philosophy, Psychiatry, & Psychology,* 2(3): 277–280.

Sundström, P. (1987). *Icons of Disease: A Philosophical Inquiry into the Semantics, Phenomenology and Ontology of the Clinical Conceptions of Disease.* Linköping University, Sweden: Department of Health and Society.

Suppes, P. (2002). Linguistic markers of recovery: underpinnings of first person pronoun usage and semantic positions of patients. (Commentary on Van Staden, 2002). *Philosophy, Psychiatry, & Psychology,* 9(2): 127–130.

Sutherland, S. (1998). *Breakdown: A personal crisis and a medical dilemma.* Oxford: Oxford University Press.

Svenaeus, F. (1999). Alexithymia: a phenomenological approach. *Philosophy, Psychiatry, & Psychology,* 6(2): 71–82.

Svenaeus, F. (1999). Response to the Commentaries. *Philosophy, Psychiatry, & Psychology,* 6(2): 105–108.

Svensson, T. (1990). *On the notion of mental illness: problematizing the medical–model conception of certain abnormal behaviour and mental afflictions.* Linköping, Sweden: Department of Health and Society.

Sverdlik, S. (2002). Unconscious evil principles. (Commentary on Ward, 2002). *Philosophy, Psychiatry, & Psychology,* 9(1): 13–14.

Swinton, J. (2001). *Spirituality in Mental Health Care: rediscovering a forgotten dimension.* London: Jessica Kingsley Publishers.

Sykes, S. (2002). Commentary: The borderlands of psychiatry and theology. *Philosophy, Psychiatry, & Psychology,* 9(4): 381–382.

Sykes, S. (2002). The borderlands of psychiatry and theology. (Commentary on Marzanski and Bratton, 2002). *Philosophy, Psychiatry, & Psychology,* 9(4): 381–382.

Szasz, T.S. (1960). The myth of mental illness. *American Psychologist,* 15: 113–118.

Szasz, T.S. (1972). The myth of mental illness. *The Myth of Mental Illness.* St Albans, England: Paladin reprinted as (1974). *The Myth of Mental Illness.* New York: Harper and Row.

Szasz, T.S. (1976). *Schizophrenia: The Sacred Symbol of Psychiatry.* New York: Basic Books.

Szasz, T.S., (1987). *Insanity: The Idea and its consequences.* Chichester: Wiley.

Szasz, T.S. (1998). Commentary: Aristotle's function argument and the concept of mental illness. *Philosophy, Psychiatry, & Psychology,* 5(3): 203–208.

Szasz, T.S. (2000). Second Commentary: Aristotle's function argument. *Philosophy, Psychiatry, & Psychology,* 7(1): 3–16.

Szmukler, G. and Holloway, F. (1998). Mental health legislation is now a harmful anachronism. *Psychiatric Bulletin,* 22: 662–665.

Szmukler, G. and Holloway, F. (2001). Confidentiality in community psychiatry. In *Confidentiality and Mental Health* (ed. C. Cordess). London: Jessica Kingsley Publishers, Chapter 3.

Tam, H. (1996). *Punishment, Excuses and Moral Development.* Aldershot: Avebury Press.

Tan, J. (2005). Bridging the gap between fact and values. *World Psychiatry,* 4: 2, p 92.

Tan, J.O.A., Hope, T. and Stewart, A. (2003). Anorexia nervosa and personal identity: The accounts of patients and their parents. *International Journal of Law and Psychiatry,* 26: 533–548

Tanney, J. (1995). Why reasons may not be causes. *Mind and Language,* 10: 105–128.

Taylor, C. (1985). *Philosophical Papers*: Vol. 2, *Philosophy and the Human Sciences.* Cambridge: Cambridge University Press.

Taylor, R. (1997). Chisholm's idea of a person. In *The Philosophy of Roderick Chisholm* (ed. L. Hahn). Chicago: Open Court, pp. 45–51.

Temerlin, M.K. (1968). Suggestion effects in psychiatric diagnosis. *Journal of Nervous and Mental Disease,* 147, 349–353.

Tengland, P.-A. (1998). *Mental Health: a philosophical analysis.* Linköping, Sweden: Department of Health and Society.

Thornton, T. (1997). Reasons and causes in philosophy and psychopathology. *Philosophy, Psychiatry, & Psychology*, 4(4): 307–318.

Thornton, T. (1998). *Wittgenstein on Language and Thought.* Edinburgh: Edinburgh University Press.

Thornton, T. (2000). Mental illness and reductionism: can functions be naturalized? *Philosophy, Psychiatry, & Psychology*, 7(1): 67–76.

Thornton, T. (2002). Thought insertion, Cognitivism and inner space. *Cognitive neuropsychiatry* 7: 237–249

Thornton, T. (2003). Psychopathology and two kinds of narrative account of the self. (Commentary on Wells, 2003, Kennett and Matthews, 2003, Phillips, 2003 and Wooding, 2003). *Philosophy, Psychiatry, & Psychology*, 10(4): 361–368.

Thornton, T. (2004). Wittgenstein and the limits of empathic understanding in psychopathology. *International Review of Psychiatry*, 16, 3: 216–224.

Thornton, T. (2004). *John McDowell.* Chesham: Acumen.

Thornton, T. (2004). Reductionism/antireductionism. In *The Philosophy of Psychiatry: a companion* (ed. J. Radden). New York: Oxford University Press, pp. 191–204.

Thornton, W.L. (1997). Primitive mental processes: psychoanalysis and the ethics of integration. (Commentary on Hinshelwood, 1997) *Philosophy, Psychiatry, & Psychology*, 4(2): 155–158.

Toombs, K. (1993). The body. In *The Meaning of Illness: a phenomenological account of the different perspectives of physician and patient.* Dordrecht: Kluwer Academic, pp. 51–71.

Toulmin, S. (1980). Agent and patient in psychiatry. *International Journal of Law and Psychiatry*, 3: 267–278.

Toulmin, S. (1982). How medicine saved the life of ethics. *Perspectives on Biology and Medicine*, 25 (4): 736–750.

Toulmin, S. and Jonsen, A.R. (1988). *The Abuse of Casuistry.* Berkeley, CA: University of California Press.

Tröhler, U. (2002). Human research: from ethics to law, from national to international regulations. In *Historical and Philosophical Perspectives in Biomedical Ethics: from Paternalism to Autonomy?* (ed. A.-H. Maehle and J. Geyer-Kordesch). Aldershot: Ashgate, pp. 95–117.

Tyreman, S. (2003). Likening strikes twice: psychiatry, osteopathy, and the likeness argument. (Commentary on Pickering, 2003). *Philosophy, Psychiatry, & Psychology*, 10(3): 267–272.

Tyrer, P. and Steinberg, D. (1993). *Models for Mental Disorder: conceptual models in psychiatry* (2nd edn). Chichester: Wiley.

Unger, P. (1979). There are no ordinary things. *Synthese*, 14: 117–154.

Unger, P. (1979). I do not exist. In *Perception and Identity* (ed. G.F. MacDonald). Ithaca, NY: Cornell University Press, pp. 235–251.

Urfer, A. (2001). Phenomenology and psychopathology of schizophrenia: the views of Eugene Minkowski. *Philosophy, Psychiatry, & Psychology*, 8(4): 279–290.

Urmson, J.O. (1950). On grading. *Mind*, 59: 145–169.

Urmson, J.O. (1982). *Berkeley.* PastMasters Series. Oxford: Oxford University Press.

Urmson, J.O. and Warnock, G.J. (eds) (1961, revised 1989) *J.L. Austin: Philosophical Papers.* (Third edition). Oxford: Oxford University Press.

Van Fraassen, B. (1980). *The Scientific Image.* Oxford: Oxford University Press.

Van Fraassen, B. (1999). The pragmatics of explanation. In *The Philosophy of Science* (ed. R. Boyd, P. Gasker, and J.D. Trout). Cambridge, MA: MIT Press, pp. 317–327.

Van Fraassen, B.C. (1999). To save the phenomena. In *The Philosophy of Science* (ed. R. Boyd, P. Gasker, and J.D. Trout). Cambridge, MA: MIT Press, pp. 187–194.

Van Gulick, R. (1994). Deficit studies and the function of phenomenal consciousness. In *Philosophical Psychopathology* (ed. G. Graham and G.L. Stephens). Cambridge, MA: MIT Press. 25–50

Van Inwagen, P. (1990). *Material Beings.* Ithaca, NY: Cornell University Press.

Van Staden, C.W. (2002). Linguistic markers of recovery: theoretical underpinnings of first person pronoun usage and semantic positions of patients. *Philosophy, Psychiatry, & Psychology*, 9(2): 105–122.

Van Staden, C.W. (2002). Language mirrors relational positions in recovery: a response to commentaries by Falzer and Davidson, Gillett, and Suppes. *Philosophy, Psychiatry, & Psychology*, 9(2): 137–140.

Van Staden, C.W. (2005) The need for trained eyes to see facts and values in psychiatric diagnosis. *World Psychiatry*, 4(2): 94.

Van Staden, C.W. and Fulford, K.W.M. (2004). Changes in semantic uses of first person pronouns as possible linguistic markers of recovery in psychotherapy. *Australian and New Zealand Journal of Psychiatry*, 38(4): 226–232.

Varela, F.J., Thompson, E.T., and Rosch, E. (1992). *The Embodied Mind: cognitive science and human experience.* Cambridge, MA: MIT Press.

Vattimo, G. (1997). *Beyond Interpretation.* Cambridge: Polity Press.

Vesey, G. (ed) (1986) *Philosophers Ancient and Modern.* Cambridge: Cambridge University Press.

Vienna Circle (1929). *The Scientific World View: The Vienna Circle.*

von Wright, G.H. (1963). *The Varieties of Goodness.* New York: Routledge and Kegan Paul.

von Wright, G. H. (1971). *Explanation and Understanding.* London: Routledge and Kegan Paul.

Waismann, F. (1981). Verification and definition. In *Essential Readings in Logical Positivism* (ed. O. Hanfling). Oxford: Blackwell.

Wakefield, J.C. (1995). Dysfunction as a value-free concept: a reply to Sadler and Agich. *Philosophy, Psychiatry, & Psychology*, 2(3): 233–246.

Wakefield, J.C. (2000). Aristotle as sociobiologist: the 'function of a human being' argument, black box essentialism, and the concept of mental disorder. *Philosophy, Psychiatry, & Psychology*, 7: 17–44.

Wakefield, J.C. (2000). Spandrels, vestigal organs, and such: reply to Murphy and Woolfolk. The harmful dysfunction analysis of mental disorder *Philosophy, Psychiatry, & Psychology*, 7(4): 253–270.

Wakefield, J.C. (2005). On winking at the facts, and losing one's Hare: value pluralism and the harmful dysfunction analysis. *World Psychiatry*, 4(2): 88.

Walker, C. (1994). Karl Jaspers and Edmund Husserl—I: The perceived convergence. *Philosophy, Psychiatry and Psychology* 1: 117–134.

Walker, C. (1994). Karl Jaspers and Edmund Husserl—II: The divergence. *Philosophy, Psychiatry and Psychology* 1: 245–265.

Walker, C. (1995). Karl Jaspers and Edmund Husserl—III: Jaspers as a Kantian phenomenologist. *Philosophy, Psychiatry, & Psychology*, 2: 65–82.

Walker, C. (1995). Karl Jaspers and Edmund Husserl—IV: Phenomenology as empathic understanding. *Philosophy, Psychiatry and Psychology* 2: 247–266.

Walker, N. (1968) *Crime and Insanity in England*. Volume 1: the historical perspective. Edinburgh: Edinburgh University Press.

Wallcraft, J. (2003). *Values in Mental Health—the role of experts by experience*. (Available at www.connects.org.uk conferences)

Waller, B.N. (2004). Neglected psychological elements of free will. (Commentary by Lieberman, P.B. (2004, pp. 119–124) and reply Waller, B.N. (2004, 125–128)) *Philosophy, Psychiatry, & Psychology*, 11(2): 111–118.

Waller, B.N. (2004b). Comparing psychoanalytic and cognitive-behavioral perspectives on control. (Response to Lieberman, 2004) *Philosophy, Psychiatry, & Psychology*, 11(2): 125–128.

Walton, D. (1989). *Informal Logic*. Cambridge: Cambridge University Press.

Warburton, N. (2000). *Thinking from A to Z*. London: Routledge.

Warburton, N. (2004) *Philosophy: the basics (4th edition)*. London: Routledge.

Ward, D.E. (2002). Explaining evil behavior: using Kant and M. Scott Peck to solve the puzzle of understanding the moral psychology of evil people. *Philosophy, Psychiatry, & Psychology*, 9(1): 1–12.

Ward, D.E. (2002). Commentary on 'The complexity of evil behavior'. *Philosophy, Psychiatry, & Psychology*, 9(1): 23–26.

Warlow, C. (2005) Over-regulation of clinical research: a threat to public health. *Clinical Medicine: Journal of the Royal College of Physicians of London*, 5: 33–8.

Warner, M. (1999). Theory and practice: negotiating the differences. (Commentary on Widdershoven, 1999). *Philosophy, Psychiatry, & Psychology*, 6(4): 265–266.

Warnock, G.J. (1967). *Contemporary Moral Philosophy*. London: Methuen.

Warnock, G.J. (1971). *The Object of Morality*. London: Methuen.

Warnock, G.J. (1989) *J L Austin*, London: Routledge.

Warnock, M. (1970) *Existentialism*. Oxford: Oxford University Press.

Warnock, M. (1978). *Ethics Since 1900* (3rd edn). Oxford: Oxford University Press.

Warnock, M. (1998). Freedom, responsibility and determinism. In *An Intelligent Person's Guide to Ethics*, Chapter 5.

Warnock, The Baroness M. (1998). Suicide, euthanasia, and the psychiatrist (Commentary on Burgess and Hawton, 1998). *Philosophy, Psychiatry, & Psychology*, 5(2): 127–130.

Watson, G. (ed.) (2003). *Free Will*. Oxford: Oxford University Press.

Watson, J.B. (1950). *Behaviourism*. New York: Norton.

Weber, M. ([1904] 1949). 'Objectivity' in social science and social policy. In *The Methodology of the Social Sciences* (ed. and trans. E.A. Shils and H.A. Finch). New York: The Free Press, pp. 50–112.

Weber, M. ([1917] 1949). The meaning of 'ethical neutrality' in sociology and economics. In *The Methodology of the Social Sciences* (ed. and trans. E.A. Shils and H.A. Finch). New York: The Free Press, pp. 1–49.

Weber, M. (1975). *Roscher and Knies: the logical problems of historical economics* (trans. G. Oakes). New York: The Free Press.

Weber, M. (1989). The concept of 'following a rule'. In *Max Weber: selections in translation* (ed. W.G. Runciman) (trans. E. Matthews). Cambridge: Cambridge University Press, pp. 99–110.

Weiner, S. (2003). Unity of agency and volition: some personal reflections. (Commentary on articles in the Special Issue on agency, narrative, and self). *Philosophy, Psychiatry, & Psychology*, 10(4): 369–372.

Weiss, B. (2002). *Michael Dummett*. Chesham: Acumen.

Wells, L.A. (1995). True wishes. (Commentary on Dickenson and Jones, 1995). *Philosophy, Psychiatry, & Psychology*, 2(4): 315–318.

Wells, L.A. (2003). Discontinuity in personal narrative: some perspectives of patients. *Philosophy, Psychiatry, & Psychology*, 10(4): 297–304.

West Midlands Mental Health Partnership (2003) *Values in Action: Developing a Values Based Practice in Mental Health* (available from West Midlands Mental Health Partnership)

West, D.J. and Walk, A. (eds) (1977) *Daniel McNaughton: His Trial and the Aftermath*. London: Gaskell Books.

Whewell, W. (1849). *Of Induction, With Especial Reference to Mr J Stuart Mill's System of Logic*. London: Parker.

White, A.R. (ed.) (1968). *The Philosophy of Action*. Oxford: Oxford University Press.

Whitehead, A.N. and Russell, B. (1910, 1912, 1913) *Principia Mathematica*, 3 vols, Cambridge: Cambridge University Press. (2nd edn), 1925 (Vol. 1) 1927 (Vols 2,3).

Widdershoven, G.A.M. (1998). A phenomenology of dyslexia. (Commentary on Philpott, 1998). *Philosophy, Psychiatry, & Psychology*, 5(1): 29–32.

Widdershoven, G.A.M. (1999). Cognitive psychology and hermeneutics: two approaches to meaning and mental disorder. *Philosophy, Psychiatry, & Psychology*, 6(4): 245–254.

Widdershoven, G.A.M. (1999). Response to the Commentaries. *Philosophy, Psychiatry, & Psychology*, 6(4): 267–270.

Widdershoven, G.A.M. (2002) Alternatives to principleism in Fulford, K.W.M., Dickenson, D., and Murray, T.H. (eds) *Healthcare Ethics and Human Values*. Oxford: Blackwell Science.

Widdershoven, G.A.M. and Widdershoven-Heerding, I. (2003). Understanding dementia: a hermeneutic perspective. In *Nature and Narrative: an introduction to the new philosophy of psychiatry* (ed. K.W.M. Fulford, K.J. Morris, J.Z. Sadler, and G. Stanghellini). Oxford: Oxford University Press, Chapter 6.

Widdershoven, G.A.M., Hope, T., van der Scheer, L., McMillan, J. (eds.) (forthcoming) *Empirical Ethics in Psychiatry*. Oxford: Oxford University Press.

Wiggins, D. (1980). *Sameness and Substance*. Cambridge, MA: Harvard University Press.

Wiggins, O.P. (1994). Commentary on Stephens and Graham, (1994). *Philosophy, Psychiatry, & Psychology*, 1(1): 11–12.

Wiggins, O.P. and Schwartz, M.A. (1994). The limits of psychiatric knowledge and the problem of classification. In *Philosophical Perspectives on Psychiatric Diagnostic Classification* (ed. J.Z. Sadler, O.P. Wiggins, and M.A. Schwartz). Battimore, MD: Johns Hopkins University Press, pp. 89–103.

Wiggins, O.P. and Schwartz, M.A. (1995). Chris Walker's Interpretation of Karl Jaspers' phenomenology: a critique. *Philosophy, Psychiatry, & Psychology*, 2(4): 319–344.

Wiggins, O.P. and Schwartz, M.A. (1997). Edmund Husserl's influence on Karl Jaspers' phenomenology. *Philosophy, Psychiatry, & Psychology*, 4: 15–36.

Wiggins, O.P. and Schwartz, M.A. (1997). Encoding of meaning. (Commentary on Bolton, 1997) *Philosophy, Psychiatry, & Psychology*, 4(4): 277–282.

Wiggins, O.P., Schwartz, M.A., and Naudin, J. (2001). Husserlian comments on Blankenburgs psychopathology of common sense. (Commentary on Blankenburg, 2001). *Philosophy, Psychiatry, & Psychology*, 8(4): 327–330.

Wiggins, O.P., Schwartz, M.A., and Spitzer, M. (1992). Phenomenological/descriptive psychiatry: Husserl and Jaspers. In *Phenomenology, Language and Schizophrenia* (ed. Spitzer, M. et al.). New York: Springer-Verlag, p. 67.

Wilkes, K. (1988). *Real People: personal identity without thought experiments*. Oxford: Oxford University Press.

Wilkes, K. (1991). How many selves make me? In *Human Beings* (ed. D. Cockburn). Cambridge: Cambridge University Press.

Wilkes, K. (1999). Know thyself. In *Models of Self* (ed. S. Gallagher and J. Shear). Toverton, UK: Imprint Academic.

Wilkinson, G., Fahy, T., Russell, G., Healy, D., Marks, I., Tantam, D., and Dimond, B. (1995). Case reports and confidentiality: opinion is sought, medical and legal. *British Journal of Psychiatry*, 166: 555–558.

William, B. (1978). *Descartes: project of pure inquiry*. London: Penguin.

Williams, D.D.R and Garner, J. (2002). The case against 'the evidence', a different perspective on evidence-based medicine *British Journal of Psychiatry* 180: 8–12.

Williams, B. (1970). Are persons bodies? *The Philosophy of the Body* (ed. S. Spicker). Chicago, IL: Quadrant Books, pp. 137–156.

Williams, B. (1970). The self and the future. *Philosophical Review*, 79: 161–180.

Williams, B. (1978). *Descartes: the project of pure inquiry*. Brighton: Harvester Press.

Williams, B. (1985) *Ethics and the Limits of Philosophy*. London: Fontana.

Williams, B. (1985). *Ethics and the Limits of Philosophy*. Cambridge, MA: Harvard University Press.

Williams, M. (1996). *Unnatural Doubts*. Princeton: Princeton University Press

Williams, M. (2001). *Problems of Knowledge: a critical introduction to epistemology* Oxford: Oxford University Press.

Williams, R. (2004). Finding the way forward in professional practice. (Commentary on Fulford and Colombo, 2004). *Philosophy, Psychiatry, & Psychology*, 11(2): 151–158.

Williams, R., and Kerfoot, M. (eds) (2005). *Child and adolescent mental health services: strategy, planning, delivery, and evaluation*. Oxford: Oxford University Press.

Williams, W. (1985). *Ethics and the Limits of Philosophy*. London: Fontana Press/Collins.

Williamson, T. (2004). Can two wrongs make a right? (Commentary on Fulford and Colombo, 2004) *Philosophy, Psychiatry, & Psychology*, 11(2): 159–164.

Wilson, J. (1979). *Preface to the Philosophy of Education*. London: Routledge.

Wilson, P.E. (1996). Sanity and irresponsibility. *Philosophy, Psychiatry, & Psychology*, 3(4): 293–302.

Winch, P. ([1958] 1990). *The Idea of a Social Science and its Relation to Philosophy*. London: Routledge.

Winch, P. (1960). *The Idea of Social Science and its Relation to Philosophy*, (2nd edn). London Routledge & Kegan Paul.

Winch, P. (1972). *Ethics and Action*. London: Routledge and Kegan Paul.

Wing, J.K. (1978). *Reasoning about Madness*. Oxford: Oxford University Press.

Wing, J.K., Birley, J.L.T., Cooper, J.E., Graham, P., and Isaacs, A.D. (1967). Reliability of a procedure for measuring and classifying 'Present Psychiatric State'. *British Journal of Psychiatry*, 113: 499–515.

Wing, J.K., Cooper, J.E., and Sartorius, M. (1974). *Measurement and Classification of Psychiatric Symptoms*. Cambridge: Cambridge University Press.

Wise, T.N. (1994). Normal Grief: Good or Bad? Health or Disease? (Commentary on Kopelman, 1994) *Philosophy, Psychiatry, & Psychology*, 1(4): 223–224.

Wittgenstein, L. (1921) *Tractatus Logico-Philosopohicus* (trans. D.F. Pears and B.F. McGuinness). London: Routledge and Kegan Paul.

Wittgenstein, L. (1953). *Philosophical Investigations*. Oxford: Blackwell.

Wittgenstein, L. (1958). *The Blue and the Brown Books*. Oxford: Blackwell.

Wittgenstein, L. (1979). *On Certainty*. Oxford: Blackwell.

Wittgenstein, L. (1982). Conversations on Freud. In *Philosophical Essays on Freud* (eds R. Wollheim and J. Hopkins). Cambridge: Cambridge University Press.

Wolff, S. (2000). The phenomenology of abnormal emotions of happiness: a translation from the German of William Mayer-Gross doctoral thesis. *Philosophy, Psychiatry, & Psychology*, 7(4): 295–310.

Wolfram, S. (1989). *Philosophical Logic*. London: Routledge.

Wollheim, R. (1973). *Freud*. London: Fontana.

Wollheim, R. (1981) *Sigmund Freud*. Modern Masters Series. New York: Viking Press (1971). Cambridge and New York: Cambridge University Press.

Wollheim, R. and Hopkins, J. (1982). *Philosophical Essays on Freud*. Cambridge and New York: Cambridge University Press.

Wolpert, L. (1999). *Malignant Sadness: the anatomy of depression*. London: Faber and Faber.

Woodbridge, K. (2003). The forgotten self: training mental health and social care workers to work with service users (Commentary on articles in the Special Issue on agency, narrative, and self) *Philosophy, Psychiatry, & Psychology*, 10(4): 373–378.

Woodbridge, K. and Fulford, K.W.M. (2003). Good practice? Values-based practice in mental health. *Mental Health Practice*, 7(2): 30–34.

Woodbridge, K. and Fulford, K.W.M. (2004). Right, wrong and respect. *Mental Health Today*, September: 28–30.

Woodbridge, K. and Fulford, K.W.M. (2004). *Whose values? A workbook for values-based practice in mental health care*. London: Sainsbury Centre for Mental Health

Woods, J. and Walton, D. (1982) *Argument: the logic of the fallacies*. New York: McGraw-Hill Ryerson.

Woody, J.M. (2003). When narrative fails. *Philosophy, Psychiatry, & Psychology*, 10(4): 329–346.

Woody, J.M. and Phillips, J. (1995). Freud's Project for a scientific psychology after 100 years: the unconscious mind in the era of cognitive neuroscience. (Commentary by Mohl, 1995, pp. 135–136) *Philosophy, Psychiatry, & Psychology*, 2(2): 123–134.

Woolfolk, R. (2003). On the border: reflections on the meaning of self-injury in borderline personality disorder. (Commentary on Potter, 2003). *Philosophy, Psychiatry, & Psychology*, 10(1): 29–32.

Woolhouse, R.S. (1988). *The Empiricists*. Opus series: *A History of Western Philosophy*, Vol. 5. Oxford: Oxford University Press.

World Health Organization (1948). *Manual of the International Statistical Classification of Diseases, Injuries, and Causes of Death* (ICD-6). Geneva: World Health Organization.

World Health Organization (1967). *Manual of the International Statistical Classification of Diseases, Injuries, and Causes of Death* (ICD-8). Geneva: World Health Organization.

World Health Organization (1973). *International Pilot Study of Schizophrenia*. Geneva: World Health Organization.

World Health Organization (1974). *Glossary of Mental Disorders and Guide to their Classification, for use in Conjunction with the International Classification of Diseases*, 8th revision. Geneva: World Health Organization.

World Health Organization (1978). *International Classification of Diseases*, (9th edn). Geneva: World Health Organization.

World Health Organization (1978). *Mental disorders: glossary and guide to their classification in accordance with the ninth revision of the International Classification of Diseases*. Geneva: World Health Organization.

World Health Organization (1992). ICD-10. *International Classification of Diseases and Related Health Problems* (10th edn). Geneva: World Health Organization.

World Health Organization (2001). *International Classification of Functioning, Disability and Health*. Geneva: World Health Organization.

World Psychiatric Association (1996). *Declaration of Madrid*. Geneva: World Psychiatric Association.

World Psychiatric Association (1996) *Declaration of Madrid* (reproduced with a brief commentary in the Appendix – Codes of Ethics, 511–531, in Bloch, S., Chodoff P., and Green S.A., (1999) *Psychiatric Ethics* (3rd Edition). Oxford: Oxford University Press.

Wright, C. (ed.) (1986). *Realism Meaning and Truth*. Oxford: Blackwell.

Wright, C. (1987). On making up one's mind: Wittgenstein on intention. In *Logic, Philosophy of Science and Epistemology: Proceedings of the 11th international Wittgenstein symposium* (ed. P. Weingartner and G. Schurz). Vienna: Holder Pichler Tempsky.

Wright, C. (1992). *Truth and Objectivity*. Cambridge, MA: Harvard University Press.

Wright, C. (1991). Wittgenstein's later philosophy of mind. In *Meaning Scepticism* (ed. Puhl) Berlinide Gruyter.

Wulff, H.R., Pedersen, S.A. and Rosenberg, R. (1986) *Philosophy of Medicine, an introduction*. Oxford: Blackwell Scientific Publications.

Yalom, I.D. (1981). *Existential Psychotherapy*. New York: Basic Books.

Young, A. and de Pauw, K.W. (2002). One stage is not enough. (Commentary on Gerrans, 2002). *Philosophy, Psychiatry, & Psychology*, 9(1): 55–60.

Youngner, S.J. (1998). Commentary on 'Is Mr Spock mentally competent? (Commentary on Charland, 1998) *Philosophy, Psychiatry, & Psychology*, 5(1): 89–92.

Zahavi, D. (2001). Schizophrenia and self-awareness. (Commentary on Bin, 2001). *Philosophy, Psychiatry, & Psychology*, 8(4): 339–342.

Zilboorg, G. and Henry, G.W. (1941). The second psychiatric revolution. In *A History of Medical Psychology*. London: George Allen and Unwin, pp. 479–510.

Zimmerman, D. (1998). Criteria of identity and 'identity mystics'. *Erkenntnis*, 48: 281–301.

Zubin, J. (ed) (1961) *Field Studies in the Mental Disorders*. New York: Grune and Stratton.

Readings

Reading 2.1   EXERCISE 6

From: page 9 of The Empiricist Background, Chapter 1 in *The Collapse of the Fact/Value Dichotomy and other Essays* by Putnam, H., Cambridge, MA: Harvard University Press, 2002.

A Distinction is not a Dichotomy:

The point of view concerning the relation between "facts" and "values" that I shall be defending in this book is one that John Dewey defended throughout virtually all of his long and exemplary career. Dewey's target was not the idea that, for certain purposes, it might help to draw a distinction (say, between "facts" and "values"); rather his target was what he called the fact/value "dualism." It is one of a great many such philosophical dualisms that Dewey was concerned to identify, diagnose, and exorcise from our thinking. A misunderstanding that his work always tends to provoke (as I have learned by teaching it) is the misunderstanding that when Dewey attacks what he called "dualisms" he is thereby attacking all allied philosophical *distinctions*. Nothing could be further from the truth.

Reading 6.4

EXERCISE 3

Extract from: Williams, B. (1985) *Ethics and the Limits of Philosophy*. London: Fontana Press/Collins, page 23.

The writers' note of urgency suggests . . . that what will happen could turn on the outcome of these arguments, that the justification of the ethical life could be a *force*. If we arc to take this seriously, then it is a real question, who is supposed to be listening. Why are they supposed to be listening? What will the professor's justification do, when they break down the door, smash his spectacles, take him away?

Reading 13.14

EXERCISE 16

Extract from: Van Fraassen, B.C. (1999). To save the phenomena. In *The Philosophy of Science* (eds. R. Boyd, P. Gasker, and J.D. Trout). Cambridge, MA: MIT Press, pp. 187–194 (Extract pp 187–8).

After the demise of logical positivism, scientific realism has once more returned as a major philosophical position. I shall not try here to criticize that position, but rather attempt to outline a comprehensive alternative.

I

What exactly is scientific realism? Naively stated, it is the view that the picture science gives us of the world is true, and the entities postulated really exist. (Historically, it added that there are real necessities in nature; I shall ignore that aspect here.) But that statement is too naive; it attributes to the scientific realist the belief that today's scientific theories are (essentially) right.

The correct statement, it seems to me, must indeed be in terms of epistemic attitudes, but not so directly. The aim of science is to give us *a literally true story of what the world is like*; and the proper form of acceptance of a theory is to believe that it is true. This is the statement of scientific realism: "To have good reason to accept a theory is to have good reason to believe that the entities it postulates are real," as Wilfrid Sellars has expressed it. Accordingly, all antirealism is a position according to which the aims of science can well be served without giving such a literally true story, and acceptance of a theory may properly involve something less (or other) than belief that it is true.

The idea of a literally true account has two aspects: the language is to be literally construed; and, so construed, the account is true. This divides the antirealists into two sorts. The first sort holds that science is or aims to be true, properly (but not literally) construed. The second holds that the language of science should be literally construed, but its theories need not be true to be good. The antirealism I advocate belongs to the second sort.

II

When Newton wrote his *Mathematical Principles of Natural Philosophy* and *System of the World*, he carefully distinguished the phenomena to be saved from the reality he postulated. He distinguished the "absolute magnitudes" that appear in his axioms from their "sensible measures" which are determined experimentally. He discussed carefully the ways in which, and extent to which, "the true motions of particular bodies [may be determined] from the apparent," via the assertion that "the apparent motions . . . are the differences of true motions."

The "apparent motions" form relational structures define by measuring relative distances, time intervals, and angles of separation. For brevity, let us call these relational structures *appearances*. In the mathematical model provided by Newton's theory, bodies are located in Absolute Space, in which they have real or absolute motions. But within these models we can define structures that are meant to be exact reflections of those appearances and are, as Newton says, identifiable as differences between true motions. These structures, defined in terms of the relevant relations between absolute locations and absolute times, which are the appropriate parts of Newton's models, I shall call *motions*, borrowing, Simon's term.

When Newton claims empirical adequacy for his theory, he is claiming that his theory has some model such that *all actual appearances are identifiable with (isomorphic to) motions in that model*.

Newton's theory goes a great deal further than this. It is part of his theory that there is such a thing as Absolute Space, that absolute motion is motion relative to Absolute Space, that absolute acceleration causes certain stresses and strains; and thereby deformations in the appearances, and so on. He offered, in addition, the hypothesis (his term) that the center of gravity of the solar system is at rest in Absolute Space. But, as he himself noted, the appearances would be no different if that center were in any other state of constant absolute motion.

Let us call Newton's theory (mechanics and gravitation) TN, and $TN(v)$ the theory TN plus the postulate that the center of gravity of the solar system has constant absolute velocity. By Newton's own account, he claims empirical adequacy for $TN(0)$; and also claims that, if $TN(0)$ is empirically adequate, then so are all the theories $TN(v)$.

Recalling what it was to claim empirical adequacy, we see that all the theories $TN(v)$ are empirically equivalent exactly *if all the motions in a model of $TN(v)$ are isomorphic to motions in a model $TN(v + w)$*, for all constant velocities v and w. For now, let us agree that these theories are empirically equivalent, referring objections to a later section.

Reading 26.3
EXERCISE 4

From: Davidson, D. (1980a). Actions, reasons and causes. In *Essays on Actions and Events*. Oxford: Oxford University Press, pp. 3–19. (Extract pp. 11–17).

IV

In order to turn the first 'and' to 'because' in 'He exercised *and* he wanted to reduce and thought exercise would do it', we must, as the basic move,[1] augment condition C1 with:

C2. A primary reason for an action is its cause.

The considerations in favour of C2 are by now, I hope, obvious; in the remainder of this paper I wish to defend C2 against various lines of attack and, in the process, to clarify the notion of causal explanation involved.

A. The first line of attack is this. Primary reasons consist of attitudes and beliefs, which are states or dispositions, not events; therefore they cannot be causes.

It is easy to reply that states, dispositions, and conditions are frequently named as the causes of events: the bridge collapsed because of a structural defect; the plane crashed on takeoff because the air temperature was abnormally high; the plate broke because it had a crack. This reply does not, however, meet a closely related point. Mention of a causal condition for an event gives a cause only on the assumption that there was also a preceding event. But what is the preceding event that causes an action?

In many cases it is not difficult at all to find events very closely associated with the primary reason. States and dispositions are not events, but the onslaught of a state or disposition is. A desire to hurt your feelings may spring up at the moment you anger me; I may start wanting to eat a melon just when I see one; and beliefs may begin at the moment we notice, perceive, learn, or remember something. Those who have argued that there are no mental events to qualify as causes of actions have often missed the obvious because they have insisted that a mental event be observed or noticed (rather than an observing or a noticing) or that it be like a stab, a qualm, a prick or a quiver, a mysterious prod of conscience or act of the will. Melden, in discussing the driver who signals a turn by raising his arm, challenges those who want to explain actions causally to identify 'an event which is common and peculiar to all such cases' (87), perhaps a motive or an intention, anyway 'some particular feeling or experience' (95). But of course there is a mental event; at some moment the driver noticed (or thought he noticed) his turn coming up, and that is the moment he signalled. During any continuing activity, like driving, or elaborate performance, like swimming the Hellespont, there are more or less fixed purposes, standards, desires, and habits that give direction and form to the entire enterprise, and

there is the continuing input of information about what we are doing, about changes in the environment, in terms of which we regulate and adjust our actions. To dignify a driver's awareness that his turn has come by calling it an experience, or even a feeling, is no doubt exaggerated, but whether it deserves a name or not, it had better be the reason why he raises his arm. In this case, and typically, there may not be anything we would call a motive, but if we mention such a general purpose as wanting to get to one's destination safely, it is clear that the motive is not an event. The intention with which the driver raises his arm is also not an event, for it is no thing at all, neither event, attitude, disposition, nor object. Finally, Melden asks the causal theorist to find an event that is common and peculiar to all cases where a man intentionally raises his arm, and this, it must be admitted, cannot be produced. But then neither can a common and unique cause of bridge failures, plane crashes, or plate breakings be produced.

The signalling driver can answer the question, 'Why did you raise your arm when you did?', and from the answer we learn the event that caused the action. But can an actor always answer such a question? Sometimes the answer will mention a mental event that does not give a reason: 'Finally I made up my mind.' However, there also seem to be cases of intentional action where we cannot explain at all why we acted when we did. In such cases, explanation in terms of primary reasons parallels the explanation of the collapse of the bridge from a structural defect: we are ignorant of the event or sequence of events that led up to (caused) the collapse, but we are sure there was such an event or sequence of events.

B. According to Melden, a cause must be 'logically distinct from the alleged effect' (52); but a reason for an action is not logically distinct from the action; therefore, reasons are not causes of actions.[2]

One possible form of this argument has already been suggested. Since a reason makes an action intelligible by redescribing it, we do not have two events, but only one under different descriptions. Causal relations, however, demand distinct events.

Someone might be tempted into the mistake of thinking that my flipping of the switch caused my turning on of the light (in fact it caused the light to go on). But it does not follow that it is a mistake to take. 'My reason for flipping the switch was that I wanted to turn on the light' as entailing, in part, 'I flipped the switch, and this action is further describable as having been caused by wanting to turn on the light'. To describe an event in terms of its cause is not to confuse the event with its cause, nor does explanation by redescription exclude causal explanation.

The example serves also to refute the claim that we cannot describe the action without using words that link it to the alleged cause. Here the action is to be explained under the description: 'my flipping the switch', and the alleged cause is 'my wanting to turn on the light'. What relevant logical relation is supposed to

---

[1] I say 'as the basic move' to cancel any suggestion that C1 and C2 are jointly *sufficient* to define the relation of reasons to the actions they explain. For discussion of this point, see the Introduction and Essay 4.

[2] This argument can be found in one or more versions, in Kenny, Hampshire, and Melden, as well as in P. Winch, *The Idea of a Social Science*, and R. S. Peters. *The Concept of Motivation*. In one of its forms, the argument was of course inspired by Ryle's treatment of motives in *The Concept of Mind*.

hold between these phrases? It seems more plausible to urge a logical link between 'my turning on the light' and 'my wanting to turn on the light', but even here the link turns out, on inspection, to be grammatical rather than logical.

In any case there is something very odd in the idea that causal relations are empirical rather than logical. What can this mean? Surely not that every true causal statement is empirical. For suppose 'A caused B' is true. Then the cause of B = A; so substituting, we have 'The cause of B caused B', which is analytic. The truth of a causal statement depends on *what* events are described; its status as analytic or synthetic depends on *how* the events are described. Still, it may be maintained that a reason rationalizes an action only when the descriptions are appropriately fixed, and the appropriate descriptions are not logically independent.

Suppose that to say a man wanted to turn on the light *meant* that he would perform any action he believed would accomplish his end. Then the statement of his primary reason for flipping the switch would entail that he flipped the switch—'straightway he acts' as Aristotle says. In this case there would certainly be a logical connection between reason and action, the same sort of connection as that between, 'It's water-soluble and was placed in water' and 'It dissolved'. Since the implication runs from description of cause to description of effect but not conversely, naming the cause still gives information. And, though the point is often overlooked, 'Placing it in water caused it to dissolve' does not entail 'It's water-soluble'; so the latter has additional explanatory force. Nevertheless, the explanation would be far more interesting if, in place of solubility, with its obvious definitional connection with the event to be explained, we could refer to some property, say a particular crystalline structure, whose connection with dissolution in water was known only through experiment. Now it is clear why primary reasons like desires and wants do not explain actions in the relatively trivial way solubility explains dissolvings. Solubility, we are assuming, is a pure disposition property: it is defined in terms of a single test. But desires cannot be defined in terms of the actions they may rationalize, even though the relation between desire and action is not simply empirical; there are other, equally essential criteria for desires—their expression in feelings and in actions that they do not rationalize, for example. The person who has a desire (or want or belief) does not normally need criteria at all—he generally knows, even in the absence of any clues available to others, what he wants, desires, and believes. These logical features of primary reasons show that it is not just lack of ingenuity that keeps us from defining them as dispositions to act for these reasons.

C. According to Hume, 'we may define a cause to be an object, followed by another, and where all the objects similar to the first are followed by objects similar to the second'. But, Hart and Honoré claim, 'The statement that one person did something because, for example, another threatened him, carries no implication or covert assertion that if the circumstances were repeated the same action would follow' (52). Hart and Honoré allow that Hume is right in saying that ordinary singular causal statements imply generalizations, but wrong for this very reason in supposing

that motives and desires are ordinary causes of actions. In brief, laws are involved essentially in ordinary causal explanations, but not in rationalizations.

It is common to try to meet this argument by suggesting that we do have rough laws connecting reasons and actions, and these can, in theory, be improved. True, threatened people do not always respond in the same way; but we may distinguish between threats and also between agents, in terms of their beliefs and attitudes.

The suggestion is delusive, however, because generalizations connecting reasons and actions are not—and cannot be sharpened into—the kind of law on the basis of which accurate predictions can reliably be made. If we reflect on the way in which reasons determine choice, decision, and behaviour, it is easy to see why this is so. What emerges, in the *ex post facto* atmosphere of explanation and justification as *the* reason frequently was, to the agent at the time of action, one consideration among many, *a* reason. Any serious theory for predicting action on the basis of reasons must find a way of evaluating the relative force of various desires and beliefs in the matrix of decision; it cannot take as its starting point the refinement of what is to be expected from a single desire. The practical syllogism exhausts its role in displaying an action as falling under one reason; so it cannot he subtilized into a reconstruction of practical reasoning, which involves the weighing of competing reasons. The practical syllogism provides a model neither for a predictive science of action nor for a normative account of evaluative reasoning.

Ignorance of competent predictive laws does not inhibit valid causal explanation, or few causal explanations could be made. I am certain the window broke because it was struck by a rock—I saw it all happen; but I am not (is anyone?) in command of laws on the basis of which I can predict what blows will break which windows. A generalization like, 'Windows are fragile, and fragile things tend to break when struck hard enough, other conditions being right' is not a predictive law in the rough—the predictive law, if we had it, would be quantitative and would use very different concepts. The generalization, like our generalizations about behaviour, serves a different function: it provides evidence for the existence of a causal law covering the case at hand.[3]

We are usually far more certain of a singular causal connection than we are of any causal law governing the case; does this show that Hume was wrong in claiming that singular causal statements entail laws? Not necessarily, for Hume's claim, as quoted above, is ambiguous. It may mean that 'A caused B' entails some particular law involving the predicates used in the descriptions 'A' and 'B', or it may mean that 'A caused B' entails that there exists a causal law instantiated by some true descriptions of A and B.[4] Obviously,

---

[3] Essays 11, 12, and 13 discuss the issues of this paragraph and the one before it.

[4] We could roughly characterize the analysis of singular causal statements hinted at here as follows: 'A caused B' is true if and only if there are descriptions of A and B such that the sentence obtained by putting these descriptions for 'A' and 'B' in 'A caused B' follows from a true causal law. This analysis is saved from triviality by the fact that not all true generalizations are causal laws; causal laws are distinguished (though of course this is no analysis) by the fact that they are inductively confirmed by their instances and by the fact that they support counterfactual and subjunctive singular causal statements. There is more on causality in Essay 7.

both versions of Hume's doctrine give a sense to the claim that singular causal statements entail laws, and both sustain the view that causal explanations 'involve laws'. But the second version is far weaker, in that no particular law is entailed by a singular causal claim, and a singular causal claim can be defended, if it needs defence, without defending any law. Only the second version of Hume's doctrine can be made to fit with most causal explanations; it suits rationalizations equally well.

The most primitive explanation of an event gives its cause; more elaborate explanations may tell more of the story, or defend the singular causal claim by producing a relevant law or by giving reasons for believing such exists. But it is an error to think no explanation has been given until a law has been produced. Linked with these errors is the idea that singular causal statements necessarily indicate, by the concepts they employ, the concepts that will occur in the entailed law. Suppose a hurricane, which is reported on page 5 of Tuesday's *Times*, causes a catastrophe, which is reported on page 13 of Wednesday's *Tribune*. Then the event reported on page 5 of Tuesday's *Times* caused the event reported on page 13 of Wednesday's *Tribune*. Should we look for a law relating events of these *kinds*? It is only slightly less ridiculous to look for a law relating hurricanes and catastrophes. The laws needed to predict the catastrophe with precision would, of course, have no use for concepts like hurricane and catastrophe. The trouble with predicting the weather is that the descriptions under which events interest us—'a cool, cloudy day with rain in the afternoon'—have only remote connections with the concepts employed by the more precise known laws.

The laws whose existence is required if reasons are causes of actions do not, we may be sure, deal in the concepts in which rationalizations must deal. If the causes of a class of events (actions) fall in a certain class (reasons) and there is a law to back each singular causal statement, it does not follow that there is any law connecting events classified as reasons with events classified as actions—the classifications may even be neurological, chemical, or physical.

Reading 27.2

From: Malcolm, N. (1958). Knowledge of other minds. *Journal of Philosophy*, 55. (Reprinted in Rosenthal, D (ed.) (1991). *The Nature of Mind*. Oxford: Oxford University Press, pp. 92–97. (Extract pp. 92–3).

I believe that the argument from analogy for the existence of other minds still enjoys more credit than it deserves, and my first aim in this paper will be to show that it leads nowhere. J. S. Mill is one of many who have accepted the argument and I take his statement of it as representative . . .

Suppose this reasoning could yield a conclusion of the sort `it is probable that that human figure' (pointing at some person other than oneself) `has thoughts and feelings'. Then there is a question as to whether this conclusion can *mean* anything to the philosopher who draws it, because there is a question as to whether the sentence `That human figure has thoughts and feelings' can mean anything to him. Why should this be a question? Because the assumption from which Mill starts is that he has no *criterion* for determining whether another `walking and speaking figure' does or does not have thoughts and feelings. If he had a criterion he could apply it, establishing with certainty that this or that human figure does or does not have feelings (for the only plausible criterion would lie in behaviour and circumstances that are open to view), and there would be no call to resort to tenuous analogical reasoning that yields at best a probability. If Mill has no criterion for the existence of feelings other than his own then in that sense he does not understand the sentence `that human figure has feelings' and therefore does not understand the sentence `It is *probable* that the human figure has feelings'.

There is a familiar inclination to make the following reply: `Although I have no criterion of verification still I understand, for example, the sentence `He has pain'. For I understand the meaning of `I have pain' and `He has pain' means that he has the *same* thing I have when I have a pain.' But this is a fruitless manoeuvre. If I do not known how to establish that `someone has a pain' then I do not know how to establish that he has the *same* as I have when I have a pain. You cannot improve my understanding of `He has a pain' by this recourse to the notion of `the same', unless you give me a criterion for saying that someone *has* the same as I have. If you do this you will have no use for the argument from analogy; and if you cannot then you do not understand the supposed conclusion of that argument. (pp. 92–93)

Name Index

Stich, S. 684, 685, 756, 757
Stocker, M. 157, 159, 532, 538
Stone, T. 750
Storr, A. 17, 256, 280
Straus, E.W. 44
Strawson, P. 201, 618–19, 722, 733–34
Sturdee, P.G. v, vi, xxvi, 24, 157, 159, 176, 179, 494, 497, 532, 536, 538, 619
Styron, W. 38
Sullivan, M.D. 58
Sundstrom, P. 24, 30
Suppes, P. 84, 88, 136, 137
Sutherland, S. 51, 58
Svenaeus, F. 176, 179
Svensson, T. 30
Sykes, S. 58, 582, 584
Swinburne, R. 766
Szasz, T. 11, 14–17, 19–21, 42, 73, 74, 117, 118, 124, 141, 244, 292, 341, 344–46, 486, 575–76
Szmukler, G. 483, 502, 555

T
Tan, J. 599
Tanney, J. 731–32
Tarski, A. 294, 703
Taylor, P.J. 22, 28
Taylor, R. 766
Templeman, Lord 553
Tengland, P.-A. 24, 30
Thomas, P. 26, 665
Thomasma, D.C. 527
Thornton, T. 23, 30, 52, 59, 88, 135, 136, 137, 158, 159, 236, 237, 287, 314, 315, 381, 428, 432, 463, 494, 497, 532, 538, 605, 684, 685, 714, 715
Thorpe, Mr Justice 548
Toombs, K. 130–31
Toulmin, S. 472, 507, 512
Tröhler, U. 499
Trout, J.D. xxxvi
Tuke, W. 151
Tyreman, S. 25, 30
Tyrer, P. xxxvi

U
Unger, P. 760, 762
Urmson, J.O. 124
Üstün, B. 321

V
Van Fraassen, B.C. 352, 353–56, 361, 362–63, 370, 389, 394–96, 419
Van Gulick, R. 646
Van Inwagen, P. 763, 766
van Voren, Robert 599
Varela, F.J. 176, 178, 179
Vaughn, C. 17
von Neumann, J. 2294
von Wright, G.H. 12
Vygotsky, L. 688

W
Waismann, F. 294
Wakefield, J.C. 393
Wakefield, J.E. 573, 576
Walk, A. 487
Walker, C. v, xxvi, 205–6
Walker, N. 490
Wallcraft, J. 603, 607
Walton, D. 107
Ward, D.E. 533, 538
Warlow, C. 538
Warner, M. xxvi, 85, 88, 176, 179
Warnock, G.J. 71, 122, 124, 125–26, 576–77
Warnock, M. xxxii–xxxiii, 126
Watson, J.B. 154, 634
Weber, M. 167, 168, 212, 217, 219, 223, 224–25, 226, 229, 230–31, 233, 234, 426
Weierstrass, K. 192, 193
Weiss, B. 94
Wells, L.A. 52, 59, 88, 136, 138, 532
Wernicke, C. 152, 167, 189
Wertheimer, M. 305
West, D.J. 487
Whewell, W. 460, 461
Whitehead, A.N. 77, 114
Widdershoven, G. 528, 599

Widdershoven-Heerding, I. 599
Wiggins, D. 766
Wiggins, O.P. xxxvi, 205, 224
Wilkes, K. xxxvii, 72, 82, 448, 614, 762
Williams, B. 117, 118, 341–42, 347–49, 434, 458, 472, 516, 627, 766
Williams, M. 740
Williams, R. 17
Williamson, T. 17, 524
Wilson, G.D. 256
Wilson, J. 473
Winch, P. 423, 426–27
Windelband, W. 167, 168, 172, 219
Wing, J.K. 16, 41, 290, 292–93, 313, 333, 377, 486, 567, 751–52, 770
Wing, L. 751, 752
Winterton, R. xxvii, 527
Wittgenstein, L. xxxii, 15, 67, 70, 71, 77, 82, 95, 115, 116, 117, 118, 119, 185, 264, 294, 301, 305–7, 308, 400–402, 426, 449–57.476, 459, 625, 634, 635, 687, 705, 742–45, 754–55
Wolff, S. 158, 159
Wollheim, R. 272, 280
Wolpert, L. 38
Woodbridge, K. xxxvi, 524, 526–27
Woods, J. 109, 110
Woody, M.J. 256
Woolfolk, R.L. 84, 87, 559, 563
Wright, C. 343, 344, 373, 692–94, 695
Wulff, H.R. 24, 30
Wundt, W. 153, 614

Y
Yalom, I. 38

Z
Zahavi, D. 55, 176, 179
Zilboorg, G. 156
Zilsel, E. 294
Zimmerman, D. 767
Zubin, J. 325, 331, 380, 383

Subject Index